Hazards and Complications of Anaesthesia

For Churchill Livingstone

Publisher Geoff Nuttall
Project Editor Lowri Daniels
Production Controller Mark Sanderson
Sales Promotion Executive Marion Pollock

Hazards and Complications of Anaesthesia

Edited by

T. H. Taylor MBBS FRCA

Consultant Anaesthetist
The Royal London Hospital, Whitechapel, London;
Member of Council, Medical Protection Society, London

Edward Major MBBS FRCA

Consultant in Intensive Therapy and Anaesthesia
Morriston Hospital, Swansea

Foreword by
W. D. Wylie

SECOND EDITION

CHURCHILL LIVINGSTONE
EDINBURGH LONDON MADRID MELBOURNE NEW YORK AND TOKYO 1993

CHURCHILL LIVINGSTONE
Medical Division of Longman Group UK Limited

Distributed in the United States of America by Churchill Livingstone Inc., 650 Avenue of the Americas, New York, N.Y. 10011, and by associated companies, branches and representatives throughout the world.

First edition 1987
Second edition 1993
Reprinted 1994

ISBN 0-443-04259-4

British Library Cataloguing in Publication Data
A catalogue record for this book is available from the British Library.

Library of Congress Cataloging in Publication Data
A catalog record for this book is available from the Library of Congress.

The publisher's policy is to use **paper manufactured from sustainable forests**

Produced by Longman Singapore Publishers (Pte) Ltd.
Printed in Singapore

Contents

SECTION 4
Hazards related to anaesthetic drugs

SECTION 5
Hazards of anaesthesia procedures

SECTION 6
Equipment hazards

SECTION 7
The law

Foreword

For many years there has been a need for a definitive textbook concerned with the hazards and complications of anaesthesia, and not only with those problems that are of sufficient gravity to disrupt the long-term health of the patient. Major sequelae of anaesthesia such as death or permanent neurological disability are very exceptional but they inevitably and rightly lead to investigation. Minor complications may easily be forgotten by the anaesthetist but to the individual patient they are significant, and they too should be considered with view to prevention in the future.

Doctors are to some extent the victims of their own successes, and anaesthetists are no exception. The media – press, television and radio – have ensured that patients, potential as well as actual, can be as up to date in many aspects of specialized care as the average medical practitioner. As a consequence, there has been an increasing interest in medical litigation. Unhappily in this area the spotlight has all too frequently been turned on anaesthesia, not because anaesthetists are more prone to error than any other group of specialists but because in their practice a seemingly minor misjudgement or mistake may lead to a catastrophic outcome for the patient. There is a theory that suggests the need for living with a certain amount of tension to ensure the highest standards of medical practice. If this theory has any merit then public interest in anaesthetic practice will prove to be of value because a substantial proportion of the complications of anaesthesia are preventable.

I wrote the previous paragraphs during 1987 for the first edition of this textbook and I believe that they are as apposite now as they were then. I also wrote that the book was uniquely comprehensive, valuable and a necessary work for practising anaesthetists seeking to provide safe anaesthesia. The great success of the first edition and the need for a second larger and more comprehensive successor so soon after the first is a deserved tribute to Drs Taylor and Major and their team of contributors.

W. D. Wylie

Preface

Some accidents and errors are inevitable in the practice of medicine. Litigation alleging negligence by doctors as a result is increasing and many arise after anaesthesia. Claims sometimes originate as a result of a true accident, but often they are the result of errors which are not only avoidable, but which have been previously reported in the literature. Anaesthetic mishaps often have tragic consequences for the patient, including death or severe brain damage, but even in the most minor cases, adding to the discomfort of operative procedures.

The simplest routine anaesthetic may give rise to a dangerous or life-threatening situation, but experienced anaesthetists are often able to foresee the consequences of their actions and are therefore better able, almost unknowingly, to avoid complications. This ability is difficult to define and therefore not always imparted to trainees, who may in turn only learn of the hazards by bitter experience, as indeed their seniors may have done before them. We asked our contributors to analyse their daily practice, and try to distil the years of experience into these pages, so that trainees and even experienced anaesthetists working outside their normal sphere are made aware of the pitfalls. We also wanted even the commonest hazard and the most minor complications to be listed. This book contains then, as far as possible, a catalogue of the known hazards, risks and complications of anaesthesia and a description of the means of avoiding them. We do not include material on anaesthetic techniques or on the patho-physiology of disease, unless it is imperative to explain a particular hazard, since these are best dealt with in standard anaesthetic texts.

In this the second edition we have tried to incorporate many of the excellent suggestions made by readers of the first, whilst at the same time updating the text throughout. New chapters are added on anaesthetic safety, malignant hyperpyrexia, specific drug contraindications, pseudocholinesterase deficiency, reversal of neuromuscular blockade, adverse excitatory responses to anaesthetic agents, induced hypotension and avoiding hazards by monitoring. In addition some 17 new contributors have become involved. The overall outline remains unchanged however, with sections on safety, physical status of the patient, surgical factors, anaesthetic drugs, anaesthetic procedeures, equipment and monitoring and the law.

It is intended that this edition will be of assistance to anaesthetists of all experience levels, and that ultimately it will benefit their patients. If that were to be the case, then the efforts of our co-contributors will have been rewarded.

T. H. Taylor
E. Major

Contributors

Alan R. Aitkenhead BSc MD FRCA
Professor of Anaesthesia, University of Nottingham, Queen's Medical Centre, Nottingham, UK

Cindy S. T. Aun MBBS FRCA
Senior Lecturer, Department of Anaesthesia and Intensive Care, The Chinese University of Hong Kong, Hong Kong

David R. Bevan MB MRCP FRCA
Professor & Head, Department of Anaesthesia, University of British Columbia, Vancouver, Canada

Colin E. Blogg MBBS DObstRCOG FRCA
Consultant Anaesthetist, Nuffield Department of Anaesthetics, Radcliffe Infirmary, Oxford; Clinical Lecturer, University of Oxford; Associate Professor of Anesthesiology, University of Texas, Southwestern Medical School, Dallas, USA

Nicholas Osburn Boheimer MBBS FRCA
Consultant Anaesthetist, South Devon Healthcare NHS Trust; Former Senior Registrar, West and South Glamorgan Area Health Authorities, UK

J. G. Bovill MD PhD FFARCSI
Professor of Experimental Anaesthesiology, Department of Anaesthesiology, University Hospital Leiden, Netherlands

David E. R. Burt MB ChB FRCA
Senior Lecturer, The London Hospital Medical College; Honorary Consultant Anaesthetist, Newham General Hospital, London, UK

V. Chopra MBBS FRCA
Staff Anaesthesiologist, University Hospital Leiden, Netherlands

B. T. Colvin MA FRCP FRCPath
Senior Lecturer in Haematology, The London Hospital Medical College, London, UK

M. P. Colvin BSc MBBS FRCA
Consultant Anaesthetist, The Royal London Hospital, UK

Griselda M. Cooper MB ChB FRCA
Senior Lecturer in Anaesthesia, University of Birmingham; Honorary Consultant Anaesthetist, Birmingham Maternity Hospital, Queen Elizabeth Medical Centre, Birmingham, UK

M. V. Copp MBBS FRCA
Senior Registrar in Anaesthesia, Southampton General Hospital and Queen Alexandra Hospital, Portsmouth, UK

Jerome Cotter MBBS FRCA
Consultant Anaesthetist, The Royal London Hospital, London, UK

Judith M. Dunnet BSc MB ChB MRCP FRCA
Consultant Anaesthetist, Frenchay Hospital, Bristol, UK

F. Richard Ellis PhD MB ChB FRCA DObs RCOG
Professor of Anaesthesia, University of Leeds; Director of Malignant Hyperthermia Unit and

Honorary Consultant Anaesthetist, St James's University Hospital, Leeds, UK

R. O. Feneck MBBS LRCP MRCS FRCA
Consultant Anaesthetist, The London Chest Hospital, London, UK

David R. Goldhill MA MBBS FRCA
Senior Lecturer and Honorary Consultant, The Royal London Hospital, London, UK

Ronald A. Green MA MB BChir FRCA
Former Consultant Anaesthetist, St George's Hospital and Royal Free Hospital, London, UK

Geraldine Holt MRCPsych BSc
Consultant Psychiatrist, Greenwich Health Authority and Section of Mental Handicap, U.M.D.S. (Guy's), London

C. J. Hull MBBS DA FRCA
Professor of Anaesthesia, University of Newcastle Upon Tyne; Honorary Consultant Anaesthetist, Royal Victoria Infirmary, Newcastle upon Tyne, UK

George C. Jenkins PhD FRCP(Ed) FRCPath
Professor of Haematology, The London Hospital Medical College, London, UK

Frank Samsoe Jensen MD
Resident, Department of Anaesthesia, Rigshospitalet, University of Copenhagen, Denmark

J. Gareth Jones MB FRCP FRCA FANZCA
Professor of Anaesthesia, University of Cambridge, Addenbrooke's Hospital, Cambridge, UK

J. Lumley MBBS DA FRCA
Consultant Anaesthetist, Hammersmith Hospital; Honorary Senior Lecturer, Royal Postgraduate Medical School, University of London, London, UK

Edward Major MBBS FRCA
Consultant in Intensive Therapy and Anaesthesia, Morriston Hospital, Swansea, UK

A. G. Marshall BSc MBChB FRCA
Consultant Anaesthetist, The Royal London and Royal Brompton National Heart and Chest Hospitals, London, UK

Rosemary A. Mason MB ChB DObstRCOG FRCA
Consultant Anaesthetist, Singleton Hospital, Swansea, UK

Barbara M. Morgan MB ChB FRCA
Senior Lecturer and Consultant Anaesthetist, Institute of Obstetrics and Gynaecology, Queen Charlotte's Hospital, London, UK

Maldwyn Morgan MBBS DA FRCA
Reader in Anaesthetic Practice, Royal Postgraduate Medical School; Honorary Consultant Anaesthetist, Hammersmith Hospital, London, UK

A. C. Newland MA FRCP FRCPath
Professor of Haematology, Department of Haematology, The London Hospital Medical College and Royal London Hospital, London, UK

P. K. T. Nichols FRCA
Consultant Anaesthetist, Royal Gwent Hospital, Newport, UK

P. J. O'Shea MBBS FRCA
Consultant Anaesthetist, The Royal London Hospital, London, UK

R. N. Palmer LLB MBBS DObstRCOG
of Middle Temple, Barrister at Law; Secretary and Medical Director, The Medical Protection Society, London, UK

Mark B. Patrick MBBS BSc FRCA
Consultant and Anaesthetist, Wythenshawe Hospital, Manchester, UK

J. Payan MBBS(Lond) FRCP
Consultant Clinical Neuro-physiologist, Guy's and King's College Hospitals; Consultant in Electromyography, The Hospitals for Sick Children, London, UK

Anthony P. Rubin MB BChir FRCA
Consultant Anaesthetist, Charing Cross Hospital, London, UK

Peter Saunders MBChB FRCA DRCOG
Consultant Anaesthetist, St Bartholomew's Hospital, London

J. W. Sear MA BSc MBBS PhD FRCA
Clinical Reader in Anaesthetics, Nuffield

Department of Anaesthetics, University of Oxford; Honorary Consultant Anaesthetist, Oxfordshire Health Authority, UK

D. S. Selsby MB ChB FRCA
Consultant Paediatric Anaesthetist, Leeds General Infirmary, Leeds, UK

J. H. Sheldrake MA FRCA
Consultant Anaesthetist, Good Hope Hospital, Sutton Coldfield, UK

Anne J. Sutcliffe BSc MBChB FFRACSI FRCA ARPS
Consultant Anaesthetist, Birmingham Accident Hospital, Birmingham, UK

T. H. Taylor MBBS FRCA
Consultant Anaesthetist, Royal London Hospital; Member of Council, Medical Protection Society, London, UK

Jorgen Viby-Morgensen MD DMS FRCA
Professor and Chairman, Department of Anaesthesia, Rigshospitalet, University of Copenhagen, Denmark

Carl S. Waldmann MA MB BChir DA FRCA
Consultant Anaesthetist and Director of Intensive Care, Royal Berkshire and Battle Hospitals, Reading, UK

Bryan Walton MBBS FRCA
Consultant Anaesthetist, The Royal London Hospital, London, UK

Cheryl Lynn Westmoreland MD
Assistant Professor of Anesthesiology. Emory University Hospitals, Atlanta, USA

Kathleen Wilkinson FRCA DCH MRCP
Senior Registrar (Anaesthesia), Royal London Hospital, London, UK

Norton E. Williams MB ChB FRCA
Consultant Anaesthetist, St Helens and Knowsley Trust; Lecturer in Clinical Pharmacology, University of Liverpool, UK

P. M. Yate MBBS FRCA
Consultant Anaesthetist, The Royal London Hospital, London, UK

D. A. Zideman QHP BSc MBBS FRCA
Consultant Anaesthetist, Hammersmith Hospital; Honorary Senior Lecturer, Royal Postgraduate Medical School, University of London, London, UK

Safety of anaesthesia

1

Anaesthetic deaths and near misses

E. Major

INTRODUCTION

The overwhelming majority of anaesthetics proceed uneventfully and leave no serious ill effects, but the administration of anaesthesia does carry with it a measurable risk of death or serious brain injury. The need for anaesthesia arises only out of a need for surgery, so both surgical and anaesthetic factors must be included in the assessment of all perioperative deaths since both may be contributory. It is important, therefore, to define what is meant by an anaesthetic death and a symposium entitled 'Preventable anaesthetic mortality and morbidity', held in Boston in 1984, produced workable definitions of both mortality and morbidity (Lunn 1985).

Mortality was defined as 'death which occurred before recovery from the effects of a drug or drugs given to facilitate a procedure, or to relieve the pain of a condition, or arising from an incident which occurred while the drugs were effective'.

Morbidity was defined as an 'unplanned, unwanted, undesirable consequence of anaesthesia'. Three types of morbidity were described:

- major morbidity causing permanent disability
- intermediate morbidity causing serious distress and/or prolongation of hospital stay but no permanent sequelae
- minor morbidity causing moderate distress but no prolongation of hospital stay and no permanent sequelae.

ANAESTHETIC MORTALITY

In the past, authors have used varying definitions of anaesthetic death. Some have included mention of a death only if it occurred within a specified postoperative time-interval. Harrison (1978) chose 24 h, Turnbull et al (1980) chose 48 hours, and Lunn & Mushin (1982) studied all deaths occurring within 6 postoperative days. Harrison has reported regularly on deaths due to anaesthesia at the Groote Schuur Hospital, (1968, 1978), but a summary of 30 years' data (Harrison 1990) suggested that anaesthesia contributed to death at an overall rate of 0.19 per 1000 administrations. Although he concentrated mainly on the first 24 postoperative h, patients failing to regain consciousness following anaesthesia were included regardless of the time of death. Turnbull et al (1980) found a very similar mortality rate while limiting their reporting to the first 48 h. Clearly it is not correct to ignore mortality occurring outside the survey period if anaesthesia was contributory, but in very large studies there has to be some cut-off point to facilitate data collection.

Harrison (1978) in his report of 250 000 administrations at the Groote Schuur Hospital reported that only 2.2% of the total mortality from surgery was due to anaesthesia, but a survey of UK practice (Lunn & Mushin 1982) suggested that the figure was nearer 16%. This large discrepancy is unlikely to be due solely to differences of interpretation and it seems likely that the choice of a 6-day survey period might have picked up many more anaesthesia-related deaths than did Harrison's 24-h survey.

The 1987 Report of the Confidential Enquiry into Perioperative Deaths included more than 4000 postoperative deaths (an overall mortality rate of about 0.7%). Of these, anaesthesia was considered to have been the sole cause of death in 0.1% and a contributory factor in some 14% of deaths.

Bradley et al (1988) reported a very similar overall mortality rate of 0.68% when reviewing deaths occurring in the first 7 postoperative days in Queensland, Australia. Data from Cohen et al (1988) based on 100 000 patient procedures performed between 1975 and 1984 also settle on an overall mortality rate of around 7 per 1000. Major identifiable risk factors for mortality included patient and surgical factors and procedures performed in the first half of the 10-year period.

While comparisons of performance between different departments and different countries are most interesting, there are likely to be many confounding factors preventing meaningful interpretation. Not least of these will be differing patient populations and patterns of disease. Standards of training among anaesthetists will also be variable. It is for these reasons that comparisons of the same patient base over time are invaluable.

The triennial reports on Maternal Mortality in the UK contain information dating back to 1952, so it is possible to observe changes over 4 decades. Fortunately the mortality rate due to anaesthesia in pregnancy appears to be declining. From 1970 to 1972 mortality solely due to anaesthesia was found to be 12.8 per million pregnancies, while in the 1985–1987 report the figure was down to 1.9 deaths per million (Department of Health 1991). The anaesthetic contribution to maternal mortality also declined in relation to other causes from over 10% in the years between 1970 and 1984 (Department of Health 1991) to 4.4% in the latest report. It is to be hoped that this trend will be maintained.

Harrison has also reported a 6-fold improvement in anaesthetic mortality rates (1990), but over three decades from 1956 to 1987. Since Harrison's audit included information on 750 000 anaesthetic procedures, the improvement from a mortality rate solely due to anaesthesia of 0.43 per 1000 administrations in the first 5 years to a mortality rate of 0.07 per 1000 in the last 5 years represents a considerable advance. Nevertheless he is careful to point out that as many as 86% of the anaesthetic deaths were preventable. Put another way, if the experience of the Groote Schuur Hospital is typical, Harrison calculates that at least 100 patients die each year in South Africa because they are anaesthetized. If it is remembered that almost 90% of deaths in his survey were preventable, 'death solely due to anaesthesia must continue to be of concern'. This has always been the case. Almost 40 years ago Beecher & Todd (1954) identified errors of 'anaesthetic technique, choice or management' in almost 80% of 384 anaesthetic deaths collected from a multicentre audit of some 600 000 anaesthetic administrations.

AIRWAY PROBLEMS

Difficulty in placing an endotracheal tube is mentioned by many authors as a cause of perioperative mortality. This is particularly so in obstetric anaesthesia. Intubation difficulty is not the prerogative of obstetric anaesthetists, however. Green & Taylor (1984) reported on deaths and severe brain damage resulting in claims against members of the Medical Protection Society in the years 1977–82 inclusive. The annual rate of claims increased over the 5 years and both consultant and trainee anaesthetists were involved, although trainees were implicated almost twice as often as their seniors. This may reflect the number of difficult emergency cases trainees attempt, perhaps inappropriately. The increasing rate of claims possibly reflects the changing attitudes of the legal profession and the general public, rather than an alarming trend toward more frequent complications. It is important to note, however, that 30 of the 71 patients suffered death or serious brain damage as a direct result of respiratory obstruction or intubation difficulty.

All too frequently failure of technique is related to care of the airway, and whereas the underlying mortality rate due to anaesthesia may be declining, there is little evidence for improvement in airway management when measured by crude mortality statistics. In a retrospective survey of maternal deaths at one hospital for a 20-year period, Morgan (1980) reported five anaesthesia deaths, two of which were attributable to intubation difficulty. Between 1976 and 1979 in England and Wales, thirty pregnant women died as a direct result of anaesthesia and six of these deaths were associated with difficult intubation.

The problem has not diminished over the years and intubation difficulty was the single most common problem among the 18 maternal deaths solely due to anaesthesia reported in England and Wales between 1982 and 1984 (Department of Health 1988; Table 1.1). By the next triennium (1985–87) the total number of maternal deaths solely due to anaesthesia had fortunately fallen to eight, in spite of data from Scotland and Northern Ireland being included for the first time (Department of Health 1991). Unfortunately the proportion due to intubation difficulty had increased to a massive 75% and a further death was attributed to aspiration of gastric contents. Anaesthesia contributed to death in a further 16 cases and the anaesthetic care in all of these was considered to be below accepted standards.

The problem is apparently international. Holland (1984) reported from Australia that 69% of 109 anaesthesia-related deaths up to 1979 were due to airway catastrophes, 40% were due to aspiration of gastric contents, 12% were due to failure to maintain an airway, and 3% involved oesophageal intubation. Airway difficulty was also by far the most common cause of damage in the American Society of Anesthesiologists' Closed Claims Study (Cheney et al 1989), accounting for 522 of 1541 claims (34%). Death or brain damage occurred in 85% of these airway cases and a total of 94 patients had been oesophageally intubated.

Table 1.1 Factors involved in deaths solely due to anaesthesia in pregnancy

	1982–84	1985–87
Inhalation of gastric contents	7	1
Intubation difficulty	10	6
Failure of postoperative care	5	–
Haemorrhage	4	–
Drug misuse	1	–
Apparatus misuse	1	–
Epidural anaesthesia	1	1

It seems from an editorial by Newton (1991) that we are even incapable of giving oxygen to patients in the postoperative period without causing deaths. Four cases (two fatal) of barotrauma from direct application of pipeline or cylinder pressure to the airway had been reported to the Safety Committee of the Association of Anaesthetists in the UK. In three cases patients had been given oxygen from a face mask although intubated and 'by chance the inlet port of the oxygen mask . . . had impacted onto the 15 mm male connector of the tracheal tube causing a flow of oxygen of some 5 l/min to be delivered directly to the trachea'. In another incident ambulance personnel had connected the oxygen supply directly to an endotracheal tube because of difficulty keeping the mask in place.

Management of the airway is the basis of anaesthetic practice and it is of serious concern that this aspect should cause so many deaths, especially since in the view of the assessors in the American Society of Anesthesiologists' Closed Claims Study (Cheney et al 1989) most adverse outcomes (72%) were considered preventable with better monitoring. Three mechanisms of injury accounted for three-quarters of the respiratory adverse events. These were inadequate ventilation, oesophageal intubation and difficult intubation, in descending order of frequency. In 90% of cases labelled 'inadequate ventilation' care was considered to be substandard. Auscultation of breath sounds proved to be a poor test for identifying oesophageal intubation since auscultation led to the erroneous belief that the tube was correctly sited in 48% of cases. This highlights the need for improved training of anaesthetists specifically in these crisis situations. One way in which we may focus on these events is to develop incident monitoring systems which pick up the much more frequent near misses which can prove so instructive to trainees. Unless we do so it seems that we are destined to make the same mistakes over and over again.

Airway problems are also discussed in Chapter 31.

INFLUENCE OF PRE-EXISTING DISEASE

In most operative deaths both surgical and anaesthetic factors are involved as well as patient factors. Death due solely to anaesthesia is rare. It becomes important, therefore, to distinguish not only between surgical and anaesthetic causes, but also between patients who are at very high risk and those who should certainly survive. Patients classified as ASA V (ASA: American Society of Anesthesiologists physical scoring system) have no chance of survival regardless of anaesthesia or surgery. Conversely, patients classified ASA I have no pre-existing disease to increase the risk of anaesthesia and this group should have a nil mortality rate from anaesthesia alone.

The 12 chapters in Section 2 of this book deal in considerable detail with specific diseases and conditions which make anaesthesia more hazardous in patients who would be classified ASA II, III and IV. Consequently this aspect needs little mention here. It is, however, essential to understand the relationship between overall mortality from elective and emergency surgery and factors such as site of operation, age, preoperative condition and type of surgery. Vital data on these relationships have been collected over many years in Cardiff, and Lunn et al (1982) reported on a series of more than 100 000 anaesthetics administered between 1972 and 1977. The end point of study for each patient was discharge from hospital or death, so that all patients dying in hospital following anaesthesia and surgery were included, but no attempt was made to differentiate between anaesthetic and surgical causes of death. The overall mortality rate was 2.2% and almost two-thirds of deaths had occurred within 2 weeks of surgery. In a second report on the data Farrow et al (1982) demonstrated that the mortality in males was higher than that in females and that the risk was greatest in patients over 65 years of age. Mortality rate varied according to site of operation and, perhaps not surprisingly, intracranial surgery carried the greatest risk (9.7% mortality). Intrathoracic procedures were also high risk (8.6%), as were upper abdominal operations (6.6%). In contrast there were no deaths associated with caesarean sections or surgery on the ear. Patients treated as emergencies were 35 times more likely to die than those dealt with electively. Even simple routine surgery was associated with a measureable mortality rate and repair of inguinal hernia (0.4%), cystoscopy (0.6%), and even dilatation and curettage (0.1%) proved not to be immune from risk.

The third and final report on this data (Fowkes et al 1982) concentrated on the influence of coexisting disease. Each preoperative condition was associated with a higher mortality rate than occurred in patients with no preoperative condition. For example the overall risk of death in hospital was 0.5% for healthy individuals, but the mortality rate in patients with ischaemic heart disease or diabetes was much greater (7% and 5.7%, respectively). A combination of emergency surgery and preoperative disease increased the mortality rate by a factor of 18, but, interestingly, the influence of pre-existing disease diminished with increasing age. It was not stated to what extent anaesthesia may have contributed to the deaths reported in this series, but it is reasonable to assume that the relative contribution of anaesthesia would be much smaller than that of surgery.

This information is now rather old, but the principles remain unchallenged. As techniques and available agents improve, no doubt we will see a gradual lowering of the anaesthetic risk to patients with serious underlying disease, and it is tempting to speculate that better techniques of postoperative care will also reduce the surgical-risk component. Anaesthesia-related deaths are not, however, limited to sick patients, for many disasters occur in previously healthy individuals. Obviously no blame can be attached to the patient and often the surgery will have been straightforward. The issues are simple: How did anaesthesia cause the death? Did the anaesthetist make an error? Was the death the result of an unexpected severe reaction to an anaesthetic drug or a failure of equipment? If so could the anaesthetist reasonably have been expected to treat it more effectively? The answers to these questions may be difficult to ascertain, but the influence of human error cannot be ignored.

Mistakes that prove fatal need to be subjected to peer review and this is now increasingly the case. Of course, disclosure of the facts may well be facilitated if the review is anonymous, such as is the case with the triennial reports on maternal mortality in the UK. There is inevitably a delay in the publication of such audits and, while this does not soften the message, there is considerable potential for other similar disasters in the interim. The other problem is that anaesthetic deaths may well be the tip of a very large iceberg of anaesthetic mishaps. There is consequently much merit in systems that identify mishaps not causing damage.

ANAESTHETIC INCIDENTS

It is easy for individual anaesthetists to dismiss the conclusions from large audits of anaesthetic death or morbidity as not being applicable to them. Anaesthetic deaths are, after all, comparitively rare. It is, however, more difficult for us to ignore near misses and incidents occuring in our own departments. Various systems of incident reporting have been devised, starting with the so-called 'Critical Incident' (CI) Reporting System adapted by Cooper et al (1978) from the original work of Flanagan (1954). Unfortunately, to limit reporting to so-called 'critical' incidents ignores many other incidents of value in the education of trainees, and it is for this reason that many departments have expanded their reporting systems to include any incident involving patient care occurring in the operating theatre or recovery room.

Our confidence in incident reporting systems will of course be greatly enhanced if such systems identify many of the problems which have in the past proved damaging to patients. But the final proof of efficacy of incident reporting will only come when the number of patients suffering serious morbidity or death decreases as a direct consequence of such initiatives. In the first instance it is important that an incident reporting system is seen to be non-threatening, for it is then much more likely to pick up a high percentage of the problems. The additional effort of data collection must not become burdensome or interest will be short-lived. This latter aspect is vital since a successful incident reporting system will presumably need to continue indefinitely if new recruits to the specialty are to be taught correctly. Unfortunately, response rate seems to fall with time (Currie 1989) and continual effort from the data collector is necessary to maintain the system.

Cardiac arrests

Cardiac arrests (CAs) are, of course, CIs in their own right, but an arrest may be preceded by another CI which, if treated promptly, could have avoided the need for cardiopulmonary resuscitation (CPR) and possible damage to the patient. Of course, not all CAs result in morbidity or mortality, and it might be supposed that CAs occurring under anaesthesia would be attended by better results than arrests occurring in ordinary wards or casualty departments. Sadly, inspite of monitoring and the presence of an anaesthetist, there is little evidence to suggest that patients suffering CA in the operating room do any better than patients arresting elsewhere. This may well be because so many such episodes are accompanied by identifiable errors of anaesthetic management.

In an audit of CAs over a 15-year period Keenan & Boyan (1985) reported that almost half the anaesthetic CAs were caused by failure to provide adequate ventilation and a third resulted from an absolute overdose of inhalational agent. They identified errors of management in 75% of cases. In all, 449 patients suffered CA (a rate of 2.7 per 1000), but the majority of arrests were ascribed to the patient's condition or type of surgery. The overall incidence of CA solely due to anaesthesia was 27 out of 163 240 procedures (1.7 per 10 000), but this figure is probably an underestimate since it does not appear to include CAs from anaesthetic causes occurring in the recovery room or postoperative ward. The survival rate was less than 50% and only 12 patients out of the 27 survived without long-term damage.

Factors associated with increased risk of CA were emergency surgery (6.5 per 10 000; see also Ch. 39), age less than 12 years (4.7 per 10 000; see also Ch. 12) and ASA classes III and IV. Significantly, 15 patients arrested due to drug-related problems but 12 patients were labelled 'failure to ventilate' due either to inability to intubate or to ventilate (4), oesophageal intubation (4), displaced endotracheal tube (1), or bronchospasm (1). Two of the 12 were victims of ventilator disconnection. Only one CA was considered to have been unavoidable, 20 were labelled avoidable and the remaining six were questionable. This survey yet again points to the human factor as being the most common cause of problems, with equipment failure totally unrepresented as a cause of CA. Equipment hazards are discussed fully in Section 6.

Olsson & Hallen (1988) reported an incidence of 6.8 per 10 000 procedures for CA during anaesthesia at the Karolinska Institute in Sweden between 1967 and 1984. Like Keenan's data, these figures also appear to exclude CAs occuring in the postoperative ward. In all there were over 250 000 cases, including 170 CAs of which 115 were due to anaesthesia. This incidence of 4.6 per 10 000 anaesthetics appears to be much higher than that quoted by Keenan, but the rate reduced more than 10-fold over the period of the audit from an alarmingly high level of more than 20 per 10 000 in 1967 to less than 2 per 10 000 in 1984. Non-anaesthetic factors associated with increased risk of CA included ASA III and IV, age less than 9 years, emergency surgery and age more than 60 (see also Ch. 13). Drug-related problems were the most common cause of CA, but ventilatory problems were the cause of 27 cases. Perhaps most significant, two-thirds of the CAs occurred with non-specialist anaesthetists and the authors point out that the decreasing incidence of CA over the years coincided with the employment of an increasing number of trained anaesthetists. The figures presented by Olsson & Hallen (1988) may therefore reflect a local problem (i.e. inadequate training), particularly in the early years of the study, but the message is one that we can ill afford to ignore.

Critical incidents

There is no doubt that the same problems feature commonly both in CI reports and in mortality statistics. Currie (1989) analysed 167 CIs occurring in Sydney over a 2½-year period and he reported human error to be a contributory factor in 82% of cases. There were 102 reports involving the airway, including 47 episodes of non-ventilation of the patient, 17 disconnections or leaks, and a further 14 reports of oesophageal or failed intubation, none of which appeared to be associated with morbidity. This is very much in keeping with studies reporting a high incidence of airway problems and human error resulting in death or serious injury. However, Currie also reported a high incidence of drug-related and equipment-related CIs which rather contradicted a report of an earlier pilot study from the same department (Currie et al 1988). In general, drug and equipment incidents are not common causes of anaesthetic deaths. Could it be that we all find it easier to report equipment failure than human failure?

Does critical incident reporting improve safety?

Cooper et al (1987) have attempted to relate incident reporting and feedback of data to improvement in standards using an incident monitoring system called Recovery Room Impact Event (RRIE). An RRIE was defined as 'an unanticipated, undesirable, possibly anaesthesia-related effect that required intervention, was pertinent to recovery room care, and did or could cause mortality or at least moderate morbidity'. The study lasted 65 weeks and was divided into three phases. In the first phase of 17 weeks, information on RRIEs was collected and anaesthetic staff were regularly encouraged to participate but were given no feedback. From weeks 18 to 28, staff were given intensive feedback on complications, and at the beginning of week 29 pulse oximeters were placed in all anaesthetizing locations. Over the study period 12 088 patients were treated and the most commonly reported RRIEs were hypotension (4.4%), arrhythmia

(3.9%), hypertension (1.5%), unanticipated intubation difficulty (0.82%), hypoventilation (0.76%), hypovolaemia (0.62%) and bronchospasm (0.58%). Other RRIEs had individual incidences of less than 0.5%. This list differs somewhat from that reported by Currie et al (1988) and this may reflect the fact that RRIEs are specifically designed to be pertinent to recovery staff.

Intensive feedback did not alter the rate of reporting of RRIEs, and no single complication was identified as having a significantly different incidence for the feedback period versus the control period. The impact of pulse oximetry was also somewhat disappointing in that the incidence of RRIEs in the operating room remained unchanged when compared to the immediately preceding feedback-period alone. There was, however, an overall decline in the number of patients suffering at least one RRIE in operating rooms and recovery rooms combined, following the introduction of pulse oximetry. No single complication seemed to be significantly reduced in frequency by the new technology when the pulse oximetry period was compared to the feedback period, and, although there was a trend towards fewer reports as the study progressed, it was not clear whether this was due to apathy or a genuine reduction in rate of complications.

Rhoton (1989) used an incident monitoring system to evaluate anaesthesiology trainees in an American teaching hospital. Over a period of 6 years teachers were encouraged to complete Clinical Anaesthesia System of Evaluation (CASE) forms each day on each trainee. These were then analysed weekly by a senior staff member. Every 6 weeks, trainees met the head of department to discuss their progress and receive feedback on their own CASE data. Positive and negative comments were recorded in 13 categories such as pre/postoperative evaluation, patient management, efficiency and organisation, composure, eagerness to learn, interpersonal relationships, knowledge, technical skills and so on. In addition, CIs were recorded, as were examples of unprofessional behaviour. From a response rate of 75%, the highest number of positive and negative comments was made in the first 3 months of each 2-year training period for each of the six training intakes. The categories with the highest proportion of negative comments were technical skills, efficiency and organisation, management, knowledge and CIs. Of the CIs, drug, airway and monitoring incidents were common for all six intakes, but, most interestingly, the frequency of CIs decreased over the first four training intakes before rising again for the last two. Perhaps more important, the frequency of CIs did not decrease for individual groups as training progressed; in fact, quite the reverse. The highest incidence of CIs overall was between months 16 and 18 of training. This was in spite of a quite intensive programme of monitoring and individual feedback. This is somewhat disappointing in view of the enormous effort involved, but is not altogether unexpected since, in the author's words, the trainees may have been 'vigorously testing their increasing freedom to manage difficult cases'.

ANAESTHETIC SIMULATION

Rather than allowing trainees to test their abilities on patients with all the attendant risks, some workers have developed anaesthesia simulations as training tools. DeAnda & Gaba (1990) have developed a simulation system based on real monitors in a real operating room, complete with simulated waveforms and patient information. The patient is replaced by a mannequin with palpable veins for intravenous access. The simulation is run in real time and trainees are encouraged to think aloud while the whole process is videotaped for immediate debriefing after the session. From a total of 19 simulations, 132 unplanned incidents were documented (6.9 per case) of which 36 were considered 'critical'. The majority (87) were due to human error and of these, monitor usage, airway management, and ventilation and circuitry problems were the most numerous. In addition, drug administration errors accounted for more than 10% of this total, while equipment failure, such as failure of the laryngoscope light, was relatively uncommon (3%). Such a preponderance of human error incidents fits in well with data from real situations (Cooper et al 1978, 1984), but the simulation may itself have caused either increased vigilance or decreased standards of practice depending on the personality of the trainee.

Schwid & O'Donnell (1990) have developed a simulation running on an IBM compatible computer which is clearly, therefore, more easily accessible to trainees than is the comprehensive simulation devised by DeAnda & Gaba, described above. Schwid & O'Donnell's system was found to be easily understood even by those trainees without computer experience, and since it simulates CIs, such as oesophageal intubation, obstructed endotracheal tube, bronchospasm, anaphylaxis and myocardial ischaemia, it offers the promise of educating trainees in the correct thought processes to deal with such events. Whether or not such simulations will ultimately translate into safer anaesthesia remains to be seen, but the potential role of simulators in training anaesthetists is discussed in detail in Chapter 2.

STANDARDS OF PRACTICE

In the UK, at least in legal terms, good standards of practice might be defined as those which 'would receive support from a responsible body of professional opinion' (see Ch. 46). Standards continue to improve, but thus far the standards taken as acceptable by the courts have been those that would have been appropriate at the time of the alleged negligence, which is likely to have been several years earlier. Proof of medical negligence is necessary before judgement can be given against the doctor, and negligence has not usually been proved when expert medical opinion has been supportive of the method of treatment, regardless of any injury the patient might have suffered. In other words, no negligence, no financial settlement. Increasingly, however, cases are settled out of court without admission of liability since the costs of the legal process are so very high. Whether this will distort the picture remains to be seen.

The situation in the USA is very different, in that a good standard of anaesthetic practice may be insufficient defence against a claim for medical malpractice. Data from 1004 closed malpractice claims (Cheney et al 1989) suggest that while payment to the injured patient or his estate was made in 80% of cases, judged by the Committee on Professional Liability of the American Society of Anesthesiologists to have received substandard care, payment was also made in 40% of cases where anaesthetic care was considered appropriate. In other words, the courts appear to be setting standards of practice that are at odds with expert opinion.

Clearly neither of the above systems is satisfactory, but a system of no-fault-compensation also has problems. The New Zealand system removes the right of an injured person to bring an action for negligence (Laurenson & Gibbs 1988). Instead, an independent body assesses the case and makes an award if appropriate. The only method of complaint against a doctor is, therefore, through the General Medical Council, and there has been a significant increase in complaints of this type. Since hospital administrators are very unlikely to be held accountable in a court of law in New Zealand, they are apparently less inclined to replace outdated equipment which is, of course, a strategy not in the best interests of the patient either. This is particularly so if the findings of Medical Malpractice Underwriting Associations in the USA are representative. In 1988 it was reported (Pierce 1988) that at least three of the major malpractice insurance companies in the USA had reduced rates to anaesthetists as a result of reduced morbidity following the introduction of the Harvard Minimum Monitoring Standards (Eichhorn et al 1986).

Brahams (1989b) pointed out that three anaesthetic fatalities in the UK in 1988 might not have occurred if the Harvard Minimum Monitoring Standards had been in operation and she went on to recommend that 'Defence societies and health authorities in Britain should take greater note of the US experience.'

STANDARDS OF TRAINING

In criticizing the conduct of the resuscitation of two unfortunate patients suffering cardiac arrest in the dental chair, Brahams (1989a), a barrister at law, suggested that health authorities in Britain 'should take note of the US experience' and that formal training in resuscitation was essential. In another article, Brahams (1988) commented on a case of irreversible brain damage resulting from an anaesthetic incident involving an overseas trainee unfamiliar with the anaesthetic ventilator. In discussing the question of supervision of trainees, Brahams (1988) stated that 'if mistakes occur through ignorance and lack of skill the health authority and the doctor may both be liable'. She also criticized the General Medical Council in the UK for supporting the sponsorship system whereby overseas trainees may be appointed without the necessary language skills: 'Sponsorship may be valuable but should the Professional Linguistics Assessment Board (PLAB) exam be avoided as a consequence?' In the event of a medical accident involving a trainee, therefore, it may be incumbent on the supervising consultant and the employing health authority to show that adequate supervision and training were given.

REFERENCES

Beecher H K, Todd D P 1954 A study of the deaths associated with anaesthesia and surgery. Ann Surg 140: 2–35

Bradley J P, Beem M F, O'Donnell J E, Van De Meene A H 1988 Mortality audit in a large teaching hospital. Anaesth Intensive Care 16: 94–97

Brahams D 1988 Lessons from an anaesthetic accident. Lancet 2(8599): 1408

Brahams D 1989a Death in the dentist's chair. Lancet 2(8669): 991–992

Brahams D 1989b Monitoring equipment and anaesthetic failures. Lancet (8629): 111–112

Cheney F W, Posner K, Caplan R A, Ward R J 1989 Standard of care and anaesthesia liability. J Am Med Assoc 261(11): 1599–1603

Cohen M M, Duncan P G, Tate R B 1988 Does anaesthesia contribute to operative mortality? J Am Med Assoc 260(19): 2859–2863

Cooper J B, Newbower R S, Long C D, McPeek B 1978 Preventable anaesthesia mishaps: a study of human factors. Anesthesiology 49: 399–406

Cooper J B, Newbower R S, Kitz R J 1984 An analysis of major errors and equipment failures in anaesthesia management: considerations for prevention and detection. Anesthesiology 60: 34–42

Cooper J B, Cullen D J, Nemeskal R, Hoaglin D C, Gevirtz C C, Csete M, Venable C 1987 Effects of information feedback and pulse oximetry on the incidence of anaesthesia complications. Anesthesiology 67: 686–694

Currie M 1989 A prospective survey of anaesthetic critical incidents in a teaching hospital. Anaesth Intensive Care 17: 403–411

Currie M, Pybus D A, Torda T A 1988 A prospective survey of anaesthetic critical events: a report on a pilot study of 88 cases. Anaesth Intensive Care 16: 103–107

DeAnda A, Gaba D M 1990 Unplanned incidents during comprehensive anaesthesia simulation. Anesth Analg 71: 77–82

Department of Health 1988 Report on confidential enquiries into maternal deaths in England and Wales 1982–84. HMSO, London

Department of Health 1991 Report on confidential enquiries into maternal deaths in the United Kingdom 1985–87. HMSO, London

Eichhorn J H, Cooper J B, Cullen D J, Maier W R, Philip J H, Seeman R G 1986 Standards for patient monitoring during anaesthesia at Harvard Medical School. J Am Med Assoc 256(8): 1017–1020

Farrow S C, Fowkes F G R, Lunn J N, Robertson I B, Samuel P 1982 Epidemiology in anaesthesia II. Br J Anaesth 54: 811–817

Flanagan J C 1954 The critical incident technique. Psychol Bull 51: 327–358

Fowkes F G R, Lunn J N, Farrow S C, Robertson I B, Samuel P 1982 Epidemiology in anaesthesia III. Br J Anaesth 54: 819–824

Green R A, Taylor T H 1984 An analysis of anaesthesia medical liability claims in the United Kingdom, 1977–1982. In: Pierce C E (ed) Analysis of anaesthetic mishaps. Little, Brown, Boston, pp 73–89

Harrison G G 1968 Deaths associated with anaesthesia: a classification and autopsy evaluation. J Forensic Med 5: 71–83

Harrison G G 1978 Death attributable to anaesthesia. Br J Anaesth 50: 1041–1046

Harrison G G 1990 Death due to anaesthesia at Groote Schuur Hospital, Cape Town: 1956–1987. S Afr Med J 77: 412–415

Holland R 1984 Anaesthesia related mortality in Australia. Int Anesthesiol Clin 22: 61–71

Keenan R L, Boyan C P 1985 Cardiac arrest due to anaesthesia. J Am Med Assoc 253(16): 2373–2377

Laurenson V G, Gibbs J M 1988 The New Zealand scene: implications of no fault accident compensation. Anaesth Intensive Care 16: 89

Lunn J N 1985 Preventable anaesthetic mortality and morbidity. Anaesthesia 40: 79

Lunn J N, Farrow S C, Fowkes F G R, Robertson I B, Samuel P 1982 Epidemiology in anaesthesia I. Br J Anaesth 54: 803–809

Lunn J N, Mushin W W 1982 Mortality associated with anaesthesia. Nuffield Provincial Hospitals Trust, London

Morgan B M 1980 Maternal death. Anaesthesia 35: 334–338

Newton N I 1991 Supplementary oxygen: potential for disaster. Anaesthesia 46: 905–906
Olsson G L, Hallen B 1988 Cardiac arrest during anaesthesia: a computer aided study in 250543 anaesthetics. Acta Anaesthesiol Scand 32: 653–664
Pierce E C 1988 Monitoring instruments have significantly reduced anaesthetic mishaps. Journal Clin Monit 4: 111–114
Rhoton M F 1989 A new method to evaluate clinical performance and critical incidents in anaesthesia: quantification of daily comments by teachers. Med Educ 23: 280–289
Schwid H A, O'Donnell D 1990 The anesthesia simulator–recorder: a device to train and evaluate anesthesiologists' responses to critical incidents. Anesthesiology 72: 191–197
Turnbull K W, Fancourt-Smith P F, Banting G C 1980 Death within 48 hrs of anaesthesia at the Vancouver General Hospital. Can Anaesth Soc J 27: 159–163

2

Improving anaesthesia safety

V. Chopra and J. G. Bovill

LESSONS TO BE LEARNED FROM AVIATION

The past four decades have seen a remarkable decrease in the risk associated with anaesthesia and, in particular, the risk of death. The risk of death attributable to anaesthesia in the period 1948–1952 was reported as 1 in 2680 (Beecher & Todd 1954). However, in the recent report of a confidential enquiry into perioperative deaths in the UK (Buck et al 1987), only three deaths in 555 258 anaesthetics were directly attributable to anaesthesia, an incidence of 1 in 185 056. In the USA 13-fold reduction in anaesthetic mortality has been reported from 2.16 deaths per 10 000 anaesthetics in the period 1955–1964 to 0.16 deaths per 10 000 anaesthetics in the period 1977–1984 (Zeitlin 1989). This remarkable increase in anaesthetic safety has come about as the result of improvement in anaesthetic drugs, better apparatus and a general increase in our understanding of the physiological and pharmacological aspects of anaesthesia. Although these advances have undeniably increased our ability to anaesthetize successfully and safely even the most sick patient, they also bring with them potential disadvantages. In particular, our reliance on often complex equipment brings with it its own risks and potentials for danger. These risks lie not so much in the machines themselves, but in how we use them.

There remains a significant morbidity associated with anaesthesia (Cooper et al 1984, Cohen et al 1986, Chopra et al 1990). A major factor contributing to anaesthetic morbidity, or to the occurrence of incidents that have the potential for morbidity, is human error involving either equipment or drugs. Anaesthetists rightly place considerable emphasis on making the correct choice of anaesthetic drugs and technique for a particular patient to ensure that patient's optimum safety. A major part of the training of an anaesthetist is devoted to developing these professional skills. Much less attention is given to other aspects of general anaesthetic safety such as the careful and disciplined checking of apparatus, drugs, etc. By contrast this aspect of safety is given considerable attention during pilot training, and indeed throughout a pilot's professional career. This is one of several ways in which we in anaesthesia can profit from the experience of our counterparts in aviation.

Errors

The Oxford dictionary describes an error as 'something incorrectly done through ignorance or inadvertence; a flaw or malformation'. In anaesthesia, errors can either be the result of human or equipment failings. Human error contributes to 65–80% of all errors in anaesthesia (Utting et al 1979, Craig & Wilson 1981, Cooper et al 1984). Three types of human error can be distinguished: slips, mistakes and omissions (Schreiber & Schreiber 1989). Slips are errors in which the intended action was correct but the actual action was wrong. Inadvertent turning off the oxygen instead of the nitrous oxide at the end of surgery is an example of a slip. A mistake is an error, where the intention itself was wrong. Inducing anaesthesia with thiopentone in a patient in whom there were reasonable grounds to suspect porphyria is a mistake. An omission is the failure to act when an action is required. Failure to check the equipment before use or failure to turn on the monitor is an omission.

Equipment failure plays a relatively minor role as a cause of anaesthetic mishaps. Cooper et al (1984) reported that equipment failure accounted for only 11% of all critical incidents and that only 4% of the incidents with substantive negative outcomes involved equipment failure. The majority of these incidents involved breathing circuits and monitoring devices. The results of a prospective study of unsafe practices and working conditions during anaesthesia show that equipment error was responsible for 21% of all reported incidents and the majority of these involved monitoring devices (Chopra et al 1992).

Human errors involving drug administration, airway management and ventilation are the most common (Cooper et al 1984, Chopra et al 1992). These factors have also been identified as the major contributors to anaesthesia-related cardiac arrests (Table 2.1). Most of the errors in drug administration involve picking up the wrong syringe, drawing up a drug from the wrong ampoule and inadvertent or relative drug overdosage. Faults in drug administration during anaesthesia are listed below (Chopra et al 1990):

- 100% N_2O instead of 100% O_2 at the end of anaesthesia
- intramuscular suxamethonium instead of ketamine to a child
- isoprenaline instead of atropine to treat bradycardia
- intravenous sodium citrate instead of potassium chloride
- intravenous sufentanil instead of alfentanil during general anaesthesia
- administration of saline solution which was not intended for intravenous use
- adrenaline given instead of atropine
- overdose of fentanyl during neurolept anaesthesia
- wrong concentration of lignocaine during cardiorespiratory resuscitation
- interchange of inlet and outlet of halothane vaporizer leading to overdose
- rapid intravenous injection of potassium chloride during general anaesthesia
- ketamine overdose as a result of calculation based on wrong weight of a child.

Errors of airway management and ventilation include breathing-circuit disconnections, gas-flow setting errors, oesophageal intubation, circuit leaks, hypoventilation and unintentional extubation.

Table 2.1 Summary of preventable cardiac arrests in patients with an ASA classification 1–3 (modified from Chopra et al 1990)

Age (years)	ASA	Fatal outcome	Description
26	2	No	Overdose of halothane due to unintentionally open vaporizer
54	2	No	Overdose of neurolept anaesthesia leading to postoperative respiratory arrest in the recovery room
54	2	No	Hypotension leading to cardiac arrest during epidural anaesthesia
57	2	No	Hypoxia due to accidental bronchial intubation
58	3	No	Hyperkalaemia because of rapid i.v. injection of potassium chloride
68	3	No	Hypoventilation in spontaneously breathing patient, and hypokalaemia treated with rapid intravenous administration of potassium chloride during general anaesthesia, leading to ventricular fibrillation
72	3	Yes	Cardiac arrest during epidural plus general anaesthesia; history of preoperative myocardial infarction; possible cause, intraoperative hypotension and myocardial infarction
73	3	Yes	Ventilator disconnection with alarms switched off in the postoperative period

Of the factors associated with human errors during anaesthesia, failure to perform a proper check is the most frequently reported (Craig & Wilson 1981, Cooper et al 1984). Lack of vigilance, carelessness, distraction, inadequate experience and haste are other commonly associated factors (Table 2.2). Vigilance during anaesthesia, defined as a state of clinical awareness whereby dangerous conditions are anticipated or recognized and promptly corrected, has been investigated by Gravenstein & Weigner (1986) and Mackie (1987). Paget et al (1981) reviewed factors that influence the vigilance of an anaesthetist. Sleep deprivation, time sharing, the signal frequency, the strength and mode of presentation of information by monitors, noise and environmental pollution were the most important factors that they identified. The interaction between the anaesthetist and equipment also influences vigilance. Kay & Neal (1986) found that automated blood pressure devices had a negative influence on vigilance as compared to manual measurement of blood pressure. Parker (1987) reviewed the effect of fatigue on performance and suggested that anaesthetists should be relieved for short periods every 2 h when responsible for long (more than 3 h) procedures. He also recommended that an anaesthetist should not work for more than 16 h at a stretch without a full 12 h recovery period, and no anaesthetist should be on call for more than 24 h without a full 24 h recovery period. When fatigued, one is less likely to detect important changes in monitored variables than when rested and mentally alert. This was shown by Denisco et al (1987) who measured the effect of fatigue on 21 anaesthesia residents in a simulated monitoring situation. The beneficial effect of intraoperative exchanges of anaesthesia personnel in discovering errors, or causes of errors, during anaesthesia has been demonstrated (Cooper et al 1982).

Table 2.2 Commonly associated factors with misadventures during anaesthesia (from Craig & Wilson 1981)

Associated factors	Number
Failure to perform a normal check	27
Emergency case	12
Distraction	10
Inattention	10
Hurry	9
Lack of skilled assistance	8
Fatigue	7
Lack of experience with equipment	6
Lack of experience with technique	4
Restricted access to patient	2
Boredom	1
Failure to assess the situation preoperatively	1
Failure of planning	1
Confusion over equipment	1

ANAESTHESIA AND AVIATION

Anaesthesia and aviation have much in common, not least in the extensive use of modern technology to control and monitor the functioning of the respective patient or aeroplane. There are many similarities between the workspace of a pilot in the cockpit of an aeroplane and that of an anaesthetist in a modern operating theatre. Both systems are undeniably complex, with many human and technical elements interacting with each other (Figs 2.1 & 2.2). The ultimate aim of both anaesthesia and aviation is to maintain a high standard of customer (patient or passenger) safety. Both tend to achieve this goal by utilizing the concept of team work (crew concept).

Checklist procedures

For many years the routine and disciplined use of checklists has formed an integral part of standard operating procedures in aviation. Considerable time is spent on teaching and practising these procedures during pilot training so that their use becomes automatic. A pilot, during routine and emergency procedures, backs up his memory with standard checklists. In contrast, an anaesthetist in similar circumstances relies heavily on his memory alone.

In aviation, standard checklists are applied before all critical events, such as engine start up, take off, descent, landing, etc. (Table 2.3). Items on the list are called out by one of the crew, while the other performs the specific check procedure. If one of them has doubts about an item on the checklist, reading stops until both agree that it is safe to proceed. This minimizes the possibility of

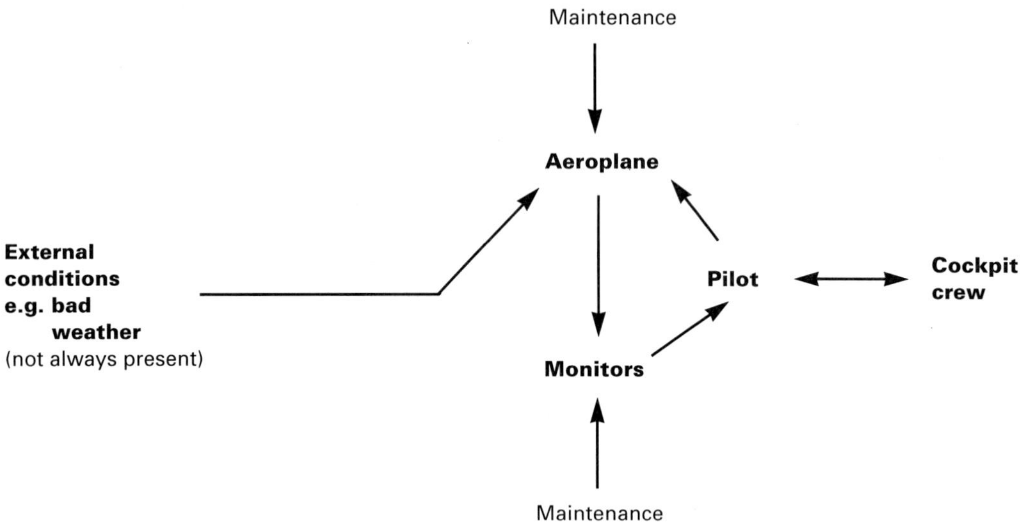

Fig. 2.1 Some important interactions that influence aviation safety.

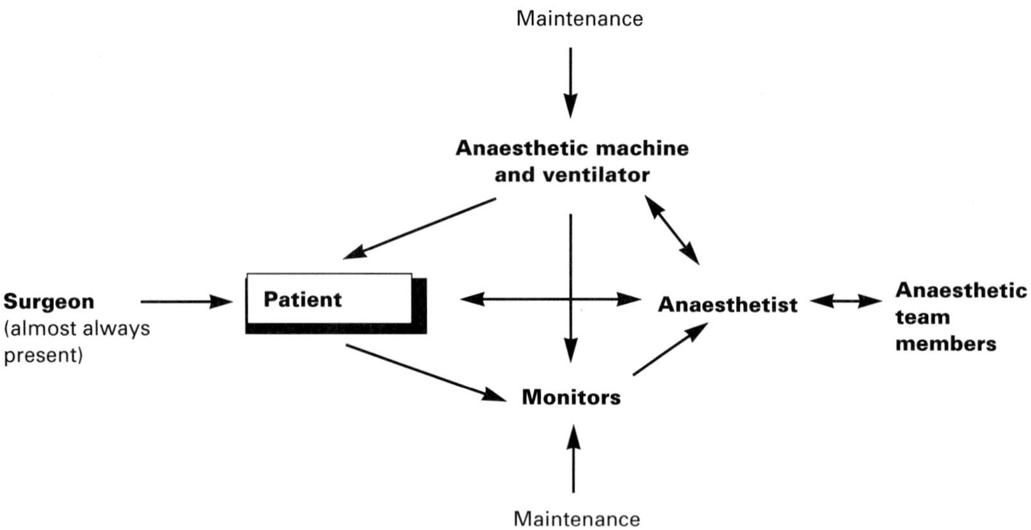

Fig. 2.2 Some important interactions that influence anaesthesia safety.

Table 2.3 Part of the preflight checklist used by pilots of Boeing 747

Nav. equipment	Checked
Oxygen and interphone	Checked
Grd. prox. warning	Checked
Marker beacon lights	Checked
Instrumental warning	Checked
Radio altimeters	Checked
FMAs	Checked
ADIs	Checked
Heading indicators	Checked and set
Clocks	Checked and set
PMS preflight check	Completed
INS	Checked
Waypoints	Loaded and Checked
Cockpit lights	Set
Airspeed bugs	Set
FD Computer selectors	C and B
Altimeter bug	Set . . . ft
Speedmode selector	Off
FD pitch wheels	Set . . . ° up
Altimeter	Set . . .

misinterpreting or overlooking an item. Such a disciplined approach to the checking of equipment is essential when operating a complex piece of modern technology, such as a Boeing 747, where the lives of passengers and crew depend totally on the proper functioning of all its many systems.

Many of the items on the checklist will have been preset before carrying out the checklist procedure. Take-off speed will have been calculated according to total aircraft weight, number of passengers and prevailing weather, and set on the airspeed indicators by means of coloured pointers or 'bugs' set into the rim of the instruments. Engine settings will have been calculated and preset, and the correct frequencies chosen for communication and navigation equipment. These actions are the equivalent of an anaesthetist presetting tidal volume and ventilation frequency on a ventilator, adjusting alarm limits on monitoring equipment, etc. The checklist procedures serve as a double check that these preset items have been correctly set.

Although checklists are used in anaesthesia (Cundy & Baldock 1982, Kilian 1987), these have not been standardized and a structured and disciplined approach to their routine use is often lacking. In the department of anaesthesia in Leiden we have been using checklists analogous to those used in aviation (Table 2.4). As in the

Table 2.4 Part of the preanaesthetic checklist used in the University Hospital, Leiden. The complete checklist procedure also covers monitoring equipment, drugs, intubation materials and the patient

Anaesthetist 1 (Call)		Anaesthetist 2 (Response)	
A	Anaesthesia machine Dräger AV 1		
1	Check electrical connections	Electricals	OK
2	Check alarm limits	Alarm	OK
3	Check gas connections (Please attach artificial lung)	Gas	OK
4	Check and set O_2 meter	Oxymeter	OK and set
5	Check spirolog calibration	Spirolog	Calibrated
6	Check fresh gas flow	Flow	OK
7	Check vaporizer	Vaporizer	OK
8	Check suction	Suction	OK
9	Check circle system	Circle	OK
10	Check O_2 bypass	Bypass	OK
11	Leakage test	Test	OK
12	Check function control IPPV	IPPV	OK
13	Check and set volume	Volume	OK and set . . .
14	Check and set frequency	Frequency	OK and set . . .
15	Check and set PEEP	PEEP	OK and set zero
16	Check and set trigger	Trigger	OK and set off
17	Set selector 'IPPV/SPONT–MAN/MAN (FLOW+)'	Selector	Set for . . .
18	Set selector 'O_2–N_2O/O_2–AIR'	Selector	Set for . . .

Table 2.5 Effect of checklist procedures on critical incidents in anaesthesia (modified from Kumar et al 1988)

Category	Type of incident	Period A (before checklists)	Period B (after checklists)
Transmission of anaesthetic gases and vapours	Vaporizer problems	17	5
	Tracheal tube problems	10	1
	Disconnections	8	2
	Inadvertent gas flow changes	4	0
	Malfunctioning evacuation	4	2
	Leaks	4	3
	Ventilator problems	2	3
	Problems with ventilation	2	1
Drug administration	Syringe swap	16	5
	Relative overdosage	6	4
	Other		2
Miscellaneous		13	15
	Total number of incidents	86	43

cockpit, the checklist procedures are carried out by two people, usually an anaesthetist and an anaesthetic nurse. One calls out the individual items on the checklist, the other is responsible for performing the check. Each has a joint responsibility for the proper carrying out of the procedure. If a fault is found this must be corrected before proceeding with the remaining items on the checklist. The procedure covers not only the anaesthesia and monitoring equipment, but also the identification of drugs that have been drawn up prior to induction of anaesthesia, checking of intubation materials, and finally, and very importantly, the patient is checked. Though initially developed for a specific anaesthesia machine, the list can be modified easily for other anaesthetic apparatus.

Working through the complete checklist at the beginning of an operating session lasts about 6–7 min. Shorter checklists are used between patients. These checklist procedures have been in use for more than 2 years and have had a very high acceptance rate, both from anaesthetists and nurses. Checklists have also been developed for specific emergencies, such as cardiac arrest and malignant hyperthermia. These are used, once the emergency situation has been brought under control, as a back-up for the anaesthetist to ensure that important items that might have been forgotten during the crisis are not overlooked.

Evidence that the use of checklists, and in general better awareness of the relevance of critical incidents and the factors associated with them, can improve safety was provided by a study by Kumar et al (1988) at the University of Iowa. They carried out a prospective study into two 1-year periods; 1 year before and 1 year after the introduction of checklist procedures. In the first period 86 incidents were reported, the majority of which (80%) were attributed to human error. The most common mishaps involved transmission of anaesthetic gases and vapours or errors in drug administration. There was a significant decrease in the number of incidents during the second 1-year period, with an overall reduction in the total number of incidents reported from 86 to 43 (Table 2.5).

The use of checklist procedures is, however, only one of the lessons that we as anaesthetists can learn from our aviation counterparts.

Equipment design

As in anaesthesia, human error is largely responsible for the majority of accidents or near accidents in aviation. Hence it is more often the user, rather than the machine, that fails. How can we reduce the frequency of user errors? One approach is the improvement of equipment design and presentation of information by monitors. In the cockpit the instruments are so arranged that the attention of the pilot is never distracted from the main monitors. The most important instruments are situated in front of the pilot in his direct line of vision. In contrast, in the operating theatre, equipment is often situated so that the anaesthetist is forced to turn his head and usually look away from the patient in order to read the monitors. Arranging instruments so that the most important ones are placed in a direct line of vision, as in the cockpit, would help to improve safety and also reduce fatigue.

Until recently, the designers of anaesthetic equipment have paid little attention to the difficulties of anaesthetists in assimilating and acting upon the multitude of information that is presented to them and there was little incentive to carry out ergonomic studies (Rendell-Baker 1982, Cooper 1985). Rendell-Baker (1982) suggested that the electrocardiograph, flowmeters, vaporizers, respiratory pressure gauge, and valves should be mounted closest to the user's line of vision, and the controls for the ventilator, the blood pressure apparatus and the oxygen analyser should be close at hand. Failure to achieve good ergonomic design in operating theatres is largely due to the fragmentation of existing anaesthetic equipment between many different manufacturers. This situation is likely to change with the introduction of integrated anaesthetic workstations in which a ventilator, gas-delivery systems, vaporizers and monitors are incorporated into one machine. Integration of data acquisition and presentation has become standard in the new generation of aeroplanes and has been advocated for anaesthesia (Saunders & Jewett 1983, Cooper 1985).

The amount of visual information that the pilot of a previous generation of aircraft, for example the Boeing 747-200, is required to scan is quite enormous. There are over 20 sq. ft of dials, switches, levers and lights. In the new generation of aircraft the majority of information is presented on one computer screen. Under normal conditions, only information that is currently of direct relevance is displayed. In anaesthetic terms that might be, for example, heart rate, blood pressure and oxygen saturation data from a pulse oximeter. Other data are only displayed when it becomes relevant or the parameter deviates outside the normal limits, in which case suitable warnings are displayed on the screen. The development of such a system for the anaesthetist would undoubtedly be beneficial. With a small display screen placed at the head end of the operating table, interfaced to a suitable computer system, the anaesthetist could be presented with all relevant patient information at one focal point.

In spite of all these improvements, the safety of anaesthetic equipment will, in practice, depend on the user's understanding and implementation of them, reliable and regular maintenance, the avoidance of local modifications and the development of effective international standards for equipment (Thompson 1987).

Alarms

Another area where anaesthesia and aviation can be compared is the use of alarms. Alarms are an essential feature of, and cannot be separated from, any useful monitoring system. In recent years the monitoring devices used during anaesthesia have increased considerably, both in number and complexity. This, in turn, has lead to a multiplicity of alarms. Every item of modern anaesthetic equipment has one or more built-in alarms. Some give only a visual indication when an alarm is activated, others give only an audible indication, while the majority give both types of signal when activated. Kestin et al (1988) evaluated the significance of auditory alarms during routine anaesthesia in 50 patients. Of all alarms, 75% were spurious, while only 3% indicated risk to the patient. Meijler (1987) analysed warnings generated by a statistical disturbance algorithm during cardiac surgery by linking them to the responses of the anaesthetist. Of the 731 warnings analysed, only 7% turned out to be useful, and another 13% followed some intervention where the triggering of an alarm could have been anticipated. A haphazard combination of alarms and a high incidence of 'false' alarms reduces their effectiveness. When multiple alarms are triggered by some accidental interference, unrelated to the status of the patient, the resulting cacophony distracts the attention of both the anaesthetist and the surgical staff from their proper attention to the patient. The common response of the anaesthetist in this situation is to disable the alarm (McIntyre 1985, Sury et al 1986). McIntyre surveyed 852 Canadian anaesthetists and found that over half of them had at some time deliberately deactivated audible alarms at the start of the anaesthetic. The most common reason given was the high incidence of false alarms. Other reasons were that confusion between different audible signals made the alarm useless and actually hindered patient care.

The acceptability of an alarm system is increased if the alarm can be temporarily deactivated. This is common in ventilators so that the low-pressure alarm can be deactivated for periods of 30–60 s during, for example, suctioning of the trachea, when the presence of an alarm-generating condition can be predicted. The other situation is when an audible alarm signal has succeeded in capturing the attention of the anaesthetist to a potentially hazardous situation. At this point it is no longer needed and indeed becomes a hindrance. However, one should not be able to deactivate an alarm permanently, either directly with an on–off switch or by bypassing the alarm mechanism by setting alarm thresholds at unrealistic levels, for example high and low heart rates of 0 and 200 beats/min. Ideally, threshold limits for alarms should be automatically set when a piece of equipment is switched on, although these limits must be adjustable by the operator as conditions change during anaesthesia. Failure to preset, or to set appropriately low-pressure alarm thresholds in a ventilator, can result in failure to recognize a partial disconnection (McEwan et al 1980, Reynolds 1983). For signals that are expected to change gradually during the course of a procedure, some form of automatic scaling of alarm threshold limits would be a worthwhile option (Beneken & van der Aa 1989).

In the aviation industry, graded alarm functions are becoming standard. For example when an instrument or facility is activated, this is indicated to the pilots by a blue background light in the appropriate switch. Should the monitored signal or function deviate outside a defined normal limit, then the background light changes first from blue to yellow when the deviation is not immediately threatening. When the deviation is such that a real threat is posed, the background light changes from yellow to red. Usually these changes are also accompanied by an audible alarm. This may also be graded in frequency and/or amplitude. Such principles could be applied to our anaesthetic equipment.

From studies in civil aviation, Patterson (1982) proposed that alarm sounds should consist of a sequence of notes composed of at least four harmonics. This would improve localization of the sound. In addition, the alarm should sound once, followed by a period of silence of 20–30 s. If the cause had not been corrected within this period, the alarm would be repeated and urgency indicated by shorter periods of silence and an increase in pitch rather than amplitude.

The current situation in anaesthesia involves alarms that are scattered widely around the anaesthetist's workstation. When, as is often the case, several alarms become activated simultaneously, the anaesthetist can waste valuable time in deciding which alarms have sounded; time that should be spent in recognizing and solving the problem that initiated the alarm condition. Ideally we should have only one, centrally situated alarm annunciation, coupled with a screen on which messages indicating the source of the alarm, and possibly probable causes of the alert condition, are displayed. This calls for the implementation of an 'intelligent' monitoring and alarm system. Such systems are being introduced in aviation, in which trends in several parameters are monitored and the results collated and interpreted by computer, so that a warning can be given of a potential adverse incidence. This allows corrective action to be taken before the development of serious consequences. A commonly quoted situation where intelligent monitoring could be of value is the interpretation of changes in heart rate, arterial blood pressure and pulmonary capillary wedge pressure in a patient developing left ventricular failure. Such a system would also reduce the number of false alarms by utilizing the redundancy that is often present in current, and presumably also in future, monitoring systems. A good example is the monitoring of heart rate. This is universally derived from the ECG signal, but can often also be derived from an invasive arterial or other pressure waveform, a plethysmogram or oxygen-saturation monitor. An intelligent monitoring system would not activate an alarm state when the ECG-derived heart rate deviated outside the 'safe limits' provided the rate derived from one or, preferably, two other monitors indicated that the heart rate had not changed.

Data acquisition and storage

The digital flight data recorder or the 'black box' is an integral part of modern aviation. It is mandatory for any aeroplane certified for flying above 25 000 ft altitude or that is turbine-engine powered to have one or more approved flight recorders that continuously record the flight parameters. Data on time, altitude, speed, etc. are recorded as long as the aeroplane is airborne. Voice recordings in the cockpit are collected continuously in a separate recorder, but only the last 30 min of the record is preserved after termination of electrical power (e.g. at crash impact). In contrast the digital flight data recorders are capable of retaining 25 hours of flight information on a recycling magnetic tape, and recorded data are preserved even after electrical power has been disconnected.

In case of an accident or incident, recorders have to be turned over to the investigating authorities. During an accident investigation, the tapes are fed into a computer system. This gives a numerical and graphical print-out of the data. From these data the events leading to the accident can be reconstructed and analysed.

More recently, Aircraft Integrated Data Systems (AIDS) are being used by many airlines. This system monitors engine and aeroplane performance and provides important maintenance data. These data are regularly analysed for engine operation maintenance and fault detection. This helps to identify and correct problems before they can lead to major failures.

Attempts are being made to collect data automatically during anaesthesia, but the major aim until now has been to generate an automatic anaesthesia record (Mitchell 1982, Zissos & Strunin 1982, Meijler & Beneken 1987). Several commercial automatic anaesthesia records systems are available. These can be interfaced with the anaesthesia machine, ventilator and monitoring equipment. Data can be recorded automatically at user-specified intervals and/or during specified events, and there is provision for manual entry of data and comments. Attempts have also been made to enter such data using speech recognition systems (Sarnat et al 1982). Automated anaesthesia records have certain advantages compared with the normal handwritten records (van Kessel et al 1987). They are clearer and more complete. Readability is greatly improved. They are more objective and trend detection is facilitated. For example trends in a parameter are easier to detect when the data are plotted rather than listed numerically. An additional advantage is a reduction of the workload of the anaesthetist. Because of better clarity and completeness, an automatically generated anaesthesia record can be a valuable tool for retrospective analysis of an anaesthetic mishap. Those with experience of anaesthesia accident analysis know how unreliable and uninformative handwritten records can be. Most of the important information is either missing or was reconstructed from memory after the event (Schneider 1982).

Education and training

After initial flight training, the further training of an airline pilot involves three distinct steps (Beach 1988). The first step involves at least 10 days of extensive classroom (ground school) instruction based on one type of aircraft (Fig. 2.3). Trainees proceed through the course as a crew. During this course, time is spent not only on acquiring theoretical knowledge, but also in learning the cockpit systems by the use of instructor-conducted crew sessions in a cockpit-system simulator. The completion of this step is followed by an evaluation session, which lasts for at least half a day. Next the trainee crew spends nine 4-hour periods in a full flight simulator

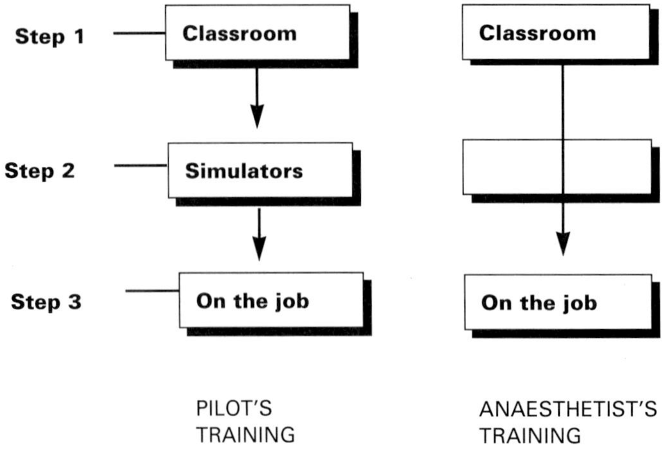

Fig. 2.3 Schematic comparison of the training procedures for pilots and anaesthetists. During anaesthesia training more use should be made of classroom instruction during the initial phase. Simulators are likely to play an important role in training anaesthetists in the future.

(Step 2). Here they are presented with many of the problems with which they could be confronted during actual flights. The crew is taught how to solve these problems using established operating procedures and their own judgement. The high fidelity, full flight simulator has the ability to replicate accurately the aircraft and its environment, and lets the trainee see all the consequences of his actions. If a wrong decision leads to a catastrophe, it is allowed to happen. All events are stored on computer so that they can be recalled to demonstrate to the trainee what went wrong. The exercise can be restarted from the point of deviation and the trainee given another chance to solve the problem. A 28-hour simulator instruction period is followed by evaluation. If successful, the candidate is issued with a licence to operate that particular aircraft in commercial service. Step 3 of training is accomplished with documentation of the candidate's completion of the required number of hours of actual line-operating experience under the supervision of a designated check pilot ('on the job' training).

Even after full certification the commercial pilot is still required to undergo regular evaluation checks, generally every 6 months. This usually involves time in a simulator. A typical simulator session may involve exposure to many emergency situations, such as engine failure at critical periods, for example take-off, engine fire, etc., which are fortunately uncommon in real life. The pilot is judged on his ability to cope with these situations according to predefined standard procedures. This mandatory regular evaluation applies equally to junior copilots and senior captains. In addition, pilots are subjected to regular 'line checks' by specially trained operational captains during routine flights. When a new instrument or device is introduced into the cockpit, pilots must also undergo training in its use in order to maintain competence. A move from one aircraft type to another requires that pilots undergo intensive retraining or conversion.

Compared with pilots, anaesthetists are trained largely 'on the job'. Anaesthesia training requires 4–6 years of postgraduate experience in which 1000–2000 supervised anaesthetics are given. Several life-threatening anaesthetic complications have an incidence of less than 1 in 10 000 cases. Thus most trainees will never be exposed to some anaesthetic emergencies and, while one may read about them, the ability to deal with them expertly in real life requires practical experience. The incidences of some emergencies are even more rare, so that an anaesthetist in the course of his/her career may only come across them a few times, if at all. Aviation has similar problems. A pilot may clock up hundreds of flying hours but never experience an engine failure. Simulators are extensively used in aviation to maintain the pilot efficiency in dealing with these rare situations.

In anaesthesia, as in aviation, simulators and training devices have many advantages. Regular use of simulators will not only maintain an anaesthetist's efficiency, but will also assist him/her in dealing with those rare events that demand quick and appropriate action to prevent them escalating into disaster. With the advent of modern and sophisticated computer technology it is now possible to develop a comprehensive anaesthesia simulation device that will recreate critical incidents in anaesthesia. Such devices have recently been described (Schwid 1987, Gaba & DeAnda 1988, Good et al 1988) and evaluated (Gaba & DeAnda 1989). However, much fundamental research is still needed to achieve the tremendous potential of simulators in our speciality.

In comparison with airline pilots, anaesthetists are not compelled to undergo any form of retraining. It is perfectly possible for someone to qualify in his early thirties and to continue a career in anaesthesia to retirement age without ever attending a postgraduate course or other form of postgraduate education. In anaesthesia, when a new piece of apparatus is introduced, the anaesthetist more often than not learns how to use this 'on the job' with the instruction manual in his hand. This is a far from ideal situation. Clearly, sound training, retraining and education of anaesthetists will help reduce the incidence of mishaps. Perhaps formal retraining, proficiency checks and recertification should be made mandatory, say once a year. A proficiency test, for example, could be conducted in a suitable anaesthesia simulator.

CONCLUSIONS

There are many similarities between anaesthesia and aviation, including the potentially fatal consequences of slips, errors and mistakes. Even though both anaesthetists and pilots make extensive use of complex technology, human error continues to play a major and approximately equal role in the causation of accidents and near accidents in both professions. Although both have long recognized the importance of safety, their approaches to the implementation of safety procedures has been very different. Aviation has for many decades adopted a very structured and disciplined approach to this problem, and this is universally accepted within the aviation industry. The approach to safety in anaesthesia, however, has been much more individually orientated and, in general, poorly structured. In contrast to the acceptance of mandatory checklist procedures, regular retraining and proficiency checking by pilots, these have frequently been opposed by individual members of the anaesthetic profession. Fortunately there is evidence that attitudes in our profession are changing (Charlton 1990).

There are many ways that we can benefit from the experiences and approaches to safety of our counterparts in aviation, particularly their widespread use of mandatory checklist procedures and their approach to continuing education, including the use of simulators. There are, however, important differences between flying and giving anaesthetics. Modern aircraft are examples of high-precision engineering with individual components manufactured to narrow tolerance limits. By contrast the anaesthetist has to contend with considerable biological variability, even in healthy patients. A pilot knows that when he sets the thrust lever of an engine for a given power output he will get that power within a fraction of a per cent. An aeroplane with controls that had a coefficient of variation of even 5% would be unmanageable. As anaesthetists we readily accept that, for example, the sleep dose of thiopentone can vary between 2 and 6 mg/kg. Imagine trying to fly an aeroplane where those tolerance limits were accepted as normal. Another important difference between pilots and anaesthetists is that the pilot can assume that his aeroplane is 'healthy', whereas we almost always have to deal with 'sick' patients. Finally, there is one fundamental difference between pilots and anaesthetists that makes flying easier than giving anaesthetics. This is that a pilot does not have to contend with a surgeon messing about with his aeroplane.

REFERENCES

Beach B E 1988 A case for simulation in cost effective training. In: Gravenstein J S, Holzer J F (eds). Safety and cost containment in anesthesia. Butterworths, Boston, pp 201–206

Beecher H K, Todd D P 1954 A study of the deaths associated with anesthesia and surgery based on a study of 599, 548 anesthesias in 10 institutions. Ann Surg 140: 2–35

Beneken J E W, van der Aa J J 1989 Alarms and their limits in monitoring. J Clin Monit 5: 205–210

Buck N, Devlin H B, Lunn J N 1987 The report of a confidential enquiry into perioperative deaths. Nuffield Provincial Hospitals Trust and the Kings Fund, London

Charlton J E 1990 Checklists and patient safety. Anaesthesia 45: 425–426

Chopra V, Bovill J G, Spierdijk J 1990 Accidents, near accidents and complications during anaesthesia: a retrospective analysis of a 10-year period in a teaching hospital. Anaesthesia 45: 3–6

Chopra V, Bovill J G, Spierdijk J, Koornneef F 1992 A prospective analysis of reported significant observations during anaesthesia. Br J Anaesth 68: 13–17

Cohen M M, Duncan P G, Pope W D B, Wolkenstein C 1986 A survey of 112,000 anaesthetics at one teaching hospital (1975–83). Can Anaesth Soc J 33: 22–31

Cooper J B 1985 Anesthesia can be safer: the role of engineering and technology. Med Instrum 19(3): 105–108

Cooper J B, Long C D, Newbower R S, Philip J H 1982 Critical incidents associated with intraoperative exchanges of anesthesia personnel. Anesthesiology 56: 456–461

Cooper J B, Newbower R S, Kitz R J 1984 An analysis of major errors and equipment failures in anesthesia management: consideration for prevention and detection. Anesthesiology 60: 34–42

Craig J, Wilson M E 1981 A survey of anaesthetic mishaps. Anaesthesia 36: 933–936

Cundy J, Baldock G J 1982 Safety check procedures to eliminate faults in anaesthetic machines. Anaesthesia 37: 161–169

Denisco R A, Drummond J N, Gravenstein J S 1987 The effect of fatigue on the performance of a simulated anesthetic monitoring task. J Clin Monit 3: 22–24

Gaba D M, DeAnda 1988 A comprehensive anesthesia simulation environment: re-creating the operating room for research and training. Anesthesiology 69: 387–394

Gaba D M, DeAnda A 1989 The responses of anesthesia trainees to simulated critical incidents. Anesth Analg 68: 444–451

Good M L, Lampotang S, Gibby G L, Gravenstein J S 1988 Critical events simulation for training in anesthesiology. J Clin Monit 4: 140

Gravenstein J S, Weinger M B 1986 Why investigate vigilance? J Clin Monit 2: 145–147

Kay J, Neal M 1986 Effect of automatic blood pressure devices on vigilance of anesthesia residents. J Clin Monit 2: 148–150

van Kessel H M, Meijler A P, Hennis P J, Cluitmans P J M 1987 Comparison between a handwritten and automated anesthesia record. In: Gravenstein J S, Newbower R S, Ream A K, Smith N T (eds) The automated anesthesia record and alarm systems. Butterworths, Boston, pp 143–150

Kestin I G, Miller B R, Lockhart C H 1988 Auditory alarms during anesthesia monitoring. Anesthesiology 69: 106–109

Kilian J 1987 Safety check procedures and maintenance. Eur J Anaesthesiol 4: 211–213

Kumar V, Barcellos W A, Mehta M P, Carter J G 1988 An analysis of critical incidents in a teaching department for quality assurance: a survey of mishaps during anaesthesia. Anaesthesia 43: 879–883

McEwen J A, Small C F, Saunders B A, Jenkins I C 1980 Hazards associated with the use of disconnect monitors. Anesthesiology 53: S391

McIntyre J W R 1985 Ergonomics: anaesthetists' use of auditory alarms in the operating room. Int J Clin Monit Comput 2: 47–55

Mackie R R 1987 Vigilance research – are we ready for counter-measures? Hum Factors 29: 707–723

Meijler A P 1987 Automation in anesthesia: a relief? Springer–Verlag, Berlin

Meijler A P, Beneken J E W 1987 Data acquisition and display: a system with centralized display, automatic record keeping and intelligent alarms. In: Gravenstein J S, Newbower R S, Ream A K, Smith N T (eds) The automated anesthesia record and alarm systems. Butterworths, Boston, pp 229–238

Mitchell M M 1982 Automated anesthesia data management and keeping. Med Instrum 16: 279–282

Paget N S, Lambert T F, Sridhar K 1981 Factors affecting an anaesthetist's work: some findings on vigilance and performance. Anaesth Intensive Care 9: 359–365

Parker J E R 1987 The effect of fatigue on physician performance: an underestimated cause of physician impairement and increased patient risk. Can J Anaesth 34: 489–495

Patterson R 1982 Guidelines for auditory warning systems on civil aircraft. Civil Aviation Authority Report 82017. Department of Transport, London, pp 67

Rendell-Baker L 1982 Problems with anesthetic gas machines and their solutions. Int Anesthesiol Clin 20(3): 1–82

Reynolds A C 1983 Disconnect alarm failure. Anesthesiology 58: 488

Sarnat A J, Quinn M L, Smith N T 1982 A computerized speech recognition system for anesthesia record keeping. Anesthesiology 57: A165

Saunders R J, Jewett W R 1983 System integration: the need in future anesthesia delivery systems. Med Instrum 17: 389–392

Schneider A J L 1982 The validity of data from anesthesia records. In: Grundy B L, Gravenstein J S,(eds) The quality of care in anesthesia. Charles C Thomas, Springfield Illinois, pp 100–113

Schreiber P, Schreiber J 1989 Diagnosis and prevention of operator error and equipment failure. Semin Anesth 8: 141–148

Schwid H A 1987 A flight simulator for general anesthesia training. Comput Biomed Res 20: 64–75

Sury M R, Hinds C J, Boustreal M 1986 Accidental disconnection following inactivation of Servoventilator alarm. Anaesthesia 41: 91

Thompson P W 1987 Safer designs of anaesthetic equipments. Br J Anaesth 59: 913–921

Utting J E, Gray T C, Shelley F C 1979 Human misadventures in anaesthesia. Can Anaesth Soc J 26: 472–478

Zeitlin G L 1989 Possible decrease in mortality associated with anaesthesia: a comparison of two time periods in Massachusetts, USA. Anaesthesia 44: 432–433

Zissos A, Strunin L 1982 A micro-computerized anaesthetic record system. Can Anaesth Soc J 29: 168–173

SECTION 2

Hazards related to the physical status of the patient

3

Cardiovascular function and the safety of anaesthesia

M. V. Copp and R. O. Feneck

INTRODUCTION

For many years only the healthiest of patients were considered to be acceptable risks for general anaesthesia. In particular, those patients suffering from pre-existing cardiovascular disease were regarded as a high-risk group, and anaesthesia and surgery in these patients was known to carry both a high morbidity and high mortality.

In recent years, advances in medicine and surgery, as well as in anaesthesia, have resulted in the development of anaesthetic techniques that now readily permit the safe management of such patients. Over this same period the incidence of cardiovascular disease, especially of ischaemic heart disease (IHD), appears to have risen dramatically.

It is impossible to know precisely the incidence of all forms of cardiovascular disease occurring in the general population. However, it may be possible to understand the scale of the problem by considering the published mortality figures (Table 3.1). In England and Wales, circulatory diseases have consistently accounted for 40–60% of all yearly deaths since 1969. Analysis of recent data suggests that the figures remain similarly high, although there are, perhaps, some signs of a small reduction in deaths from circulatory disease since 1985 (Office of Population Censuses and Surveys 1969–73, 1981–89).

The trend in mortality from IHD has remained constant since 1985. Over 150 000 deaths annually are caused by IHD. This is the highest single cause of death and is responsible for over 70% of deaths due to heart disease. In the USA the annual mortality for cardiovascular disease is 1 million. This exceeds that of all other diseases and accounts for 50% of deaths (US National Center for Health Statistics 1988).

Thus the mortality from circulatory disease is massive and, although it is difficult to quantify the incidence of such disease, the available data make depressing reading. Cardiovascular disease has been estimated to affect one in four

Table 3.1 Mortality from circulatory disease in England and Wales (from the Office of Population Censuses and Surveys 1969–73, 1981–89)

Year(s)	Number of deaths from circulatory disease	% total mortality	Number of deaths from ischaemic heart disease	% of deaths from all circulatory disease
1969–1973	1 480 000	51	720 000	46
1981	286 225	49	155 196	54
1983	282 815	49	156 550	55
1985	287 054	49	163 104	57
1987	271 061	48	155 235	57
1989	264 600	46	150 794	57

Americans (US National Center for Health Stastistics 1988), and it has been estimated that approximately 5% of all patients over the age of 35 may be expected to have symptomless IHD (Master & Geller 1969). These data clearly have implications for the anaesthetist since we must assume from them that the incidence of cardiovascular disease in the general population is high. The medical significance of cardiovascular disease is obvious, both in terms of morbidity and mortality. For the anaesthetist an awareness of these factors must be complemented by an understanding of their implications for safe anaesthesia, including an appreciation of the haemodynamic effects that anaesthetic drugs and techniques have on the patient, and whether these effects can be suitably modified.

AVOIDABLE HAZARDS IN PATIENTS WITH CARDIOVASCULAR DISEASE

The safe conduct of anaesthesia in a patient with significant cardiovascular disease will demand great attention to detail, since virtually every drug and action of both surgeon and anaesthetist will have an impact on the circulation. Safety will only be ensured if three hazards are avoided. These are:

- myocardial oxygen imbalance and consequent ischaemia
- cardiac failure
- haemodynamically or prognostically significant arrhythmia.

Myocardial oxygen imbalance

For normal aerobic cardiac metabolism to be maintained, the myocardial oxygen supply must be adequate to meet the demand. Those factors that affect myocardial oxygen supply and demand are shown in Table 3.2. As can be seen, the myocardial oxygen supply is dependent on an adequate oxygen content of the coronary blood and on adequate coronary blood flow. These in turn are influenced by many factors, but among the most important are adequate coronary perfusion pressure (diastolic aortic pressure minus left ventricular end-diastolic pressure [LVEDP]) and adequate diastolic coronary perfusion time. Thus hypotension, which will reduce coronary perfusion pressure, and tachycardia, which will shorten the diastolic interval, will both have adverse effects on myocardial oxygen supply. Increases in left ventricular wall stress due to hypertension, increases in preload (LVEDP), increases in contractility and tachycardia will increase myocardial oxygen demand. Unless these increases in demand can be met appropriately, the oxygen supply will become inadequate and the heart will convert from aerobic to anaerobic metabolism, with the risk of ischaemia and subsequent perioperative infarction. From the foregoing it is evident that tachycardia may be a particularly potent hazard in a patient with ischaemic heart disease, since both myocardial oxygen supply and demand are adversely affected. Published data (Slogoff & Keats 1985) suggest that tachycardia is the haemodynamic abnormality that most clearly correlates with

Table 3.2 Determinants of myocardial oxygen supply and demand

Oxygen supply		Oxygen demand	
Heart rate		Heart rate	
Oxygen content:	Haemoglobin	Contractility	
	O_2 saturation	Wall tension:	Afterload (impedance)
	PaO_2		Preload (LVEDP)
Coronary blood flow:	CPP = DP – LVEDP		
	CVR		

CPP: coronary perfusion pressure, DP: diastolic blood pressure, LVEDP: left ventricular end-diastolic pressure, CVR: coronary vascular resistance.

an adverse outcome in patients with IHD, and should therefore be treated as a serious hazard.

Cardiac failure

Cardiac failure may be defined as a state of the circulation that is inadequate to meet the oxygen requirements of the body tissues. Cardiac function is dependent on preload, afterload and contractility. If we further stipulate that cardiac failure occurs when metabolic oxygen requirements cannot be met, despite optimal loading conditions, then the terminology may be more accurate in that it specifically relates to cardiac contractility. However, it should be remembered that optimal loading conditions may vary widely between patients, dependent on both the severity and the chronicity of cardiac disease.

As we shall see later, many anaesthetic drugs have depressant effects on cardiac contractility. Cardiac failure may develop if anaesthetic drug dosage is not carefully controlled. It is also more likely to occur in the patient with pre-existing poor ventricular function, although even young and fit patients may suffer from a degree of pump failure if very high concentrations of cardiodepressant volatile agents are used for prolonged periods. Fortunately, in these patients recovery is usually swift following termination of the anaesthetic. Cardiac failure may also be exacerbated by inadequate gas exchange or poor acid–base and electrolyte control.

The presence of cardiac failure at the outset of an anaesthetic is a clearly identified outcome determinant and every effort should be made to optimize cardiac function prior to surgery (Goldman et al 1977, Larsen et al 1987).

Arrhythmia

The factors that may promote the development of perioperative arrhythmias are dealt with on page 50. However, the significance of perioperative arrhythmia may be defined in either functional or prognostic terms. Functionally significant arrhythmias are often less difficult to deal with, since they usually produce haemodynamic effects which are easy to identify (hypotension and tachycardia) and successful treatment is easy to monitor. However, prognostically significant arrhythmias are more complex since they may produce little haemodynamic upset initially, but lead to severely abnormal functioning during the perioperative period. Furthermore, assessment of the prognostic significance of an arrhythmia will be substantially influenced by the underlying cardiac pathology. Thus brief episodes of rapid atrial fibrillation are of far greater significance in a patient with aortic stenosis than in a patient with congestive cardiac failure.

The risks of anaesthesia in a patient with circulatory disease are thus lessened by the preservation of myocardial oxygen balance, the maintenance of optimal cardiac performance and the avoidance of factors likely to promote the development of arrhythmias. The following text (pp. 31–41) will consider the effects that anaesthetic drugs and techniques may have on the circulation, and how the hazards to safe anaesthesia may be minimized.

EFFECTS OF ANAESTHETIC DRUGS AND TECHNIQUES ON THE CIRCULATION

Most drugs used in anaesthetic practice have effects on the circulation, and these may occur as a result of actions of the drug at more than one site. The principal sites of action are on venous and arteriolar tone, cardiac contractile proteins, and cardiac innervation and conduction tissue.

Even in a normal patient population the magnitude of the circulatory response to an anaesthetic drug is subject to individual variation. The response may vary in its magnitude, but its nature and direction are predictable. On occasion the haemodynamic response to an anaesthetic drug may be substantially different not only in its magnitude, but also in its nature. When an anaesthetic drug produces a substantial haemodynamic effect it is important to be able to differentiate between an augmented but qualitatively normal pharmacological effect, and a bizarre response qualitatively different to the effect normally seen (Rawlins 1981). These latter reactions may occur as a result of inherited abnormalities (i.e. disorders of pharmacogenetics) or immunological processes (i.e. Type 1 IgE-mediated anaphylactic reactions or activation of complement) and will constitute a substantial hazard to the safe conduct of anaesthesia.

Effect of intravenous agents

The administration of an induction dose of thiopentone produces a mild fall in systemic arterial blood pressure and a compensatory increase in heart rate. Measurements of cardiac output show a small reduction both in normals and in patients with heart disease (Flickinger et al 1961). This effect may occur either as a result of a direct depressant effect on myocardial contractility, or following a decrease in cardiac filling pressure due to venous pooling, or due to a decrease in sympathetic outflow from the central nervous system (Hug 1979). Systemic vascular resistance (SVR) is usually little altered, but may increase substantially following endotracheal intubation (Patrick et al 1986).This effect may be important in patients with IHD. This is because the increase in SVR and also in heart rate may result in an increase in myocardial oxygen consumption (MVO_2) that cannot be adequately met by a parallel increase in coronary blood flow. Ischaemia may, therefore, ensue.

Thiopentone was first used by Lundy in 1934 and since that time has become the most widely used intravenous induction agent in anaesthetic practice (Reeves & Kissin 1983). It is difficult to envisage absolute contraindications to its use apart from porphyria and barbiturate intolerance. Nevertheless, since it may reduce arterial and venous tone, thiopentone should be used with extreme caution in situations where sudden reductions in vascular tone may prove catastrophic. These would include patients with hypovolaemic hypotension, cardiac tamponade or constrictive pericarditis. However, even in these patients the effects of thiopentone can be minimized by substantially reducing the total dose and by slowing the rate of administration. Rapid injection of large doses may cause severe hypotension and myocardial depression even in normals.

Methohexitone produces circulatory effects similar to thiopentone. In normals a small decrease in cardiac output and compensatory tachycardia occur (Dundee et al 1961). In patients with cardiac disease it would appear that doses of methohexitone that are equipotent with thiopentone produce a similar degree of myocardial depression (Conway & Ellis 1969).

The effects of etomidate on the circulation, both in patients with heart disease and in normals, suggest that the drug is associated with a marked degree of haemodynamic stability. Arterial blood pressure remains unchanged in normals, but in patients with valvular heart disease, arterial blood pressure has been shown to be slightly reduced (Colvin et al 1979). There is evidence that etomidate produces the least change in the balance of myocardial oxygen supply and demand when compared to thiopentone and ketamine (Kettler et al 1977).

The favourable haemodynamic profile of etomidate coupled with its short duration of action may make it suitable as an induction agent for short surgical procedures in patients with a high cardiovascular risk factor. Unfortunately, the effects of etomidate on steroidogenesis clearly contraindicate its use as a continuous infusion (Ledingham & Watt 1983).

Early studies with propofol showed that arterial hypotension may occur both in normals and in patients with heart disease (Stephan et al 1986, Claeys et al 1988). One recent review of the literature has suggested that the main effect of propofol on the circulation is systemic vasodilatation (Sebel & Lowdon 1989). This conclusion is controversial, as others believe there is a significant negative inotropic effect (Merin 1990). Vasodilatation may be beneficial in that it may reduce left ventricular impedance and thus also MVO_2. Clearly, however, if hypotension is severe enough to reduce coronary perfusion pressure significantly, then adequate coronary blood flow and hence myocardial oxygen supply may not be maintained, even in the presence of a reduction in MVO_2. If severe hypotension occurs then coronary perfusion pressure will be substantially reduced. In the presence of coronary artery disease and altered vascular reflexes this will lead to a substantial reduction in coronary blood flow, such that ventricular perfusion is seriously impaired with adverse effects on left ventricle (LV) function. These effects will occur irrespective of any direct negative inotropic effect. Thus induction with propofol in hypertensive patients with IHD may be hazardous and is probably best avoided. However, in most patients, even in those with significant circulatory disease, propofol may be used safely (Sebel & Lowdon 1989). The decision to use or avoid propofol will then probably be more correctly based on other considerations, including recovery.

Continous infusion of propofol for the maintenance of anaesthesia appears to be an acceptable technique and well-tolerated by high-risk patients (Russell et al 1989). Hypotension appears to be less of a problem in this situation. Slow infusion regimes for the induction of anaesthesia have been described that may reduce the incidence and severity of adverse haemodynamic effects, since they recommend substantially less propofol than previously described (Manara et al 1991). Overall it would appear that the other properties of propofol continue to make it an attractive intravenous induction agent, and may do so even when pre-existing cardiovascular disease causes concern.

Ketamine differs from other induction agents in most respects, and its haemodynamic effects are no exception. Uniquely, ketamine causes an increase in blood pressure, and in systemic and pulmonary vascular resistance (PVR), as well as an increase in heart rate. Despite small reductions in stroke volume (SV), cardiac output is usually increased secondary to the tachycardia (Tweed et al 1972). The mechanisms responsible for these haemodynamic effects are unclear. However, two factors emerge: firstly, ketamine has a directly acting negative inotropic effect on the myocardium; secondly, centrally mediated sympathetic responses override this depressant effect (Gooding et al 1977). Interestingly, a second dose of ketamine frequently appears to produce depressant effects on the circulation, as does the administration of ketamine to patients anaesthetized with halothane or enflurane. It may be that in both these situations the direct negative inotropic effects of ketamine predominate.

Following the identification of specific benzodiazepine receptors and the synthesis of the antagonist drug flumazenil, benzodiazepine drugs such as diazepam, midazolam, lorazepam and flunitrazepam have become much more widely used as intravenous induction agents. The haemodynamic effects of benzodiazepines appear to be minimal in normal patients when these drugs are given either for intravenous sedation or as an induction agent. The main haemodynamic effects appear to be mild vasodilation and hypotension. These are greatest with flunitrazepam in comparison with other benzodiazepines, but are still less than those associated with induction doses of thiopentone, even in patients with circulatory disease (Clarke et al 1977).

The advent of cardiac surgery has necessitated the development of anaesthetic techniques that ensure circulatory stability. Since the early work of Lowenstein, opioid drugs have played a major part in achieving that goal (Lowenstein et al 1969). Extensive use of a variety of drugs, especially fentanyl and its derivatives, has shown that anaesthetic sequences based around the use of opioids are associated with minimal hypotension or tachycardia, and small increases in cardiac output (Dubois-Primo et al 1979, de Lange et al 1980). Hypotension may occur with morphine, and the effects of morphine on the brainstem may result in vagal activity and bradycardia. The development of a bradycardia is common to many opioid drugs, including fentanyl, and appears to be related to both a rapid rate of administration and a large total dose. Opioids may cause a reduction in vasomotor tone, and this effect has been partially responsible for their therapeutic use in patients suffering from acute LV failure.

In general the circulatory effects of opioids during anaesthesia are relatively benign. Haemodynamic problems are usually manifest in the failure to prevent haemodynamic responses to anaesthetic or surgical stimuli, particularly in patients with well-preserved LV function. This may lead to a hyperdynamic circulation, and the risk of myocardial oxygen imbalance and ischaemia (Sonntag et al 1989). These hyperdynamic responses can be obtunded by opioids, but often very large doses are necessary that create other difficulties, such as prolonged respiratory depression in the postoperative period. For this reason the use of lower doses of opioids, supplemented with volatile anaesthetic agents, is now more popular, and high-dose opioid techniques are reserved for the most sick patients.

The effect of gases and volatile anaesthetic agents

Haemodynamic effects

The haemodynamic effects of nitrous oxide in normal volunteers have been studied using N_2O alone and in combination with other anaesthetics. Substitution of 40% N_2O and O_2 for 40% N_2 in O_2 causes a 15% reduction in cardiac output, with decreases in heart rate and contractility. Systemic vascular resistance increases and there is little overall effect on blood pressure. Similar effects are seen when N_2O is used in conjunction with morphine (Wong et al 1973).

The addition of N_2O to a stable concentration of halothane or enflurane may cause a slight variation in blood pressure by increasing SVR. In practice, however, the addition of N_2O will usually permit a reduction in the required concentration of volatile agent, and thus the dose-related cardiovascular depression caused by the more potent volatile agent may be reduced. Similarly, the direct myocardial depressant effect of N_2O is often overshadowed by the effects of the more potent volatile anaesthetics. However, the depressant effects of N_2O may become more evident if patients with poor cardiac function are anaesthetized with an opioid-based technique which has minimal haemodynamic effects, and then N_2O is subsequently added. Such a situation may occur following withdrawal of cardiopulmonary bypass support during cardiac surgery, and in this highly specialized setting the use of N_2O may be hazardous.

The addition of N_2O to a volatile anaesthetic will permit a reduction in the inspired concentration of volatile agents, resulting in less depression of cardiovascular function. In contrast the addition of N_2O to patients receiving large doses of opioids given as the main agent may result in greater cardiovascular depression. It should be said, however, that in healthy patients neither of these situations is critical. The haemodynamic effects of halothane have been studied using human volunteers maintained at normal body temperature, ventilated to maintain normocarbia and given no other anaesthetic drugs. In these subjects an end-tidal concentration of 1–2.5% results in dose-dependent decreases in cardiac output of up to 50%, with reductions in SV and contractility. Heart rate does not change, right atrial pressure (RAP) increases and arterial blood pressure falls in parallel with the reduction in cardiac output (Eger et al 1970). However, halothane is a potent respiratory depressant, causing an elevation of the arterial carbon dioxide (CO_2) tension during anaesthesia under spontaneous ventilation and depression of the carbon dioxide response curve. Although carbon dioxide has a direct depressant effect on the isolated myocardial cell, the effect of hypercapnia on the subject is to cause sympathoadrenal stimulation resulting in an increase in arterial blood pressure, heart rate, pulmonary artery pressure (PAP) and cardiac output. Thus in the spontaneously breathing patient the depressant haemodynamic effects of halothane are to some extent offset by the haemodynamic effects of hypercapnia. However, in patients taking beta blockers the sympathoadrenal response due to hypercapnia may be severely impaired since beta-adrenergic activity is substantially obtunded. Therefore, hypercapnia produces little sympathoadrenal stimulation, but may produce further cardiovascular depression as a consequence of the effects of the developing respiratory acidosis and the direct depressant effect of a low pH.

The haemodynamic effects of enflurane would appear to be similar to those of halothane. Enflurane administration is associated with dose-dependent reduction in blood pressure, SVR, SV and contractility, and the addition of N_2O to enflurane anaesthesia in patients has been shown to further reduce cardiac output and blood pressure (Smith et al 1978). The haemodynamic effects of isoflurane have been studied in fit volunteers and patients both with and without cardiac disease. Although there are quantitative response differences between these groups, the pattern of response would appear to be similar. Isoflurane anaesthesia appears to leave LV function better preserved than halothane, enflurane or enflurane/N_2O (Calverley et al 1978, Bastard et al 1982). Arterial blood pressure and SVR show small falls, SV and cardiac output are relatively well preserved being only slightly reduced, and heart rate is increased. These data are well-established and uncontroversial, in contrast to the data regarding the effects of isoflurane on the coronary circulation.

EFFECTS ON CARDIAC CONDUCTION, CORONARY HAEMODYNAMICS AND CARDIAC METABOLISM

A schematic representation of a cardiac cell action potential is shown in Figure 3.1. After rapid depolarization (Phase 0) there is a short period of rapid repolarization (Phase 1) followed by a plateau (Phase 2) and then another rapid phase completing repolarization (Phase 3). Slow diastolic depolarization occurs (Phase 4) until a critical threshold is reached, whereupon rapid (Phase 0) depolarization commences and the cycle is repeated. During depolarization (Phase 0) the opening of fast-response sodium (Na^+) channels is responsible for the massive influx of Na^+ ions which increase the transmembrane potential from –90 to +20 mV. The terminal notch (Phase 1) is caused by deactivation of the sodium current and an inward chloride (Cl^-) current. Slow calcium (Ca^{2+}) channels open during depolarization (Phase 0) at about –40 mV. These remain open for 30–300 ms and are thus responsible for the plateau (Phase 2). This slow inward calcium current is inactivated (Phase 3) and the outward potassium (K^+) current is activated, thereby causing a reduction in transmembrane potential. The Na^+/K^+ pump re-establishes the baseline concentration gradient of the relative cations with two K^+ ions moving into the cell for every three Na^+ ions moving out (Phases 3 and 4).

Pacemaker cells have a much less negative resting membrane potential (–50 to –60 mV) and at this level fast sodium channels are refractory. Thus slow calcium channels are responsible for depolarization resulting in a slow-rising action potential. At –40 mV a secondary phase of rapid depolarization occurs associated with inward sodium currents. The prolonged repolarization phase is associated with the termination of inward cation movement and the efflux of K^+ ions.

Halothane causes a decrease in the rate of depolarization (Phase 4) in sinoatrial (SA) node fibres and raises the threshold for further depolarization (Phase 0). This results in a reduced beating frequency (Fig. 3.2). These effects are similar to those seen with acetylcholine, the vagal neurotransmitter, and help to explain the development of a sinus bradycardia during halothane anaesthesia. Atrioventricular (AV) nodal rhythm

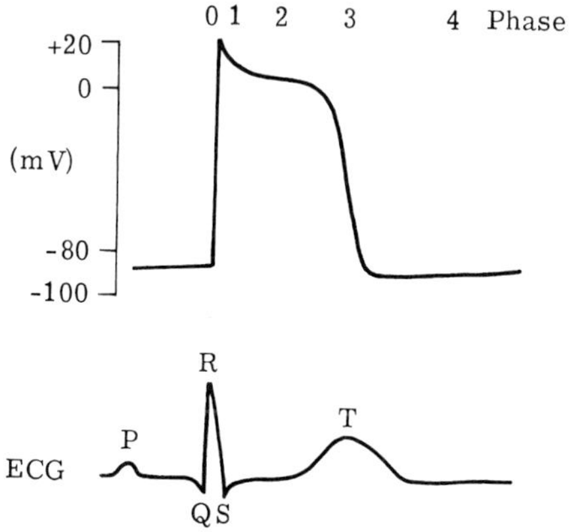

Fig. 3.1 Cardiac pacemaker cell action potential events timed against the ECG. See text for description.

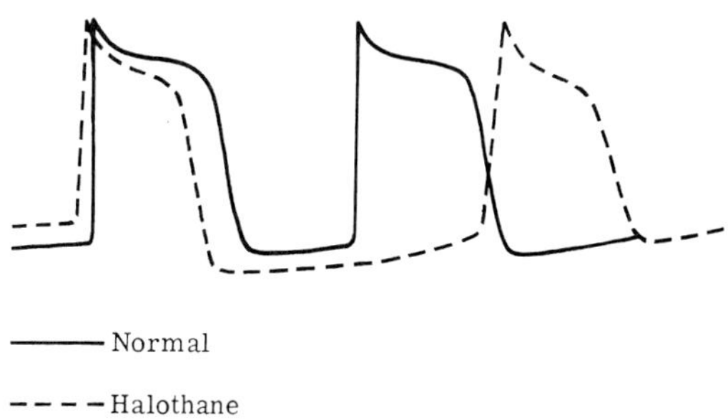

Fig. 3.2 Effects of halothane on action potential of SA node fibres.

may also be explained in part by a reduction in SA nodal activity, but it may also be relevant to consider the effects of halothane on electrical conduction within atrial tissue (Fig. 3.3). If transatrial electrical conduction of an SA nodal impulse is slowed sufficiently, AV nodal cells will spontaneously discharge before the incoming wave of depolarization has arrived. This AV nodal depolarization is rapidly conducted through the His–Purkinje system and thence to ventricular muscle, resulting in ventricular systole before atrial systole is complete.

Alterations of cardiac rate and/or rhythm are not uncommon during halothane anaesthesia, and the mechanisms responsible for bradycardia and nodal rhythm are those described above. Ventricular extrasystoles are also commonly seen, particularly during spontaneous breathing. Catecholamine secretion during hypercarbia is a potent stimulus for the development of automatic pacemaker activity below the AV node. Thus the combination of the effect of halothane to depress atrial pacemaker activity, and of hypercarbia to increase ventricular automaticity, may increase the tendency to develop ventricular extrasystoles. Also, the dose of adrenaline required to produce experimental ventricular extrasystoles with halothane is less than in awake controls (Andersen et al 1963). Thus halothane would appear to sensitize the myocardium to the arrhythmic effects of catecholamines.

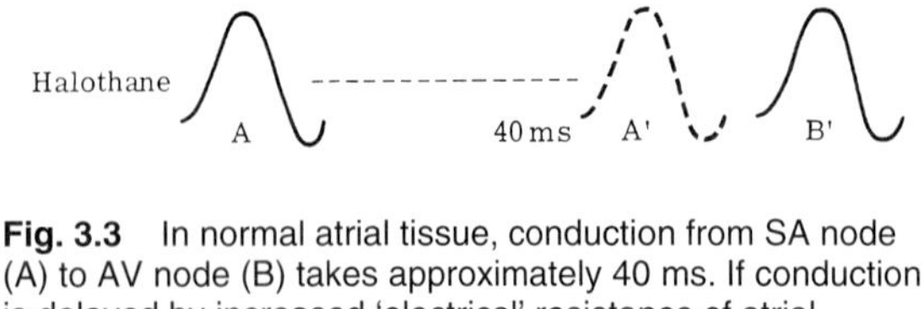

Fig. 3.3 In normal atrial tissue, conduction from SA node (A) to AV node (B) takes approximately 40 ms. If conduction is delayed by increased 'electrical' resistance of atrial muscle, the wave of depolarization only reaches (A[1]) after 40 ms. Spontaneously depolarizing AV node cells (B[1]) reach critical threshold and generate an action potential, resulting in a nodal beat.

Enflurane causes a similar reduction in AV conduction to halothane, but in contrast it does not cause an increase in conduction time in Purkinje fibres or in ventricular muscle. This may have a protective effect on the development of re-entry arrhythmias. There is a greater dose requirement of adrenaline for the experimental production of ventricular extrasystoles with enflurane than with halothane (Lippman & Reisner 1974).

The dose of adrenaline required to produce ventricular extrasystoles is more during isoflurane anaesthesia than during halothane anaesthesia (Johnston et al 1976), thus isoflurane would appear to be less of a hazard in that respect. Other effects on conduction would appear also to be relatively benign.

Isoflurane has no significant effect on His–Purkinje conduction times and a protective effect on the arrhythmogenic potential of cardiac glycosides (Blitt et al 1979). The effects of isoflurane on cardiac rate appear to be variable, and at least in part related to the degree of systemic vasodilatation produced. Early studies showed that the heart rate was unchanged or reduced (Blitt et al 1979), but more recent data, including one large multicentre trial, suggest that isoflurane anaesthesia is more likely to be associated with tachycardia than other volatile agents (Forrest et al 1990).

The effects of volatile agents on the coronary circulation in patients will be substantially affected by numerous indirect factors, as well as by the direct effects of the agents themselves. In particular, systemic vasodilation resulting in a reduction in diastolic blood pressure will directly lower coronary perfusion pressure, and a reflex tachycardia will shorten diastolic time. Both may result in coronary blood flow being reduced. Also, surgical stimulation and a hyperdynamic circulation will increase myocardial oxygen requirements, causing a reflex increase in coronary blood flow to meet this increased demand. These physiological responses of the coronary circulation may override the direct pharmocological effect of drugs, including volatile anaesthetics.

Because of these and other factors, it may be difficult to interpret studies evaluating the effects of intravenous or volatile anaesthetics on coronary haemodynamics in patients undergoing surgery. However, a number of factors emerge, as follows.

It is difficult to ensure adequate protection against myocardial oxygen imbalance when using opioids alone, even in very large doses (Rao et al 1983, Sonntag et al 1989). Thus it may be preferable to combine the use of opioids with volatile anaesthetics if myocardial oxygen balance is to be preserved during anaesthesia and surgery. Which volatile is best for this purpose?

Data from studies with both halothane and enflurane suggest that, as the concentration of volatile agent is increased, myocardial work and oxygen requirements are reduced. Thus coronary blood flow and myocardial oxygen consumption are reduced. However, there is usually little or no evidence of the production of myocardial lactate or other metabolites, suggestive of the conversion from aerobic to anaerobic cardiac metabolism and the consequent risk of ischaemia. Coronary flow autoregulation is well preserved with both halothane and enflurane (Moffit & Sethna 1986). However, isoflurane is a potent coronary vasodilator and may, therefore, affect coronary flow autoregulation. As the concentration of isoflurane increases, coronary vasodilatation increases and thus total coronary blood flow becomes pressure dependent. Studies of isoflurane anaesthesia in man have shown that myocardial oxygen imbalance may occur. This has been particularly evident when either diastolic blood pressure and hence coronary perfusion pressure has been reduced, or tachycardia is apparent (Reiz et al 1983, Sahlman et al 1989). The potent coronary vasodilator effects of isoflurane may produce preferential vasodilation of the non-ischaemic bed, thus a coronary steal phenomenon has been postulated as a possible mechanism (Priebe 1989). This concept, once thought to be largely theoretical, is a practical reality. Indeed, one large survey of coronary angiography has shown that 23% of patients with coronary artery disease awaiting surgery may have coronary lesions, making them susceptible to coronary steal syndrome (Buffington et al 1988).

In conclusion it would appear to be difficult to quantify the relative hazards of different anaesthetics in patients with cardiovascular disease. However, a simple approach is possible, particularly if one concentrates of the importance of preserving myocardial oxygen balance, and avoiding cardiac failure and arrhythmia, as described on page 50.

All intravenous anaesthetics except ketamine reduce vascular tone, and thus may precipitate both myocardial oxygen imbalance and cardiac failure in those patients in whom maintenance of vasomotor tone is of critical importance. In contrast, ketamine may produce a hyperdynamic circulatory response. This may prove deleterious in patients at severe risk from myocardial ischaemia due to increased cardiac work and myocardial oxygen demand.

The negative inotropic effect of volatile anaesthetics will generally protect against myocardial oxygen imbalance. However, these anaesthetics may precipitate cardiac failure and should therefore be used intermittently and in low dosage in patients with poor LV function. In this group of patients the effects of halothane and enflurane on cardiac conduction may be significant, since it may be critically important to preserve sinus rhythm.

The effects of isoflurane on the coronary circulation are interesting, but are unlikely to be an outcome determinant, particularly if other, more simple haemodynamic aspects of the anaesthetic are well controlled. However, the data regarding isoflurane and the coronary circulation cannot simply be ignored; it is likely that isoflurane anaesthesia may prove hazardous in some patients (Priebe 1989). It is worth stressing that isoflurane anaesthesia is more clearly identified with tachycardia than other agents (Forrest et al 1990), that tachycardia with isoflurane has been shown to provoke anaerobic cardiac metabolism (Reiz et al 1983), and that tachycardia is generally associated with the development of ischaemic episodes which, in turn, have been shown to correlate with perioperative infarction (Slogoff & Keats 1985). This sequence excludes any of the effects that isoflurane may have on the generation of coronary steal. Nonetheless, it is salutary to remind ourselves that a number of studies, no doubt provoked by the isoflurane controversy, have shown that the type of anaesthetic used does not appear to influence outcome, whereas outcome may be influenced by the demonstrable competence of the anaesthetist (Slogoff & Keats 1985, Mangano 1989).

EFFECTS OF IPPV

There are two factors to take into account in considering the effects of IPPV:

- the haemodynamic effects of neuromuscular blocking drugs
- the mechanical effects of IPPV and the effects of changing $Pa\text{CO}_2$.

Neuromuscular blocking drugs

Suxamethonium (succinylcholine) is the only depolarizing neuromuscular blocking drug in common use. The administration of suxamethonium usually produces small and often inconsistent effects on the circulation. However, one predictable effect is the bradycardia seen occasionally following a single dose and frequently seen following repeated administration. This occurs as a consequence of stimulation of the muscarinic receptors of the SA node either by suxamethonium itself or by a metabolite (i.e. choline or succinylcholine). The muscle fasciculations following suxamethonium may cause muscle damage and an increase in plasma K^+ concentration, which could theoretically have adverse circulatory effects. In practice this only occurs in certain patients, that is those suffering from burns, massive injuries or chronic wasting neuromuscular disease, since in these the increase in serum K^+ may be large enough to cause serious arrhythmias. Suxamethonium should be avoided in these cases and used with extreme caution in any patient with high serum potassium.

The haemodynamic effects of the non-depolarizing neuromuscular blocking drugs are usually mild, although differences do exist between the different compounds. Early drugs, such as gallamine, had mild vagolytic effects. These effects are also seen with pancuronium (Brown et al 1973). Thus heart rate, blood pressure and cardiac output may be increased, and the vagolytic effects may help to protect against sudden bradycardia during surgery, which could occur as a result of parasympathetic stimulation or the use of volatile anaesthetics, as discussed on page 40. The vagolytic effects of pancuronium and the resulting tachycardia may be a theoretical disadvantage to this drug's use in patients with IHD, since tachycardia may provoke myocardial oxygen imbalance and ischaemia. There are some data to support this (Thompson & Putnins 1985). However, current practice of maintaining preoperative beta blockade and the use of large doses of opioids may serve to maintain good control of heart rate in patients with IHD, so that pancuronium produces only a very small increase in heart rate. D-tubocurarine causes a dose-dependent fall in arterial blood pressure and cardiac output with only a small increase in heart rate. The mechanism for these effects has been hotly debated over the years. Larger doses of D-tubocurarine may produce ganglion blockade (certainly in animals) and histamine release is known to occur. There is some evidence that a direct negative inotropic effect may be implicated. Alcuronium also causes a slight fall in blood pressure and a reflex tachycardia. Although the mechanism remains unclear, these effects do not appear to be related to histamine release.

Vecuronium and atracurium are two compounds synthesized in an attempt to produce an ultra-short-acting non-depolarizing relaxant. They are also free of vagolytic effects, which means that parasympathetic stimulation or other mechanisms provoking bradycardia will be free to act unopposed. Reports of bradycardia abound in the recent literature (Baraka & Chaya 1986, Starr et al 1986), although there is controversy as to whether bradycardia occurs as a primary effect, particularly with vecuronium (Wierda et al 1989). Whatever the mechanism, it is clear that bradycardia is a hazard and may be protected against with muscarinic antagonists.

A reversal of non-depolarizing neuromuscular blockade is achieved using an anticholinesterase such as neostigmine, and a muscarinic antagonist to block the vagal effects of the anticholinesterase. However, the duration of action of these drugs may be dissimilar. A tachycardia is frequently seen following atropine, then a return to baseline levels of heart rate, followed by a bradycardia as neostigmine acts relatively unopposed. The bradycardia may be attenuated if pyridostigmine is used instead of neostigmine. Both the initial tachycardia and later bradycardia can be avoided if glycopyrollate is used instead of atropine.

Mechanical effects of IPPV and alterations in $Pa\text{CO}_2$

During spontaneous ventilation the transpulmonary pressure gradient increases but intrapleural pressure decreases with respect to atmospheric pressure. During controlled ventilation the changes in the transpulmonary pressure gradient parallel those seen during spontaneous ventilation, but the intrapleural pressure becomes positive with respect to atmospheric pressure during inspiration. It is this latter change that is of importance in causing a reduction in cardiac output during controlled ventilation, particularly as it affects the pressure gradient for venous return. The development of a positive mean intrathoracic pressure during controlled ventilation will reduce the pressure gradient for venous return, thus reducing it and also reducing cardiac output.

In practical terms this is compensated for by an increase in peripheral venous tone, thus maintaining the pressure gradient and restoring venous return. The reduction of right ventricular (RV) stroke volume seen during the inspiratory phase of IPPV is compensated by an increased SV during the expiratory phase, thus cardiac output is maintained. (This phenomenon is of interest to those who wish to use thermodilution techniques to measure cardiac output, since the timing of the administration of cooled injectate becomes important.) Another interesting phenomenon often seen is the effect that passive inspiration (i.e. during IPPV) has on right and left stroke output; the former is reduced and the latter is increased. Thus cyclical variations in arterial blood pressure may be visible during IPPV, especially in those patients with low cardiac filling pressures.

Other factors involved in the cardiovascular depression seen with mechanical ventilation, and particularly with positive end-expiratory pressure (PEEP) include: increased pulmonary artery resistance (PAR) due to compression of small-diameter vessels in the pulmonary vascular bed, alteration of the shape of the interventricular septum due to increased RV pressure with resulting 'tamponade' effect on the LV, and the release of humoral factors with a negative inotropic effect.

The effect of potent volatile agents on the normal circulation is to attenuate the vascular reflexes that would normally lead to compensation, thus reducing venous return and cardiac output.

The effect of the application of PEEP is to reduce venous return and cardiac output, unless venomotor tone is increased to compensate. When this response is poor due to deep anaesthesia, or when venomotor tone is already maximal, as in patients suffering from severe haemorrhage, then hypotension will ensue. The application of PEEP may lead to an improvement in cardiovascular function when impairment is due to hypoxia secondary to pulmonary oedema or atelectasis – a situation not found in healthy patients.

The cardiovascular effects of high-frequency positive-pressure ventilation or high-frequency jet ventilation appear to be related solely to the changes seen in mean intrathoracic pressure, assuming effective oxygenation and carbon dioxide homeostasis. Mean intrathoracic pressure is usually reduced, as is peak airway pressure, although there is inevitably an increasing amount of inadvertent PEEP as the ventilatory rate is increased. Naturally, at higher frequencies augmentation and restriction of left and right stroke output during the inspiratory/expiratory phases is not seen.

Hypercapnia causes a sympathoadrenal response resulting in a hyperdynamic circulation. The direct effect of CO_2 on the myocardium is a negative inotropic action. Hyperventilation of the lungs during anaesthesia may cause blood pressure and other indices to fall. This is due to the cessation of the sympathomimetic effect allowing the cardiodepressant effects of the volatile agents to predominate, and due to the rise in mean intrathoracic pressure associated with the increase in tidal and minute volume.

EFFECT OF POSTURE

The effect of a steep head-down tilt in the anaesthetized patient is to increase venous return and thus right atrial (RA) filling pressure. Unless the myocardium has been poisoned by excessive concentrations of negative inotropes such as volatile anaesthetic agents, this increase in filling pressure will cause an increase in stroke output, and restoration of cardiac output and blood pressure. In those patients breathing spontaneously, and especially in the obese, however, steep head-down tilt may cause ventilatory insufficiency resulting in hypoxia (see Ch. 34).

A steep head-up tilt will have the reverse effect, that is to reduce filling pressures and thence reduce blood pressure and cardiac output. Normally, vascular reflexes would compensate by increasing vascular tone, but in the deeply anaesthetized patient this compensatory reflex will be attenuated. Thus a steep head-up tilt is successfully employed as part of a technique for elective hypotensive anaesthesia in normal adults undergoing head and neck surgery. A lighter plane of anaesthesia, and slow and careful positioning of the patient will allow a head-up tilt or even sitting posture to be used with minimal haemodynamic disturbance.

The lateral position has minimal effects on the circulation, although the initial movement and positioning of the patient may produce transient hypotension. The reason for this is unclear, but may be related to sudden mediastinal shift.

THE EFFECTS OF ANAESTHETIC AND SURGICAL STIMULATION

Anaesthetic manoeuvres and surgical stimulation provoke some degree of pain and an accompanying sympathoadrenal response, resulting in effects on the circulation similar to a small dose of adrenaline, that is tachycardia, an increase in systemic and pulmonary arterial pressures, an increase in cardiac filling pressures and an increase in cardiac output. Classical anaesthetic teaching has emphasized that these and other signs of sympathetic activity denote an inadequate depth of anaesthesia, and may therefore be prevented by increasing the depth of anaesthesia appropriately. However, the haemodynamic responses to certain stimuli, such as instrumentation of the upper respiratory tract during laryngoscopy or bronchoscopy, are only prevented with difficulty, although it could be argued that these circulatory responses are of little concern to the healthy patient. In this regard it is interesting to note that the concept of minimum alveolar concentration (MAC) has been extended to include the concentrations of volatile anaesthetic neccessary to prevent responses to certain potent simuli (Table 3.3). From Table 3.3 it can be seen that the concentration of anaesthetic gases required to prevent the responses described in 95% of healthy individuals is high. The supposition must therefore be that, during a straightforward anaesthetic, in a healthy patient, the circulatory state of the patient is partly a result of the effects (usually depressant effects) of anaesthetic drugs and manoeuvres on the patient, and partly the result of a sympathoadrenal response caused by surgical stimulation. In addition, surgical and anaesthetic manoeuvres may cause parasympathetic stimulation, resulting in a bradycardia that is responsive to anticholinergic drugs. The most common example follows surgical

Table 3.3 Concentrations of halothane and enflurane required to prevent responses to certain stimuli (comparison of MAC, MACEI and MACBAR)

	Halothane	Enflurane
MAC_{50}	1.0 MAC (0.74 ± 0.03%)	1.0 MAC (1.68 ± 0.04%)
$MACEI_{50}$	1.3 MAC	1.4 MAC
$MACBAR_{50}$	1.5 MAC	1.6 MAC
MAC_{95}	1.2 MAC	1.1 MAC
$MACEI_{95}$	1.7 MAC	1.9 MAC
$MACBAR_{95}$	2.1 MAC	2.6 MAC

These values have been age-adjusted. MACEI: concentration of volatile agent permitting laryngoscopy and intubation without untoward movement, MACBAR: concentration of volatile agent required to block adrenergic response to skin incision, 50 and 95: percentages of individuals in whom above responses are blocked at concentrations stated.

traction on the peritoneum or abdominal viscera, or on the extraocular muscles.

CARDIOVASCULAR DISEASES THAT AFFECT THE SAFETY OF ANAESTHESIA

Assessing the risk

Adverse cardiac events in the perioperative period are the leading causes of death following anaesthesia and surgery. This observation, coupled with an increasing incidence of cardiovascular disease in an increasingly older population, strongly suggests that it is essential to identify groups at risk as early and effectively as possible. It is also important to avoid whatever factors have been shown to increase cardiac risk and therefore to ensure hazard-safe anaesthesia. Factors that predict the risk of perioperative cardiac morbidity and outcome have been extensively studied in recent years, and lately these studies have been comprehensively reviewed by Mangano (1990). The relevant factors may be identified as preoperative (historical), intraoperative and postoperative predictors of cardiac morbidity. These have been further subdivided and are considered in turn below.

Historical predictors

A number of predictive factors have been identified that may indicate an increased risk based simply on a patient's medical history. Since the incidence of cardiovascular disease rises with age, it may be reasonable to assume that with increasing age cardiac risk is greater. In fact, data from different sources substantially support and refute age as a predictor of cardiac risk (Goldman et al 1977, Steen et al 1978). This controversy may be explained by the need to evaluate whether the patient's overall physiological condition is appropriate for their age. A history of prior myocardial infarction would appear to be a significant predictive risk factor, particularly if surgery occurs within 6 months of the infarction. Perioperative infarction is both more frequent and more serious in patients with pre-existing cardiac infarction (Steen et al 1978). However angina, despite being clear evidence of symptomatic IHD, is a less certain predictor and one substantial study has found that a history of stable angina has no predictive value whatever (Foster et al 1986).

Studies have attempted to determine whether a history of hypertension or diabetes is able to predict cardiac risk, but without conclusion for or against, although in both these instances the severity of the disease may be more important than the simple diagnosis (Prys-Roberts 1979). However, the data regarding congestive heart failure are less at issue, and evidence of active cardiac failure at the time of surgery clearly correlates with poor outcome (Goldman et al 1977, Larsen et al 1987). What is less clear is which specific signs of cardiac failure are best for identifying both the severity of the disease and an increased risk.

Both cigarette smoking and high serum cholesterol are factors known to be associated with an increased incidence of IHD but, in the absence of any other factors, there is no evidence that these factors per se increase perioperative cardiac risk (Foster et al 1986). Previous cardiac intervention (coronary artery bypass graft surgery or percutaneous coronary angioplasty) would appear to confer protection against adverse perioperative cardiac events, and the continuation of effective cardiovascular drug therapy has been shown to reduce the incidence of perioperative infarction (Miller et al 1975). Also, the presence of peripheral vascular disease and valvular heart disease have been shown to be influential, especially in the latter group of patients undergoing non-cardiac surgery (Goldman et al 1977). The value of preoperative diagnostic tests have also been studied. The potential benefit of highly specific, sensitive and preferably simple preoperative testing is clear. However, equally clear is the potential for misuse or waste of resources if large numbers of preoperative tests are carried out that have no predictive value whatever.

Clearly the 12-lead ECG remains the 'gold standard' non-invasive diagnostic test, and it has the advantage of being cheap and widely available. Computer analysis is possible that will permit reliable and reproducible assessment of abnormalities. However, not all studies confirm its predictive value (Goldman et al 1978). Similarly, the predictive value of exercise stress testing and ambulatory ECG monitoring are also controversial, although greater interest is now focusing on the latter (Chierchia et al 1983). Continuous Holter monitoring has been used successfully to evaluate the incidence of ischaemia in patients with risk factors for IHD but with no direct evidence of the disease (Knight et al 1979). Precordial and transoesophageal echocardiography are useful methods of identifying wall-motion abnormality and perioperative ventricular dysfunction, but their use as preoperative tests to predict perioperative risk has not been evaluated.

The use of radionuclear imaging techniques has been extensively studied and there are data both supporting and refuting their value as predictive tests (Eagle et al 1989). One problem with their use is the high number of false positives suggesting increased risk. However, the specificity of a negative test is 100%.

Other imaging modalities include MRI and modern CT scanning. No doubt these will be evaluated in due course, although cost implications are likely to restrict their use to small identifiable subgroups. Similarly the cost and invasive nature of cardiac catheterization restricts its use as a predictor test, although clearly this remains the best method for evaluating cardiac performance and the presence of cardiac lesions.

Intraoperative predictors

A number of studies have been carried out in an attempt to identify whether choice of anaesthetic influences outcome in patients at risk of perioperative cardiac morbidity. Clearly, a safe anaesthetic technique should be designed to reduce to a minimum the risk factors described earlier (pp. 35–38), that is, myocardial oxygen imbalance, cardiac failure and significant arrhythmia. However, the data from outcome studies are conflicting, suggesting that choice of anaesthetic is a poor determinant of perioperative cardiac outcome. Regional anaesthesia does not appear to confer any advantage in comparison with general anaesthesia, although certain types of surgery (e.g. prostate resection) or specific patients (those in cardiac failure) may benefit (McGowen & Smith 1980). The use of high-dose opioid techniques has not been shown to be preferable to inhalational anaesthesia; indeed, there is one study that clearly suggests the opposite (Rao et al 1983). Furthermore, despite evidence that isoflurane may provoke ischaemia, there is no suggestion that perioperative infarction or mortality in cardiac patients is increased by isoflurane (Slogoff & Keats 1989). The differences between studies may represent a failure to identify the relevant at-risk subgroups. However, surgical factors have been shown to be important in evaluating risk. Emergency surgery, major vascular surgery and prolonged upper abdominal or thoracic surgery have all been shown to be relevant (Larsen et al 1987).

Evaluation of those factors associated with myocardial oxygen imbalance suggests that hypertension, hypotension and tachycardia may all be associated with an increased incidence of perioperative cardiac morbidity. Individual studies have confirmed this, but the clearest relationship exists between tachycardia and perioperative ischaemia in comparison with other haemodynamic abnormalities (Slogoff & Keats 1985). The incidence of ischaemia itself and its relationship to perioperative infarction have also been studied using a range of methods. The most important of these are the studies based on ECG analysis, since this is a widely available and well validated method of ischaemia detection. Recent data have shown that analysis of perioperative ST segment change is able to identify ischaemic episodes, that multilead ECG monitoring is far more effective than single-lead monitoring, that ischaemic episodes so detected are associated with an increased incidence of perioperative infarction, and that silent ischaemia is often present in at-risk groups in the preoperative period (Lierberman et al 1983, Slogoff & Keats 1986, Knight et al 1989). Thus the potential use of the ECG for detection of perioperative ischaemic events would appear to be increasing, and the widespread use of new technology such as real-time ST-segment trend analysis may help further.

Other methods of detecting perioperative ischaemia do exist (transoesophageal echocardiography (TOE), pulmonary artery catheter monitoring, and cardiac biochemical and nuclear imaging techniques), but these all suffer from a number of drawbacks. Of these methods, TOE appears to be the most promising as a practical method of intraoperative monitoring.

Postoperative predictors

Many of the haemodynamic abnormalities described above are particularly prevalent in the postoperative period, so this may represent a period of serious risk. However, little outcome data exists based on the analysis of events in the postoperative period, although ischaemic episodes, frequently silent, have been shown to occur. This clearly represents an area of interest for future study.

Conclusions

Most studies agree that recent myocardial infarction and current cardiac failure are important predictors of perioperative cardiac morbidity. Emergency and/or prolonged major surgery are also proven predictors. Other factors, such as age, hypertension and diabetes may be relevent in selected subgroups, but, as yet, these have not been fully defined. The importance of choice of anaesthetic may prove to be relevant in selected subgroups, but this is also not yet clear. Haemodynamic disturbances including hypertension, severe hypotension and especially tachycardia do correlate with adverse outcome.

Several guides have been developed in order to facilitate a quick and accurate preoperative assessment of risk. The most widely used, devised by Goldman et al (1977), is shown in Table 3.4. This table clearly identifies recent myocardial infarction, cardiac failure and arrhythmia as important events, together with age, general preoperative condition and major or emergency surgery. Furthermore, 28 of the 53 points in the cardiac-risk index are potentially controllable, and the possibility exists that overall risk might be lower if surgery is delayed until the patient is on optimum medical therapy.

Table 3.4 Computation of cardiac risk index

Criteria*	'Points'
1. History:	
(a) Age > 70 years	5
(b) MI in previous 6 months	10
2. Physical examination:	
(a) S_3 gallop or JVD	11
(b) Important VAS	3
3. Electrocardiogram:	
(a) Rhythm other than sinus or PAC on last preoperative ECG	7
(b) >5 PVC/min documented at any time before operation	7
4. General status:	
P_{O_2} <60 or P_{CO_2} >50 mmHg, K <3.0 or HCO_3 <20 mEq/litre, BUN >50 or C_R >3.0 mg/dl, abnormal SGOT, signs of chronic liver disease or patient bedridden from non-cardiac causes	3
5. Operation:	
(a) Intraperitoneal, intrathoracic or aortic operation	3
(b) Emergency operation	4
Total possible	53

* MI: myocardial infarction, JVD: jugular venous distension, VAS: vascular aortic stenosis, PAC: premature atrial contractions, ECG: electrocardiogram, PVC: premature ventricular contractions, P_{O_2}: partial pressure of oxygen, P_{CO_2}: partial pressure of carbon dioxide, K: potassium, HCO_3: bicarbonate, BUN: blood urea, C_R: creatinine, SGOT: serum glutamine oxaloacetic transaminase.

Ischaemic heart disease

Clearly, recent myocardial infarction is a significant factor in determining perioperative cardiac morbidity and outcome. When recent infarction is complicated by cardiac failure and arrhythmia, there exists a major hazard to safe anaesthesia. In patients who have already suffered previous infarction, further perioperative infarction is both more frequent and more severe (Goldman 1983). Also, evidence suggests that the development of perioperative ischaemia correlates with perioperative infarction. Thus it is essential that the anaesthetic management of these patients is directed to minimize risk of myocardial oxygen imbalance, cardiac failure and arrhythmia. However, a number of controversies remain, as described below.

The value of continuing myocardial protection through antianginal medication into the perioperative period is well established, although the data are more convincing for continuing Beta blockade than calcium channel blockade (Miller et al 1975, Slogoff & Keats 1988). However, now the onus is more correctly placed on the need to justify withdrawing any cardiac medications rather than the need to justify continuing them. One recent controversy surrounds the use of heavy premedication in patients with IHD. The justification for this technique lies in the value of minimizing haemodynamic disturbance immediately before and during induction of anaesthesia. However, studies have shown that heavy premedication may be associated with relative oxygen desaturation, although there is no confirmatory evidence to suggest that this provokes ischaemic episodes (Marjot et al 1990).

Although the appropriate haemodynamic management of IHD patients is based on identification and avoidance of those factors known to disturb myocardial oxygen balance, it should be stressed that perioperative ischaemic episodes often occur without any significant haemodynamic disturbance. The data regarding choice of anaesthetics remain inconclusive, although a question mark still exists against the use of narcotic techniques without volatile supplements and against the use of high concentrations of isoflurane.

The postoperative management of patients with significant IHD continues to be the subject of debate. In many ways the patient who has undergone myocardial revascularization may suffer less risk than patients with IHD undergoing other major surgery. The latter should be offered at least as much intensive monitoring and care, including a period of postoperative intermittent positive pressure ventilation (IPPV), as cardiac surgical patients.

Congestive cardiac failure

Congestive cardiac failure is a term used to describe combined left and right heart failure, characterized by dependent oedema, jugular venous distension, hepatomegaly, poor effort tolerance usually provoking attacks of dyspnoea, and pulmonary oedema. In congestive heart failure the right heart failure is secondary to chronic left ventricular failure and is usually, but not exclusively, due to diffuse coronary artery disease. Medical treatment is directed towards correction of salt and water retention with diuretics, and improvement of cardiac performance with cardiac glycosides, angiotensin converting enzyme (ACE) inhibitors and vasodilators.

Patients in stable chronic congestive heart failure usually tolerate general anaesthesia and surgery well, but great care must be taken to prevent acute exacerbations of cardiac failure in the perioperative period. In particular, attention should be paid to preoperative electrolyte balance and fluid loading. Hypokalaemia, if left uncorrected, may provoke the development of serious arrhythmias in the perioperative period.

Chronic treatment with diuretics and especially vasodilators serves to reduce cardiac filling pressures, thereby reducing LA pressure and the generation of pulmonary oedema. Hypoxia is reduced, but cardiac output may be reduced also, and these patients may be vulnerable to the vasodilator side-effects of most intravenous induction agents.

Regional techniques have been advocated for patients with congestive heart failure, although there is no clear evidence that such techniques are superior; indeed, the risks and hazards may simply be different, not less. Adequate oxygenation, a period of IPPV, close attention to the fluid and electrolyte balance, and a mild degree of sympathoadrenal activation during general anaesthesia may all serve to enhance myocardial function and cardiac output, and to minimize risk. However, these patients tolerate even minor setbacks poorly, and great care must be taken in the postoperative period lest serious heart failure develops.

Hypertension

Although essential hypertension is the most common cause of pathologically raised blood pressure, many renal, endocrine, neurological and other causes of hypertension exist. Affected patients may present an increased anaesthetic risk related to the primary disease, as well as to the consequences of secondary hypertension. Whatever the cause, hypertension is a common and potent cause of mortality, chiefly from cerebrovascular haemorrhage, LV failure, IHD and renal disease.

Previously it was accepted that patients with hypertension have blood-vessel walls that are abnormally hyperreactive to the effects of neurotransmitters, such that large increases in vascular tone occur. However, it is now well established that the changes seen in hypertension are due not to hyperactive blood vessels, but to adaptive hypertrophy of the arterial media such that the diameter of the arteriolar lumen is profoundly reduced without there being any alteration in the resting tone of vascular smooth muscle (Folkow 1971). Examination of the arterial wall in hypertensives reveals hypertrophy and hyperplasia of muscle cells in the media, an increase in the deposition of mucopolysaccharides and collagen, and an increase in the sodium chloride and water content of the arterial wall. Any reduction in the internal luminal diameter will have profound effects on flow–pressure relationships: the effect of reducing the luminal radius (r) by 50% is to cause considerable opposition to flow, since resistance to flow will be increased 16-fold. Such an increase necessitates the development of raised LV systolic pressures, the increase in systolic wall tension, and thus MVO_2 may cause myocardial oxygen imbalance.

There are a number of other considerations regarding added risk to safe anaesthesia posed by the existance of hypertension. Many patients will be on antihypertensive drugs, that is beta blockers, diuretics, vascular smooth muscle relaxants and other vasodilators. There has been much anxiety about the possible interaction of such drugs with anaesthetics. However, the need to maintain adequate control of hypertension up to and during surgery is now regarded to be of overriding importance.

Due to the changes in morphology of the arterioles discussed above, excessive hypotension may follow even moderate doses of intravenous induction agents. Drugs should therefore be used in reduced dosage and administered slowly. Conversely, excessive hypertension and tachycardia may occur following anaesthetic and surgical stimuli, in particular, laryngoscopy and intubation (Prys-Roberts et al 1971). The consequences of this are dealt with earlier (p. 40).

Many drugs have been used to prevent this pressor response to laryngoscopy; indeed, one instinctively feels that if such patients were anaesthetized 'properly', such untoward responses would not occur. The problem of successful management lies in the fact that the amount of anaesthetic required to prevent such a response is considerably in excess of that required to continue anaesthesia under the circumstances. Table 3.3 outlines the concentrations of volatile anaesthetic agents required to suppress well-defined responses to endotracheal intubation, and to suppress a haemodynamic response to a surgical stimulation. As can be seen, they are considerably greater than 1.0 MAC; at such concentrations, cardiovascular depression becomes likely in the patient with cardiovascular disease, including hypertension. This is especially likely in the severe hypertensive, taking very large doses of beta blockers. In these patients, should hypotension and cardiovascular depression occur due to injudicious use of anaesthetic agents, unusually large doses of pressor drugs and/or inotropes may be needed to reverse the situation.

These patients are also particularly susceptible to the consequences of dysrhythmias, including nodal or junctional rhythm. Normocapnic controlled ventilation and the avoidance of high concentrations of volatile agents will minimize this risk.

Finally, the risk does not end with the termination of surgery. Rebound hypertension may occur in the postoperative period, due either to pain and anxiety or to poor hypertensive control medication, or both.

Atherosclerotic disease

Atheromatous deposits may affect sites other than the coronary arteries, in particular, peripheral arteries, the brain, kidneys and other vital organs may be affected. The disease may occur in the aorta and predispose to aneurysmal dilatation.

Atherosclerosis is a generalized disease of blood vessels, therefore evidence of localized disease (e.g. in the coronary arteries) is a warning that disease may exist elsewhere (e.g. in the carotids and intracerebral circulation). The reduction in diameter of major arteries, and the weakened and dilated arterial wall, render the patient at risk from large alterations in perfusion pressure. Hypotension may cause a significant reduction in blood flow through the stenosed vessel, whereas hypertension may cause aneurysmal rupture and catastrophic haemorrhage. As in patients with other circulatory disorders, anaesthesia associated with minimal disturbance of haemodynamics is essential.

In patients with vertebrobasilar disease, movements (e.g. extension of the neck) may cause dizziness or fainting. This should alert the anaesthetist to the possibility of embarrassing cerebral perfusion during anaesthesia, particularly during laryngoscopy and intubation when the neck may be inadvertently hyperextended. Systemic blood pressure may fall to very low levels during cardiopulmonary bypass. Patients undergoing these procedures may be at increased risk from tissue hypoperfusion unless periods of hypotension are kept to a minimum and adequate perfusion pressure on bypass is maintained. Whether pulsatile perfusion is perferable over non-pulsatile is not fully clear.

Atheroma in a carotid artery is especially worrying since it may predispose to cerebral hypoxia during bypass. A preoperative history of transient ischaemic attacks and the presence of carotid bruits are indicators of significant disease. Confirmation may be obtained by ultrasound or, if necessary, carotid angiography. Significant carotid stenosis may require surgical treatment, which usually involves a short period of clamping the carotid artery. The risk of anoxic brain damage during periods of occlusion is minimized by maintaining arterial blood pressure in the normal or low–normal range, and by achieving normocapnic or mild hypocapnic ventilation of the lungs. Patients known to have stable coronary artery disease may have carotid artery surgery carried out before myocardial revascularization. In poor risk or unstable coronary patients both carotid artery surgery and myocardial revascularization may be undertaken as a combined procedure, with carotid endarterectomy carried out first. However, bypass procedures are increasingly being undertaken without surgical correction of the carotid lesion, but with great care taken to preserve cerebral perfusion without uncoupling flow/metabolism, thereby minimizing operative risk. These strategies appear to be successful, thus carotid surgery can be carried out at a later date if necessary.

Valvular heart disease

Any of the valves of the heart may be affected, but in practice aortic and mitral valve disease are the most common. All patients with valvular heart disease are at risk from subacute bacterial endocarditis following even trivial surgical procedures, and appropriate antibiotic prophylaxis should be given. In cases of valvular heart disease the extent to which disease presents a hazard to safe anaesthesia is determined by the severity of the lesion, the presence of mixed univalvular disease, the presence of more than one affected valve, the duration of the disease, and thus whether secondary and non-reversible changes have taken place (i.e. pulmonary hypertension, LV dilation and hypertrophy), and the presence of other cardiopulmonary pathology (i.e. IHD and chronic bronchitis). A number of more specific aspects are covered below.

Aortic valve disease

The volume of blood ejected from the LV is governed by the equation:

$$SV = Ts \times AVA \times LV\text{–}Ao \times k$$

where SV = stroke volume, Ts = duration of systole, AVA = aortic valve area, LV–Ao = mean pressure gradient from the left ventricle to the aorta, k = constant.

Therefore, as the aortic valve area decreases, stroke volume will fall unless there is a compensatory increase either in the duration of systole, or in the mean LV to aorta pressure gradient. In practice, SV is maintained mostly by increasing left ventricular systolic pressure (LVSP) and hence the transvalvular gradient, which leads to concentric hypertrophy of the LV wall. LV dilatation occurs late in aortic stenosis as LV failure develops.

The concentric hypertrophy of the LV produces a stiff chamber, which fills both slowly and poorly unless ordered atrial contraction is present. Indeed, atrial contraction (active filling) contributes more to LV volume in aortic stenosis patients than in normals, since early diastolic (passive) filling is so ineffective. The patient with aortic stenosis is extremely sensitive to the loss of sinus rhythm or tachycardia (due to less time for passive diastolic filling). Peripheral vasoconstriction may be poorly tolerated since LV impedance is increased, necessitating a further increase in LV systolic pressure in order to maintain SV.

Symptoms of angina in patients with severe aortic stenosis do not necessarily indicate the coexistence of coronary artery disease. Myocardial ischaemia may occur owing to the increased myocardial oxygen consumption (MVO_2) of the hypertrophied ventricle and to decreased subendocardial perfusion. Peripheral vasoconstriction and tachycardia may exacerbate the problem, and should be avoided.

The anaesthetic technique should therefore be designed to minimize the onset of dysrhythmias, preserve LV contractile power and avoid overlight anaesthesia with vasoconstriction and tachycardia. Great care must be taken, particularly in the dose and rate of administration of intravenous induction agents. The presence of aortic stenosis contributes significantly to the risks of anaesthesia. The presence of severe aortic stenosis is a profound hazard to safe anaesthesia.

Patients with aortic valve regurgitation (AR) suffer from volume overloading of the LV in contrast to the pressure overloading seen in pure aortic stenosis. The regurgitation volume is determined by the valve area, the mean diastolic pressure gradient from aorta to LV, and the duration of diastole.

Tachycardia is better tolerated in AR since diastolic duration is shortened (less time for regurgitation to occur). In theory this may potentiate the development of ischaemia since coronary perfusion time is reduced, but in practice the increase in mean aortic diastolic pressure associated with the tachycardia provides adequate compensation. LV dilatation occurs earlier than in patients with aortic stenosis and, although left ventricular contractility is usually well preserved until late, any reduction in power may cause a severe reduction in forward flow and hence reduce SV. Peripheral vasoconstriction, which will increase the pressure gradient for regurgitation, is obviously to be avoided, but the effects of vasodilators vary, depending on whether pre-existing SVR is high or normal, and whether LV function is impaired. In general, these patients with a high LVEDP, high SVR and low (forward) SV are likely to benefit from vasodilators.

In mixed aortic valve disease, significant regurgitation may occur even though there is a very small valve orifice, thus increasing the work needed to achieve an adequate (forward) SV. Both ischaemia and failure may occur in mixed valve disease.

Mitral valve disease

Stenosis of the mitral valve results in a small valve area through which the LV may fill in diastole. Thus the problems of mitral valve stenosis are those consequent upon a reduced SV, and upon the higher mean left atrial pressure (LAP) necessary to overcome the stenosis. When tissue oxygen demands are increased, for example during exercise, the stenosed valve may constitute a significant barrier to blood flow and to LV filling, and LAP may rise steeply. Thus dyspnoea is a valuable sign in patients with mitral stenosis, and the level of exercise required to produce dyspnoea is a useful indication of the severity of the stenosis.

Although the left atrium (LA) is often large, LV dilatation is not common in pure stenosis and may indicate the presence of mixed mitral valve disease, or concomitant AR or coronary artery disease. In patients with tight mitral stenosis the duration of diastole is an important determinant of left ventricular end diastolic volume (LVEDV). Tachycardia will reduce diastolic filling time, and the absence of sinus rhythm may also reduce ventricular filling since there is no late diastolic atrial filling component. This problem, although real, would appear to be of less significance to patients with mitral stenosis than to those with aortic stenosis. Atrial fibrillation is common in patients with mitral stenosis, and in this situation SV becomes even more dependent on the preceding diastolic filling time. Adequate digitalization may be necessary to control the ventricular response.

Peripheral vasoconstriction is detrimental to patients with mitral stenosis, but the use of vasodilators will produce a varied response. A useful reduction in PAP and pulmonary capillary wedge pressure (PCWP) may be seen, but there may also be a reduction in transvalvular gradient causing a reduction in LV filling. Provided that LVEDV is not too low to start with (i.e. severe mitral stenosis), the reduction in LV impedance may be of benefit.

Worsening mitral stenosis will produce increasingly high LA pressures with pulmonary venous congestion, an increase in pulmonary extravascular water (interstitial oedema) and pulmonary arterial hypertension with RV hypertrophy. With critical mitral stenosis (LAP >25 mmHg at rest), PVR rises secondary to pulmonary arteriolar constriction, potentiating RV failure and tricuspid regurgitation.

Despite the foregoing, patients with mild or moderate mitral stenosis usually do remarkably well during general anaesthesia and surgery. A mildly enhanced inotropic state, careful acid–base balance and well-controlled gas exchange may improve LV performance, provided that dysrhythmias (including tachycardia) are avoided and pulmonary venous congestion is not potentiated by overenthusiastic transfusion. Small increments of volatile agents may be useful in serving to blunt the sympathoadrenal response, but in patients with severe mitral stenosis these should be avoided owing to the myocardial depressant effects. Many factors associated with poor-quality anaesthesia cause PVR to be elevated, that is hypoxia, hypercapnia, acidosis and hypothermia. These should be avoided in all patients, including those with mitral stenosis.

Patients with severe disease or following major surgery will benefit from a period of postoperative IPPV, since the effects of high resting pulmonary venous and arterial pressure, decreased lung compliance, increased airway resistance and the increased work of breathing may precipitate respiratory failure.

The volume of blood regurgitating through the mitral valve during LV systolic depends on the valve area, the duration of LV systolic and the LV–LA pressure gradient (influenced in turn by LV function, LA compliance and LV impedance).

There are important functional differences depending on whether the mitral regurgitation is acute or chronic, or whether it is associated with mitral stenosis or other cardiac disease. For example, the myocardial energy cost of pure mitral regurgitation is low in comparison to aortic stenosis or aortic regurgitation, and therefore ischaemia is rare unless coexisting IHD is present. Acute mitral regurgitation may occur in association with IHD or following actual infarction. In this situation, atrial hypertrophy without dilatation may result in a poorly compliant chamber leading to early pulmonary hypertension and RV failure. Vasodilators may help by lowering PAP and by decreasing LV impedance, hence promoting forward LV ejection.

Classically, patients with chronic mitral regurgitation have a large dilated LA into which blood regurgitates freely but without any great increase in LAP, or without the development of pulmonary venous congestion or RV failure. In practice most patients demonstrate haemodynamics in between the acute and chronic groups.

Patients with mixed mitral valve disease often have an enlarged LA, with pulmonary hypertension and RV failure, and are in atrial fibrillation. Those with severe mitral stenosis do not develop significant mitral regurgitation.

Anaesthetic factors that decrease systemic vascular resistance and thus reduce LV impedance would be useful in promoting forward flow, although any significant reduction in LV contractility would offset this advantage. Thus the place of volatile agents is controversial. Tachycardia is better tolerated in mitral regurgitation than mitral stenosis and, since pulmonary congestion is a late feature, there is less risk of overtransfusion.

Tricuspid valve disease

Since the RA and vena cavae are very compliant structures, tricuspid regurgitation is usually well tolerated (even total tricuspid valve removal is tolerated for a time). Pure RV volume overload is acceptable, but if RV pressure overload is added (i.e. following an increase in PVR), then RV forward flow is reduced and cardiac output decreased. Those anaesthetic factors that increase RV impedance or PVR should be avoided.

Cardiomyopathy and carditis

Cardiomyopathy is usually divided into three pathological entities: congestive, obstructive and constrictive cardiomyopathy. Congestive cardiomyopathy is usually associated with IHD and the sequelae of congestive cardiac failure. Valvular lesions may be present, especially regurgitation of the AV valves. The risk to safe anaesthesia is dependent on the severity of the disease. Cardiomyopathy may also be a feature of other conditions with anaesthetic implications, for example Friedreich's ataxia and dystrophia myotonica.

Obstructive cardiomyopathy may be a profound hazard to safe anaesthesia. Hypertrophic obstructive cardiomyopathy, obstructive asymmetric septal hypertrophy, or idiopathic hypertrophic subaortic stenosis presents with symptoms secondary to LV outflow tract obstruction, increased diastolic stiffness (poor compliance) of the hypertrophied myocardium, and an increase in myocardial oxygen consumption (MVO_2). Conduction problems may occur and may be partly responsible for the significant incidence of sudden death.

Outflow tract obstruction is worsened by decreasing aortic pressure, decreasing LV volume and increasing LV ejection velocity. Hypovolaemia should be avoided and care must be taken to keep the circulatory volume sufficiently expanded. Vasodilators, including nitrates, may be counterproductive since LV volume decreases, aortic pressure decreases and LV ejection velocity reflexly increases.

Isoprenaline, which causes an increase in LV ejection velocity and a decrease in aortic pressure, should be avoided. Indeed, propanolol is used to treat patients up to the time of corrective surgery and beyond. Halothane may be particularly useful in these patients since it reduces myocardial contractility and has been shown to reduce the outflow tract gradient. However, the concentration used must be judged with great care since the poorly compliant ventricle will fill incompletely in any rhythm but sinus.

Patients with hypertrophic obstructive cardiomyopathy frequently have mitral regurgitation. However, drugs may have the opposite effect on mitral regurgitation with coexisting hypertrophic obstructive cardiomyopathy in comparison to pure mitral regurgitation. Since vasodilators may increase outflow tract obstruction, they will increase mitral regurgitation in those patients with coexisting hypertrophic obstructive cardiomyopathy. Vasoconstrictors may lessen the regurgitation flow, in direct contrast to those patients with pure mitral regurgitation.

Constrictive cardiomyopathy is rare and resembles constrictive pericarditis in that the myocardium is abnormally stiff, and the LV is poorly compliant and therefore difficult to fill. Constrictive cardiomyopathy may be associated with leukaemia, haemochromatosis or amyloidosis, and occasionally may only be differentiated from constrictive pericarditis at thoracotomy.

The anaesthetic implications of constrictive pericarditis, acute pericarditis with pericardial effusion, acute cardiac tamponade and constrictive cardiomyopathy are essentially qualitatively similar. The use of anaesthetic drugs, including many intravenous induction agents, results in vasodilatation and a reduction in cardiac filling pressure in a patient when filling pressure needs to be kept high in order to achieve adequate ventricular end-diastolic volume, and hence SV. Cardiac output falls and hypotension may be profound, especially in patients with acute postoperative tamponade or severe constrictive disease. Many workers have suggested that inhalation agents provide the safest management in this situation, but, in practice, intravenous agents can be used, provided that great care is taken to limit total dosage and rate of administration. Ketamine may be particularly useful in these patients.

Viral myocarditis may rarely complicate acute pericarditis. Although frequently unremarkable, it may be associated with tachyarrhythmias and cardiac failure. Whenever possible, anaesthesia should be postponed until recovery is complete. When incomplete recovery occurs, the anaesthetic problems are usually those of congestive cardiac failure, although if the acute is still in the acute phase, low-output arrhythmias may occur.

Arrhythmias

Sinus rhythm is not an essential prerequisite for safe anaesthesia. Nevertheless, the presence of a preoperative arrhythmia may increase the risk of anaesthesia since it may indicate the presence of significant circulatory disease, and the arrhythmia may be liable to further exacerbation during anaesthesia with consequent reduction in cardiac output. Clearly it is important to consider the clinical setting in which the arrhythmia occurs, and to that end it is useful to consider four categories of patient:

1. Patients with no previous arrhythmia who develop benign arrhythmias during anaesthesia.
2. Patients with a preoperative chronic stable arrhythmia who undergo no change during anaesthesia.
3. Patients with no significant arrhythmia who develop haemodynamically or prognostically significant arrhythmias during anaesthesia.
4. Patients with preoperative arrhythmia who develop either exacerbations of the previous arrhythmia or who develop new significant arrhythmia during anaesthesia.

Many patients with no previous history of arrhythmia and no circulatory disease may develop benign arrhythmias during anaesthesia, simply as a result of the effects of anaesthetic agents on cardiac conduction. These benign arrhythmias may require some fine-tuning of the anaesthetic, but little else in the way of therapy. However, it is vital to understand that it is not simply the arrhythmia that is benign, but the combination of the arrhythmia and the clinical context. Thus AV nodal rhythm in a normal patient is a benign and common arrhythmia during anaesthesia; the same arrhythmia in a patient with severe aortic stenosis may be lethal.

Patients with chronic stable arrhythmia frequently undergo anaesthesia and surgery uneventfully, provided that no new arrhythmia develops. The degree of hazard posed is related more to the cause of the chronic arrhythmia (cardiac valve disease, IHD, hypertension, thyrotoxicosis, etc.) than to the arrhythmia itself. There are a number of arrhythmias that are potentially hazardous in any patient (Table 3.4). These include severe disorders of rate, some ventricular ectopic activity and many conduction abnormalities. The significance of the latter defects is that they may progress to complete heart block with no ventricular activity and thus effective ventricular asystole. Complete heart block rarely occurs without any warning, and preoperative investigation may reveal a more benign conduction abnormality (e.g. 1st-degree block) which might progress to complete heart block in adverse circumstances.

How are such arrhythmias provoked and how are they prevented? Anaesthesia involves the use of a variety of drugs, all of which have both antiarrhythmic and proarrhythmic potential. This, coupled with the large degree of alteration in autonomic nervous system activity associated with both anaesthesia and surgery, suggests that the perioperative period should be regarded as essentially proarrhythmic (Feneck 1990). Alterations in blood gases, acid–base status and electrolytes, the effects of mumerous drugs used in anaesthesia, and the autonomic consequences of anaesthesia and surgical stimulation may all influence the development of arrhythmias. It is clearly logical to minimize the proarrhythmic effects of surgery by properly conducted, balanced anaesthesia. In those patients with preexisting heart disease prone to arrhythmia and taking chronic antiarrhythmic therapy, this will be especially important as correction of proarrhythmic factors alone may not lead to reversion to a stable rhythm. Acute preoperative withdrawal of antiarrhythmic therapy may be deleterious, indeed it is difficult to conceive of a situation where withdrawal of therapy would be advisable other than during antiarrhythmia surgery. Thus antiarrhythmic therapy should normally be continued, and the anaesthetic planned to be as stable (or non-proarrhythmic) as possible. Continuation of antiarrhythmia therapy in the postoperative period should be considered, if necessary by the intravenous route, although frequently the half-life of oral therapy will be sufficiently prolonged to cover the postoperative period until oral medication can be resumed.

How important is the development of arrhythmia as an outcome determinant? Perioperative diagnosis of arrhythmia is not difficult, so this should be an easy question to answer. However, since perioperative arrhythmia may reflect both preoperative disease and/or anaesthetic factors to a variable degree, the simple diagnosis of an arrhythmia is often less relevant than its chronicity, controlling drug therapy, underlying pathophysiology and many other factors. Some data suggest that 'any rhythm but sinus' indicates an increased risk (Goldman et al 1977, Olsen et al 1975), but this is controversial. Clearly some arrhythmias will increase the hazard to safe anaesthesia in any patient, but it is not yet clear whether or not the development of a benign arrhythmia in an otherwise normal patient constitutes any added risk.

Congenital heart disease

The incidence of congenital heart disease (CHD) is approximately 0.8% of live births. If left untreated, 20% of babies with CHD will die in the first year of life, and half of these within the first month. Around 30–40% of children with trisomy 21 have CHD, and many other chromosomal abnormalities are associated with coexisting cardiac anomalies. The presence of CHD constitutes a major hazard to the safe conduct of any anaesthetic and the degree of risk is determined by the nature, severity and multiplicity of the lesions. It is not intended to provide a comprehensive account of the anaesthetic management of each condition here. Only the broadest outline of the hazards involved will be discussed. It is important to understand the physiological consequences of congenital lesions before surgery. All patients should be fully evaluated to assess their current clinical status, prior to any surgery for either correction of the defects or incidental non-cardiac surgery. It may be necessary to have corrective or palliative surgery before any non-cardiac surgery. Patients with surgically corrected defects may still have residual lesions present, compromising their degree of cardiac reserve.

A good assessment of cardiac reserve can be made from the history. Exercise tolerance is a good indicator of the patient's ability to tolerate anaesthesia. The ability of babies to feed and suckle without breathlessness, and information concerning growth and development are useful in assessing the patient's current clinical state. The majority of patients with CHD will require suitable antibiotic prophylaxis against the development of subacute bacterial endocarditis. All patients who have a right-to-left shunt are at increased risk of microemboli entering the systemic circulation. Meticulous intravenous technique is required to prevent inadvertent injection of air.

The implications of anaesthesia are determined by the nature of the underlying congenital defect. Patients with excessive pulmonary blood flow (i.e. septal defects, patent ductus arteriosus or pulmonary venous congestion) or obstruction to forward flow (i.e. coarctation of the aorta, aortic or mitral stenosis or atresia, or certain cases of total anomalous venous pulmonary venous drainage) are prone to develop congestive heart failure early. Indeed, some patients (i.e. aortic stenosis or preductal coarctation of the aorta) present with severe life-threatening LV failure. Patients with left-to-right intracardiac shunts are usually acyanotic. However, if PVR increases in the presence of systemic hypotension, the shunt may reverse right-to-left with the subsequent development of cyanosis. This may occur at induction or at any time during anaesthesia. Hypoxia, hypercapnia, acidosis, excessive catecholamine secretion, excessive pressures generated by IPPV or the injudicious use of vasodilators may all potentiate this.

Patients with reduced pulmonary blood flow often have severe cyanosis and polycythaemia (i.e. Fallot's tetralogy, pulmonary stenosis or atresia, and tricuspid atresia). Any increase in PVR or right outflow-tract obstruction may cause cyanosis to worsen. This is classically seen in patients with Fallot's tetralogy who develop infundibular spasm. Survival is dependent on the patency of the ductus arteriosus, and patients benefit from preoperative prostaglandin therapy. Cyanosis can also occur due to intracardiac mixing of pulmonary and systemic venous blood (e.g. AV canal, common chamber defects), or when systemic blood is returned to the aorta bypassing the lungs (transposition of the great arteries).

Many of the lesions referred to above have a mortality of 80% if left untreated, therefore anaesthesia is likely to be for corrective or palliative surgery rather than coincidental surgery. Meticulous anaesthetic technique is called for. There is also no doubt now that overall results favour the establishment of specialized centres to deal with these complex problems.

HEART AND HEART–LUNG TRANSPLANTATION

In recent years the number of heart and heart–lung transplant procedures has increased dramatically. This has followed advances in preoperative care and surgical technique, and, in particular, has been achieved as a result of the successful introduction of cyclosporin A. Patients undergoing cardiac transplantation will be in New York Heart Association Class IV cardiac failure, as a result of either ischaemia or cardiomyopathy. Heart–lung transplantation is usually carried out on patients with either severe irreversible pulmonary vascular disease or severe parenchymal disease (i.e. fibrosing alveolitis or cystic fibrosis).

The risks of anaesthesia in such patients are considerable, and are related, in particular, to cardiac failure and arrhythmia, haemorrhage and infection. Multisystem organ failure may be present preoperatively and appropriate supportive therapy will be needed. In such circumstances the risk of a poor outcome is very high. Anaesthesia for general surgical procedures in successful transplant recipients is becoming more common. Such patients may not only have abnormal haemodynamics, but may also demonstrate abnormal responses to drugs. In particular, the denervated heart is unresponsive to vagolytic agents, but sympathetic denervation may increase cardiac B-receptor density and thus enhance the sensitivity of cardiac tissue to circulating cathecholamines (White & Latimer 1991). Thus the arrhythmogenic effects of anaesthetics and catecholamines, and the risks of perioperative cardiac failure, may all be increased. To this must be added the risk of infection and therefore the absolute need for sterility in all immunosuppressed patients.

REFERENCES

Andersen N, Johansen S J 1963 Incidence of catecholamine induced arrhythmias during halothane anaesthesia. Anesthesiology 24: 51–56

Baraka A, Chaya L 1986 Haemodynamic effects of vecuronium in patients with coronary artery disease. Acta Anaesthesiol Scand 30: 28–29

Bastard O G, Carter J G, Moyer J R et al 1982 A comparison of the circulatory effects of isoflurane and halothane in patients with ischaemic heart disease. Anaesth Analg 61: 170–171

Blitt C D, Raessler K L, Wightman et al 1979 Atrioventricular conduction in dogs during anaesthesia with isoflurane. Anesthesiology 50: 210–212

Brown E M, Smiler B G, Plaza J A 1973 Cardiovascular effects of pancuronium. Anesthesiology 38: 597–599

Buffington C W, Davis K B, Gillespie S, Pettinger M 1988 The prevalence of steal prone coronary anatomy in patients with coronary artery disease: an analysis of the coronary artery surgery study registry. Anesthesiology 69: 721–727

Calverley R K, Smith N T, Prys-Roberts C 1978 Cardiovascular effects of enflurane anaesthesia during controlled ventilation. Anaesth Analg 57: 619–628

Chierchia S, Lazzari M, Freedman B, Brunelli C, Maseri A 1983 Impairment of myocardial perfusion and function during painless myocardial ischaemia. J Am Coll Cardiol 1: 924–930

Claeys M A, Gepts E, Gamu F 1988 Haemodynamic changes during anaesthesia induced and maintained with propofol. Br J Anaesth 60: 3–9

Clarke R S J, Lyons S M 1977 Diazepam and flunitrazepam as induction agents for surgical operations. Acta Anaesthesiol Scand 21: 282–292

Colvin M P, Savege T M, Newland P E et al 1979 Induction of anaesthesia with etomidate in patients with cardiac disease. Br J Anaesth 51: 551–556

Conway C M, Ellis D B 1969 The haemodynamic effects of

short acting barbiturates. Br J Anaesth 41: 534–542
deLange S, Stanley T H, Boscoe M J 1980 Fentanyl-oxygen anaesthesia: comparison of anaesthetic requirements and cardiovascular responses in Salt Lake City and Leiden, Holland. 7th World Congress of Anaesthesiologists, Abstracts, Hamburg, FRG p 313
Dubois-Primo J, DeWachter B, Massaut J 1979 Analgesic anaesthesia with fentany (F) and sufentanil (SF) in coronary surgery. A double blind study Acta Anaesthesiol Belg 30: 113–126
Dundee J W, Moore J 1961 Thiopentone and methohexitone: a comparison of main anaesthetic agents for a standard operation. Anaesthesia 16: 50
Eagle K A, Coley C M, Newell J B et al 1989 Combining clinical and thallium data optimizes preoperative assessment of cardiac risk before major vascular surgery. Ann Intern Med 110: 859–866
Eger E I, Smith N T, Stoelting R K et al 1970 Cardiovascular effects of halothane in man. Anesthesiology 32: 396–409
Feneck R O 1990 Anti arrhythmics. Curr Opin Anaesthesiol 3: 110–116
Flickinger H, Fraimow W, Cathcart R T et al 1961 Effect of thiopental induction on cardiac output in man. Anaesth Analg 40: 694–700
Folkow B 1971 The haemodynamic consequences of adaptive structural changes of the resistance vessels in hypertension. Clin Sci 41: 1–7
Forrest J B et al 1990 Multicentre study of general anaesthesia 2: results. Anesthesiology 72: 262–268
Foster E D, Davis K B, Carpenter J A, Abele S, Fray D 1986 Risk of non cardiac operation in patients with defined coronary disease: the Coronary Artery Surgery Study (CASS) Registry Experience. Ann Thorac Surg 41: 42–50
Goldman L 1983 Cardiac risks and complications of non cardiac surgery. Ann Intern Med 98: 504–513
Goldman L, Caldera D L, Nussbaum S R et al 1977 Multifactorial index of cardiac risk in non cardiac surgical procedures. N Engl J Med 297: 845–850
Goldman L, Caldera D L, Southwick F S et al 1978 Cardiac risk factors and complications in non cardiac surgery. Medicine 57: 357–370
Gooding J M, Dimick A R, Tavakoli M et al 1977 A physiologic analysis of cardiopulmonary responses to ketamine anaesthesia in non cardiac patients. Anaesth Analg 56: 813–816
Hug C C Jr 1979 Pharmacology of Anaesthetic drugs. In: Kaplan J A (ed) Cardiac anaesthesia. Grune & Stratton, New York, pp 3–37
Johnston R R, Eger E I, Wilson C 1976 A comparative interaction of epinepherine with enflurane, isoflurane and halothane in man. Anaesth Analg 55: 709–712
Kettler D, Sonntag H, Wolfram-Donath U et al 1977 Haemodynamics, myocardial function, oxygen requirement, and oxygen supply of the human heart after administration of etomidate. In: Doenicke A (ed) Anaesthesiology and resuscitation. Springer-Verlag, Berlin, pp 81–94
Knight A A, Hollenburg M, London M J et al 1979 Perioperative myocardial ischaemia: importance of the preoperative ischaemic pattern. Anesthesiology 51: 393–397
Knight A A, Hollenburg M, London M J, Mangano D T 1989 Myocardial ischaemia in patients awaiting coronary artery bypass grafting. Am Heart J 117: 1189–1196
Larsen S F, Olesen K H, Jacobsen E et al 1987 Prediction of cardiac risk in non cardiac surgery. Eur Heart J 8: 179–185
Ledingham I M, Watt I 1983 Influence of sedation on mortality in critically multiple trauma patients. Lancet 1: 1270
Lierberman R W, Orkin F K, Jobes D R, Schwartz A J 1983 Haemodynamic predictors of myocardial ischaemia during halothane anaesthesia for coronary artery revascularization. Anesthesiology 59: 36–41
Lippman M, Reisner L S 1974 Epinephrine injection with enflurane anaesthesia: incidence of cardiac arrhythmias. Anaesth Analg 53: 886–889
Lowenstein E, Hallowell P, Levine F H et al 1969 Cardiovascular response to large doses of intravenous morphine in man. N Engl J Med 281: 1389–1393
Lundy J S, Tovell R M 1934 Some of the newer local and general anaesthetic agents. Methods of their administration. Northwest Medicine (Seattle) 33: 308–311
McGowen S W, Smith G F N 1980 Anaesthesia for transurethral prostatectomy: a comparison of spinal intradural analgesia with two methods of general anaesthesia. Anaesthesia 35: 847–853
Manara A R, Monk C R, Bolsin S R, Prys-Roberts C 1991 Total i.v. anaesthesia with propofol for coronary artery bypass grafting. Br J Anaesth 66(6): 716–718
Mangano D T 1989 Anaesthetics, coronary artery disease, and outcome: unresolved controversies (editorial). Anesthesiology 70: 175–178
Mangano D T 1990 Perioperative cardiac morbidity. Anesthesiology 72: 153–184
Marjot R, Valentine S J 1990 Arterial oxygen saturation following premedication for cardiac surgery. Br J Anaesth 64: 737–740
Master A M, Geller A J 1969 The extent of completely asymptomatic coronary artery disease (editorial). Am J Cardiol 23: 73
Merin R 1990 Propofol causes cardiovascular depression. Anesthesiology 72(2): 393
Miller R R, Olsen H G, Amsterdam E A, Mason D T 1975 Propranol withdrawl rebound phenomenon. Exacerbation of coronary events after abrupt cessation of anti anginal therapy. N Engl J Med 293: 416–418
Moffit E A, Sethna D H 1986 The coronary circulation and myocardial oxygenation in coronary artery disease: effects of anaesthesia. Anaesth Analg 65: 395–410
Office of Population Censuses and Surveys 1969–73, 1981–89 Mortality statistics: cause (England and Wales, 1969–1989). HMSO, London, DH2 Nos 9–16
Olsen G N, Block A J, Swenson E W et al 1975 Pulmonary function evaluation of the lung resection candidate: a prospective study. Am Rev Respir Dis 3: 379–386
Patrick M R, Blair I J, Feneck R O, Sebel P S 1986 A comparison of the haemodynamic effects of propofol and thiopentone in patients with coronary artery disease. Postgrad Med J Suppl 3 61: 23–28
Priebe J H 1989 Isoflurane and coronary haemodynamics. Anesthesiology 71: 960–976
Prys-Roberts C 1979 Hypertension and anaesthesia: fifty years on (editorial). Anesthesiology 50: 281–284
Prys-Roberts C, Greene L T, Meloche R, Foex P 1971 Studies of anaesthesia in relation to hypertension 2: haemodynamic consequences of induction and endobronchial intubation. Br J Anaesth 43: 531–546

Rao T L K, Jacobs K H, El-Etr A A 1983 Reinfarction following anaesthesia in patients with myocardial infarction. Anesthesiology 59: 499–505
Rawlins M D 1981 Clinical pharmacology: adverse reactions to drugs. Br Med J 282: 974–976
Reeves J G, Kissin I 1983 Pharmacology of anaesthetic drugs intravenous anaesthetics. In: Kaplan (ed) Cardiac anaesthesia. Grune & Stratton, New York, vol 2 pp 3–31
Reiz S, Balfors E, Sorenson M B et al 1983 Isoflurane: a powerful coronary vasodilator in patients with coronary disease. Anesthesiology 59: 91–97
Russell G N, Wright E L, Fox M A et al 1989 Propofol-fentanyl anaesthesia for coronary artery surgery and cardiopulmonary bypass. Anaesthesia 44: 205–208
Sahlman L, Milocco I, Appelgren L et al 1989 Control of intraoperative hypertension with isoflurane in patients with coronary artery disease: effects on regional myocardial blood flow and metabolism. Anaesth Analg 68: 105–111
Sebel P S, Lowdon J D 1989 Propofol: a new intravenous anaesthetic. Anesthesiology 71(2): 260–277
Slogoff S, Keats A S 1985 Does perioperative myocardial ischaemia lead to post operative myocardial infarction? Anesthesiology 62: 107–114
Slogoff S, Keats A S 1986 Further observations on perioperative myocardial ischaemia. Anesthesiology 65: 539–542
Slogoff S, Keats A S 1988 Does treatment with calcium entry blocking drugs reduce perioperative myocardial ischaemia? Anesthesiology 68: 676–680
Slogoff S, Keats A S 1989 Randomized trial of primary anaesthetic agents on outcome of coronary bypass operations. Anesthesiology 70: 179–188
Smith N T, Calverley R K, Prys-Roberts C et al 1978 Impact of nitrous oxide on the circulation during enflurane anaesthesia in man. Anesthesiology 48: 345–349
Sonntag H, Stephan H, Lange H et al 1989 Sufentanil does not block sympathetic responses to surgical stimuli in patients having coronary artery revascularization surgery. Anaesth Analg 68: 584–592
Starr N J, Sethna D H, Estafanous F G 1986 Bradycardia and asystole following the rapid administration of sufentanil with vecuronium. Anesthesiology 64: 521–523
Steen R A, Tinker J H, Tarhan S 1978 Myocardial reinfarction after anaesthesia and surgery. J Am Med Assoc 239: 2566–2570
Stephan H, Sonntag H, Schenk H D et al 1986 Effects of propofol on cardiovascular dynamics, myocardial blood flow, and myocardial metabolism in patients with coronary artery disease. Br J Anaesth 58: 969–975
Thompson I R, Putnins C L 1985 Adverse effects of pancuronium during high dose fentanyl anaesthesia for coronary artery bypass grafting. Anesthesiology 62: 708–713
Tweed W A, Minuck M, Mymin D 1972 Circulatory responses to ketamine anaesthesia. Anesthesiology 37: 613–619
US National Center for Health Statistics 1988 United States annual mortality statistics. US Government Printing Office, Washington, DHSS Publication No. PHS 89–1232
White D A, Latimer R D 1991 Cardiac transplantation. Curr Opin Anaesthesiol 4: 83–89
Wierda J M K H, Maestrone E, Bencini A F et al 1989 Haemodynamic effects of vecuronium. Br J Anaesth 62: 194–198
Wong K C, Martin W E, Hombein T F et al 1973 The cardiovascular effects of morphine sulphate with oxygen and with nitrous oxide in man. Anesthesiology 38: 542–549

4

Respiratory function and the safety of anaesthesia

D. S. Selsby and J. G. Jones

INTRODUCTION

General anaesthesia exerts a variety of deleterious effects on pulmonary function. Some of the problems that have been recognized for many years are: airway obstruction, impaired pulmonary gas exchange, the inefficiency of intermittent positive pressure ventilation, and the susceptibility to post-operative chest complications.

Most general anaesthetics impair ventilation and gas exchange to a minor degree in the majority of patients and the effects are often undetectable using conventional clinical examination. Because of this, and prior to the widespread use of pulse oximeters, an increased inspired oxygen concentration was usually employed to compensate for these effects and to give a greater margin of safety. The routine use of oximetry showed that, while in many patients there was little or no change in oxygen saturation during anaesthesia, a considerable proportion did have episodes of hypoxaemia, many of which could be attributed to partial upper airway obstruction.

Additional factors that may contribute to a severe impairment of pulmonary function during anaesthesia are:

- impaired control of ventilation and the upper airway
- change in function of the chest wall
- bronchospasm
- pulmonary oedema
- lung injury (aspiration, sepsis)
- pulmonary infection
- pulmonary embolus.

Many of the mechanisms responsible for these and other aspects of deterioration in lung function have now been elucidated. A thorough understanding of these principles, combined with a knowledge of the specific hazards in high-risk patients, is essential in reducing perioperative respiratory morbidity and mortality. The use of up-to-date monitoring and appropriate choice of physiotherapy will also further improve patient outcome.

THE EFFECTS OF ANAESTHESIA ON RESPIRATORY FUNCTION

Control of ventilation

Ventilation is regulated by neurones in the brainstem that depend upon feedback from receptors in the chest wall, joints and lung, as well as chemoreceptors in the brainstem and carotid bodies. Thus there is neural and chemical control of ventilation; the former dominates during wakefulness, the latter in the unconscious state. The addition of anaesthetic agents and opioid drugs not only induces unconsciousness, but also leads to a marked impairment of the chemical control of ventilation. Of particular importance is the effect of anaesthetic and analgesic drugs on the brainstem neurones which, in addition to their effects on the respiratory muscles, have an important controlling influence on the muscles and thus the patency of the upper airway. Thus an impairment of ventilatory control is often accompanied by a loss of patency of the upper away, which almost invariably leads to hypoxaemia.

An increase in Pa_{CO_2} normally produces a linear increase in ventilation, which is heightened in the presence of hypoxia. Hypoxia alone becomes a significant protective reflex only when the Pa_{O_2} falls below 8 kPa. The specific actions of different anaesthetic drugs may be compared by assessing either the pattern of resting ventilation or the ventilatory responses to various challenges using different inspired concentrations of CO_2 and O_2, or to the imposition of a load.

Premedication

Opiates depress ventilatory responses to CO_2 and hypoxia (Weil et al 1975), and raise the apnoeic threshold for Pa_{CO_2}. The degree of change is dose dependent for pure agonists such as morphine (Gal et al 1982), but a ceiling may exist for opiates with partial antagonist properties, for example nalbuphine when used in premedicant doses (Pugh et al 1989). Normally the increased ventilatory response to a rising Pa_{CO_2} is mediated mainly by an increase in rib-cage activity. This effect is markedly depressed by morphine (Rigg & Rondi 1981) and by halothane (Tusiewicz et al 1977), and indicates a common site of interference with the neural chemical feedback control of ventilation, possibly at spinal cord level. A similar mechanism may also explain the decreased ability to respond to added inspiratory loads following the administration of a number of analgesic drugs (Jordan et al 1979).

The alteration in phasic rib-cage tone produced by opiates is most likely to be secondary to disordered activity in brainstem respiratory nuclei. Tabatabai et al (1989) found that fentanyl in decerebrate cats generated a continuous discharge in one group of medullary inspiratory neurones, while activity in a second group was abolished. Medullary activity was restored to normal by nalbuphine. Similarly, in patients following coronary artery surgery, nalbuphine reversed the respiratory depression caused by fentanyl, but this was accompanied by an unacceptably high incidence of both cardiovascular side effects and inadequate analgesia (Jaffe et al 1988). Arunasalam et al (1983) showed that a morphine premedication had the same depressant effects on ventilation in young (28–37 years) and old (65–82 years) subjects (Fig. 4.1). However, seven of the 13 old subjects showed periods of apnoea and periodic breathing, whereas only three of the 13 younger subjects had this phenomenon at much less frequent intervals.

While opiate-induced respiratory depression is offset by preoperative anxiety or pain, exacerbation is also likely with the concomitant use of drugs, such as hyoscine or diazepam (Bailey et al 1984). Sedative doses of midazolam or diazepam used alone maintain minute volume, but at the expense of shallow breathing with an increased respiratory rate. The addition of opiates further compromises alveolar ventilation (Berggren et al 1987).

Benzodiazepines inhibit the ventilatory response to CO_2 to an extent similar to that seen with

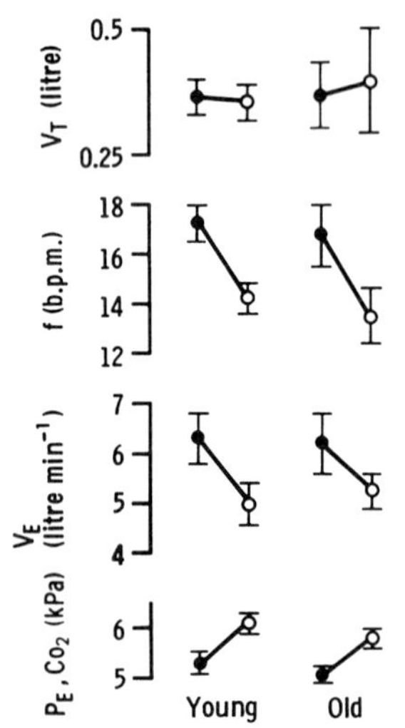

Fig. 4.1 The effect of morphine premedication (10 mg/70 kg) on ventilation in young and old subjects. Tidal volume (Vt), rate of respiration (f), minute volume (VE) and end-tidal carbon dioxide tension (kPa), before (•) and 30 min after (o) morphine (10 mg/70 kg; mean + SEM; from Arunasalam et al 1983).

morphine premedication, and in sedative doses also impair the hypoxic ventilatory response (Alexander & Gross 1988). However, in contrast to opiates there is no depression of the ventilatory response to added inspiratory loads (Jordan et al 1981). A possible explanation for this may be the fact that benzodiazepines decrease tidal volume by an effect on the diaphragm rather than the rib-cage component of ventilation (Berggren et al 1987).

Therefore, premedicant doses of opiates, and to a lesser extent benzodiazepines, should be used with caution in patients with severe respiratory disease, excessive secretions accompanied by a decreased cough reflex, raised intracranial pressure, and upper airway obstruction. Combined premedication should only be used if the risks of respiratory depression are outweighed by the likelihood of anxiety-induced complications, for example in patients with severe ischaemic heart disease. In such cases preoperative oxygen administration and respiratory monitoring should be employed to prevent hypoxaemia (Marjot & Valentine 1990).

Induction of anaesthesia

Most of the intravenous induction agents in current use, with the exception of ketamine, can cause marked respiratory depression, often manifest as apnoea. Knill et al (1978) observed that thiopentone depresses both the hypercapnic and hypoxic ventilatory responses; propofol results in even greater respiratory depression (Taylor et al 1986). Goodman et al (1987) intended to assess the ventilatory effects of propofol as a sole anaesthetic agent, but most of their patients developed apnoea, sometimes lasting more than 3 min. An early evaluation of etomidate also demonstrated a 40% incidence of apnoea on induction (Morgan et al 1977).

During anaesthesia with spontaneous ventilation this apnoeic period can be a testing time and, not surprisingly, many anaesthetists opt to hand ventilate soon after induction. However, this usually results in hypocarbia and hyperoxia and abolishes any residual ventilatory reflexes, especially in the presence of opiates and additional inhalational agents. The anaesthetist may now find himself assisting ventilation throughout the surgical procedure. In view of the ease with which most patients can be ventilated in such circumstances, the use of neuromuscular blockade to maintain paralysis for ventilatory purposes is often unnecessary.

Maintenance of anaesthesia

Nitrous oxide administered in sedative concentrations causes a fall in resting $P\text{aCO}_2$, and CO_2 responsiveness remains normal or is slightly increased, but hypoxic responses are dulled to approximately one-third of normal (Yacoub et al 1976). The addition of a volatile anaesthetic results in a marked diminution of ventilation and an elevated $P\text{aCO}_2$, although the combination is less depressant than an equivalent concentration of volatile alone (Hornbein et al 1969). Isoflurane and enflurane have similar effects to halothane and cause a dose related increase in resting $P\text{aCO}_2$, flattening of the ventilation/$P\text{aCO}_2$ response curve, and a rise in the apnoeic threshold to CO_2.

We mentioned earlier (p. 56) that volatile anaesthetics decrease both tidal volume and $P\text{aCO}_2$ responsiveness by an inhibitory effect on rib-cage excursions (Tusiewicz et al 1977). In children an increase in the level of halothane from 0.5% to 1.5% depresses airway occlusion pressures (Lindahl 1987). This is the pressure drop measured in the occluded airway 100 ms after the start of inspiration (P 0.1) and indicates an inhibitory effect of anaesthesia on chest-wall activation. In addition to severely reducing phasic rib-cage movement, inhalational anaesthesia also reduces tone in rib-cage muscles. Jones et al (1979) demonstrated that this can result in greatly increased paradoxical movement of the chest on the addition of small inspiratory loads, for example that due to a narrow-bore nasotracheal tube. Furthermore, Pietak et al (1975) found that patients with chronic obstructive pulmonary disease (COPD), but without CO_2 retention, were much less able to mount a response to an increase in $P\text{aCO}_2$ than a normal control group during halothane anaesthesia. This may be explained by the fact that anaesthesia increases the resistance to breathing by lowering functional residual capacity. Another important factor is that, because of the Laplace equation, the flattened diaphragm in patients with emphysema works at a considerable mechanical disadvantage compared to a diaphragm with a normal curvature.

A major difference between the inhalational agents is the effect on respiratory rate; a decrease with enflurane, tachypnoea with halothane, and a more normal rate with isoflurane (Murat et al 1987). Therefore, ventilatory depression is considered to be most marked with enflurane, but the difference between the other two agents is less clearcut. For example, Alagesan et al (1987) found that despite the effects on respiratory rate, $PaCO_2$ was consistently lower with isoflurane due to a greater preservation of tidal volume. However, the $PaCO_2$ ranged from 7.2 to 8.6 kPa, a very high level in the presence of surgical stimulation which offsets the rise by about 1.3 kPa at various MAC (minimum alveolar concentration) values of isoflurane anaesthesia (Eger et al 1972). Nevertheless, high levels of $PaCO_2$ are well tolerated in the presence of good oxygenation, and even with halothane and surgical stimulation the threshold for cardiac arrhythmias is as high as 9 kPa (Robertson et al 1981).

Of much greater concern is the effect of volatile anaesthetics on the ventilatory responses to hypoxaemia. It is well known that patients with COPD and CO_2 retention may rely solely on a hypoxic drive. Additional oxygen is given to such patients only with great caution, and the presence of subanaesthetic concentrations of volatile agents will also switch off the hypoxic drive. Even in normal subjects MAC levels of halothane, enflurane or isoflurane will block hypoxic ventilatory responses, and severe attenuation is likely even with subanaesthetic concentrations (Knill & Gelb 1982). Inhibition of the hypoxic response occurs within 30 sec of inhalation of halothane, suggesting a direct action on peripheral chemoreceptors (Knill & Clement 1984). Therefore, within 1 min from induction the patient's ventilatory reflexes are severely handicapped, and it becomes essential to maintain a clear airway, and to monitor ventilation and oxygenation. In theatre the anaesthetist should be well equipped to carry out these tasks, but the effects of most anaesthetic agents may well extend into the postoperative period, making continued monitoring just as essential. It has been argued that the very high blood flow of the carotid bodies leads to a rapid washout of anaesthetic from the chemosensors. Nevertheless, it is becoming increasingly well recognized that abnormalities of ventilatory control are frequently encountered during the emergence from anaesthesia.

Postoperative period

Catley (1984) has pointed out the important interactions between the effects of sleep, opiate analgesia, surgery and the waning effects of general anaesthetics in the postoperative period (Fig. 4.2). The application of recently developed, continuous monitoring techniques to study ventilation in this period has revealed a high incidence of remarkably episodic ventilatory disturbances, often accompanied by profound hypoxia. Local anaesthetic nerve blocks used for postoperative pain relief cause little disturbance of ventilation, whereas parenteral opiate administration frequently results in severe oxygen desaturation when the patient falls asleep, and this is associated with upper airway obstruction rather than central apnoea (Catley et al 1985). For this reason the intermittent monitoring of ventilatory function by measuring the respiratory rate is quite inadequate for evaluating the safety of postoperative analgesia.

It is also worth noting that parenteral fentanyl can cause delayed respiratory depression 1–3 hours postoperatively when ventilation has previously been well maintained (Becker et al 1976). A variety of pharmacodynamic factors have been proposed to account for this, but increases in plasma levels of fentanyl during this period are very slight, and other workers have been unable to demonstrate this effect. The most likely explanation is that patients in the immediate postoperative period are exposed to a generally high level of stimulation from pain and from nursing procedures. These factors increase patient alertness, which has a stimulant effect on

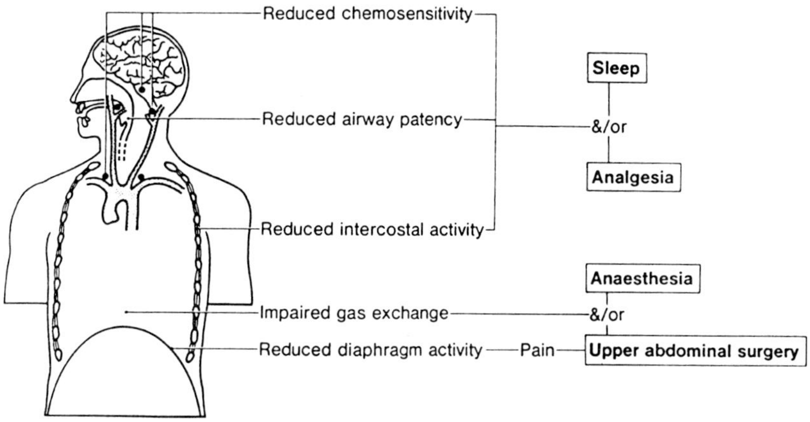

Fig. 4.2 To show the interaction of anaesthesia, site of surgery, analgesia and sleep on oxygen saturation in the postoperative period (from Catley 1984).

ventilation. As vigilance is relaxed, light levels of sleep are seen. The combination of sleep and opiates results in a very abnormal pattern of breathing, in which apnoeic episodes are common, and arterial oxygen desaturation can occur if the patient is breathing air.

Reports of the efficacy of opiates administered via the epidural and spinal routes led to their enthusiastic and indiscriminate use, although this was soon tempered by evidence of late, and often profound, depression of respiration. After a single injection of epidural morphine, respiratory depression can persist for 24 hours (Knill et al 1981), and is characterized by apnoeic periods and ventilation at low tidal volumes. Interestingly, Jones & Jones (1980) found that intravenous naloxone can reverse respiratory depression following intrathecal morphine while leaving analgesia intact. However, since most of the widely used opiates have longer durations of action than a bolus of naloxone, respiratory depression may recur as the effect of the latter declines. Admittedly this danger can be overcome by repeated dosage or by using an infusion, but cautious titration is necessary to avoid causing distress to the patient. Other problems associated with the use of naloxone include occasional cardiovascular effects, such as hypertension, arrhythmias, pulmonary oedema and even sudden death.

In contrast to epidural morphine, the use of epidural fentanyl has only rarely been associated with severe respiratory depression (Etches et al 1989). However, regardless of the route of administration, all opiates will have some effect on the ventilatory responses to $P\text{aCO}_2$ and hypoxia. For example, Wheatley et al (1990) compared the effects of different modes of administration of postoperative analgesia on ventilatory control by using a novel method of monitoring oxygen saturation (Fig. 4.3). They demonstrated that epidural diamorphine tended to produce more prolonged episodes of oxygen desaturation than when using a Patient Controlled Administration system.

Respiratory mechanics and gas exchange

Functional residual capacity and diaphragmatic effects

Bergman (1963) was the first to observe that anaesthesia decreases functional residual capacity (FRC), an effect subsequently shown to be related both to a reduction in rib-cage volume and to a cephalad movement of the diaphragm (Hedenstierna et al 1985). An additional mechanism may be a central shift of blood into the chest and abdomen (Jones 1987). With the exception of ketamine, these volume displacements occur regardless of the type of anaesthetic employed, and are little affected by the use of

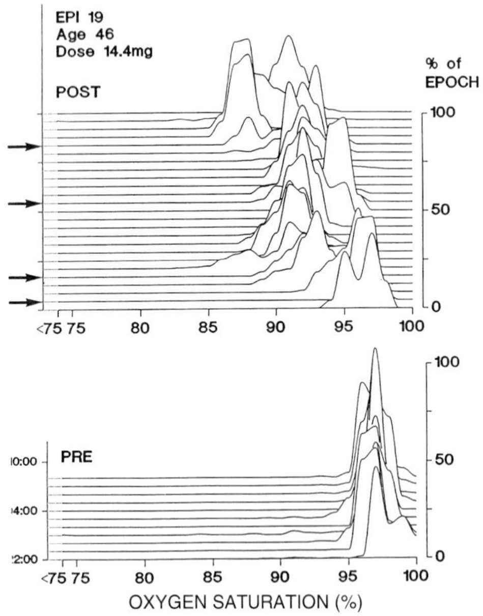

Fig. 4.3 Shows the pattern of oxygen saturation PRE and POST lower abdominal surgery using repeated doses of epidural diamorphine for postoperative pain relief (→). One curve shows the oxygen saturation distribution in each hour. The upper panel shows the result of a 25 h monitoring period starting at 14 00 hrs, 1 h after completion of surgery (from Wheatley et al 1990).

relaxants and intermittent positive pressure ventilation (IPPV) (Hedenstierna 1988). Ketamine not only preserves lung volumes, but even increases chest wall excursions (Mankikian et al 1986).

The fall in FRC is approximately 500–700 mls, occurs soon after induction, and is secondary to an acute reduction in both rib cage (Drummond 1987) and diaphragmatic tone (Muller et al 1979). As discussed on page 56, anaesthesia markedly curtails movement of the rib cage (Tusiewicz et al 1977), while having a lesser effect on diaphragmatic motion. For example, Froese & Bryan (1974) demonstrated that despite a cephalad shift, diaphragmatic excursions were maintained, but with a greater displacement of the dependent diaphragm during spontaneous respiration and more marked movement of the uppermost part of the diaphragm with IPPV. However, in a recent investigation by Krayer et al (1989) of diaphragmatic function in both prone and supine positions, the dorsal portion exhibited greater mobility in both positions while awake. Anaesthesia with paralysis and IPPV were associated with greater dorsal movement in the prone position, but piston-like movement in the supine position. Therefore, anatomical differences between costal and crural fibres may exist to augment Froese & Bryans' (1979) earlier hydrostatic theory of diaphragmatic motion. Interestingly, Heneghan & Jones (1985) found that electrical stimulation of the phrenic nerve resulted in greater movements of the dorsal diaphragm and more effective gas exchange than an equal increase in lung volume produced by positive end-expiratory pressure (PEEP).

A decrease in FRC leads to changes in lung compliance, airway resistance, the FRC-closing capacity disparity and, ultimately, gas exchange with a variable but consistent increase in the A–aPO_2 gradient.

Lung compliance and airway calibre

Because of the effect of gravity, the top and bottom of the lung lie on different parts of the sigmoid-shaped compliance curve. When the FRC falls, the dependent lung moves onto the flat, lowermost portion of this curve, so that its recoil pressure, compliance, ventilation and ventilation/perfusion (V/Q) ratio are all very low. In contrast the upper lung moves from the flat, upper part of the curve, so that its effective compliance increases, as does its ventilation and V/Q.

The efficacy of elimination of CO_2 is lowered by anaesthesia, and this is conveniently expressed as an increase in the ratio of physiological dead space to tidal volume (Vd/Vt). Conscious healthy young subjects have a Vd/Vt below 30%. With anaesthesia this can rise to as much as 60%, being similar for either spontaneous or mechanical ventilation. The exact mechanisms are not clear, although the V/Q mismatch inherent to anaesthesia must be a contributory factor. Systemic hypotension, accompanied by lowered pulmonary artery pressures, decreases perfusion of the uppermost parts of the lung causing additional increases in dead space. Air embolism is an obvious cause during head and neck surgery. Dead space is also known to increase with advancing age, smoking and lung disease.

A very important effect of a reduced lung volume is a generalized passive narrowing of airways, rather than active bronchoconstriction. This is because lung recoil pressure, which is a major factor maintaining airway patency, falls as lung volume is reduced. In obese patients both the reduction in lung volume and the associated rise in airway resistance are proportional to the patient's weight. Additional bronchoconstriction due to either histamine or airway instrumentation will magnify the effects of anaesthesia on airway resistance (Fig. 4.4A). However, this increase in airway resistance is offset to some extent by halothane or enflurane anaesthesia with IPPV, and there is a small rise in FRC (Lehane et al 1980). Similar results can be demonstrated during isoflurane anaesthesia (Fig. 4.4B). In the case of halothane, the effect on airway resistance is due to bronchodilatation, a shift of blood from the thoracic cavity and a change in lung tissue resistance (Vetterman et al 1989). Nevertheless, the overall effect of anaesthesia is an increase in resistance and a fall in compliance, which results in an increased work of breathing.

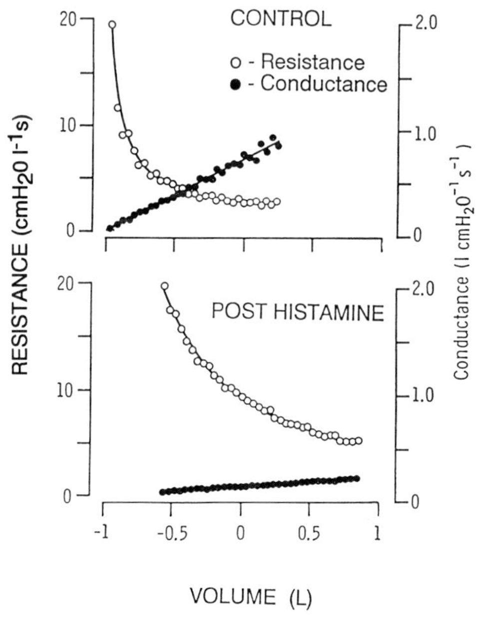

Fig. 4.4A To show the effect of histamine release on bronchomotor tone in man. Note the curvilinear relationship between airway resistance (R) and lung volume (V), and the linear relationship between conductance and volume. FRC is at zero volume. With induction of anaesthesia FRC falls, say by 0.5 l, causing a much greater rise in R after histamine than before.

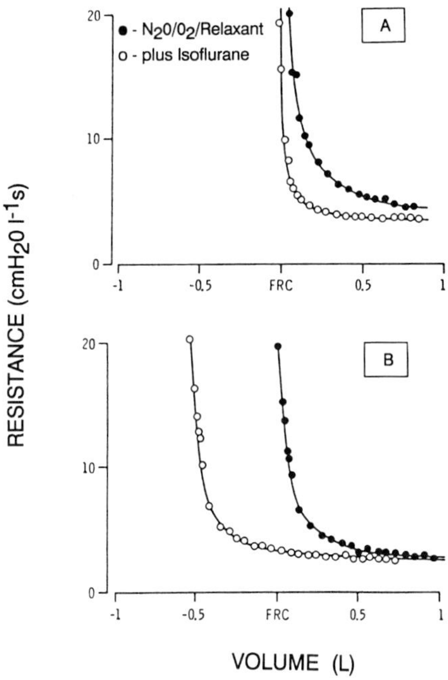

Fig. 4.4B To show the effect on airway resistance of adding isoflurane to a N_2O/O_2/relaxant anaesthetic. In patient A the resistance falls dramatically, whereas in Patient B there is an increase in FRC of 0.5 l. The net effect is a large fall in airway resistance.

Gas mixing in the lung

Inspired gas mixes rapidly with alveolar gas by molecular diffusion. In contrast a breath from an aerosol taken into the lung does not mix with alveolar gas because diffusion of large aerosol particles is so slow. Mass movement of gas along the airway to the alveoli undergoes marked slowing as the total cross-sectional area of the airways rapidly increases towards the alveoli. In the normal lung the transition from mass movement to molecular diffusion occurs only a few millimetres from the end of the airway. In chronic obstructive pulmonary disease (COPD) the lung architecture is often disordered and the diffusion distance is increased. This, together with regional abnormalities of airway resistance and compliance, causes a considerable impairment of efficiency of intrapulmonary gas mixing. This can be most easily demonstrated using the nitrogen washout technique. If expired nitrogen is measured during oxygen breathing on open circuit there is an exponential decline in nitrogen concentration. This usually takes about 7 min to fall from 78% to 2%. In patients with COPD this time might be increased to more than 30 min, and is inversely related to the peak expiratory flow rate (PEFR). This clearly has practical implications for the time needed for both preoxygenation, inhalational induction, and the elimination of nitrogen and gaseous anaesthetics from the lungs. The decreased uptake and elimination of gas from these 'slow alveoli' is caused by impaired mixing. This is a result of either distorted lung architecture (emphysema, bronchiectasis), or impaired ventilation per unit volume due to high airway resistance.

Closing capacity: FRC relationship and gas exchange

As lung volume falls there comes a point where airways in the dependent lung begin to narrow critically or close. The lung volume at this point is called the closing capacity (CC) (Fig. 4.5), and it is increased in old age, the obese, smokers and following bronchospasm. It is not clear whether CC is affected by anaesthesia. Studies have shown that there is either no change (Hedenstierna et al 1976), or CC falls in line with FRC following anaesthesia (Bergman & Tien 1983). In healthy young non-smokers the FRC is greater than CC in the supine position when awake, and may remain so even following anaesthesia. However, FRC equals CC at age 66 years in the erect posture, and at 44 years in the supine position. The subsequent fall in FRC with anaesthesia in these and other high risk patients may entail tidal breathing within the CC. For example, Hedenstierna et al (1976) demonstrated that CC was already larger than FRC in six of 20 patients prior to anaesthesia, and in as many as 17 patients following induction.

This change in the CC–FRC relationship during anaesthesia contributes to an abnormal V/Q distribution and the development of a shunt causing an increased A–aP_{O_2} gradient. Some regard a shunt as an extreme form of V/Q maldistribution (i.e. when V/Q = 0), but the effect of increasing the inspired oxygen in the presence of a shunt has a different effect than with a V/Q abnormality (Fig. 4.6, p. 66). Note that the Pa_{O_2} will suddenly start to increase in patients with a low V/Q, whereas with a shunt there is only a slight improvement. This differing effect can be seen in patients during one-lung anaesthesia.

The close correlation between the CC–FRC difference and shunt following anaesthesia was amply highlighted by Dueck et al (1988). They showed that the average shunt during anaesthesia was only 2% if FRC remained above awake CC, but increased to 11% when FRC fell below CC. Furthermore, the size of shunt was associated with increases in 'body mass index', and smokers developed greater shunts for any given CC–FRC difference compared to non-smokers. The reduction in FRC during anaesthesia creates not only regions with a low V/Q ratio, but also causes atelectasis in dependent lung regions. Computerized tomography shows that basal lung collapse occurs within minutes of either intravenous or inhalational anaesthesia, and during both spontaneous and mechanical ventilation. Furthermore, the degree of atelectasis correlates well with the size of shunt and arterial oxygenation (Hedenstierna 1988).

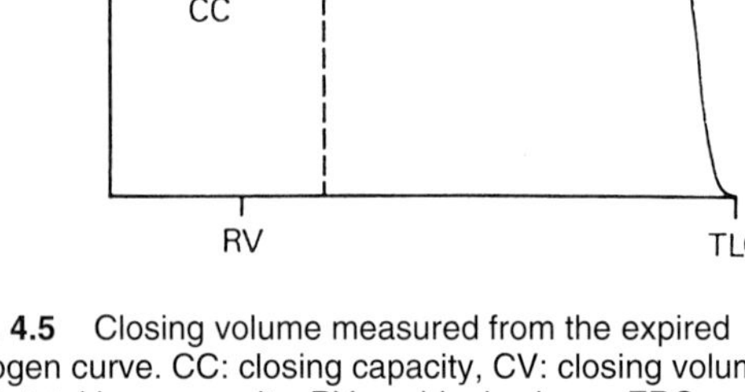

Fig. 4.5 Closing volume measured from the expired nitrogen curve. CC: closing capacity, CV: closing volume, TLC: total lung capacity, RV: residual volume, FRC: functional residual capacity (see text).

Hypoxic pulmonary vasoconstriction

Hypoxic pulmonary vasoconstriction (HPV) is an important mechanism in matching perfusion to ventilation and, until recently, was thought to limit the decrease in $Pa\text{O}_2$ during anaesthesia. HPV is generally not impaired by intravenous anaesthetics, but animal studies have demonstrated a marked reduction in HPV with inhalational agents, particularly in isolated lungs (Marshall et al 1984), and this effect is potentiated by the concomitant administration of calcium-channel blockers (Kjaeve & Bjertnaes 1989). However, such as dramatic impairment of HPV is not evident in human studies employing clinical concentrations of inhalational agents. For example, during thoracotomy with one-lung anaesthesia, a change from inhalational to intravenous anaesthesia produced minimal effects on $Pa\text{O}_2$ and shunt following isoflurane and only slight improvements after halothane (Benumof et al 1987a). Similarly, the introduction of isoflurane or enflurane, following one lung hypoxic challenges in patients prior to elective surgery, resulted in minimal alteration of cardiac output, pulmonary vascular resistance, pulmonary blood flow, and arterial oxygenation (Carlsson et al 1987a, 1987b). This highlights the dangers of extrapolating from animal data, and isoflurane in clinical concentrations may not be contraindicated during one lung anaesthesia.

Lung defence mechanisms

Mucociliary clearance

Anaesthesia compromises mucociliary clearance via several mechanisms. With the inhalational of dry, cold anaesthetic gases, especially if the warming and humidifying function of the nose is bypassed, mucus will become more viscous. Ciliary beating is depressed by lowered temperatures, and mucociliary flow is also reduced by various drugs, including atropine, opiates, barbiturates, halothane, enflurane and nitrous oxide. Oxygen breathing reduces tracheal mucus velocity, but this takes several hours at high concentrations, while hypoxia also causes disordered beating of cilia and poor mucociliary transport. A tracheal tube slows mucociliary clearance if the cuff is inflated to provide a gas-tight seal. Mucus clearance ceases altogether after about 90 min of general anaesthesia, utilizing endotracheal intubation and mechanical ventilation with oxygen, nitrous oxide and halothane.

Cough reflex

In the postoperative period the cough reflex may also be depressed, either centrally by sedation or opiates, or peripherally by pain from abdominal or thoracic wounds. Coughing effects mucus clearance by causing dynamic compression of the airways, which creates localized regions of maximum gas velocity and shears mucus from the bronchial wall by a 'two-phase flow' mechanism (Selsby & Jones 1990). If the patient has a weak cough then inadequate pressure is generated to cause dynamic airway compression and the gas velocity is insufficient to detach mucus. Alternatively, if mucus viscosity is high, because of excessive drying during inhalational anaesthesia with impaired humidification, then mucus may not be detached even with a normal cough mechanism.

Not surprisingly, patients with excessive secretions, such as smokers and those with chronic lung disease, are at greater risk of developing postoperative chest complications, especially following upper abdominal surgery. In a study in which radio-opaque tantalum powder was insufflated into patients' lungs, the powder was retained for nearly a week in the lungs of patients who had just undergone major abdominal surgery. Powder was seen to pool in dependent bronchi, and this was followed by atelectasis. In contrast, patients undergoing limb operations of shorter duration showed complete clearance of tantalum powder within 2 days postoperatively (Gamsu et al 1976).

ANAESTHESIA AND RESPIRATORY FUNCTION IN HIGH-RISK GROUPS

The previous section describes the numerous mechanisms by which anaesthesia consistently compromises lung function. Young healthy patients tolerate these changes remarkably well, but there are many high-risk groups that require special attention perioperatively, both to limit the detrimental effects of anaesthesia on lung function and to decrease postoperative respiratory complications.

Patients with deranged respiratory control

Abnormalities of the control of breathing induced by anaesthesia may be superimposed on a pre-existing disorder to produce a life-threatening condition.

Premature infants

Episodes of central apnoea are common in premature babies, and more frequent with increasing prematurity. Following general anaesthesia the majority of premature infants less than 44 weeks conceptual age will experience periodic breathing (Wellborn et al 1986). The risk of postoperative apnoea then decreases with conceptual age, but may persist until 60 weeks (Kurth et al 1987). Such apnoeas may be life-threatening and require intubation and mechanical ventilation. Accordingly, non-urgent surgery should be delayed until 44 weeks, and postoperative apnoea monitoring for 12 hours or longer should be employed up to 60 weeks conceptual age. The use of intravenous caffeine has also been advocated. In a recent study a high-dose regime dramatically reduced the incidence of postoperative apnoea and desaturation in infants with a mean gestational age of 30 weeks, and postconceptual age under 44 weeks at the time of surgery (Wellborn et al 1989). Alternatively, spinal or caudal analgesia should be considered for inguinal hernia repair.

Sleep apnoea syndromes

Sleep apnoea syndromes may be subdivided into either central, obstructive or mixed types. Central apnoea is defined as a cessation of breathing due to a transient abolition of drive to the respiratory muscles. Periodic breathing refers to a regular waxing and waning of ventilation as a result of fluctuation in central respiratory drive. The congenital form of central apnoea, known as Ondine's Curse, is extremely rare, and usually presents shortly after birth with cyanosis or apnoea (Mather 1987). More commonly, central apnoea is due to acquired causes, for example encephalitis, neurosurgical trauma, head injury or when patients are given substantial doses of opiates, either for induction of anaesthesia or postoperatively.

Obstructive apnoea is defined as cessation of airflow at the nose and mouth because of complete occlusion of the upper airway despite continued activation of the respiratory muscles. Muscles of the upper airway normally show phasic activity synchronous with respiratory movement, and by increasing their tone resist closure of the pharynx during inspiration. However, like the intercostals, they lose tone and occlude the airway more easily during sleep and after the administration of alcohol, sedative and anaesthetic drugs. Obstructive sleep apnoea may result from chronic narrowing of the upper airway due to obesity, tracheal stenosis, micrognathia and hypertrophied tonsils or adenoids. The success of nasal continuous positive airway pressure (CPAP) in patients with obstructive sleep apnoea is noteworthy (Remmers et al 1990).

Disturbed sleep, snoring or daytime somnolence should alert the anaesthetist to the possibility of sleep apnoea in the postoperative period. The diagnosis is confirmed by sleep studies which include monitoring of SaO_2 with pulse oximetry, EEG, airflow measurements and thoracic plethysmography. Central and obstructive apnoea are differentiated by the analysis of airflow and thoracic cage movement.

These patients present three main problems: firstly, chronic hypoxaemia may result in pulmonary hypertension and cor pulmonale; secondly, both intubation and airway maintenance may be difficult; and thirdly, either central or obstructive apnoea is very likely in the postoperative period. Preoperative management includes the treatment of heart failure, polycythaemia and coincidental lung disease. Premedication is avoided since it may precipitate severe respiratory obstruction (Rafferty et al 1980), although temazepam was used uneventfully in a recent case report (Tierney et al 1989). If possible, local anaesthesia is employed, otherwise anaesthetic drugs with fast recovery characteristics should be used. Postoperatively, close monitoring of respiratory pattern and oxygen saturation is vital, and elective ventilation or CPAP on the ITU may be required until the effects of anaesthetic agents have cleared. Elective tracheostomy should be held in reserve for severe cases of obstructive sleep apnoea.

Respiratory tract infections

Upper respiratory tract infection

Airways remain hyperactive for at least 3 weeks after an upper respiratory tract infection (URTI) (Empey et al 1976). A potential hazard in such patients is that protracted coughing due to endotracheal intubation may lead to a sharp decrease in FRC (Bickler et al 1987), with the consequent deleterious effects on airway resistance and gas exchange. Furthermore, excessive mucus secretion, mediated by the same vagal reflex as airway hyperactivity, may also sufficiently soil the tracheobronchial tree and interfere with ventilation. This problem is compounded by the fact that mucociliary clearance is impaired following most respiratory tract infections, particularly those that cause cell destruction, such as influenza virus.

However, studies are lacking as regards the risks of anaesthesia in adult patients with URTIs, and there are conflicting reports from research in paediatric patients (Fenelly & Hall 1990). For example, in children, endotracheal intubation is a more common stimulus for bronchospasm than respiratory infection (Olsson 1987), and mask anaesthesia for minor surgery in the presence of URTI also results in comparatively few perioperative respiratory complications (Tait & Knight 1987). In contrast, DeSoto et al (1988) demonstrated an increased incidence of recovery room hypoxaemia in children aged 1–4 years with an active or recent URTI. Therefore, in the presence of URTI it would seem prudent to postpone a non-urgent operation, especially if endotracheal intubation is necessary.

Lower respiratory tract infection

There are two considerations: the immediate problem of impaired gas exchange; and the subsequent problem of exacerbation of the infection.

Oxygenation may already be poor in patients with pneumonia, and may worsen following induction of anaesthesia. Spontaneous ventilation may be difficult due to a decrease in lung compliance. IPPV may be indicated, but leads to preferential ventilation and excessive alveolar distension of normal lung units, thus encouraging the diversion of blood flow towards abnormal lung. After upper abdominal or thoracic surgery, shallow breathing, pain, decreased mucus clearance and attenuation of the cough reflex all contribute to a prolonged recovery and impaired oxygenation.

Lung abscess and bronchopleural fistula

Of paramount importance is the prevention of contamination of normal lung by the control of the movement of infective fluid within the lung. This is achieved by posture, suction and the use of double-lumen tracheal tubes, in preference to single-lumen tubes with bronchus-blockers. Until a large bronchopleural fistula (BPF) has been isolated, IPPV should be avoided, since most of the tidal volume may be lost via the fistula. The successful treatment of a BPF by high frequency jet ventilation (HFJV) led to the suggestion that this is the optimum mode of ventilation for such patients (Carlon et al 1980). Controlled trials in patients are lacking, and an animal study showed that at 10 cmH_2O levels of PEEP, fistula flow was increased during HFJV as compared to conventional positive pressure ventilation (Spinale et al 1989). A similar increase in fistula flow-rate was demonstrated in a case report by Roth et al (1988), and was possibly due to the fact that HFJV resulted in higher mean airway pressures. It is essential to monitor pressure in the central airways during HFJV. Fistula flow-rate is also dependent on the frequency of jet ventilation (Orlando et al 1988). The use of dual-mode ventilation via a double-lumen tracheal tube may be useful because it allows HFJV of the diseased lung at low pressures, while maintaining conventional high minute-volume ventilation of the normal lung (Feeley et al 1988).

Bronchiectasis

In this disorder there is chronic infection within the lung and distortion of bronchial anatomy with considerable right-to-left shunt and hypoxaemia. Quite commonly there is associated chronic obstructive pulmonary disease and CO_2 retention. Bronchography under general anaesthesia may be necessary to make the diagnosis. The contrast medium is viscid and can interfere with ventilation, so that it is safer to outline only one lung at a time. The use of pulse oximetry is mandatory. Remember that there may be a considerable shunt and that a high inspired oxygen may be necessary (Fig. 4.6).

Before elective surgery the patient should be free of infection, and sputum should be cleared using up-to-date physiotherapy procedures in combination with bronchodilators (Selsby & Jones 1990). It may be unwise to admit the patient to hospital for too long beforehand, since this may increase the risk of acquiring a new variety of chest infection. Despite adequate preparation, a postoperative chest infection is more likely than in a normal individual, and appropriate respiratory therapy may be necessary for several days after the operation.

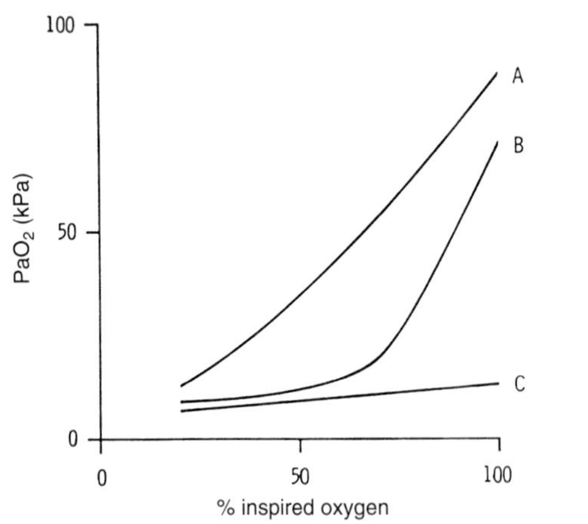

Fig. 4.6 To show the effect of increasing inspired oxygen on $Pa\text{O}_2$ with (A) normal lungs (B) impaired gas exchange with a predominant V/Q abnormality and (C) predominant shunt. Note the considerable improvement in $Pa\text{O}_2$ as the inspired oxygen approaches 100% when V/Q abnormality predominates. This degree of improvement is not seen with a pure shunt.

Pneumothorax, bullae, lung cysts and lobar emphysema

These conditions present a particular hazard because they all involve relatively large air-containing spaces that communicate to a variable degree with the tracheobronchial tree. During anaesthesia they can expand dramatically, compressing surrounding lung and mediastinal structures, just like a tension pneumothorax, causing impairment of gas exchange and cardiac output. The causes of expansion in any of these conditions may be summarized as:

- coughing and straining
- IPPV
- diffusion of nitrous oxide.

Pneumothorax

Pneumothorax may be classified as a tension, open, or closed pneumothorax, the size of which correlates well with the magnitude of right-to-left shunt.

Tension pneumothorax is the most serious type of disturbance, since it becomes inexorably larger and fatally impairs heart and lung function, unless urgently decompressed by whatever means is available. It can occur during anaesthesia or resuscitation, either by alveolar rupture due to excessive inflation pressure, or by direct damage to the lung by the surgeon or anaesthetist. The diagnosis of a tension pneumothorax during anaesthesia is sometimes difficult. Severe bronchospasm with lung hyperinflation is the main alternative diagnosis, and both of these conditions impair spontaneous ventilation or cause a rising airway pressure during IPPV. Displacement of the trachea away from the side of a tension pneumothorax is a valuable sign in such circumstances.

Open pneumothorax is seen occasionally after violent trauma to the chest wall, and as a regular feature of every thoracotomy. Spontaneous ventilation is inefficient as air may be drawn in and out of the wound instead of the trachea. During anaesthesia these problems are largely solved by the use of IPPV, although spontaneous ventilation can be satisfactorily maintained by some patients.

Closed pneumothorax should be managed with a chest drain prior to anaesthesia for several reasons. Firstly, nitrous oxide can diffuse into an air space within the body over 30 times more quickly than nitrogen can diffuse out. Eger & Saidman (1965) demonstrated that if 75% nitrous oxide were used for anaesthesia, the volume of air in a pneumothorax could double in 10 min and triple in 30 min. Secondly a rise in airway pressure, with coughing, straining or IPPV, can aggravate an air leak, expanding a closed pneumothorax and even converting it to a tension type. Finally, lung mechanics may be affected by the combination of pneumothorax and anaesthesia, resulting in a severe impairment of gas exchange. Concomitant disease of the lung adds to the problem. For example patients with emphysema may have a very small pneumothorax, radiographically, which can produce very severe respiratory embarrassment. This is because the loss of elastic recoil is so great that widespread airway closure is caused by a small reduction in lung volume, as may occur with a pneumothorax, and the induction of anaesthesia. However, if the pneumothorax is small and the patient is asymptomatic, anaesthesia can be undertaken provided that full monitoring is available and there would be no delay in inserting a chest drain should this become necessary during surgery. Nitrous oxide and IPPV would be best avoided in these circumstances.

Bullae and lung cysts

Bullae and lung cysts are large, poorly ventilated regions of lung with virtually no perfusion. Some patients have only one or two cysts and remaining normal lung, but more commonly underlying lung disease COPD is also present. The most severely affected patients have multiple bullae and generalized emphysema, and are greatly incapacitated. It is preferable to avoid general anaesthesia altogether, but if it is necessary then coughing, straining and vigorous IPPV probably present more of a hazard than the use of nitrous oxide. In unilateral lung disease a double-lumen tracheal tube can be used to prevent hyperinflation of the affected side during IPPV. If the patient's condition deteriorates during anaesthesia and no alternative explanation is likely except massive enlargement of such an air space, it may be necessary to insert an intercostal drain. This should be reserved as a life-saving measure, since the end-result is often a prolonged air leak which is difficult to control.

Lobar emphysema

Lobar emphysema can be congenital, or secondary to a ball-valve type of bronchial obstruction, caused, for example, by a foreign body or tumour. The affected lobe can enlarge dramatically with anaesthesia as gas is pushed past the obstruction and nitrous oxide diffuses in.

Restrictive lung disease

There are three categories of disease that result in this defect in ventilatory capacity. Firstly, disease processes, such as fibrosis, oedema and infiltrates which reduce lung compliance. Secondly, stiffness of the pleura and chest wall, for example due to kyphoscoliosis. Thirdly, a large volume lesion within the thorax or abdomen may result in a decrease in volume of ventilatable lung. This includes pleural effusions, pneumothorax, pain from an 'acute abdomen' or abdominal incision, plus distension due to gas or ascites, all of which may result in a restrictive pattern of breathing.

Lung fibrosis

Lung fibrosis can be idiopathic, or can accompany various connective tissue or allergic disorders. The carbon monoxide transfer coefficient is diminished and patients are commonly hypoxaemic, but arterial oxygenation can be maintained at adequate levels during anaesthesia by increasing the inspired oxygen. PEFR can be above the normal range which may confer an effective cough mechanism, and postoperative retention of secretions is unlikely. With increasing severity of disease, vital capacity and PEFR fall, and patients may eventually begin to retain CO_2. Problems are then much more severe.

Pulmonary oedema

The factors that influence the development of alveolar oedema are shown in Figure 4.7. Starling (1896) described the balance of hydrostatic and colloid osmotic pressures, and more recently the importance of surface forces and active transport have also been reported (Hills 1990). Pulmonary oedema may occur during anaesthesia because of fluid overload, myocardial depression or aspiration of gastric contents. Careful control of pulmonary artery wedge pressure in patients with severe cardiac disease is required if pulmonary oedema is to be avoided.

The term 'adult respiratory distress syndrome' (ARDS) defines those patients in whom pulmonary oedema is due to abnormal leakiness of the alveolar–capillary barrier, rather than cardiac failure or fluid overload. The diagnosis of ARDS is usually confirmed by means of pulmonary artery catheterization. However, a more satisfactory method of diagnosis and quantification is to measure the lung clearance of a water-soluble radiolabelled tracer, which will clear more rapidly the leakier are a patient's lungs (Barrowcliffe & Jones 1989). Patients with ARDS are cared for in the intensive care unit, but they sometimes need anaesthesia for drainage of intraabdominal sepsis. Patients with pancreatitis or septicaemia from abdominal pathology may demonstrate impaired oxygenation despite a normal chest X-ray. This may be due to incipient ARDS, which is often averted by treatment of the underlying disorder. Important measures to prevent worsening of pulmonary oedema include the avoidance of overhydration and a greater readiness to employ inotropes to boost cardiac output. However, renal function is also likely to be impaired in these patients. Therapy is then best undertaken with full monitoring of cardiac function and in consulation with the renal physicians.

During anaesthesia in a patient with pulmonary oedema mechanical ventilation is mandatory. High levels of oxygen and PEEP may be necessary, and the distribution of ventilation and oxygenation can be improved by employing a long inspiratory time or end-inspiratory pause. In such patients, in whom oxygenation is critical, great care must be taken during postoperative physiotherapy with airway suction, since a dangerous fall in oxygenation may be precipitated (Selsby 1989).

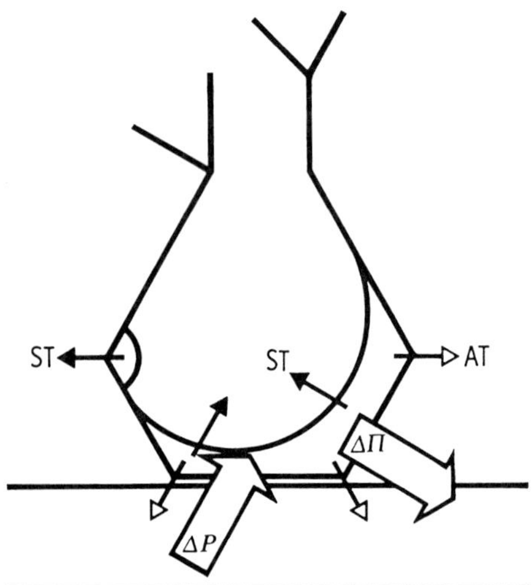

$$\text{flux} = \text{Kf}\,[\Delta P - \Sigma\sigma\Delta\Pi]$$

Fig. 4.7 Factors that influence the development of alveolar oedema. ΔP: hydrostatic pressure gradient from pulmonary capillary to alveolus. $\Delta\Pi$: gradient of colloid osmotic pressure in the opposite direction. σ: reflection coefficient, which is a measure of permeability to colloid of the alveolar wall. ST: surface tension. AT: active transport. Kf: hydraulic conducting factor.

Restrictive disease of the rib cage

Kyphoscoliosis or ankylosing spondylitis may present with an alarming chest radiographic appearance, but pulmonary complications are generally uncommon in the absence of any additional disorder of lung parenchyma. A raised $Paco_2$ and a reduced Pao_2 or SaO_2 are important prognostic factors, as is a reduced exercise tolerance. Almost all the tidal volume may depend upon diaphragmatic movement, so that these patients are at most risk in the postoperative period following upper abdominal surgery. They should derive benefit from local anaesthetic techniques which permit deeper diaphragmatic inspiration. However, the spinal abnormality may make it particularly difficult to perform thoracic epidural analgesia.

Pleural effusion

A pleural effusion compresses lung tissue, potentiates the fall in lung volume that is associated with anaesthesia, and leads to a sharp increase in both airway resistance and closure following induction. Accordingly, a sizable or symptomatic effusion should be drained before anaesthesia. However, this should not be done so long beforehand that fluid has time to accumulate, but enough time should be allowed to exclude the possibility of pneumothorax. In a malignant pleural effusion a chemical pleurodesis should be considered. Tetracycline is the agent of choice. 20 mg/kg of tetracycline diluted to 50 ml is injected into the pleural space, left for 2 hours, then suction is applied for at least 48 hours.

An effusion can be drained after the induction of anaesthesia, but until this is done spontaneous ventilation may be inadequate. The safest course is thus to intubate and assist or control ventilation. IPPV also helps to expel fluid from a pleural drain. Sometimes when large volumes of fluid are removed by this means cardiovascular disturbances occur, related to loss of colloid in the effusion or perhaps to movements of the mediastinum, which can be averted by using one-lung anaesthesia.

Obstructive lung disease

Asthma

Optimal therapy should be established before elective surgery, and be continued into the immediate preoperative period. The major problem during anaesthesia is hyper-reactivity of the airways, so that bronchoconstriction is more easily induced than in a normal patient. This is most likely to be a reflex triggered by instrumentation of the upper airway, mediated by the vagus, and is less commonly due to an adverse drug reaction. Therefore, deep levels of anaesthesia are indicated, while both unnecessary instrumentation of the airway and drugs, such as thiopentone, curare and morphine, known to release histamine are best avoided. Ketamine is a bronchodilator and may occasionally be useful as an induction agent. The volatile agents also have good bronchodilating properties (Fig. 4.4B, p. 61), and have been used successfully in the management of bronchospasm complicating anaesthesia.

In the treatment of severe bronchospasm, ventilation with full muscle relaxation (pancuronium) may be necessary and B_2 agonists are much more effective than aminophylline (Jones et al 1987, Tobias & Hirshman 1990). If there is generalized anaphylaxis and cardiovascular collapse adrenaline is the drug of choice, given either directly into the airway (1 mg of adrenaline in 10 ml saline) or a similar dose intravenously in a controlled manner with monitoring of the blood pressure.

The optimum mode of ventilation in severe airflow obstruction is controversial, with proponents of both increased inspiratory to expiratory (I:E) ratios (Branthwaite 1990) and PEEP (Smith & Marini 1988). Cautious adjustment of the I:E ratio would appear logical, firstly, because the time constant, which is a function of compliance and resistance, is prolonged with the presence of many 'slow lung compartments'. Secondly, some degree of hyperinflation will be encouraged and may counteract the fall in lung volume induced by anaesthesia, and thus return the lung to a more favourable position on the resistance–lung volume curve (Fig. 4.4B). However, the patient must be closely observed for signs of overinflation and barotrauma, and a pneumothorax may even be mistaken for bronchospasm. During anaesthesia the first indication that this is occurring may be hypotension, secondary to decreases in venous return and cardiac output.

Chronic obstructive pulmonary disease

Excessive sputum production and a reduced FEV_1 and PEFR typify chronic bronchitis;

extensive loss of alveolar structure and flattened diaphragms are implied by a diagnosis of emphysema. Numerically they represent the largest category of patients with respiratory disease, at least in the UK. The problems and hazards invoked by anaesthesia will be considered below.

Abnormal respiratory control is present in patients with loss of sensitivity to CO_2, and dependence upon a hypoxic drive for resting ventilation. In these patients, who have developed CO_2 retention, the sensitivity to hypoxia is also much reduced (Anthonisen et al 1977), and compensation to imposed loads is impaired. It is often safest to omit preoperative sedation, but in the presence of pain the titration of intravenous opiates may be necessary but difficult. Benzodiazepines in cautious dosage are preferable for the relief of anxiety. Intravenous induction agents should be given slowly in reduced dosage if the aim is to retain spontaneous ventilation. However the dramatic effect of volatile agents in attenuating the hypoxic ventilatory responses is obviously disastrous for patients with CO_2 retention who survive on a hypoxic drive. Even in patients not dependent on hypoxic drive, halothane anaesthesia causes more depression of resting ventilation than in normal individuals, mainly by a fall in tidal volume (Pietak et al 1975). Postoperatively, parenteral opiates should be given very cautiously with continuous SaO_2 monitoring. Naloxone or doxapram may be useful if breathing becomes excessively depressed, especially if epidural opioids are employed. Local anaesthetic techniques rarely disturb central control of breathing, and should be strongly considered for postoperative pain relief (Catley et al 1985). Such patients will need prolonged postoperative monitoring of oxygen saturation using a system similar to that described by Wheatley et al (1990). Patient-controlled analgesia combined with epidural local anaesthesia may be the best method of achieving safe postoperative pain relief.

Mechanical problems, for example bronchospasm, may occur since many patients with COPD have irritable airways, although they are not as labile as asthmatics. The stimulus is usually either airway manipulation or irritant gases and, as with asthma, gas trapping and progressive hyperinflation may occur if insufficient time is allowed for the emptying of lung units during expiration. It should be possible to improve this situation by an appropriate adjustment of the pattern of ventilation.

Gas exchange in heavy smokers with COPD is impaired both before and during anaesthesia (Dueck et al 1980). Poor V/Q matching accounts for most of this abnormality in conscious subjects, and the additional deterioration during anaesthesia is due to the frequent development of intrapulmonary shunts. This is likely to be secondary to a reduction in FRC, so that tidal breathing occurs within the closing capacity and creates lung regions with little or no ventilation.

Choice of anaesthetic technique in COPD is based on three main approaches: general anaesthesia with either spontaneous ventilation or IPPV, or local anaesthesia.

Spontaneous ventilation is feasible in mild disease using inhalational anaesthetics, but it is advantageous not to depress ventilation by opiate premedication. However, increasing severity of the disease is accompanied by increasing sensitivity to the ventilatory depressant effect of the anaesthetic drugs. General anaesthesia with spontaneous ventilation is *not* an option in patients dependent on a hypoxic drive to ventilation, because both opiates and volatile agents (as well as oxygen) inhibit hypoxic drive. If surgery is attempted under such conditions the profound inhibitory effect of anaesthesia on ventilation may make it impossible to reach a deep enough level of anaesthesia to permit the operation.

Regional anaesthesia or IPPV are the only practical ways of providing anaesthesia in such cases. Many patients with COPD have barely adequate blood gases when breathing spontaneously, but gas exchange can improve markedly during IPPV, particularly in emphysematous patients. There are good reasons not to seek a rapid reduction in $P\text{aCO}_2$ by hyperventilating patients with CO_2 retention. This can lead to instability of cardiac rhythm, a lowered cardiac output and excessive reduction of cerebral blood flow.

The re-establishment of spontaneous ventilation at the end of surgery may be difficult, and one approach to this problem is to continue mechanical ventilation for the first few postoperative hours in selected cases. This usually necessitates admission to an intensive care unit, and allows adequate analgesia and good oxygenation to be maintained, while many residual anaesthetic effects decline. Dyspnoea at rest and a low preoperative PaO_2 of less than 70% of normal for age were found to be the best prognostic factors for postoperative ventilation in a series of patients with severe COPD and FEV_1 values between 1 and 0.3 l (Nunn et al 1988). This was, however, a retrospective study and may thus be an unreliable prospective guide.

Local anaesthesia as the sole anaesthetic is particularly suitable for lower abdominal and limb operations, and even respiratory cripples can be anaesthetized by this means. In one retrospective study of patients with COPD, spinal anaesthesia for such surgery had no associated mortality, whereas general anaesthesia resulted in a 5% mortality attributable to postoperative respiratory dysfunction (Tarhan et al 1973). However, problems may still arise. Not all patients (or surgeons) are sufficiently phlegmatic to tolerate local anaesthesia. Benzodiazepines, in small divided doses intravenously, help to allay anxiety, as can the inhalation of sedative concentrations of nitrous oxide. The posture necessary for operation may be poorly tolerated, an extreme example being a head-down tilt in the lithotomy position, but some patients may not even cope with the supine position. Care must also be taken to ensure that the local block does not significantly weaken the respiratory muscles or destroy their coordination. This is quite likely with high spinals or epidurals, and perhaps with bilateral intercostal nerve blocks. The phrenic nerve, and thus the diaphragm, may be affected by blocks around the neck, for example those directed at the stellate ganglion and brachial plexus. Any block around the thorax carries a risk of pneumothorax.

Thoracic surgery

If patients who present for pulmonary resection are not carefully selected, they may have insufficient residual lung function so that postoperative respiratory failure and death are inevitable. Although no single pulmonary function test can predict this possibility, the result of a number of tests can provide a satisfactory indication. The criteria for operability vary from centre to centre, and depend on the amount of lung it is planned to resect, but general guidelines can be given (Brindley et al 1982, Gothard & Branthwaite 1982), as in Table 4.1.

An elevated $PaCO_2$ (>6 kPa) contraindicates resection since there will inevitably be further deterioration, whereas a depressed PaO_2 may actually rise after surgery if sufficient shunting were occurring in the resected lung. Even if the patient fails to meet the above criteria he may still survive the operation. This possibility is assessed by measuring regional lung function. Radionuclide perfusion scanning has replaced differential bronchospirometry, and enables an index of operability to be derived. The fractional perfusion to the normal lung is multiplied by the FEV_1: a value more than 0.8 indicates a reasonable operative risk. Furthermore, unimpaired preoperative perfusion of the diseased lung is also a strong predictor for hypoxaemia during one-lung anaesthesia (Hurford et al 1987). The safety of isoflurane in this situation has been demonstrated by a minimal effect on HPV (Benumof et al 1987a).

More specialized texts should be consulted for further details of anaesthesia for thoracic surgery, but one particular aspect merits special attention, namely the positioning of disposable PVC double-lumen tracheal tubes. The margin of

Table 4.1 Criteria suggesting survivability after pneumonectomy

Lung function test	Level indicating survivability
FVC	>50% predicted
FEV_1	>50% predicted or > 2 l
RV/TLC	<50% predicted
Diffusing capacity	>50% predicted
Exercise tolerance	Climb two flights of stairs without difficulty

safety in positioning both left- and right-sided disposable tubes was investigated by Benumof et al (1987b). Although this was found to be much greater using left-sided tubes, it was still poor enough for the authors to advise rechecking tube position after patient movement and the use of fibre-optic bronchoscopy. Right-sided disposable Mallinckrodt and Robertshaw red rubber tubes have also been directly compared using fibre-optic bronchoscopy: 90% of the red rubber tubes were correctly positioned blindly, whereas this was only possible in 11% of patients with disposable tubes (McKenna et al 1988). Therefore, fibre-optic bronchoscopy is desirable for any double-lumen tube placement, but is essential when employing modern disposable tubes, especially right-sided.

Other factors that exacerbate the deleterious effect of anaesthesia upon lung function

Site of surgery

Upper abdominal and thoracic surgery are important contributory factors for postoperative pulmonary complications (PPC), especially in the elderly and patients with preoperative lung disease (Enberg & Wiklund 1988). Consistent changes in ventilatory pattern occur following both types of surgery, resulting in rapid shallow breathing, and a fall in FRC and impaired oxygenation which may last for several days (Craig 1981). The residual effects of anaesthesia are partly responsible for some of these changes for the first few hours after the operation. Subsequently the influence of the surgical procedure predominates, for example after upper abdominal surgery diaphragmatic movements are inhibited more than those of the rib cage (Ford et al 1983). In contrast, lower abdominal operations are much less stressful to the respiratory system, while limb surgery offers little insult.

It is uncertain to what extent the deterioration in lung function after upper abdominal surgery is pain related, since studies assessing the effects of different analgesic regimens on postoperative pulmonary function have produced conflicting results. For example, intercostal nerve block for subcostal incision both reduced PPC (Enberg & Wiklund 1988) and improved forced vital capacity (FVC), FEV_1 and PEFR (Enberg 1985). Similarly, interpleural bupivacaine following cholecystectomy increased FEV_1 and reduced the requirement for patient-controlled morphine analgesia (VadeBoncouer et al 1989). Mankikian et al (1988) employed thoracic extradural block after upper abdominal surgery, and demonstrated improvements not only in Vt and FRC, but also in the abdominal contribution to Vt and gastric pressures, reflecting an increase in diaphragmatic function. In contrast, Jayr et al (1988) found no correlation between improved pain-relief with extradural morphine and the incidence of PPC, while Scott et al (1989) achieved total alleviation of pain, with a combination of thoracic extradural bupivacaine and morphine, in patients following upper abdominal surgery, but PEFR, FEV_1 and FVC were unaltered and remained markedly lower than preoperative values.

Therefore, mechanisms other than pain exist to compromise lung function after upper abdominal surgery, and good analgesia should be supplemented by adequate monitoring and physiotherapy. This is particularly vital both in the elderly and in patients with pre-existing pulmonary disease.

Duration of surgery

Several studies have shown that an anaesthetic time in excess of 2–3 hours results in a significant increase in the incidence of complications, such as atelectasis and infection. This may relate to depression of mucociliary clearance, neutrophil phagocytosis and other defence mechanisms.

Age

Pulmonary function becomes progressively poorer with increasing age, illustrated by worsening performance in a variety of pulmonary function tests. Respiratory muscles weaken, the rib cage becomes stiffer and lung architecture steadily deteriorates, so that the surface area for gas exchange falls. The elastic recoil of the lung also declines, resulting in airway closure at larger lung volumes. In normal subjects lying supine, Leblanc et al (1970) found that CC exceeds FRC by about 44 years of age, while Mansell et al (1972) found a similar situation in children below the age of about 6 years. This implies airway closure during normal tidal breathing, which may then be exacerbated by anaesthesia with a detrimental effect on oxygenation.

Obesity

Perioperative respiratory complications are more frequent in the obese for several reasons. Total compliance is reduced to approximately one-third of normal due to the weighty chest wall, which increases the work of breathing and contributes to the abnormally high oxygen consumption. The FRC is reduced in proportion to increasing obesity, while the CC is increased and easily encroaches on FRC. Hypoxaemia can be found at rest, especially when lying supine, since this leads to an additional reduction in FRC.

Not surprisingly, overweight patients are also prone to develop a greater degree of basal atelectasis during anaesthesia (Strandberg et al 1987), since induction decreases FRC by about 50% to a level often below awake residual volume (Damia et al 1988). An interesting finding was that FRC returned to preinduction levels following laparotomy incision, indicating that pressure on the vena cava and changes in thoracic blood volume may have contributed to the initial fall in FRC (Jones 1987).

Induction of anaesthesia in the morbidly obese patient is hazardous with the potential for both arterial desaturation and aspiration. Either preoxygenation with rapid sequence induction or awake intubation is indicated. During anaesthesia 50% oxygen is often required to prevent hypoxaemia, which may be aggravated by a head-down tilt or even retraction of the abdominal wound. Postoperatively a semi-sitting position has beneficial effects on gas exchange, and should be encouraged if the circulation is stable. The duration of postoperative hypoxaemia justifies prolonged oxygen therapy in the obese patient. Epidural local analgesia has been advocated as a means of reducing pulmonary complications, although in one study this failed to improve pulmonary function after upper abdominal surgery in very obese patients (Gelman et al 1980). A further consideration is that placement of an epidural catheter may prejudice the willingness to use subcutaneous heparin; deep vein thrombosis is twice as common in the obese as is usual in the perioperative period and pulmonary embolism is the major cause of postoperative death in this group.

Smoking

Smokers exhibit small airways disease, irritable airways and increased mucus production, but with decreased clearance. The hyper-reactive tracheobronchial tree in smokers may lead to coughing and bronchospasm following airway manipulation, unless a greater depth of anaesthesia is employed than in non-smokers. These factors, combined with an elevated closing capacity, predispose smokers to increased V/Q inequality and impaired oxygenation during anaesthesia (Dueck et al 1980), and greater respiratory morbidity postoperatively.

At least 6–8 weeks of smoking cessation are required to detect improvements in either small airways disease or tracheobronchial clearance. Similarly, a non-smoking period of 2 months was necessary to influence the incidence of PPC in patients undergoing coronary artery bypass grafts (Warner et al 1983). A 6-week abstinence prior to surgery has been recommended (Jones et al 1987), but is difficult to achieve. However, a period of 12–24 hours cessation will benefit most patients as regards the effect on COHb and oxygen transport, and is especially desirable for patients with ischaemic heart disease.

Upper airway obstruction

The anaesthetic management of patients with upper airway obstruction is discussed in detail in Chapter 31. Ventilation in these patients is already compromised and the use of premedicant and anaesthetic drugs will not only depress respiratory drive, but will also increase the work of breathing

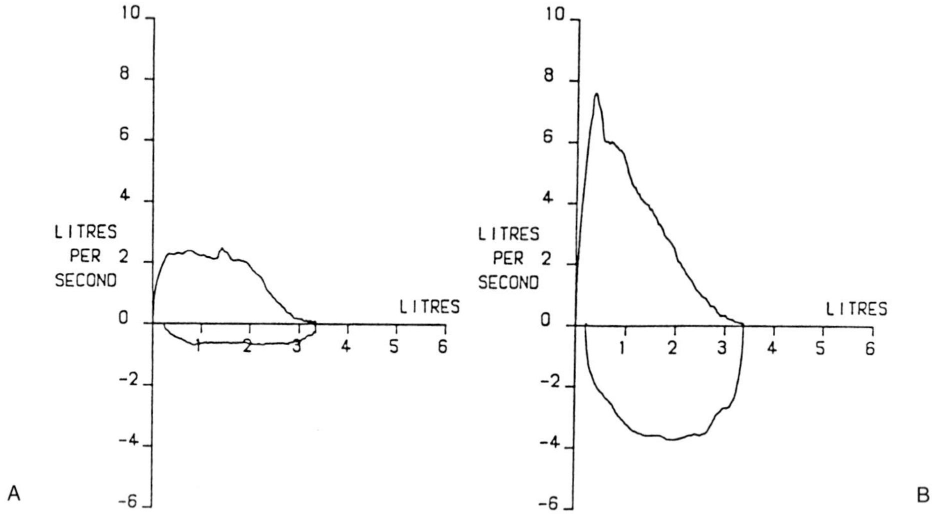

Fig. 4.8 To show the effect of a thyroid adenoma in compressing the upper airway. The flow-volume curve (A) shows the characteristic flat top of severe upper airway obstruction. Compare this with the curve following surgical removal of the thyroid (B). A flat-top flow-volume curve suggests difficulty in tracheal intubation (from Miller et al 1990).

by an adverse effect on both lower and upper airway resistance. In particular a decrease in the tone of pharyngeal muscles during inspiration will potentiate upper airway obstruction.

Stridor at rest or on minimal exertion will alert the anaesthetist to these problems, but many patients may have upper airway obstruction not evident on clinical examination. For example, upper airway obstruction was detected by flow–volume loops in about one third of patients presenting for surgery with symptomatic goitre (Fig. 4.8), and only three of the 26 patients had stridor (Miller et al 1990). Flow–volume loops are a very sensitive and accurate investigation for upper airway obstruction and should routinely be performed in any patient in whom the diagnosis is suspected.

MEASURES TO IMPROVE RESPIRATORY FUNCTION AND THE SAFETY OF ANAESTHESIA

Anaesthetic technique

Preoperative preparation

Any remedial disorders should be treated. Bronchitics are more likely to be fit in summer than in winter, and elective surgery should be arranged accordingly. Chest physiotherapy combined with bronchodilator therapy can dramatically reduce the incidence of PPC in patients with COPD. It is also of benefit in patients with bronchiectasis and cystic fibrosis, and being taught the appropriate manoeuvres preoperatively facilitates patient cooperation in the post-operative period.

Intraoperative considerations

Anaesthesia depresses ventilatory responses to hypoxia, hypercapnia and added loads that may strip the patient bare of defence mechanisms. At the same time it induces other changes in lung mechanics that also place the patient in danger. Furthermore, an increase in A-aP_{O_2} following induction of anaesthesia is so common that it is almost universal practice to employ an FiO_2 more than 0.3. Even greater inspired concentrations may be necessary in high-risk groups to maintain adequate oxygenation, although the possibility of inducing lung damage with an FiO_2 as low as 50% should not be forgotten (Register et al 1987).

Pulse oximetry is useful in determining the lowest FiO_2 that will allow reasonable saturation.

Large tidal volumes during IPPV may reduce the A–aPo_2. It is important to consider circulatory changes that may accompany a raised intrathoracic pressure. This can reduce cardiac output and thus oxygen delivery to tissues, even though the Pao_2 is higher.

No benefit has been shown in the prophylaxis of postoperative chest infections by the use of bacterial filters or sterile anaesthetic circuits. This may be because the causative organisms are already present in the lungs at the beginning of the operation. Warming and humidifying inspired gases has been shown to reduce slightly the incidence of chest complications, presumably by preserving mucociliary clearance (Chalon et al 1979). For short operations there are unlikely to be any benefits, but for lengthy procedures in high-risk groups there may be some, and disposable condenser-humidifiers are recommended for cheapness and convenience.

Postoperative period

Respiratory disturbances are common in the postoperative period and are particularly marked when pain necessitates sizable doses of parenteral opiates. Patients in high-risk groups, for example after thoracic or upper abdominal surgery or those with COPD, are likely to experience greater deterioration in respiratory pattern and oxygenation than normal subjects. In high-risk patients undergoing lower abdominal and limb surgery, the use of both general anaesthesia and opiates may be avoided by employing local anaesthetic techniques, and may result in little disturbance to ventilation. In contrast, perioperative thoracic epidural bupivacaine for cholecystectomy improved postoperative oxygen saturation (Catley et al 1985) and almost halved the incidence of atelectasis compared to general anaesthesia combined with parenteral opiates (Hendolin et al 1987). However, the local analgesia group still showed a 20% deterioration in postoperative lung function tests, and 25% developed atelectasis.

Perioperative respiratory therapy

The detrimental effects of anaesthesia on lung volume, basal atelectasis, mucociliary clearance and coughing create an ideal setting for the development of postoperative respiratory complications. Most patients with previously healthy lungs will tolerate these changes with little respiratory morbidity. However, in patients with pre-existing lung disease the basal atelectasis induced by anaesthesia is not only likely to persist postoperatively, especially after upper abdominal surgery, but may evolve and become infected.

Patients in high-risk groups, for example smokers and the elderly, require good postoperative analgesia, an appropriate use of antibiotics, and physiotherapy. The importance of coughing exercises and brondhodilator therapy during chest physiotherapy have recently been reviewed, together with the merits of 'external chest-wall oscillation' and the 'forced expiration technique' (Selsby & Jones 1990). Even patients with previously normal lung function, but undergoing upper abdominal surgery, benefit from breathing exercises (Roukema et al 1988). There is no evidence of benefit from incentive spirometry (O'Connor et al 1988).

Respiratory monitoring and anaesthesia

Until the recent widespread use of pulse oximetry and capnography, anaesthetic monitoring relied mainly on the anaesthetist's powers of observation, combined with ventilator disconnect alarms and airway pressure gauges. Capnography and pulse oximetry now enable the anaesthetist to monitor more reliably the effects of anaesthesia on ventilation and oxygenation, but the problem of postoperative monitoring has not been resolved.

Capnography

Capnography is valuable in detecting both oesophageal intubation and apnoeic episodes. Although pulse oximetry can also diagnose these events, there will be an inevitable time delay, especially after preoxygenation (Guggenberger et al 1989). End-tidal CO_2 serves as a guide to $PaCO_2$. It is used to maintain hypocapnia in patients with raised intracranial pressure and normocapnia in both the elderly and patients with coronary artery disease. A sudden drop in end-tidal CO_2 reflects a decreased pulmonary blood flow, which may occur following an air embolism or other cause of decreased cardiac output. In contrast a sharp increase in end-tidal CO_2 will precede temperature changes in malignant hyperpyrexia.

Pulse oximetry

Many studies using oximetry have demonstrated varying degrees and lengths of hypoxaemia during induction, maintenance and recovery from anaesthesia. Pulse oximetry alerts the anaesthetist to the presence of hypoxaemia sooner than clinical signs (McKay & Moble 1988). Pulse oximetry also performs an important role in advancing our knowledge about the impact on oxygenation of different techniques of anaesthesia and postoperative pain relief. In children, halothane induction preserves SaO_2, whereas isoflurane often results in desaturation (Sampaio et al 1989). Patient-controlled analgesia, extradural opiates and intramuscular opiates all give rise to periods of desaturation following either caesarean section (Brose & Cohen 1989) or hysterectomy (Wheatley et al 1990).

Therefore, pulse oximetry is indispensable in a variety of settings, but in the presence of an increased FiO_2 a considerable A-aPO_2 will already have developed before the oximeter starts to alarm. In many cases this ‘predesaturation phase’ may be anticipated, and possibly prevented, by an understanding of the effects of anaesthesia on respiratory function in high-risk patients.

REFERENCES

Alagesan K, Nunn J F, Feeley T W, Heneghan C P H 1987 Comparison of the respiratory depressant effects of halothane and isoflurane in routine surgery. Br J Anesth 59: 1070–1079

Alexander C M, Gross J B 1988 Sedative doses of midazolam depress hypoxic ventilatory responses in humans. Anesth Analg 67: 377–382

Anthonisen N R, Bradley C A, Dhingra S 1977 Control of ventilation in chronic respiratory failure. Clin Res 25: 711A

Arunasalam K, Davenport H T, Painter S, Jones J G 1983 ventilatory response to morphine in young and old subjects. Anaesthesia 38: 529–533

Bailey P L, Andriano K P, Pace N L, Westenskow D R, Stanley T H 1984 Small doses of fentanyl potentiate and prolong diazepam induced respiratory depression. Anesth Analg 63: 183A

Barrowcliffe M P, Jones J G 1989 Pulmonary clearance of 99m Tc-DTPA in diagnosis and evolution of increased permeability pulmonary oedema. Anaesth Intensive Care 17: 422–432

Becker L D, Paulson B A, Miller R D, Severinghaus J W, Eger E I 1976 Biphasic respiratory depression after fentanyl-droperidol or fentanyl alone used to supplement nitrous oxide anesthesia. Anesthesiology 44: 291–296

Benumof J L, Augustine S D, Gibbons J A 1987a Halothane and isoflurane only slightly impair arterial oxygenation during one-lung ventilation in patients undergoing thoracotomy. Anesthesiology 67: 910–915

Benumof J L, Partridge B L, Salvatierra C, Keating J 1987b Margin of safety in positioning modern double-lumen endotracheal tubes. Anesthesiology 67: 729–738

Berggren L, Erikkson I, Mollenholt P 1987 Changes in breathing pattern and chest wall mechanics after benzodiazepines in combination with meperidine. Acta Anaesthesiol Scand 31: 381–386

Bergman N A 1963 Distribution of inspired gas during anaesthesia and artificial ventilation. J Appl Physiol 18: 1085–1089

Bergman N A, Tien Y K 1983 Contribution of the closure of pulmonary units to impaired oxygenation during anesthesia. Anesthesiology 59: 395–401

Bickler P E, Dueck R, Prutow R J 1987 Effects of barbiturate anesthesia on functional residual capacity and ribcage/diaphragm contributions to ventilation. Anesthesiology 66: 147–152

Branthwaite M A 1990 An update on mechanical ventilation for severe acute asthma. Clinical Intensive Care 1: 4–6

Brindley G V, Walsh R E, Schnarr W T, Allen G W, Mendenhall M K, Ahlgren E W 1982 Pulmonary resection in patients with impaired pulmonary function. Surg Clin North Am 62: 199–214

Brose W G, Cohen S E 1989 Oxyhemoglobin saturation following caesarian section in patients receiving epidural morphine, PCA, or i.m. meperidine analgesia. Anesthesiology 70: 948–953

Carlon G C, Ray C Jr, Klain M 1980 High frequency positive pressure ventilation in management of a patient with bronchopleural fistula. Anesthesiology 52: 160–162

Carlsson A J, Bindslev L, Hedenstierna G 1987a Hypoxia-induced pulmonary vasoconstriction in the human lung. Anesthesiology 66: 312–316

Carlsson A J, Hedenstierna G, Bindslev L 1987b Hypoxia-induced vasoconstriction in the human lung exposed to enflurane anaesthesia. Acta Anaesthesiol Scand 31: 57–62

Catley D M 1984 Postoperative analgesia and respiratory control. In: Jones J G (ed) Effects of anaesthesia and surgery on pulmonary mechanisms and gas exchange. Little Brown, Boston, pp 95–112

Catley D M, Thornton C, Jordan C, Lehane J R, Royston D, Jones J G 1985 Pronounced episodic oxygen desaturation in the post-operative period: its association with ventilatory pattern and analgesic regimen. Anesthesiology 63: 20–28

Chalon J, Patel C, Ali M, Ramanathan S, Capan L, Tang C, Turndorf H 1979 Humidity and the anesthetized patient. Anesthesiology 50: 195–198

Craig D B 1981 Postoperative recovery of pulmonary function. Anesth Analg 60: 46–52

Damia G, Mascheroni D, Croci M, Tarenzi L 1988 Perioperative changes in functional residual capacity in morbidly obese patients. Br J Anaesth 60: 574–578

DeSoto H, Patel R I, Soliman I E, Hannallah R S 1988 Changes in oxygen saturation following general anaesthesia in children with upper respiratory infections signs and symptoms undergoing otolaryngological procedures. Anesthesiology 68: 276–279

Drummond G B 1987 Reduction of tonic ribcage muscle activity by anesthesia with thiopentone. Anesthesiology 67: 695–700

Dueck R, Young I, Clausen J, Wagner P D 1980 Altered distribution of pulmonary ventilation and blood flow following induction of inhalational anesthesia. Anesthesiology 52: 113–125

Dueck R, Prutow R J, Davies N J H, Clausen J L, Davidson T M 1988 The lung volume at which shunting occurs with inhalation anesthesia. Anesthesiology 69: 854–861

Eger E I, Saidman L J 1965 Hazards of nitrous oxide anesthesia in bowel obstruction and pneumothorax. Anesthesiology 26: 61–66

Eger E I, Dolan W M, Stevens W C 1972 Surgical stimulation antagonizes the respiratory depression produced by forane. Anesthesiology 36: 544–549

Empey D W, Laitinen L A, Jacobs L, Gold W M, Nadel J A 1976 Mechanisms of bronchial hyperreactivity in normal subjects after upper respiratory tract infection. Am Rev Respir Dis 113: 131–139

Enberg G 1985 Respiratory performance after upper abdominal surgery: a comparison of pain relief with intercostal blocks and centrally acting analgesics. Acta Anaesthesiol Scand 29: 427–433

Enberg G, Wiklund L 1988 Pulmonary complications after upper abdominal surgery: their prevention with intercostal blocks. Acta Anaesthesiol Scand 32: 1–9

Etches R C, Sandler A N, Daley M D 1989 Respiratory depression and spinal opioids. Can J Anaesth 36: 165–185

Feeley T W, Keating D, Nishiwura T 1988 Independent lung ventilation using high-frequency ventilation in the management of a bronchopleural fistula. Anesthesiology 69: 420–421

Fennelly M E, Hall G M 1990 Anaesthesia and upper respiratory tract infections: a non-existent hazard? Br J Anaesth 64: 535–536

Ford G T, Whitelaw W A, Rosenal T W, Cruse P J, Guenter C A 1983 Diaphragm function after upper abdominal surgery in humans. Am Rev Respir Dis 127: 431–436

Froese A B, Bryan A C 1974 Effects of anesthesia and paralysis on diaphragmatic mechanisms in man. Anesthesiology 41: 242–255

Gal T J, DiFazio C A, Moscicki J 1982 Analgesic and respiratory depressant activity of nalbuphine: a comparison with morphine. Anesthesiology 57: 367–374

Gamsu G, Singer M M, Vincent H H, Berry S, Nadel J A 1976 Postoperative impairment of mucus transport in the lung. Am Rev Respir Dis 114: 673–679

Gelman S, Laws H L, Potzick J, Strong S, Smith L, Erdemir H 1980 Thoracic epidural versus balanced anesthesia in morbid obesity: an intraoperative and postoperative haemodynamic study. Anesth Analg 59: 902–908

Goodman N W, Black A M S, Carter J A 1987 Some ventilatory effects of propofol as sole anaesthetic agent. Br J Anaesth 59: 1497–1503

Gothard J W W, Branthwaite M A 1982 Anaesthesia for thoracic surgery. Blackwell, Oxford, pp 8–27

Guggenberger H, Lenz G, Federle R 1989 Early detection of oesophageal intubation: pulse oximetry versus capnography. Acta Anaesthesiol Scand 33: 112–115

Hedenstierna G 1988 Causes of gas exchange impairment during general anaesthesia. Eur J Anaesthesiol 5: 221–231

Hedenstierna G, McCarthy G, Bergstrom M 1976 Airway closure during mechanical ventilation. Anesthesiology 44: 114–123

Hedenstierna G, Strandberg A, Brismar B, Lundquist H, Svensson L, Tokics L 1985 Functional residual capacity, thoracoabdominal dimensions, and central blood volume during general anesthesia with muscle paralysis and mechanical ventilation. Anesthesiology 62: 247–254

Hendolin H, Lahtinen J, Lansimies E, Tuppurainen T, Partanen K 1987 The effect of thoracic epidural analgesia on respiratory function after cholecystectomy. Acta Anaesthesiol Scand 31: 645–651

Heneghan C P H, Jones J G 1985 Pulmonary gas exchange and diaphragmatic position: effect of tonic phrenic stimulation compared with that of increased airway pressure. Br J Anaesth 57: 1161–1166

Hills B A 1990 The role of lung surfactant. Br J Anaesth 65: 13–29

Hornbein T F, Martin W E, Bonica J J 1969 Nitrous oxide effects on the circulatory and respiratory responses to halothane. Anesthesiology 31: 250–260

Hurford W E, Kolker A C, Strauss H W 1987 The use of ventilation/perfusion lung scans to predict oxygenation during one-lung anesthesia. Anesthesiology 67: 841–844

Jaffe R S, Moldenhauer C C, Hug C C, Finlayson D C, Tobia V, Kopel M E 1988 Nalbuphine antagonism of fentanyl-induced ventilatory depression: a randomized trial. Anesthesiology 68: 254–260

Jayr C, Mollie A, Bourgain J L, Alarcon J, Masselot J, Lasser P 1988 Postoperative pulmonary complications: general anesthesia with postoperative parenteral morphine compared with epidural analgesia. Surgery 104: 57–63

Jones J G 1987 Anaesthesia, and atelectasis: the role of V_{TAB} and the chest wall. Br J Anaesth 59: 949–953

Jones J G, Faithfull D, Jordan C, Minty B 1979 Rib cage movement during halothane anaesthesia in man. Br J Anaesth 51: 399–407

Jones J G, Jordan C, Scavin B, Lehane J R 1987 Prophylactic effect of aminophylline and salbutamol on histamine-

induced bronchoconstriction. Br J Anaesth 59: 498–502
Jones R D M, Jones J G 1980 Intrathecal morphine: naloxone reverses respiratory depression but not analgesia. Br Med J 281: 645
Jones R M, Rosen M, Seymour L 1987 Smoking and anaesthesia. Anaesthesia 42: 1–2
Jordan C, Lehane J R, Robson P J, Jones J G 1979 A comparison of the respiratory effects of meptazinol, pentazocine and morphine. Br J Anaesth 51: 497–502
Jordan C, Lehane J R, Jones J G, Altman D G, Royston J P 1981 Specific conductance using forced airflow oscillation in mechanically ventilated human subjects. J Appl Physiol 51: 715–724
Kjaeve J, Bjertnaes L J 1989 Interaction of verapamil and halogenated anesthetics on hypoxic pulmonary vasoconstriction. Acta Anaesthesiol Scand 33: 193–198
Knill R L, Bright S, Manninen P 1978 Hypoxic ventilatory responses during thiopentone sedation and anaesthesia in man. Can Anaesth Soc J 25: 366–372
Knill R L, Clement J L, Thompson W R 1981 Epidural morphine causes delayed and prolonged ventilatory depression. Can Anaesth Soc J 28: 537–543
Knill R L, Gelb A W 1982 Peripheral chemoreceptors during anesthesia: are the watchdogs sleeping? Anesthesiology 57: 151–152
Knill R L, Clement J L 1984 Site of selective action of halothane on the peripheral chemoreflex pathway in humans. Anesthesiology 61: 121–126
Krayer S, Rehder K, Vetterman J, Didier E P, Ritman E L 1989 Position and motion of human diaphragm during anesthesia-paralysis. Anesthesiology 70: 891–898
Kurth C D, Spitzer A R, Broennle A M, Downes J J 1987 Postoperative apnea in preterm infants. Anesthesiology 66: 483–488
Leblanc P, Ruff F, Milic-Emili J 1970 Effects of age and body position on airway closure in man. J Appl Physiol 28: 448–451
Lehane J R, Jordan C, Jones J G 1980 Influence of halothane and enflurane on respiratory airflow resistance and specific conductance in anaesthetized man. Br J Anaesth 52: 773–780
Lindahl S G E, Yates A P, Hatch D J 1987 Respiratory depression in children at different end tidal halothane concentrations. Anaesthesia 42: 1267–1275
McKay W P S, Moble W H 1988 Critical incidents detected by pulse oximetry during anaesthesia. Can J Anaesth 35: 265–269
McKenna M J, Wilson R S, Bothello R J 1988 Right upper lobe obstruction with right-sided double-lumen endotracheal tubes: a comparison of two tube types. J Cardiothorac Anesth 2: 734–740
Mankikian B, Cantineau J P, Sartene R, Clergue F, Viars P 1986 Ventilatory pattern and chest wall mechanics during ketamine anesthesia in humans. Anesthesiology 65: 492–499
Mankikian B, Cantineau J P, Bertrand M, Kieffer E, Sartens R, Viars P 1988 Improvement of diaphragmatic function by a thoracic extradural block after upper abdominal surgery. Anesthesiology 68: 379–386
Mansell A, Bryan A C, Levison H 1972 Airway closure in children. J Appl Physiol 33: 711–714
Marjot R, Valentine S J 1990 Arterial oxygen saturation following premedication for cardiac surgery. Br J Anaesth 64: 737–740
Marshall C, Lindgren L, Marshall B E 1984 Effects of halothane, enflurane and isoflurane on hypoxic pulmonary vasoconstriction in rat lung in vitro. Anesthesiology 60: 304–308
Mather S J 1987 Ondine's curse and the anaesthetist. Anaesthesia 42: 394–403
Miller M R, Pinock A C, Oates G D, Wilkinson R, Skene-Smith H 1990 Upper airway obstruction due to goitre: detection, prevalence and results of surgical management. Q J Med 274: 177–188
Morgan M, Lumley J, Whitwam J G 1977 Respiratory effects of etomidate. Br J Anaesth 49: 233–235
Muller N, Volgyesi G, Becker L, Bryan M A, Bryan A C 1979 Diaphragmatic muscle tone. J Appl Physiol 47: 279–284
Murat I, Chaussain M, Hamza J, Saint-Maurice C1 1987. The respiratory effects of isoflurane, enflurane and halothane in spontaneously breathing children. Anaesthesia 42: 711–718
Nunn J F, Milledge J S, Chen D, Dore C 1988 Respiratory criteria of fitness for surgery and anaesthesia. Anaesthesia 43: 543–551
O' Connor M, Tatershall M P, Carter J A 1988 An evaluation of the incentive spirometer to improve lung function after cholecystectomy. Anaesthesia 43: 785–787
Olsson G L 1987 Bronchospasm during anaesthesia. A computer-aided incidence study of 136,929 patients. Acta Anaesthesiol Scand 31: 244–252
Orlando R, Gluck E H, Cohen M, Mesologitis C G 1988 Ultra-high-frequency jet ventilation in a bronchopleural fistula model. Arch Surg 123: 591–596
Pietak S, Weenig C S, Hickey R F, Fairley H B 1975 Anesthetic effects on ventilation in patients with chronic obstructive pulmonary disease. Anesthesiology 42: 160–166
Pugh G C, Brown D T, Drummond G B 1989 Effect of nalbuphine hydrochloride on the ventilatory and occlusion pressure responses to carbon dioxide in volunteers. Br J Anaesth 62: 601–609
Rafferty T D, Ruskis A, Sasaki C, Gee J B 1980 Perioperative considerations in the management of tracheotomy for the obstructive sleep apnoea patient. Br J Anaesth 52: 619–621
Register S D, Downs J B, Stock M C, Kirby R R 1987 Is 50% oxygen harmful? Crit Care Med 15: 598–601
Remmers J E, Issa F G, Suratt P M 1990 Conference report: sleep and respiration. J Appl Physiol 68: 1286–1289
Rigg J R A, Rondi P 1981 Changes in rib cage and diaphragm contribution to ventilation after morphine. Anesthesiology 55: 507–514
Robertson B J, Clement J L, Knill R L 1981 Enhancement of the arrhythmogenic effect of hypercarbia by surgical stimulation during halothane anaesthesia in man. Can Anaesth Soc J 28:342–349
Roth M D, Wright J W, Bellamy P E 1988 Gas flow through a bronchopleural fistula: measuring the effects of high-frequency jet ventilation and chest-tube suction. Chest 93: 210–213
Roukema J A, Carol E J, Prins J G 1988 The prevention of pulmonary complications after upper abdominal surgery in patients with non-compromised pulmonary status. Arch Surg 123: 30–34
Sampaio M M, Crean P M, Keilty S R, Black G W 1989 Changes in oxygen saturation during inhalation induction of anaesthesia in children. Br J Anaesth 62: 199–201

Scott N B, Mogenson T, Bigler D, Lund C, Kehlet H 1989 Continuous thoracic extradural 0.5% bupivacaine with or without morphine: effect on quality of blockade, lung function and the surgical stress response. Br J Anaesth 62: 253–257

Selsby D S 1989 Chest physiotherapy may be harmful in some patients. Br Med J 298: 541–542

Selsby D S, Jones J G 1990 Some physiological and clinical aspects of chest physiotherapy. Br J Anaesth 64: 621–631

Smith T C, Marini J J 1988 Impact of PEEP on lung mechanics in severe airflow obstruction. J Appl Physiol 65: 1488–1499

Spinale F G, Linker R W, Crawford F A, Reines H D 1989 Conventional versus high frequency jet ventilation with a bronchopleural fistula. J Surg Res 46: 147–151

Starling E H 1896 On the absorption of fluids from the connective tissue spaces. J Physiol 19: 312–326

Strandberg A, Tokics L, Brismar B, Lundquist H, Hedenstierna G 1987 Constitutional factors promoting atelectasis during anaesthesia. Acta Anaesthesiol Scand 31: 21–24

Tabatabai M, Kitahata L M, Collins J G 1989 Disruption of the rhythmic activity of the medullary inspiratory neurons and phrenic nerve by fentanyl and reversal with nalbuphine. Anesthesiology 70: 489–495

Tait A R, Knight P R 1987 The effects of general anesthesia on upper respiratory tract infections in children. Anesthesiology 67: 930–935

Tarhan S, Moffit E A, Sessler A D 1973 Risk of anesthesia and surgery in patients with chronic bronchitis and chronic obstructive pulmonary disease. Surgery 74: 720–726

Taylor M B, Grounds R M, Molrooney P D, Morgan M 1986 Ventilatory effects of propofol during induction of anaesthesia. Anaesthesia 41: 816–820

Tierney N M, Pollard B J, Doran B R H 1989 Obstructive sleep apnoea. Anaesthesia 44: 235–237

Tobias J D, Hirshman C A 1990 Antagonism of histamine-induced bronchoconstriction. Anesthesiology 72: 1103

Tusiewicz K, Bryan A C, Froese A B 1977 Contributions of changing rib cage-diaphragm interactions to the ventilatory depression of halothane anesthesia. Anesthesiology 47: 327–337

VadeBoncouer T R, Riegler F X, Gautt R S, Weinberg G L 1989 A randomized, double-blind comparison of the effects of interpleural bupivacaine and saline on morphine requirements and pulmonary function after cholecystectomy. Anesthesiology 71: 339–343

Vetterman J, Warner D O, Brichant J, Rehder K 1989 Halothane decreases both tissue and airway resistances in excised canine lungs. J Appl Physiol 66: 2698–2703

Warner M A, Tinker J H, Divertie M B, 1983 Preoperative cessation of smoking and pulmonary complications in pulmonary dysfunction. Anesthesiology 59: A60

Weil J V, McCullogh R E, Kline J S, Sodal I E 1975 Diminished ventilatory response to hypoxia and hypercapnia after morphine in normal man. N Engl J Med 292: 1103–1106

Wellborn L G, Ramirez N, OH T E, Ruttimann U E, Fink R, Guzzetta P, Epstein B S 1986 Postanesthetic apnea and periodic breathing in infants. Anesthesiology 65: 658–661

Wellborn L G, Hannallah R S, Fink R, Ruttimann U E, Hicks J M 1989 High-dose caffeine suppresses postoperative apnea in former preterm infants. Anesthesiology 71: 347–349

Wheatley R G, Somerville I D, Sapsford D J, Jones J G 1990 Postoperative hypoxaemia: comparison of extradural, i.m. and patient-controlled opioid analgesia. Br J Anaesth 64: 267–275

Yacoub O, Doell D, Kryger M H, Anthonisen N R 1976 Depression of hypoxic ventilatory response by nitrous oxide. Anesthesiology 45: 385–389

5

Nervous system disorders and the safety of anaesthesia

P. J. O'Shea

INTRODUCTION

This chapter deals with the problems and safety of anaesthesia in patients with pre-existing nervous system disorders, starting with the central nervous system (CNS) and progressing towards the peripheral nervous system. It also covers some disorders of muscle.

PROBLEMS DUE TO RAISED INTRACRANIAL PRESSURE

Because of the rigid cranium, any change in the volume of one of the three components it contains – brain, cerebrospinal fluid (CSF) or blood – must be reflected by a reciprocal change in one or both of the others if intracranial pressure (ICP) is to remain unaltered. Raised intracranial pressure will occur if the increase in volume of one of the components is greater than can be accommodated. If intracranial pressure is low or normal, then a small increase in intracranial volume may produce either no change or a very small increase in ICP. If, however, intracranial pressure is already raised, then the small increase in volume within the rigid cranium will cause gross elevation of ICP (Fig. 5.1). Elevation of ICP without a change in blood pressure will reduce cerebral perfusion pressure (CPP) according to the equation below:

$$mCPP = mAP - mICPP$$

where mCPP = mean cerebral perfusion pressure, mAP = mean arterial pressure and mICP = mean intracranial pressure.

Under normal circumstances cerebral blood flow is kept constant over a wide range of blood pressure (Fig. 5.2). In conditions of raised ICP, autoregulation is absent and the intracranial pressure is more than usually dependent on the three main factors affecting the cerebral circulation, namely arterial pressure, carbon dioxide tension and oxygen tension.

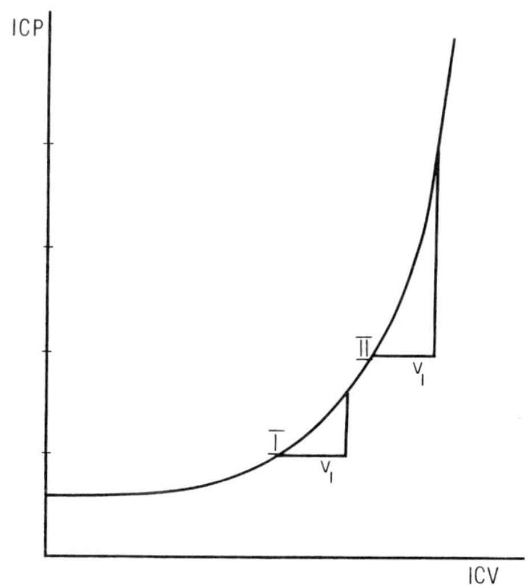

Fig. 5.1 The relationship between intracranial pressure (ICP) and intracranial volume (ICV).

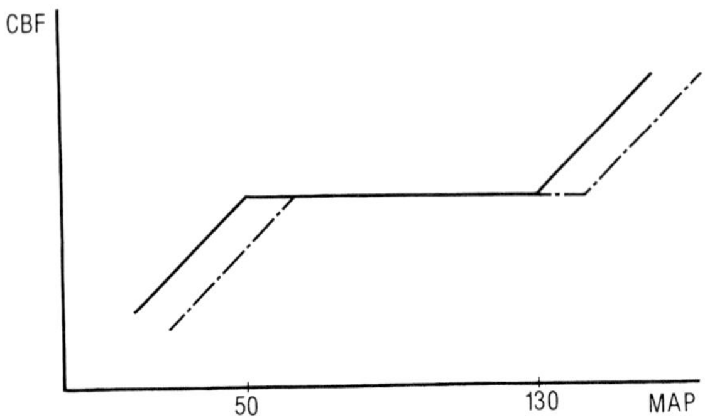

Fig. 5.2 Autoregulation of cerebral blood flow (CBF) over the normal range of mean arterial pressure (MAP). The dotted lines show the shift of the autoregulatory curve to the right in consequence of systemic hypertension or haemorrhage.

Cerebral blood flow and systemic blood pressure

The cerebral circulation autoregulates within a range of mean blood pressure from 50–130 mmHg in awake normotensive and normocapnic subjects, thus maintaining a constant flow as shown in Figure 5.2. In hypertensive patients, or following acute haemorrhage, the autoregulatory curve is shifted to the right (Fitch 1976), and the cerebral blood flow may fall to a critical level at a higher mean arterial pressure compared to normotensive and normovolaemic patients. In the presence of raised ICP a fall in blood pressure may produce an even greater decrease in blood flow. Such patients are therefore more vulnerable to general or localized cerebral ischaemia due to inadequate cerebral perfusion, especially in the 'boundary zones' where the final branches of the vascular supply from the major cerebral arteries meet. Ischaemic damage will cause further cerebral oedema and this in turn will raise the ICP. The importance of maintaining CPP under anaesthesia in patients with intracranial hypertension cannot be overemphasized.

At the other end of the cerebral blood flow curve, it can be seen that increases in mean arterial pressure above the upper limit of autoregulation will cause a 'breakthrough', where cerebral blood flow is directly proportional to blood pressure. Excessive pressure will over-distend the vessel walls. This will allow the exudation of proteinaceous fluid into the interstitial space, thus giving rise to vasogenic oedema. This is the mechanism of cerebral oedema formation in hypertensive crisis. In the presence of intracranial hypertension, ICP is dependent on blood pressure and acute excessive blood pressure elevation must be avoided. Surges in blood pressure can occur on laryngoscopy and following a painful stimulus if anaesthesia is inadequate. Many methods of preventing hypertension in these circumstances have been recommended, but the use of a short-acting opiate, such as fentanyl, prior to intubation is simple and effective.

Arterial carbon dioxide tension and cerebral blood flow

Cerebral blood flow is sensitive to changes in the arterial carbon dioxide tension within the physiological range shown in Figure 5.3. This effect is due to the local hydrogen ion concentration affecting the vascular resistance. The curve is flattened at either end, for at the lower end of the curve the cerebral vessels are maximally constricted and at the other end they are maximally dilated. The vasoconstrictive effect of hypocapnia is maximal at around 2.6 kPa, but this effect is overcome by hypoxia, due to the severely reduced blood flow, so if hyperventilation is used as a part of the anaesthetic technique the carbon dioxide

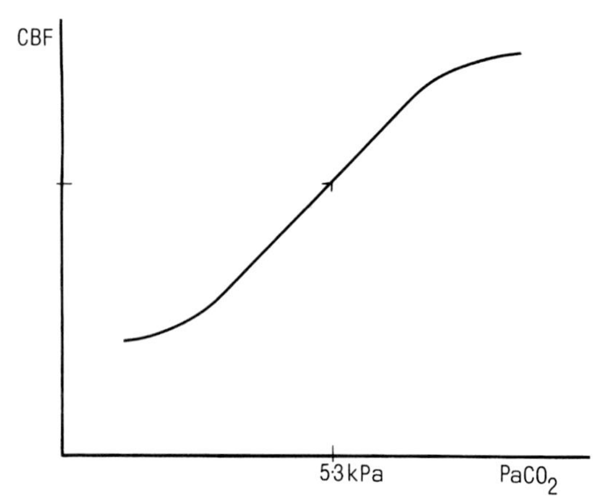

Fig. 5.3 The effect of change in the arterial carbon dioxide tension ($Paco_2$) on cerebral blood flow (CBF).

tension (or end-tidal carbon dioxide) should be monitored and kept at around 4 kPa. A rise in the arterial carbon dioxide tension will cause cerebral vasodilation and increased cerebral blood volume. In the normal situation this effect would be insignificant but in the presence of raised ICP hypercapnia will increase the intracranial pressure further and may reduce cerebral perfusion to critical levels. Control of arterial CO_2 is therefore vitally important during anaesthesia for patients with raised ICP.

Intracerebral 'steal'

In the presence of hypercarbia, blood may be diverted away from vessels in the region of cerebral pathology, where there is local tissue hypoxia, to vessels in normal regions of the brain. Two mechanisms are proposed to explain this phenomenon:

1. In the pathological region, local tissue hypoxia ensures maximally dilated vessels, but in the surrounding areas the vasculature retains the normal response to carbon dioxide tension. If hypercapnia occurs, the normal vasculature dilates and in the presence of a finite perfusion pressure there is a loss or 'steal' of blood away from the vessels of the pathological area, thus promoting further local hypoxia.
2. The other mechanism is thought to be due to hypercapnia causing vasodilatation, and so an increase in the cerebral blood volume with consequent increased intracranial pressure. This, in the presence of low intracranial compliance, will reduce the CPP and therefore the blood flow in the pathological area devoid of autoregulation.

In either case, hypercapnia by means of mechanical ventilation will reverse the situation because vasoconstriction of the normal vasculature will divert blood into the vasculature of the pathological area. This is referred to as 'inverse steal'. It is therefore obvious that control of the arterial carbon dioxide tension is an important part of the management of these patients.

Arterial oxygen tension and the cerebral blood flow

Changes in the arterial oxygen tension do not produce any changes in cerebral blood flow unless the tension falls to 7 kPa or less, when rapid cerebral vasodilation occurs with a concomitant increase in the cerebral blood flow. If at the same time the carbon dioxide tension is raised above normal, the increase in cerebral blood flow and blood volume (and hence the increase in intracranial pressure) is greater than that produced by either hypoxia or hypercarbia alone. The anaesthetist should prevent extreme fluctuation in blood pressure and endeavour to maintain adequate CPP. The difficulty is defining exactly what the CPP should be in the presence of raised intracranial pressure.

ANAESTHETIC DRUGS ADVERSELY AFFECTING INTRACRANIAL PRESSURE

Nitrous oxide

Although nitrous oxide is a cerebral vasodilator, cerebral blood flow remains constant because it reduces the cerebral metabolic rate. Nitrous oxide does not affect autoregulation and it is an acceptable agent in neuroanaesthesia. Any rise that does occur can be prevented by prior administration of thiopentone and limited by hyperventilation. However, there are two situations where nitrous oxide should be avoided. The first is where air persists in the ventricles following pneumoencephalography. The administration of nitrous oxide to such a patient, especially if the intracranial compliance is low, would raise the intracranial pressure due to the nitrous oxide entering the air-filled space faster than the nitrogen leaves. Following pneumoencephalography, air persists for 48 hours but has occasionally been found for 5 days. The second situation is where a patient is suffering from severe intracranial hypertension. In these circumstances, nitrous oxide administration would raise the intracranial pressure even higher. It is therefore better to avoid nitrous oxide until after intubation and the institution of hyperventilation.

Halogenated anaesthetics

All volatile agents cause cerebral vasodilatation and an increase in the cerebral blood volume, and this causes an increase in ICP. The extent of the rise in ICP depends upon the concentration of the agent and, its effects on the arterial carbon dioxide tension and the cardiovascular system. Even if normocarbia is maintained, volatile agents such as halothane, trichloroethylene, methoxyflurane and enflurane produce greater increases in intracranial pressure in patients with space-occupying lesions than in patients with normal intracranial pressure (Shapiro 1975). If spontaneous respiration with a volatile agent is permitted in the presence of intracranial hypertension, any concomitant rise in the arterial carbon dioxide tension would lead to further serious increases in the intracranial pressure. Furthermore, a concomitant fall in the systemic blood pressure reduces the CPP to critical or inadequate levels. Hyperventilation, osmotic agents and hypothermia may attenuate the increase in intracranial pressure due to the administration of a volatile agent, but should not be relied upon.

It is better, therefore, that halogenated volatile agents are avoided in patients with extensive head injuries and tumours, and in patients with impaired consciousness following an ischaemic episode. If a volatile agent is required it should not be introduced before the bone flap and dura have been raised (so that the brain is exposed to atmospheric pressure), the 'tightness' of the brain or the intraventricular pressure has been assessed and CSF drainage has, if necessary, been performed. It has been recommended that if a volatile agent is to be used, at least 10 min hyperventilation should first be carried out to reduce the cerebral vasodilatation, but, even then, rises in ICP may occur. Of the volatile agents, isoflurane is the agent of choice since it does not produce seizure activity and, provided hyperventilation has been instituted, a comparatively smaller increase in intracranial pressure will occur.

The role of isoflurane in neurosurgical anaesthesia is not yet fully settled as rises in intracranial pressure have been observed, despite prior institution of hyperventilation in some patients with head injuries and with tumours causing lateral shift of midline structures (Grosslight et al 1985).

Adverse effects of intravenous anaesthetic agents

Ketamine increases ICP, cerebral blood flow and cerebral metabolic rate with reduced CPP (Takeshita et al 1971), and these untoward effects have been demonstrated in patients with intracranial lesions (Shapiro et al 1972). Although contraindicated in neuroanaesthesia generally, ketamine has been used for diagnostic procedures in patients with intracranial lesions, and intramuscularly for radiotherapy in children undergoing treatment for medulloblastoma. Other methods of anaesthesia are probably more appropriate but, if ketamine is to be used, ready access to CSF drainage should be available.

Narcotic analgesics

Morphine has little effect on the cerebral blood flow in normocarbic patients and neurolept anaesthesia is a recommended technique for patients with low intracranial compliance. Problems may arise if the opiate is allowed to cause respiratory depression with carbon dioxide retention, thus increasing the cerebral blood volume and ICP. Hence, long-acting opiates should be avoided altogether and, if there is any question of opiate-induced respiratory depression, mechanical ventilation should be employed immediately.

Muscle relaxants

Non-depolarizing muscle relaxants should not affect the ICP provided the patient is normocarbic and no histamine release occurs. Suxamethonium may cause a transient rise in the ICP due to the muscle fasciculations raising the intraabdominal and intrathoracic pressure which, in turn, will raise the central and intracerebral venous pressures. It is therefore recommended that a small dose of non-depolarizing muscle relaxant is administered beforehand.

PRE-ANAESTHETIC PROBLEMS PECULIAR TO PATIENTS WITH RAISED ICP

Deficient airway protection occurs in patients who are unconscious or where there is cranial nerve deficit. There is a danger of respiratory obstruction or lack of protection of the airways against aspiration of gastric contents.

Respiratory tract infection may be present in the unconscious patient either due to absent cough reflex or following inhalation of gastric contents.

Dehydration and electrolyte disturbance may occur following deliberate fluid restriction or induced osmotic diuresis to reduce intracranial pressure by the reduction of brain water content.

Dexamethasone may have been received by patients with raised ICP, especially those with intracranial tumours. It is important that precautions are taken against the potential problem of gastric erosions by the administration of antacids and a histamine receptor antagonist. This therapy may need to be prolonged. Hyperglycaemia may also be noted.

PROBLEMS ASSOCIATED WITH HEAD INJURIES

The anaesthetist has an important role to play in the immediate care of head injuries. Aggressive treatment reduces the mortality rate without increasing the number of patients in a vegetative or severely disabled state (Becker et al 1977). Following the primary brain injury, secondary effects often occur. An obstructed airway, hypotension and epileptic fits are the chief secondary effects that are amenable to anaesthetic management. About 30% of head-injured patients have extracranial injuries and these may require surgical treatment under general anaesthesia.

The most severe brain injury is due to the formation of intracranial haematoma with cerebral oedema and ischaemia, due either to vascular disruption or to severely raised tissue pressure. There are three types of intracranial haematoma, the least severe of which is the **extradural haematoma**. This is a result of rupture of the meningeal vessels or middle meningeal artery due to a fracture. **Subdural haematomata** are due to the rupture of the bridging vessels causing a haematoma between the dura and arachnoid. If acute, there is usually severe primary brain injury, but symptoms and signs may develop over several days. This may happen in the elderly or in patients taking oral anticoagulants. **Intracerebral haematoma** occurs when severe primary brain injury has been sustained and, as with severe acute subdural haematoma, the outcome is often poor.

Both 'cytotoxic' and 'vasogenic' cerebral oedema occur in head injuries and both raise the intracranial pressure. The former is due to cellular swelling following trauma or ischaemia, the latter to the disruption of the blood–brain barrier with exudation of proteinaceous fluid into the interstitial space. If hypotension should occur after injury, cerebral perfusion will fall and the brain is rendered more ischaemic.

Autoregulation is impaired regionally in the first week following severe injury. This means that the cerebral blood flow varies passively with the MAP or CPP. At the same time the response of the cerebral circulation to carbon dioxide is impaired. The anaesthetist may become involved with the head-injured patient in many ways. The role of the anaesthetist in the management of head injury in the accident and emergency department or intensive therapy unit is outside the scope of this book, but the sequence – **airway, breathing, circulation** – is as important here as in any other emergency.

Airway

A clear airway must be maintained and this may prove difficult in patients with complicating spinal or maxillofacial injury. Thiopentone in hypovolaemic patients may cause severe hypotension and should therefore be used with care. Before using succinylcholine the patient must be pretreated with a small dose of non-depolarizing muscle relaxant to prevent fasciculations, which will cause a rise in the central venous pressure and thus increase cerebral venous pressure. Even so, anaesthesia must be adequate as laryngoscopy may increase blood pressure and heart rate which, in the absence of autoregulation, will cause a further increase in intracranial pressure, haemorrhage and/or further 'vasogenic' oedema. To prevent this hypertensive response to laryngoscopy, 1.5 mg/kg lignocaine has been advocated (Wilson et al 1991). Although beta blockers have been used to prevent this effect of laryngoscopy in elective neuroanaesthetic practice, these are best avoided in a situation where there may be hypovolaemia or dehydration.

Breathing

Controlled hyperventilation will induce vasoconstriction in the cerebral vasculature that has retained the CO_2 response, thus reducing the intracranial pressure and creating an 'inverse steal'. The respiratory alkalosis will also help against the regional cerebral acidosis as a pool for the acid ions. If in spite of intermittent positive pressure ventilation (IPPV) there is persistent hypoxaemia, positive end-expiratory pressure (PEEP) up to 10 cmH_2O is well tolerated if the patient's head is raised 30 degrees. If there is poor pulmonary compliance, due to pulmonary contusions or neurogenic pulmonary oedema, the effect of PEEP on the venous pressure is reduced.

Circulation

The cardiovascular system should be maintained as close to physiological normality as possible. Hypertension may occur as a reaction to maintain cerebral perfusion in the presence of intracranial hypertension. If the systolic blood pressure rises above 170–180 mmHg, this should be treated as further intracranial bleeding may occur. Hypotension is rare in closed-head injuries, so if present it should be aggressively treated and associated injuries sought, even if not apparent.

Anaesthesia in the head-injured patient

Even for minor extracranial procedures, anaesthesia with muscular relaxation and hyperventilation must be used, as this technique reduces the intracranial pressure. Anaesthesia using spontaneous ventilation with a volatile agent is contraindicated as this will raise ICP because of cerebral vasodilation due to effects of the volatile agent and the raised arterial carbon dioxide tension.

Transporting the head-injured patient

Initial resuscitation should provide a safe airway, adequate respiration, good intravenous access, cardiovascular stability and an empty stomach. If the patient requires transfer, the admitting team should be consulted after summarizing the history and treatment so far, so that any further necessary measures can be taken. Patients with severe head injuries should be intubated and ventilated prior to transfer. For the actual transfer there must be adequate means of ventilation with sufficient amounts of diazemuls, thiopentone, and non-depolarizing muscle relaxant to prevent any coughing and bucking and for treating epileptiform convulsions should they occur. The anaesthetist should also ensure that appropriate monitoring, life-support systems and drugs are available.

Anaesthesia in the X-ray department for the head-injured patient

Requests are often made for the sedation of restless patients in the X-ray department or CAT scanning room. Often it is suggested that only sedation is required, but this can be dangerous. Sedation may turn out to be inadequate with the danger that too much drug may be given leading to depression of consciousness. Respiratory obstruction may follow and intubation be required. It is far better to give a light anaesthetic with intubation, neuromuscular paralysis and hyperventilation which can easily be reversed. In other words anaesthesia is indicated if any of the following apply:

- the Glasgow coma scale is less than 12
- there is any doubt about the airway
- the patient is restless and uncooperative.

Although Gelb et al (1984) warn that extra precautions are required in the X-ray department due to the lack of anaesthetic equipment, this situation should not be tolerated by those in charge of anaesthetic departments. It is true, however, that there is often a lack of space, great distance between the patient and the anaesthetic machine and the potential for complications with angiographic dyes and catheters. Furthermore, the anaesthetist is more often without assistance in the X-ray department. The anaesthetist must be wary of undiagnosed injury at all times.

Neurogenic pulmonary oedema

Neurogenic pulmonary oedema has been recognized for a long time and carries with it a mortality rate that may be as high as 90%. This subject has recently been discussed by Casey (1983), Wauchob et al (1984) and Demling & Riessen (1990). Neurogenic pulmonary oedema occurs in patients with raised ICP and may therefore occur in those with head injuries, subarachnoid haemorrhage, cerebral tumour, cerebral emboli and chronically raised ICP. It may be triggered by a painful stimulus if anaesthesia is inadequate. In patients with head injury, neurogenic pulmonary oedema will usually present within 24 hours of the insult. Sometimes the patient will also have had periods of lucidity but then deteriorates, with pulmonary oedema following shortly afterwards. The mechanism seems to be that following the hypothalamic disturbance, due to the raised ICP, there is a massive sympathetic discharge with an increase in both the systemic and pulmonary blood pressures, resulting in a shift of blood from the systemic to the pulmonary circulation. This causes engorgement of pulmonary veins and the left atrium.

Endothelial damage to the pulmonary vessels occurs due to the massive increase in the pulmonary capillary pressure, with consequent leakage of proteinaceous fluid thus forming pulmonary oedema. The fact that the protein concentration of the oedema fluid is almost that of plasma supports the evidence for capillary damage. Treatment of neurogenic pulmonary oedema is directed not only towards the pulmonary problems, but also to the raised intracranial pressure and any concomitant cardiovascular instability.

Respiratory treatment

IPPV with raised inspired oxygen should be instituted with PEEP of 10 cmH_2O pressure (PEEP + 10). Due to poor lung compliance PEEP + 10 will not affect the ICP through venous back-pressure.

Reduction of intracranial pressure

Hyperventilation will help to reduce the ICP. Ventriculostomy, CSF drainage and/or surgical decompression would be performed if necessary. Steroids and mannitol will almost certainly have been given already. Further administration of mannitol may be deleterious. This is because there will be an initial increase in the circulating blood volume and mannitol molecules may pass through the damaged pulmonary capillary endothelium, thus increasing pulmonary oedema. It may be more prudent to give diuretics, such as frusemide, in large doses (e.g. 2 mg/kg). Even this may not be effective, since the action of this drug is dependent on renal blood flow and this may be reduced due to the intense sympathetic vasoconstriction. Intravenous sedation will be required, although the choice of drug is now limited. If not required continuously, sedatives should certainly be given before manoeuvres such as physiotherapy.

Adrenergic receptor blockade

Various alpha-adrenergic blocking agents have been used to reverse the vasoconstriction, including chlorpromazine, phentolamine and droperidol. Sodium nitroprusside, although not an adrenergic receptor blocker, may be used in the acute stage. If tachycardia or dysrhythmias occur, beta-receptor blockade may be required, but it should be noted that *prior* treatment with beta blockers may worsen the function of the already strained myocardium (Wauchob et al 1984). If the myocardium is strained due to the sympathetic vasoconstriction then inotropic support may be required. The drugs of choice for controlled infusion are isoprenaline or dobutamine as these have no alpha-agonist activity.

Fluid restriction

Intravenous crystalloid fluids should be restricted to prevent further cerebral oedema and pulmonary oedema, but must be adequate to maintain renal function.

Pulmonary dysfunction following head injury

Apart from neurogenic pulmonary oedema, there are other causes of pulmonary dysfunction causing hypoxaemia that appear related to the degree of head injury. Hypoxaemia in the head-injured must be treated aggressively. The hypermetabolic state that occurs after severe head injury will also compound hypoxaemia and should be managed with nutritional support (Demling & Riessen 1990).

Hyperkalaemia in closed-head-injury patients without paresis following succinylcholine

Hyperkalaemia may occur following succinylcholine administration in patients with closed-head injury without appreciable skeletal muscle weakness but with evidence of upper motor neurone disease, that is present Babinski responses (Stevenson & Birch 1979, Frankville & Drummond 1987). The exact mechanism in this situation is not known as it does not seem to be the same as that in patients with prolonged immobility and paraplegia. Hyperkalaemia may also occur in patients with ruptured cerebral aneurysm who are given succinylcholine (Iwatsuki et al 1980).

SPINAL CORD INJURY

The anaesthetist is frequently involved in the immediate management of patients with spinal cord injury in the Accident and Emergency department. As there is a significant association between head injuries and neck injuries, it is important that the anaesthetist always suspects spinal cord injury in the head-injured patient until this has been excluded both clinically and radiologically. Spinal cord injuries may be missed because of:

- the circumstances surrounding the accident (including alcohol) or ambiance
- the absence of any initial serious neurodeficit
- multiple injuries
- radiographic/diagnostic errors
- failure to appreciate the mechanism of injury (Ravichandran 1989).

The anaesthetist must therefore be aware of these possibilities, especially if there are physiological disturbances which may be due to spinal shock or paralysis.

Injury to the spinal cord follows severe extension, flexion, rotation, or a combination of these severe movements, with or without fracture of vertebrae and disruption of ligaments. Herniation of an intervertebral disc may occur. The severity depends on the nature of the accident and the region of the vertebral column that suffers trauma. Obviously the cervical spine, which supports and allows mobility of the head, is the most vulnerable. The upper thoracic spine is more stable due to the splinting effect of the rib cage, but further down, at the thoracolumbar junction, is the most common site for cord transection. Fraser & Edmonds-Seal (1982) in their review article on spinal cord injuries discuss the mechanism of injury in greater detail.

Unless transection occurs, the anterior and posterior spinal arteries, which supply blood to the spinal cord, dura mater and arachnoid mater, remain intact. However, even minor cord compression may damage the intramedullary vasculature causing haemorrhage into the central grey matter. The accumulation of thrombus, and the joining and spreading of the haemorrhages over the next 4–6 hours, leads to oedema formation and ischaemia of the cord. Trauma also disrupts the autoregulation of cord blood flow which, together with hypotension due to spinal shock, leads to further hypoperfusion and ischaemia. Increased quantities of noradrenaline in the traumatized region may be an additional cause for vasospasm and cord hypoxia. For these reasons spinal lesions often ascend progressively over several hours. It is therefore important that therapeutic measures are directed towards preventing such spread and further trauma to the cord in the early stages.

As CNS neurones do not regenerate, the resulting neurological deficit depends on the severity of the intitial trauma and the success or failure of treatment in preventing the extension of cord damage. A complete cord lesion will block all neurological function below the lesion site. However, there are incomplete cord lesions, such as the Brown-Sequard syndrome, and anterior/posterior and central cord syndromes, in which different sensory and motor deficits occur.

If a cervical fracture is suspected, it should be immobilized by holding the neck in a neutral position with the aid of a collar. Conservative or early surgical treatment depends on the degree of instability. Conservative treatment may consist of traction applied via a halo or Crutchfield tongs. In the absence of neurological deficit or neurological deterioration, traction may be maintained for 3 months, but this poses considerable problems if the patient requires general anaesthesia for any other injury. In some patients, muscle spasm may prevent the reduction of a cervical dislocation which will then require induction of anaesthesia and muscle relaxation (Duke & Spreadbury 1983, Doolan & O'Brien 1985). Operative treatment is required if there is disc disruption with pain, spinal compression or instability.

Patients with thoracolumbar spine injuries are usually treated conservatively until spinal shock has passed. However, the trend is now for early posterior spinal fusion and insertion of Harrington rods, in order to obtain early stabilization of the spine and mobilization of the patient. This may mean anaesthetizing a patient who is in 'spinal shock'. Apart from this, the operation is associated with considerable blood and heat loss and a tendency to inferior vena cava obstruction. As the Harrington rods are used to distract the fractured spine, overdistraction may occur. The anaesthetic technique used should be one where the patient is woken intraoperatively to check the neurological status. Complete paraplegia due to overdistraction will recover if the distraction is immediately reduced.

Anaesthetic hazards in spinal injury

Spinal cord transection or injury from the anaesthetic point of view should be considered in two phases: Phase I, or 'spinal shock', from the time of injury to 3 weeks postinjury, and Phase II, or 'chronic stage', of spinal cord injury (Babinski 1987).

Early phase of spinal injury

Airway problems. An unstable cervical spine is a severe hazard if the airway is obstructed. Upper airway obstruction may follow facial injuries, or depressed consciousness due to head injury. Intubation may be indicated even at this hazardous stage. Intubation is best carried out in the presence of the surgeon, who stabilizes the head and, especially in the case of a flexion dislocation, controls the limited extension allowable for intubation. Intubation may be carried out with the patient awake or anaesthetized. Suxamethonium may cause fasciculations of the neck muscles which, if uncontrolled, may cause further damage to the cervical cord. Fasciculation may cause regurgitation of stomach contents and Sellick's manoeuvre may be difficult to apply adequately in stable flexion rotation injuries. The safest technique for those with expertise is probably using a fibre-optic bronchoscope in an awake or lightly sedated patient. Care must be taken to avoid oversedation and sleep, as the epiglottis will fall backwards into the oropharynx making even fibre-optic intubation difficult. Topical anaesthesia with lignocaine must be applied, otherwise the patient may cough and buck as the bronchoscope passes through the larynx. Tracheostomy with local anaesthesia has been suggested, but is hazardous in the presence of neck and head injury. In a dire emergency transtracheal ventilation via laryngostomy may be required.

Ventilatory problems. The effect of spinal cord injury depends on the segmental level at which the injury has occurred. Severe damage between C2 and C5 leads to diaphragmatic paralysis in addition to intercostal muscle paralysis. This necessitates IPPV. If the lesion is below C4 level, diaphragmatic action remains but not without an element of paradoxical respiration, as the intercostal muscles remain paralysed and on expiration the chest wall expands. The paradoxical movement of the chest wall disappears after a few weeks or months when the intercostal muscles pass into a phase of spastic paralysis. Luce (1984) has described the respiratory changes in paraplegic and quadriplegic patients in detail. Respiration rapidly becomes inadequate with hypoxia and hypercarbia, and secretions accumulate due to the ineffective cough. Thus in patients with high cervical cord injury early intervention with mechanical ventilation and physiotherapy is mandatory.

Body position in quadriplegic patients is important due to the abdominal muscle paralysis. If the body is positioned head-up, the abdominal contents will gravitate to the pelvis thus lowering the diaphragm. This will shorten the descent of the diaphragm in inspiration with no diaphragmatic rebound in expiration. Conversely, the head-down position will cause the abdominal contents to push up against the diaphragm restricting movement. The optimum position in these patients is therefore supine.

Pulmonary oedema. Pulmonary oedema may occur in up to 50% of cases of spinal cord injury and may be present immediately or during the first 48 hours after the injury. It is similar to neurogenic pulmonary oedema following head injury. The mechanism seems to be that following trauma there is short but massive autonomic discharge with systemic hypertension, bradycardia and dysrhythmias. Unlike neurogenic pulmonary oedema following head injury, the mechanism is independent of the brain but requires an intact cord between the site of trauma and the thoracic outflow, and seems to be due to direct mechanical stimulation of the sympathetic outflow tract. The extreme systemic and pulmonary vasoconstriction with high vascular pressures shifts blood into the central circulation increasing pulmonary capillary permeability, with proteinaceous pulmonary oedema or even alveolar haemorrhage, as in neurogenic pulmonary oedema following head injury. These events may also precipitate left ventricular failure. Subendocardial myocardial infarction may occur and in itself may cause heart failure.

Cardiovascular problems. There are two phases of cardiovascular response to spinal cord trauma. Compression of the cord causes an initial transient period of autonomic hyperactivity causing a hypertensive period, and this is soon followed by hypotension following paralysis of the autonomic system below the level of the trauma. By the time the patient reaches hospital he is usually in the hypotensive phase. If the trauma is above the segment of T4, the sympathetic outflow is totally paralysed and there is hypotension due to absence of vasomotor tone, and sinus bradycardia due to absence of sympathetic supply to the heart. Consequently, venous pooling with failure of venous return may occur with repositioning the patient or use of IPPV, both of which may therefore be hazardous. There have been reports of sudden death following change of patient position (Silver 1968). If the trauma is below T4 there is enough sympathetic outflow to control venous tone.

Abnormal respiratory tract reflexes. The usual response of the upper and lower respiratory tract to stimulation, such as laryngoscopy and intubation, is a rise in blood pressure accompanied by a tachycardia. In the normal situation the sympathetic response dominates the opposing vagal response, hence the tachycardia and hypertension. In patients with high cord transection or trauma the vagal nervous supply to the heart remains intact but the sympathetic outflow is lost, so the vagal stimulation causes bradycardia. As these patients may already have a bradycardia and a tendency to hypoxia due to inadequate ventilation, stimulation of the trachea may produce a vasovagal cardiac arrest. Therefore oxygen and atropine should be given prior to laryngoscopy and intubation or tracheobronchial suctioning (Dolfus & Frankel 1965, Frankel et al 1975).

Gastric aspiration and gastrointestinal problems. Patients with these problems are at risk of aspiration of gastric contents, especially if laryngeal reflexes are impaired and the supine position is required because of a cervical fracture. Gastric distension may be present due to pain, abdominal or spinal trauma, etc. Intubation will protect the airways from aspiration. However, even in those patients who do not require intubation, it is prudent to pass a nasogastric tube, and to give metoclopramide to encourage gastric emptying and alkali to lower the gastric acidity. Histamine (H_2) receptor antagonists are also widely used in such patients. The gastric atony that accompanies spinal cord trauma may lead to abdominal distension and this will compromise respiration as there is upward pressure on the diaphragm. This gastric distension may even progress to rupture. It is therefore important that the nasogastric tube is left in situ to keep the stomach decompressed. Following thoracolumbar fracture, paralytic ileus may last for 1–2 weeks and parenteral feeding may be required.

Long-term anaesthetic problems

Postural hypotension. In patients with lesions above T4, postural hypotension may be severe as described earlier. Those with lesions below this level may have postural hypotension to a lesser degree depending on how much of the cardiovascular reflexes remain. Sudden changes of posture may cause cardiac arrest due to lack of tone in capacitance vessels and consequently reduced venous return. Vascular tone will return to the capacitance vessels eventually, but this takes months.

Autonomic hyper-reflexia. After 10–14 days, due to changes in the spinal cord, autonomic hyper-reflexia, spasticity and involuntary muscle spasm occur. Spinal shock arises due to the absence of facilitatory impulses in presynaptic nerves from higher centres to the anterior horn cells. The endings of these divided presynaptic fibres become disorganized and there is a sympathetic and similar disorganization in neighbouring endings. Over the next 2 weeks the neighbouring presynaptic nerve-endings multiply and cover the area of postsynaptic membrane previously occupied by those of the damaged fibres. This arrangement is disorganized and so gives rise to inappropriate connections, and creates incoordinate reflexes with autonomic hyper-reflexia, spasticity and involuntary muscle spasm. This occurs most frequently in those patients with cord lesions above T7.

Classically, bladder distension is the mechanism that will trigger a massive autonomic response. In the segments below the level of injury there is massive vasoconstriction and hypertension. In response to this there is vasodilation, bradycardia, and facial flushing due to stimulation of aortic arch and carotid sinus baroreceptors. In this phase of hypertension there may be electrocardiogram (ECG) evidence of subendocardial ischaemia which may proceed to myocardial infarction and heart failure. Retinal, subarachnoid and intracerebral haemorrhage may occur, the latter being a common cause of death in these patients. In consequence of this, simple procedures and especially cystoscopy become hazardous. In the case of cystoscopy it should be realized that local anaesthesia to the mucosa does not prevent the problem.

Denervation sensitivity. Following spinal cord injury, denervated muscle becomes very sensitive to non-depolarizing muscle relaxants, and depolarization following suxamethonium administration causes rapid potassium efflux with a high incidence of dysrhythmias and cardiac arrest. This increased sensitivity to non-depolarizing muscle relaxants is due to the sensitivity to the muscle relaxant spreading from the motor endplate to the whole surface of the muscle fibre. This is in contrast to patients who have suffered a stroke (an upper motor neurone lesion) where there is reduced sensitivity to non-depolarizing muscle relaxants (Azar 1984). In clinical practice the important implications are whether or not the respiratory muscles are involved. Obviously if the respiratory muscles are involved then there is an increased risk of respiratory failure postoperatively. It is therefore important to reduce the dose of muscle relaxant. Monitoring of neuromuscular conduction will assist in this respect. This period of hypersensitivity develops over 8–10 days postinjury and lasts for 8–9 months (Fraser & Edmonds-Seal 1982).

Administration of suxamethonium to these patients immediately after trauma does not produce the high potassium efflux (but beware of suxamethonium administration in patients with multiple injuries). The period of vulnerability to hyperkalaemia seems to be present between 21 and 85 days postinjury, but this period has not been clearly defined (Azar 1984). Babinski (1987) gives a good and detailed account of the anaesthetic considerations in patients with spinal cord injury.

NEUROLOGICAL DISEASES INCREASING THE RISK OF ANAESTHESIA

Amyotrophic lateral sclerosis

Amyotrophic lateral sclerosis is a degenerative disease that affects motor neurones throughout the brain and the spinal cord. When it occurs it mainly affects males between 40 and 60 years of age. If limited to the motor cortex the disease is called primary lateral sclerosis, but pseudobulbar palsy if limited to the brain stem. Another condition similar to amyotrophic lateral sclerosis is Werdnig-Hoffmann disease which occurs in the first 3 years of life. The hazards associated with this type of condition are:

- pulmonary aspiration which may occur due to dysphagia and poor protective laryngeal reflexes as the bulbar involvement is an early manifestation of the disease
- hyperkalaemia following suxamethonium administration
- increased sensitivity to non-depolarizing muscle relaxants.

These patients have an electromyogram resembling that of patients suffering from myasthenia gravis. Carcinoma of the lung may also occur in association with the amyotrophic lateral sclerosis.

Friedreich's ataxia

This familial condition is due to degeneration of the spinocerebellar and pyramidal tracts. Apart from the presenting symptoms of ataxia, and associated symptoms of dysarthria and nystagmus, there is muscular weakness, atrophy and spasticity. There may also be scoliosis and/or cardiomyopathy. Cardiomyopathy is characterized by a hypertrophied and poorly compliant left ventricle (causing heart failure and death in adulthood). All the above problems increase the hazard of anaesthesia. These patients are sensitive to non-depolarizing muscle relaxants, and may develop chest infections and respiratory failure postoperatively. The cardiomyopathy makes intravenous induction of anaesthesia hazardous and the thiopentone dosage should be drastically reduced.

Huntington's chorea

Huntington's chorea is an inherited disease in which there is degeneration with atrophy of the caudate nucleus and, to a lesser degree, the putamen and globus pallidus. There are also biochemical abnormalities which include reduced gamma aminobutyric acid (GABA) concentrations, and increased dopamine and histamine concentrations, in the basal ganglia. The symptoms and signs are those of choreoathetosis and progressive dementia. The pharyngeal muscles are involved, so these patients may be susceptible to pulmonary aspiration.

There is a case report of delayed awakening and generalized tonic spasms following the administration of thiopentone (Davies 1966). Another case report concerns the prolonged effect of suxamethonium in one of these patients due to reduced plasma cholinesterase activity (Propert 1979). These patients may also be sensitive to non-depolarizing muscle relaxants (Lamont 1979).

Shy–Drager syndrome

The Shy-Drager syndrome was first described in 1960 (Shy & Drager 1960). It is characterized by disturbance of the autonomic nervous system with widespread nerve cell loss involving the CNS and spinal cord as well as multiple system atrophy. It usually presents in the 50–70 age group and progresses slowly to death, often due to syncope with cerebral ischaemia. This syndrome and the anaesthetic management have been described by Bevan (1979) and Hutchinson & Sugden (1984).

The main problems are related to hypotension, which has two main causes: failure of the sympathetic nervous system and reduced plasma volume due to abnornal renal function. Vocal cord paralysis with respiratory obstruction is another potential complication. This feature of the syndrome is not described in the original article by Shy & Drager (1960). Drury & Williams

(1991) describe a patient where vocal cord paralysis, with respiratory obstruction, occurred postoperatively and they discuss vocal cord paralysis in these patients. It may even be a presenting feature in some cases.

Hypotension due to pathology of the sympathetic nervous system causes orthostatic hypotension without a rise in pulse rate and venous pooling due to failure to respond normally to the valsalva manoeuvre. Therefore anaesthetic drugs that tend to lower the systemic blood pressure should be avoided. Controlled ventilation will cause hypotension. In order to counteract this effect a G-suit or, more conveniently, elastic stockings are recommended. Vasoconstrictors of the directly acting type have been used, but should be used with caution as denervation sensitivity with hypertension could occur. Indirect vasoconstrictors are of little value. Change of patient position must be carried out with great care, especially under anaesthesia, because of the risk of hypotension, and blood loss must be carefully replaced as the sympathetic response to haemorrhage is absent.

Hypotension due to reduced plasma volume is due to nocturnal or recumbent polyuria and nocturesis causing an exaggerated fluid loss and hence more severe postural hypotension in the morning. In other words, there is postural variation in renal function (Bevan 1979). This problem can be overcome by the use of elastic stockings, the preoperative administration of 9-fluorohydrocortisone and careful administration of crystalloids and/or colloids. If the patient is regularly on 9-fluorohydrocortisone the beneficial effect lessens over a year or so. Fluid loading with crystalloids and/or colloids will lessen the chance of hypotension. Hutchinson & Sugden (1984) described a patient very sensitive to fluid imbalance who easily moved from fluid underload to overload with consequent heart failure. They therefore used a balloon-tipped flotation catheter to monitor the pulmonary artery wedge pressure.

Riley–Day syndrome (dysautonomia)

Riley–Day syndrome (familial dysautonomia) is a rare autosomal recessive neurological disease presenting from birth and usually involving Jewish children. Although most of the nervous system is involved, the autonomic and peripheral neuronal elements are of most concern to the anaesthetist. A decrease in activity of sympathetic, parasympathetic and sensory neurones, a decrease in synthesis of noradrenaline (but with a normal adrenal medulla) and a sensitivity to exogenous catecholamines have been shown. Emotional lability is common, but the IQ is normal.

There is autonomic dysfunction with postural hypotension and lability of blood pressure, increased vagal reflexes, swallowing difficulties with excess salivation, gastric reflux, reduced gastrointestinal motility, absent sweating and impaired temperature control. Sensitivity to pain and temperature is decreased. Muscle hypotonia occurs, with incoordination and reduced tendon reflexes. Kyphosis, scoliosis or a combination of both is common, presumably due to inadequate muscle tone and impaired muscle proprioception. Crowded teeth, malocclusion and a smooth tongue are characteristic. Dysautonomic and emotional crises may be precipitated by stress and can be associated with elevated plasma noradrenaline and dopamine levels. During these there may be nausea, vomiting, hypertension, tachycardia, sweating and the appearance of erythematous skin lesions.

Anaesthetic implications

General problems. Surgery may be required to treat complications of the condition. Operations most often recorded are fundoplication, gastrostomy and orthopaedic procedures. Chronic dehydration is common and intravenous fluid therapy should be started preoperatively. Anxiety may precipitate a dysautonomic crisis, so prophylactic measures should be taken. Diazepam has been found to be effective in controlling such crises, and cimetidine reduces gastric secretions. Premedication with both drugs has been suggested (Axelrod et al 1988). Opiates should be avoided if possible, as marked sensitivity to respiratory depression may occur. The use of atropine is controversial. Reports exist of sensitivity to cholinergic agents and, conversely, of pronounced reactions to vagal stimulation. Both its cautious use and its avoidance have been advocated.

Impaired cardiovascular responses. Autonomic nervous system dysfunction, apparently due to reduced endogenous catecholamine release, means that the patient is unable to respond to hypovolaemia or to drugs causing myocardial depression (Meridy & Creighton 1971, Foster 1983). Several cases in which either cardiac arrest or severe hypotension occurred during general anaesthesia have been reported (Kritchman et al 1959, Axelrod et al 1988). This cardiovascular instability may be compounded by chronic dehydration due to dysphagia for fluids.

Monitoring of arterial pressure and temperature should be started preferably before induction of anaesthesia. Vascular access is facilitated by the relative sensory deficit. Blood and fluid loss must be replaced promptly. The use of high-dose fentanyl as an alternative to inhalation agents, in order to reduce hypotension, has been suggested (Beilin et al 1985), although ventilatory support may be required after the operation.

Sensitivity to catecholamines. Exaggerated responses to exogenous noradrenaline have occurred, therefore catecholamines should be administered with caution. However, successful control of intraoperative hypotension with both adrenaline and dopamine infusions have been reported (Stenqvist & Sigurdsson 1982). Close monitoring is required so that the blood pressure is raised but an unacceptable tachycardia prevented.

Respiratory complications. Patients may have pre-existing lung disease secondary to episodes of pulmonary aspiration. The situation is compounded by muscle hypotonia and kyphoscoliosis. Respiratory responses to hypercarbia and hypoxia are impaired, so marked sensitivity to opiates may occur.

Muscular hypotonia and incoordination. Intraoperative IPPV is required, even for short cases, because of the impaired response to hypoxia and hypercarbia. The uneventful use of both depolarizing and non-depolarizing myoneural blockers has been reported. However, the presence of hypotonia will reduce the requirement for them. Residual blockade superimposed on hypotonia may necessitate IPPV after surgery, particularly for abdominal procedures. For operations in which major analgesics are needed, it has been suggested that IPPV should be continued postoperatively until opiates are no longer required (Axelrod et al 1988).

Postoperative problems. Major problems have occurred in the postoperative period (Meridy & Creighton 1971, Albanese & Bobechko 1987, Axelrod et al 1988). Complications include fever, pulmonary atelectasis or infection, aspiration, cardiovascular instability and vomiting crises. Axelrod et al (1988) have analysed 127 procedures in 81 patients. A high incidence of atelectasis after gastric surgery prompted a policy of elective artificial ventilation. If severe vomiting occurs, it should be treated with gastric decompression, diazepam and cimetidine.

Diabetic neuropathy

The incidence of diabetic neuropathy increases with age and duration of the disease. It may affect not only motor and sensory nerves, but also the autonomic nervous system which is when the main problems arise. The parasympathetic system is the more commonly affected, in which case there are less opposing influences against the sympathetic system. The problematic effects are those of tachycardia at rest and dysrhythmias. Page & Watkins (1978) have described twelve patients with diabetic autonomic and peripheral neuropathy who suffered cardiac arrest. They suggested that the cardiac arrest was of respiratory rather than cardiac origin, and five of these patients died following anaesthesia. These patients tend to show reduced ventilatory responses to hypoxia due to vagal blockage. High oxygen concentrations may also induce apnoea, and respiratory depression responds to doxapram.

Sympathetic neuropathy is associated with orthostatic hypotension, bradycardia and lack of cardiovascular response to the Valsalva manoeuvre or IPPV. Gastric stasis may increase the risk of regurgitation of gastric contents. Although patients with this problem may complain of vomiting, gustatory sweating and epigastric discomfort, some patients may be asymptomatic and thus difficult to identify preoperatively. It is recommended that patients who have diabetic neuropathy with autonomic nervous system involvement should be starved for a longer period than usual and given metoclopramide or domperidone preoperatively. Suitable precautions against inhalation of gastric contents will be needed at induction of and arousal from anaesthesia.

Neuralgias

Trigeminal neuralgia

There is no specific anaesthetic hazard related to trigeminal neuralgia except that attempts to thermocoagulate the ganglion may be accompanied by hypertension due to the strong stimulus.

Glossopharyngeal neuralgia

In glossopharyngeal neuralgia intense pain in the throat may be triggered by swallowing, chewing, coughing or talking. The important problem in this condition, apart from pain, is the effect on the cardiovascular system due to the proximity of and consequent excitation of the motor nucleus of the vagus. This will cause bradycardia, hypotension and syncopal attacks. It has even been known for cerebral ischaemic seizures and cardiac arrest to occur in these patients. As these patients are vulnerable to sudden death, treatment should be aggressive. This will include such measures as atropine, isoprenaline infusion or insertion of a cardiac pacemaker.

In the preoperative period, the patient's state of hydration should be assessed as some patients may avoid swallowing and hence reduce fluid intake. Further fluid loss may occur due to drooling of saliva. A transvenous cardiac pacemaker may be considered if there is a history of syncope. The ECG should be monitored before induction is started. It is recommended that atropine or glycopyrronium is given and topical lignocaine applied to the oropharynx in order to prevent bradycardia and hypotension on laryngoscopy.

The surgical treatment of this condition is glossopharyngeal nerve section and upper vagal nerve-root section via craniotomy. The section of these nerves can cause hypertension, tachycardia, premature beats and even ventricular fibrillation. The hypertension is usually transient but may persist into the postoperative period and is due to the unopposed sympathetic activity. If this occurs, vasodilator therapy will be required. Lastly, if respiratory obstruction occurs postoperatively this is likely to be due to vocal cord paralysis consequent upon sectioning of the vagus nerve. It is therefore important to see that the patient is able to maintain a clear airway after the operation.

Multiple (disseminated) sclerosis

Patients with multiple sclerosis are often receiving steroids, so steroid cover may be required. Muscle spasms are often treated chronically with diazepam, dantrolene or baclofen. Long-term dantrolene therapy may cause hepatic damage and liver function should be checked. Increase in body temperature should be avoided as this may cause further demyelination.

Regional anaesthesia is usually avoided in case it be incriminated should the disease worsen. However there is no hard evidence to support this approach. General anaesthesia is preferred and there seems to be no particular 'dos or don'ts'. Non-depolarizing muscle relaxants are well tolerated and there are no reports of abnormal response to this type of muscle relaxant, but Azar (1984) quotes one report of hyperkalaemia following suxamethonium administration. In the absence of other reports, however, he suggests that the vulnerability to suxamethonium is low.

Muscular denervation

Suxamethonium-induced hyperkalaemia will occur in patients with denervated muscles. After the first week postinjury, suxamethonium should be avoided in patients with a significant denervated muscle mass. Although the potassium release in these patients is attenuated by the prior administration of a small dose of non-depolarizing muscle relaxant (Tobey et al 1972), this does not totally protect the patient. Complete protection requires 0.5 mg/kg of tubocurarine (Baraka 1981).

Acute idiopathic polyneuritis

The cause of acute idiopathic polyneuritis (Guillain–Barré syndrome) is unknown but could be viral in origin. Vaccinations and immunosuppressive therapy have also been implicated. The syndrome is characterized by rapid onset of weakness or paralysis in the legs, spreading upwards to include the trunk, upper limbs and head. There is both sensory and motor neurone involvement. The sensory manifestations usually precede the motor, hence there is the symptom of paraesthesia before the flaccid paralysis due to lower motor neurone involvement. Autonomic nervous system dysfunction also occurs. The problems that may be encountered by the anaesthetist with these patients are therefore those concerned with paralysis, autonomic dysfunction and sensory disturbances. The most common surgical procedure is probably tracheostomy to aid management, but surgical emergencies may, of course, occur.

Muscular weakness or paralysis

Muscular weakness becomes problematic when there is intercostal muscle and bulbar involvement. If the intercostal muscles are involved respiratory insufficiency may well occur, and if the vital capacity is less than 15 ml/kg or there are other signs of respiratory insufficiency (e.g. blood gases, etc.) IPPV should be commenced. If there is bulbar involvement, this is manifested as bilateral facial paralysis. There may then be pharyngeal muscle weakness with difficulty in protecting against pulmonary aspiration, therefore intubation or tracheostomy may be required.

Autonomic nervous system dysfunction

Autonomic nervous system dysfunction can be severe and may be associated with sudden death. The signs of autonomic dysfunction are due to an imbalance between the parasympathetic and sympathetic parts of the autonomic nervous system. Therefore the signs of autonomic dysfunction include wide systemic blood-pressure fluctuations, resting tachycardia, cardiac conduction abnormalities and orthostatic hypotension. It is important that the anaesthetist is prepared to deal with any untoward cardiovascular changes before the patient suffers harm.

Sensory disturbances

Patients with sensory disturbances often suffer with pain such as headache, backache and skeletal muscle tenderness on pressure, so extra gentleness in handling the patients is essential.

Anaesthetic management

Anaesthesia with spontaneous respiration is probably best avoided as the anaesthetic drugs will cause some depression of respiration. If there is already weakness of the trunk muscles this method of anaesthesia may cause respiratory insufficiency. Suxamethonium should be avoided as this may induce hyperkalaemia due to muscle denervation. The non-depolarizing muscle relaxant used should be one with the least effect on the cardiovascular system in order to avoid hyper/hypotension. The drug of choice at the present time is vecuronium. Laryngoscopy may cause excessive hypertension if anaesthesia is inadequate. Orthostatic hypotension may be a problem, so careful fluid replacement will be necessary. If vasoconstrictors are deemed necessary, these must be used cautiously as they may cause hypertension due to denervation sensitization. Postoperatively, IPPV may be required due to respiratory insufficiency. Bulbar involvement may prevent the removal of the cuffed endotracheal tube or tracheostomy.

Neurofibromatosis

Neurofibromatosis is associated with orthopaedic disorders, cancers, mental retardation, congenital heart disease, endocrine disturbances and seizures. Neurofibromata may occur in the mediastinum or cervical region and cause distortion or obstruction of the trachea. Kyphoscoliosis is well known to be associated and this may cause respiratory problems. Intubation may be difficult. Endocrine disorders associated with this condition include phaeochromocytoma, medullary thyroid carcinoma and hyperparathyroidism, the anaesthetic problems of which are dealt with elsewhere (Ch. 9). These patients require no particular anaesthetic technique. Azar (1984) quotes two patients with neurofibromatosis and sensitivity to non-depolarizing muscle relaxants, but problems with muscle relaxants seem to be rare.

MUSCULAR DISORDERS

Myasthenia gravis and the myasthenic syndrome are covered in detail in Chapter 22 and will not be discussed here. Details of specific drug contraindications in Duchenne muscular dystrophy are also covered in Chapter 22, although a general discussion follows.

Myotonic dystrophies

Myotonic dystrophies (myotonias, dystrophia myotonica) are inherited degenerative disorders of skeletal muscles characterized by prolonged contracture of the muscles after stimulation. A diagnostic test is the inability to relax the muscle after voluntary contractions. The site of the lesion is in the muscle fibre distal to the neuromuscular junction. Neuromuscular blocking agents and local nerve blocks do not affect the contracture, although infiltration of the muscles with local anaesthetic agents may induce relaxation.

Myotonic contractures may be precipitated by shivering, and 'percussion' myotonia is the term used for myotonic contracture triggered by the surgeon handling the patient's muscle. There are three types of myotonia: myotonia dystrophica, myotonia congenita and paramyotonia. Aldridge (1985) has described in detail the problems involved when anaesthetizing these patients.

Dystrophia myotonica

Dystrophia myotonica (myotonia atrophica or Steinert's disease) is the most common and most serious form, with onset in the 20–40 age-group and death due to cardiac failure or respiratory infection in the sixth decade. The treatment is symptomatic, so the patient may be taking phenytoin, procainamide or quinidine. All types of muscle are eventually involved and anaesthetic hazards are as follows:

1. Cardiac dysrhythmias and cardiomyopathy. First-degree heart block is a common finding on the ECG before the clinical onset of the disease. About 20% of patients may have mitral valve prolapse and sudden death may be due to third-degree heart block. Even if the patient is asymptomatic, cardiomyopathy should be assumed and the anaesthetic dosage reduced accordingly.
2. Respiratory muscle weakness may become obvious in the postoperative period. This is due either to associated central respiratory dysfunction or to the fall off in the diaphragmatic component during the REM phase of sleep, that is actual respiratory muscle weakness (Hannon et al 1986). If infection occurs these patients may have difficulty expectorating. Respiratory function tests ought to be carried out preoperatively to assess respiratory reserve.
3. Associated endocrine problems include diabetes mellitus, hypothyroidism and adrenal insufficiency.
4. Response to muscle relaxants. Suxamethonium administration may cause prolonged generalized myotonia with ventilatory embarrassment. The limbs become flexed, and the back and neck become extended with a tight abdomen and rigid jaw. Under these conditions intubation may not be possible. The contraction will last for 2–3 min with slow gradual relaxation after this. The response is unpredictable. The effect of non-depolarizing muscle relaxants is either normal or prolonged, but here again the response seems to be unpredictable. If there are associated dystrophic muscular changes with wasting, the dose of non-depolarizing agent should be reduced accordingly. Since the lesion is distal to the neuromuscular junction, surgical relaxation can be a problem. The spasm cannot be relieved by muscle relaxants, regional anaesthesia or nerve blocks and surgical manipulation may trigger 'percussion'

contracture. Reversal of relaxants with neostigmine may cause generalized contracture in some patients, although it has been given without ill-effect in other cases. Atracurium has been used successfully, producing good operating conditions without sensitivity and neostigmine was not required (Nightingale et al 1985).

5. Other causes of myotonic contractures. Hypothermia and shivering may induce generalized contracture so it is imperative that these patients are kept warm and the operating theatre environment is not allowed to become cold. Potassium may also provoke generalized myotonia and therefore should only be given in the situation of life-threatening hypokalaemia.
6. Sensitivity to respiratory depressant drugs. These patients can be very sensitive to the respiratory depressant effects of barbiturates, diazepam and narcotics (Mudge et al 1980). If there is already respiratory muscle weakness, the respiratory depressant effect of these drugs will enhance respiratory infection, including aspiration pneumonia or failure in the postoperative period (Hannon et al 1986). There is no statistical evidence of a definite association with malignant hyperthermia, although it has been known to occur in these patients (Mudge et al 1980).

Myotonia congenita

Myotonia congenita (Thomsen's disease) is an inherited disease which occurs at birth or in early childhood. It affects muscles generally, but other organs are unaffected. Precautions are the same as for myotonia dystrophica. Laryngospasm and cyanosis have been reported in one case of this type of myotonia following suxamethonium administration (Paterson 1962).

Paramyotonia

Paramyotonia is the most rare of the three and appears only when the patient becomes cold. Otherwise it is identical to myotonia congenita.

Muscular dystrophy

Muscular dystrophy is an inherited condition in which the primary disorder is of muscle degeneration and atrophy. Some believe that it follows pathological changes in the neuromuscular junction. The disease is classified into four types: pseudohypertrophic, facioscapulohumeral, limb-girdle and ocular muscular dystrophy.

Pseudohypertrophic dystrophy (see also pp. 346–348). Pseudohypertrophic dystrophy (Duchenne's dystrophy) starts between the ages of 2 and 5 years, and usually the patient is in a wheelchair by the age of 12 years. The serum creatinine phosphokinase is raised and this is in parallel with the degree of muscle necrosis. The calf muscles are hypertrophied and there is general muscular weakness, but particularly so in the lower limbs and pelvic girdle. Anaesthetic problems are described below:

1. Muscular weakness. When intercostal muscles are involved there is a significantly reduced ability to expectorate so the patient is subject to chest infections, particularly in the postoperative period.
2. Response to muscle relaxants. Non-depolarizing muscle relaxants may last longer than normal, but the response may be normal (Azar 1984). There are reports of both normal responses to suxamethonium and cardiac arrest following its administration (Azar 1984). The cardiac arrests were assumed to be due to hyperkalaemia, but serum potassium levels were not measured. Suxamethonium is therefore better avoided in these patients.
3. Cardiac problems. When there is degeneration of cardiac muscle there may also be mitral regurgitation due to papillary muscle dysfunction. Reduced myocardial contractility eventually leads to heart failure and death.
4. Possibility of malignant hyperthermia. There have been reports of atypical malignant hyperthermia associated with this condition, but it is now considered unlikely that these patients are more susceptible to malignant hyperthermia than the normal population.

However, it has been recommended that such patients should be regarded as susceptible to malignant hyperthermia and that dantrolene is immediately available (Sethna & Rockoff 1986, Chalkiadis & Branch 1990). A number of cases of cardiac arrest have been reported following suxamethonium, halothane and isoflurane. These seem to be associated with rhabdomyolysis, subsequent hyperkalaemia followed by hyperthermia (Chalkiadis & Branch 1990). For successful treatment of the cardiac arrest in these patients, resuscitation should be undertaken with perserverance as correction of the hyperkalaemia and hyperthermia may take 2–3 hours.

Smith & Bush (1985) have given a detailed account of this condition and the anaesthetic implications, and Blumgart et al (1990) have reported the successful management of two patients with dystrophia myotonica presenting for urgent caesarean section using general anaesthesia. Further discussion of specific drug contraindications in Duchenne muscular dystrophy is to be found in Chapter 22.

Facioscapulohumeral dystrophy. Facioscapulohumeral dystrophy occurs later in adolescence and involves those muscles suggested by the name. The heart muscles are not involved and the creatinine phosphokinase is not raised. No particular anaesthetic problems should be encountered except muscle weakness.

Limb-girdle dystrophy. Limb-girdle dystrophy occurs later in life and is relatively benign.

Ocular dystrophy. In ocular dystrophy the patients are very sensitive to non-depolarizing muscle relaxants, rather akin to patients with myasthenia gravis. The added problem is that the muscular weakness does not respond to neostigmine (Azar 1984).

Parkinson's disease

Parkinson's disease (paralysis agitans) is a degenerative disease of the extrapyramidal CNS in which there is a loss of dopaminergic fibres in the basal ganglia and thus dopamine depletion. Dopamine is thought to be the neurotransmitter inhibiting the firing rate of neurones controlling the extrapyramidal system. If dopamine depletion occurs, this tends to allow the extrapyramidal system to be uninhibited and the action of acetylcholine in this region to remain unopposed. This gives rise to muscular rigidity, weakness and tremor. Dopamine does not cross the blood–brain barrier, but levodopa (L-dopa) does and is converted to dopamine by a decarboxylase enzyme. This enzyme is found in the tissues and the increase in dopamine concentration will cause systemic side effects. Carbidopa is therefore often prescribed as well to inhibit the decarboxylase in the systemic circulation. Anticholinergic drugs are also prescribed to reduce the effects of unopposed acetylcholine in the region of the basal ganglion.

The side effects of levodopa give rise mainly to cardiovascular changes. Firstly, levodopa, by being converted to dopamine, may give rise to inotropic and chronotropic effects, and even cardiac dysrhythmias. High dosage may cause peripheral vasoconstriction. Chronic administration may lead to reduced noradrenaline stress in the heart and reduce the concentration of noradrenaline systemically, due to the negative feedback by increased circulating dopamine. This may lead to orthostatic hypotension. Another side effect of levodopa is the effect on the kidneys when administered in lower doses over a long period. This will lead to increased renal blood flow, glomerular filtration and sodium excretion. Renin secretion will also be reduced and, because of the reduced intravascular volume, orthostatic hypotension may occur. Other side effects include nausea and vomiting (probably due to stimulation of the chemoreceptor trigger zone), psychiatric symptoms of agitation, confusion and depression. Dyskinesia occurs in 80% of patients who have been taking levodopa for more than a year.

Problems in the anaesthetic management of patients with Parkinson's disease who are treated with L-dopa

In spite of the adverse cardiovascular effects of L-dopa it is better to continue the drug in the perioperative period. If withdrawn, muscle rigidity may occur and this may interfere with mechanical ventilation or spontaneous respiration. Drugs to be avoided are phenothiazines, butyrophenones and ketamine. Phenothiazines and butyrophenones antagonize the effects of dopamine at the basal ganglion. Ketamine, on the other hand, may cause exaggerated sympathetic nervous system responses in the presence of increased dopamine concentrations. At induction of anaesthesia, hypotension may occur because of reduced intravascular volume due to the side effects of L-dopa, therefore crystalloids and/or colloids may be required. Non-depolarizing muscle relaxants may be used and seem to have no untoward effects. As far as suxamethonium is concerned, Gravelee (1980) has reported suxamethonium-induced hyperkalaemia. However, Azar (1984) in a review on the response of patients with neuro-muscular disorder to muscle relaxants, could find no other reports similar to this in Parkinsonian patients. Dysrhythmias may especially occur with halothane if L-dopa has been given within the previous 4 hours.

REFERENCES

Albanese S A, Bobechko W P 1987 Spine deformity in familial dysautonomia (Riley-Day syndrome). J Pediatr Orthop 7: 179–183

Aldridge L M 1985 Anaesthetic problems in myotonic dystrophy: A case report and reviews of the Aberdeen experience. Br J Anaesth 57: 1119–1130

Axelrod F B, Donenfeld R F, Danziger F, Turndorf H 1988 Anesthesia in familial dysautonomia. Anesthesiology 68: 631–635

Azar I 1984 The response of patients with neuromuscular disorders to muscle relaxants: a review. Anesth Analg 61: 173–187

Babinski M 1987 Anaesthetic considerations in patient with acute spinal cord injury. Crit Care Clin 3: 619–636

Baraka A 1981 Antagonism of succinylcholine-induced contracture of denervated muscles by D-tubocurarine. Anesth Analg 60: 605–607

Becker D P, Miller J D, Ward J D, Greenberg R P, Young H F, Sakalas R 1977 The outcome from severe head injury with early diagnosis and intensive management. J Neurosurg 47: 491–502

Beilin B, Maayan C H, Vatashsky E, Schulman D, Vinograd I, Aronson H B 1985 Fentanyl anesthesia in familial dysautonomia. Anesth Analg 64: 72–76

Bevan D R 1979 Shy-Drager syndrome: a review and description of the anaesthetic management. Anaesthesia 38: 866–873

Blumgart C, Hughes D, Redfern N 1990 Obstetric anaesthesia in dystrophia myotonica. Anaesthesia 45: 26–29

Casey W F 1983 Neurogenic pulmonary oedema. Anaesthesia 38: 985–988

Chalkiadis G, Branch K 1990 Cardiac arrest after isoflurane anaesthesia in a patient with Duchenne's muscular dystrophy. Anaesthesia 45: 22–25

Davies D D 1966 Abnormal response to anaesthesia in a case of Huntington's chorea. Br J Anaesth 38: 490–491

Demling R, Riessen R 1990 Pulmonary dysfunction after cerebral injury. Crit Care Med 18: 768–774

Dolfus P, Frankel H L 1965 Cardiovascular reflexes in tracheotomised tetraplegics. Paraplegia 2: 227–232

Doolan L A, O'Brien J F 1985 Safe intubation in cervical spine injury. Anaesth Intensive Care 13: 319–324

Drury P M E, Williams E G N 1991 Vocal cord paralysis in the Shy-Drager syndrome. A cause of post-operative respiratory obstruction. Anaesthesia 46: 466–468

Duke R F N, Spreadbury T H 1983 Spinal cord injuries. Anaesthesia 38: 507

Fitch W, Mackenzie E T, Jones J V, Harper A M 1976 Effect of halothane on the autoregulation of the cerebral blood flow in the normotensive and chronically hypertensive baboons. Anaesthesia 48: 1123

Foster J M G 1983 Anaesthesia for a patient with familial dysautonomia. Anaesthesia 38: 391

Frankel H L, Mathias C F, Spalding J M K 1975 Mechanisms of reflex cardiac arrest in tetraplegic patients. Lancet 2: 1183–1185

Frankville D, Drummond J 1987 Hyperkalaemia after succinlycholine administration in a patient with closed head injury without paresis. Anesthesiology 67: 264–266

Fraser A, Edmonds-Seal J 1982 Spinal cord injuries: a review of the problems facing the anaesthetist. Anaesthesia 37: 1084–1098

Gelb A W, Mannuen P H, Mezon B J, Durward G J 1984 The anaesthetist and the head-injured patient. Can Anaesth Soc J 31: 98–108

Gravelee G P 1980 Succinylcholine-induced hyperkalaemia in a patient with Parkinson's disease. Anesth Analg 59: 444–446

Grosslight K, Foster R, Colohan A R, Bedford R 1985 Isoflurane for neuroanaesthesia: risk factors for increases in intracranial pressure. Anesthesiology 63: 533–536

Hannon V, Cunningham A, Hutchinson M, McNicholas W 1986 Aspiration pneumonia and coma: an unusual presentation of dystrophia myotonica. Can Anaesth Soc J 33: 803–806

Hutchinson R C, Sugden J C 1984 Anaesthesia for Shy-Drager syndrome. Anaesthesia 39: 1229–1231

Iwatsuki N, Kuroda N, Amaha K, Iwatsuki K 1980 Succinylcholine induced hyperkalaemia in patients with ruptured cerebral aneurysms. Anesthesiology 53: 64–67

Kritchman M M, Schwartz H, Papper E M 1959 Experiences with general anesthesia in patients with familial dysautonomia. J Am Med Assoc 170: 529–533

dysautonomia. J Am Med Assoc 170: 529–533
Lamont A M S 1979 Brief report: anaesthesia and Huntington's chorea. Anaesth Intensive Care 7: 189–190
Luce J M 1984 Medical management of spinal cord injury. Int. Care Med. 13: 126–133
Mudge B J, Taylor P B, Vanderspek A F L 1980 Perioperative hazards of myotonic dystrophy. Anaesthesia 35: 492–495
Meridy H W, Creighton R E 1971 General anaesthesia in eight patients with familial dysautonomia. Can Anaesth Soc J 18: 563–570
Nightingale P, Healey T E J, McGuiness K 1985 Dystrophia myotonica and atracurium: a case report. Br J Anaesth 57: 1131–1135
Page M M, Watkins P J 1978 Cardiorespiratory arrest and diabetic autonomic neuropathy. Lancet 1: 14–16
Paterson I S 1962 Generalised myotonia following suxamethonium. Br J Anaesth 34: 340–342
Propert D N 1979 Pseudocholinesterase activity and phenotypes in mentally ill patients. Br J Psychiatry 134: 477–481
Ravichandran G 1989 Errors and omissions in the acute management of spinal cord injury. Journal of the Medical Defence Union 14–16
Sethna N, Rockoff M 1986 Cardiac arrest following inhalation induction of anaesthesia in a child with Duchenne's muscular dystrophy. Can Anaesth Soc J 33: 799–802
Shapiro H M 1975 Intracranial hypertension 43: 445–471
Shapiro H M, Wyte S R, Harris A B 1972 Ketamine anaesthesia in patients with intracranial pathology. Br J Anaesth 44: 1200–1209
Shy G M, Drager G A 1960 A neurologic syndrome associated with orthostatic hypotension. Arch Neurol 2: 511–527
Silver J A 1968 Chest injuries and complications in the early stages of spinal cord injury. Paraplegia 5: 196–209
Smith C L, Bush G H 1985 Anaesthesia and muscular dystrophy. Br J Anaesth 57: 113–118
Stenqvist O, Sigurdsson J 1982 The anaesthetic management of a patient with familial dysautonomia. Anaesthesia 37: 929–932
Stevenson P, Birch A 1979 Succinylcholine induced hyperkalaemia in a patient with closed head injury. Anesthesiology 51: 89–90
Takeshita H, Okudi Y, Sari A 1971 The effects of ketamine on the cerebral circulation and metabolism in man. Anesthesiology 36: 69–77
Tobey R E, Jacobsen P M, Kahle R T, Chibb R J, Dear M A 1972 The serum potassium response to muscle relaxants in neural injury. Anesthesiology 37: 69–77
Wauchob T D, Brooks R J, Harrison K M 1984 Neurogenic pulmonary oedema. Anaesthesia 39: 529–534
Wilson I, Meiklejohn B, Smith G 1991 Intravenous lignocain and sympathoadrenal responses to laryngoscopy and intubation: the effect of varying time of injection. Anaesthesia 46: 177–180

6

Renal function and the safety of anaesthesia

D. R. Bevan

What is man when you come to think upon him, but a minutely set, ingenious machine for turning, with infinite artfulness, the red wine of Shiraz into urine.

K Blixen-Fincke

INTRODUCTION

Renal function is altered during anaesthesia and surgery. In particular, urine volume and solute excretion are reduced, although this may be concealed by administration of large quantities of fluid and diuretics. Characteristically, the induction of anaesthesia is associated with minor changes unless cardiovascular alterations occur. However, the commencement of surgery is followed by a sudden decrease in urine volume, even when a preoperative diuresis has been induced (MacKenzie & Donald 1969), and the small amount of urine is poorly concentrated (Fig. 6.1; Zideman et al 1978). These changes should not be considered hazards of anaesthesia but rather the physiological response of the kidney to stress. In the normal patient, renal function returns to normal rapidly after surgery, although the changes may persist in the presence of hypovolaemia or sepsis.

The excretory data of Figure 6.1 can be used as the physiological norm. They demonstrate that after major surgery solute output is approximately 10 mOsm/kg/day. Thus, to prevent solute retention and accumulation of urea and creatinine, a 70 kg patient must excrete 700 mOsm/day. This can be achieved by the production of urine of either high volume and low concentration (e.g. 2000 ml/day, 350 mOsm/kg) or low volume and high concentration (e.g. 500 ml, 1400 mOsm/kg). However,

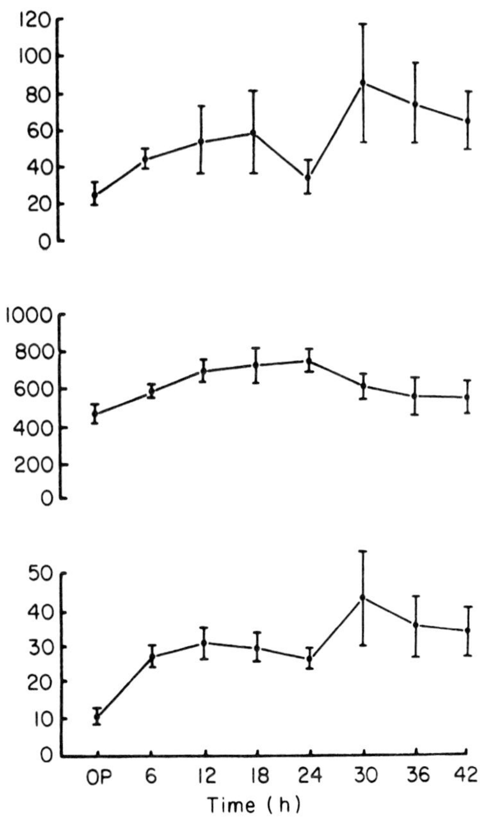

Fig. 6.1 Mean values (+ SEM) of the operative and 6-hourly postoperative samples of urine volume (ml/h), urine osmolality (mmol/kg) and solute output (mmol/h) (from Zideman et al 1978).

urine concentration in the postoperative patient seldom exceeds 1000 mOsm/kg, so that the minimal urine volume to excrete adequate solute is 700 ml/day (approximately 30ml/hour). Clearly, it is important to establish the relationship between urine volume and concentration before impaired renal function can be identified. Equally, the manipulation of fluid and diuretic therapy to produce an 'ideal' urine output is illusory (Alpert et al 1983): oliguria during surgery does not predict impaired renal function if blood volume is maintained.

The aetiology of the renal changes during surgery is multifactorial (Bevan 1979). Most patients are deprived of food and water for several hours before induction of anaesthesia. In addition, many exhibit marked anxiety. Consequently the kidney is under the influence of antidiuretic hormone and sympathetic stimulation before anaesthesia and surgery commence. Most anaesthetic agents produce further depression of renal function, revealed by reductions in urine volume, glomerular filtration and blood flow. In addition, positive pressure ventilation, deliberate or accidental hypotension and changes in Po_2 and Pco_2 may all compromise renal function secondary to cardiovascular changes. While anaesthesia may initiate these disturbances, operative trauma is necessary to perpetuate them. Alteration in the excretion of water and solute follows activation of the hormonal barrage to the kidney by catecholamines, corticosteroids, antidiuretic hormone, renin, angiotensin and several others. Certain anaesthetic techniques, including regional anaesthesia, high-dose narcotics, or halothane and enflurane in high concentrations, decrease or inhibit the neurohumoral accompaniment of surgery, but sometimes at the cost of cardiopulmonary instability. In most patients renal function returns to normal soon after surgery. Nevertheless, the kidney is vulnerable and poorly prepared to defend against additional disturbances, such as hypovolaemia, sepsis or exposure to nephrotoxins.

PRESERVATION OF RENAL FUNCTION

The avoidance of renal failure and the prevention of deterioration of function in the patient with pre-existing disease depend upon the recognition of worsening function and its early treatment. Several indices have been recommended (Table 6.1), but most are too slow for acute corrections. Only two – fractional sodium excretion and osmolar excretion – are useful in acute care. Fractional sodium excretion (FE_{Na}; the urine:plasma sodium concentration ratio divided by the urine:plasma creatinine concentration ratio expressed as a percentage) is a useful discriminant of hypovolaemic prerenal dysfunction and acute renal failure (Espinel 1976), but is worthless after the administration of diuretics. The importance of osmolar excretion has been discussed already, and the relationship between urine output and concentration in the recognition of renal failure is shown in Figure 6.2.

Renal function is preserved best by maintenance of blood volume and urine solute excretion and, perhaps, with active restoration of renal blood flow. Thus when renal dysfunction is identified its management is non-specific (Table 6.2). Fluid replacement should be guided by the use of central venous pressure (CVP) and/or pulmonary artery catheterization. Frusemide can be given in small doses to maintain solute output, but massive doses (3 g/day) do not appear to give further improvement (Brown et al 1981). The effectiveness of specific renal vasodilators is unproven, but low-dose dopamine infusion may be considered after fluid volume has been restored.

In the patient with pre-existing renal disease no prophylactic therapy has been proved effective. However, uncontrolled studies suggest that deterioration in renal function after major surgery may be prevented by fluid-loading with normal saline (Tasker et al 1974). Similarly, retrospective analysis suggests that the early function of renal transplants is improved by maximal hydration

Table 6.1 Indices of postoperative renal failure

Urine volume	<500 ml/day
Blood urea increase	>5 mmol/day
Urine:blood urea ratio	<14
Urine:blood creatinine ratio	<10
Urine:osmolality	<400 mOsm/kg
Urine:blood osmolality	<1.05
Urine:sodium concentration	>40 mmol/1
Fractional excretion of sodium	>1%
Osmolar excretion	<25 mOsm/h

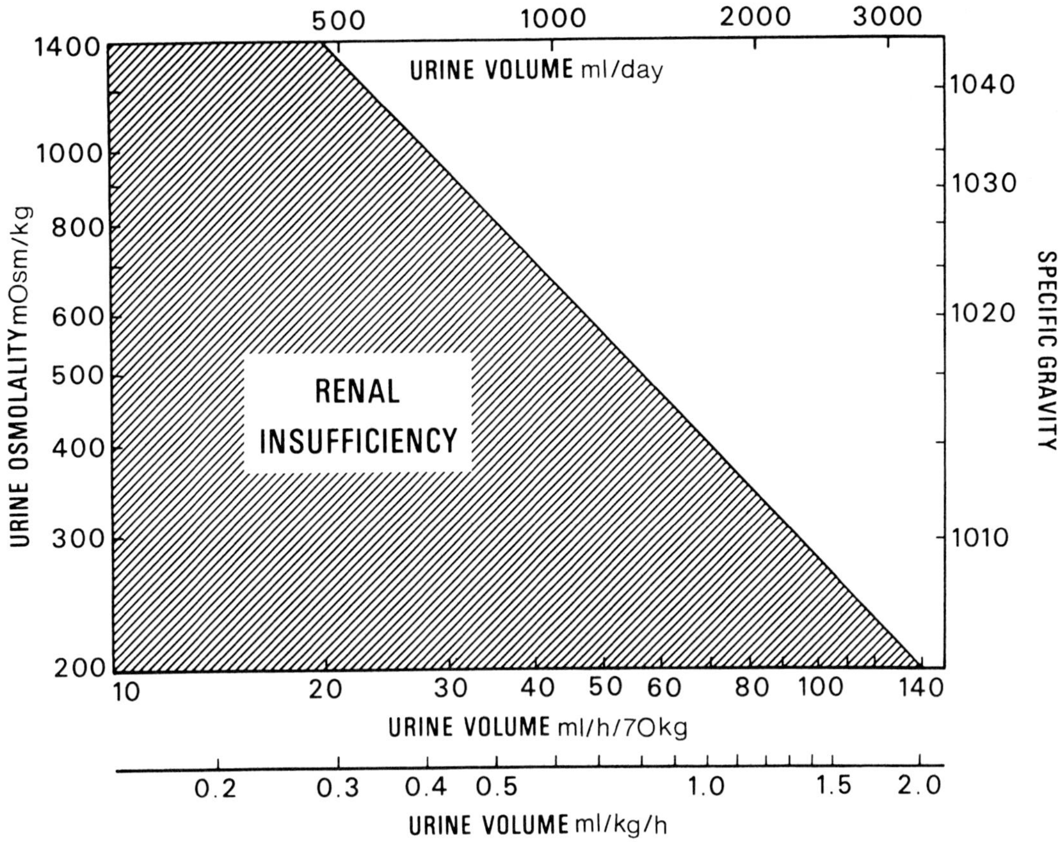

Fig. 6.2 Relationship between urine volume and concentration, expressed as osmolality and specific gravity, in the recognition of renal insufficiency.

during anaesthesia (Carlier et al 1982). However, these conclusions should be accepted with reservation until controlled studies provide more reliable data. Clearly, the avoidance of hypovolaemia and hypotension is important, but recommendations to uncontrolled, excessive hydration may lead to fluid overload in these patients whose control of intravascular volume is impaired.

Table 6.2 Management of postoperative renal dysfunction

Fluid load	500 ml normal saline in 15 min and maintain normovolaemia
Diuretics	Frusemide 0.25–1.00 mg/kg 1–2 hourly
Vasodilators	Dopamine 2–5 μg/kg/min

ANAESTHESIA IN END-STAGE RENAL FAILURE

Anaesthetic considerations

Anaemia

The renal failure patient is usually severely anaemic, but values for haemoglobin concentration of 7–9 g/dl at surgery are higher than previously because it was found that graft survival is improved by repeated transfusion (Opetz & Terasaki 1978). However, the improvement in the results of renal transplantation since the introduction of cyclosporine (Showstack et al 1989) has been substantial, so that the need for pretransplant transfusion has been questioned (Lancet 1988). The anaemia is the result of impaired erythropoiesis, haemolysis, haemorrhage, folate deficiency and chronic loss of iron. The removal of 20 ml of blood represents the loss of 5 mg of iron, which is twice the daily alimentary absorption of iron. Despite the anaemia, oxygen delivery is maintained by an increase in cardiac output and by a shift to the right of the haemoglobin dissociation curve from an increase in the concentration of 2,3 diphospholglycerate. Recombinant erythropoietin is effective in producing a dose-related increase in haematocrit and obviates the need for blood transfusion (Eschbach et al 1987).

Potassium

Hyperkalaemia is uncommon in the recently dialysed patient. The arrhythmias that occur during surgery are more often associated with hyperkalaemia and hyperglycaemia (Charters 1981), administration of suxamethonium, or as a consequence of release of renal preservative fluid after removal of the vascular clamps (Soulillou et al 1977). Collins' and Sack's solutions resemble intracellular fluid in electrolyte composition and are used in the rapid cooling of the donor kidney after harvesting. If the serum potassium concentration exceeds 5.5 mmol/1, suxamethonium should be avoided and non-urgent surgery postponed. When surgery is essential the potassium concentration can be reduced rapidly by infusion of glucose, insulin and calcium using 25 ml boluses from a solution of 50% dextrose (100 ml), containing insulin (24 units) and 10% calcium gluconate (10 ml).

Sodium

Mild hyponatraemia, 120–130 mmol/1, is common. It is usually the result of dilution and requires no treatment. Rapid shifts of water within the body are possible with the use of efficient, ultrafiltrating dialysis membranes and the rapid osmolar changes that this produces may be responsible for the fatigue, lethargy and occasional seizures seen in the dialysis disequilibrium syndrome. Comparison of the patient's actual weight with his known dry weight may be useful in assessing fluid status.

Acid-base

Metabolic acidosis is rare in the controlled patient. However, acid-base monitoring is seldom performed because if the arteries were damaged they would not be available later for vascular access and fistula creation.

Bone disease

About 15% of patients receiving chronic dialysis develop bone disease secondary to hyperparathyroidism. This may cause disseminated calcification and bone pain with pathological fractures. Treatment is with vitamin D analogues, aluminium antacids and diet. Magnesium for enemas or antacids is avoided to prevent its cerebral effect. Care must be taken to avoid damage to brittle bones while the patient is anaesthetized.

Glucose

Renal transplantation is now performed more frequently in the diabetic patient, although the transplanted kidney may develop diabetic changes later. Diabetes presents additional challenges in the control of fluid and potassium administration.

Cardiovascular

Hypertension is common, but is usually volume-dependent and can be controlled by careful dialysis. Rarely it is the result of renin-angiotensin hypersecretion and requires therapy which should be continued during the operative period. The occurrence of hypertension and arrhythmias during surgery may herald the release of renin from the graft (Levine & Blaufox 1978) or of catecholamines from the attached adrenal gland (Freilich et al 1984). Myocardial function is often impaired. Cardiac output is increased to compensate for the anaemia, but coronary artery disease is common and up to 20% may have a pericardial effusion (Lazarus 1980). Frequently, in addition to systemic hypertension and increased cardiac output, the CVP and pulmonary wedge pressure are increased in patients with end-stage renal failure. This may represent fluid overload or reduced left ventricular compliance. Whatever the cause, fluid therapy needs careful control. The practice of giving a fluid load to increase the 'firmness' of the kidney is dangerous. It does not increase cardiac output or arterial pressure and is of questionable benefit in ensuring adequate perfusion of the transplant (Cronnelly et al 1983).

Neurological

Uraemic encephalopathy is common in the elderly patient receiving dialysis. The cause is uncertain but may be related to the rapid movement of osmotically active substances or to persistent uraemia. Peripheral neuropathy is more frequent in the diabetic patient. It is usually sensory, seldom motor, but commonly may affect the autonomic nervous system and produce cardiovascular instability.

Sepsis

The frequency of infection is increased in renal failure as a result of immune deficiency. It tends to improve with dialysis but the institution of immunosuppressive therapy after transplantation may reveal occult infection. Haemodialysis patients have increased cytomegalovirus titres, and an incidence of type B hepatitis of up to 50% has been reported. Exposure of nurses, doctors and patients to blood from patients with chronic antigenaemia poses a major health problem.

Drug therapy

It can be seen that such patients may be receiving a wide array of drugs. In particular, digitalis, antihypertensive and antiarrhythmic agents, diuretics and nitrates are common, while corticosteroids and immunosuppressive agents are added after transplantation.

Pharmacokinetics

Renal failure reduces the excretion of ionized, water-soluble compounds. For anaesthesia the clearance of muscle relaxants and their antagonists will be prolonged, while there will be no excretory impairment of the lipid-soluble anaesthetic vapours or narcotics. However, they may appear to be more potent as a result of decreased protein binding producing an increase in free drug, or by an increase in receptor sensitivity. In addition, the volume of distribution of some agents may be altered as a result of fluid shifts.

Anaesthetic considerations

Despite the catalogue of severe disorders, it is surprising how infrequently problems arise during anaesthesia in renal failure. If fluid therapy is controlled carefully with appropriate monitoring the major problems are concerned with the use of neuromuscular relaxants.

General

The patient in renal failure needs to be handled carefully during anaesthesia. He should be moved gently to avoid damage to his skeleton. Precautions should be taken for a full stomach, in part because the surgical procedures including transplantation may be emergencies, but also because gastric emptying is delayed. If aspiration occurs, pulmonary damage and infection are more likely because of the susceptibility to sepsis. Monitoring of ECG, blood pressure and, often, CVP are essential, but blood pressure cuffs should not be applied to limbs with shunts or fistulae. Inspired oxygen concentration should be maintained at 40–50% to compensate for the decrease in oxygen-carrying capacity. Sterile precautions should be taken while making intravenous access. This is usually difficult and it is better to avoid forearm veins which may be required for arteriovenous fistulae. The principles for fluid replacement are no different from those in the normal patient. Fluid is necessary for maintenance and to replace losses of extracellular fluid and blood. Transfusion should be started early to aim for a higher haemoglobin concentration at the end of surgery than at the beginning.

Premedication

Most patients are anxious before surgery, and this applies particularly to the renal transplant recipient who recognizes the importance of the procedure for his future. Benzodiazepines and narcotics have been used successfully. If narcotics are used the dose should be reduced because of increased sensitivity. Problems are unlikely after a single dose, but repeated postoperative use may require naloxone treatment for several days to reverse cerebral and respiratory depression (Don et al 1975). Vagal blockade is usually achieved with atropine or hyoscine, although glycopyrrolate may be more appropriate to avoid tachycardia in the patient with heart disease.

General anaesthesia

Induction. Anaesthesia in renal failure is induced most commonly with thiopentone, although only small doses are required. The sensitivity to barbiturates may result from decreased protein binding (Ghonheim & Pandya 1975), qualitative albumen abnormalities (Shoeman & Azarnoff 1972), increased permeability of the blood–brain barrier (Freeman et al 1962) or abnormal cerebral metabolism (Richel et al 1970).

Maintenance – inhalational agents. If inhalational agents are to be used, equipotent concentrations of halothane, enflurane or isoflurane are equally safe and effective. Although there are three reports of deterioration in renal function after enflurane in surgical patients (Eichhorn et al 1976), the connection between enflurane and renal failure was tenuous in two of them. More recently, no differences in postoperative renal function could be detected between patients who had received either halothane or enflurane (Mazze et al 1984). Also, de Temmerman & Gribomont (1979) reported the successful use of enflurane in 375 transplant operations. Earlier fears of inducing fluoride polyuric nephropathy after enflurane seem to have been unjustified. Thus any of these inhalational agents may be used. Care must be taken to avoid cardiovascular depression and slow awakening can be anticipated (Casthely & Vollaneuva 1983). Despite the small amount of inorganic fluoride produced during the metabolism, potentially nephrotoxic fluoride concentrations were found in a patient who received about 107 MAC hours of isoflurane anaesthesia to control postoperative chorea (Truog & Rice 1989). However, no change in renal function was seen.

Narcotics. Narcotics may be used to replace or supplement the anaesthetic vapours. Although the clearance of morphine, and probably other opioids (Chauvin et al 1987a), is not altered in renal failure, morphine metabolites accumulate (Chauvin et al 1987b). This may cause prolonged action if morphine is given in large doses or over a prolonged period. Thus, large doses should be avoided and the rapid clearance of fentanyl, and the absence of active metabolites, make it a suitable choice compared with morphine or pethidine. The combination of droperidol and fentanyl neurolept anaesthesia is attractive to provide sedation and analgesia, and has been used successfully in some cases (Morgan & Lumley 1975). In patients with normal kidneys a fluid load can be tolerated better using neuroleptanaesthesia than halothane, although this is probably irrelevant in the patient with advanced renal disease.

Neuromuscular relaxants. All neuromuscular blocking drugs (NMBD) are ionized, water-soluble compounds that are normally excreted passively by the kidney. Consequently their action will be prolonged in renal failure. For gallamine and metocurine the kidney is the principal route of excretion, so that their use is contraindicated in severe renal disease. Others are less affected because they are either metabolized (succinylcholine and atracurium) or are also excreted by the liver (d-tubocurarine, pancuronium and vecuronium). Profound muscle relaxation is required to provide optimal conditions for endotracheal intubation. After that, less intense paralysis is necessary to provide surgical relaxation. Thus, ideal conditions for anaesthetist and surgeon may be achieved by choosing the appropriate relaxant in the appropriate dose for the appropriate time. Also, supplementation of anaesthesia with enflurane or isoflurane may be particularly useful to intensify the paralysis, which will recover when they are eliminated.

Suxamethonium. In a dose of 1 mg/kg succinylcholine produces excellent intubating conditions within 2 min, and this is particularly appropriate to isolate the respiratory tract in the patient with a full stomach. Unfortunately, suxamethonium has particular problems for the renal failure patient. Serum potassium concentration increases by about 0.5 mmol/l and this cannot be prevented by precurarization (Koide & Waud 1972). Thus its use is contraindicated if the potassium concentration exceeds 5.5 mmol/l. The duration of action of suxamethonium depends upon plasma cholinesterase activity, and this may be reduced for 1–2 weeks after renal transplantation (Ryan 1979). Earlier reports that plasma cholinesterase was reduced by haemodialysis (Holmes et al 1958) appear to be exaggerated (Ryan 1977). The action of suxamethonium may also be potentiated after transplantation by the action of azathioprine. This is a phosphodiesterase inhibitor which increases acetylcholine release and prolongs the action of depolarizing relaxants, while tending to antagonize competitive relaxants (Dretchen et al 1976).

Non-depolarizing relaxants. The plasma clearance of tubocurarine, pancuronium (Fig. 6.3) and vecuronium is decreased in renal failure, although the time of onset of action and the potency

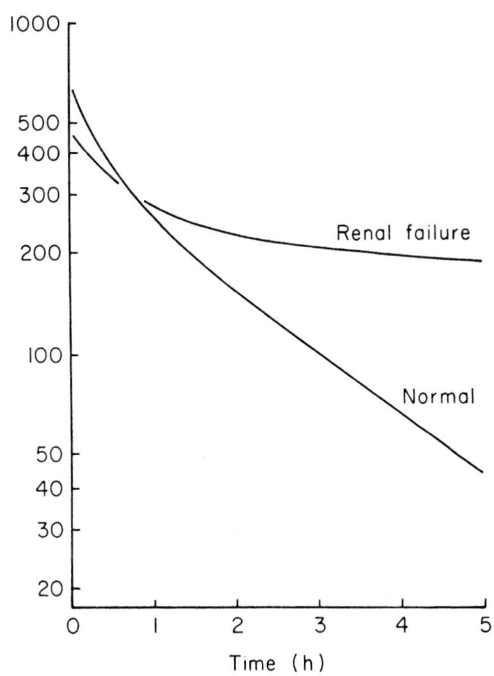

Fig. 6.3 The influence of renal failure on plasma clearance of pancuronium (from McLeod et al 1976).

are not affected. Consequently the onset is too slow to provide good inhibiting conditions rapidly, unless large doses are given which, for pancuronium and tubocurarine, would be associated with an unnecessarily prolonged duration of action. There is some dispute about which of pancuronium and tubocurarine is more affected in renal failure. Unfortunately the three pharmacokinetic studies examined one drug each in San Francisco, USA (Miller et al 1977), Newcastle, England (McLeod et al 1976) and Sydney, Australia (Somogyi et al 1977). It seems from the heterogeneous data that both drugs have similar reductions in plasma clearance. Vecuronium is affected like pancuronium in renal failure, but as the duration of action of equipotent doses is only one-third that of pancuronium, small changes in pharmacokinetic behaviour have little clinical effect (Bevan et al 1984). The action of atracurium is unaffected by renal failure because of rapid metabolism by Hofmann elimination. The duration of action of single and repeated doses is not prolonged (Hunter et al 1982). Thus it seems that the shorter-acting, newer relaxants are associated with fewer postoperative ventilatory consequences. Unfortunately the short duration of action requires frequent 'top-up' to maintain relaxation. One hopes that if anaesthetists are encouraged to use larger doses they will also be guided by more frequent measurement of neuromuscular transmission.

There are many reports of renal failure patients requiring reintubation and ventilation some time after surgery (Miller & Cullen 1976). It is now clear that this syndrome is not the result of reoccupation of the receptors with relaxant after the anticholinesterase has been excreted. The clearance of anticholinesterase is also decreased in renal failure, matching that of pancuronium and curare (Cronnelly et al 1979, Morris et al 1981). Thus there is no reason to use pyridostigmine to prolong reversal (Cronnelly et al 1980). If neuromuscular transmission is measured carefully, administration of neostigmine is followed by progressive recovery of function over the succeeding 2–3 hours (Bevan et al 1982). Thus the syndrome of apparent recurarization may be the result of clinically adequate ventilation when the partially paralyzed patient is stimulated and moved at the end of surgery. Left in peace and given additional analgesia in the recovery room, respiration is reduced. The incidence of such problems would be diminished if neuromuscular monitoring were used routinely, so that persistent paralysis could be recognized at the end of surgery and antagonized with the appropriate dose of anticholinesterase.

Regional anaesthesia

The problems of general anaesthesia could be avoided by more frequent use of regional anaesthesia. Indeed, brachial plexus block is ideal for the creation of atrioventricular (AV) fistulae in the forearm, and field block is usually adequate for the insertion of Tenckoff catheters for chronic ambulatory peritoneal dialysis. However, the duration of action of local anaesthetic block appears to be reduced in renal failure (Bromage & Gertel 1972), perhaps because the increased cardiac output produces quicker wash-out of the solution.

The use of spinal analgesia (Vandam et al 1962) or epidural analgesia (Wyant 1967) has been recommended for abdominal surgery, and is probably safe as long as any significant bleeding tendency has been excluded by a coagulation screen and bleeding time. High blocks may be associated with sympathetic blockade, which may result in considerable hypotension in the presence of autonomic blockade (Trudnowski et al 1971).

Patients on long-term haemodialysis programmes are asked to tolerate considerable discomfort and inconvenience in the control of their disease. We assume that they can tolerate more pain and discomfort than other patients. Often they cannot, and general anaesthesia is indicated to avoid the extreme anxiety of situations, particularly when their future may be altered so greatly by successful renal transplant.

CONCLUSION

The patient with end-stage renal failure is at particular risk during anaesthesia. However, safe anaesthesia can be provided if care is given to cardiovascular support and the judicious use of neuromuscular relaxants. Both aspects require appropriate monitoring to be successful.

REFERENCES

Alpert R A, Roizen M F, Hamilton W K et al 1983 Intraoperative urinary output does not predict postoperative renal function. Anesthesiology 59: A157

Bevan D R 1979 Renal function in anaesthesia and surgery. Academic Press, London

Bevan D R, Archer D, Donati F, Ferguson A, Higgs B D 1982 Antagonism of pancuronium in renal failure: no recurarization. Br J Anaesth 54: 63–68

Bevan D R, Donati F, Gyasi H, Williams A 1984 Vecuronium in renal failure. Can Anaesth Soc J 31: 491–496

Bromage P R, Gertel M 1972 Brachial plexus anesthesia in chronic renal failure. Anesthesiology 36: 488–493

Brown C B, Ogg C S, Cameron J S 1981 High dose frusemide in acute renal failure. Clin Nephrol 15: 90–96

Carlier M, Squifflet J-P, Pivson Y, Gribmont B, Alexandre G P J 1982 Maximal hydration during anaesthesia increases pulmonary arterial pressure and improves early function of human renal transplants. Transplantation 34: 201–204

Casthely P A, Villanueva R 1983 Level of consciousness after cadaveric kidney transplant under halothane anaesthesia. Can Anaesth Soc J 30: 587–592

Charters P 1981 Renal transplantation in diabetes mellitus. Anaesthesia 35: 199–204

Chauvin M, Lebrault C, Levron J C, Duvaldestin P 1987a Pharmacokinetics of alfentanil in chronic renal failure. Anesth Analg 66: 53–56

Chauvin M, Sandouk P, Scherrmann J M, Farinotti R, Strumza P, Duvaldestin P 1987b Morphine pharmacokinetics in renal failure. Anesthesiology 66: 327–221

Cronnelly R, Stanski D R, Miller R D, Sheiner L B, Sohn Y J 1979 Renal failure and the pharmacokinetics of neostigmine in anesthetized man. Anesthesiology 51: 222–226

Cronnelly R, Stanski D R, Miller R D, Sheiner L B 1980 Pyridostigmine kinetics with and without renal function. Clin Pharmacol Ther 28: 78–81

Cronnelly R, Kremer P F, Beaupre P N, Cahalan M K, Salvatierra O, Feduska N 1983 Hemodynamic response to fluid challenge in anesthetized patients with end-stage renal disease. Anesthesiology 59: A49

deTemmerman P, Gribomont B 1979 Enflurane in renal transplantation: report of 375 cases. Acta Anaesthesiol Scand supplement 71: 24–31

Don H F, Dieppa R A, Taylor P 1975 Narcotic analgesics in anuric patients. Anesthesiology 42: 745–747

Dretchen K L, Morgenroth V H, Standaert F G, Walts L F 1976 Azathioprine: effects on neuromuscular transmission. Anesthesiology 45: 604–609

Eichhorn J H, Hedley-White J, Steinman T I, Kaufman J M, Aasberg L H 1976 Renal failure following enflurane anesthesia. Anesthesiology 45: 557–560

Eschbach J W, Egrie J C, Downing M R, Browne J K,

Adamson J W 1987 Correction of the anemia of end-stage renal disease with recombinant human erythropoietin. N Engl J Med 316: 73–78

Espinel C H 1976 The Fe_{Na} test: use in the differential diagnosis of acute renal failure. J Am Med Assoc 236: 579–581

Freeman B B, Sheff M F, Maher J F, Schreiner G E 1962 The blood–cerebrospinal fluid barrier in uremia. Ann Intern Med 56: 233–240

Freilich J D, Waterman P D, Rosenthal J T 1984 Acute hemodynamic changes during renal transplantation. Anesth Analg 63: 158–160

Ghonheim M M, Pandya H 1975 Plasma protein binding of thiopental in patients with impaired renal or hepatic function. Anesthesiology 42: 545–549

Holmes J H, Makamoto S, Sawyer K C 1958 Changes in blood composition before and after dialysis with the Kolff twin coil kidney. Trans Am Soc Artif Intern Organs 4: 16–21

Hunter J M, Jones R S, Utting J E 1982 Use of atracurium in patients with no renal function. Br J Anaesth 54: 1251–1258

Koide M, Waud B E 1972 Serum potassium concentration after succinylcholine in patients with renal failure. Anesthesiology 36: 142–145

Lancet 1988 (Editorial) Time to abandon pre-transplant blood transfusion? Lancet 1: 567–568

Lazarus J M 1980 Complications in hemodialysis: an overview. Kidney Int 18: 783–796

Levine R D, Blaufox M D 1978 Hyperreninemia during renal transplantation. Nephron 22: 226–231

MacKenzie A I, Donald J R 1969 Urine output and fluid therapy during anaesthesia and surgery. Br Med J 2: 619–621

McLeod K, Watson M J, Rawlins M D 1976 Pharmacokinetics of pancuronium in patients with normal and impaired renal function. Br J Anaesth 48: 341–345

Mazze R I, Sievenpiper T S, Stevenson J 1984 Renal effects of enflurane and halothane in patients with abnormal renal function. Anesthesiology 60: 161–163

Miller R D, Cullen D J 1976 Renal failure and postoperative respiratory failure: recurarization? Br J Anaesth 48: 253–256

Miller R D, Matteo R S, Benet L Z, Sohn Y J 1977 The pharmacokinetics of d-tubocurarine in man with and without renal failure. J Pharmacol Exp Ther 202: 1–6

Morgan M, Lumley J 1975 Anaesthetic considerations in chronic renal failure. Anaesth Intensive Care 3: 218–226

Morris R B, Cronnelly R, Miller R D, Stanski D R, Fahey M R 1981 Pharmacokinetics of edrophonium in anephric and renal transplant patients. Br J Anaesth 53: 1311–1314

Opetz G, Terasaki P I 1978 Improvements of kidney-graft survival with increased numbers of blood transfusions. N Engl J Med 299: 799–803

Richel G, De Novales E L, Verrdust P 1970 Drug intoxication and neurological episodes in chronic renal failure. Br Med J 2: 394–395

Ryan D W 1977 Preoperative serum cholinesterase concentration in chronic renal failure. Br J Anaesth 49: 945–949

Ryan D W 1979 Postoperative serum cholinesterase activity following successful renal transplantation. Br J Anaesth 51: 881–884

Shoeman D W, Azarnoff D L 1972 The alteration of plasma protein in uremia as reflected in their ability to bind digitoxin and diphenylhydantoin. Pharmacology 7: 169–174

Showstack J, Kay P, Amend W, Bernstein L, Lipton H, O'Leary M, Birdman A, Salvatierra O 1989 The effect of cyclosporine on the use of hospital resources for kidney transplantation. N Engl J Med 321: 1086–1092

Somogyi A A, Shanks C A, Triggs E J 1977 The effect of renal failure on the disposition and neuromuscular blocking action of pancuronium bromide. Eur J Clin Pharmacol 12: 23–29

Soulillou J P, Fillaudeau F, Keribin J P, Guenel J 1977 Acute hyperkalaemia risks in recipients of kidney graft cooled with Collins' solution. Nephron 19: 301–304

Tasker P R W, MacGregor G A, de Wardemer H E 1974 Prophylactic use of intravenous saline in patients with chronic renal failure undergoing major surgery. Lancet 2: 911–912

Trudnowski R J, Mostert I W, Hobika G H, Rico R 1971 Neuroleptanalgesia for patients with kidney malfunction. Anesth Analg 50: 679

Truog R D, Rice A A 1989 Inorganic fluoride and prolonged isoflurane anesthesia in the Intensive Care Unit. Anesth Analg 69: 843–845

Vandam L D, Harrison J H, Murray J E, Merrill J P 1962 Aspects of renal homotransplantation in man. Anesthesiology 23: 783–792

Wyant G M 1967 The anaesthetist looks at tissue transplantation: three years' experience with kidney transplants. Can Anaesth Soc J 14: 255–275

Zideman D A, Dudley H A F, Bevan D R 1978 Osmolar output in the perioperative period. Anaesthesia 33: 788–793

7

Liver function and the safety of anaesthesia

B. Walton

INTRODUCTION

This chapter is intended to provide a brief practical review of the hepatic complications of anaesthesia. The main topics are the approach of the anaesthetist to the patient with liver disease and the problem of postoperative jaundice. It seems apposite, however, to preface such a review with a resume of the factors affecting hepatic blood flow (HBF) and the interpretation of liver function test results.

HEPATIC BLOOD FLOW

Of the 1500 ml/min of blood passing through the liver, 25% derives from the hepatic artery and 75% from the portal vein. Flow studies involve either continuous infusion or single-injection techniques, using markers such as indocyanine green, bromsulphthalein or labelled chromic phosphate. It has been shown that, at least in patients with normal liver function, there is reasonable correlation between these indirect methods and direct flow probe measurements. Hepatic arterial and portal venous blood passes (via intralobular arterioles and intralobular veins, respectively) into hepatic sinusoids. These drain into the hepatic vein and finally into the inferior vena cava. Sphincters control flow within the liver, allowing diversion of blood between the two systems. The main differences between the two sources of blood supply are:

- the relatively poor oxygen saturation of portal blood (70% at best)
- the very low pressure head driving the portal system (about 6 mmHg).

That the liver derives 75% of its blood supply from a system with these 'inadequacies' explains to some extent the vulnerability of the organ to hypoxia, and the dramatic reduction in HBF caused by relatively minor elevations in hepatic outflow tract pressure.

Anaesthesia, surgery and HBF

Hepatic blood flow may be expected to fall by some 20–25% during anaesthesia and surgery, irrespective of the agents and techniques used. Superimposed on this 'baseline' reduction are factors that may reduce flow further, some of which may be avoided by the choice of agents and careful attention to technique. Intermittent positive pressure ventilation (IPPV), by raising mean intrathoracic pressure, raises pressure in the inferior vena cava and, therefore, in the hepatic venous outflow tract. As the portal system operates at such a low pressure head, the rise in outflow tract pressure which accompanies *excessive* IPPV may greatly reduce HBF. HBF is profoundly affected by alterations in sympathetic tone, with alpha activity increasing vascular resistance and reducing flow, and beta activity having opposite effects. An increase in alpha sympathetic tone is responsible for the reduction in HBF associated with hypercarbia. Poor venous return due to excessive IPPV, pooling of blood in splanchnic areas during surgical manipulation, and haemorrhage, will all reduce cardiac output and HBF will decrease further.

Effects of anaesthetic agents on HBF

In general, any transient alterations in HBF associated with intravenous anaesthetic agents and muscle relaxants are relatively minor, and reflect changes in cardiac output and peripheral vascular tone. Of the inhalational agents, the most dramatic reduction in HBF (90%) is seen with cyclopropane, with splanchnic vascular resistance increasing in response to an increase in alpha sympathetic tone. Methoxyflurane, now only of historical interest, reduces HBF by some 50%, due in part to hepatic arterial constriction as well as a general reduction in perfusion pressure. Exposure to nitrous oxide, halothane, enflurane or isoflurane is associated with a 20–25% 'baseline' fall in HBF mentioned above. Similar reductions are seen with regional techniques (as a corollary of reduced perfusion pressure). It has been shown that, at least in some species, the reduction in HBF seen with isoflurane is somewhat less than that seen with either halothane or enflurane. However, the clinical significance (at least in patients with ostensibly normal liver function) of such differences remains in some doubt! In any event, it is important to ask whether or not the liver is embarrassed by these reductions in HBF. Clearly, if the oxygen consumption by the liver falls to the same extent as HBF, embarrassment would be avoided, as the reduced blood supply would remain adequate for the reduced metabolic rate. Comparisons between reductions in hepatic oxygen consumption and reductions in HBF have shown that with *all* commonly used techniques, the (to some extent) unavoidable reductions in HBF *are* associated with a degree of hepatic hypoxia.

The metabolic difficulty manifests itself as a rise in hepatic venous blood lactate, and may also be responsible for the minor alterations in liver function test results seen *routinely* during the perioperative period. Although such changes in HBF and hepatic metabolism may well be insignificant in patients with normal liver function, patients with pre-existing liver disease may be ill-served by exposure to agents and/or techniques that reduce HBF more than the unavoidable minimum.

LIVER FUNCTION TESTS

A preoperative liver function test (LFT) screen not only allows assessment of the degree of liver dysfunction, but also provides a 'baseline' for comparison with serial postoperative test results. It must be stressed that patients presenting for anaesthesia and surgery with severe pre-existing liver disease will be *expected* to show a post-operative deterioration in liver function. Thus, in the patient with, for example, acute viral hepatitis, surgery must be postponed unless absolutely essential. It should be the aim of the anaesthetist to choose agents and techniques which (as far as possible) minimize the deterioration. A brief review of some common LFTs may be of value here.

Serum bilirubin

The normal concentration of serum bilirubin is less than 18 μmol/l. Some 80% of bilirubin is derived from the catabolism of haemoglobin from old red blood cells. The haem moiety is transported to the liver (bound to albumin), where it is conjugated to a water-soluble derivative which can then be excreted in the bile. Conjugated bilirubin is not reabsorbed from the gut, although bacterial action converts some to urobilinogen which is absorbed into the portal system and returned to the liver. Urobilinogen is then excreted into the bile. Predominantly unconjugated (indirect) hyperbilirubinaemia is associated with an increased bilirubin load (as in haemolysis or the breakdown of old transfused blood cells), or with impaired uptake and conjugation of bilirubin (as in congenital deficiency states, such as Gilbert's and Crigler–Najjar syndromes). Conversely, high levels of conjugated (direct) bilirubin are seen when the excretion of bilirubin is impaired. Thus hepatocellular disease and/or hepatic obstruction (both cholestatic and extrahepatic obstructive jaundice) are associated with predominantly conjugated hyperbilirubinaemia. Only conjugated bilirubin appears in the urine.

Serum alkaline phosphatase

Normal values 20–90 IU/l, 5–13 KA units. This is produced mostly by bone, and liver alkaline phosphatase is excreted in the bile. Raised levels imply impaired hepatic excretion. A slight rise is often seen in patients with parenchymal or metastatic liver disease, moderately high levels are associated with varying degrees of intrahepatic obstruction, and very high levels usually relate to severe cholestasis or posthepatic obstruction (cholelithiasis or malignancy). Various bone diseases (e.g. Paget's) also feature high alkaline phosphatase levels.

Aminotransferases (transaminases)

Normal values <20 IU/l, Aspartate aminotransferase (SGOT, AST) and alanine aminotransferase (SGPT, ALT) levels are raised in patients with hepatocellular damage, although damage to other organs rich in these enzymes (e.g. the heart) should be excluded. Extensive hepatic necrosis (as, for example, in severe viral hepatitis) may be associated with levels greater than 1000 IU/l, and serial estimations help chart the course of the disease. Fulminant hepatic failure may, late, be associated with falling enzyme levels, presumably as the cells become depleted.

Lactic dehydrogenase

Normal values 30–90 IU/l. Lactic dehydrogenase (LDH) is present widely and, although moderately raised levels are seen in hepatitis and cirrhosis, identification of organ-specific isoenzyme fractions may be necessary.

Gamma glutamyl transpepidase

Normal values <24 IU/l. Gamma glutamyl transpeptidase (γ-GT) is a sensitive indicator of liver damage.

PROBLEMS TO BE ANTICIPATED IN PATIENTS WITH SEVERE LIVER DISEASE

Abnormal blood coagulation

Abnormalities result from both inadquate absorption of vitamin K from the gut (in the face of a reduced supply of bile salts) and reduced clotting factor synthesis. A preoperative clotting screen is mandatory. Parenteral vitamin K may be of value (if time allows and the liver can utilize it!), and abnormalities can be at least partially corrected with fresh frozen plasma. Clearly, if transfusion is indicated, very fresh blood will be preferable (in terms of both coagulation and potassium levels; see later). Blood should be liberally cross-matched and, if the surgery is expected to be associated with considerable loss, two intravenous infusions should be set up. It could be argued that, as central venous pressure monitoring may well be of value during and after surgery, one of the venous lines should be central. In the face of abnormal coagulation the anaesthetist must weigh the relative disadvantage of the poor flow possible with a long line inserted via the antecubital fossa, against the risks associated with inexpert internal jugular puncture. In these circumstances it might also be even more advisable to avoid the subclavian approach! Frequent postoperative re-evaluation of coagulation status may indicate the need for further fresh frozen plasma.

Renal failure

Although most commonly associated with obstructive jaundice and extreme hyperbilirubinaemia, renal failure is a well-recognised corollary of severe liver disease in general. The causes of the so-called 'hepatorenal syndrome' are unclear, although circulating endotoxins, reduced renal blood flow (related to hypovolaemia), renal cortical vasoconstriction (of unknown aetiology) and renal vein obstruction (due to ascites and raised intra-abdominal pressure) have been suggested as contributory factors. A tendency to develop acute renal failure in these patients may be accelerated by any reduction in renal blood flow associated with anaesthesia and surgery, and certainly hypotension is to be avoided at all costs. Preoperative rehydration may be necessary to correct hypovolaemia induced by long-term diuretic therapy, and fluid balance must be monitored closely throughout. Hypoalbuminaemia (with levels <25 g/l suggesting a serious problem) should be corrected in order to encourage administered fluids to remain in the appropriate compartment. Urinary catheterization will allow early recognition and treatment of oliguria. Intravenous mannitol (say, 20 g, repeated as necessary) is often advocated as useful prophylaxis (particularly in patients with very high bilirubin levels), although close attention to central venous pressure is necessary to avoid an excessive rise in intravascular volume and the precipitation of cardiac failure. I have found that incipient postoperative renal failure (not only in patients with hepatic disease!) may be averted by a 'renal' dose of dopamine (say, 3–5 μg/kg/min by intravenous infusion), which may increase renal blood flow without ostensibly causing generalized cardiovascular changes.

Blood sugar abnormalities

Severe liver disease is often associated with alterations in glucose metabolism. Hypoglycaemia is common, resulting from long-term reductions in glucose intake and uptake, glycogen storage and gluconeogenesis. On the other hand, in fulminant hepatic failure, hyperglycaemia, associated with high circulating insulin levels, may be a feature, reflecting reduced insulin sensitivity. Repeated blood-sugar estimations are essential, with dextrose and/or insulin infusions as necessary.

Acid-base and potassium changes

A distinction can be drawn between patients with chronic hepatic disease, in whom long-term diuretic therapy may result in whole-body potassium depletion, hypokalaemia and metabolic alkalosis, and those with acute severe disease in whom metabolic acidosis and hyperkalaemia may be major features. Normal lactate levels (<2 mmol/l) reflect the balance between lactate production from normal metabolizing muscle and red blood cells and, predominantly, lactate consumption (for gluconeogenesis) by the liver. In severe liver disease (particularly in the presence of hypoxia), lactate is produced rather than consumed, a situation referred to as Type A lactic acidosis. If poor peripheral tissue perfusion is a complicating factor, the switch from aerobic to anaerobic metabolism results in a greatly increased lactate load, referred to as Type B lactic acidosis. Hypoglycaemia may further exacerbate the problem, as lactate metabolism requires adequate blood-sugar levels. Lactic acidosis in severe liver disease is marked by an increased anion gap. The normal gap $(Na^- + K^-) - (Cl^- + HCO^{3-})$, reflecting usually unmeasured anions, lies between 15 and 20 mmol/l.

The advisability of correcting a metabolic acidosis with infusions of sodium bicarbonate is now widely debated. It is believed that, in some circumstances, rapid infusions can exacerbate *intracellular* acidosis. I believe that at least partial correction, with, say, 100 mmol of sodium bicarbonate intravenously over 30 min, can be of benefit. Certainly, myocardial responses to infusions of inotropes often improve with correction of the acidosis in this way. In any event, frequent monitoring is essential, as rehydration and improvements in peripheral tissue perfusion may have dramatic effects on acid-free states and potassium levels.

Notwithstanding the chronic potassium depletion associated with long-term diuretic therapy mentioned above, in patients with severe acute disease and metabolic acidosis, hyperkalaemia may be a problem. This may be exacerbated in patients with poor renal function and those given old stored blood (in which potassium levels of 20 mmol/l are not uncommon). Preoperative enteral ion exchange resins may be of value if time allows and levels are only moderately raised, although very high levels are more effectively treated with infusions of glucose and insulin (initially 25 g glucose and 10 units insulin). Frequent potassium estimations must be made as violent swings may occur, particularly in long-term potassium-depleted patients in whom hyperkalaemia has resulted from shifts from the intracellular compartment associated with metabolic acidosis. It should be remembered that only 5% of whole-body potassium resides in the extracellular compartment. An initially high extracellular fluid (ECF) potassium level may become dangerously low in response to, say, glucose and insulin if a metabolic acidosis is being corrected at the same time. ECG monitoring is mandatory to allow early recognition and treatment of dysrhythmias.

Hypoxia

Decompensated cirrhosis is associated with hypoxia reflecting alterations in pulmonary ventilation/perfusion relationships. Intrapulmonary shunting and arteriovenous anastomoses may develop. Further mismatching results from dilatation of small pulmonary vessels (seen in both cirrhosis and fulminant hepatic failure), and thickening of pulmonary capillary walls further limits gas exchange. A tendency towards arterial hypoxaemia may be exacerbated by poor basal lung expansion in the face of ascites, raised intra-abdominal pressure and 'splinting' of the diaphragm. Clearly, systemic hypotension can only cause further deterioration in oxygenation as the associated pulmonary hypotension increases ventilation/perfusion mismatching.

In summary, the approach to the patient with severe liver disease must be characterized by awareness of the problems to be anticipated, comprehensive monitoring of glucose and potassium levels, acid-base status, oxygenation, fluid balance, peripheral perfusion and renal function, and correction of abnormalities as far as possible before surgery. It should be restated that, however fastidious the anaesthetist and whatever agents and techniques are employed, liver function in patients with severe liver disease may be *expected* to deteriorate in response to the 'insult' of exposure to anaesthesia and surgery. Surgery should only be undertaken if essential and, if possible, delayed to allow at least partial correction of the abnormalities discussed.

ANAESTHESIA FOR PATIENTS WITH PRE-EXISTING LIVER DISEASE

Choice of agents

Relevant factors in the choice of agents include: alterations in protein binding and drug availability in hypoalbuminaemic, hyperglobulinaemic patients; reduced hepatic metabolism; associated renal impairment.

Premedication with a small dose of benzodiazepine seems reasonable. Less thiopentone is protein-bound if albumin levels are low. Less may be needed at induction, and the dose should be titrated against the patient response. Opiates and sedatives should be used sparingly, as encephalopathy may be precipitated in patients with severe liver failure. In addition, as opiates may cause spasm of the sphincter of Oddi, it could be argued that they should be used sparingly in patients with intrahepatic cholestasis or posthepatic obstruction. Reduced pseudocholinesterase levels may increase sensitivity to suxamethonium.

Patients with liver disease have variable requirements for non-depolarizing muscle relaxants. There may be initial resistance to globulin-bound drugs such as tubocurarine and pancuronium, although, as 25% of pancuronium is metabolized in the liver, its action may be prolonged. On the other hand, alcuronium is predominantly albumin-bound and lower doses may be adequate. Associated renal impairment may prolong the action of alcuronium and, to a lesser extent, pancuronium and tubocurarine, as these drugs are, at least in part, excreted in the urine. It could be argued that these more or less 'cerebral' discussions of preferred non-depolarizing relaxants in severe liver disease have been rendered obsolete by the advent of atracurium. This drug, by virtue of non-enzymatic hydrolysis, can be considered to be, in some respects, the relaxant of choice in the anhepatic (and anephric) patient.

Reduced metabolism of local anaesthetic agents may render normally acceptable large doses more toxic.

With regard to the inhalational agents, while it is clear that HBF will reduce by a minimum of 25% the effects of whatever agents or techniques are used, it seems sensible to avoid those known to reduce HBF more dramatically. Thus, if agents such as cyclopropane or methoxyflurane were still available, their use in this context would be discouraged. As mentioned earlier, some studies have suggested that isoflurane reduces HBF somewhat less than enflurane or halothane. Such minor differences between these agents are unlikely to have clinical significance when viewed in the context of the many other factors influencing choice of inhalational agent, in any event likely to be used in low concentrations as part of a 'balanced' anaesthetic technique.

It may be that, as free fluoride levels rise during enflurane anaesthesia (although not, of course, to the same degree as with methoxyflurane) this agent is best avoided if renal failure is a complicating factor.

The use of halothane in a patient with pre-existing liver disease (*unrelated* to previous exposure to anaesthesia and surgery) raises interesting questions. The *relatively* minor reduction in HBF associated with the use of halothane (25% and comparable with, for example, N_2O/relaxant techniques) suggests that, in patients with compromised liver function (who must benefit if anaesthesia avoids unnecessary reduction in HBF and metabolic embarrassment), halothane remains a most suitable agent. It must be stressed that there is *no* evidence that the use of halothane in such patients is associated with a greater degree of deterioration of liver function than that seen with other agents and techniques. On the other hand, some authorities may advise that, in the light of the halothane toxicity clearly demonstrable in carefully prepared animal models (the relevance of which will be discussed later), it is safer to avoid halothane in these patients. Whether such advice addresses itself to overall (or even hepatic) patient safety or to the medico-legal well-being of the practitioner is an entirely different matter! As always, it remains the responsibility of the anaesthetist to choose agents and techniques which, in his hands, he considers best serve the overall interests of his patient. If his choice includes agents known to minimize HBF reduction and metabolic embarrassment, in my view, at the present state of knowledge he cannot be faulted.

In general, the choice of acceptable anaesthetic agents in patients with liver disease is of secondary importance when compared with the need for attention to detail and the avoidance of aspects of technique which unnecessarily reduce HBF and adversely affect the liver. As in so many areas of anaesthesia, it is much more important to choose the anaesthetist! The chosen technique should avoid the following:

1. Hypoxia. Portal blood is only 70% saturated at best and centrilobular areas are particularly at risk. Concern for adequate oxygenation must extend to the recovery room and beyond.
2. Hypercarbia. Increased sympathetic activity is associated with splanchnic vasoconstriction and reduced HBF. Halothane to some extent protects the splanchnic circulation from the constrictive effects of hypercarbia because, by limiting the expected increase in sympathetic tone, it allows carbon dioxide to act directly as a vasodilator.
3. Hypocarbia. This implies excessive IPPV with unnecessary reduction in HBF. Hyperventilation should be avoided, and a ventilatory pattern should be chosen with a view to achieving the lowest possible mean intrathoracic pressure. This will minimize the rise in hepatic outflow tract pressure. Infrequent large tidal volumes with a short inspiratory time are preferable in this respect, although the higher *peak* pressures required may not be thought advisable in patients with concomitant pulmonary disease. As always, the benefits of any technique must be balanced against the potential hazards in other areas. End-tidal CO_2 or blood gas monitoring will allow adjustment of IPPV to achieve normocarbia.
4. Hypotension. The 25% of HBF supplied by the hepatic artery carries some 65% of the oxygen supply to the liver, and hypotension may increase metabolic embarrassment. Thus consideration should be given to the myocardial depression caused by various agents, and blood loss (often increased due to abnormal coagulation) should be carefully monitored and replaced. Excellent venous access is mandatory, with facilities for central venous pressure monitoring if appropriate. The ventilatory pattern advised above will

also minimize the adverse effects of IPPV on venous return (and therefore cardiac output), effects that may be particularly marked if venous return is already compromised by the raised intra-abdominal pressure of ascites.

The importance of close monitoring has been repeatedly stressed throughout this review and attention to detail in the postoperative period may avoid further deterioration in liver function.

POSTOPERATIVE JAUNDICE

Of all controversial topics in anaesthesia, the question of whether or not there is a direct cause-and-effect relationship between exposure to halothane and postoperative liver damage has been the subject of the most bitter, vitriolic and long-lasting debate. The following discussion concentrates on halothane-associated hepatitis, but includes references to other inhalational agents as appropriate. For many years, opposing groups adopted sharply polarized positions. On the one hand, several 'authorities' (usually non-anaesthetists) clearly identified the syndrome of 'halothane hepatitis' as a serious problem, accepted the evidence at face value, and even advocated very severe limitation of halothane usage. On the other hand, some anaesthetists refused to countenance even the possibility of a direct relationship, staunchly defended (against all-comers) a very valuable agent, and objected fundamentally to what they saw as an attempt by those far removed from the 'sharp end' to dictate anaesthetic practice. After all, many anaesthetists quite rightly felt that overall anaesthetic safety had been revolutionized by the advent of halothane. Between these extreme views, attempts were being made to scrutinize the 'evidence' scientifically and encourage a perspective view of the problem in the context of modern anaesthetic practice. Now, while there is general agreement on the existence of the entity, debate continues on the mechanism(s) involved and, perhaps more importantly, the relevance of a 'syndrome' that remains ostensibly very rare.

At the height of the controversy a newcomer might have been excused the misapprehension that postoperative jaundice was a problem almost exclusively related to the use of halothane. Such was the heat of the debate that it was often forgotten that unexplained postoperative jaundice had been reported in association with almost all anaesthetic agents and techniques. The literature includes cases following regional and neuroleptic anaesthesia and even thiopentone alone, with, in many cases, the 'syndrome' appearing remarkably similar to 'halothane hepatitis'.

When halothane was first introduced (Raventos 1956) it was expected that, in the light of experience with carbon tetrachloride and chloroform, the use of this new halogenated hydrocarbon would be associated with liver damage. Somewhat surprisingly, the extensive animal work which preceded its introduction and early studies in man failed to demonstrate a problem. However, within a few years isolated case reports of 'halothane hepatitis' started to appear, not only in the medical press, but also (perhaps reflecting the sharp public polarization of views) in the media. These reports prompted a number of retrospective reviews of anaesthetic records, in both the UK (Committee on Safety of Medicines 1986) and the USA. Relatively little emerged, even from the massive 856 000 case US National Halothane Study (Bunker et al 1969). Overall, halothane was pronounced a safe anaesthetic (which was news indeed!), but a direct cause-and-effect relationship between its use and liver damage could not be excluded. Of particular interest was a study from Toronto comparing two 4-year periods before and after the introduction of halothane (Henderson & Gordon 1964). A four-fold increase in the overall postoperative jaundice rate was demonstrated, although further analysis of the results for the second period showed that, from this point of view, halothane compared favourably with even nitrous oxide/relaxant techniques. It was suggested that the apparent increasing incidence of postoperative jaundice was attributable to a variety of non-anaesthetic factors. These included an increasing tendency to perform major heroic surgery with associated massive blood transfusions, and the increasing use of potentially 'hepatoxic' drugs such as steroids and certain antibiotics. The problem is by no means uncommon. It has been reported that, following major surgery, some 20% of patients will become jaundiced, although the majority of these will suffer only mild transient disturbances of liver function.

The most common abnormal postoperative liver-function test picture suggests an element of intrahepatic cholestasis, with predominantly conjugated hyperbilirubinaemia, mildly raised serum alkaline phosphatase and normal or minimally raised aminotransferases. These changes, possibly reflecting perioperative alterations in HBF, may be more pronounced in patients in whom hypoxia and/or hypotension further embarrass liver function, or if haemolysis of transfused blood presents an increased bilirubin load, or in patients in whom congestive cardiac failure (with raised hepatic outflow tract pressure) exacerbates the 'normal' reduction in HBF associated with anaesthesia and surgery. Variable changes are associated with cirrhosis, intra-abdominal sepsis, and shock with, quite often, moderately raised aminotransferases. Higher levels of alkaline phosphatase may well suggest more severe intrahepatic cholestasis as seen, for example, with fucidic acid or erythromycin. In patients with very high alkaline phosphatase levels, unsuspected cholelithiasis or other causes of posthepatic obstruction (e.g. malignancy) must be excluded.

Thus the liver function test profile will suggest, in most cases, that parenchymal liver cell damage is not a dominant feature, that the mild degree of liver dysfunction probably reflects the non-specific perioperative changes in HBF and that uneventful resolution is to be expected. Some authorities believe that even the minor transient alterations in liver function test results described are, in fact, manifestations of mild hepatotoxicity of the inhalational agent concerned, rather than merely reflecting the alterations in HBF and possible minor degree of associated metabolic embarrassment to be expected as a corollary to anaesthesia and surgery. I find the evidence for this point of view unconvincing and prefer to consider these minor changes to be non-specific. The many reports of minor alterations in liver function tests following both inhalational and intravenous anaesthetic techniques support the non-specificity of these changes.

The very few patients who present with a liver function test picture suggesting moderate or severe hepatocellular disease (in the absence of apparent alternative causative factors, such as intra-abdominal sepsis, pre-existing liver disease, etc. [see later]) are those in whom a diagnosis of anaesthetic-agent-associated hepatitis must be seriously entertained. It is these patients, with variable hyperbilirubinaemia, normal or minimally raised alkaline phosphatase and moderately or severely raised aminotransferases who are of most concern in this context. In general terms the diagnosis of halothane, enflurane or isoflurane hepatitis remains one of exclusion.

Until recently, the exclusion of viral causes for an episode of postoperative jaundice was impossible. The development of tests for serum markers for virus A and virus B hepatitis, and for other possible causative viruses (including cytomegalo, Epstein–Barr and herpes viruses), and the recent detection of antibodies to hepatitis C virus (Zuckerman 1989) allows the exclusion of viral causes with increasing confidence. However, it remains impossible to exclude such agents with absolute certainty. The exclusion of viral hepatitis from the differential diagnosis is important for several reasons. Firstly, the syndrome of anaesthetic agent associated hepatitis appears clinically, biochemically and histologically virtually indistinguishable from acute viral hepatitis. Minor differences have been reported under both light and electron microscopy by some authors, but such claims (mostly without the obvious benefits of 'double blind' assessment) are not universally accepted. Secondly, it has been estimated that annually in the USA alone some 4000 patients are exposed to anaesthesia and surgery while coincidentally incubating viral hepatitis (Dykes et al 1972). Presumably in at least some of these patients the viral illness will become manifest in the immediate postoperative period. The suggestion that patients with possible 'halothane hepatitis' are unlikely to be suffering from viral hepatitis because viral hepatitis has a very low mortality rate is unconvincing. As exposure to anaesthesia and surgery is associated with alterations in immunocompetence (Walton 1979), it would come as no surprise to learn that coincidental viral hepatitis is more likely to pursue a fulminant course postoperatively than if the infection were contracted in the absence of the stress of anaesthesia and surgery. On the other hand, the age group predominantly at risk from 'halothane hepatitis' does seem somewhat older than that most commonly associated with viral hepatitis. Unsuspected preoperative hepatic dysfunction may be more common than generally realized, and financial considerations may preclude the routine preoperative liver function test screening necessary to identify such patients. It has been reported that 1 in 700 surgical patients may have unsuspected problems of this nature and 1 in 2500 may become jaundiced *without* exposure to anaesthesia and surgery (Wataneeyawech & Kelly 1975, Schemel 1976)! As exposure to anaesthesia and surgery may exacerbate previously subclinical hepatic insufficiency (from whatever cause), such an incidence may well be relevant to this discussion of an ostensibly rare clinical problem.

The mechanism by which halothane (or, for that matter, methoxyflurane or enflurane) produces liver damage remains far from clear. The evidence used to support the various current theories may be worth closer scrutiny.

The direct hepatotoxicity theory

A theory claiming increasing support suggests that halothane (or, more likely, a metabolite thereof) is a direct hepatotoxin, causing variable degrees of liver dysfunction *very commonly*. For a drug to be labelled a direct hepatotoxin, several criteria should ideally be satisfied. For example the damage should be dose-related and occur in all recipients (if enough of the drug is given) after a predictable brief latent period. Furthermore, the distinct histological pattern should be easily recognizable and should be easily reproducible in animals. 'Halothane hepatitis' seems to satisfy few of these criteria. The lesion is *not* dose-dependent, indeed, many severe cases follow very brief exposures. The problem (at least clinically) is rare although, as mentioned above, some authorities interpret minor postoperative alterations in liver function test results as evidence for minor degrees of hepatotoxicity and consider mild 'halothane hepatitis' to be very common. The latent period is very variable, with jaundice appearing at any time within 3 weeks of exposure. The histological picture is variable and, as mentioned earlier, there is some doubt whether 'halothane hepatitis' and acute viral hepatitis can be differentiated (double-blind) by either light or electron microscopy.

Early attempts to produce an animal model for 'halothane hepatitis' were unconvincing, with the drug often administered by inappropriate (intraperitoneal or intragastric) routes to a wide variety of species. The results were very variable and the histological picture often bore little resemblance to that seen in man. However, the research scene was transformed by the work of Sipes & Brown (1976). They showed that, in rats pretreated with a powerful hepatic microsomal enzyme-inducing agent (pentachlorobiphenol), the inhalation of halothane reliably results in massive hepatic necrosis. Since that pioneering study, innumerable reports have confirmed that hepatic necrosis can be produced in rats, particularly if they are pretreated with enzyme-inducing agents and rendered hypoxic during halothane administration or, alternatively, if they are rendered thyrotoxic before receiving the drug. Under similar rather artificial circumstances, hepatic necrosis can also be produced by methoxyflurane, enflurane and even isoflurane, although with the latter agents often to a lesser degree. These models suggest that techniques that encourage reductive metabolism of halogenated agents tend to produce most liver damage.

Research has, most laudably, been directed towards the development of an inhalational agent which approaches the 'ideal' of being totally inert within the body. Whereas some 20% of an inhaled dose of halothane is metabolized, the figures for enflurane (2%) and isoflurane (0.15%) suggest that, if metabolism is a primary mechanism responsible for the liver damage, these latter agents may have progressively less potential for producing this postoperative problem. However, although many of these animal experiments clearly incriminate metabolism as the mechanism involved, it is far from certain whether or not these experiments provide reliable pointers to the mechanism(s) in man. Extrapolation from animals to man is notoriously unreliable. Interspecies differences in hepatic metabolic pathways and pharmacodynamics render conclusions very difficult to draw with confidence. There are several anomalies that cast doubt on the validity of the various animal models. For example there are major differences in the results achieved with different strains of rats. Massive hepatic necrosis occurs predominantly in hypoxic male rats or in females given testosterone, a finding which contrasts sharply with the apparent predominance of females among patients with 'halothane' and 'methoxyflurane' hepatitis. Furthermore, in fasted rats pretreated with phenobarbitone, liver damage can be produced by hypoxia *alone* (i.e. without exposure to anaesthetic agents). Doubt has also been cast on the relevance of the thyrotoxic rat model by a study of patients with thyrotoxicosis anaesthetized with either halothane or fentanyl. Similar transient changes in LFT results were demonstrated in both groups, with no evidence of increased toxicity in the halothane group. There is increasing evidence that the phenobarbitone/hypoxic and the thyrotoxic rat models are very different. For example, fasting increases toxicity in the former model (in association with an increase in free fluoride ions, i.e. more reductive metabolism), whereas in the thyrotoxic rat, fasting reduces toxicity. Furthermore, hypoxia seems unnecessary in the latter case, and free fluoride ion levels do not rise. It is of interest that N_2O exacerbates the liver damage in the phenobarbitone/hypoxic rat. Recently, attention has been redirected towards the guinea-pig, in which hepatic necrosis can be produced by halothane administration in the absence of enzyme induction and hypoxia (Lunam et al 1985). It seems that, although both halothane and isoflurane reduce mean arterial blood pressure in this species to a similar degree, hepatic necrosis is not seen in the isoflurane group. It remains to be seen whether this animal model proves to be relevant to the syndrome in man, but it does seem likely that the arcane rat models described above will eventually be acknowledged as of very limited value.

It is clear, therefore, that although animal models for 'halothane hepatitis' have been developed (with considerable difficulty), their relevance to the syndrome in man remains in some doubt. These difficulties contrast strikingly with the relatively simple production of animal models for chloroform- and fluroxene-associated liver damage. The hepatotoxicity of these drugs in animals has been very clearly correlated with hepatic metabolism, with microsomal-enzyme-inducing agents increasing both metabolism and damage, and enzyme inhibitors producing opposite results. Microsomal enzyme inhibition also reduces halothane-associated liver damage in the guinea-pig model mentioned above, suggesting that, at least in that species, metabolism and liver damage *are* directly related. In fluroxene-associated hepatitis in man, those patients who died in fulminant hepatic failure tended to be those on long-term enzyme-inducing agents (such as phenobarbitone). There has been little such correlation reported in patients with 'halothane hepatitis'. Nomura et al (1986) have reported that patients taking phenobarbitone before neurosurgery are more likely to suffer halothane-related liver damage than those not 'pretreated' with microsomal-enzyme-inducing agents. One study of children taking long-term phenobarbitone and exposed to halothane failed to demonstrate an increase in postoperative liver dysfunction, although the relevance of this study must be diminished by the apparent extreme rarity of 'halothane hepatitis' in children.

Trichloroethylene-associated hepatitis has excited little interest among anaesthetists, although isolated case reports have been produced. Its use in anaesthesia has almost ceased, but the problem remains relevant in the context of the increasingly popular pastime of glue sniffing. Glue sniffers' hepatitis is thought often to be directly related to the metabolism of trichloroethylene, the vapour of which is a major constituent of favoured brands. Repeated exposure in rats results in an increase in both metabolism and toxicity.

It has been shown that the capacity to metabolize halothane may be, to some extent, genetically predetermined (Cascorbi et al 1971). It has been argued, therefore, that as the clinical syndrome of 'halothane hepatitis' seems rare, if metabolism is responsible an abnormal metabolite may be involved – produced only occasionally in genetically predisposed individuals. It is of interest that there have, indeed, been very few reports suggesting that 'familial halothane hepatitis' is an entity (Hoft et al 1981). HLA typing has produced confusing results, although studies in in vitro lymphocyte susceptibility to electrophylic metabolites, in patients with 'halothane hepatitis' and some of their relatives, raise the *possibility* that familial factors may be relevant (Farrell et al 1985). However, it seems likely that, had genetic factors been relevant, a clear picture would have emerged from the myriad of reports and studies in the literature.

The hypersensitivity theory

Although research into possible metabolic mechanisms for halothane hepatitis continues unabated, despite the questionable relevance of various animal models, much interest remains in the concept that the syndrome has an immunological basis. The 'evidence' quoted in support of the hypersensitivity theory falls into four main categories: clinical stigmata of hypersensitivity reported in some patients; autoantibodies found in some cases; evidence for cell-mediated immunity; and, finally, reports of in vitro cytotoxicity and circulating antibodies.

The relevance of some of the clinical stigmata of hypersensitivity reported in association with 'halothane hepatitis' remains in some doubt. For example, leucocytosis and pyrexia are very common non-specific postoperative findings; arthralgia is very rare (and I have seen painful drip sites at the wrist and elbow reported as arthralgia and, therefore, evidence for hypersensitivity); a skin rash may very often be related to concomitant drug therapy; and bronchospasm, although mentioned in early reviews, is not a feature. Potentially of greater interest is the suggestion that pyrexia following *previous* exposure to halothane might indicate a mild hypersensitivity reaction to the agent and, some authorities believe, that this should preclude its further use. Unfortunately, temperature records relating to previous surgery are often difficult to find. Postoperative pyrexia is *very* common indeed, and in 55% of patients with postoperative pyrexia no cause can be found (Dykes 1971). Despite attempts to eliminate these 'normal' early postoperative pyrexias by attaching significance only to unexplained 'spikes' during the second postoperative week, the importance of such a finding must remain in some doubt. It is of concern that the Committee on Safety of Medicines' statement on halothane hepatotoxicity once again restated that: 'A history of unexplained jaundice or pyrexia in a patient following exposure to halothane is an absolute contraindication to its future use in the patient.' (CSM 1986). This seems to disregard the published evidence on the non-specifity of the mild pyrexia almost always seen after exposure to anaesthesia and surgery, and makes no attempt to highlight the possibly increased significance of late pyrexia. On the other hand, eosinophilia is a common finding. The 'syndrome' is clearly associated with rapidly repeated exposures, and reports of positive 'challenge' experiments in personnel with liver dysfunction associated with exposure to halothane (Klatskin & Kimberg 1969, Johnston & Mendelsohn 1971) are considered by some reviewers to be convincing evidence in support of the 'hypersensitivity theory'. More recently, further cases have been described in which circulating halothane-related antibodies were demonstrated (Neuberger et al 1981).

The association of liver, kidney, microsomal and thyroid autoantibodies with 'halothane hepatitis' led to the suggestion that patients with autoimmune disease might be more vulnerable. However, a study of liver function in such patients receiving halothane failed to detect evidence of toxicity.

Attempts to provide in vitro evidence of cell-mediated immunity have had mixed results. Early reports of positive lymphocyte transformation tests in patients with 'halothane hepatitis' were not reproducible by most other workers, while positive migration inhibition results from another group seemed somewhat more promising. However, these early workers used halothane itself as the potential antigen in their in vitro studies and, as halothane is a relatively small molecule (immunologically speaking), not shown to combine covalently with protein, it seems unlikely that the parent molecule is capable of being antigenic in its own right. Much more likely is the explanation that a reactive metabolite of halothane might combine with a protein and thus achieve antigenic status.

Recently, various techniques have been developed to demonstrate the presence of circulating antibodies in patients with halothane hepatitis. Early unreliable cell-based cytotoxicity studies (Vergani et al 1980) have been supplanted by more elegant techniques. Both immunoblotting (using microsomal proteins from halothane treated rabbits or rats as antigen) and enzyme-linked immunosorbent assays (ELISA; using halothane treated rabbit microsomes or trifluoracetate-rabbit serum albumin complexes as antigen) have produced positive results in up to 80% of patients (Kenna et al 1984). Apparent specificity is improving and it has been suggested that similar techniques may be applicable in patients with suspected enflurane- or isoflurane-associated hepatitis (Martin et al 1990).

Just as the metabolic toxicity theory cannot easily be seen to explain this clinically rare syndrome, the hypersensitivity theory also leaves many questions unanswered. For example, what of those patients who have multiple, rapidly repeated halothane exposures uneventfully some years previously and then develop severe hepatic dysfunction after one further exposure? This anomaly is, of course, equally difficult to explain on direct hepatotoxicity grounds. It is possible that such early reports were actually describing patients with coincidental viral hepatitis, for which no markers were available at that time. Patients who ostensibly develop halothane hepatitis after a single exposure are most unlikely to be hypersensitive to the agent, and it is possible, of course, that different mechanisms are responsible in some patients.

It is clear, therefore, that both theories are attractive in some respects, but remain less than completely convincing. Apparent predisposing factors seem to lead in different directions. The association between halothane hepatitis and obesity might be explained by the increased likelihood of obese patients becoming relatively hypoxic in the recovery room, with a resultant increase in potentially damaging reductive metabolism. However, one study of postoperative LFT changes in obese patients found similar alterations following exposure to N_2O/fentanyl, halothane or enflurane. On the other hand, as a history of allergy is frequently found, could it be that patients with such a history are more likely to develop an immunological response to a metabolite-protein complex?

It has recently been shown that in an adult surgical population the *reductive* metabolism of halothane is greater in females than in males. It is possible that such differences contribute to the apparent increased incidence of the syndrome in females (Jenner et al 1990).

It seems to me that the most likely sequence of events is: metabolism (producing reactive intermediate metabolites); combination of a metabolite with protein (achieving antigenic status); and, finally, an immunological component resulting in liver damage. The suggestion that direct metabolite toxicity is wholly responsible for damage which is *not* dose-related and seems to be very rarely of *clinical* relevance seems less than convincing. After all, innumerable patients must become relatively hypoxic (at least briefly) during the immediate postoperative period without developing serious hepatic sequelae.

Incidence of and mortality rate from 'halothane hepatitis'

It is difficult to have confidence in any published figures for incidence or mortality. Neither the numerator (i.e. the total number of patients with 'halothane hepatitis') nor the denominator (i.e. the total number of patients exposed (to halothane) are more than educated guesswork! Nevertheless, figures of 1 in 10 000 for single exposure and 1 in 1100 for multiple exposure have been suggested. Of course, if one believes that the transient minor alterations in LFT results referred to above are indeed minor episodes of 'halothane hepatitis', then the incidence becomes very high. Reports of death rates vary widely, presumably reflecting the differing patient populations under review. Rates of 50–80% have been reported from specialist liver failure units, although the rate falls to 20% when the whole spectrum of the clinical syndrome is considered.

Halothane in present-day anaesthetic practice

The syndrome of 'halothane hepatitis' appears more common in obese, middle-aged women with a history of allergy. The increased usage of enflurane and isoflurane has seen a dramatic reduction in the administration of halothane. In many centres the agent has been abandoned altogether, or its use has been severely restricted. It would appear that, as halothane use has diminished in favour of the newer agents, case reports of inhalational-agent-associated hepatitis have diminished also. While many anaesthetists continue to believe that halothane still has a place in adult anaesthesia (with due regard, of course, to previous anaesthetic history), rather more retain the agent solely for use in children. As rare as the *clinical* syndrome appears in adults, 'halothane hepatitis' is very rare indeed in children. Cases have been reported (Kennal et al 1987), but with an apparent incidence of between 1 in 82 000 (Wark 1983) and 1 in 200 000 (Warner & Beach 1984). It is widely believed that, once again with appropriate concern for anaesthetic history, halothane remains very valuable for the inhalational induction of children. In this area at least it has considerable advantages when compared with its widely used 'replacements'. It is of interest that a recent study of halothane metabolism in normal children suggested that both quantitative and qualitative metabolism (by oxidative and reductive pathways) are comparable to that seen in adults, thus shedding no light on the apparent difference in incidence between the two groups (Wark et al 1990).

Although 'halothane hepatitis' can apparently occur following single exposure to the agent, the syndrome is clearly associated with multiple, rapidly repeated exposures. In recent years, conflicting evidence has been presented regarding the minimum advisable period between exposures to halothane. Early suggestions of 'not within a month' based on reports to CSM (Inman & Mushin 1974) were subsequently 'updated' (Inman & Mushin 1978). More recently, recommendations have appeared, firstly in the British Medical Journal and then from the CSM, for minimum 'recommended' intervals between exposures of 6 months and 3 months, respectively. The former asked the question: 'Are there now any absolute indications for the repeated use of halothane within six months?' (Blogg 1986). One might wonder whether there are *ever* any *absolute* indications for the use of *any* anaesthetic drug under *any* circumstances! Anaesthetic drugs are used, or not, depending on the perceived balance between their merits and demerits in a particular clinical situation. Nonetheless the concerned anaesthetist might infer that, were he to administer halothane twice within this new arbitrary 'unsafe period' (despite no evidence of problems following previous exposure), he would do so at his medico-legal peril! The advice that 'repeated exposure to halothane within a period of at least 3 months should be avoided unless there are overriding clinical circumstances (CSM 1986) suggests that the onus of responsibility rests with the anaesthetist to be able to *prove conclusively* that previous exposure to halothane produced no problems, and even *that* may be unacceptable if the agent is used for perfectly valid reasons within this newly advised 'unsafe period' and problems ensue! The irrationality of this blanket restriction, and the possible detriment to a patient who might benefit from the use of halothane but does not receive it for perceived medico-legal reasons, was highlighted by a timely letter from 13 professors of anaesthesia in the British Medical Journal (Adams et al 1986) commenting on the CSM statement.

It remains the responsibility of the anaesthetist to choose an anaesthetic regimen which best suits the *overall* interests of the patient. The conscientious anaesthetist is, obviously, at least as keen to avoid anaesthesia-related complications as are hepatologists and others far removed from the 'sharp end' of clinical anaesthesia. It is in the interest of both anaesthetists and their patients that the choice of agent or technique should be based on sound clinical criteria (with an awareness of possible problems), rather than unduly influenced by medico-legal fears (Weis & Engelhardt 1989).

Realistically, the prudent anaesthetist may feel that his own professional health will best be served by observing the 'not within 3 months' directive. However, he should be satisfied that the alternatives are equally appropriate. If he decides that they are not and that halothane would be the best agent for his purposes, he would be well advised to follow the advice of the 13 professors and record his reasons. Of course, all the above relates to a patient previously uneventfully exposed to halothane (etc.). If the previous exposure (however long ago) was followed by jaundice (whatever the supposed cause), it must be good practice to avoid the same agent. The basic medical tenet that no patient should be re-exposed to a drug to which he has previously had an apparent adverse response applies no less forcibly to anaesthesia. If in *any* doubt about the cause, it *must* be sensible to assume the worst.

Cross-sensitivity

There is relatively little convincing evidence for 'cross-sensitivity' between inhalational agents, although occasional reports suggesting the possibility have been made (Sadove & Kim 1974, Sigurdsson & Hreidarsson 1985). A mechanism has been suggested involving an immunological response to metabolite–protein complexes (Christ et al 1988). It could be argued that, until the position becomes clear, patients with a history of inhalational-agent-associated hepatitis should not be exposed to alternative inhalational agents. On the other hand, the anaesthetist may feel that either a regional technique would be inappropriate or a totally intravenous approach would be inadvisable. If so, he could argue that the use of an alternative halogenated agent would be very much in the best *overall* interests of the patient and therefore, medico-legally, an entirely appropriate course of action. As always, the anaesthetist must balance the risks.

The approach to the patient with a history of jaundice

Preoperative anaesthetic assessment should always include a specific question about previous jaundice (or 'liver trouble'). If a previous episode of jaundice was **not** chronologically related to exposure to anaesthesia, it can be ignored. There is no evidence to suggest that patients with a history of, for example, viral hepatitis some years earlier should not receive halothane or any other agent. However, if the previous episode *was* related to exposure to anaesthesia, despite the fact that, in most cases, no details of the anaesthetic or the suspected cause of the jaundice are available, it seems sensible to assume 'the worst' and avoid halothane. A patient's contention that he had a previous attack of 'viral hepatitis' should not be accepted at face value without confirming that the episode was unrelated to exposure to anaesthesia.

The case for halothane-free machines

It has been suggested that, should a patient with a history of 'halothane hepatitis' require anaesthesia, a 'halothane-free machine' should be used. There is little evidence that such advice serves anything but medico-legal self-interest. Although it is clear that a patient anaesthetized with a machine on which halothane has recently been used will receive a minute dose of the agent, the possible significance of such minimal exposure is extremely doubtful. I have seen 19 patients with apparent 'halothane hepatitis' who were subsequently uneventfully anaesthetized on standard 'halothane-contaminated' machines (Walton et al 1976). One could argue that a minimal dose of halothane cannot result in sufficient reactive metabolite either directly to damage the liver or (if one supports the hypersensitivity theory) to trigger an immunological response. Very rare reports suggesting that patients suffer by such halothane contamination are far from convincing.

Enflurane- and isoflurane-associated hepatitis

Reports of enflurane-associated hepatitis have been made, and analysis of such cases suggests a clinical, biochemical and histological picture similar to that seen with halothane (Lewis et al 1983). The validity of many of these isolated reports has been questioned (Eger et al 1986).

The mechanism by which enflurane may cause hepatitis is, once again, far from clear, although recent studies have suggested the possibility that metabolites of enflurane may combine with hepatic proteins and achieve antigenic status (Christ et al 1988). The lesser extent to which enflurane and isoflurane are metabolized should render them less likely than halothane to cause hepatitis, whether direct metabolic injury or combined metabolic/ immunological mechanisms are involved. The increasing popularity of enflurane has not, apparently, been associated with widespread reporting of suspicious cases! If enflurane hepatitis exists, it seems to be rare.

A somewhat similar picture emerges with isoflurane. Despite its immense popularity in some areas, only very few isolated case reports have appeared (Gregoire & Smiley 1986, Carrigan & Straughen 1987), and doubts have been expressed regarding their validity (Stoetling et al 1987). Recent reports of rat hepatocyte monolayer cell culture damage by hypoxia, enzyme induction and halothane showed that such damage could not be reproduced in the presence of isoflurane. As isoflurane is minimally metabolized, its potential for hepatotoxicity (in the rat, and *possibly* in the human) may be negligible.

Sevoflurane and desflurane

These two recently developed inhalational agents are of some interest as potential replacements for those currently popular. Some authors have reported (in some species) liver damage with sevoflurane similar to that seen with isoflurane (Strum et al 1987). Desflurane has not been shown to produce hepatic damage in rats despite hypoxia and enzyme induction (Eger et al 1987). In pigs, neither desflurane nor isoflurane was shown to cause elevation of hepatic enzyme levels (Holmes et al 1990). Preliminary evidence suggests that both these newer agents have minimal hepatotoxic potential.

REFERENCES

Adams A P, Campbell D, Clarke R S J et al 1986 Halothane and the liver. Br Med J 293: 1023

Blogg C E 1986 Halothane and the liver: the problem revisited and made obsolete. Br Med J 292: 1691–1692

Bunker J P, Forrest W H, Mosteller F 1969 A study of the association between halothane anesthesia and post-operative hepatic necrosis. In: National Halothane Study. US Government Printing Office, Washington

Carrigan T W, Straughen W J, 1987 A report of hepatic necrosis and death following isoflurane anaesthesia. Anesthesiology 67: 581–583

Cascorbi H F, Vesell E S, Blake D A, 1971 Genetic and environmental influence on halothane metabolism in twins. Clin Pharmacol Ther 12: 50–55

Christ D C, Kenna J G, Kammerer W 1988 Enflurane metabolism produces covalently bound liver adducts recognised by antibodies from patients with halothane hepatitis. Anesthesiology 69: 833–838

Committee on Safety of Medicines 1986 Halothane hepatotoxicity. Curr Probl 18: 1–2

Dykes M H M 1971 Unexplained post-operative fever: its value as a sign of sensitisation. J Am Med Assoc 216: 641–644

Dykes M H M, Gilbert J P, McPeek B 1972 Halothane in the United States. Br J Anaesth 44: 925–935

Eger E I, Smuckler E A, Ferrell L D 1986 Is enlurane hepatotoxic? Anesth Analg 65: 21–30

Eger E I, Johnson B H, Strum D P 1987 Studies of the toxicity of 1–653, halothane and isoflurane in enzyme-induced hypoxic rats. Anesth Analg 66: 1227–1229

Farrell G, Prendergast D, Murray M 1985 Halothane hepatitis: detection of a constitutional susceptibility factor. N Engl J Med 313: 1310–1314

Gregoire S, Smiley R K 1986 Acute hepatitis in a patient with mild factor IX deficiency after anaesthesia with isoflurane. Can Med Assoc J 135: 645–646

Henderson J C, Gordon R A 1964 The incidence of post-operative jaundice with special reference to halothane. Can Anaesth Soc J 11: 453–459

Hoft R H, Bunker J P, Goodman H I 1981 Halothane hepatitis in three pairs of closely related women. N Engl J Med 304: 1023–1024

Holmes M A, Weiskopf R B, Eger E I 1990 Hepatocellular integrity in swine after prolonged desflurane (1–653) and isoflurane anaesthesia: evaluation of plasma alanine aminotransferase activities. Anesth Analg 71: 249–253

Inman, W H N, Mushin W W 1974 Jaundice after repeated exposure to halothane. Analysis of reports to the Committee on Safety of Medicines. Br Med J 1: 5–10

Inman W H N, Mushin W W 1978 Jaundice after repeated exposure to halothane. Br Med J 2: 1455–1456

Jenner M A, Plummer J L, Cousin S M J 1990 Halothane reductive metabolism in an adult surgical population. Anaesth Intensive Care 18: 395–399

Johnston C I, Mendelsohn F 1971 Halothane hepatitis in a laboratory technician. Aust N Z J Med 1: 171–173

Kenna J G, Neuberger J, Williams R 1984 An enzyme-linked immunosorbent assay for detection of antibodies against

halothane-altered hepatocyte antigens. J Immunol Methods 75: 3–14
Kenna J G, Neuberger J, Mieli-Vergani G 1987 Halothane hepatitis in children. Br Med J 294: 1209–1211
Klatskin G, Kimberg D V 1969 Recurrent hepatitis attributable to halothane sensitisation in an anesthetist. N Engl J Med 280: 515–522
Lewis J H, Zimmerman H J, Ishak K G 1983 Enflurane hepatotoxicity: a clinico-pathological study of 24 cases. Ann Intern Med 98: 984–992
Lunam C A, Cousins M J, Hall P 1985 Guinea-pig model of halothane associated hepatotoxicity in the absence of enzyme induction and hypoxia. J Pharmacol Exp Ther 232: 802–809
Martin J L, Kenna J G, Pohl L R 1990 Antibody assays for the detection of patients sensitised to halothane. Anesth Analg 70: 154–159
Neuberger J, Vergani D, Mieli-Vergani G 1981 Hepatic damage after exposure to halothane in medical personnel. Br J Anaesth 53: 1173–1177
Nomura F, Hatano H, Ohnishi K 1986 Effects of anticonvulsant agents on halothane-induced liver injury in human subjects and experimental animals. Hepatology 6: 952–956
Raventos J 1956 The action of flurothane: a new volatile anaesthetic. Br J Pharmacol 11: 394–410
Sadove M S, Kim S I 1974 Hepatitis after use of two different fluorinated anaesthetic agents. Anesth Analg 53: 336–340
Schemel W H 1976 Unexpected hepatic dysfunction found by multiple laboratory screening. Anesth Analg 55: 810–812
Sigurdsson J, Hreidarsson A B 1985 Enflurane hepatitis: a report of a case with a previous history of halothane hepatitis. Acta Anaesthesiol Scand 29: 495–496
Sipes I G, Brown B R 1976 An animal model of hepatotoxicity associated with halothane anaesthesia. Anesthesiology 45: 622–628
Stoetling R K, Blitt C D, Cohen P J 1987 Hepatic dysfunction after isoflurane anaesthesia. Anesth Analg 66: 147–153
Strum D P, Eger E I, Johnson B H 1987 Toxicity of sevoflurane in rats. Anesth Analg 66: 769–773
Vergani D, Mieli-Vergani G, Albert A 1980 Antibodies to the surface of halothane-altered rabbit hepatocytes in patients with severe halothane-associated hepatitis. N Engl J Med 303: 66–71
Walton B 1979 Effects of anaesthesia and surgery on immune status. Br J Anaesth 51: 37–43
Walton B, Simpson B R, Strunin C 1976 Unexplained hepatitis following halothane. Br Med J 1: 1171–1176
Wark H J 1983 Post-operative jaundice in children: the influence of halothane. Anaesthesia 38: 237–242
Wark H, Earl J, Chau D D 1990 Halothane metabolism in children. Br J Anaesth 64: 474–481
Warner L O, Beach T P 1984 Halothane and children: the first quarter century. Anesth Analg 63: 838–840
Wataneeyawech M, Kelly K A 1975 Hepatic diseases: unsuspected before surgery. N Y State J Med 75: 1278–1281
Weis K H, Engelhardt W 1989 Is Halothane obsolete? Two standards of judgement. Anaesthesia 44: 97–100
Zuckerman A J 1989 The elusive hepatitis C virus. Br Med J 299: 871–872

8

The endocrine response to surgery and the modifying effects of anaesthesia

P. S. Sebel and C. L. Westmoreland

INTRODUCTION

Imagine being attacked by a masked person with a large knife in a poorly lit street late at night. The neuroendocrine response that prepares an organism for 'fight or flight' is essentially the same as that a patient undergoes during elective surgery. There may be more light, and the attacker may be dressed in green, but the response is the same. This endocrine response, however appropriate in the poorly lit street, may be inappropriate in the controlled conditions of a hospital environment. The 'fight or flight' mechanism, also known as the general adaptation syndrome, is a response controlled by the central nervous system and mediated via endocrine and autonomic responses. This response enables the body to retain its integrity in response to a threatening stimulus. Apart from local responses to trauma (swelling, vasoconstriction, etc.) there is a set of general reactions which occur following trauma, burns or surgical insults. Part of this response was noted by Bauer (1872), who observed that an increased urinary nitrogen concentration occurred following haemorrhage.

Cannon (1929) demonstrated the importance of the autonomic nervous system in the homeostatic responses to trauma. He showed that cats that had undergone total sympathectomy were able to survive in a protected environment, but were unable to defend themselves against haemorrhage, hypoxia or fluid restriction and to respond normally to exercise or alterations in environmental temperature. He introduced the concept of a 'neuroendocrine response to stress'. Selye (1946) suggested that the adrenal cortex is the initiator and controller of this neuroendocrine response. Hume & Egdahl (1959) observed that, both in man and the dog, trauma resulted in increased corticosteroid output, and if this response failed, then the individual died. The late response to trauma of weight loss, negative nitrogen balance and hypermetabolism was described by Cuthbertson (1976). The peak effect of these metabolic changes occurred during the third and eighth day after the injury.

The stress response has three phases: the initial 'fight or flight' response, associated with increased sympathetic tone and catecholamine secretion; an 'ebb phase', associated with a reduction in body weight and fatigue; and a 'flow phase' of recovery with hypermetabolism, a negative nitrogen balance and glucose intolerance. It does not appear possible to reduce the catabolic state that produces large nitrogen losses by giving high protein nutrition. In fact, the cachectic patient will conserve nitrogen much better than a well-nourished patient after major stress.

The potential adverse effects of a stress response in a hospital environment have been reviewed by Savege (1978). The catecholamine and sympathetic response will cause an increase in both heart rate and blood pressure, which may be damaging to the patient with an ischaemic myocardium. Dysrhythmias and the results of vasoconstriction, namely tissue hypoxia and acidoses, are other potential problems. From the metabolic viewpoint the increased protein catabolism may lead to impaired tissue repair. There will be sodium and water retention, and potassium loss. There is increased mobilization and metabolism of fats leading to ketone production. Both the inflammatory and immune responses may be reduced, possibly leading to depressed protection against infection and tumour growth.

There are many factors that may initiate the metabolic response to injury. These can be due to external stimuli or originate within the organism itself. The most important environmental factors are probably extremes of temperature. Psychic stimuli of rage, anxiety and fear have also been demonstrated to be of importance. It has been suggested that, in surgical patients, waiting for anaesthesia may cause greater metabolic disturbances than anaesthesia itself (Allison 1971). One of the most potent stimuli producing the stress response is fluid loss, whether actual loss from the body in the form of haemorrhage, vomiting, etc., or redistribution into the gut or other tissues. Various other pathological processes can cause or enhance the response. These include myocardial infarction, thermal injury and infection, especially endotoxins and exotoxins.

Whatever the initiating stimulus, the metabolic response is uniform and the hypothalamus appears to be the integrating centre for the response. It is here that the hormonal and neuroendocrine responses are initiated. Although uniform, the response is graded: the more stressful the episode the greater the metabolic response. Quantitative relationships between pain intensity and beta endorphin levels were shown to occur during uncomplicated vaginal deliveries. Statistically significant relationships were found between plasma beta endorphin and cortisol levels, and the degree of pain subjectively perceived by patients with increasing cervical dilatation (Bacigalupo et al 1990).

In sum, various factors may modify the neuroendocrine response. We have already seen that patients who are cachectic conserve nitrogen better than the well-nourished. Immobility will also induce protein breakdown. Underlying metabolic disorders such as diabetes and thyroid disease will modify the response, as will drug therapy, particularly agents such as beta blockers and others acting on the sympathetic nervous system. We will now consider the endocrine response to surgery in more detail, discussing each metabolic response in turn and then the modifying effects of anaesthesia.

ENDOCRINE RESPONSE TO INJURY

Hypothalamic–hypophyseal axis

Pain, anaesthesia and surgical stress cause beta endorphin release in the region of the hypothalamus. This is one of the initiating factors that cause the various hypothalamic nuclei to secrete releasing factors into the hypothalamo–hypophyseal circulation. This will cause release of the various trophic and other hormones from the anterior and posterior hypophysis. Marschall et al (1989) studied plasma levels of beta endorphins in patients undergoing minor elective surgery. On arrival at the operating room it was found that there were increases in beta endorphin but not ACTH levels. This change was independent of the administration of a preoperative medication. In the post-surgical period there were increases in both beta endorphin and ACTH. These results indicate that, while beta endorphin and adrenocorticotrophic hormone are neuropeptides produced from the pituitary and derived from the same precursor, pre- and post-surgical stress may differentially affect plasma levels (Marschall et al 1989).

Antidiuretic hormone (vasopressin) is increased after anaesthesia and surgery, and is markedly elevated during traction on abdominal viscera (Zimmerman 1965). Cardiopulmonary bypass will also cause an increase in antidiuretic hormone secretion (Stanley et al 1979). Antidiuretic hormone induces water reabsorption from the collecting ducts and distal convoluted tubules, and is partly responsible for the oliguria and urinary concentration that occurs after surgery (Dudley et al 1954). Oxytocin is released from the posterior hypophysis at the same time as antidiuretic hormone and causes vasoconstriction. This response may be inappropriate following surgery.

All the hypophyseal hormones are increased following stress. The level of adrenocorticotrophic hormone (ACTH) increases rapidly after surgical stimulus. This leads to the release of both cortisol and aldosterone. Previously, studies of hormonal response during the perioperative period were difficult to interpret. This was because they relied on measurements using different anaesthetic techniques at intervals that were greater than the plasma half-life of an episodically secreted hormone, such as ACTH. In a recent study by Udelsman et al (1987), ACTH, cortisol and adrenaline levels were measured at regular intervals preoperatively, intraoperatively and postoperatively in patients undergoing neck surgery. During surgery, ACTH, cortisol, and adrenaline were mildly elevated, and glucocorticoid secretion appeared to be maintained primarily by continuous rather than pulsatile ACTH secretion. Even more interesting, however, were the profound elevations in the plasma ACTH, cortisol and adrenaline concentrations post-anaesthesia, with extubation, and in the immediate postoperative period. These data suggest that anaesthetic reversal may be a major determinant of stress hormone secretion, rather than surgical stimulus as previously suggested (Udelsman et al 1987).

Propofol, a relatively new anaesthetic agent gaining wide acceptance in induction and maintenance of anaesthesia, appears to attenuate ACTH and cortisol release (Mitchell et al 1990). The clinical importance of these findings has yet to be determined.

Growth hormone, a polypeptide secreted by the anterior pituitary, is elevated during surgery (Newsome & Rose 1971) and especially during cardiopulmonary bypass. Growth hormone secretion produces hyperglycaemia, release of free fatty acids thus inducing ketogenesis, and cellular uptake of amino acids. The release of growth hormone is known to be stimulated by hypothalamic growth hormone releasing factor.

In an effort to determine the site of action of fentanyl in attenuating the pituitary-adrenal response to surgery, serum concentrations of growth hormone and cortisol were compared for two groups of patients. The growth hormone response and serum cortisol concentration were significantly greater in the group receiving concomitant administration of releasing factors (corticotrophin releasing factor, arginine vasopressin and growth hormone releasing hormone) than in the fentanyl-alone group. This suggested that the primary site of action of fentanyl during surgery is hypothalamic, either directly or indirectly, rather than pituitary (Hall et al 1990).

Because high-dose opioids alone currently appear unlikely to eliminate hormonal changes associated with cardiopulmonary bypass, opioids in combination with specific hormonal blocking agents have been tried in attempts to produce complete suppression. Somatostatin, formed in the hypothalamus and the pancreatic D cells, and known to inhibit the secretion of growth hormone and glucagon secretion, was given to patients undergoing elective valve replacements using sufentanil and trimethaphan. This combination did prevent increases in the cortisol, glucagon and growth hormone responses, as well as decreasing serum catecholamine concentrations, although this latter change was not statistically significant (Desborough et al 1990).

There is little information about thyroid stimulating hormone (TSH) secretion during surgery, and until recently assays of TSH levels were insufficiently sensitive to detect changes occurring during surgery. Thus, while the impact of surgical trauma on thyroid function had been well defined for some time, little was known about the relationship of thyreotropin (TSH) secretion during surgery. Recently, highly sensitive and specific monoclonal-antibody-based methods permitted the study of peri- and postoperative changes in the concentration of TSH under general anaesthesia. Noreng et al (1987) recorded an immediate rise in plasma TSH (similar to other anterior pituitary hormones) with skin incision. Nevertheless, such changes in TSH serum levels may be due to discrepancies in TSH measurements using different assays, as no significant increase in TSH was found in a later study (Shigemasa et al 1988).

Adrenal medulla

Detailed information on the catecholamine response to stress has been limited, until recently, by a lack of a suitable assay method for the individual catecholamines in plasma at picogram levels.

Newly introduced radioenzymatic and high-pressure liquid chromatography techniques are much more sensitive and specific than the older fluorometric techniques. There are two other problems when assessing catecholamine responses. Firstly, the catecholamines are very evanescent and their plasma concentrations may decrease very rapidly, thus if a blood sample is taken 2 min after a stimulus, the response may have already evaporated. Secondly, when investigating responses such as tachycardia, it is difficult to determine whether a response is mediated via catecholamine release from the adrenal medulla or via the sympathetic nervous system. There are also many factors that will affect catecholamine responses, for instance, changing from the supine to the erect posture will cause marked elevations in catecholamines (Kothary & Zsigmond 1980).

Increases in catecholamine production have immediate and marked systemic effects, and produce the early part of the 'fight or flight' response. Stimulation of alpha receptors, which are present at the postsynaptic effector sites of smooth muscle, will lead to vasoconstriction, contraction of the iris in the eye and sphincter contraction. Clonidine, a partial alpha-adrenergic agonist with antihypertensive, antinociceptive and sedative properties, has been used for its potential benefits in minimizing the increases in arterial hypertension related to intubation, and after cardiopulmonary bypass graft surgery. Pouttu et al (1987) tested the efficacy of orally administered clonidine in reducing stress responses related to anaesthesia and surgery in breast surgery patients. On finding clonidine to be a potent suppressor of sympathoadrenal activity, they proposed that clonidine could theoretically reduce stress responses in patients with coronary heart disease. During elective cardiac surgery, intravenous clonidine was found to lower plasma catecholamine concentrations during and after surgery (Halbo-Hansen et al 1986). Intraoperatively, clonidine did have a moderate hypotensive effect. However, in the postoperative period, arterial hypertension was not reduced in the clonidine patients compared with the controls, indicating that factors other than sympathoadrenal hyperactivity are important for the development of systemic arterial hypertension post-cardiopulmonary bypass graft (Halbo-Hansen et al 1986, Quintin et al 1991).

Beta-receptor stimulation results in increased cardiac activity as demonstrated by increased ventricular ejection fraction, decreased ejection time, an increase in coronary artery blood flow and an increase in heart rate. Beta stimulation will also result in bronchodilatation, an increase in blood flow to skeletal muscle and relaxation of intestinal smooth muscle. The subsequent effect of catecholamine secretion and increasing sympathetic activity is to 'shut down' parts of the body not required for immediate escape and to provide the skeletal muscle with more oxygen (as a result of increased blood flow).

Until recently the actions of dopamine were thought to be due to its effects at the adrenoreceptors. There is now an accumulating body of evidence that suggests the existence of a separate dopamine receptor (Iversen 1975). Such dopamine receptors exist in the brain, and dopamine depletion is known to be involved in the production of Parkinson's disease. Dopamine receptors have also been found in blood vessels, particularly in renal and mesenteric systems.

Adrenal cortex

Corticosteroid production is increased at times of stress. Moore et al (1955) discovered the relationship between the negative nitrogen balance that occurs after stress and the increased excretion of metabolites of corticosteroids. Corticosteroid production is thought to be the main factor in postoperative protein catabolism.

Aldosterone production also increases after surgery. Since aldosterone causes an increase in blood pressure and increased absorption of sodium from the renal tubules, it is likely that increased aldosterone production contributes to postoperative sodium retention. Control of aldosterone production is multifactorial. It is affected by ACTH, alterations in sodium:potassium ratio and changes in the circulating blood volume. However, activation of the renin-angiotensin system is a major factor controlling aldosterone production. Reductions in afferent renal arteriolar pressure (caused by decreased blood pressure or reduced circulating blood volume) result in increased renin production from the juxtaglomerular apparatus. This results in the conversion of angiotensinogen to angiotensin, which is subsequently converted to angiotensin II and stimulates aldosterone production in the adrenal cortex. The resultant sodium retention and increased blood pressure suppress further renin production by a negative feedback mechanism.

The pancreas

Insulin and glucagon exert major influences on carbohydrate metabolism. Insulin enhances glucose uptake by muscle and also increases glycogen formation by the liver. Glucagon increases glycogenolysis, amino acid utilization and free fatty acid mobilization. During surgery, insulin secretion is unchanged, but there is a decreased responsiveness to a glucose load (Allison 1971). It is surprising that even major surgery, for example cardiac surgery, has no effect on insulin production (Sebel et al 1981). Glucagon secretion is increased during surgery and remains elevated for up to 8 days postoperatively. There are many factors controlling the blood glucose concentration: insulin, glucagon, catecholamines, thyroid hormones and growth hormone. The net effect is for surgical stress to be accompanied by hyperglycaemia.

Thyroid

Thyroid hormone production in relation to stress has not been conclusive. There are a number of reports illustrating a reduction of total triiodothyronine (TT3) and sometimes total thyroxine (TT4) in patients with acute and chronic nonthyroidal diseases (Imberti et al 1988). Known as a Low T3 syndrome, this state seems to be a nonspecific response to stress. A similar state was documented in 25 patients without thyroid linked pathology (Imberti et al 1988). In seven of these patients, TT3 levels were below the normal limit. The lowest levels of TT3 and TT4 occurred on the first postoperative day. Changes in TT4 and FT4 were significant but smaller. One patient in this series with persistently low levels of TT3 died after 30 days of hospitalization. Whether or not these reported reductions can be used as a prognostic indicator in patient management remains to be seen, as it is not clear that the aforementioned changes contribute to patient morbidity. It is possible that they represent a reflection of the normal response to injury (Mogensen & Hjortso 1988).

THE MODIFYING EFFECT OF ANAESTHESIA

The endocrine metabolic response to surgery is related to the type of surgery and the level of stimulation. The response after body-surface surgery is relatively small, compared with abdominal surgery or cardiopulmonary bypass when marked increases in catecholamine secretion occur (Bovill et al 1983). Two anaesthetic techniques are effective in blocking metabolic responses to some degree: regional analgesia and large doses of opioid analgesics. Local analgesic techniques are probably effective because they block afferent input into the nervous system, although efferent blockade may be important. Ophthalmic surgery in elderly patients did provide additional new information on the hormonal and metabolic responses of local versus general anaesthesia. A significant decrease in glucose and lactate concentrations occurred in the local anaesthetic group, suggesting a reduced catecholamine secretion (Barker et al 1990). The mechanism of action of opioid analgesics is uncertain, but may be related to the inhibition of hypothalamic function (George et al 1974, Lacoumenta et al 1987). An alternative approach to modifying the stress response is to minimize the effects of the altered hormonal balance after it has occurred. This may be done by infusing appropriate substrates, administering anabolic hormones such as insulin, or nursing the patients in a thermoneutral environment (Traynor & Hall 1981).

Regional analgesia

It is well established that epidural analgesia either abolishes or decreases the ACTH and cortisol response to surgery. However, the effects are somewhat variable, and this variation may relate to incomplete blockade of all afferent pathways. When all afferent pathways were blocked by epidural analgesia, complete inhibition of the cortisol response was demonstrated (Enquist et al 1977). Effective regional analgesia will block the catecholamine, growth hormone and glucagon response to surgery. However, in cases where pain relief is significantly improved but incomplete, as with post-thoracotomy patients with various pain control methods (single intercostal block, repeated intercostal block, epidural morphine, and epidural bupivacaine infusions), endocrine responses proved difficult to ablate (Scheinin et al 1987).

It appears that regional anaesthesia exerts no effect on thyroid hormone secretion, and data on the renin–angiotensin–aldosterone axis are conflicting: some suggest increased aldosterone production, others suppression. The blood pressure and circulating blood volume are likely to be as important as regional analgesia, and regional variations in these factors may explain the conflicting data. Epidural analgesia will produce a less negative nitrogen balance in the first 5 days following hysterectomy than a general anaesthetic technique (Brandt et al 1978). Lipolysis and increases in both plasma lactate and ketone levels are suppressed by effective regional analgesia.

The benefits to the patient from modifying the stress response by regional analgesic techniques remain to be proven. Theoretically, a decrease in protein catabolism as demonstrated by Brandt et al (1978) should be beneficial in reducing substrate mobilization and breakdown of muscle tissue. It has been suggested that regional analgesic techniques will decrease the overall mortality after surgery (McLaren et al 1978), but whether this is related to the suppression of endocrine responses remains a matter for conjecture.

Opioid analgesics

Because of the cardiovascular stability obtained, opioid analgesics given in large doses have achieved considerable popularity as sole anaesthetic agents for cardiac surgery. They are also effective in suppressing hormonal responses. Morphine (4 mg/kg) suppresses both the cortisol and growth hormone responses to cardiac surgery (George et al 1974), but it has no effect on the antidiuretic hormone response (Philbin et al 1976) and catecholamine levels may be elevated following morphine anaesthesia (Hasbrouk 1970). Morphine therefore provides partial attenuation of the endocrine response to surgery.

Fentanyl (50 μg/kg), compared with halothane used as an anaesthetic supplement, was found to suppress the metabolic and endocrine responses to tubal surgery in young healthy women (Hall 1978). Fentanyl used as the sole anaesthetic for cardiac surgery suppresses all metabolic responses, including increases in catecholamine production in the period before cardiopulmonary bypass. During bypass, however, marked elevations in catecholamine secretion occur (Sebel et al 1981). Sufentanil, a more potent derivative than fentanyl in a dose of 20 μg/kg, is also ineffective in blocking stress responses during cardiopulmonary bypass (Bovill et al 1983, Lacoumenta et al 1987). If fentanyl were effective in blocking stress responses, then continuing fentanyl administration into the postoperative period should reduce the negative nitrogen balance. However, this does not occur (Walsh et al 1981). Therefore the metabolic benefits of large-dose opioid anaesthetics are debatable. As with regional analgesic techniques, short-term metabolic benefits can be proven with opioids, but no longer term reduction in morbidity or mortality has ever been demonstrated.

Etomidate

Etomidate, an anaesthetic induction agent, was extensively used by infusion for sedation in intensive therapy units. Following a suggestion that this was associated with an increase in mortality (Ledingham & Watt 1983), the metabolic effects of etomidate have been extensively investigated and this subject has been reviewed (Owen & Spence 1984). In essence, etomidate blocks cortisol production by inhibiting the action of mitochondrial 17-alpha and 11-beta hydroxylase activity in the adrenal cortex. Thus, the mechanism of cortisol suppression after etomidate is different from that obtained by regional analgesia and opioid analgesics, and may be harmful.

SUMMARY

Surgical stress is accompanied by a metabolic response consisting of increased production of most hormones. This response can be blocked by regional analgesia or large doses of opioid analgesics, without proven benefit to the patient.

REFERENCES

Allison S P 1971 Changes in insulin secretion during open heart surgery. Br J Anaesth 43: 138

Bacigalupo G, Riese S, Rosendahl H, Saling E 1990 Quantitative relationships between pain intensities during labor and beta-endorphin and cortisol concentrations in plasma. Decline of the hormone concentrations in the early postpartum period. J Perinat Med 18: 289

Barker J P, Robinson P N, Vafidis G C et al 1990 Local analgesia prevents the cortisol and glycaemic responses to cataract surgery. Br J Anaesth 64: 442

Bauer J 1872 Ueber die Zersdetzungsvorgange im Thierkorper under dem Einglusse von Blutenziehungen. Z Biol 8: 567

Bovill J G, Sebel P S, Fiolet J W T, Touber J L, Kok K, Philbin D M 1983 The influence of sufentanil on endocrine and metabolic responses to cardiac surgery. Anesth Analg 62: 391

Brandt M R, Fernandes A, Mordhorst R, Kehlet H 1978 Epidural analgesia improves postoperative nitrogen balance. Br Med J 121: 1106

Cannon W B 1929 Bodily changes in pain, hunger, fear and rage. Appleton Century Crofts, New York

Cuthbertson D 1976 In: Wilkinson A W, Cuthbertson D (eds) Metabolism and the response to injury. Pitman, Tunbridge Wells

Desborough J P, Hall G M et al 1990 Hormonal responses to cardiac surgery: effects of sufentanil, somatostatin and ganglion block. Br J Anaesth 64: 688

Dudley H A F, Boling E A, Quesne L P, La Moore F D 1954 Studies on antidiuresis during surgery: effects of anaesthesia surgery and postoperative pituitary antidiuretic hormone on water metabolism in man. Ann Surg 140: 354

Enquist A, Brandt M R, Fernandes A, Kehlet H 1977 The blocking effect of epidural analgesia on the adrenocortical and hyperglycaemic responses to surgery. Acta Anaesthesiol Scand 21: 330

George J M, Reier C E, Lanese R R, Rower J M 1974 Morphine anaesthesia blocks cortisol and growth hormone response to surgical stress in humans. J Clin Endocrinol Metab 38: 736

Halbo-Hansen S, Fletcher R, Lundberg D et al 1986 Clonidine and the sympatico-adrenal response to coronary artery by-pass surgery. Acta Anaesthesiol Scand 30: 235

Hall G M 1978 Analgesia and the metabolic response to surgery. Stress Free Anaesthesia. International Congress Symposium Series No. 3. Royal Society of Medicine, London, 22

Hall G M, Lacoumenta S, Hart G R, Burrin J M 1990 Site of action of fentanyl in inhibiting the pituitary-adrenal response to surgery in man. Br J Anaesth 65: 251–253

Hasbrouk J D 1970 Morphine anaesthesia for open heart surgery. Ann Thorac Surg 10: 364

Hume D M, Egdahl R H 1959 The importance of the brain in the endocrine response to injury. Ann Surg 150: 697

Imberti R, Maira G, Confortini M C et al 1988 Effect of fentanyl-oxygen anesthesia during cardiac surgery on serum thyroid hormones. Acta Anaesthesiol Belg 39: 217

Iversen L L 1975 Dopamine receptors in the brain. Science 188: 1084

Kothary S P, Zsigmond E K 1980 Plasma cortisol and norepinephrine after pain relief. Excerpta Medica International Congress Series 533: 1010

Lacoumenta S, Yeo T H, Burrin J M, Hall G M 1987 Beta-endorphin infusion fails to modulate the hormonal and metabolic response to surgery. Clin Endocrinol 26: 657

Lacoumenta S, Yeo T H, Paterson J L, Burrin J M, Hall G M 1987 Hormonal and metabolic responses to cardiac surgery with sufentanil-oxygen anaesthesia. Acta Anaesthesiol Scand 31: 258

Ledingham I McA, Watt I 1983 Influence of sedation on mortality in critically ill multiple trauma patients. Lancet 2: 1270

McLaren A D, Stockwell M C, Reid V T 1978 Anaesthetic techniques for surgical correction of fractured neck of femur: a comparative study of spinal and general anaesthesia in the elderly. Anaesthesia 33: 10

Marschall K, Schlesinger M D, Turndorf H, Puig M M 1989 Beta-endorphin and ACTH levels in the perioperative period. Gen Pharmacol 20: 399

Mitchell P, Smythe G, Torda T 1990 Effect of the anesthetic agent propofol on hormonal responses to ECT. Biol Psychiatry 28: 315

Mogensen T, Hjortso N–C 1988 Acute hypothyroidism in a severely ill surgical patient. Can J Anaesth 35: 74

Moore F D, Steenberg R W, Ball M R, Wilson G M, Myrden J A 1955 Studies in surgical endocrinology. Ann Surg 141: 145, 174

Newsome H H, Rose J C 1971 The response of human adrenocorticotrophic hormone and growth hormone to surgical stress. J Clin Endocrinol Metab 33: 481

Noreng M F, Jensen P, Thellden N U 1987 Peri- and postoperative changes in the concentration of serum thyreotropin under general anaesthesia, compared to general anaesthesia with epidural analgesia. Acta Anaesthesiol Scand 31: 292

Owen H, Spence A A 1984 Etomidate. Br J Anaesth 56: 555

Philbin D M, Wilson N E, Sokoloski J, Coggins C 1976 Radioimmunoassay of antidiuretic hormone during morphine anaesthesia. Can Anaesth Soc J 23: 290

Pouttu J, Scheinin B, Rosenberg P H, Viinanaki O, Scheinin M 1987 Oral premedication with clonidine: effects on stress responses during general anaesthesia. Acta Anaesthesiol Scand 31: 730

Quintin L, Roudot F, Roux C et al 1991 Effect of clonidine on the circulation and vasoactive hormones after aortic surgery. Br J Anaesth 66: 108

Savege T 1978 Stress-free anaesthesia. Academic Press, London, p 11
Scheinin B, Scheinin M, Asantila R, Lindberg R, Viinamaki O 1987 Sympatho-adrenal and pituitary hormone responses during and immediately after thoracic surgery: modulation by four different pain treatments. Acta Anaesthesiol Scand 31: 762
Sebel P S, Bovill J G, Schellekens A P M, Hawker C D 1981 Hormonal responses to high-dose fentanyl anaesthesia. Br J Anaesth 53: 941
Selye H 1946 The general adaptation syndrome. J Clin Endocrinol 6: 117
Shigemasa C, Adachi T, Igawa O et al 1988 Sequential changes in serum thyroglobulin, triiodothyronine, and thyroxine following partial thyroidectomy for nontoxic nodular goiter. Metabolism 37: 677
Stanley T H, Philbin D M, Coggins C H 1979 Fentanyl-oxygen anaesthesia for coronary artery surgery: cardiovascular and antidiuretic hormone responses. Can Anaesth Soc J 26: 168
Traynor C, Hall G M 1981 Endocrine and metabolic changes during surgery: anaesthetic implications. Br J Anaesth 53: 153
Udelsman R, Norton J A, Jelenich S E et al 1987 Responses of the hypothalamic-pituitary-adrenal and renin-angiotensin axes and the sympathetic system during controlled surgical and anesthetic stress. J Clin Endocrinol Metab 64: 986
Walsh E S, Paterson J L, O'Riordan J B A, Hall G M 1981 Effect of high dose fentanyl anaesthesia on the metabolic and endocrine response to cardiac surgery. Br J Anaesth 53: 1155
Zimmermann B 1965 Pituitary and adrenal function in relation to surgery. Surg Clin North Am 45: 299

9

Endocrine disorders and the safety of anaesthesia

C. E. Blogg and J. M. Dunnet

INTRODUCTION

Patients suffering from endocrine disorders may require surgery to ablate the gland involved and thus correct the condition. They can also be at risk from the disorders or their complications during anaesthesia and surgery for unrelated conditions. This chapter attempts to record the hazards encountered from both these causes. Its aim is not to provide a full clinicopathological explanation of the diseases themselves, for this is beyond the range of the book.

DISORDERS OF THE PITUITARY

Anaesthesia is required for operations on the pituitary when surgery or chemical ablation is performed for primary pituitary disease, or for hormone-dependent problems. Anaesthesia may also be required for patients with other diseases or conditions with a concomitant pituitary problem.

There are two surgical approaches to the pituitary, transfrontal and trans-sphenoidal, depending on the site and spread of the lesion. The hazards and complications of the transfrontal approach are similar to those of any frontal craniotomy and considerably higher than the trans-sphenoidal approach; postoperative mortality is four times greater, and other complications (pulmonary embolism, respiratory disturbances, hypothalamic disorders and diabetes insipidus) are reported as more frequent (Kiss et al 1982; Table 9.1). The trans-sphenoidal approach to the pituitary gland allows chemical destruction of the pituitary by injection with a neurolytic agent, such as ethyl alcohol, or destruction by local radiation with radioactive yttrium implants. Alternatively, direct surgical ablation may be required.

Primary hyperpituitarism

Acromegaly results, in the adult, from hyperfunction of the pituitary gland. The facies of the patient are unmistakable: the jaw is prognathic, the patient's bite may have altered such that the lower teeth protrude in front of the upper, the tongue is enlarged and thickened, and the hands are spade-like with large fingers. The patient may complain of weakness, but there is no direct evidence of impaired neuromuscular trans-

Table 9.1 Hazards of pituitary disorders

Complication	Implication
Hyperfunction	
Gigantism	No special precautions
Acromegaly	Airway difficulties Osteoporosis Insulin resistance
Hypofunction	
Adrenal cortical suppression	Hypotension
Diabetes insipidus	Dehydration
Surgical complications	
Proximity of optic nerves	Blindness
Operative trauma	
Hyperthermia	

mission. Insulin resistance is common, and hyperglycaemia should be anticipated and treated with oral hypoglycaemic agents, or insulin if necessary. Regular finger-stick blood glucose estimations should initially be made at 1-hourly intervals until stability is achieved.

Intubation

Intubation is particularly hazardous in acromegaly. A preoperative lateral X-ray of the head and neck will show whether there are osteoporotic lesions of bone, and will establish the degree of distortion of the airway. A poorly penetrated film may show that the epiglottis, pharyngeal mucosa and vocal cords are also thickened. Vocal cord paralysis may occur and the resulting hoarseness may mistakenly be attributed to stretching of the recurrent laryngeal nerve. Intubation may also be difficult because of the excessive distance from the front teeth to larynx, and the longest available laryngoscope blade will be necessary. It may even be difficult to achieve an airtight fit with a face mask. Tracheostomy may be necessary under local anaesthesia before undertaking hypophysectomy, and an experienced tracheostomist should be ready at the time of induction of anaesthesia.

Pupil reaction

The surgical hazards of operating on the pituitary are principally of damage to the nearby optic chiasma or optic nerves. Whatever anaesthetic is chosen, drugs that alter the pupillary reactions should be avoided. Thus atropine, hyoscine or ganglion-blocking drugs which may dilate the pupil, or narcotic analgesics which cause pupillary constriction, should not be used, or, if they are, the surgeon should be prewarned to avoid his alarm at finding apparent pupillary changes. This is especially important if chemical ablation of the hypophysis is used.

Hormone functions

Most postoperative problems that result from the removal of the hormone-secreting functions of the pituitary can be anticipated and managed prospectively.

Acute adrenal corticoid deficiency. This should be anticipated preoperatively. A long-acting steroid (methyl prednisolone, 40 mg) given intramuscularly with the premedication will provide cover for the operative period. Adequate cover postoperatively will be provided by 100 mg hydrocortisone hemisuccinate intramuscularly, then 8-hourly and reduced by one-half every 24 hours until a maintenance dose of 20–30 mg per 24 hours is achieved. At this point, 25–37.5 mg oral cortisone acetate in divided doses can be substituted. Subsequently the requirement for steroid replacement will depend on how much functioning anterior pituitary tissue has been removed. If a radical hypophysectomy has been performed, oral replacement therapy will be required for the rest of the patient's life.

During surgery, otherwise unexplained hypotension should first be blamed on inadequate steroid replacement and managed by 100 mg intravenous hydrocortisone and intravenous infusion of crystalloid solutions to maintain the central venous pressure. Hyponatraemia from reduced ability to excrete water is also common.

Diabetes insipidus. This occurs in about 50% of patients subjected to operation, and becomes apparent when careful monitoring of fluid balance in the early postoperative period shows polyuria and polydipsia. If untreated, diabetes insipidus results in severe dehydration, but simple observation of the continuing profuse urine output will be misleading until cardiovascular collapse occurs. Daily weighing is a reliable, if gradual, method of following changes in fluid balance. Substitution therapy with vasopressin is required if the fluid demands are unreasonable (in excess of 5 l/day). Intranasal pitressin snuff (lysin-vasopressin [LVP]) is the most convenient preparation but each administration lasts only 4 hours. Non-vasoconstrictor vasopressin, desmopressin (1-desamino-8-p-arginine vasopressin) can be given intranasally (10–20 μg once or twice a day). Immediately after the surgery, injected aqueous or oily depot preparations of vasopressin should be used to avoid placing the snuff into the healing surgical wound.

Allergic reactions to the injected preparation are common, therefore a small test dose should be given before using the oily preparations (lysine-vasopressin, duration 6–8 hours or desmopressin, duration 12 hours). Because coronary vasoconstriction may result from all except desmopressin, extreme caution and minimal doses of other preparations should be given to patients with myocardial ischaemia.

Intracerebral tumours, trauma, surgery or cerebrovascular accidents may rarely cause primary central diabetes insipidus. Vasopressin therapy and preoperative correction of dehydration, hypotension or electrolyte derangement are necessary.

Hypophysectomy for secondary malignant disease

If hypophysectomy is used in the management of advanced metastatic disease, such as carcinomatosis from breast cancer, other systemic problems may be present. The prudent anaesthetist will search for signs of pleural effusions or metastases, and will expect the patient to be anaemic. Pleural effusions large enough to cause respiratory symptoms should be drained preoperatively but, since they tend to reaccumulate rapidly, the relief is transient. Blood transfusion 48 hours preoperatively should be considered if haemoglobin levels are 10 g/dl or less. Care in positioning osteoporotic bones will reduce the risk of fractures.

THYROID DISORDERS

Hyperthyroidism

Medical management of hyperthyroidism has greatly reduced the need for surgery on the thyroid gland. The major complications of thyroid surgery for excessive thyroid function are intraoperative or postoperative bleeding, obstruction of the airway by tumour or haematoma and dysrhythmias resulting from increased myocardial irritability. The main hazards of thyroid surgery are summarized in Table 9.2.

Table 9.2 Hazards of thyroid disorders

Complication	Implication
Hyperfunction	
Exophthalmos	Conjunctival damage, pressure damage
Enlarged gland	Airway difficulties
Increased metabolic rate	Excessive bleeding
Myocardial excitability	Dysrhythmias
Catecholamine sensitivity	Ventricular ectopics, atrial fibrillation
Congestive cardiac failure	Worsened by beta blockers
Myopathy, myasthenia	Increased sensitivity to non-depolarizing relaxants
Thyroid storm	Tachycardia, hyperpyrexia, hypotension
Hypofunction	
Airway obstruction or coma	Reduced anaesthetic requirement
Cardiomyopathy	Congestive cardiac failure, bradycardia
Surgical complications	
Excessive bleeding	Neck haematoma, tracheal compression
Trauma to recurrent laryngeal nerves	Airway obstruction, acute aphonia
Hypoparathyroidism	Hypoparathyroidism

Exophthalmos

Exophthalmos is common in Graves' disease. The problem of potential compression of the protuberant eye and the risk of corneal abrasion remain until the patient is awake and cooperative. Sterile bland ointment should be instilled in the conjunctival sac once anaesthesia has been induced and, after taping the eyes shut with a non-irritant tape (Micropore, 3M), soft pads should be fixed over the eyes and taped to the forehead and temples. Strabismus may confuse the clinical picture and falsely suggest pre-existing damage to the cranial nerves or persistent neuromuscular block.

Preoperative medication

Hyperthyroid patients usually exhibit signs suggestive of excessive catecholamine secretion and increased metabolic rate, such as tachycardia, ventricular dysrhythmias, sweating, tremor, weight loss and increased body temperature. These signs should be reduced preoperatively by suppression of thyroid function by propylthiouracil, up to 800 mg daily for 6 weeks, and then potassium iodide, 5–10 drops each day for 10 days until surgery. Intraoperative bleeding will be increased by hypertension, hypercarbia, raised venous pressure, constriction around the neck and failure to make the patient euthyroid preoperatively. Preoperatively, beta blockers (propranolol up to 160 mg daily in divided doses, or labetalol 100–200 mg twice daily) should reduce the excessive oxygen consumption and the signs of hyperthyroidism, as well as blunt the hypertensive response to laryngoscopy and intubation.

If a thyrotoxic patient requires emergency anaesthesia, beta blockers should be given cautiously while monitoring heart rate, until a normal heart rate is restored. Fluid and electrolyte balance should also be corrected. Beta blockers are contraindicated if the patient is in atrial fibrillation and has congestive cardiac failure. Digitalis preparations are then preferable. Premedication should be aimed to produce freedom from anxiety and a reduction in the increased metabolic rate in hyperthyroid states. A combination of a benzodiazepine and narcotic analgesic is appropriate. Hyoscine, or glycopyrrolate which results in less tachycardia, is preferable to atropine to reduce secretions. Phenothiazines may produce undue hypotension. Experimental evidence from rats (Berman et al 1983) suggests that the propensity for anaesthesia-related liver necrosis is enhanced by the hypermetabolic state resulting from either thyrotoxicosis or thyroxine administration, and may be associated with the use not only of halothane, but also of enflurane or isoflurane. However, evidence is lacking in man.

Retrosternal extension

The thyroid may be grossly enlarged and extend behind the sternum in Graves' disease or other proliferative disorders, such as Hashimoto's thyroiditis or carcinoma. For this reason all patients in whom the thyroid is enlarged in the neck should have a preoperative lateral X-ray of the thoracic inlet to determine whether there is extension of the gland. Preoperative symptoms may include hoarseness resulting from involvement of the recurrent laryngeal nerve. A sternal splitting procedure or one-lung anaesthesia may be required in the rare situation of massive retrosternal enlargement of the thyroid.

Airway problems

All patients should be intubated with a non-kinking oral tracheal tube (latex armoured, Oxford or disposable plastic). Local anaesthesia from spraying the cords and larynx with lignocaine will reduce the incidence and severity of sore throat and coughing or bucking on the tube. When the anaesthetist views the larynx at laryngoscopy, the position and reaction of the cords should be noted.

At the end of the operation, during extubation, the cords should again be inspected and their movement noted. If one or both cords fails to move, it is likely that the recurrent laryngeal nerve has been traumatized on the non-moving side. The surgeon should be informed immediately and anaesthesia maintained until the decision has been made to re-explore the wound to inspect, and possibly repair, the damaged nerve. If the cord paralysis is not immediately recognized the patient may have difficulty in breathing past unmoving vocal cords, may develop stridor and asphyxiate. Immediate reintubation is life-saving.

A haematoma in the neck is another potential cause of early postoperative respiratory embarrassment by compression of the larynx and trachea from without. If this complication is suspected the sutures should be removed immediately and the clot evacuated. Delay results in such gross distortion of the upper airway that immediate cricothyrotomy or tracheostomy is necessary.

Maintenance of anaesthesia

Intermittent positive pressure ventilation and a combination of neuromuscular blocking drugs with narcotic analgesics should be used to prevent hypercarbia and the associated increased risk of dysrhythmias and bleeding. Thus the use of a thyroid mask is to be condemned, as is spontaneous ventilation in the anaesthetized patient. Pancuronium should be avoided because of the effects on myocardial catecholamine uptake. During surgery the head of the operating table should be raised by about 15–20° to aid venous drainage and improve surgical access. Ketamine is contraindicated because of its propensity to increase blood pressure, heart rate and bleeding.

Myasthenia gravis or a myopathy is relatively commonly associated with thyrotoxicosis, therefore a test dose of non-depolarizing neuromuscular blocking drugs should be used before a full dose.

After operation

Acute hypoparathyroidism may occur postoperatively (see p. 142) due to excision or damage to the parathyroid glands. 'Thyroid storm' is the term used to describe an acute hyperthyroid crisis which may occur 6–24 hours into the postoperative period. It is recognized by the combination of change in consciousness, tachycardia, hyperpyrexia and hypotension. Vomiting, diarrhoea and nausea may also occur. The management consists of increasing intravenous crystalloid fluids, oxygen by face mask, suppression of thyroid oversecretion with Lugol's iodine (0.1–0.3 ml 8-hourly), hydrocortisone hemisuccinate (100 mg i.v. 2-hourly), surface cooling, propylthiouracil (350–400 mg orally, to reduce the storage of thyroid hormones in the remaining gland) and, if tachycardia persists, titration of intravenous beta blockers is required until an acceptable heart rate is achieved. In resistant cases, reserpine (2.5–5 mg i.m.) will reduce sympathetic overactivity, and droperidol (5–10 mg 6–12 hourly i.m.) will maintain sedation and produce some alpha adrenergic blockade. Intravenous dextrose should be infused because of the increased metabolic demand. Thyroid storms may also develop in response to the stresses of surgery and anaesthesia in any patient with a history of thyrotoxicosis when undergoing unrelated procedures. Failure to recognize this as a 'thyroid storm' may result in confusion of the clinical syndrome with malignant hyperpyrexia.

Hypothyroidism

Patients suffering from hypothyroidism may, coincidentally, present for surgery. Inadequate secretion from the thyroid gland results in myxoedema, characterized by lethargy, bradycardia, hoarseness, and generalized thickening and coarsening of the tissues resulting in characteristic facies. In severe cases, especially if untreated, pericardial effusions may be found, and congestive cardiac failure may result from myocardial involvement and anaemia. S-T segment abnormalities may be mistaken for myocardial infarction. The ventilatory response to hypoxia may be blunted, and the maximum breathing capacity and lung compliance are reduced. Hyponatraemia is common. Amyloidosis may also occur, resulting in an enlarged tongue, cardiac conduction defects and renal disease. Surgery should be delayed until replacement treatment is effective. Liothyronine sodium (10–20 μg) should be given daily for 1–2 weeks until the serum thyroid stimulating hormone (TSH) level reaches the normal range. Hypothyroidism then rarely causes problems.

If there is insufficient time, intravenous thyroxine (300–500 μg) or triiodothyronine (25–50 μg) can be given to reduce the potential sensitivity to central nervous system depressant drugs. There may be a conflict of interest with patients who are both significantly hypothyroid and have angina, since treatment of hypothyroidism may worsen the angina. In patients with hypothyroidism secondary to hypopituitarism, adrenocortical steroids will also be necessary to reduce the sequelae of adrenal hyposecretion. The perioperative management of the airway is otherwise as for thyroid problems.

PARATHYROID DISORDERS

Parathyroidectomy may be carried out as a simple curative procedure, either for hyperplasia and tumours of the four parathyroid glands or as part of another associated procedure, such as thyroidectomy for carcinoma or a radical neck dissection for head and neck cancer. The main hazards of parathyroid surgery are summarized in Table 9.3.

Hyperparathyroidism

Hyperparathyroidism results in, and is diagnosed by, elevated serum calcium levels above the normal range of 2.12–2.62 mmol/l. Confirmation of the diagnosis is made by the presence of elevated parathyroid hormone blood levels. The severity of the disease is related to the degree of elevation of the serum calcium levels.

Before operation

Preoperative evaluation should include assessment of the patient for other signs of hypercalcaemia, such as anorexia, nausea, vomiting, abdominal pain, polyuria, tachycardia and dehydration. There may be a history of calcium-containing renal stones or crush fractures of osteoporotic vertebrae. If the preoperative serum calcium value is in excess of 3.49 mmol/l, urgent treatment is needed to increase urinary excretion using normal saline diuresis, frusemide and replacement of whole-body potassium depletion by infused potassium chloride at 10–20 mmol/h until serum potassium values are maintained in the normal range. If the hypercalcaemia is refractory, corticosteroids (40–60 mg prednisone i.m.) will aid calciuresis. There is otherwise considerable risk of cardiac dysrhythmias, especially sinus tachycardia or heart block. Digitalis preparations increase these hazards and must be withheld. The electrocardiogram appearance of hyperparathyroidism is characterized by a shortened Q–T interval. If these measures fail, recalcitrant hypercalcaemia will eventually respond by falling at about 2 mg/dl for 36–48 hours if mithramycin (25–50 μg/kg), a cytotoxic antibiotic, is used.

Table 9.3 Hazards of parathyroid disease

Complication	Implication
Hyperfunction	
Hypercalcaemia	Heart block, ventricular dysrhythmias, cardiac sensitivity, tachycardia, hypertension
Osteoporosis	Intubation difficulty
Hypovolaemia	Infusion colloid solutions
Hypertension	Monitor frequently
Association with chronic renal failure	
Hypofunction	
Hypocalcaemia	Muscle irritability and spasm
	Airway difficulties, convulsions, congestive cardiac failure, prolonged Q–T interval, hypotension
Surgical complications	
Neck haematoma	Airway compression

Anaesthetic technique

There is no necessity for special premedication or general anaesthetic technique for patients with hyperparathyroidism, and the anaesthetic management is identical to that described for thyroidectomy. Preoperative X-rays of the neck may demonstrate cervical osteoporosis, necessitating extreme care during laryngoscopy and intubation to avoid causing damage to the vertebrae. Intraoperative dysrhythmias may result from increased serum calcium levels when the glands are handled. Antidysrhythmic drugs should, therefore, be to hand and include potassium chloride to restore the potassium/calcium ratio.

Hypoparathyroidism

Acute hypocalcaemia may develop after surgical removal of the parathyroid glands. If untreated, the patient may develop convulsions and laryngeal stridor from muscular irritability. Treatment consists of intravenous calcium chloride (1 g) via a large cannula. It is wise to have the calcium placed ready at the bedside of patients at risk. Subsequently such patients require vitamin D derivatives and oral calcium supplementation to maintain the serum calcium within the normal range.

ADRENAL DISEASE

The adrenal glands have two areas of hormone secretion: the medulla and the cortex. Surgical excision of the adrenal may be necessary to remove destructive lesions of the gland, or to remove the hormone secretion in the hope of relieving malignant conditions. The main hazards of adrenal surgery are summarized in Tables 9.4 and 9.5.

Hypersecretion

Preoperative problems in Cushing's syndrome include diabetes mellitus with hyperglycaemia, hypocalcaemia and hypertension, the management of which is described on pages 147 and 142. Osteoporosis is common. A careful history, followed by the appropriate X-ray, will often reveal significant osteoporosis in the cervical spine. This may make the manoeuvres associated with laryngoscopy and intubation hazardous.

Before operation

Premedication should take account of concurrent hypertension or diabetes, but otherwise no special management is necessary other than anticipating that the patient will acutely develop adrenal hypofunction after the glands are removed. It is wise to give 100 mg hydrocortisone hemisuccinate with the premedication, a further 100 mg intravenously at induction and subsequently 100 mg intramuscularly 6-hourly until oral cortisone (25 mg 12-hourly) can be substituted. The anaesthetist should liaise with the surgeon to anticipate adverse pressure effects from awkward positioning of the patient. The possibility of fragile bones and vertebral fractures in these osteoporotic patients must be remembered. Also, the skin tends to be thin, so will bruise with minor trauma.

Table 9.4 Hazards of adrenal cortical diseases

Complication	Implication
Hyperfunction	
(Cushing's syndrome)	
Diabetes mellitus	Hyperglycaemia
Obesity	Airway difficulties
Lax skin	Ready bruising
Hypertension	Hypotension when gland removed
Osteoporosis	Cervical damage at intubation, lumbar damage with positioning
Polycythaemia	Congestive cardiac failure
Hypocalcaemia	Muscular irritability, convulsions
Gastric ulceration	Haematemesis
Hypofunction	
(Addison's disease)	
Steroid replacement	Hypotension if inadequate
Hyponatraemia	Hypotension
Hypovolaemia	Infuse colloid solutions
Hypoglycaemia	Coma, sensitivity to CNS depressants
Surgical complications	
Delayed, impaired wound healing	Wound infection

Table 9.5 Hazards of adrenal medulla diseases

Complication	Implication
Hyperfunction	
(Phaeochromocytoma)	
Increased catecholamine secretion	Tachycardia, hypertension, hypovolaemia, myocardial irritability, ventricular dysrhythmias
Cardiomyopathy	Congestive cardiac failure, myocardial ischaemia
Hyperglycaemia	Low cardiac output if
Hypotension	excessive preoperative preparation
Hypofunction	
Surgical excision	Acute hypotension, low cardiac output
Special complications	
Handling tumour	Releases catecholamines, precipitates hypertension and dysrhythmias
Acute adrenal cortical insufficiency if excess adrenal tissue removed	Hypotension

After operation

Insulin requirements may vary widely after adrenalectomy, and the regimen of infused glucose and potassium balanced with intravenous insulin may need frequent adjustments, preferably with an hourly sliding scale. Polycythaemia is common and incipient cardiac failure may worsen at operation. A central venous line will ease the task of fluid balance and, if left in place after the operation, will spare the patient multiple bruises. An acute decrease in blood pressure unresponsive to increasing the rate of infusion of intravenous crystalloid is an indication for a bolus dose of 100 mg intravenous hydrocortisone.

Adrenalectomy

Acute hyposecretion obviously occurs at adrenalectomy carried out for concomitant problems. In this situation the clinical features of Addison's disease are absent. The preoperative assessment is concerned with the presence of metastatic disease (usually with primary carcinoma of the breast). A regimen of intramuscular steroid supplementation (hydrocortisone hemisuccinate, 100 mg i.m., with premedication, and 6-hourly until oral cortisone acetate, 25 mg 12-hourly, can be substituted) is usually all that is required. A decrease in blood pressure, usually with hypothermia, is an indication for 100 mg intravenous hydrocortisone. Supplementation with steroids may, rarely, cause aggravation of hypertension and fluid retention, encourage gastric stress ulcers and precipitate psychiatric disorders. The suggestion has been made that wound healing may be delayed and local infection is more common, but conclusive evidence is lacking.

Phaeochromocytoma

Phaeochromocytoma, an uncommon catecholamine-secreting tumour of the adrenal medulla, can present a considerable challenge to the anaesthetist, who should be consulted in the preoperative preparation. Preoperative problems include hypertension, tachycardia, sweating, cardiomyopathy, angina and, sometimes, severe postural hypotension. Blood sugar may be raised due to suppression of insulin by the catecholamines. A high proportion of phaeochromocytomata are remote from the adrenal glands, and may lie in the area of the embryonic neural crest and extend into the thorax or even the bladder. Therefore preoperative localization of the tumour is vital, if necessary by computerized tomography or selective venous sampling along the vena cava to establish where blood containing raised catecholamine levels in the effluent from the overactive gland joins the venous circulation. The tumour may also extend into the vena cava and increase the risk of distal venous thrombus.

Before operation

Preoperative preparation is directed principally to the reduction of the effects of catecholamine secretion and thus to open up the constricted arterioles and venules, to reduce heart work by reducing peripheral vascular resistance, thereby decreasing systemic arterial pressure and allowing the re-expanded intravascular space to be adequately perfused. Ventricular ectopy should also be suppressed.

Initially an alpha-adrenergic blocker is given to cause peripheral vasodilation. Phenoxybenzamine is used (10 mg 8-hourly initially, and increased at 2–3-day intervals to as much as 250 mg/day in divided doses if hypertension is particularly refractory; Hull 1986). When the supine blood pressure is reduced to 155 mgHg systolic and 90 mmHg diastolic, a beta-blocking agent is added to the regimen (propanolol 20 mg b.d., increasing to 100 mg daily) until the heart rate is reduced to close to 90 bpm in patients with myocardial ischaemia or below 120 bpm for others. Repeated careful monitoring of blood pressure is required at this time so that, if undue postural or supine hypotension occurs, intravenous fluids can be immediately infused to maintain an adequate intravascular volume, aided by central venous pressure measurement. Crystalloid solutions are temporarily useful, but colloid solutions, human albumen solution or packed red cells will remain longer in the intravascular space. Caution is advised in volume loading if the myocardial reserve is poor as congestive cardiac failure may be precipitated.

Patients with phaeochromocytoma are particularly liable to wild and dangerous swings in blood pressure. Hypotension may result from overtreatment. Excessive hypertension can occur with trivial provocation. Rapid reduction in excessively high blood pressure is best achieved by a carefully controlled and monitored dilute infusion of nitroprusside (25–50 mg/500 ml), unless there is evidence of ischaemic heart disease when nitroglycerine infusion (50 mg/500 ml) would be more appropriate. Invasive monitoring of central venous, systemic arterial, pulmonary artery and wedge pressures is essential, and should ensure that the dose of vasodilator drug is carefully titrated against the response.

By the time the patient presents for surgery, the anaesthetist should expect to find that the patient is effectively alpha- and beta-blocked. The systemic blood pressure will be close to the normal range with some postural hypotension and the heart rate stable at around 90 bpm. The patient's peripheral perfusion and urinary output will be good. A preoperative electrocardiogram (ECG) may show signs of ischaemic heart disease and dysrhythmias which may have been reduced by preoperative beta- and alpha-adrenergic blockade. There are disadvantages, however, to such preparation, since all cardiovascular depressant anaesthetic drugs will have a more profound effect. Furthermore the final location of aberrant phaeochromocytoma tissue may require the surgeon to manipulate the gland to induce an elevation of blood pressure or heart rate. Some patients also have abnormal glucose tolerance and elevated fasting blood glucose due to the predominant alpha-adrenergic effects of catecholamines.

Preoperative medication

It is important that premedication should reduce anxiety and produce sedation to decrease the risk of further rise in catecholamine secretion. Drugs that may raise heart rate (such as atropine) or further reduce blood pressure (phenothiazine, chlorpromazine and, possibly, narcotics by their histamine-releasing properties) are best avoided. Droperidol, an alpha-adrenergic blocking agent, may paradoxically raise blood pressure in patients with phaeochromocytoma (Blitt 1981). Temazepam (20 mg) by mouth 2 hours preoperatively is advocated by Hull (1986).

Anaesthesia

Intraoperative monitoring of ECG, heart rate, central venous pressure and intra-arterial pressure is mandatory and best initiated before induction of general anaesthesia. If there is evidence of cardiomyopathy or ischaemic heart disease, a balloon-tipped flow-directed pulmonary artery catheter will also be useful for following changes in pulmonary capillary wedge pressure. Before induction of anaesthesia, drugs to reduce blood pressure should be prepared and ready for use. Suitable agents include intravenous infusion of nitroprusside 50 mg/500 ml 5% dextrose or infusion of nitroglycerine 50 mg/500 ml 5% dextrose, or phentolamine 5 mg or labetalol 50–200 mg. To restore blood pressure calcium chloride 13.3 mmol, ephedrine 30 mg in 20–30 ml normal saline or an infusion of dilute noradrenaline 4 mg/500 ml 5% dextrose may be used. Irritant drugs, such as calcium chloride and noradrenaline, must be administered via the central venous line to reduce the risk of skin sloughing, and to ensure that the effects of the infusion are independent of the state of the peripheral perfusion.

Propranolol (1–2 mg) and intravenous lignocaine (1.0–1.5 ml/kg) should be at hand for the management of intraoperative ventricular dysrhythmias. Nifedipine (5–10 mg 8-hourly) is the drug of choice for supraventricular dysrhythmias. Since there is no intravenous formulation of nifedipine, verapamil (5–10 mg) given slowly intravenously should be used if the oral route is inappropriate.

Induction of anaesthesia aiming for cardiovascular stability with high-dose fentanyl (0.5–1.0 mg) and minimal thiopentone is satisfactory, although etomidate (0.2–0.3 mg/kg) is theoretically the more logical choice of induction agent since it has minimal cardiovascular effects. The dose of fentanyl should be generous to reduce the possibility of an undue increase in heart rate and blood pressure, or dysrhythmias during laryngoscopy and intubation. The drug of choice to produce neuromuscular block for intubation and abdominal relaxation is vecuronium, as this is unlikely to alter the cardiovascular state. Intermittent positive pressure ventilation is required to avoid hypercarbia and the associated increased risk of dysrhythmia. Monitoring of expired carbon dioxide will help to ensure that mild hypocarbia is maintained. The arterial blood gases should be analysed and the ventilation adjusted appropriately when anaesthesia is stable. Maintenance of anaesthesia with analgesics, nitrous oxide and addition of a halogenated agent is usually appropriate. Halothane, and to a lesser extent enflurane, are relatively contraindicated because of the increased risk of dysrhythmias. Isoflurane appears to offer advantages due to its low blood-gas solubility, which allows the effect to be modified readily. It also has vasodilating properties which reduce blood pressure, and there is little risk of dysrhythmias.

Intraoperative problems principally involve acute changes in blood pressure. The blood pressure may fall precipitously when the tumour is removed. If so, intravenous fluids should be given rapidly until the central venous pressure is restored, while support for the myocardium is given by calcium chloride and dobutamine. Peripheral resistance is temporarily increased by infusion of dilute phenylephrine (5 mg/500 ml 5% dextrose). Colloid infusion or blood transfusion should be used if there is significant surgical bleeding or if the central venous and systemic arterial pressures cannot easily be maintained or restored by crystalloid solutions. Dopamine or dobutamine infusions may also be useful.

Acute hypertension may also be associated with dysrhythmias and ECG signs of myocardial ischaemia, and should be treated as described on page 145.

After operation

The patient remains at risk of developing hypo- or hypertensive episodes postoperatively, and should be closely observed in an intensive care unit for 2–3 days while the adrenergic blocking drugs are gradually reduced. Fluid replacement must be adequate to maintain urine output. Undue somnolence and hypoglycaemia attributable to loss of accustomed activating catecholamines may occur for the first 48 hours after surgery. Occasionally some of the phaeochromocytoma tissue may not have been removed, and this should be suspected if hypertension persists. Urgent re-exploration may be necessary. It is rare for the adrenal cortex to be sufficiently damaged during removal of a phaeochromocytoma for acute adrenal cortical insufficiency to occur. However, if both adrenals have been explored, prophylactic steroid cover is advisable lest the hypotension of adrenal cortical hypofunction is wrongly attributed to overtreatment of the phaeochromocytoma.

Undiagnosed phaeochromocytoma

The alert anaesthetist may be able to indicate the presence of an otherwise undiagnosed phaeochromocytoma if, during an unrelated surgical procedure, he notices that a particular manipulation is associated with a transient and dramatic increase in systemic blood pressure or heart rate. Unless adequate monitoring and therapeutic or resuscitative measures are ready, it would be prudent to advise the surgeon to avoid further manipulation of the offending tissue. Surgical clips placed locally with enable easier location when re-exploration is attempted after better preparation. If continued surgical exploration is unavoidable, alpha and beta blockade with labetalol can be used, carefully titrated against the response while intravascular lines are established. Thereafter the management is as described for an elective excision of phaeochromocytoma (p. 145).

CARCINOID TUMOURS

Carcinoid tumours may first present with episodes of flushing, tachycardia and hypertension resulting from intermittent excess secretion of histamine, serotonin and bradykinin. Hypotension, bronchospasm, valvular heart disease and congestive cardiac failure may also be associated. The main hazards of the carcinoid syndrome are summarized in Table 9.6.

Most attempts to reduce the sequelae of intraoperative excessive secretion by the carcinoid tumour have had little success. Corticosteroids (hydrocortisone hemisuccinate, 100 mg i.m. 6-hourly for 3 days, or oral cortisone acetate, 40 mg 2-hourly) may reduce the formation of bradykinin. Serotonin inhibitors (fenclonine,

Table 9.6 Hazards of carcinoid tumours

Hormone	Effect
Histamine release provoked by drugs	Tachycardia
Serotonin	Hypertension
Bradykinin	Congestive cardiac failure

methyltrimeprazine) may be effective but are not readily available. Aprotinin, a kallikrein trypsin inhibitor (Trasylol, 200 000 units by slow intravenous infusion), may also be effective in reducing the hazards of peripheral vasodilation and a fall in blood pressure associated with excess bradykinin secretion.

Before operation

Premedication should consist of drugs that are unlikely to release histamine or cause cardiovascular effects which may confuse the clinical picture. Both H1 and H2 histamine-receptor-blocking agents are advisable. Monitoring before induction of anaesthesia *must* include displays of ECG, central venous and direct arterial pressure monitoring. Pulmonary artery pressure measurements may be particularly useful if liver metastases are present. A decrease in core: peripheral temperature ratio may usefully indicate the vasodilation due to bradykinin.

Anaesthesia

Induction of anaesthesia is most appropriately achieved with etomidate, fentanyl and vecuronium, that are unlikely to release histamine. Enflurane is probably a more appropriate inhalation agent to choose than isoflurane, in view of its minimal vasodilator effect on muscle blood vessels and relative lack of dysrhythmogenic effect compared to halothane. Any intraoperative decrease in blood pressure is better managed with intravenous fluids, calcium chloride and dobutamine than with catecholamines that may also activate kallikrein and release vasoactive substances from the tumour.

DIABETES MELLITUS

Diabetes mellitus is the most common of the endocrine disorders and affects 1–2% of the population. In the past, diabetic patients were subdivided into two groups: juvenile or insulin-dependent diabetes mellitus (IDDM) and maturity onset or non-insulin dependent diabetes mellitus (NIDDM). The groups were subsequently renamed Type 1 and Type 2, respectively. Most Type 2 patients are controlled by diet alone or diet and oral hypoglycaemic agents. However, as physicians strive for better control of plasma glucose, increasing numbers of Type 2 elderly patients are being treated with insulin, particularly with the longer-acting depot preparations. The method of treatment will obviously influence the management during surgery.

The reported additional risk of mortality during surgery among diabetics ranges from no greater than in age-matched controls (Hjortrup et al 1985) to a three- or four-fold increase in those receiving renal transplants (Kjellstrand et al 1973). However, for those diabetic patients with the serious complications of their disease such as chronic renal failure, ischaemic heart disease or autonomic neuropathy, or those whose disease is difficult to control, the risks of anaesthesia and surgery, both in terms of morbidity and mortality, must be considerably higher than for the general population.

The preoperative assessment of the patient with diabetes determines the perioperative management of the patient and also gives warning of the presence of potentially hazardous complications. Other important factors are the degree of control, as shown by regular blood sampling (often performed by the patients themselves at home), and overt symptoms of ischaemic heart disease or autonomic neuropathy. The main hazards of diabetes mellitus are summarized in Table 9.7.

Current drug therapy that might include beta blockers and calcium-channel blockers should also be noted. Examination may be completely normal but special attention should be paid to the cardiovascular system, particularly looking for poorly controlled hypertension. The presence of

Table 9.7 Hazards of diabetes mellitus

Hazard	Implication
Hyperglycaemia	Coma, ketosis, acidosis, hyperkalaemia hypokalaemia, dehydration, osmotic diuresis
Hypoglycaemia	Confusion with signs of light anaesthesia
Chlorpropramide	Long half-life, so hypoglycaemia provoked by perioperative starvation
Peripheral vascular disease	Tourniquets may cause vascular or neurological damage
Increased susceptibility to infection	
Infection	May precipitate hypo- or hyperglycaemia
Autonomic neuropathy	Hypotension
Hypertension	Monitor carefully
Chronic renal failure	Avoid lactate solutions
Proliferative retinopathy	Impaired vision

retinopathy and signs of peripheral neuropathy may infer the coexistence of autonomic neuropathy.

Investigations should include serum electrolytes and glucose, and an ECG. The former will give early warning of renal impairment by elevations of potassium, urea and creatinine. The most sensitive bedside test of autonomic compensatory mechanisms is the increase in heart rate that is part of the normal response to a change of position from lying to standing (Fig. 9.1). Absence of the normal increase in heart rate by more than 1.11 times measured at 15 beats after changing to a standing position, then a compensatory bradycardia at 30 beats is very suggestive of autonomic neuropathy (Ewing et al 1978; Fig. 9.2). Other problems associated with autonomic neuropathy include gastric atony, acute urinary retention, sweating, diarrhoea, silent myocardial infarction and unexpected cardiac arrest.

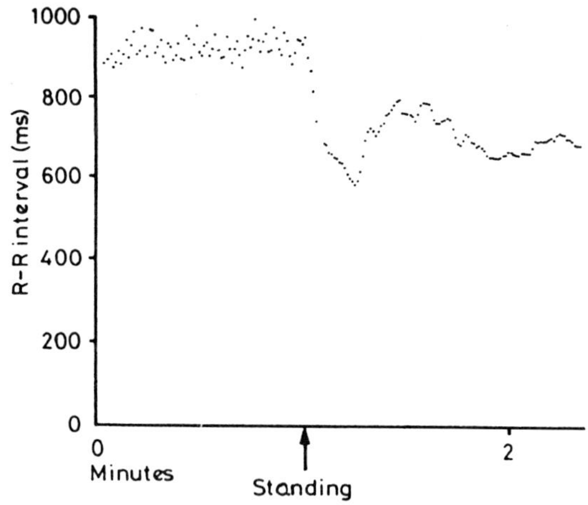

Fig. 9.1 Response of R–R interval to standing in normal 31-year-old man (from Ewing et al 1978, with permission).

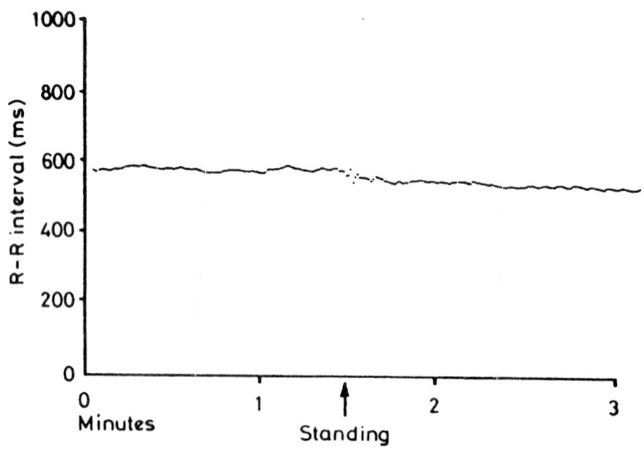

Fig. 9.2 Response of R–R interval to standing in 30-year-old man with diabetic autonomic neuropathy (from Ewing et al 1978 with permission).

Local and regional anaesthesia

Local and regional anaesthesia are useful alternatives for diabetic patients to avoid the problems posed by prohibiting oral intake of food and attempting to balance insulin therapy to meet an intravenous carbohydrate load. Patients must still be starved for an appropriate time to avoid the risks of a full stomach if general anaesthesia is required. However, if general anaesthesia is avoided the postoperative management is simplified because the patient should soon be able to eat and drink again. It should be stressed that patients with proven autonomic neuropathy may have impaired compensatory mechanisms in response to hypotension and any technique in which this may occur should be carried out with great caution.

Intraoperative management for general anaesthesia

The choice of management regimen depends primarily on the severity of the diabetes and the nature of the proposed surgery. Patients with a history of poor control may require admission some days before surgery for stabilization. Management may be considered under two groupings:

1. Well-controlled patients, whether by diet alone, oral hypoglycaemic agents, or insulin, who are due to have a minor surgical procedure that is unlikely to upset the normal control regimen.
2. Insulin-treated patients or those poorly controlled by other means, who are due to have any surgery that will interfere with normal diet for more than 24 hours. This group should include all patients having emergency surgery.

Well-controlled patients should be scheduled for surgery in such a way that they are able to maintain their usual regimen of diet and therapy while being appropriately starved. That is, first case on a morning list: delay breakfast and therapy until after surgery; or first on an afternoon list: give breakfast and normal therapy. It is unlikely that these patients will develop hypoglycaemia, but an hourly check of blood glucose using capillary blood and BM stix until the normal diet is recommenced is a sensible precaution. If the blood glucose falls below 4 mmol/l, an intravenous infusion of 5% dextrose should be started, but this is probably otherwise unnecessary as a routine. The anaesthetic technique used should allow as rapid a return to normal activity as possible and the use of antiemetics should be encouraged.

Insulin-treated patients or those whose control is inadequate may be treated in a variety of ways, but the method first described by Alberti & Thomas (1979) has gained increasing acceptance (Dunnet et al 1988), although there have also been criticisms (Hall 1984). The technique consists of an intravenous infusion of glucose, potassium and insulin (GKI) commenced on the morning of surgery and continued until normal diet is resumed. The recommended protocol consists of 1000 ml of 10% dextrose to which has been added 32 units of insulin (Actrapid or Leo Neutral) and 20 mmols of potassium chloride, run at 100 ml/hour from a burette. Blood glucose estimations by capillary stab or venous sampling should be performed 2-hourly and the insulin content of the infusion altered according to the scheme in Table 9.8. The advantage of this regimen is that insulin and glucose are given simultaneously avoiding the possibility (where separate intravenous lines are used) that one may be given without the other.

Table 9.8 Regimen for insulin management of diabetes. Infusion, 1-hourly, of 10% dextrose in 100 ml aliquots based on: 1 litre 10% dextrose containing potassium chloride (20 mmol) and 32 units insulin (modified from Alberti & Thomas 1979)

Blood glucose (mmol/l)	Insulin dose (units/l)
< 4.5	Reduce by 8
< 7.0	Reduce by 4
7.1–10.0	Leave unchanged
> 10.0	Add 4
> 15.0	Add 8

Alternative methods include a variety of protocols for intravenous insulin, or giving the insulin subcutaneously (usually one-half to two-thirds of the usual total daily dose) in conjunction with intravenous glucose. Glycaemic control with all of the intravenous regimens has proved reasonable and has tended to be better than with subcutaneous insulin (Pezzarossa et al 1988). However, whichever method is used, the aim is to achieve good control of blood glucose, that is between 7 and 10 mmol/l.

Specific problems

Hypoglycaemia. In the past, hypoglycaemia was considered a major hazard of anaesthesia in the diabetic patient as the clinical signs may be masked by general anaesthesia. However, with the increased availability and reliability of finger-prick sampling, this is no longer the case. Similarly, it is no longer justified to allow moderate hyperglycaemia, that is greater than 12 mmol/l, in an attempt to avoid hypoglycaemia.

Diabetic ketoacidosis. If this is suspected, or if the patient's general condition is poor, arterial blood gas analysis will aid in the management of pH variation and correction of the acid-base state. The general principle should be followed of achieving the best preoperative preparation of the patient within the time available before surgery becomes mandatory. Local anaesthetic techniques may be preferable but the same strictures apply.

Emergency surgery

Emergency surgery may require giving a general anaesthetic to a patient with severe fluid and electrolyte imbalance. Serious infections often precipitate diabetic ketoacidosis and active management must be started prior to surgery. Large volumes of fluid and potassium, as well as intravenous insulin, will be required. For a precise treatment regimen the reader is referred to any current text on medical emergencies. Only overwhelming surgical urgency should necessitate anaesthetizing a patient whose restoration to normal values for glucose and electrolytes is incomplete. Measurement of central venous pressure is often of value in assessing fluid replacement, particularly in the elderly. As always, resuscitation should precede surgery unless the condition is truly life-threatening, when the two should proceed simultaneously.

Autonomic neuropathy

Autonomic neuropathy occurs in 20–40% of diabetics and is more common in Type 2 diabetics. It is manifested by dysrhythmias and unexpected cardiac arrest, readily provoked by hypoxia. It may be first suspected by loss of R–R interval variation in the ECG (Fig. 9.3). Various tests have been proposed to demonstrate the presence of parasympathetic or sympathetic involvement. Vickers (1984) suggested that observation of the ECG while the patient takes six slow, deep breaths, when positive, demonstrates a failure of the heart rate to change. Other tests rely on demonstration of a lack of or

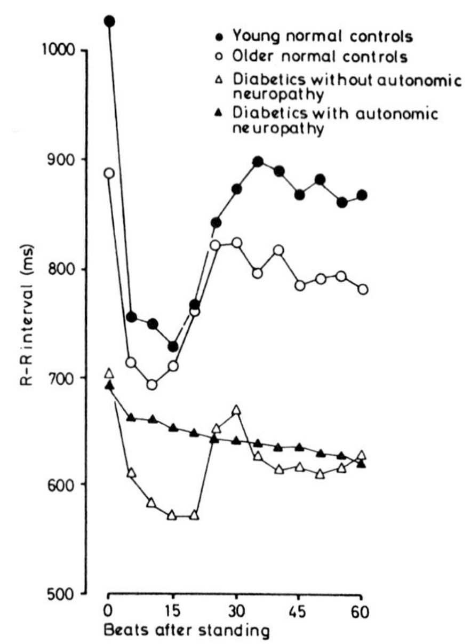

Fig. 9.3 Response of R–R intervals on standing. Mean R–R intervals in four groups (young normal controls older normal controls, diabetics with and without diabetic autonomic neuropathy) measured every fifth beat for 60 beats (from Ewing et al 1978 with permission).

reduced increase in heart rate on standing from lying, grip testing, or during a Valsalva manoeuvre (Ewing & Clarke 1982).

A history of syncope is another preoperative clue to the presence of an autonomic neuropathy. The anaesthetic management then consists of a cardiovascularly stable anaesthetic with avoidance of hypotension. Continuous ECG monitoring, including the induction period, is recommended.

Cardiac surgery in diabetics

Cardiac surgery presents particular difficulties to the anaesthetist when autonomic neuropathy coexists with ischaemic heart disease. The fluid shifts caused by coronary bypass procedures are poorly tolerated by these patients and special care is required both going on and coming off bypass. For this reason, and also to avoid loading the patient with glucose or lactate-containing fluids, a colloid pump prime is preferred. The use of cardiopulmonary bypass increases the insulin requirements due to absorption onto the tubing, so frequent measurements of blood glucose are especially important during this time. After bypass a standard glucose insulin potassium infusion may be used.

Renal transplantation

Diabetics have a relatively high incidence of end-stage renal failure. Their management differs from the non-diabetic by virtue of their inability to metabolize lactate-containing solutions and their requirement for larger volumes of crystalloid when the transplanted kidney becomes viable and the hyperosmolar state produces an osmotic diuresis. Frequent BM stix measurements allow close control (Thomas & Pollard 1989).

REFERENCES

Alberti K G M M, Thomas D J B 1979 The management of diabetes during surgery. Br J Anaesth: 51: 693–710

Alberti K G M M, Marshall S M 1988 In: Alberti K G M M, Krall L P (eds) The Diabetes Annual 4. Elsevier, Amsterdam, pp. 248–271

Berman M L, Kuhnert L, Phythyon J M, Holaday D A 1983 Isoflurane and enflurane-induced hepatic necrosis in triiodothyronine-pretreated rats. Anesthesiology 58: 1–5

Blitt C D 1981 Droperidol and pheochromocytoma. Anesth Analg 60: 770–771

Dunnet J M, Holman R R, Turner R C, Sear J W 1988 Diabetes mellitus and anaesthesia. Anaesthesia 43: 538–542

Ewing D J, Campbell I W, Murray A, Neilson J M H, Clarke B F 1978 Immediate heart-rate response to standing: simple test for autonomic neuropathy in diabetes. Br Med J 1: 145–147

Ewing D J, Clarke B F 1982 Diagnosis and management of diabetic autonomic neuropathy. Br Med J 255: 916–918

Hall G M 1984 Diabetes and anaesthesia: a promise unfulfilled? Anaesthesia 39: 627

Hjortrup A, Sorensen C, Dyremose E, Hjortson N-C, Kehlet H 1985 Influence of diabetes mellitus on operative risk. Br J Surg 72: 783–785

Hull C J 1986 Phaeochromocytoma. Diagnosis, preoperative preparation and anaesthetic management. Br J Anaesth 58: 1453–1468

Kiss I, Eggert H R, Schulz B 1982 Anaesthetic considerations in the transsphenoidal and transcranial pituitary surgery. Proceedings of the Sixth European Congress of Anaesthesiology, Anaesthesia pp. 185

Kjellstrand C M, Simmons R L, Goetz F C et al 1973 Renal transplantation in patients with insulin-dependent diabetes. Lancet 2: 4–8

McGuinness C, Vickers M D 1982 Advances in medicine relevant to anaesthesia. In: Kaufman L (ed) Anaesthesia review I. Churchill Livingstone, Edinburgh, p. 3

Pezzarossa A, Taddei F, Cimicchi M C et al 1988 Perioperative management of diabetic subjects. Diabetes Care 11: 52–58

Thomas A N, Pollard B J 1989 Renal transplantation and diabetic autonomic neuropathy. Can J Anaesth 36: 590–592

Vickers M D 1984 Diabetes and the anaesthetist. WFSA lectures, p. 41

Brown B R (ed) 1980 Anesthesia and the patient with endocrine disease. F A Davis, Philadelphia
Katz J, Benumof J, Kadis L B (eds) 1981 Anesthesia and uncommon diseases: pathophysiologic and clinical correlations, 2nd edn. W B Saunders, Philadelphia
Kjellstrand C M, Simmons R L, Goetz F C et al 1973 Renal transplantation in patients with insulin dependent diabetes. Lancet 2: 4–8
Roizen M 1984 Endocrine abnormalities and anesthesia. Annual Refresher Course Lectures. American Society of Anesthesiologists, p. 218
Scherpereel Ph 1983 Adrenalectomy and anesthesia. In: Oyama T (ed) Endocrinology and the anaesthetist. Elsevier, Amsterdam, p. 123
Slowey H F, Vickers M D 1984 Advances in medicine relevant to the anaesthetists. In: Kaufman L (ed) Anaesthesia Review 3. Churchill Livingstone, Edinburgh, p. 1
Verner I 1984 Management of pheochromocytoma. Annual Refresher Course Lectures. American Society of Anesthesiologists, p. 216
Vickers M D (ed) 1977 Medicine for anaesthetists. Blackwell Scientific, Oxford

10

Blood disorders and the safety of anaesthesia

G. C. Jenkins, B. T. Colvin and A. C. Newland

GENERAL HAEMATOLOGY

Anaemia

Tissue hypoxia is a direct result of anaemia. However, oxygen delivery depends also on the oxygen saturation of arterial blood and the regional blood flow. The only practical clinical measurement of total oxygen-carrying capacity of the blood is the haemoglobin level. Normally about 30% of the oxygen carried by the blood is released in the tissues; but if the oxygen tension of the periphery falls this figure will be significantly higher. This adjustment is achieved by reducing the affinity of haemoglobin for oxygen when the tissues have a higher carbon dioxide tension and a lower pH. With increasing severity of anaemia the oxygen dissociation curve shifts progressively to the right, and at a haemoglobin level of 10 g/dl this is clearly detectable. For blood with a haemoglobin concentration of 15 g/dl, at pH 7.4 and 37°C, 50% haemoglobin saturation is reached at a partial pressure of oxygen (PO_2) of 3.5 kPa. However, with an anaemia of 7.5 g haemoglobin/dl the affinity of oxygen is reduced and a PO_2 of 4.0 kPa is needed to achieve 50% saturation. This degree of shift of the dissociation curve to the right means that at the PO_2 of mixed venous blood, approximately 5.0 kPa, the haemoglobin of an anaemic patient will be only 60% saturated compared with 70% in the normal.

As the haemoglobin concentration falls, the total available supply of oxygen to the tissues is reduced, even though the haemoglobin in the pulmonary capillaries is usually saturated. Under these circumstances progressive tissue hypoxia will occur with a reduction in the tissue PO_2 and increased desaturation of the capillary blood.

Clinical features

If oxygen delivery to the tissues is inadequate, a compensatory increase in cardiac output takes place. As oxygen needs are increased by physical activity, even moderate anaemia may be accompanied by symptoms related to compensatory cardiovascular adjustment, such as dyspnoea and palpitations, and to tissue hypoxia, such as weakness and lassitude. These symptoms and signs are more or less apparent depending on the speed of onset of anaemia, the severity of anaemia and the age of the patient. The effects of vascular insufficiency, particularly in the elderly, will be exacerbated by the oxygen lack so that angina, claudication and symptoms of cerebral ischaemia are accentuated. Mild anaemia, with a haemoglobin about 9–10 g/dl, may be virtually symptom-free when the onset has been gradual in a young, otherwise healthy, patient. On clinical examination, pallor is the only general sign as judged by the appearance of the conjunctiva, mucous membranes of the tongue and mouth, and the nail beds and skin creases.

Investigation of anaemia

Regrettably it is common practice for all patients entering hospital to be subjected to a full blood-count as part of the routine 'work up'. There is no necessity for a patient to have a blood count automatically simply because he is about to undergo general anaesthesia, unless the clinical history indicates a likely cause for anaemia or there is clinical evidence of it. This is particularly so if the surgical procedure is only of limited extent. With the help of modern equipment it is possible to measure accurately the size and haemoglobin content of a patient's red cells and to classify the type of anaemia accordingly. Microcytic, hypochromic cells usually indicate iron deficiency but are also found in thalassaemia. Cells that are normochromic and normocytic may occur after acute blood loss, in haemolytic anaemias and secondary anaemias or bone marrow failure. Macrocytic anaemia usually indicates vitamin B_{12} or folate deficiency.

Correction of anaemia

There are few data on the incidence of morbidity or mortality attributable to anaemia, however it must be an advantage to restore the haemoglobin level preoperatively once the cause of deficiency has been established. A reasonable working value to set as the lower limit prior to elective surgery is 10 g/dl, though obviously this must be related to the condition of the patient, the extent of the surgical procedure and the blood loss that might be expected. When possible, in cases planned for elective surgery, appropriate replacement or corrective therapy will have been instituted preoperatively.

Iron deficiency

Most cases of iron deficiency will have been treated with oral iron therapy over some weeks, and parenteral iron in the form of intramuscular sorbitol or dextran provides no advantage over oral iron in rate of haemoglobin response. Furthermore, there is a contraindication to the administration of iron sorbitol in patients with urinary infection, for the excreted iron may encourage the growth of organisms in the urinary tract. However, a total dose infusion of iron dextran in 0.9% sodium chloride over a period of hours may be used to correct the total body iron deficit. Toxic effects may be troublesome, especially in subjects with an allergic history. Total dose infusion should be preceded by a test dose, and the full dose administered under close supervision, with antihistamine and hydrocortisone available. Iron dextran has been used most frequently for non-compliance or poor tolerance of oral iron, for correction of severe iron deficiency in late pregnancy or in patients requiring surgery who have continuing excessive blood loss.

If urgent or extensive surgery is required the transfusion of packed red cells is indicated. Preferably this should be carried out at least 24 hours preoperatively to avoid overloading the circulation, and to permit the patient's oxygen dissociation curve to return to normal. Due to the circulatory hyperdynamic state in patients still deprived of red cells, the administration of intravenous narcotic drugs may result in an accelerated induction time.

Macrocytic anaemia

When macrocytic anaemia is due to a deficiency of vitamin B_{12} or folate (or both) it may be severe enough to be accompanied by incipient or overt heart failure. In addition to vitamin replacement, digoxin and diuretics may be indicated. Blood transfusion is usually avoided if possible, as death from circulatory overload may result. If urgent surgery is indicated, the patient is in late pregnancy, or if the severity of the anaemia is itself causing cardiac distress, transfusion may be essential. Up to 500 ml of packed red cells may be administered slowly with diuretics under careful clinical observation for signs of heart failure. When possible, surgery should be postponed until the anaemia has been corrected by medical treatment.

Nitrous oxide effects. Nitrous oxide anaesthesia causes rapid inactivation of body vitamin B_{12} by oxidizing the reduced cobalt atom of methyl B_{12}. Megaloblastic marrow changes occur within several days and prolonged N_2O administration can cause pancytopenia. Chronic exposure, as experienced by anaesthetists and dentists, has been associated with neurological damage resembling vitamin B_{12} deficiency neuropathy (Hoffbrand 1989).

Haemolytic anaemias

Patients with excessive red cell destruction may require a cholecystectomy due to long-standing excess bile pigment and stone production or a therapeutic splenectomy. Blood transfusion may be required, and in the case of autoimmune haemolysis the antibody in the serum may complicate the cross-matching procedures so that additional time may be required to produce donor blood. Cold agglutinin disease can cause severe intravascular haemolysis during anaesthesia unless the patient is kept warm throughout the procedure. It is also important to warm intravenous and irrigation fluids before use. This should be done in a water jacket, carefully regulated to 37°C.

Glucose 6-phosphate dehydrogenase (G6PD) deficiency. Different genetic variants of this condition affect black (especially west African), Mediterannean and southwest Asian races, apart from sporadic groups in other populations, such as the Middle East and the Indian subcontinent. G6PD in the red cell enables the oxidation of glucose via the pentose phosphate pathway. This chain of reactions produces glutathione, necessary to prevent oxidative denaturation of haemoglobin by a variety of compounds. If the deficient red cells are exposed to oxidizing agents, haemolysis occurs. Important drugs in the present context which may be responsible are analgesics, such as phenacetin, paracetamol, acetanilide and aspirin, and antibiotics, such as the sulphonamide and sulphone preparations, trimethroprim and nitrofurantoins. Because the normal reduction of methaemoglobin is impaired in this condition, prilocaine is contraindicated as it may result in an alarming degree of cyanosis.

Abnormal haemoglobins

Sickle-cell haemoglobin (HbS) may be inherited from one parent and combined with normal adult (A) haemoglobin from the other parent (sickle trait HbAS), or inherited from both parents (HbSS), or combined with any of the other variants of clinical importance (HbSC, HbSD, HbSE or HbSβ thalassaemia). These genetically distinct conditions are known as the sickle syndromes.

When sickle-cell haemoglobin is in the oxygenated form it is a soluble protein. However, when the pigment is in the reduced form it becomes, compared with normal adult haemoglobin, highly insoluble, 'crystallizing' out of solution and distorting the red cells into their characteristic sickle form. Sickle cells tend to tangle within capillaries and vessels, obstructing the flow through nutrient vessels and producing infarcted areas in different tissues (the infarctive crisis). The most important factor that exacerbates the sickling phenomenon is a reduction in oxygen tension.

Haemoglobin C, D and E, and beta thalassaemia. The common haemoglobin variants, haemoglobin C, D and E, do not show the phenomenon of insolubility and consequent distortion of the erythrocyte when in the deoxygenated state. Beta thalassaemia is characterized by an inherited defect in beta polypeptide chain synthesis in the globin part of the haemoglobin molecule. The peripheral blood picture of beta thalassaemia minor looks very similar to that of iron deficiency, and it is important to distinguish it by haemoglobin analysis and plasma iron studies. Some patients may need preoperative blood transfusion. In beta thalassaemia major, transfusion dependency is the rule and iron overload occurs unless adequate chelation therapy is given. Splenectomy is often necessary in childhood, when it should be preceded by pneumococcal vaccine and followed by prophylactic antibiotics. Despite these measures, overwhelming pneumococcal infection can still occur, either in the immediate postoperative period or in the long term. Iron overload may affect cardiac function, especially during early adult life, in inadequately chelated patients.

Geographic and ethnic distribution. Sickle-cell haemoglobin has its highest incidence in the black populations of Central Africa, the West Indies and North America. Haemoglobin C is also predominantly a black variant, particularly in northern Ghana. Haemoglobin D Punjab and

E, the other two common haemoglobin variants, are found respectively in subjects from northwest India (and Pakistan) and the Far East. Beta thalassaemia is largely confined to populations in a broad band running through the countries along the Mediterranean, the Middle East, India and into China.

Screening procedures. For most operative procedures it might seem unnecessary to screen all patients of black African origin for sickle-cell haemoglobin. It is reasonable to accept that, if a person has a normal haemoglobin level and has reached the age of 20 years without any clinical incident suggestive of a sickling attack, he is extremely unlikely to suffer from a good anaesthetic procedure. However, the combination of sickle haemoglobin and haemoglobin C (HbSC) may be potentially more hazardous, in that cases have been recorded of infarctive crises in such subjects following operative procedures, even though the preoperative haemoglobin level was normal. It is therefore wise to screen for HbS most patients who are candidates for sickle cell syndrome. Screening may be carried out in outpatients and, if general anaesthesia is given to dental patients, screening of possible 'sicklers' should be conducted using a simple technique such as Sickledex, which requires only a fingerprick blood sample. Full typing by electrophoresis and a general haematological assessment are necessary in positive cases. Hospital admission is indicated for patients requiring general anaesthesia if sickle-cell disease or haemoglobin SC disease is confirmed.

Sickle-cell trait. Depending on the amount of HbS present the patient may be little affected clinically or, most likely, not at all. Under conditions of reduced inspired oxygen an HbS concentration of 40% may not produce significant sickling until an oxygen tension of approximately 2.5 kPa is reached. During anaesthesia simple precautions ensuring adequate oxygenation from induction to full postoperative recovery are important. Dehydration, lengthy application of tourniquets and circulatory stasis must be avoided. Under special circumstances, such as major thoracic surgery, even patients with HbAS may need preoperative exchange transfusion (see below).

Sickle-cell disease. The term 'sickle-cell disease' covers the disorders (sickle-cell anaemia, sickle-cell beta thalassaemia and sickle-cell haemoglobin C disease) in which the presence of HbS commonly results in clinical disability, varying in severity from mild anaemia to lethal crisis. The major factors liable to provoke infarctive crises are low blood oxygen tension, vascular stasis and low blood pH. In sickle-cell anaemia (HbSS) the cells will sickle at a Po_2 of about 5.5 kPa. General anaesthesia for patients with sickle-cell disease is a hazardous undertaking. Where possible, hypotensive techniques and cooling procedures should be avoided. Surgeons and anaesthetists should be aware that abdominal pain in patients with sickle-cell disease may be caused by an infarctive crisis, and surgical intervention is almost certainly contraindicated at such a time. If general anaesthesia is necessary when surgery is essential a planned procedure should be followed.

Preoperative management of sickle-cell syndromes. Whenever possible, operations should be carried out electively when the patient is in the 'steady state', that is when the patient is in the best clinical condition and not in crisis. Infections should be treated and prophylactic antibiotic therapy given to avoid postoperative pulmonary infection which may give rise to poor ventilation. Depending on the amount of the HbS component in the blood, a variable quantity of donor blood should be transfused. Patients only moderately anaemic (say 9.0 g/dl) may be sufficiently corrected by a slow infusion of packed red cells. More often it is necessary to perform exchange transfusion prior to operation. The aim should be to ensure that at least 60% of the patient's red cells are replaced by normal, newly donated red cells. By doing so the HbS component of the blood should be reduced to 10% or less. Blood donated within 24 hours should be used because blood stored for longer not only has a low pH, but also has a low 2–3 diphosphoglycerate content, which makes it extremely avid for oxygen for some hours. Old blood thus increases the blood volume and viscosity without increasing the oxygen-carrying capacity.

The administration of alkali, frequently advocated to inhibit sickling by raising the blood pH, is more controversial in that it results in a left shift of the oxygen dissociation curve and again oxygen is less available to the tissues. Obviously premedication must not cause respiratory depression.

During the surgical procedure. The temperature of the operating theatre should be controlled so that neither sweating nor excessive cooling of the patient occurs. Tissue blood flow should be maintained by avoiding cardiac depression or any degree of vasoconstriction. Care in positioning the patient on the table is essential. If the application of a tourniquet is unavoidable it should be applied after exsanguination of the extremity and then only for the shortest possible time. Unless it is minimal, blood loss should be replaced with the freshest blood available and hydration maintained by appropriate intravenous fluids. Dextrose (5%) encourages swelling of the red cells and thus may retard the sickling process. Adequate oxygenation must be given and again drugs likely to cause respiratory depression should be avoided.

Postoperative care. The immediate postoperative period is the time when sickling complications are most likely to occur. Close supervision of oxygen therapy must be maintained until full clinical recovery occurs, and oxygen should be available for a further 24 hours. Early mobilization should be encouraged and infections should be energetically treated. Hydration must be maintained. The onset of severe bone pain may herald marrow infarction, and pulmonary infarction may also occur. This complication is particularly frequent in postpartum patients with HbSC. Anticoagulant therapy should be considered if the patient's surgical condition permits.

Disorders of white cells

Neutropenia

A lack of sufficient granulocytes may be part of a general pancytopenia, usually due to bone marrow failure or hypersplenism, or it may represent a selective neutropenia, drug-induced, idiopathic or familial. Mild asymptomatic low neutrophil counts are found as a genetic feature of some African peoples. Patients with a neutrophil count below 1.0×10^9/l are likely to present with fever and foci of infection, and are particularly vulnerable to postoperative infection. Full supporting therapy is necessary in the form of barrier nursing, antibiotic cover and, if necessary, leucocyte transfusions.

Acute leukaemias

Acute leukaemias commonly present with the features of pancytopenia due to a disorganized bone marrow: anaemia, haemorrhage and infection. Aggressive combined chemotherapy also contributes to the low cell counts until full remission is achieved. Supportive measures again need to include antibiotic regimes and isolation with platelet and possibly granulocyte transfusion, as well as red cell transfusions. During periods of thrombocytopenia, if an anaesthetic is required, every effort should be made to prevent the least endothelial trauma, and intramuscular injections should be avoided. Patients with acute leukaemia and a very high leucocyte count producing sludging in the cerebral capillaries may present with hyperviscosity syndromes (see also p. 158), including unsteady gait, visual disturbances and coma, sometimes leading to fatal cerebral anoxia. Blood transfusions should be avoided at this stage, and efforts should be made in the first instance to reduce the leucocyte count as rapidly as possible by leucopheresis and cytotoxic drugs.

Chronic leukaemias

In both of the more common types of chronic leukaemia, very high white cell counts and very large spleens may be present with a variable degree of anaemia and thrombocytopenia, although platelet counts may be high in the early stages of chronic granulocytic leukaemia. In chronic lymphocytic leukaemia, autoimmune haemolytic anaemia may occur with its attendant possible delay in providing compatible blood for transfusion as previously mentioned (p. 155). In this condition hypogammaglobulinaemia may also reduce resistance to infection.

Hypersplenism and splenectomy

Many patients with enlargement of the spleen, from whatever cause (of which there are many), have a resulting reduction of one or more of the cellular elements of the blood with anaemia, neutropenia and thrombocytopenia, and their attendant complications. There is an increase in the plasma volume which exaggerates the anaemia. In some cases splenectomy is indicated. Preoperatively, patients who are to undergo splenectomy may require platelet transfusions in addition to blood transfusions. After the operation there is usually a sharp increase of platelets which in some cases may rise to over 1000×10^9/l after 7 days. There is therefore considerable increase in the risk of thromboembolism and it may be advisable in some cases to treat the patient with antiplatelet drugs or anticoagulants until the thrombocytosis subsides.

There is an increased risk of overwhelming pneumococcal infection after splenectomy and it is important, particularly in children, to make sure that prophylactic pneumococcal vaccine is administered preoperatively. This does not altogether remove the risk, so oral penicillin should be given for at least 3 years post-splenectomy.

Hyperviscosity

Erythrocytosis

Polycythaemia vera. In the peripheral blood all types of blood cells are usually increased in polycythaemia vera so that, although clinically the emphasis is that of erythrocytosis, in most cases granulocytosis and thrombocytosis also result from the overall excessive marrow activity. The raised blood viscosity, sluggish blood flow and increased platelet count predispose to the occlusion of major vessels and peripheral vasculature. Defective platelet function and vascular distension may, however, also produce a haemorrhagic tendency. Cerebral vascular accidents are therefore a frequent operative or postoperative complication. The incidence of major haemorrhage or thrombosis during operations on patients with uncontrolled polycythaemia vera is over 80%, and in one series a postoperative mortality of 18% was recorded (Wasserman & Gilbert 1963). Even in controlled patients no surgical procedure should be carried out that is not strictly essential, and then only after complete haematological assessment. When elective surgery is planned it is important to give a cytotoxic agent, such as radioactive phosphorus, or chemotherapy until the blood count is near normal. When emergency surgery is indicated, however, rapid haemodilution may be effected by venesection or erythrapheresis with a cell separator, accompanied, if necessary, by infusion of low molecular weight dextran or plasma protein fraction. During the operation vascular stasis must be avoided. Since the circulation time may be considerably slowed, induction of anaesthesia may be affected in these patients. Fresh blood containing normal platelets may be required to control bleeding.

Hypoxia and excessive erythropoietin production. These are other causes of erythrocytosis that may cause complications. The total red cell mass in hypoxic emphysema has been found to be as high as 34% above normal. The increased blood viscosity provides serious hazard of thrombosis and cautious venesection may be required preoperatively. Congenital heart disease, which results in a right-to-left shunt so that deoxygenated blood enters the systemic circulation, produces erythrocytosis. Venesection is a reasonable preoperative measure prior to surgical repair or any other operative procedure.

A variety of neoplasms, such as renal carcinoma, hepatocellular carcinoma, cerebella haemangioblastoma or uterine fibromyoma, as well as an assortment of renal disorders, such as simple and multiple cysts and occlusive vascular disease, can cause serious erythrocytosis due to inappropriate erythropoietin secretion. Venesection or erythrapheresis may well be indicated prior to operation followed by anticoagulant therapy. Complete surgical removal of the tumour or lesion, if it is possible, usually results in reduction of the erythropoietin levels to normal with remission of the erythrocytosis.

Hyperglobulinaemia

Myelomatosis and macroglobulinaemia. Myelomatosis results from a neoplastic proliferation of plasma cells that produces bone destruction and bone marrow failure. In most cases the proliferating cells produce large amounts of one of the serum globulins with reduction in the normal immunoglobulins. Myelomatosis is frequently associated with a variable degree of renal failure, largely due to the excretion of Bence–Jones protein which damages the renal tubules. In addition, patients are often dehydrated, and have hypercalcaemia and hyperuricaemia, all of which contribute to renal dysfunction. Surgery is sometimes necessary to assist in the repair of a pathological fracture or to relieve spinal cord compression by laminectomy. It is very important to ensure that the patient is well hydrated preoperatively and that a high serum calcium or uric acid is controlled, if possible, before an anaesthetic is given. These patients are particularly prone to chest infections due to neutropenia and reduced immunoglobulins, especially if there are rib fractures present that limit the normal cough mechanism. Blood transfusion is necessary to rectify anaemia, and platelet transfusion for thrombocytopenia. Rarely the high serum proteins cause a hyperviscosity syndrome with visual disturbance, drowsiness, confusion, heart failure and purpura, due to the abnormal protein interfering with coagulation and platelet function. Plasmapheresis, usually on two or three successive days, may be required to control these complications.

Primary macroglobulinaemia may produce similar changes and effects due to high serum proteins and hyperviscosity, but there is no bone destruction. The high level of paraprotein may increase intravascular oncotic pressure with a concomitant expansion of plasma volume. In these patients anaemia may be spurious and blood transfusion inappropriate. Anaemia will usually be corrected following plasma exchange when excess protein is removed.

DISORDERS OF HAEMOSTASIS

General precautions

Abnormal bleeding is of more immediate importance than thrombosis in patients with haemostatic disorders who are given an anaesthetic. If an abnormal bleeding tendency is suspected then, until the cause has been established and corrected, the following precautions should be observed:

1. No intramuscular injections should be given and oral premedication should be used.
2. Intubation should be avoided if possible, nasotracheal intubation being particularly dangerous.
3. Venous access should be obtained through readily controllable peripheral sites, and cutting down onto a vein should be avoided, except in an emergency. Blind puncture of the internal jugular or subclavian vein is especially hazardous, and if access to a central vein is essential the femoral site is preferred.
4. Arterial sampling should be avoided or kept to a minimum.
5. Regional anaesthesia should not be performed.

Patients with an increased risk of thrombosis or evidence of existing thrombosis are sometimes given antithrombotic drugs before surgery. Most of these drugs increase the risk of bleeding and, in general, the guidelines given above apply. Those receiving low dose subcutaneous heparin (5000 units 8- or 12-hourly), and warfarin-treated patients whose International Normalised Ratio (INR) does not exceed 2.0, have only a modest increase in bleeding tendency. Even small doses of aspirin can contribute to abnormal bleeding and treatment with fibrinolytic agents is an absolute contraindication to invasive procedures or surgery.

Preoperative investigations

Clinical assessment remains a vital part of any haemostatic investigation. Important aspects of this are shown in Table 10.1. Laboratory investigation involves a small number of routine screening tests (Table 10.2). most of which can be quickly performed even outside normal working hours. When the results are available other tests can be performed, if necessary with the help of a haematologist.

The PTR and KCCT/PTT assess the extrinsic and intrinsic coagulation pathways respectively. The TT tests the final reaction between thrombin

Table 10.1 Disorders of haemostasis: clinical assessment

Severity / Frequency / Nature	of abnormal bleeding
Response to:	dental extraction tonsillectomy
Previous blood transfusion	
Family history	
Drug history	
Purpura or telangiectasia	
Jaundice	
Ascites	
Hepatic or splenic enlargement	
Joint damage	
Untidy scars	

and fibrinogen which results in fibrin formation, and it is therefore sensitive to hypofibrinogenaemia, dysfibrinogenaemia, FDPs and the antithrombin, heparin. The reptilase test works in a similar way, but the snake venom used is insensitive to heparin so that the test is valuable in excluding heparin's presence. The ELT is shortened in the presence of fibrinolytic activator and the bleeding time is an in vivo measure of platelet numbers and function (Chanarin 1989).

Table 10.3 is a brief guide to the interpretation of the data obtained from screening tests of haemostasis, together with some management options.

Table 10.2 Disorders of haemostasis: laboratory assessment

Test	Normal range
Peripheral blood film	—
Platelet count	150–450 × 10^9/l
Prothrombin ratio (PTR)	1.0–1.3
Kaolin cephalin clotting test (KCCT) or partial thromboplastin test (PTT)	35–45 s
Thrombin test (TT)	10–12
Other tests	
Bleeding time	3–9 min
Reptilase test	17–19 s
Fibrinogen concentration	2–4 g/l
Fibrin(ogen) degradation products (FDP)	<10 mg/l
Euglobulin lysis time (ELT)	>2 h

Pre-existing haemostatic defects

Thrombocytopenia

A platelet count above 100 × 10^9/l is not usually associated with a bleeding tendency, but between 50 and 100 × 10^9/l trauma or surgery may result in haemorrhage. Below this level bleeding may be severe.

If time allows, the cause of the thrombocytopenia should be determined and corrected. This may require haematinic assay, tests of autoimmunity and bone-marrow examination. Possible treatments include folic acid or other vitamin supplements, withdrawal of drugs, immunosuppression, splenectomy and specific treatment for bone-marrow disorders. Drugs known to affect platelet function, especially aspirin, should be avoided.

If the platelet count cannot be corrected then platelet transfusion may be required. The antifibrinolytic drug, tranexamic acid, can help to reduce bleeding after dental extraction or prostatectomy, but is contraindicated in the presence of liver disease, consumption coagulopathy or bleeding within the renal pelvis. During splenectomy, platelet transfusion should be withheld until after the splenic pedicle has been tied. Patients with disorders of platelet function may require platelet infusions despite a normal or near-normal platelet count, and tranexamic acid is often given as well.

Thrombocytosis

Patients with high platelet counts, especially those with myeloproliferative disease, may develop thrombosis or haemorrhage in response to surgery. If possible the count should be brought down before surgery as antithrombotic treatment is likely to exacerbate bleeding (Kessler et al 1982).

Haemophilia and allied disorders

The great majority of congenital disorders of haemostasis are due to haemophilia A (factor VIII deficiency), haemophilia B (factor IX deficiency) and von Willebrand's disease (factor VIII-determined coagulation and functional platelet defect). These conditions should only be treated

Table 10.3 A brief guide to data interpretation in disorders of haemostasis (modified from Dunnill & Colvin 1989)

Abnormality	Possible diagnosis	Possible management
Platelets reduced; clotting tests normal	Bone marrow failure, e.g. aplasia, malignancy, vitamin deficiency consumption of platelets, e.g. ITP, hypersplenism	Specific therapy, e.g. folic acid, withdrawal of causative drugs, platelet infusions, corticosteroids, immunosuppression.
PTR only abnormal	Exclude presence of oral anticoagulants and liver disease. Factor VII deficiency rare	If presence of oral anticoagulants confirmed then consider vitamin K, factor concentrates and/or FFP
PTT only abnormal	Probable inherited defect of intrinsic pathway, e.g. haemophilia, or von Willebrand's disease. In the latter, platelet function is defective with long bleeding time	After confirming with specific factor assays give specific factor concentrates, DDAVP or other treatment as advised by a haematologist
PTR, PTT abnormal; TT and platelets normal	Typical of oral anticoagulants, liver disease, vitamin K deficiency. Exclude CC and inherited defects of II, V, X which are rare	Vitamin K, factor concentrates and/or FFP
PTR, PTT abnormal; TT normal, platelets reduced	Massive blood transfusion. Exclude CC and liver disease	Platelet concentrates, especially when platelets < 50 × 9/l FFP and/or cryoprecipitate when PTR > 1.8 (see text)
PTR, PTT, TT abnormal; reptilase and platelets normal	Typical of heparin therapy (or see below)	Consider withdrawal of heparin or use of protamine
All clotting tests abnormal; Platelets normal or reduced; Red cells fragmented on film	Typical of severe liver disease or CC	Avoid factor concentrates if possible.[a] In liver disease use vitamin K and FFP. In CC use FFP, cryoprecipitate, platelet concentrates and possibly heparin, after trying to treat the underlying condition[b]

ITP: idiopathic thrombocytopenic purpura, FFP: fresh frozen plasma, CC: consumption coagulopathy.
[a] Factor concentrates may be dangerous because of the possibility of exacerbating CC.
[b] Antifibrinolytic agents should be confined to those patients who show abnormal proteolytic activity in the absense of CC. They are generally contraindicated in bleeding from the upper renal tract.

in haemophilia centres designated by the Department of Health. Major surgery, joint replacement and the management of difficult cases, such as those with inhibitors to factor VIII, should be confined to the larger regional centres.

All patients should be screened for inhibitory activity before any surgical procedure. Liver function tests should be performed together with a test for the hepatitis-associated antigen (HBsAg) and the antibody to Human Immunodeficiency Virus (HIV). The main principle of management is intravenous factor replacement therapy, but patients with mild haemophilia A or one of most types of von Willebrand's desease may be suitable for treatment with the vasopressin analogue DDAVP, usually combined with tranexamic acid. DDAVP releases factor VIII from available stores giving a useful haemostatic effect which is limited by a reduced response to repeated doses (Mannucci et al 1977). The choice of treatment is the responsibility of the haemophilia centre director, and very significant financial savings can be made by avoiding the use of factor concentrates. It is particularly important to remember the general precautions outlined earlier (p. 159) when treating patients with haemophilia, and to collaborate with the haemophilia centre so that invasive procedures and replacement therapy can be coordinated.

Anticoagulants

Heparin rarely causes abnormal bleeding, except following an overdose or cardiac bypass surgery when heparin rebound can be a problem (Kamath & Fozard 1980). If a patient being treated with full dose heparin (30 000–40 000 units/24 hours) requires surgery, the dose should be reduced, preferably to a low-dose subcutaneous regimen (5000 units, 8- or 12-hourly). At this level the PTT or TT should be within normal limits and the correction should occur quite rapidly as the half-life of heparin in vivo is only 90 min. If necessary, protamine sulphate can be given intravenously, 1 mg neutralizing 100 units of heparin. Dosage can be calculated by an in vitro protamine neutralization test, but this is rarely necessary.

Warfarin does not usually compromise haemostasis until the INR rises above 2.0, and it has been used to prevent thrombosis following surgery (Taberner et al 1978). Its value in this context is limited by the absence of a parenteral preparation, interaction with other drugs, and the effect of surgery itself on warfarin control, so that it is usual to change to a low-dose subcutaneous heparin regimen. The approach to the patient with an INR greater than 2.0 who requires an operation depends on the urgency of surgery, the value of the INR, the importance of the anticoagulation and the condition of the patient. If there is no immediate need to operate, warfarin can be stopped for a few days until the INR is acceptable.

If surgery is necessary within about 12 hours, but there is no active bleeding, a very small dose of vitamin K can be given intravenously in an attempt to bring about a partial correction of the warfarinization. Not more than 1 mg should be given at a time and the INR should be repeated after 6 hours. Subsequent warfarinization may be difficult. If surgery is urgent, or the patient is bleeding, warfarin should be stopped and the INR corrected with prothrombin complex concentrate or fresh frozen plasma (FFP), the dose being repeated as necessary under the direction of a haematologist (British Committee for Standards in Haematology 1990). Where there is no indication to continue warfarin a full dose of vitamin K should be given intravenously, and this would be effective in about 6 hours.

Fibrinolytic agents. The use of these agents is an absolute contraindication to surgery, and invasive procedures should be performed only if essential and then with extreme care.

Liver disease. Patients with severe hepatic dysfunction may bleed as a result of vitamin K deficiency, failure of clotting factor synthesis, consumption coagulopathy, portal hypertension with oesophageal varices and thrombocytopenia due to hypersplenism or folic acid deficiency. Deficiency states are easily corrected by a slow intravenous injection of the appropriate vitamin, but management is otherwise very difficult. Active blood loss should be treated with red cells, FFP and platelets, together with appropriate medical or surgical measures. Prothrombin complex concentrates have been used in an attempt to correct the haemostatic defect in liver disease (Mannucci et al 1976) but, although they are now free of the risk of viral infection, anxieties remain about their potential for causing thrombosis or even consumption coagulopathy. Antifibrinolytic drugs are usually avoided for similar reasons.

Renal disease. Haemorrhage in patients with renal failure is probably partly due to platelet dysfunction, but may be controlled by the use of arginine vasopressin (DDAVP; 0.3 μg/kg in 20 ml of saline over 15 min) or by cyroprecipitate infusion. The mechanism of the effect is not clear but is probably related to the interaction of factor VIII, platelets and the endothelium (Remuzzi 1988).

Consumption coagulopathy

Consumption coagulopathy may present before, or arise during or after, surgery, and has many causes, most of which involve tissue death. It represents a failure of control of haemostasis and can cause a very serious mixture of shock, loss of consciousness, hypoxia, renal failure, microangiopathic haemolytic anaemia, purpura and uncontrollable haemorrhage. In addition to the abnormalities listed in Table 10.3 there may be evidence of hypofibrinogenaemia and abnormal fibrinolysis (Larcan et al 1987).

Management should be a cooperative effort between haematologist, physician and anaesthetist. Any known cause, such as placental abruption or infection, should be corrected if possible, and careful attention should be paid to oxygenation, perfusion, electrolyte balance and the avoidance of further trauma. Replacement of missing factors using red cells, FFP, cryoprecipitate and platelet concentrates is generally accepted as being worthwhile, despite the theoretical risk of making matters worse. The value of anticoagulation with heparin is still not clearly defined and each case has to be treated on its merits. Prothrombin concentrates carry the potential risk of exacerbation of the thrombotic tendency, the latter also being the reason for not giving antifibrinolytic agents.

Bleeding during and after anaesthesia

Excessive operative haemorrhage may be due to:

- an unrecognized haemostatic defect
- surgical problems
- surgery in an area where haemostasis is difficult to secure
- local factors, such as urine flow, which interfere with normal haemostatic mechanisms
- some unexpected event, such as hypotension or an incompatible blood transfusion, during surgery which causes consumption coagulopathy.

Once bleeding is established it may be self-perpetuating unless steps are taken to correct its cause. Underlying haemostatic defects can be very difficult to diagnose against the background of the postoperative state where hepatic and renal dysfunction, often with an element of consumption coagulopathy, may arise. Repeated haemostatic screens, as outlined in Table 10.2, are valuable in planning treatment, a guide to which is given in Table 10.3.

In the past, FFP and platelet concentrates were often given to patients who have received massive blood transfusion in an attempt to prevent the consequences of dilutional depletion of labile clotting factors and viable platelets. This practice has been discontinued because of the lack of scientific evidence that it is beneficial, since it is wasteful of scarce resources and because it carries some hazards. The issue is addressed by Jones (1987) who gives the following indications for FFP:

- isolated factor deficiences where specific concentrates are not available
- reversal of warfarin effect and vitamin K deficiency (but see alternatives of vitamin K and prothrombin complex concentrates)
- consumption coagulopathy
- liver disease where there is bleeding or before major surgery
- thrombotic thrombocytopenic purpura.

In patients who have had massive blood transfusions and are bleeding abnormally, platelet concentrates are more likely to be beneficial than FFP. If the platelet count falls below 50×10^9/l the use of prophylactic platelet concentrates is justifiable. If the PTR exceeds 1.8 or the fibrinogen concentration falls below 0.8 g/l, cryoprecipitate and FFP are indicated (Ciavarella et al 1987). Fresh whole blood is unsafe and has numerous disadvantages. Organization may be difficult, there is a greater risk of clerical or laboratory error and there may be no time to perform the usual tests for syphilis, hepatitis or HIV on the donor blood.

While there is a theoretical risk of citrate anticoagulant toxicity, this almost never causes a problem in clinical practice and it is easy to inject 5 mmol calcium chloride intravenously if an otherwise unexplained fall in blood pressure should occur.

Post-transfusion hepatitis

Hepatitis A virus causes infectious hepatitis, is transmitted by the faecal–oral route and is hardly ever transfusion associated. The first important measure to reduce the transmission of hepatitis B by blood transfusion (post-transfusion hepatitis [PTH]) was the introduction of routine screening for hepatitis B markers nearly two decades ago. Since the incubation period is variable, ranging from 36 to 150 days, a number of infectious donor units could slip through, but the risk has been further reduced by donor selection procedures and less than 0.2% of potential new donors in the UK are infected. Anaesthetists should be immunized against hepatitis B and there is good evidence that the vaccine is both safe and effective (Joint Committee on Immunisation and Vaccination 1988).

During the 1980s there was a growing interest in the problem of non-A non-B hepatitis in which no laboratory markers were available and diagnosis relied on clinical hepatitis, elevated transaminases and the exclusion of other causes. It was thought that a number of different viruses were involved because of incubation periods which seemed to separate cases into short (2–4 weeks) and long (6–15 weeks) incubation periods. Some infections were asymptomatic, but it was realized that the clinical course could be acute or chronic and that chronic persistent or chronic active hepatitis or cirrhosis could occur. The risk of transmission was particularly high in pooled preparations of factor VIII, factor IX and fibrinogen, but safer donor selection procedures and concentrate production techniques have eliminated concentrate-mediated infection.

It is now apparent that the newly described hepatitis C virus (HCV) is the chief cause of transfusion-associated non-A non-B hepatitis and that about 90% of blood donors with anti-HCV antibodies have infectious virus in their blood (Esteban et al 1990). Routine screening of blood donors for anti-HCV antibodies has now been introduced in the UK. HCV seroconversion in a surgeon following a needle-stick injury has been reported (Vaglia et al 1990).

Human albumin solution and salt-poor albumin are rendered non-infective by heating to 60°C for 10 hours. Cytomegalovirus and Epstein–Barr virus are readily transmitted by fresh blood, but the virus becomes non-viable after storage at 4°C for a few days. These infections are commonly associated in bypass surgery with a post-perfusion syndrome, developing several weeks after transfusion with large quantities of fresh blood.

The immunocompromised patient is particularly susceptible to transfused micro-organisms. Immunosuppression following transplantation and treatment of leukaemia, and the use of many blood components increase the risk.

All cases of hepatitis must be reported to the regional transfusion director so that the donors can be traced and investigated, and all other possible contaminated products withdrawn.

Acquired immune deficiency syndrome

Human immunodeficiency virus (HIV) is spread by sexual activity and the transfusion of blood or blood products. In the USA and UK those most affected have been homosexual or bisexual men, intravenous drug abusers and haemophiliacs. By contrast, in sub-Saharan Africa the disease affects men and women equally and acquired immune deficiency syndrome (AIDS) has now become a world-wide problem.

The risk of the HIV transmission by blood or blood products collected in the UK is now very small because of the introduction of donor selection and screening techniques, together with improvements in concentrate preparation and viral inactivation (UK Haemophilia Centre Directors 1988). Human albumin solution is safe because it has been pasteurized and the processes involved in the preparation of intravenous immunoglobulin inactivate the virus. Large pool clotting factor concentrates are now being heat treated or virally inactivated in other ways, and there is the prospect of genetically engineered factor VIII concentrate being commercially available in the near future (Schwartz et al 1990).

Unfortunately the use of unheated clotting factor concentrates in the past, before heat treatment became available, has resulted in transmission of the virus to a high proportion of haemophiliacs throughout the developed world. Those with severe haemophilia A are particularly commonly affected, and about a quarter of those infected in the UK had developed AIDS by the end of 1990. After 10 years of infection it is anticipated that approximately 50% will develop AIDS, and this proportion is very similar to that expected for other high-risk groups (Rutherford et al 1990).

The risk of transmission of HIV infection from patients to hospital personnel by contact with their blood or secretions is very low, and large numbers of needlestick injuries have been reported without HIV infection occurring. A number of isolated seroconversions have, however, been reported, usually following needlestick injuries, but there is no evidence of a risk of spread by aerosol (Advisory Committee on Dangerous Pathogens 1990).

The precautions used in the management of patients positive for hepatitis B_e antigen will be more than adequate to prevent infection with HIV. Gloves should be worn when handling blood or secretions from patients known to be anti-HIV positive, and suitable protective clothing is sensible when splashing is likely to occur. Mouth and eye protection is only advisable where the distribution of fluid particles is possible, and a suitable airway should be used to avoid mouth-to-mouth contact during resuscitation.The majority of patients can be nursed in the open ward, but where blood is being lost or secretions are difficult to contain a single room is desirable.

There is continuing interest in the issue of HIV testing for patients undergoing surgery, especially in an emergency. It has been proposed that, where there is a perceived risk, testing should be performed without consent. A large study in San Francisco found no evidence to suggest that preoperative testing for HIV infection would reduce the frequency of accidental exposure to blood, but supported the practice of double gloving, and the increased use of waterproof garments and face shields to prevent mucocutaneous exposure to blood (Gerberding et al 1990). No vaccine for the prevention of HIV infection is likely to be available in the immediate future.

BLOOD TRANSFUSION HAZARDS IN ANAESTHESIA

The purpose of transfusion therapy is the temporary replacement of a blood component that the patient lacks. Transfusion is only justified if the physician believes that the patient will suffer without such treatment. One unit of whole blood contains a variety of components, many of which the average patient undergoing transfusion does not require, and some of which may even be harmful. Transfusion therapy should be undertaken only after careful assessment of the patient's clinical condition with due regard to the nature and quantity of the fluid required to be transfused.

A transfusion should never be given without a definite indication. Not only is this in the interests of the patient involved in view of the small but definite risk associated with transfusion of all blood products, but supplies of blood and blood components are limited and with increasing demand it is important that blood is not used unnecessarily.

Compatibility testing

After routine ABO and Rhesus (D) grouping of the patient's blood, a compatibility test should be performed between the donor's red cells and the patient's serum before transfusion. In an emergency, when delay caused by performing a comprehensive crossmatch might endanger the patient's life, an abbreviated emergency crossmatch can be performed to provide blood urgently, and may be followed by the fuller tests later.

To tide the patient over, either a plasma volume expander can be used or blood that is group-compatible can be issued. The latter course can be followed with sufficient confidence if the patient has been grouped and antibody-screened prior to transfusion. For this reason it is vital that all patients who may require transfusion are studied as early as possible prior to possible transfusion. The correct tests can then be performed in the course of time and abnormal results repeated. This does not replace the need for a crossmatch, but if the patient has no abnormal antibodies it makes the possibility of an incompatible group-match blood unlikely. Patients who have abnormal antibodies should have blood ordered well in advance of proposed use. This will then usually be held in store in the transfusion laboratory until required.

With extensive antibody screening of recipient serum it has been suggested that the need to crossmatch has been eliminated. However, this procedure should always be retained as it:

- reveals antibodies against low-frequency antigens
- will identify weak antibodies that may not react in the panel of cells used for screening
- is a final check on ABO compatibility.

Each request for blood transfusion should be accompanied by a written request. Adequate identification of the patient should be given on the form and on the sample of blood. These should both be filled out at the time of venesection of the patient by the person who has taken the blood sample. The minimum information required is the full name of the patient, date of birth, ward and hospital number. Previous transfusion history should be given, in particular whether a reaction occurred and whether irregular antibodies were present. Where appropriate, drug history and previous obstetric history should be given. In antenatal patients the estimated date of delivery is helpful. This information helps in selection of the appropriate tests. Finally, the form should be signed legibly and dated.

Emergency crossmatching

Blood grouping and modified compatibility testing can be performed in 20–30 min. The risk of errors increases with speed, but if the patient has been studied previously these are minimized. It is the responsibility of the doctor requiring blood to contact the transfusion laboratory and explain the need. If the patient has had a previous group and antibody screen, a telephone call is usually sufficient to activate an emergency crossmatch. A written form can follow when the blood is collected. It is rare that the clinical urgency is such that even limited compatibility testing cannot be done. Massive life-threatening haemorrhage, or haemorrhage occurring when laboratory facilities are remote or outside the 'normal' working day, are such instances. 'Out of hours' there may not be a scientific officer available to perform an emergency crossmatch at once, and this should be taken into account when considering blood requirements for urgent, elective surgery, for example caesarean section.

For transfusion of uncrossmatched blood, selected group O Rhesus (D) negative units should be used unless the patient is known to have antibodies against the Rhesus group. If the patient's group is known then blood of that group can be used. The crossmatch should still be performed while the blood is being given.

Repeated transfusions

When repeated transfusions are given at short intervals, immune antibodies may develop during the course of treatment. It is essential, therefore, to take a fresh sample of blood for compatibility testing if more than 3 days have elapsed since the previous sample was taken. The ABO and Rhesus groups are also checked on each sample of blood to minimize labelling error.

Red cell therapy

The main indication for transfusion is to reverse a state of anaemic hypoxia in which the patient's oxygen-carrying capacity is reduced to such an extent as to produce symptoms or jeopardize other treatment. The average adult male carries approximately 900 ml of oxygen in his blood. Symptoms related to reduced oxygen carriage occur at a level of 650 ml (9.0 g/dl) but, if anaemia occurs slowly, capacities as low as 300 ml (4.5 g/dl) can be tolerated. Each unit of blood contains 66 g of haemoglobin. Each gram can transport 1.34 ml of oxygen at normal arterial $P\text{O}_2$. Therefore a single unit of blood can carry only 90 ml of oxygen. It is therefore unlikely that a single-unit transfusion is ever justified. Reduction in oxygen-carrying capacity per se is not an indication for transfusion. The clinical state of the patient should be considered and, in general, blood loss of up to 800 ml can be replaced by colloid and crystalloid solutions. Table 10.4 indicates which blood products should be chosen for different types of patient.

Whole blood

Whole blood is specifically indicated in massive haemorrhage where all blood components are required in large amounts. It is not good practice to use whole blood where known single-component deficiencies are present that could be more effectively treated with concentrates.

In practice the need to provide blood components has meant that, in the common groups, whole blood is in short supply due to fractionation, and often additional solutions need to be

Table 10.4 Red cell preparations

Types of cell	Indication	Comments
Washed red cells	For patients who react to plasma proteins	Must be used within 12 h of preparation
Microaggregate-free red cells	For patients who react to white cells or platelets Microaggregates affect pulmonary function and are undersirable in acutely ill patients receiving large transfusions	In-line filters are relatively inefficient and slow blood flow rates
Leucocyte-poor blood	For use in patients who have white cell antibodies and react severely to other preparations	Prepared by an open process and need to be used within 12 h
Frozen red cells	For long-term storage of very rare blood groups For storage of blood for autotransfusion in patients with multiple antibodies For patients who have severe transfusion reactions	Not available on an acute basis and have to be used within 12 h
Genotyped red cells	For patients with sickle-cell disease and those with multiple cell antibodies	Not available acutely

given in conjunction with plasma reduced blood to replace larger volumes.

Fresh whole blood

Fresh whole blood has in the past been recommended in conditions requiring the labile coagulation factors (V and VIII) and platelets. This does not, however, allow screening for anti-HIV, HBsAg and syphilis, and should not now be used. The appropriate components can be used instead or, by arrangement with the Regional Transfusion Centre, blood from the current day's bleed may be released after appropriate safety tests. This would not be possible for patients with rare blood groups or irregular antibodies because of the difficulty in providing sufficient compatible units.

Blood less than 5-days old

Blood less than 5-days old is useful if it is necessary to avoid the effects of storage on the blood. These include an increase in plasma potassium and ammonium, and a decrease in labile coagulation factors and pH. The loss on storage of 2,3-diphosphoglyceric acid (2,3-DPG) from the red cells can be very important to the seriously ill patient. Loss of 2,3-DPG is associated with a left shift in the oxygen dissociation curve of haemoglobin and reduces the efficiency of oxygen delivery to the tissues.

Concentrated red cells

Plasma-reduced blood is the form of red cell concentrate most widely available, and in its production approximately 200 ml of plasma plus anticoagulant is removed from whole blood. The contents of each pack have a haematocrit of 60–65%. The viscosity of the blood is greater than whole blood and in massive haemorrhage it may be difficult to achieve the flow rates desirable to replace volume.

Autologous blood transfusion

The likelihood of being infected by a blood transfusion is now almost negligible. However, the risk factor is very important because the consequences of infection with HIV are disastrous and those associated with hepatitis can be very serious.

Lack of communication with the patient about possible adverse effects would potentially be negligent, particularly if safer alternative treatments or procedures are available, even though more difficult to apply. It could be argued, therefore, that all patients requiring a planned transfusion should be offered autologous transfusion, or at least transfusion from a known related donor. However, the latter is recorded as carrying no less risk than blood from the general population (Cordell et al 1986), and this practice is not endorsed by the blood transfusion service.

Two principal methods of autologous transfusion are possible. Blood is best collected from the patient up to 35 days before an elective operation and stored at 4°C, or blood lost from the operation area is recovered and processed for reinfusion. The latter procedure is known as 'blood salvage'.

Many surgical procedures can be supported with cyrstalloid solutions only, or synthetic plasma substitutes such as gelatins and dextrose, provided that the haematocrit remains above 0.3. When the blood volume is reduced by 20% or more, anaemia becomes an important factor. Replacement should contain a proportion of red cells and, if necessary, blood products and platelets to ensure haemostasis.

A large number of patients needing blood could readily supply their own. Some operations, such as orthopaedic and cardiothoracic operations, and gynaecological procedures, are predictable in their transfusion requirements and are therefore particularly appropriate for the use of autologous blood.

It is now regular practice for patients about to undergo cardiac surgery to have one or two units of blood removed by the anaesthetist immediately before insertion of the bypass. The reduced volume is restored with a plasma substitute, such as a gelatin preparation. The units of blood secured preoperatively are then returned to the patient after coming off bypass, when required. This procedure has a number of advantages in providing normal amounts of most coagulation factors and functioning platelets, as well as lowering the haematocrit by haemodilution, thus reducing blood viscosity and improving oxygen delivery to the tissues.

However, because autologous predeposit blood collection is carried out on an individual basis, the potential hazards of the procedure may be greater than those arising from the use of volunteer donations unless clear instructions about techniques and clerical practices are laid down.

Having determined the number of units of blood required, these should be collected over the 5 weeks before operation at intervals of about a week, and stopping at least 4 days preoperatively. The haemoglobin level should be at least 12 g/dl for men and 11 g/dl for women (10 g/dl in pregnancy), and oral iron supplements should be prescribed. The patient's informed consent must be obtained and, having ensured that the collecting containers are correctly labelled, these should be signed by the patient before collection begins. A sample of the patient's blood should be tested for ABO and Rhesus (D) grouping, screened for atypical antibodies in case additional donor blood is required (the possible need for which should be communicated at the time of consent), and also screened for hepatitis B surface antigen and HIV antibodies (see Standard Haematology Practice 1991). It is important to establish liaison between the haematologist, the surgeon and the anaesthetist, as well as the Blood Transfusion Centre if necessary.

It will be evident that, apart from isolated autologous transfusions for rare medical indications, appropriate funding needs to be set aside in the local revenue development programme if this practice is to be offered widely within a hospital service.

Blood salvage procedures

Various devices have been developed that enable blood released during an operation to be salvaged and returned to the patient. The operative site must be free of bacterial contamination and tumour cells. A popular machine is the Haemonetic cell saver. This collects and anticoagulates the blood from a surgical cavity, then washes the red cells in a centrifugal washing system several times within 3–4 min before they are resuspended at a packed cell volume of about 0.50 for reinfusion (Lee & Napier 1990).

Automated cell-salvage equipment is particularly useful in operations associated with substantial blood losses, such as cardiothoracic, vascular, orthopaedic and transplant procedures, and also major trauma cases. It is of greatest value when operative losses are unexpectedly high and cause a heavy drain on blood-bank stocks.

Artificial blood substitutes

In view of the increasing demand for blood and blood products, and the strain this has put on available resources, much effort has been put into finding a physiological gas-transporting red-cell substitute. Stroma-free haemoglobin has been used, but its intravascular life is of the order of 90 min and it therefore unsatisfactory. The use of perfluorocarbon compounds seems more promising. These have a circulation time of 1–4 days and in experiments maintain oxygenation of isolated organs. They have been used to cover surgical procedures in Jehovah's Witnesses, but there remains a number of problems:

1. Batch variability between different emulsions affects clearance time.
2. Microembolism formation: platelet clumping is encouraged.
3. There is reduced binding of calcium and other cations during perfusion. This is further complicated by changing albumin concentration.

This is an area that will expand over the next few years.

Anticoagulant solutions for stored blood

Anticoagulant solutions are usually citrate or heparin solutions. The function of the anticoagulant is threefold:

- to maintain the whole blood in solution
- to maintain red cell viability, equated to adenosine triphosphate (ATP) generation by glucose and adenine
- to maintain normal haemoglobin function, related to 2,3-DPG concentration.

Heparin is seldom used as an anticoagulant for donor whole blood. The major disadvantage is that there is no glucose in the anticoagulant solution, thus limiting RBC viability and reducing shelf-life to 48 hours. A variety of citrate solutions have been used. In the past, acid citrate dextrose (ACD) was used as the main anticoagulant. The glucose concentration was adequate to maintain red cell ATP for a shelf-life of 21 days. However, the 2,3-DPG levels rapidly decrease, shifting the oxygen dissociation curve to the left, so that after 5 days there is a significant increase in oxygen affinity. Most centres now use citrate phosphate dextrose (CPD) or one of its derivates. CPD maintains the anticoagulated blood at a higher pH than ACD, and also contains additional phosphate. Adequate ATP levels are maintained and the 2,3-DPG levels are normal for at least a week. The oxygen affinity remains normal over this period.

The addition of adenine to CPD results in an increase in survival of stored blood for up to 35 days. The addition of these purine nucleotides maintains the ATP levels, although they do not prevent depletion of the 2,3-DPG. This depletion can be rapidly reversed by the addition of inosine. Potential hazards in the use of these compounds include renal tubular crystal formation, which has been produced in experimental animals given adenine, and hyperuricaemia induced by the catabolism of inosine. In clinical practice, however, human toxicity appears very low. With increasing demand for blood it seems likely that the use of these nucleotides will become more widespread.

The citrate iron in the anticoagulant solution acts by complexing or chelating the ionized calcium in the blood. Reduction in this inhibits the coagulation cascade. The ability of the liver to metabolize citrate is such that it is unnecessary to give ionized calcium to patients receiving a large amount of blood, except in two instances:

1. The premature infant with its immature liver requires supplementation to prevent tetany during exchange transfusion.
2. In acute liver failure the citrate will not be metabolized and supplemental calcium in the form of 5 mmol calcium chloride solution should be given.

Citrated blood shows a progressive tendency during storage to develop clumping and aggregation of white cells, platelets and some red cells. The standard-giving sets will only retain the larger clumps (>170 μm) and it should be remembered that in acutely ill patients, particularly those with pulmonary failure, these microaggregates may block the pulmonary circulation.

'In line' microaggregate filters should be used when large amounts of older blood are being transfused. In general, if the blood is greater than 7 days old and when more than four units are being given, a filter should be considered.

Additive solutions for red cell concentrates

An important side effect of the use of red cell concentrates has been the presentation of units of variable haematocrit, some quite high, with a resulting high viscosity which can greatly slow the infusion rate. A better standardized product is obtained if some plasma is transferred back to the red cells when the buffy coat has been removed, or if the red cells are suspended in a special suspension/preservative medium. One such solution, increasingly widely used, contains saline, adenine, glucose and mannitol (SAGM). The suspension has a standardized haematocrit and is of low viscosity. It also allows for a larger plasma yield which can be used for other purposes. In elective surgery no additional plasma need be given until 50% of the blood volume has been lost, and using such plasma-free products no alteration in the perioperative bleeding pattern is seen. These additive solutions increase red cell storage time for up to 35–42 days with considerable benefits in plasma procurement.

Blood storage

Whole blood is stored in a special blood-bank refrigerator designed to exact specifications. Blood is stored at 4–6°C. These limits should be rigidly observed and domestic refrigerators in wards should never be used for this purpose. Such refrigerators display variation in internal temperature beyond these strict boundaries, so that chance bacterial contamination may multiply or the blood may freeze. Transfusion of blood that has been frozen and thawed may cause death. Blood-bank refrigerators are usually under the supervision of a consultant haematologist. In general they have an automatic recording device with a battery-operated alarm system. The alarm system should be independent and continue to operate if there is a mains failure. When blood is taken for use it is imperative that:

1. The group and compatibility label on the unit correspond with the group and identity of the patient. In general, two observers should check the details before transfusion.
2. The expiry date should be checked prior to administration. In exceptional circumstances this may be overridden, but this should only be done in consultation with the haematologist.
3. All packs should be intact, with no signs of damage, leakage or haemolysis. A white layer may be seen on the surface of the plasma. This is fat and is not contraindication to use.
4. Blood must be used within 30 min of removal from the refrigerator and should not be left at room temperature, or on a radiator, prior to use. If left for longer than 30 min the blood must not be given.
5. It is safe to give blood taken directly from the refrigerator. If it is medically necessary to warm the blood this must be done in a carefully controlled sterile heat-exchanging coil in a blood warmer. Overheating results in haemolysis which can cause death.

Blood transfusion reactions

The total incidence of all reactions is probably less than 5%, and most are mild. In multitransfused patients and multiparous women pyrexial reactions are relatively common. However, in general, true incompatibility reactions with accompanying haemolysis are uncommon, and when they occur are more often related to a clerical error than to a laboratory mishap.

Reactions may be overt or silent. The latter type is usually signified by shortened red cell survival with a reduced response to transfusion, and may be missed if clinically insignificant. The former may show varying grades of response ranging from a febrile reaction to jaundice, haemoglobinuria and loin pain, occasionally leading to consumption coagulopathy with haemorrhage and renal failure.

Types and causes of reaction

There are three main types of transfusion reaction:

1. A febrile response soon after the start of transfusion. This is often related to an immune reaction involving transfused granulocytes, lymphocytes or platelets, and is an indication to use leucocyte-poor or washed cells.
2. An anaphylactoid reaction associated with skin flushing, dyspnoea and hypotension resulting from antigen-antibody complexes with complement activation and release of vasoactive amines. Filtered and washed red cells should be used subsequently.
3. Haemolysis. The chance of haemolysis is reduced if only blood of the same ABO group is used. Care should be taken in using group O blood as a universal donor since some units have high titre antibodies that will lyse group A, B or AB blood in the recipient. Intravascular haemolysis is most likely when IgM antibodies are present, such as anti-A or anti-B, as they rapidly lead to complete destruction of incompatible cells. Occasionally, mechanical damage due to overheating or freezing of the blood may be responsible. Renal failure may be precipitated by the direct toxic action of free haemoglobin and hypotension, and treatment should be aimed at preserving renal function. Extravascular haemolysis is caused mainly by IgG antibodies which do not bind complement, and is mediated by erythrophagocytosis in macrophages. The main clinical feature is a febrile reaction with an increase in indirect bilirubin. Severe reactions are less common.

The causes of transfusion reaction are listed below:

- clerical error
- thrombophlebitis
- allergy
- pyrogens
- white cell incompatibility
- red cell incompatibility (intravascular/extravascular haemolysis)
- overloading of the circulation with pulmonary oedema
- addition of medicaments to blood
- air embolus
- transfusion of infected blood
- transfusion of donor infection (syphilis, malaria, post-transfusion hepatitis).

Investigation of reactions

All reactions should be reported to the transfusion laboratory which will initiate an investigation and keep a record of the event. Samples required include:

- the pretransfusion sample which is retained in the laboratory (clotted)
- the remains of the used packs
- a clotted sample taken immediately after the reaction and with later samples as indicated
- a citrate sample for coagulation studies to exclude consumption coagulopathy and a heparinized sample to look for evidence of haemolysis (haptoglobin, bilirubin, haem pigments), if indicated
- the first voided urine sample for haemoglobin (a fluid balance sheet should be maintained)
- if the reaction is suspected to be due to infected blood, a sample should be sent for culture.

In addition the volume of blood transfused should be recorded along with the bleed date, expiry date, the giving set number and whether any drug was added to the unit. The previous transfusion history, and in women the previous pregnancy history, should be reviewed.

Further requests for blood depend on the type of reactions and the findings, and should be discussed with the haematologist.

REFERENCES

Advisory Committee on Dangerous Pathogens 1990 HIV: the causative agent of AIDS and related conditions. Second revision of guidelines. Department of Health

Blood Transfusion Task Force 1991 Autologous transfusion. In: Roberts B (ed) Standard haematology practice. Blackwell Scientific, Oxford, pp. 207–211

British Committee for Standards in Haematology 1990 Guidelines on oral anticoagulation, 2nd edn. J Clin Pathol 43: 177–183

Chanarin I (ed) 1989 Laboratory haematology. Churchill Livingstone, Edinburgh

Ciavarella D, Reed R L, Counts R B et al 1987 Clotting factor levels and the risk of diffuse microvascular bleeding in the massively transfused patient. Br J Haematol 67: 365–368

Cordell B R, Yulon V A, Cigahn-Haskell C, McDonough B P, Perkins H A 1986 Experience with 11,916 designated donors. Transfusion 26: 484–486

Esteban J I, Gonzalez A, Hernandez J M et al 1990 Evaluation of antibodies to hepatitis C virus in a study of transfusion associated hepatitis. N Eng J Med 323: 1107–1112

Dunnill R P H, Colvin M P 1989 Clinical and resuscitative data, 4th edn. Blackwell, Oxford

Gerberding J J, Littell C, Tarkington A, Brown A, Schechter W P 1990 Risk of exposure of surgical personnel to patients' blood during surgery at San Francisco General Hospital. N Engl J Med 322: 1788–1793

Hoffbrand A V 1989 Megaloblastic anaemia. In: Hoffbrand A V, Lewis S M (eds) Postgraduate haematology, 3rd edn. Heinemann, Oxford, p. 68

Joint Committee on Vaccination and Immunisation 1988 Immunisation against infectious disease. Department of Health

Jones J 1987 Abuse of fresh frozen plasma. Br Med J 295: 287

Kamath B S K, Fozard J R 1980 Control of heparinisation during cardiopulmonary by pass. Experience with the activated clotting time method. Anaesthesia 35: 250–256

Kessler C M, Klein H G, Havlik R J 1982 Uncontrolled thrombocytosis in chronic myeloproliferative disorders. Br J Haematol 50: 157–167

Larcan A, Lambert H, Gerard A 1987 Consumption coagulopathies. Masson, Paris

Lee D, Napier J A F 1990 Autologous transfusion. Br Med J 300: 737–740

Mannucci P M, Franchi F, Dioguardi N 1976 Correction of abnormal coagulation in chronic liver disease by combined use of fresh frozen plasma and prothrombin complex concentrates. Lancet 2: 542–545

Mannucci P M, Ruggeri Z M, Pareti F I, Capitanio A 1977 1-Deamino-8-D-Arginine Vasopressin: a new pharmacological approach to the management of haemophilia and von Willebrand's disease. Lancet 1: 869–872

Remuzzi G 1988 Bleeding in renal failure. Lancet 1: 1205–1208

Rutherford G W, Lifson A R, Hessol N A et al 1990 Course of HIV-1 infection in a cohort of homosexual and bisexual men: an 11 year follow up study. Br Med J 301: 1183–1188

Schwartz R S, Abildgaard C F, Aledort L M et al 1990 Human recombinant DNA-derived antihaemophilic factor (factor VIII) in the treatment of haemophilia A. N Engl J Med 323: 1800–1805

Taberner D A, Poller L, Burslem R W, Jones J B 1978 Oral anticoagulants controlled by the British comparative thromboplastin versus low-dose heparin in prophylaxis of deep vein thrombosis. Br Med J 1: 272–274

UK Haemophilia Centre Directors 1988 Effect of dry-heating of coagulation factor concentrates at 80°C for 72 hours on transmission of non-A, non-B hepatitis. Lancet 2: 814–816

Vaglia A, Nicolin R, Puro V, Ippolito G, Bettini C, de Lalla F 1990 Needlestick hepatitis C virus seroconversion in a surgeon. Lancet 2: 1315–1316

Wasserman L R, Gilbert H S 1963 Surgery in polycythaemia vera. N Engl J Med 269: 1226–1230

11

Pregnancy and the safety of anaesthesia

B. M. Morgan

INTRODUCTION

Pregnancy, from its earliest weeks, increases the risk of anaesthesia for the mother. This risk rises with the increasing gestational age of the fetus until, during labour, the risk of anaesthesia to the mother is considerable.

Postpartum changes are not well researched. The precise interval needed for the mother to return to the same degree of anaesthetic risk that she presented before pregnancy is not known.

Hazards to the healthy mother are also related to her age, being lowest in the young mother and increasing considerably with ageing (DHSS 1989). Pregnant women over the age of 40 have the greatest risk. This is often associated with degenerative conditions, especially of the cardiovascular system. The physiological changes that accompany pregnancy are widespread and make the mother incomparably different from any other patient. These changes especially affect the gastrointestinal, cardiovascular and respiratory systems. As well as this, pharmacokinetic changes alter the response to general and local anaesthetics. It is essential for the anaesthetist to understand maternal physiology if the safety of anaesthesia during pregnancy is to be assured.

This chapter is concerned with the hazards of anaesthesia, during pregnancy, to both mother and fetus. The problems of anaesthesia for operative delivery, including caesarean section, are discussed in Chapter 40.

Anaesthesia, where fetal survival is desired, must be tailored not only to safeguard the mother, but also to ensure the special milieu required for fetal well-being. It seems clear that many physiological changes reflect the mother's role as incubator, and that the chance of fetal survival might be best when these changes are maintained as accurately as possible by the anaesthetist. The increased fetal loss associated with anaesthesia for any condition is possibly at its maximum during the stage of fetal implantation and organogenesis (Beeley 1981). The risk that anaesthesia constitutes to the fetus seems to diminish with increasing gestational age until near term, when intrauterine death following anaesthesia is uncommon and premature labour is less catastrophic.

The actual rate of spontaneous abortion from all causes in early pregnancy is disputed. It has been quoted as 52% (Wilcox et al 1988) of all fertilizations but 12–15% of diagnosed pregnancies (Edmonds et al 1982, Whittaker et al 1983). As the rate of spontaneous abortion is not known the likely increase that anaesthesia may cause is unproven. Many factors influence the loss of a pregnancy: the mother's age, parity, obstetric history, the cytogenic state of the embryo and the surgical condition that requires anaesthesia. The role of different anaesthetic techniques is difficult to elucidate (Smith 1963, Shnider & Webster 1965), but fetal loss rates of 23% after laparotomy have been quoted (Saunders & Milton 1973). The onset of premature labour within 2 weeks of an anaesthetic with a live fetus may be related to the anaesthetic, the surgery, the obstetric condition or the general condition of the mother.

An estimated 2% of pregnant women have an anaesthetic for a surgical procedure before term where fetal survival is desired, commonly for cervical encirclage sutures. These are associated with a 30% fetal loss due, it seems, to the obstetric condition and the state of the cervix. It is not known what part anaesthesia plays in these losses. Ovarian cystectomy and appendicectomy are the most common intraperitoneal operations where fetal survival is planned. It seems reasonable to support the established view that all elective surgery should be postponed until after delivery. Also, all women of childbearing age should have pregnancy ruled out by questioning and tests before elective surgery. Changes in early pregnancy that affect maternal and fetal survival are summarized below.

PHYSIOLOGICAL CHANGES IN PREGNANCY WITH ANAESTHETIC IMPLICATIONS

Gastrointestinal factors

The change that constitutes the greatest increase in risk to the mother occurs in the gastrointestinal tract. The difficulty of keeping the gastric secretions within the stomach and out of the lungs of an unconscious mother becomes a problem of increasing severity, until during labour it becomes the major cause of anaesthetic maternal death (DHSS 1989). The problem is two-fold: the reduction in lower oesophageal sphincter tone and the delay in gastric emptying. There is no evidence of a lower than usual pH of the gastric contents in pregnancy.

The reduction in the lower oesophageal sphincter (LOS) tone and the resultant lessening of the barrier pressure is the reason for the common symptom of heartburn in pregnancy. Most sufferers are spontaneously cured within a few days of delivery. The complaint occurs in 70% of pregnant women (Atlay 1973). Actual histological evidence of oesophagitis has been demonstrated (Castro 1967). Lind et al (1968) have shown that women with symptoms of heartburn had decreased barrier pressures which returned to normal 6 weeks after delivery. The possible explanation for this phenomenon is likely to be increased progresterone levels, as it also occurs in women taking contraceptive pills (Van Thiel et al 1976). The role of the abdominal tumour as a causative factor has been refuted, but the reduction in the barrier pressure reaches a plateau by 36 weeks, then remains so during labour and for some time postpartum (Van Thiel & Wald 1981). The implication of this reduced barrier pressure for anaesthesia is that the risks of aspiration of gastric contents are increased. Drugs used in anaesthesia can aggravate the tendency by further reducing LOS tone. Atropine, hyoscine, and glycopyrrolate given intravenously increase the risk of gastro-oesophageal reflux, as does thiopentone, opiates, antiemetics, promethazine and droperidol (Cotton & Smith 1984). Other drugs increase LOS tone: metoclopramide, domperidone, cyclizine and prochlorperazine (Brock-Utne et al 1978), as do succinylcholine and antacids. Metoclopramide is ineffective in the presence of opiates (Nimmo et al 1975).

The second change that increases the likelihood of gastro-oesophageal reflux is the delay in gastric emptying, as large residual volumes further reduce the barrier pressure. The evidence that pregnancy itself delays gastric emptying is unclear due, perhaps, to methodological difficulties. O'Sullivan et al (1987) showed no difference between pregnant and non-pregnant females using epigastric impedance, but Lawson et al (1985), using the lactulose hydrogen breath test, found that gastrointestinal transit time was significantly prolonged in second and third trimesters, as compared to first trimester and postpartum women. Simpson et al (1988), using the paracetamol absorption rate as an indirect measure of gastric emptying, have also shown that emptying is delayed in the second trimester. Marsh et al (1984) showed that stress alone in preoperative surgical patients does not delay paracetamol absorption. However, gastric emptying has been shown to be delayed in labour in patients who have received opiate analgesia (Nimmo 1978), but not those with epidural analgesia (Holdsworth 1978). Gastric emptying is enhanced by metoclopromide but this action is abolished by opiates (Nimmo 1975, Holdsworth 1978). The gastric stasis caused by the opiates can be reversed with naloxone (Frame et al 1984). The action of narcotic analgesics in delaying gastric emptying and further reducing LOS tone makes regurgitation more likely. The Report on Confidential Enquiries into Maternal Deaths in England and Wales 1982–84 (DHSS 1989) suggested that a reduction in the use of narcotics in labour could increase maternal safety with anaesthesia.

There is no evidence that the gastric contents are at a lower pH than normal in pregnancy (O'Sullivan & Bullingham 1984). In fact, gastric acid secretion has been shown to be reduced in the first and second trimesters of pregnancy, returning to normal in the third trimester. Gastric contents with a pH greater than 2.5 and a volume less than 25 ml are thought to present the least likelihood of aspiration (Roberts & Shirley 1974). For many years it was accepted practice to administer mist. mag. trisilicate routinely in labour in an attempt to alkalinize gastric contents. Increasing doubt is cast over the efficacy of this treatment since, although it may substantially increase pH, it also increases gastric volume and thus reduces barrier pressure. Perhaps more important, it is now known that inhalation of a particulate substance itself can cause pulmonary aspiration syndrome (Bond et al 1979, Gibbs et al 1979). The use of H_2-receptor antagonists will increase the pH and diminish the gastric contents (Morgan 1984), but the effects of these drugs on the fetus early in gestation have not yet been proved safe, nor has the safety of metoclopramide and domperidone been proved in the developing fetus.

A suitable antacid regimen is given in Appendix 1 (see also Chapter 40). However it is important to realize that it is not the acidity of the gastric contents but the volume and the increased likelihood of gastro-oesophageal reflux that increases the risk of anaesthesia during pregnancy and labour.

Cardiovascular factors

The response of the mother's cardiovascular system (CVS) to pregnancy must be borne in mind when assessing the pregnant patient for anaesthesia. In the interests of the fetus, the physiological parameters of the CVS must be maintained during anaesthesia and in the interests of the mother as little extra stress as possible must be added.

The cardiovascular changes are profound. They occur early in the pregnancy and are measurable by the fifth week of gestation (Robson et al 1989). These changes are summarized as an increase in cardiac output as a result of an increase in heart rate and stroke volume, while the blood pressure remains constant or even falls slightly because of the decrease in systemic vascular resistance (Wichman & Ryden 1986).

New non-invasive techniques for measuring cardiovascular parameters, such as Doppler techniques and echocardiography, have added to the quantification of these changes and to understanding how these relate to the increasing gestational age of the fetus. Doppler ultrasound measurements of cardiac output have been validated against thermodilution techniques in pregnancy (Easterling et al 1987). These new techniques confirm that the mother's cardiac output has increased 40% by the 12th week of gestation and has increased 50% by the 32nd week of gestation. Thus the cardiac output increases from about 4.5 l/min to 6.0 l/min.

During labour the cardiac output increases with increasing cervical dilation until by 8–9 cm the cardiac output can be up to 12 l/min. This is about the maximum that can be achieved. The mother thus has very little cardiac reserve left towards the end of the first stage of labour. The increase in cardiac output is achieved by an enhanced stroke volume which is up by about 30%, and a heart rate up by about 15% so that resting pulse rates in pregnancy are around 75–85 beats/min.

The total systemic vascular resistance falls until about the 20th week of pregnancy so that the systolic blood pressure remains constant and the diastolic blood pressure falls. After 20 weeks the diastolic pressure increases until it is up to pre-pregnancy levels by about the 38th week.

The mother's cardiovascular state has been likened to a natural volume overload state or one equal to moderate exercise over a long period. (Schrier & Durr 1987). Circulating blood volume increases in the first trimester and continues to increase until at term it has expanded to about 1.25 l above non-pregnant levels (Hytten & Paintin 1963). The increase in blood volume is proportional to the size and number of the fetuses at term. The increase is largely in the plasma volume which expands by 45%, whereas the red cell mass increases by about 20% resulting in haemodilution, with a haemoglobin concentration of around 11 g/100 ml and a haemotocrit of 33% being normal. Thus a loss of about 1 l of blood at delivery and in the puerperium is already allowed for. If this is not exceeded the blood volume will return to its original level about 14 days postpartum. The plasma protein concentration is lowered giving decreased colloid oncotic pressure, however, the absolute quantity of plasma albumin also decreases (Hytten 1980).

The purpose of this increased blood volume and cardiac output is firstly to increase uterine flow, which at term can have a blood flow of 600–800 ml/min. The uteroplacental vessels are maximally dilated at term and placental flow is wholly dependent on maternal blood pressure. Secondly the kidneys benefit from the increased blood volume, and renal blood flow is increased by 400–500 ml/min by the end of the first trimester. This is essential to meet the greater needs of excretion of extra waste products. It is possible that liver blood flow is also increased to allow the greater metabolic activity required in pregnancy. A third important increase in regional flow is to the skin where peripheral vasodilation is required to eliminate heat from the fast-growing fetal tissues.

The CVS in pregnancy must be carefully protected from the side effects of most anaesthetic drugs, by accurate titration of drugs and by intense monitoring. Swings in cardiac output and blood pressure should be avoided, even in early pregnancy. The circulation time in pregnant women appears to be unchanged, thus allowing normal induction times for intravenous agents.

Aortocaval compression syndrome

Supine hypotensive syndrome is caused by the compression of the maternal aorta and inferior vena cava by the fetus (Kerr et al 1964). About 10% of normal unanaesthetized mothers will suffer hypotension when supine at term. This figure is higher in mothers who have general or conduction anaesthesia, as the cardiovascular compensatory mechanisms are altered. Compression of the inferior vena cava may occur by the 16th week of pregnancy. Compensatory mechanisms in the non-anaesthetized mother cause a rise in venous pressure below the caval obstruction and an increase in collateral venous return via the paravertebral veins to the azygos. Aortic compression also occurs to some degree with the mother supine, resulting in arterial hypotension to the lower part of the body. This reduces uterine blood flow and so placental perfusion.

This syndrome must be prevented during general and conduction anaesthesia by providing a 20° lateral tilt, usually to the left, in any patient more than 16 weeks pregnant, for the duration of the procedure. This is essential for the maintenance of the mother's cardiac output even when the fetus is not being considered. Even with a lateral tilt this syndrome may still occur. The mother's blood pressure must be carefully monitored and a continuous fetal heart monitor should be functioning with a surviving fetus. Renal plasma flow increases by 30% and glomerular filtration rate by nearly 50% at the end of the first trimester. A supine position causes a considerable decrease in urine production. Multiple pregnancy, a large fetus, or a fetus in a transverse position increases the problem of aortocaval compression considerably.

Altered response to conduction anaesthesia

Pregnancy from about the end of the first trimester is accompanied by some degree of obstruction to venous return from the lower part of the body, even when the mother is not supine. Efforts to compensate for this obstruction cause some of the altered responses seen in conduction anaesthesia. The rise in venous pressure causes the collateral channels in the paravertebral venous plexus to become enlarged. This in turn causes a reduction in the size of the epidural space and so smaller volumes of local anaesthetic solution are required for the pregnant patient to achieve the same height of block than would be necessary in the young non-pregnant woman.

Another problem associated with the venous collaterals is that there is considerably more risk of epidural venous puncture in the pregnant patient. Inadvertent injection of local anaesthetic into the paravertebral veins has a more profound effect in the pregnant patient because the bolus of local anaesthetic arrives at the heart via the azygos veins. This may be a factor causing cardiac depression and arrest apparently more readily in the pregnant woman.

Further compensation for venous obstruction is an increased sympathetic tone causing an increased systemic resistance of the lower limbs. Blocking the sympathetics with epidural or spinal conduction anaesthesia thus results in a more pronounced hypotension than occurs in the non-pregnant young woman. Venous capacitance vessels take up to 50% of the blood volume in pregnancy, and without vasomotor tone this is increased, revealing aortocaval compression. As placental blood flow is almost completely pressure-dependent, this greater tendency to a hypotensive response from conduction anaesthesia must be energetically counteracted with intravenous fluid preloading and ephedrine, when necessary, to maintain the systolic pressure above 100 mmHg in the normotensive.

Respiratory factors

Hyperventilation is the main respiratory change that occurs in pregnancy. The tidal volume is increased some 40% above non-pregnant levels by the end of the first trimester (Hytten 1980), but the respiratory rate remains unchanged at about 15 breaths/min. Tidal volume is increased by greater diaphragmatic contractions. This adds to increased movement of the lower rib cage which occurs with the diminished abdominal compliance (Gilroy et al 1988).

Minute ventilation rises from about 7.5 l to 10.5 l in late pregnancy. Alveolar ventilation is increased, and late in pregnancy respiratory alkalosis occurs. This augmented respiratory drive is possibly mediated by elevated levels of progesterone (Pernoll et al 1975). Functional residual capacity decreases because the diaphragm moves cephalad. The increase in inspiratory capacity equals the decline in expiratory reserve and vital capacity is unchanged (Weinberger et al 1980).

The Po_2 rises from 85 mmHg (11.3 kPa) early in pregnancy to 92 mmHg (12.3 kPa) at term (Lucius et al 1970). This very small rise occurs because of the shape of the haemoglobin dissociation curve. However, this appears to be essential for normal fetal growth as mothers who have chronically low Po_2 levels have growth-retarded infants (Fishburne 1979). Ventilation–perfusion inequalities are increased, especially in the supine position, by the increase in the closing volume where closure of the small airways occurs within the tidal volume. Physiological hyperventilation results in lower Pco_2 levels, arterial Pco_2 being at about 30 mmHg (4 kPa) in pregnancy compared to 35–40 mmHg (4.7–5.3 kPa) in the non-pregnant woman. This low Pco_2 level is reached in early pregnancy and is possibly essential in allowing the fetus to eliminate CO_2 down the concentration gradient (Dick et al 1977). This reduction in Pco_2 seems to be a result of high progesterone levels, and may lead to dyspnoea and giddiness in early pregnancy.

The increased minute ventilation, cardiac output, haemodilution and blood volume all result in increased perfusion of the alveoli and better gas exchange. This, together with the reduced functional residual capacity and increased CO_2 production, results in the arterial-to-end-tidal Pco_2 difference being smaller in pregnancy than in the non-pregnant woman (Shanker et al 1986). The mother maintains a normal arterial pH of 7.40 by reducing plasma bicarbonate. Venous pH changes from 7.38 to 7.35, possibly reflecting the increased peripheral venous flow (de Swiet 1980).

All central nervous system (CNS) depressant drugs, analgesics and anaesthetics can reverse the hyperventilation which will quickly hamper the elimination of CO_2 by the fetus. The fetus shows greater sensitivity to CO_2 than the adult. Premedicant and postoperative drugs must be used with caution if hyperventilation is not to be suppressed. The decreased functional residual capacity allows less dilution of inhalation agents and thus a more rapid rise in partial pressures. The increased alveolar ventilation results in more rapid uptake of inhalation agents.

Nasal mucous membranes are congested throughout pregnancy, possibly to saturate the greater tidal volume. These congested nasal mucous membranes can cause considerable bleeding when attempts are made to pass nasogastric, nasopharyngeal or nasotracheal tubes during pregnancy.

Excessive artificial ventilation reduces maternal cardiac output and, by raising maternal pH, reduces the oxygen-releasing capacity of maternal haemoglobin. Placental oxygen transfer can be reduced. Severe hypocapnia must also be rigorously prevented, as it reduces placental perfusion. This reduced placental perfusion may be detrimental to the fetus, particularly if the fetus is small for dates.

Pharmacokinetic factors

Physiological changes that occur in pregnancy influence the absorption, distribution, metabolism and excretion of drugs (Kraner & Kraner 1977, Cummings 1983, Boobis and Lewis 1983). Metabolism is altered whether it occurs by renal clearance, or oxidation or conjugation in the liver. Factors that alter pharmacokinetics are the increase in plasma volume with the resultant dilution of plasma proteins.

Further factors are the increase in hepatic activity and renal blood flow. Not all plasma proteins are equally affected. The total amount of serum albumen increases (Hytten & Paintin 1963) as well as the α_2 acid glycoprotein to which many basic drugs are bound. This is also increased by stress. Other than pregnancy, labour itself alters the pharmacokinetics of certain drugs. Pethidine and promazine are less well metabolized (Crawford & Rudofsky 1966, Morgan et al 1978), and midazolam has higher plasma levels during labour than in pregnancy. But the half-life of paracetamol is not altered in labour (Nimmo et al 1975).

Systemic toxicity of some local anaesthetics is affected by pregnancy. This is the result of the relationship between the protein-bound fraction of the drug and the free drug. Thus 73% of bupivacaine is bound to plasma proteins in non-pregnant ewes, but only 51% in pregnant ewes (Morishima et al 1985). In contrast, mepivacaine is 22% bound in pregnant and non-pregnant ewes (Santos et al 1989). The consequence of this change in protein binding is that bupivacaine is more cardiotoxic in the pregnant as compared to the non-pregnant animal (Morishima et al 1985) because of the greater amount of free bupivacaine available.

The volume of the central compartment (V1) is increased in pregnancy, but when expressed per kg body weight there is no significant change. It would seem logical therefore to increase the dose of anaesthetic induction agents to take into account the increased body weight, especially since the duration of action of such drugs given in a single dose depends on redistribution and not elimination. The duration of action of drugs given in repeated dosage or by infusion, however, will depend on the amount of drug present and the rate of elimination or clearance of the drug from the plasma. Clearance of many drugs is enhanced in pregnancy due to increased cardiac output, and increases in liver and renal blood flow. In the case of thiopentone (and presumably other highly lipid-soluble drugs), however, this increased clearance is more than compensated for by a large increase in the volume of distribution at steady state (Vdss). The result is that elimination half-life is prolonged. Whereas a single dose of thiopentone may be expected to have its usual short-lived effect, multiple doses in the pregnant patient may be expected to result in a slower than anticipated recovery.

Pseudocholinesterase is depressed by about 30% in pregnancy (Shnider & Webster 1965), but does not seem to prolong the activity of succinylcholine in non-pregnant women.

Fluid and electrolyte balance

Total body water increases by 6–8 l during normal pregnancy, about half of which is extracellular (Lindheimer & Katz 1989). There is also an increase in intravascular fluid. This increase in body water is called the 'physiological hypervolaemia' of pregnancy. The marked extracellular and plasma volume increases are associated with a marked sodium retention. Pregnancy changes the mother's ability to handle renal sodium. Several factors increase filtered sodium and also tubular reabsorption of sodium. The mother gains 2–6 mmol sodium/day during pregnancy, and this is distributed throughout maternal and fetal tissues. In spite of this sodium retention the plasma sodium level is lower in pregnancy and there is a small constant sodium leak. There is an equivalent retention of potassium and the corresponding anions.

Total body sodium is increased and sufficient sodium is retained by the mother to ensure that the concentration of sodium in the increased extracellular fluid is 2–3 mmol below non-pregnant levels. The glomerular filtration rate and effective renal plasma flow increases by as much as 50–80% above prepregnant levels, and this occurs early in pregnancy. There is an increased excretion of glucose, uric acids and proteins related to tubular function (Davison 1987). There is also a decrease in plasma urea, uric acid and creatinine, and these reductions cause a fall in plasma osmolality. This decrease in tonicity occurs early in gestation and reaches a plateau by 10 weeks, to return to normal by the second postpartum week (Davison et al 1981). Most of this decrease in osmolality is a result of a fall in plasma sodium.

Plasma atrial natriuretic peptide (ANP) is a cardiac hormone involved in blood volume homeostasis. This hormone increases due to expanding plasma volumes. It is found at greater than normal levels in the non-pregnant patient with chronic heart or renal failure and in some hypertensive states. There is no consensus as to whether it is elevated in normal pregnancy because of a wide range of normal values. Some studies have shown that it is increased, others that it is not (Hirai et al 1988). However all studies have shown it to be increased in pre-eclampsia. The increased level of ANP correlates with the severity of the disease, but does not provide an early indication of those at risk of pre-eclampsia.

ANP may be expected to increase in pregnancy because of the plasma volume expansion, but all the factors that regulate its increase are not as yet determined. It may be that the volume increase in pregnancy is too slow to trigger ANP secretion, or that any atrial stretch is offset by the fall in systemic vascular resistance. There is no evidence that atrial pressure is increased in pregnancy and increased atrial wall tension seems to be a stimulus. ANP may regulate blood volume, renal blood flow and vascular tone, and volume expansion with saline or increased salt intake elevates ANP in man. Its possible physiological role may be to increase renal blood flow and glomerular filtration rate, and it may be responsible for the altered vascular reactivity in pregnancy. Pre-eclampsia with its increased vascular resistance, decreased circulating blood volume and impaired uteroplacental perfusion may be associated with high levels of ANP as a result of compensation for the retention of water and sodium (Hirai et al 1988). The role in pregnancy of this natriuretic, diuretic and smooth muscle relaxant hormone is as yet unclear. It has been reported as being high postpartum, decreasing over 42 days, and may mediate the postpartum diuresis.

Metabolic adaptation

Preoperative starvation and postoperative increased catabolism can have important effects on the fetus. During pregnancy, fetal glucose utilization causes decreased fasting glucose levels by the 10th week, and this continues throughout pregnancy. Withholding of food and water causes the mother to use fatty acids with a rapid increase in ketone production. Periods of starvation should be restricted to the minimum, concomitant with anaesthetic safety.

Temperature

The fast-growing fetus produces much heat, and increased cutaneous blood flow in the mother allows for greater heat loss to compensate. Maintaining a body temperature of 37–37.5°C is important for the pregnant woman as high fetal wastage is reported following maternal infections of all types (Hurley 1982). Pre- and postanaesthetic pyrexia needs early active treatment.

Immunological system

Pregnancy is an immunosuppressive state, but the factors that allow the mother's immune mechanism to tolerate allograft, that is the fetus, are not understood. It has been assumed that the maternal immunological system has been suppressed and that the pregnant woman is therefore less likely to develop anaphylactic responses to drugs. However, several reports have indicated that these reactions do occur in pregnant women (Baraka & Steir 1980, Lund 1980). The combined bronchospasm and hypotension can be fatal for the fetus even if the mother is resuscitated. Alleviation of aortocaval compression in mothers requiring resuscitation from major anaphylactic reactions must receive immediate attention if mother and fetus are to recover.

Placental transfer

Autoregulation of maternal placental flow is almost non-existent. The low-resistance high-flow system is almost wholly dependent on maternal cardiac output and blood pressure. The uterine arteries are maximally dilated at term, and possibly much earlier. Although they cannot vasodilate, they can vasoconstrict in response to drugs with vasoconstrictor effects. They also constrict as part of the pathological process of pre-eclampsia.

Oxygen crosses the placenta by diffusion. Fetal haemoglobin has a greater affinity for oxygen than does maternal haemoglobin, and the former is present in high concentrations (17 g/100 ml). Although only a small partial pressure difference exists, this is adequate to transfer oxygen to the fetus in the absence of maternal hypoxia. Elimination of fetal CO_2 occurs down the concentration gradient caused by the mother's hyperventilation, allowing the fetus to remain normocapnic.

Reynolds (1989) in a review of placental drug transfer stressed that drugs cross the placenta by passive diffusion, the rate of which is governed by the same physicochemical properties of the drug that govern the crossing of the blood–brain barrier. Thus any drug that has an effect on the mother's CNS must cross the placenta as well. The drugs that cross these barriers are highly lipid-soluble, of low molecular weight and have a small degree of ionization. These include all inhalational anaesthetics, barbiturates, narcotics and sedatives. These drugs rapidly cross the placenta and reach equilibrium with the fetus. The rate of diffusion of these drugs is flow-dependent, as is that for oxygen and carbon dioxide.

Highly ionized water-soluble, large molecular weight drugs, such as muscle relaxants and mannitol, cross the placenta poorly by diffusion. When water-soluble drugs do cross the placenta, they may be excreted by the fetal kidneys and become trapped in the amniotic fluid. Usually this occurs only following prolonged exposure. Drugs such as local anaesthetics, which are highly protein-bound, do not cross in appreciable quantities since only a small proportion is available as the free drug to exert a concentration gradient. Once the plasma-protein binding-sites have been saturated by the drug, however, further doses have a disproportionate effect on the plasma concentration of the drug, and thus increase its placental transfer.

Diagnostic indices

Changes in the physiology of the mother make diagnosis of pathology particularly difficult. Anaesthetic assessment of the mother's preoperative condition must be seen in the light of what is normal for the pregnant patient, rather than trying to use criteria for the non-pregnant.

Symptoms of dyspnoea and giddiness are normal in early pregnancy because of hyperventilation. Complaints of polyuria and nocturia have no significance, nor do complaints of feeling too hot in usual ambient temperatures give any indication of disease with a normal body temperature. Tiredness or inability to carry out normal physical activity do not necessarily indicate diminished cardiac reserve. In mothers with heart disease the increased cardiac workload required in pregnancy, however, may well reveal inadequate cardiac reserves.

The heart appears clinically to be enlarged in normal pregnant women as the apex beat moves up and lateral to the axillary line. Frequently a systolic ejection murmur is heard, and at times a diastolic murmur. A third heart sound is common, or a split first heart sound may be heard. Radiologically the heart has an appearance similar to that seen in mitral stenosis. In the normal pregnant woman the ECG may show changes suggestive of ischaemic heart disease with left axis deviation, inverted T waves and a depressed S–T segment. Commonly, atrial or ventricular extrasystoles are present and ECG traces often require expert interpretation to rule out ischaemic damage.

The diagnosis of renal disease is more difficult in pregnancy as the ureters are dilated on X-ray appearance from about the 10th week. Possibly this is due to the overall smooth muscle atony seen in pregnancy, which is thought to be a progesterone effect. Proteinuria of modest degree is common in normal pregnancy, although, of course, much increased in pre-eclampsia. The haemoglobin concentration falls early in pregnancy to 11–12 g/100 ml, and the haematocrit falls to about 33%. Marked leucocytosis exists due to increases in the neutrophil polymorphonuclear cells. The erythrocyte sedimentation rate (ESR) has a mean in pregnancy of 56 mm in the first hour, with a range of 30–98 mm. This is due to the relatively high levels of plasma globulins and fibrinogens, so ESR has no value as a non-specific diagnosis of disease (Hytten & Lind 1973).

Glycosuria occurs in about a third of the pregnant population, making the diagnosis of diabetes, especially gestational diabetes, more difficult, and requiring fasting blood glucose levels to be tested. Serum alkaline phosphatase rises in normal pregnancy by as much as four times the non-pregnant level. It is produced by the placenta and is not a sign of disease.

EFFECT OF MULTIPLE PREGNANCY

The number of mothers with multiple pregnancies has increased with new treatments for infertility. These mothers are often older with long histories of infertility. Hazards to the fetus are greater than with a singleton pregnancy, and both mother and fetuses require more care during anaesthesia.

The physiological changes of pregnancy occur earlier and the alterations are greater than in a singleton pregnancy. Aortocaval compression is a particular problem, even before the 16th week of pregnancy. The mother's lateral tilt position must be tested before anaesthesia as the degree of tilt required will depend on the number of fetuses. Monitoring of the infants also presents greater problems. Stress on the mother's cardiovascular system is increased, with her plasma volume rising to 2 l with twins and 2.7 l with triplets (and presumably even higher with more fetuses). Therefore her cardiac output is also greater, adding considerably to her cardiac workload. It is thought that the oesophageal barrier pressure might be further decreased and that the incidence of heartburn is also greater. Anaesthesia must therefore be employed with even greater care in these mothers.

DRUGS IN BREAST MILK

Anaesthesia and analgesia in the puerperium cause an added concern where the mother is breast-feeding. Just under 3% of mothers undergo anaesthesia in the puerperium, usually for evacuation of retained products of conception. Concern for the effect of drugs on the neonate is sometimes an excuse for providing poor analgesia for the mother after caesarean section or forceps delivery, where associated maternal soft tissue damage can be considerable. Consideration must be given to the possibility of the drug being found in the milk and the effect that it might have on the neonate.

Analgesics and anaesthetics are all lipid-soluble drugs that are distributed throughout the body as they readily cross cell membranes. They are therefore also found in breast milk and would for similar reasons be absorbed by the baby. As a consequence of the newborn's limited capacity to metabolize drugs there is a prolonged half-life in the baby. However, if the drug is highly protein-bound the dose the baby receives will be small. The milk is at a lower pH than the plasma, so drugs that are weak bases can reach higher concentrations in the milk than can weak acids.

Although a pharmacological effect is seldom obtained in the fetus from drugs given to the mother for a short time, this is not necessarily true in long-term administration. There have been no reported cases of problems arising in the neonate with any of the commonly used anaesthetics or analgesics. Diazepam is an exception, possibly due to its very long elimination half-life. On balance it is not considered essential that the mother be deprived of adequate postoperative analgesia for the sake of the breast-feeding infant.

TERATOGENIC EFFECTS OF ANAESTHESIA

Drugs taken by the mother during pregnancy can affect the fetus in many different ways. During the first weeks after conception and before implantation, drugs and other environmental factors are more likely to have a lethal effect on the embryo than to cause developmental abnormality. The differentiation of embryonic cells into organs occurs from the second to the 10th week of fetal life. It is during this period of organogenesis that drugs can produce lasting developmental abnormalities in the fetus. However, even at this stage it seems more likely that the effect of drugs would be to cause fetal death and spontaneous abortion.

By the end of the first trimester the fetus has completed organ differentiation, and congenital malformations can no longer be caused by drugs. However, fetal death is still likely to occur and the likelihood of drugs causing spontaneous abortion in the second trimester seems great. During the second trimester it is also possible that drugs can cause fetal morbidity, such as the cerebral damage seen with warfarin.

Although the mechanisms by which teratogenic damage occurs are not understood, it seems essential for the drug to cross the placenta (Beeley 1981). All drugs that have their effect on the mother's CNS also cross the placenta and are thus treated with suspicion in early pregnancy.

It seems clear that fetal malformation must be caused by several factors. Thalidomide, for instance, only caused congenital abnormalities in a quarter of the fetuses exposed to it at the same stage of development. Naturally occurring malformations are seen in cytogenetically normal fetuses, as well as abnormal ones. Possibly some fetuses are more likely to exhibit teratogenic effects than others. Environmental factors may also play a part.

Investigating the teratogenic side effects of drugs is problematic as considerable species differences exist and drugs safe in animals are not necessarily so in man. However, when a new drug has powerful teratogenic effects on several different animal species it is assumed not to be safe for human use. Epidemiological studies in man seem to be the only way of attempting to investigate these side effects. However, very large numbers are required in prospective studies as all retrospective studies are unreliable. The collaborative perinatal project (Heinonen et al 1977) which studied over 50 000 pregnancies found no drug with the teratogenic potency of thalidomide. The number of congenital malformations has not increased in 20 years in the USA, despite the greatly increased use of drugs by pregnant women.

Some drugs are certainly teratogenic and, other than thalidomide, all cytotoxic drugs are known to cause a wide range of malformations. Many drugs, such as alcohol, phenytoin, warfarin, lithium and quinine are suspected of a lower grade of teratogenesis. Other drugs cannot be cleared of suspicion but are not definitely implicated. These include barbiturates, phenothiazines, diazepam, diphenhydramine (Benylin), Debendox and chronic low doses of inhalation anaesthetic agents, especially nitrous oxide (see Ch. 30).

Studies carried out in women working in operating theatres have been reviewed by Vessey & Nunn (1980). They concluded that there was some evidence for a rise in the spontaneous abortion rates for these women, but not in the rate of congenital abnormality. Scavenging systems have been widely introduced into operating theatres to eliminate this possible danger. Also, women undergoing anaesthetics in the first trimester of pregnancy appear to have a higher rate of spontaneous abortion, but not a greater incidence of congenital abnormality (Heinonen et al 1977). No anaesthetic drugs, other than nitrous oxide, have been implicated in causing congenital malformations.

Many factors may be involved in the increased fetal death rate associated with anaesthesia, such as diminished uteroplacental blood flow, anoxia, hypercarbia, hyperpyrexia, acidosis, and fluid and electrolyte imbalance, all of which at a critical level could cause fetal death. Direct trauma to the uterus, placenta or the fetus itself may occur during abdominal surgery. Anaesthetic drugs crossing the placental barrier may cause similar or exaggerated effects on fetal physiology, such as a reduction in fetal cardiac output resulting in inadequate perfusion of the fetal tissues, and so death.

Because the fetus is at its most vulnerable in the first trimester of pregnancy, often before its presence is known, it is advisable that all drugs given to women of childbearing age who could become pregnant are used with caution. No drug should be given to the mother in the first trimester unless it is essential. Whenever possible, all anaesthetics should be avoided in the first trimester.

New drugs that are of necessity untested for human teratogenicity should not be used. It is unwise to give a mother in early pregnancy untested drugs, such as new sedatives or H_2 antagonists, when the survival of the fetus is planned, even though the mother may derive some benefit from the use. All operating theatres and labour wards should have scavenging systems for the benefit of the staff. It is also possible that drug allergy or idiosyncratic effects may occur in the fetus and not in the mother.

CONCLUSIONS

The widespread and profound changes that occur in almost every organ system of the body during pregnancy seem likely to increase the hazards of anaesthesia. It is incorrect to assume that the preoperative healthy pregnant patient is no different from the same woman prior to pregnancy. Thus the ASA scoring (American Society of Anesthesiologists physical scoring system) is not applicable to pregnant patients.

As well as the physiological changes that increase the mother's anaesthetic risks in pregnancy, she is also likely to suffer anaesthetic hazards specific to her pregnancy, such as occur in pre-eclampsia with its extensive organ system involvement. Certain hazards are more likely to occur with anaesthesia in pregnancy, such as thromboembolism, haemorrhage and possibly more difficult endotracheal intubation. The exact time interval between delivery and the mother's return to her previous anaesthetic risk state is not known with certainty, but is more likely to be weeks than days.

REFERENCES

Atlay R D, Gillison E W, Horton A L 1973 A fresh look at pregnancy heartburn. J Obstet Gynaecol Br Commonw 80: 63–66

Baraka A, Steir S 1980 Anaphylactic cardiac arrest in a parturient. J Am Med Assoc 243(17): 1745–1746

Beeley L 1981 Adverse effects of drugs in the first trimester of pregnancy. Clin Obstet Gynecol 8(2): 261–274

Bond U K, Stoeling R K, Gupta C D 1979 Pulmonary aspiration syndrome after inhalation of gastric fluid containing antacids. Anesthesiology 51: 452–453

Boobis A P, Lewis P J 1983 Pharmacokinetics in pregnancy. In: Lewis P J (ed) Clinical pharmacology in obstetrics. Wright, Bristol, ch 4, pp 10–13

Brock-Utne J G, Rubin J, Welman S et al 1978 The action of commonly used antiemetics on the lower oesophageal sphincter. Br J Anaesth 50: 295–298

Castro L P 1967 Reflex oesophagitis as the cause of heartburn in pregnancy. Am J Obstet Gynecol 98: 1–10

Cotton B R, Smith G 1984 The lower oesophageal sphincter and anaesthesia. Br J Anaesth 56: 37–45

Crawford J S, Rudofsky S 1966 Some alteration in the pattern of drug metabolism associated with pregnancy. Br J Anaesth 38: 446–448

Cummings A J 1983 A survey of pharmocokinetic data from pregnant women. Clin Pharmacokinet 8: 344–354

Davison J M 1987 Kidney function in pregnant women. Am J Kidney Dis Apr 9(4): 248–252 (12 ref)

Davison J M, Vallotton M B, Lindheimer M D 1981 Plasma osmolality and urinary concentration and dilution during and after pregnancy. Br J Obstet Gynaecol 88: 472–479

de Swiet M 1980 The cardiovascular system. In: Hytten F, Chamberlain G (eds) Clinical physiology in obstetrics. Blackwell, London, ch 1, pp 6–9

DHSS 1989 Report on Health and Social Subjects: report on confidential enquiries into maternal deaths in England and Wales 1982–1984. HMSO, London, p 7

Dick W E, Ahnefeld F, Milewski P, Schoch G 1977 Important clinical adaptation processes of women during pregnancy. Anesthesiologic considerations. J Perinat Med 5: 103–113

Easterling T R, Watts D, Schmucker B C, Benedetti T J 1987 Measurement of cardiac output during pregnancy: validation of doppler technique and clinical observations in pre-eclampsia. Obstet Gynecol 69: 845–850

Edmonds D K, Lindsay K S, Miller J F, Williamson E, Wood P J 1982 Early embryonic mortality in women. Fertil Steril 38: 447–53

Fishburne I 1979 Physiology and disease of the respiratory system in pregnancy: a review. J Reprod Med 22(4): 177–189

Frame W T, Allison R H, Moir D D, Nimmo W S 1984 Effect of naloxone on gastric emptying during labour. Br J Anaesth 56: 263–265

Gibbs C G, Schwartz D J, Wynne J W et al 1979 Antacid pulmonary aspiration in the dog. Anesthesiology 51: 380–385

Gilroy R J, Mangura A B T, Lavietes M H 1988 Rib cage and abdominal volume displacements during breathing in pregnancy. Am Rev Respir Dis 137: 668–672

Heinonen O P, Slone D, Shapiro S 1977 In: Birth defects and drugs in pregnancy. Publishing Sciences Group, Littleton, Mass., ch 26, p 357

Hirai N, Yanaihara T, Nakayama T, Ishibashi M, Yamaji T 1988 Plasma levels of atrial natriuretic peptide during normal pregnancy and in pregnancy complicated by hypertension. Am J Obstet Gynecol 159: 27–31

Holdsworth J D 1978 Relationship between stomach contents and analgesia in labour. Br J Anaesth 50: 1145–1148

Hurley R 1982 Infections in pregnancy. In: Oxford textbook of medicine. Oxford University Press, London, ch 5, pp 484–486
Hytten F E 1980 Nutrition. In: Hytten F E, Chamberlain G (eds) Clinical physiology in obstetrics, ch 6, pp 176–178
Hytten F E, Paintin D B 1963 Increase in plasma volume during normal pregnancy. J Obstet Gynaecol Br Commonw 70: 402–406
Hytten F E, Lind T 1973 Diagnostic indices in pregnancy. Documenta Geigy 19–61
Kerr M G, Scott D B, Samuel E 1964 Studies of the inferior vena cava in late pregnancy. Br Med J 1: 532–533
Kraner B, Kraner F 1977 Drug kinetics in pregnancy. Clin Pharmacokinet 2: 167–181
Lawson M, Kern J, Everson G T 1985 Gastro-intestinal transit time in human pregnancy: prolongation in the second and third trimester followed by postpartum normalization. Gastroenterology 89: 996–999
Lind J F, Smith A M, McIver D K, Cooplan A T, Crispin J S 1968 Heartburn in pregnancy: a manometric study. Can Med Assoc J 98: 571–574
Lindheimer M D, Katz A 1989 The kidney and hypertension during pregnancy. In: Benner B M, Rector J C (eds) The kidney. W B Saunders, Philadelphia
Lucius H, Gahlenbeck H, Kleine H O, Fabel H, Bartles H 1970 Respiratory functions, buffer system and electrolyte concentrations of blood during human pregnancy. Respir Physiol 9: 311–317
Lund N 1980 Anaphylactic reaction to infusion of polygelatin (Haemacel). Anaesthesia 35: 655–659
Marsh R H K, Spencer R, Nimmo W 1984 Gastric emptying and drug absorption before surgery. Br J Anaesth 56: 161–164
Morgan M 1984 Control of intragastric pH and volume. Br J Anaesth 56: 47–57
Morgan D, Moore G, Thomas J, Triggs E 1978 Disposition of meperidine in pregnancy. Clin Pharmacol Ther 23: 288–295
Morishima H O, Pedersen H, Finster M, Hiraoka H, Tsuji A, Feldman H S, Arthur G R, Covino B G 1985 Bupivicaine toxicity in pregnant and nonpregnant ewes. Anesthesiology 63: 134–139
Nimmo W S 1978 The measurement of gastric emptying during labour. J Int Med Res 6: 52–53
Nimmo W S, Wilson J, Prescott I F 1975 Narcotic analgesics and delayed gastric emptying during labour. Lancet 1: 890–893
O'Sullivan G M, Bullingham R E S 1984 The assessment of gastric acidity and antacid effect in pregnant women by a non-invasive radiotelemetry technique. Br J Obstet Gynaecol 91: 973–978
O'Sullivan G M, Sutton A J, Thompson S A, Carrie L E 1987 Non-invasive measurement of gastric emptying in obstetric patients. Anesth Analg 66: 505–511
Pernoll M L, Metcalfe J, Kovach P A, Wachtel R, Dunham M J 1975 Ventilation during rest and exercise in pregnancy and postpartum. Respir Physiol 25: 295–310
Reynolds F 1989 Placental transfer of drugs used by anaesthetists. In: L Kaufman (ed) Anaesthesia review 6. Churchill Livingstone, London, pp 151–183
Roberts R B, Shirley M A 1974 Reducing the risk of acid aspiration during caesarean section. Anesth Analg 53: 859–868
Robson S C, Hunter S, Boys R J, Dunlop W 1989 Serial study of factors influencing changes in cardiac output during human pregnancy. Am J Physiol 2256 (P+2) 1060–1065
Santos A C, Pedersen H, Harmon T W, Morishima H O, Fiuster M, Arthur R, Covino B G 1989 Does pregnancy alter the systemic toxicity of local anesthetics? Anesthesiology 70: 991–995
Saunders P, Milton P J D 1973 Laparotomy during pregnancy: an assessment of diagnostic accuracy and fetal wastage. Br Med J 3: 165–167
Schrier R W, Durr J A 1987 Pregnancy: an overfill or underfill state. Am J Kidney Dis 9(4): 284–289
Shankar K B, Moseley H, Kumar Y, Verrula V 1986 Arterial to end tidal carbon dioxide tension difference during Caesarean section anaesthesia. Anaesthesia 41: 698–702
Shnider S M, Webster G M 1965 Maternal and fetal hazards of surgery during pregnancy. Am J Obstet Gynecol 92(7): 891–900
Simpson K H, Stakes A F, Miller M 1988 Pregnancy delays paracetamol absorption and gastric emptying in patients undergoing surgery. Br J Anaesth 60: 24–27
Smith B E 1963 Fetal prognosis after anesthesia. Anesth Analg Curr Res 45(5): 521–526
Van Thiel D H, Gavaler J S, Stremple J 1976 Lower oesophageal sphincter pressure in women using sequential oral contraceptives. Gastroenterology 71: 232–234
Vessey M P, Nunn J F 1980 Occupational hazards of anaesthesia. Br Med J 281: 696–698
Weinberger S E, Weiss S T, Cohen W R, Weiss J W, Johnson T S 1980 Pregnancy and the lung. Am Rev Respir Dis 121: 559–81
Whittaker P G, Taylor A, Lind T 1983 Unsuspected pregnancy loss in healthy women. Lancet 1: 1126–1127
Wichman K, Ryden G 1986 Blood pressure and renal function during normal pregnancy. Acta Obstet Gynecol Scand 65: 561–566
Wilcox A J, Weinberg C R, O'Connor J F et al 1988 Incidence of early loss of pregnancy. N Engl J Med 319: 189–194

12

Safety of anaesthesia in childhood

Cindy S. T. Aun

INTRODUCTION

The concepts of paediatric anaesthesia are basically no different from those that apply to adult anaesthesia. However, differences in anatomy, physiology, psychology, biochemistry, and pharmacology, that are at their greatest in the neonatal period, have a significant impact on the practice and safety of paediatric anaesthesia. Safety of anaesthesia in this group of patients depends, in essence, on understanding these differences.

A report by Graff et al (1964) implicated anaesthesia as contributing to 17% of paediatric deaths in the perioperative period. The actual anaesthetic mortality rate was 3.3 per 10 000 operations, which was five times greater than that for young adults. Recently, Tiret et al (1988) reported in his prospective series of 40 240 anaesthetics in children, there was only one death. Despite this reduction in mortality, the incidence of life-threatening complications, including cardiac arrest, had not improved during the intervening 25 years (Lancet editorial 1988). The complication rate as reported by Tiret et al (1986, 1988) is significantly higher in infants (4.3 per 1000) than in older children (0.5 per 1000) and adults (1.5 per 1000).

Paediatric anaesthesia is best managed in specialized centres, where staff are specially trained in handling small children. It is only by constant experience and training that complications are minimized (British Medical Journal 1978). However, the report by the Specialty Committee in Paediatric Anaesthesia of the Association of Anaesthetists of Great Britain and Ireland in 1978 showed that the vast majority of children, including almost half of all neonates, were anaesthetized outside specialist centres (Hatch 1984). Most paediatric cases are managed by anaesthetists who anaesthetize children only from time to time, the frequency being dependent on the individual's programme and practice.

The risks of anaesthesia are highest in neonates and decrease with age. Associated complications, such as prematurity and the presence of complex congenital abnormalities, further increase these hazards. The first 28 days of extrauterine life are generally considered to be the neonatal period. By the end of this period, most of the physiological systems in normal full-term infants are reasonably mature, but it may take a relatively longer time in those with a low postconceptual age. Such high-risk cases should be referred to a specialized paediatric centre (Lancet editorial 1987).

This chapter is concerned with the hazards associated with common paediatric anaesthesia, but it would not be complete without discussing the problems of neonatal anaesthesia. The chapter is divided into three parts. The first highlights the anatomical and physiological features peculiar to children which predispose them to greater anaesthetic risk. The second part covers practical anaesthesia, and the last presents some problems that are of particular concern to the anaesthetist.

ANATOMICAL AND PHYSIOLOGICAL FEATURES PECULIAR TO CHILDHOOD

Respiratory system

Various anatomical differences make the maintenance of the airway and intubation more difficult in infants than in adults. The combination of small nares, a relatively large tongue, a small mandible and a short neck increases an infant's susceptibility to airway obstruction. The vocal cords are in a more cephalad position than in the adult (C_4 vs. C_6), and the epiglottis, which lies at a 45° angle to the vocal cords, is long, narrow and U-shaped. Visualization of the larynx can be difficult, and a straight-bladed laryngoscope is frequently required to lift the epiglottis during intubation.

Unlike the adult, the narrowest part of the upper airway is at the cricoid ring, so an endotracheal tube that passes easily through the glottis may wedge here. The trachea is relatively short (approximately 4 cm in a full-term infant), and there is the hazard of bronchial intubation if the endotracheal tube is inserted too far.

The respiratory function at birth is immature, since the alveoli are incompletely developed in number and structure, and the surface area for gas exchange is relatively small. Oxygen consumption in the newborn at the neutral environmental temperature is 7 ml/kg, which is twice that of an adult. This is mainly achieved by an increased respiratory rate (30–40 breaths/min), leading to a higher dead space ventilation per minute. While the energy of normal breathing is adequately supplied, increased airway resistance or pulmonary stiffness may significantly increase the work of breathing. Small infants, therefore, easily get exhausted when allowed to breathe spontaneously through a breathing system during anaesthesia.

The breathing in neonates is primarily diaphragmatic because of immature intercostal muscles, and a very compliant chest wall with the cartilaginous ribs being placed horizontally. This mechanical disadvantage in infants increases their susceptibility to ventilatory impairment. Stomach distension, which may occur during mask ventilation, should be relieved by passing a tube into the stomach once the child is anaesthetized.

The increased tendency towards small airway closure and diminished functional residual capacity (FRC) are related to the low outward recoil of the chest wall. These factors predispose the infant to intrapulmonary shunting and hypoxia. The ventilation-to-perfusion ratio is low and the venous admixture is three-fold that of an adult (Hatch & Sumner 1986a).

Periodic breathing, defined as three or more periods of apnoea lasting 3–15 s separated by less than 20 s, or frank apnoea of 15 s or longer, are commonly observed in preterm (< 37 weeks gestational age) and ex-preterm infants (Lerman 1988). It has been suggested that immature respiratory control is responsible. Life-threatening apnoea has been reported during the postoperative period in this group of patients (Steward 1982, Liu et al 1983). Contributory factors included residual anaesthesia, hypothermia, hypoglycaemia, hypocalcaemia, reduction in functional residual capacity and airway obstruction. However, postoperative apnoea cannot be reliably predicted from the history. It is suggested, therefore, that all preterm and expreterm infants up to 60 weeks postconceptual age should be monitored for at least 12 hours postoperatively, or until 12 hours free of apnoea, whichever is the longest (Lerman 1988).

Cardiovascular system

The change from a fetal pattern of circulation to that of an adult is normally accomplished by the anatomical closure of the foramen ovale and ductus arteriosus. This occurs at about 2–3 weeks after birth, although patency may still be observed in some older children. The damaging triad of hypoxia, hypercarbia and acidosis elevates pulmonary vascular resistance and may reopen the shunt which promotes right-to-left shunting of desaturated blood.

The stroke volume in the newborn is relatively fixed and cardiac output is mainly dependent on the heart rate, which is normally faster than in the adult, ranging from 100 to 160 beats/min. Therefore, bradycardia should be rectified promptly and atropine for intravenous administration must always be ready during anaesthesia. Neonates, infants, and children in general have a greater response to vagal stimulation, and the bradycardia observed following suxamethonium and halothane, laryngoscopy, or traction on the lateral and medial rectus, is more severe than that in adults. The normal paediatric blood pressure gradually increases with age, but is usually 100 mmHg or less.

Blood

Blood volume is estimated as 100 ml/kg in the premature infant, 80 ml/kg at full term, 75 ml/kg at 2 years and 60–65 ml/kg in the adolescent and adult. The haemoglobin (Hb) concentration at birth is 16–18 g/dl, of which about 80% is HbF. It declines to 10–11 g/dl at the age of 3 months and rises to a level of 12–14 g/dl at around 1-year old. HbF also gradually decreases and is replaced by HbA during the 3 months after birth. Anaemia (Hb < 10 g/dl) compromises the oxygen-carrying capacity of the blood while polycythaemia (haematocrit > 65%) in the newborn may increase the risk of infarction of the vital organs. The HbS concentration increases after birth at the same rate as HbA, and the normal sickle-cell screening test for detecting HbS may not be positive until 3–4 months of age, whereas electrophoretic analysis is accurate at all ages (Hall 1988).

Fluid balance

The size of each fluid compartment in the body changes with age. The total body water in the newborn is approximately 75% of body weight, which is proportionately larger than that of the adult (60%). This is principally a function of a relatively larger extracellular fluid compartment. The distribution of body water begins to approach that of the adult by about 1 year (Fig. 12.1; Bush 1971).

The renal function at birth is immature with an obligatory loss of salt. A limited ability to excrete or conserve water causes the neonate to be intolerant of both fluid overload and dehydration. Functionally, the kidneys are fully developed by about a year old, but infants are less able to deal with fluid restriction, because of their larger body surface to weight ratio and water turnover as a result of their high metabolic rate.

The formulae for determining the daily maintenance fluid requirements for hospitalized paediatric patients, based on body weight as suggested by Holliday & Segar (1957), are usually used. They showed that the total body water losses, which are a function of energy expenditure, are related to body weight (Table 12.1). Infants in the first few days have a reduced

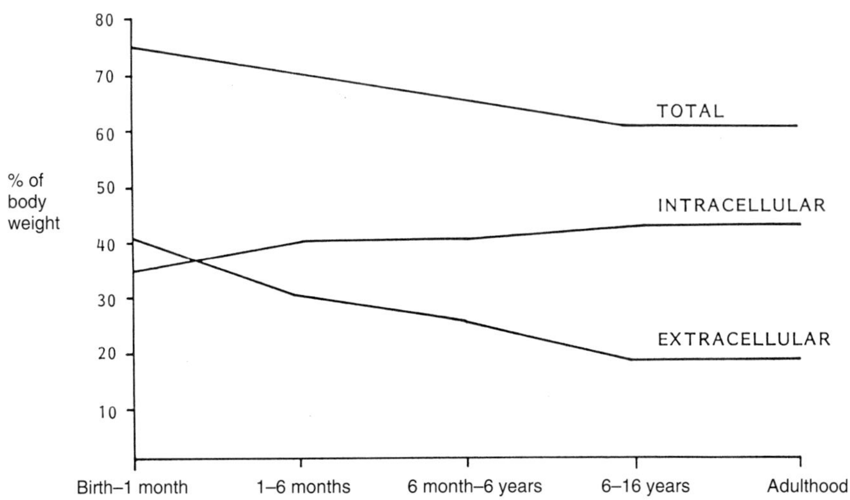

Fig. 12.1 Distribution of total, intracellular and extracellular water, expressed as a percentage of body weight related to age (from Bush 1971).

Table 12.1 Daily maintenance requirements of fluid in normal paediatric patients

Body weight	Calorific requirement	Fluid requirement
< 10 kg	100 cal/kg	100 ml/kg
10–20 kg	1000 cal plus 50 cal/kg of body weight over 10 kg	1000 ml plus 50 ml/kg of body weight over 10 kg
> 20 kg	1500 cal plus 20 cal/kg of body weight over 20 kg	1500 ml plus 20 ml/kg of body weight over 20 kg

Table 12.2 Daily maintenance requirements of electrolytes in normal paediatric patients

Electrolyte	Requirement (mmol/kg)
Sodium	3
Potassium	2
Chloride	2

water requirement, and the estimated volume should be scaled down accordingly. Hatch & Sumner (1986b) recommend 20–40 ml/kg/24 hours the first day. This is increased by 20 ml/kg/24 hours daily until the requirements reach 120 ml/kg/24 hours towards the end of the first week. Holliday & Segar's (1957) formulae can then be followed. Maintenance requirements for electrolytes are shown in Table 12.2.

Fluid therapy remains a difficult area because of the great interpatient variability in response to surgery and the disease process. The guidelines and formulae can at best only be a rough guideline, and fluid administration should be titrated against the patient's physiological status and his response to fluid.

Metabolic adaptation

The metabolic rate and energy production in children is approximately twice that of the adult, and while the carbohydrate reserves of the normal newborn are relatively low (about 11 g/kg body weight), they are even lower in premature infants. These children are therefore prone to hypoglycaemia if fasted before anaesthesia, or if there is a drop in body temperature. Hypoglycaemia is defined as 1.6 mmol/l in the term newborn and 2.2 mmol/l in those more than 3 days old.

Temperature regulation

In small infants there is an increased vulnerability to heat loss because the thermoregulatory mechanism is immature, the surface area to weight ratio is large, there is poor cutaneous vasomotor control and they are deficient in insulating subcutaneous fatty tissue. The ability to shiver in response to cold is not yet developed, so the main thermoregulatory mechanism is by means of non-shivering thermogenesis (NST). Cold exposure causes the release of noradrenaline at sympathetic nerve-endings. This stimulates heat production in the brown fat which is abundant in this age group, but this is at the expense of increased oxygen consumption. The ideal environment is a neutral thermal environment in which oxygen consumption is at its least. This can be provided by using an incubator or overhead heating devices, an increased operating theatre temperature and protective coverings. The neutral temperature range is 33–36°C for the naked newborn baby, depending on its maturity, and it is lowered with increasing age and size. The metabolic response to cold is inhibited by hypoxia, hypoglycaemia and general anaesthesia.

Psychological factor

Children vary in their responses to hospitalization and associated treatment depending on their age and maturity. The psychological effects from fears of separation from the parents, pain, being awake during operation, and even mutilation and death can make the children very difficult to deal with during the perioperative period. Sympathy, understanding and patience are the prerequisites in handling these situations. The presence of a parent during events such as induction and recovery is helpful. Psychological preparation of the patient and parents by using video programmes, pictures and interviews have also been used successfully.

Pharmacological response

The development and change of many physiological functions during childhood have contributed to the differences in pharmacokinetics and pharmacodynamics observed in paediatrics. A larger volume of distribution, related to the total and extracellular fluid to weight ratio in children, influences the effective dose. The alteration and competition of plasma-protein binding with other drugs and body products may have undesirable effects, such as kernicterus. The immature blood–brain barrier which exhibits increased permeability may contribute to the increased sensitivity to sedative and hypnotic drugs. The immature enzyme activity and excretory function may produce a prolonged duration of action and toxicity from delayed metabolism.

The uptake of inhalational agents in infants is more rapid than in adults. This is related to the differences between infants and adults in their blood gas solubility, body composition, alveolar ventilation and the distribution of cardiac output. The minimum alveolar concentration (MAC) for inhalational anaesthetic agents are inversely related to age. The incidence of bradycardia and hypotension during induction of anaesthesia is greater in infants than in adults (Friesen & Lichtor 1982, 1983).

There is an increased sensitivity to a variety of sedative and hypnotic drugs in neonates and their elimination half-life is longer. Agents such as opioids, benzodiazepines and barbiturates, should therefore be used with care in infants.

The volume of distribution for neuromuscular agents in infants is larger than that in children and adults. When allowance is made for these differences, infants appear relatively resistant to suxamethonium and relatively sensitive to non-depolarizing relaxants (Cook 1987). Goudsouzian et al (1975), from their evaluation of dose–response of tubocurarine in children, suggested that the response to non-depolarizing relaxants is unpredictable and the dose should be titrated against the response.

Recently, there has been concern about the high incidence of masseter spasm following the combination of suxamethonium and halothane anaesthesia in the paediatric population (Carroll 1987).

Drug dosage is normally calculated according to body weight, although it might be more accurate to base it on body surface area. The paediatric dosage of some commonly used drugs in anaesthesia is shown in Table 12.3. Monitoring of drug response either clinically or preferably using objective methods (e.g. a peripheral nerve stimulator) may be used to determine the appropriate dose. It is necessary to be vigilant to diagnose and treat any abnormal responses to anaesthetic

Table 12.3 Dosages of common drugs used in anaesthesia

Drug	Dosage
Premedication	
Atropine	0.02 mg/kg i.m. 30 min before operation (or) i.v. at induction (maximum 0.6 mg)
Morphine	0.05–0.20 mg/kg i.m. 1 hour before operation (maximum 10 mg)
Pethidine	1 mg/kg i.m. 1 hour before operation
Diazepam	0.2–0.5 mg/kg p.o. 1–2 hours before operation (maximum 15 mg)
Trimeprazine tartrate	2–4 mg/kg p.o. 1–2 hours before operation
Induction	
Thiopentone	4–5 mg/kg
Methohexitone	1–2 mg/kg
Ketamine	2 mg/kg i.v. 10 mg/kg i.m.
Analgesics i.v.	
Fentanyl	0.001–0.003 mg/kg i.v.
Morphine	0.1 mg/kg
Neuromuscular blocking agents	
Suxamethonium	1.0–1.5 mg/kg i.v.
Atracurium	0.5 mg/kg i.v.
Alcuronium	0.3 mg/kg
Tubocurarine	Premature 0.125 mg/kg Neonate 0.25 mg/kg >2 months 0.5 mg/kg
Pancuronium	0.05–0.10 mg/kg
Vecuronium	0.1 mg/kg (for incremental doses: ⅓–½ of initial dose)
Reversal	
Neostigmine	0.05 mg/kg
Atropine	0.02 mg/kg
Naloxone	0.005 mg/kg i.v. or i.m.
Postoperative analgesics	
Morphine	0.2 mg/kg i.m.
Pethidine	1 mg/kg i.m.
Codeine phosphate	1.0–1.5 mg/kg i.m. 4-hourly (maximum 60 mg)

agents, such as those associated with hereditary conditions which include pseudocholinesterase deficiency, myotonias and malignant hyperpyrexia.

PREOPERATIVE ASSESSMENT AND PREPARATION

Psychological preparation of the paediatric patient for surgery needs skill, experience and patience. Most children can usually be handled by direct, friendly discussion and simple explanation if they are able to communicate, but for those who cannot, a sedative may be required. Optimal sedation reduces anxiety and promotes cooperation of the patient without undue depression of his physiological function. However, preoperative sedation is normally avoided in children younger than 1 year and those with potential airway problems. Atropine or glycopyrrolate is recommended to attenuate the vagal reflex and to reduce the salivary secretions.

Unlike in the adult, congenital abnormalities such as congenital cardiac disease (8 in 1000 births) (Hatch & Sumner 1986b), craniofacial malformation with upper airway problems and myopathies are the predominant concurrent pathology observed in the paediatric surgical patient. It may be necessary to consult reference texts regarding the lesions likely to be found in unfamiliar syndromes. The presence of a cardiac murmur of undetermined origin may require preliminary cardiological evaluation. The most hazardous cardiac lesions are those with balanced shunts, such as Fallot's tetralogy, because any changes in systemic or pulmonary vascular resistance may disturb the haemodynamics and lower the arterial saturation drastically.

The decision to anaesthetize a patient who has an upper respiratory tract infection (URTI) for elective surgery is still a dilemma (Fennelly & Hall 1990). However, in view of the fact that there is an increased risk of respiratory complications during the perioperative period, it is advisable to postpone all cold surgery in a patient with an URTI (Lindahl 1985, Tait & Knight 1987, DeSoto et al 1988).

The duration of preoperative fasting is a balance between the requirements of glucose and fluids and the time needed to ensure that the 'stomach is empty' in order to reduce the risk of aspiration pneumonia. Recent reports (Splinter 1989, Schreiner 1990) have shown that there is no difference in gastric residual volume or pH between those who fasted for 8 hours or more versus those who drank clear liquids up to 2–3 hours before surgery. Furthermore surveys (Olsson 1986, Tiret 1986) have found that the incidence of aspiration pneumonia in healthy paediatric patients for elective surgery is very low. Although reports have shown that children are able to maintain their preoperative blood glucose level within the normal range after a reasonable period of fasting (Nilsson 1984, Aun 1990), prolonged fasting may result in hypoglycaemia and sometimes hypovolaemia (Cote 1990). Hence there is a dramatic change in the current views on the preoperative fasting regimen in children. Recent guidelines allow the children to take clear glucose fluid orally up to 3 hours before surgery. So far there is no delineation on the quantities of fluid based on body weight. For small infants, the usual quantities of fluid that they normally take and in older children 10–20 ml appears reasonable (Berry 1991). However, one should remember that the patient may vomit and aspirate any time during anaesthesia and care should be taken to protect the airway. It is essential to recognize the presence of risk factors during assessment of the patient and to conduct the anaesthetic accordingly.

The age and body weight of the patient should be known so that the correct dosage of drugs is prescribed. The age and weight also provide a guideline for fluid therapy and choosing an appropriately sized endotracheal tube.

ANAESTHETIC EQUIPMENT

Paediatric anaesthetic equipment may not be readily available in hospitals where paediatric anaesthesia is not performed regularly, but it is essential, at least, that a set of paediatric equipment for anaesthesia and resuscitation is checked and available at all times.

Breathing systems

Adult breathing systems should not be used for

paediatric patients, because they are bulky, heavy, and likely to have too high a resistance and dead space. For infants less than 20 kg an Ayre's T-piece (Ayre 1937) with the Jackson–Rees modification (Rees 1950) is commonly used. The features of this system are simplicity, lightness, minimal dead space and low resistance. For those patients over 20 kg, adult breathing attachments are suitable.

The end-tidal CO_2 concentration depends on CO_2 production, respiration and the fresh gas flow (FGF) into the system. In paediatrics the determination of the required FGF in terms of multiples of the estimated minute ventilation is still controversial. Many formulae have been recommended (Nightingale et al 1965, Rose & Froese 1979, Hatch et al 1987), but the dynamic physiological states associated with the growing process and the considerable variation in CO_2 production in infants make gas exchange unpredictable, and end tidal CO_2 monitoring is the most reliable method for fine-tuning the FGF and ventilation (Badgwell et al 1988).

A fresh gas flow of 2–3 times the minute ventilation is required for patients breathing spontaneously (Willis et al 1975). For controlled ventilation, Nightingale (1965) recommended 220 ml/kg/min FGF with a minimum flow of 3 l/min, while Rose & Froese (1979) recommended (1000 + 100/kg) ml/min to obtain a $Paco_2$ of 4.9 kPa, and (1600 + 100/kg) ml/min for $Paco_2$ of 4.0 kPa, and Hatch et al (1987) suggested (1000 + 200/kg) ml/min for children less than 20 kg. The use of a scavenging system is not easy with the Ayre's T-piece, although Hatch et al (1980) have described a method for its use.

Laryngoscopes

Although the Macintosh curved blade can be used in most paediatric cases, it may be difficult in small infants. Straight-bladed laryngoscopes designed to lift the epiglottis should be available, the common ones being the Seward, Robertshaw, Miller and Wisconsin blades.

Connectors

Critical incidents can easily arise from incompatibility of connections in the breathing circuit. Connectors are available in many sizes and shapes and many of them are not interchangeable. It is desirable to standardize the connectors based on the ISO standard 15 mm connectors for children.

ANAESTHESIA

Induction and intubation

Intravenous induction in children can be difficult and traumatic. Skill in venipuncture and needles or cannulae of small gauge (24–27 gauge) are required. However, intravenous induction is not advisable in patients with potential airway obstruction.

Inhalational induction is commonly used in children. Halothane is usually preferred to enflurane or isoflurane because it is less irritating and gives a smoother induction. Even so, it may be difficult in the uncooperative patient, therefore handling should be gentle to maintain rapport. In addition to frightening the conscious child, a rapid increase in inspired concentration of the inhalational agent may cause respiratory tract irritation, coughing, breath holding and laryngospasm.

Larygospasm occurs frequently during the administration of anaesthesia and intubation in paediatric patients. The incidence of 17.4 in 1000 patients aged 0–9 years reported by Olsson & Hallen (1984) was almost twice that in the general population (8.7 per 1000 patients). Airway obstruction occurs readily during induction in children. This usually responds to forward lifting of the mandible and a positive airway pressure created by applying a gentle pressure on the reservoir bag. An oral airway may help when the pharyngeal reflex has disappeared.

Intubation in normal paediatrics is potentially difficult and hazardous. These hazards are increased in patients with congenital craniofacial anomalies, emergency anaesthesia, or when awake intubation is attempted in a vigorous neonate.

It is easier to traumatize the airway in children than in adults. A thin-walled non-cuffed endotracheal tube with a small leak round the tube when a positive pressure of 30 cm H_2O is applied should be used to prevent trauma to the subglottic mucosa. A cuffed tube is only needed in older children as they approach the age of puberty. The following formulae are commonly used for estimating the size and length of endotracheal tubes (see also p. 490):

$$\text{Internal diameter (mm)} = 4.5 + \frac{\text{age in years}}{4}$$

$$\text{Length of oral tube (cm)} = 12 + \frac{\text{age in years}}{2}$$

A 1-year-old child will take a 4.5 mm tube, while a 4.0 mm tube will be appropriate for 3–9-month-old children. The full-term neonate requires a 3.5 mm tube and the premature baby may need a 2.5–3.0 mm tube. However it is wise to prepare tubes larger and smaller than the calculated size as there is individual variation.

The tip of the endotracheal tube should be in the middle of the trachea, and the chest should be auscultated routinely after intubation. Fixation of the endotracheal tube should be carried out meticulously to avoid malposition and friction of the tube in the trachea which can cause a significant degree of trauma and oedema. This may result in significant narrowing of the upper airway. About 1 mm of mucosal oedema at the cricoid level can decrease the airway diameter by about 60% in a newborn infant (Hatch & Sumner 1986a), and a reduction of 50% in airway diameter will require a 32-fold increase of pressure and work to maintain respiration (Badgwell et al 1987b).

A difficult intubation should be anticipated in a patient with congenital abnormalities. Preparation should include a selection of endotracheal tubes, laryngoscope blades and introducers. It is important to secure an intravenous access before induction or, alternatively, skilled assistance will be required to help with the airway or the intravenous cannulation. Before administration of a muscle relaxant one must ensure that control of the airway and ventilation using an oropharyngeal airway and a mask is possible. Techniques such as blind intubation, fibre-optic intubation, cricothyroid membrane puncture and the catheter or guidewire railroad method have been suggested, but these require special expertise and may be difficult in small children.

In view of the potential difficulty in securing the airway in the neonate, awake intubation before the administration of anaesthesia was traditionally taught. However, recent research has shown that the newborn baby responds to noxious stimuli with similar hormonal, metabolic and cardiorespiratory changes as the adult (Anand & Hickey 1987). Awake intubation has been implicated as one of the factors responsible for perianaesthetic intracranial haemorrhage in preterm infants (Friesen et al 1987a, 1987b). Neonates are now treated like older children, and intubation is carried out under adequate anaesthesia and analgesia, with or without muscle relaxants, unless the airway is tenuous. However, securing the airway in the newborn infant can indeed be difficult at times and clinical judgement must be used.

Maintenance

It is preferable to use an endotracheal tube and controlled ventilation in small infants, except perhaps in very short procedures, because maintenance of airway and ventilation is usually more difficult than in adults. It has been reported that the occurrence of major hypoxic events is more common in children aged 2 years or under (Cote et al 1988), and that hypoxaemia is the main factor contributing to the higher incidence of intraoperative cardiac arrest observed in children compared to adults (Keenan & Boyan 1985). On the other hand, high arterial oxygen tension is considered to be one of the prime factors in the development of retinopathy of prematurity in preterm infants less than 44 weeks post conceptual age, especially in those with a body weight of 2 kg or less. It is therefore essential to monitor and maintain an optimum oxygen saturation (90–92%) using an oximeter during anaesthesia.

For prolonged procedures, blockage of the endotracheal tube by inspissated secretions and heat loss should be prevented by humidification of the inspired air using a heat exchanger or humidifier. These systems are not without their hazards, such as an increased dead space, potential for gas leaks, thermal injury of the airway and drowning of the lungs. Mobility and malposition of the head can displace the endotracheal tube, either by flicking the tube out of the glottis or by pushing the tube further in causing endobroncheal intubation.

Fluid and blood replacement

Intraoperative fluid therapy in children can be difficult and basically depends on three factors, namely the preoperative deficit, normal fluid maintenance and the extent of tissue trauma during the operation. The preoperative fluid deficit should be corrected before surgery. If not, this must be replaced during the procedure together with the maintenance and replacement of ongoing losses. One recommendation (Gregory 1986) is to give crystalloid, such as saline or Ringer's lactate solution to which enough glucose has been added (usually 4–6 mg/kg/min) to keep the blood glucose in the normal range. The solutions commonly used are 5% dextrose in Ringer's lactate, 5% dextrose in normal saline or 4.3% dextrose in 0.18% normal saline solution. These are administered at a rate to provide the normal requirement of sugar, and additional fluid requirements are replaced with glucose-free solutions to prevent a possible hyperosmolar state and osmotic diuresis. The recommended rate is:

1. For the first hour, a hydrating solution of 10–15 ml/kg/hour.
2. For the subsequent hours, calculate the basal requirement plus that needed because of the induced trauma:

Basal: 2–4 ml/kg/hour
Trauma: mild (e.g. craniotomy) 2 ml/kg/hour
moderate (e.g. thoracotomy) 4 ml/kg/hour
severe (e.g. abdominal surgery) 6 ml/kg/hour
Blood replacement as required with either crystalloid (3:1 volume) or blood.

If the patient has been receiving intravenous fluid and is adequately hydrated on arriving in the operating theatre, no hydrating solution is needed. Intake and output balance, and the patient's clinical status should be monitored at frequent intervals to titrate the fluid administration. Fluid for flushing and drug administration should be added to the fluid balance. A burette and an electronic infusion pump system to control the rate during infusion is desirable. Meticulous care is needed to avoid the entry of any air bubbles into the intravenous delivery system because, in the presence of a vascular shunt, even a small quantity of intravenous air may cause brain damage.

Because of the small total blood volume in children, an accurate measurement of blood loss is more critical than in adults. The usual methods include weighing sponges, use of calibrated suction bottles, inspection of the surgical field and monitoring vital signs. The requirement for blood replacement will depend on the clinical condition and type of operation.

Venous access may be difficult owing to the small size of peripheral veins, and the subcutaneous fat is a particular problem in infants between 1 and 12 months old. One may have to resort to the more invasive central-line cannulation if massive and prolonged infusion is anticipated.

Monitoring

The principles of monitoring in paediatric anaesthesia are the same as in adults, but require different methodologies due to the anatomical and physiological differences.

Monitoring of oxygen saturation using pulse oximetry is now considered essential during anaesthesia. The transitional fetal circulation in neonates must be considered in the placing of the probe. The probe on the right hand (preductal oxygen saturation) monitors oxygen delivery to the brain, whereas oxygenation of other vital organs, such as the kidneys, is best monitored postductally from the feet. It is generally felt that, in preterm infants, avoiding hyperoxia is as important as preventing hypoxia. However, pulse oximetry does not monitor hyperoxia and therefore should be supplemented by oxygen-tension measurement in these cases. Fetal haemoglobin shifts the haemoglobin oxygen dissociation curve to the left. This may cause difficulty in the interpretation of oximetry in the presence of large amounts of fetal haemoglobin. Despite these limitations in paediatric pactice, it is still the best continuous non-invasive monitor of oxygenation available.

End-tidal CO_2 monitoring is being increasingly used in anaesthesia as the end-tidal CO_2 concentration closely approximates arterial PCO_2 in health. The value of end-tidal CO_2 measurement has been highlighted in a recent study of 331 children, in which 35 life-threatening incidents (disconnection, extubation, malignant hyperpyrexia) were detected by end-tidal CO_2 monitors (Cote et al 1986). However there are problems in paediatric practice. 'Mainstream' and 'sidestream' are the two types of analyser used in capnography. In the 'mainstream' analyser the sensor (cuvette) is on-line in the patient's breathing system. Although paediatric versions are available, the cuvette weight and dead space can be quite significant. In the case of 'sidestream' analysers, however, dilution of the sampled gas with fresh gas flow can occur. With the Ayre's T-piece, which permits partial rebreathing, it is critical for accuracy to sample the gas for analysis from the distal end of the endotracheal tube (Badgwell et al 1987a, 1987c).

A precordial stethoscope, which is regarded as a hallmark of the paediatric anaesthetist, allows continuous monitoring of breath and heart sounds. When this is inconvenient an oesophageal stethoscope may be used. For this purpose a disposable catheter should be positioned in the lower third of the oesophagus.

To avoid barotrauma the airway pressure should be monitored during controlled ventilation.

Blood pressure may be inaccurate if an inappropriate size of cuff is used. The cuff should be placed accurately and the width should be one-half to two-thirds the length of the upper arm. If an invasive arterial line is employed for continuous pressure reading, a fine Teflon cannula, size 22 or 24, should be used. Care must be exercised to avoid flushing the line with excessive force and flow, as blood clots and air could be propelled retrogradely into the cerebral circulation. Central venous pressure can be monitored by the internal jugular route, as in adults, but it is easy to infuse large volumes of fluid too rapidly. The ECG should be monitored, as in adults.

Temperature monitoring is necessary for all paediatric patients. The useful sites for the probes are in the oesophagus and the rectum. Because of the danger of both hypoglycaemia and hyperglycaemia, perioperative and intraoperative monitoring of blood glucose is recommended, especially in major surgery involving small infants.

POSTOPERATIVE CARE

As in the adult, the adequacy of the airway is the most common cause for concern during the emergence from anaesthesia and the immediate postoperative period in children. Although it may be safe to extubate some adult patients while they are still deeply anaesthetized, it is safer to extubate children after awakening, especially in those with a full stomach, a potentially compromised airway, or minimal cardiopulmonary reserves. Laryngospasm may occur following extubation during light anaesthesia. Lee & Downes (1983) suggested that extubation laryngospasm can be reduced by extubating the child when fully awake. Intravenous lignocaine (2 mg/kg) 1 min before extubation in high-risk cases has been suggested (Baraka 1978), although its effectiveness is questionable. Laryngospasm can usually be relieved by applying gentle continuous positive airway pressure with 100% oxygen through a tight-fitting face mask. If not, intravenous atropine and suxamethonium, with or without reintubation of the trachea, can be employed.

Agitation during the postoperative period may be difficult to manage. Hypoxaemia, hypercarbia, increased intracranial pressure or other abnormality should be excluded. Postoperative pain is one of the important causes of agitation and has often been managed inadequately. This is particularly true in paediatrics because assessment of pain is not easy, especially in those with whom communication is difficult. There was also uncertainty about the safe dosage of opioids. However, much information about pain response and pharmacokinetics of analgesics in paediatrics is now available and an increasing range of pain relief techniques, including opioids by intravenous infusions, patient-controlled analgesia, and regional analgesia using either peripheral or central blocks (intrathecal or epidural), have now been extended to infants and children (Lloyd-Thomas 1990). However, these techniques should be closely supervised and monitored for the development of complications. Sometimes an agitated, fully awake child can only be comforted by a parent.

In the immediate postoperative period the aim is to stabilize the vital signs, and to avoid or correct fluid, electrolyte and acid-base derangement. Close monitoring of the clinical condition should be coupled with laboratory data in the management of postoperative fluid therapy in complicated cases. Prediction of the 'third space' losses requires experience and knowledge of the pathophysiology of the operation involved. For the relatively straightforward case, fluid therapy is primarily based on the maintenance requirement and the replacement of abnormal losses.

Preterm infants are at increased risk of apnoeic attacks following anaesthesia. They should not undergo surgical procedures as outpatients and should be closely monitored postoperatively for 24 hours (Liu et al 1983).

OTHER PROBLEMS

Hypothermia following surgery in small infants is a major hazard, therefore every precaution should be taken to prevent heat loss. The patient should be placed in an incubator or swaddled in polyurethane-lined aluminium foil wrapping during transport to and from the operating theatre. Increasing the temperature of the operating environment by elevating the temperature or using overhead heating devices is recommended.

Giving priority to paediatric patients on the operating list helps to prevent unnecessary delay which may cause dehydration or hypoglycaemia in susceptible patients.

Loose milk-teeth which can be inhaled during anaesthesia are a particular hazard at the time of the change over from the milk to the permanent dentition.

Regional anaesthesia is increasingly used in children, usually in combination with general anaesthesia, to provide postoperative analgesia. The differences in the anatomical development should be noted, and the maximum safe dose of the local anaesthetic agent that may be used should be calculated beforehand.

SITUATIONS WITH PARTICULAR ANAESTHETIC HAZARDS

Bleeding after tonsillectomy

Continuing haemorrhage may occur after routine tonsillectomy. Davies & Steward (1977) suggested that acetylsalicylic-acid-induced platelet dysfunction may cause unexpected excessive bleeding during tonsillectomy. Surgical intervention may be required to stop the bleeding. A number of factors have made this situation particularly hazardous: the patient may still be drowsy from the initial operation and very sensitive to anaesthetics; it is difficult to gauge the amount of blood loss; the patient may be hypovolaemic, hypotensive and hypoxic, and should be resuscitated with intravenous fluid and blood transfusion; there may be an associated clotting deficiency, so clotting factors or fresh blood should be considered; the airway may be obstructed, and its view obscured by the presence of blood and blood clot in the mouth and oropharynx; blood may accumulate in the stomach, and create a risk of aspiration and regurgitation during induction of anaesthesia. Induction of anaesthesia should be conducted in such a manner that will protect the airway from aspiration of blood and stomach contents. Either an inhalational induction and intubation without the use of muscle relaxant or a rapid-sequence intravenous induction with preoxygenation, application of cricoid pressure and suxamethonium administration for intubation have been recommended. However it is wise to choose a technique with which one is experienced. Attempting awake intubation in a frightened, struggling and bleeding child is usually unsatisfactory and dangerous.

Upper airway obstruction

Upper airway obstruction may present to the anaesthetist ranging from an urgent life-threatening obstruction to stridor in children for assessment. The common cases seen in non-specialist units are acute infective upper airway obstruction. The clinical picture of acute epiglottitis is characteristically life-threatening, and may change so rapidly that urgent anaesthesia and endotracheal intubation is required once the diagnosis is made. Acute airway obstruction can easily be precipitated by any preliminary disturbing manoeuvre and should be avoided at all cost. Intubation, although usually possible, can sometimes by extremely difficult. These cases should be intubated in the operating theatre where full facilities are available. For upper airway obstruction, inhalation of oxygen and halothane is the anaesthetic of choice. There is no place for muscle relaxants until the airway is secured, or when it is known that manual ventilation can be carried out. A variety of laryngoscope blades, a range of endotracheal tube sizes, and skilled assistance are essential. Also, otolaryngological surgical and nursing staff must be notified and a bronchoscope should be ready. A smaller proportion of cases with acute laryngotracheobronchitis need airway relief. This condition is less acute, but the same principles of airway management apply. Tracheostomy, which carries a high mortality in children, especially when the upper airway is severely obstructed, is rarely required.

Bronchoscopy

Bronchoscopy is required in children for the removal of inhaled foreign bodies and for the diagnosis of upper airway obstruction. Major hazards include hypoxia from the obstruction itself and difficulty in maintaining adequate ventilation during the procedure. Removal of a foreign body can be very difficult, depending on its nature and size. Fragmentation of vegetable objects may occur during removal, causing occlusion of the airway beyond the initial site of impaction. Multiple reinsertion of the bronchoscope may be required before the foreign body is successfully removed. This may cause trauma and mucosal oedema, with postoperative stridor and respiratory distress. Trauma is more severe and common with the inexperienced endoscopist. The Sanders jet injector is seldom used in infant bronchoscopy because of the potential complication of barotrauma. The rigid ventilating bronchoscope equipped with a fibre-optic telescope is most favoured by endoscopists. Assisted or spontaneous ventilation using an Ayre's T-piece attached to the sidearm of the bronchoscope is safer in children. Spontaneous ventilation with halothane and 100% oxygen is preferred, at least until the nature and location of the foreign body is known. Manual ventilation may dislodge the foreign body further into the lung. Ventilation is difficult during suction and insertion of the telescope. Muscle relaxants should not be used during the procedure, unless one is sure of the airway and ventilation. Cardiac dysrthymias may occur during light anaesthesia, especially associated with hypoventilation and hypoxia. Adequate preoperative fasting and intramuscular atropine premedication are essential. The maximum safe dose of lignocaine used for spraying the larynx is 4–5 mg/kg. Postoperatively the child should be closely monitored for airway obstruction. Laryngospasm may develop during emergence from light anaesthesia or due to the presence of blood and secretion in the airway. Bronchoscopy may precipitate complete respiratory obstruction in marginal cases by minimal oedema caused by the instrumentation. Dexamethasone, humidified O_2, and nebulized racemic adrenaline have been recommended for prophylaxis (Hatch & Sumner 1986c).

Change of endotracheal tube

An oral tube is normally used in emergencies and for anaesthesia. It is usually changed to a nasotracheal tube for prolonged respiratory support in the intensive care unit, because nasal tubes make nursing easier, and are more secure and comfortable for the patient. The changeover procedure may be hazardous, so skilled assistance and preparation of the necessary equipment is essential. The size of the nasal tube should be at least a size smaller than the oral tube. The change is carried out with the oral tube still in place, and with the assistant ventilating the patient, while the nasal tube is passed down the nares as far as the glottis. Using the laryngoscope, and with the help of the assistant, the oral tube is removed and the nasal tube inserted through the glottis. The length of the new tube should be carefully adjusted (usually about 2 cm longer than the oral tube). Air entry to both lungs should be confirmed and a chest X-ray taken.

Transport of sick infants

Transportation of a sick child from a general adult hospital to a regional paediatric intensive care unit (PICU) may be needed from time to time. The regional PICU will usually be able to advise or assist in the transfer. The staff involved must be experienced in paediatric resuscitation as the patient may deteriorate on the way. Intravenous access should be secured, a nasogastric tube passed if gastrointestinal obstruction is suspected so that aspiration can be carried out throughout the journey, and an endotracheal tube secured if the patient is in respiratory distress so that ventilation can be assisted on the way. The condition should be reasonably stabilized before transfer. All necessary drugs, equipment, compressed gases and battery power must be checked. Continuous monitoring of the cardiovascular system, temperature, blood-glucose level and respiratory support must be organized. There should be regular communication with the receiving centre so that personnel and equipment will be ready for the arrival.

SUMMARY

Most hazards in paediatric anaesthesia can be avoided by acquiring the knowledge, careful planning and meticulous attention to detail during anaesthesia. High-risk cases are better transferred to specialized paediatric centres. In the general hospitals, where a great proportion of paediatric cases are treated, it would be useful to have a small number of staff who are specially trained in paediatric anaesthesia.

REFERENCES

Anand K J S, Hickey P R 1987 Pain and its effects in the human neonates and fetus. N Engl J Med 317: 1321–1329

Aun C S T, Panesar N S 1990 Paediatric glucose homeostasis during anaesthesia. Br J Anaesth 64: 413–418

Ayre P 1937 Endotracheal anesthesia for babies: with special reference to hare lip and cleft palate operation. Anesth Analg 16: 330–333

Badgwell J M, Heavner J E, May W S, Goldthorn J F, Lerman J 1987a End-tidal P_{CO_2} monitoring in infants and children ventilated with either a partial rebreathing or a non-rebreathing circuit. Anesthesiology 66: 405–410

Badgwell J M, McLeod M E, Friedberg J 1987b Airway obstruction in infants and children. Can J Anaesth 34: 90–98

Badgwell J M, McLeod M E, Lerman J, Creighton R E 1987c End-tidal P_{CO_2} measurements sampled at the distal and proximal ends of the endotracheal tube in infants and children. Anesth Analg 66: 959–964

Badgwell J M, Wolf A R, McEvedy B A B, Lerman J, Creighton R E 1988 Fresh gas formulae do not accurately predict end-tidal P_{CO_2} in paediatric patients. Can J Anaesth 35: 581–586

Baraka A 1978 Intravenous lidocaine controls extubation laryngospasm in children. Anesth Analg 57: 506–507.

Berry F A 1991 Preoperative fasting. Curr Opin Anaesthesiol 4: 359–362

British Medical Journal Leading Article 1978 Paediatric anaesthesia. Br Med J 2: 717

Bush G H 1971 Intravenous fluid therapy in paediatrics. Ann R Coll Surg Engl 49: 92–101

Carroll J B 1987 Increased incidence of masseter spasm in children with strabismus anaesthetized with halothane and succinylcholine. Anesthesiology 67: 559–561

Cook D R 1987 Pharmacology of pediatric anesthesia. In: Katz J, Steward D J (eds) Anesthesia and uncommon pediatric diseases. Saunders, Philadelphia, ch 2, pp 12–33

Cote C J 1990 Editorial: NPO after midnight for children: a reappraisal. Anesthesiology 72: 589–592

Cote C J, Liu L M P, Szyfelbein S K et al 1986 Intraoperative events diagnosed by expired carbon dioxide monitoring in children. Can Anaesth Soc J 33: 315–320

Cote C J, Goldstein E A, Cote M A, Hoaglin D C, Ryan J F 1988 A single-blind study of pulse oximetry in children. Anesthesiology 68: 184–188

Davies D W, Steward D J 1977 Unexpected excessive bleeding during operation: role of acetyl salicylic acid. Can Anaesth Soc J 24: 452–458

DeSoto H, Patel R I, Soliman I E, Hannallah R S 1988 Changes in oxygen saturation following general anesthesia in children with upper respiratory infections signs and symptoms undergoing otolaryngological procedures. Anesthesiology 68: 276–279

Fennelly M E, Hall G M 1990 Anaesthesia and upper respiratory tract infections: a non-existent hazard? Br J Anaesth 64: 535–536

Friesen R H, Lichtor J L 1982 Cardiovascular depression during halothane anesthesia in infants: a study of three induction techniques. Anesth Analg 61: 42–45

Friesen R H, Lichtor J L 1983 Cardiovascular effects of inhalation induction with isoflurane in infants. Anesth Analg 62: 411–414

Friesen R H, Honda A T, Theime R E 1987a Changes in anterior fontanel pressure in preterm neonates during tracheal intubation. Anesth Analg 66: 874–878

Friesen R H, Honda A T, Thieme R E 1987b Perianesthetic intracranial hemorrhage in preterm neonates. Anesthesiology 67: 814–816

Goudsouzian N G, Donlon J V, Savarese J J, Ryan J F 1975 Re-evaluation of dosage and duration of action of d-tubocurarine in the pediatric age group. Anesthesiology 43: 416–425

Graff T D, Phillips O C, Benson D W, Kelley E 1964 Baltimore Anesthesia Study Committee: factors in pediatric anesthesia mortality. Anesth Analg 43: 407–414

Gregory G A 1986 Pediatric anesthesia. In: Miller R D (ed) Anesthesia, 2nd edn. Churchill Livingstone, New York, ch 49, pp 1755–1799

Hall S C 1988 Pediatric anaesthesia. In: Dripps R D, Eckenhoff J E, Vandam L D (eds) Introduction to anesthesia: the principles of safe practice, 7th edn. Saunders, Philadelphia, ch 24 pp 315–334

Hatch D J, Miles R, Wagstaff M 1980 An anaesthetic scavenging system for paediatric and adult use. Anaesthesia 35: 496–499

Hatch D J 1984 Anaesthesia for children. Anaesthesia 39: 405–406

Hatch D J, Sumner E 1986a Perinatal physiology. In: Neonatal anaesthesia and perioperative care, 2nd edn. Current topics in anaesthesia series. Arnold, London, ch 1, pp 1–53

Hatch D J, Sumner E 1986b The surgical neonate. In: Neonatal anaesthesia and perioperative care, 2nd edn. Current topics in anaesthesia series. Arnold, London, ch 2, pp 54–84

Hatch D J, Sumner E 1986c Anaesthesia: specific conditions. In: Neonatal anaesthesia and perioperative care, 2nd edn. Current topics in anaesthesia series. Arnold, London, ch 4, pp 125–194

Hatch D J, Yates A P, Lindahl S G E 1987 Flow requirements and rebreathing during mechanically controlled ventilation in a T-piece (Mapleson E) system. Br J Anaesth 59: 1533–1540

Holliday M A, Segar W E 1957 The maintenance need for water in parenteral fluid therapy. Pediatrics 19: 823–832

Keenan R L, Boyan C P 1985 Cardiac arrest due to anesthesia: a study of incidence and causes. J Am Med Assoc 253: 2373–2377

Lancet Editorial 1987 Pain, anaesthesia, and babies. Lancet 2: 543–544

Lancet Editorial 1988 Complications of anaesthesia in infants and children. Lancet 2: 1466

Lee K W T, Downes J J 1983 Pulmonary edema secondary to laryngospasm in children. Anesthesiology 59: 347–349

Lerman J 1988 Anaesthesia in preterm and ex-preterm infants. Current Opinion in Anaesthesiology 1: 11–16

Lindahl S G E 1985 Preoperative assessment and preparation. In: Sumner E, Hatch D J (eds) Paediatric anaesthesia. Clinics in anaesthesiology, vol 3. Saunders, London, pp 487–503

Liu L M P, Cote C J, Goudsouzian N G et al 1983 Life-threatening apnea in infants recovering from anesthesia. Anesthesiology 59: 506–510

Lloyd-Thomas A R 1990 Pain management in paediatric patients. Br J Anaesth 64: 85–104

Nightingale D A, Richards C C, Glass A 1965 An evaluation of rebreathing in a modified T-piece system during controlled ventilation of anaesthetized children. Br J Anaesth 37: 762–770

Nilsson K, Larsson L E, Andreasson S, Ekstrom-Jodal B 1984 Blood glucose concentrations during anaesthesia in children: effects of starvation and perioperative fluid therapy. Br J Anaesth 56: 375–379

Olsson G L, Hallen B 1984 Laryngospasm during anaesthesia: a computer-aided incidence study in 136, 929 patients. Acta Anaesthesiol Scand 28: 567–575

Olsson G L, Hallen B, Hambraeus-Jonzon K 1986 Aspiration during anaesthesia: a computer-aided study of 185,358 anaesthetics. Acta Anaesthesiol Scand 30: 84–92

Rees G J 1950 Anaesthesia and the newborn. Br Med J 2: 1419–1422

Rose D K, Froese A B 1979 The regulation of $Paco_2$ during controlled ventilation of children with a T-piece. Can Anaesth Soc J 26: 104–113

Schreiner M S, Triebwasser A, Keon T P 1990 Oral fluids compared to preoperative fasting in pediatric outpatients. Anesthesiology 72: 593–597

Splinter W M, Steward J A, Muir J G 1989 The effect of preoperative apple juice on gastric contents, thirst and hunger in children. Can J Anaesth 36: 55–58.

Steward D J 1982 Preterm infants are more prone to complications following minor surgery than are term infants. Anesthesiology 56: 304–306

Tait A R, Knight P R 1987 Intraoperative respiratory complications in patients with upper respiratory tract infections. Can J Anaesth 34: 300–303

Tiret L, Desmonts J M, Hatton F, Vourc'h G 1986 Complications associated with anaesthesia: a prospective survey in France. Can Anaesth Soc J 33: 336–344

Tiret L, Nivoche Y, Hatton F, Desmonts J M, Vourc'h G 1988 Complications related to anaesthesia in infants and children: a prospective survey of 40240 anaesthetics. Br J Anaesth 61: 263–269

Willis B A, Pender J W, Mapleson W W 1975 Rebreathing in a T-piece: volunteer and theoretical studies of the Jackson-Rees modification of Ayre's T-piece during spontaneous respiration. Br J Anaesth 47: 1239–1246

13

Safety of anaesthesia in old age

C. S. Waldmann

INTRODUCTION

As an increasing proportion of the UK population lives on into old age, there has been a proportional increase in the number of elderly patients who are subjected to surgery and anaesthesia. There are two reasons for this. Firstly, improvements in health care in the UK have resulted in increased life expectancy. In 1975, 12% of the population was over 60 years old and by the year 2000 it is predicted that 20% of the population will be over 60 years old. At present 3 million people in the UK are over 75 years old and it will be another 20 years before a reduced birth rate affects the increase in the number of aged people. The ratio of old to young will be at its highest in year 2006 when 1 in 65 of the population will be 85 years or more (Growing older 1981). The second reason is that recent advances in anaesthesia and intensive care have enabled surgeons to operate on elderly patients who formerly would have been considered beyond surgical help. In the author's own Health Authority anaesthetic audit has recently been introduced using a Psion Organiser. Table 13.1 demonstrates that for 1991–1992 patients of 65 years and over are on average sicker as judged by their ASA classification (Saklad 1941).

Anaesthesia for elderly patients poses specific problems that set it apart from other branches of anaesthesia. The elderly differ physiologically from young adults to nearly the same extent as do neonates, yet far less attention has been directed towards the safe conduct of anaesthesia in the older patient. Only recently have publications, specifically concerned with anaesthesia in the elderly, appeared in abundance. In 1982 in Austria, the United Nations organized a world assembly on aging, from which emerged a proposal that the elderly should be cared for by practitioners with a specific interest in aging.

Recently the Age Anaesthesia Association has been formed in the UK to provide research, teaching and training in anaesthesia for older patients (Jones 1989). However, it is still all too common to find a solo junior anaesthetist struggling with a frail elderly person undergoing emergency surgery in one theatre, while next door a consultant anaesthetist and his team of assistants are concentrating their attention on a neonate with pyloric stenosis. The term Agism is used in an article published by Smith (1990). Until re-

Table 13.1

	Total No:	ASA I	ASA II	ASA III	ASA IV	ASA V
Over 65	4 507	21%	51%	23%	4.5%	0.5%
Under 65	18 426	76%	20%	3.62%	0.3%	0.08%

cently the elderly have tended to be neglected by the health and social services.

THE AGING PROCESS

It has been suggested that the aging process may involve failure to replace dead or damaged cells, resulting in a reduced reserve capacity in most organ systems. At the molecular level, Balin & Allen (1989) stated that the rate of aging is governed by amino-acid racemisation and non-enzymatic glycosylation. The result is: 'A second childishness . . . sans teeth, sans eyes, sans everything'. The following list (from Atkinson et al 1977) gives the features commonly found in elderly patients:

1. dehydration
2. tissue wasting
3. cardiomegaly
4. arteriosclerosis
   - renal
   - cerebral
   - coronary vessels
5. stiff thoracic cage
6. emphysema
7. bronchiolar narrowing
8. brain atrophy
9. dilated cerebral ventricles
10. atrophied mandible
11. brittle bones
12. decreased blood volume and haemoglobin
13. decreased cardiac reserve
14. slow circulation time
15. reduced tidal volume and vital capacity
16. impaired cough reflexes.

The word, geriatric, was coined in New York (Nascher 1914). In view of the derogatory overtones that became attached to the term many people prefer to use the word elderly. For the purposes of this chapter, elderly will be taken to apply to patients aged 65 years or over. About 50% of these patients will require surgery prior to death. However, aging and decrepitude are not synonymous, and the age at which we become physiologically old is variable, occurring prematurely in some people. The condition known as progeria (Fig. 13.1) constitutes an extreme example.

The elderly are a heterogeneous group. Dodson (1987) points out that a 75-year-old may be active, both mentally and physically, with a full social life, or may be bed-bound, confused and isolated. Physiological functions begin to deteriorate from 40 years onwards, but the worst problems arise when intellectual impairment precedes the physical decline of aging.

RISK OF ANAESTHESIA IN OLD AGE

The risk of anaesthesia and surgery increases with age. Goldman et al (1977) list age as one of nine factors increasing the cardiac risk in non-cardiac surgery (see Table 13.2).

Many past studies have consisted of uncontrolled retrospective reviews of mortality rates in the first postoperative month. Rates vary from 3% to 43%. In a recent prospective study by Palmer et al (1986), younger patients (aged 40–65) were used as controls for an over-80 group. The patients were matched for type of operation, coexisting disease and the experience of the surgeon. At 6 weeks the difference in mortality was not significant (young 10%, old 18%), but by

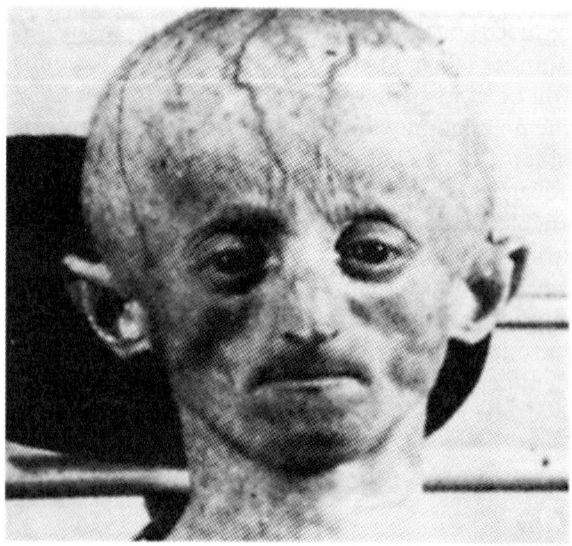

Fig. 13.1 Progeria in a 14-year-old boy (from De Busk 1972).

Table 13.2 Risk factors for calculating the Goldman cardiac risk index

Risk factor	Points
1. 3rd heart sound raised JVP	11
2. Myocardial infarct in previous 6 months	10
3. More than 5 ventricular ectopics per min	7
4. Rhythm other than sinus	7
5. Age greater than 70 years	5
6. Intraperitoneal, thoracic or aortic surgery	3
7. Emergency	4
8. Aortic stenosis	3
9. Poor general condition	3

Goldman cardiac risk index

Class	Points	Nil/Minor complications (%)	Life-threatening complications (%)	Cardiac deaths (%)
I	0–5	99	0.7	0.2
II	6–12	93	5	2
III	13–25	86	11	2
IV	25+	22	22	56

6 months the mortality for the elderly had risen to 42%, whereas that for the young was at 13%.

Kaplan et al (1972) specifically looked at the mortality associated with surgery for peptic ulcer in the aged patient. Aged 60–64, the mortality was only 7%. This rose to 18% in the 65–74 age-group and 37.5% in the over-75 group. In a reported series of 108 878 anaesthetics in Cardiff by Farrow et al (1982), the overall death rate was 2.19% (one in 46 anaesthetics), yet in the over-65 age-group the death rate was more than 6%. Interestingly there was a preponderance of women dying in this older age-group, compared to the younger age-group in which mortality was higher in men. This appears to reflect the frequency with which the elderly female population tended to undergo surgery for reduction of fractured hips, whereas elderly males had a large number of anaesthetics for less major procedures, such as cystoscopies. In the Cardiff series the overall increase in the death rate with age was associated with two factors:

1. The operation was often a major procedure
2. There was a higher proportion of emergency procedures which carried a 3.5 times greater risk.

In a more recent survey by Barlow et al (1989), these findings are confirmed. In their prospective audit of 1111 general surgical procedures they found a mortality of 3.5% in the over-64-year-olds, but mortality was twice as high in patients over 74 compared to the 65–74 age-group. There was a seven-fold increase if the procedure was performed as an emergency. In contrast to this increase in mortality with age, the relative mortality due to coexisting physical disease decreased. Relative mortality was defined as the mortality rate associated with a particular disease compared to that for healthy patients. This suggests that, in older age-groups, coexisting disease may be less important than other risk factors in determining mortality. For instance, among patients with cardiac failure over 65 years of age requiring emergency surgery, there was a mortality of 30% compared with 36% mortality in the 45–65 age-group.

Lunn & Musin (1982), in their report on mortality in anaesthesia in five regions of England and Wales, indicated that in several of the deaths associated with anaesthesia there was a failure to make a preoperative visit and there was an absence of consultation between surgeon and anaesthetist. Thorough preoperative assessment is essential to identify potential problems. Often these patients are hard of hearing and more time is required in order to complete preoperative assessment. Consultation between surgeon and anaesthetist should clarify conditions that can be treated to minimize perioperative mortality and morbidity.

In assessing the risk of anaesthesia and surgery one must take into account the patient's life expectancy and the likelihood of physical and emotional suffering if his condition is left untreated. This must then be compared with the life expectancy if surgery is successful (Table 13.3).

A high risk of death is only acceptable if the alternative is considerable suffering or impending death.

Safety related to different organ systems

Respiratory system

The following changes may occur as a result of aging:

1. Kyphosis
2. Breakdown of alveolar septa leading to emphysema
3. Reduction of vital capacity
4. Airway closure may occur during normal respiration in awake elderly patients and is one of the reasons for decreased arterial oxygen tension in the elderly. Under anaesthesia in the supine position, the functional residual capacity is often less than the closing volume, resulting in significant hypoxia. The reduction in Pa_{O_2} in mmHg can be approximately represented by the following formulae (Kitamura et al 1972):
   $Pa_{O_2} = 100 - 0.32 \times \text{age}$
   $Pa_{O_2} = 100 - 0.54 \times \text{age}$ (postoperatively)
   It is important to preoxygenate elderly patients prior to anaesthesia, administer additional oxygen perioperatively and ensure that oxygen is administered postoperatively.
5. Decreased responsiveness of the respiratory centre to carbon dioxide. This responsiveness is further decreased by the presence of opioids and anaesthetic agents, and by the incomplete reversal of muscle relaxants.
6. There is an increased potential for aspiration of stomach contents into the lungs. Pontopiddan & Beecher (1960) demonstrated a decrease in cough response to ammonia in the aged. Because of the prolonged circulation time, some very sick elderly patients are probably unsuitable for rapid sequence induction/intubation. If the stomach is full, thought should be given to alternatives such as an awake intubation.

Table 13.3 Actuarial expectation of life (years), Canada 1975–1977 from Davenport 1983

Age	Male	Female
60	17.23	21.96
65	13.95	18.00
70	11.05	14.33
75	8.55	11.03
80	6.44	8.15
85	4.73	5.81

Assessment of respiratory function is a vitally important part of preoperative assessment, but frequently old people are uncomplaining and it is easy to be misled about the true extent of a patient's respiratory disability. In some parts of the UK, chronic obstructive airways disease and/or emphysema may be almost the norm among elderly men, and often the patient will give the impression that he has no breathing problems because his disability is less than that of his acquaintances. If possible, the anaesthetist should accompany the patient for a short walk in the ward. This will reveal more about the patient's respiratory reserve than many minutes of detailed questioning and is probably more informative than bedside pulmonary function tests which do not require a sustained effort. Seymour & Pringle (1983) in a prospective study of patients aged over 65 years found that, if the patient was able to leave home unaided more than twice weekly, he was less likely to suffer respiratory or cardiac complications perioperatively. Often, of course the patient will not be mobile; it then becomes essential that the anaesthetist derives as much information as possible from chest radiographs and bedside pulmonary function tests, together with a detailed history. An estimation of preoperative arterial oxygen tension and CO_2 tension may also prove invaluable in postoperative management.

Regional anaesthesia and its continuation into the postoperative period for pain relief may well be preferable to parenteral opioid administration in the elderly patient with respiratory disease. The technique is not without its problems. Casey (1984) gives an account of an elderly patient developing respiratory failure after bilateral intercostal nerve block following laparotomy for a perforated duodenal ulcer.

Cardiovascular system

The incidence of cardiovascular disease increases with age. In Desmond's series (1970), 60% of the patients were between the ages of 70 and 90 and, of these, 67% had clinical evidence of cardiac disease. There are several cardiovascular problems that reduce the safety of anaesthesia in the elderly.

Hypertension is common in the elderly as a result of thickened elastic fibres in the walls of large arteries. This leads to a 'lead-pipe' vasculature, with an increased peripheral vascular resistance. Hypertension increases morbidity and mortality in the elderly, just as it does in the young. During anaesthesia, elderly hypertensive patients are very prone to sudden dramatic changes in blood pressure in response to stimulation and anaesthetic drugs. Because of their decreased ability to autoregulate the blood supply to various organs, these patients are at risk of strokes, myocardial ischaemic episodes and renal failure. Knight & Hantler (1986) reviewing hypertension in the elderly found 40% of patients over 65 years old to be hypertensive, compared to 30% in the 55–65 age group. They defined hypertension as blood pressure greater than 150/100. Many of the elderly patients were on reserpine, methyldopa and other 'old-fashioned' medications. Cerebrovascular accidents, congestive failure and renal failure were common in untreated patients. According to the Veterans Study (1972), these sequelae could be reduced by control of diastolic pressure, but to date there is no evidence that morbidity and mortality are improved by a reduction of systolic blood pressure. Elderly patients who suffer a stroke have a less complete recovery than younger patients.

Cardiac output decreases by about 3% per decade. Increased systemic vascular resistance, myocardial ischaemia and the presence of arrhythmias all contribute to decreased cardiac output.

Routine ECGs should be performed on all elderly patients presenting for surgery to detect arrhythmias, and 'silent' infarcts that may have occurred recently enough to increase the risk of operation. However, Davidson (1986) wrote that routine coronary angiography on a group of patients who were to undergo vascular surgery revealed a 20–30% incidence of significant coronary disease, despite the lack of cardiac symptoms and normal resting ECGs. Cooperman et al (1978) found that cardiovascular complications occurred in 33% of patients undergoing surgery if arrhythmias were present, as compared to 9% with normal ECGs.

Aortic aneurysm is present in 6% of the over-65-year-old population. The main reason for perioperative mortality is myocardial infarction. If proper preoperative evaluation of the group is carried out to exclude patients at risk from perioperative myocardial infarction in spite of normal ECG, by stress ECG, dipyridamole–thallium, scanning and ejection fraction, there is no reason why this group of patients should not do well. A recent review by Currie and his colleagues (1992) of the quality of life of octogenerians after aneurysm surgery concluded that both elective and emergency aortic aneurysm surgery can be performed with reasonable survival and a good quality of life and therefore cannot be denied to this group of patients on the basis of age alone. As long ago as 1976 O'Donnell et al reviewed aortic aneurysm surgery in 111 patients over 80 years old and found a mortality of only 2%. Elderly patients presenting for vascular surgery present specific problems and previously unnoticed cardiac decompensation may become apparent on clamping and unclamping the aorta.

Preoperative evaluation should look firstly at coronary perfusion by either exercise stress testing (EST) or more accurately by dipyridamole-thallium scanning (D-T scan) as described by Leppo (1989). Evaluation should secondly include assessment of left ventricular ejection fraction either by echocardiography or by a radioisotope technique using a gamma-camera gated to the ECG. In certain instances coronary angiography and vein grafting may be indicated prior to undertaking major vascular surgery.

In general, whenever an anaesthetist is faced with an elderly patient with significant heart disease who is about to undergo surgical procedures involving large volume shifts, Swan Ganz catheterisation should be considered (Gallo 1986). Central venous pressure lines will not give accurate information about fluid balance in elderly patients with cardiac disease. They do, however, provide very good venous access.

Shoemaker et al (1988) looked prospectively at haemodynamic indices of high risk surgical patients and determined whether this affected outcome. Merely maintaining normal values of BP, CVP and pulmonary wedge pressure was followed by a mortality of 30%. However, if patients with a Swan Ganz catheter inserted had supraoptimal values of cardiac index, oxygen delivery and oxygen consumption maintained, then mortality was reduced to 4%, average time spent on ITU fell from 16 to 10 days and time spent on the ventilator reduced from 10 to 3 days. The cost in intensive care for patients was thereby reduced by 50%.

The high mortality associated with anaesthetising patients in heart failure necessitates that heart failure should be corrected prior to operation in all but the most life-threatening conditions. Emergency surgery in the presence of heart failure in patients of 65 years or more had a 30% mortality in the Cardiff Study (Farrow et al 1982). Reduced cardiac reserve in the elderly increases the likelihood of heart failure and pulmonary oedema occurring both perioperatively and postoperatively. The monitoring of pulmonary capillary wedge pressures aids the management of elderly patients with poor cardiac reserve presenting for major surgery.

The routine use of digitalis in elderly patients prior to surgery remains controversial. On the grounds that most anaesthetic agents, including nitrous oxide, behave as myocardial depressants, digitalization should be considered if one or more of the following apply:

- The patient has radiographic and electrocardiographic evidence of heart failure.
- The patient requires major surgery.
- There is no contraindication to the patient receiving the drug.

In the elderly, the difference between inadequate digitilization and overdosage is often minimal, and blood levels should be measured (normal range at 6 h post dose should be in the range of 0.6–2.6 nmol/l). Rapid digitilization may result in cardiac irritability.

Elderly patients particularly at risk of digoxin toxicity are those on potassium-losing diuretics. Because of the drawbacks of digoxin it may be that dobutamine should be used for the control of perioperative heart failure.

Lehot et al (1989) conducted a double-blind trial in patients over 64 years old, undergoing non-cardiac surgery of 90 min duration or more. The use of dobutamine at 7 μg/kg/min prevented the perioperative reduction in cardiac output and blood pressure caused by anaesthetic agents, and might prevent perioperative neurological disorders.

The conduction system of the heart is affected by the aging process and it is not uncommon to see left bundle branch block and atrial fibrillation. Indications for temporary pacing in the perioperative period are not definite and may require a cardiological opinion, but if in doubt it is generally safer to pace.

Bifascicular block may convert to complete heart block in the presence of enflurane or halothane, which delay conduction through the atrioventricular node. Equipment for pacing should be readily at hand.

Levy (1990) describes a case of a patient developing worrying bradycardia resistant to atropine, but responding to isoprenaline and then pacing. In spite of a normal preoperative ECG the patient had a latent sick sinus syndrome and later admitted to attacks of dizziness.

If a patient already has a permanent pacemaker in situ, succinylcholine and diathermy may cause it to fail perioperatively.

Drugs such as atropine, gallamine and pancuronium must be used cautiously because the resulting tachycardia may cause increased oxygen demands that cannot be met by the aging myocardium. Gallamine and pancuronium may be replaced by some of the newer muscle relaxants, and glycopyrrolate can be substituted for atropine for reversal of muscle relaxation in combination with neostigmine.

Nervous system

With aging, the brain atrophies, particularly the frontal cortex, and by the age of 80 the weight of the brain is reduced from 1400 g to 1150 g. Cerebral blood flow (CBF) also declines with age:

CBF = [59 minus (0.34 × age)] ml/100 g/min

The brain may age much earlier in presenile dementia. One form of presenile dementia is Alzheimer's disease. This is characterized by plaques of amyloid deposited in the cerebral vessels, and the loss of neurotransmitter. A carotid bruit should be sought on preoperative examination. In the over-65 age group, asymptomatic carotid bruits are found in 7% of patients. Wolf et al (1981) found the risk of stroke doubled postoperatively in the presence of an asymptomatic bruit.

Parkinsonism affects a large number of the elderly. Problems with these patients may be enhanced by the interruption of their medication following gut surgery and worsening of their symptoms due to anaesthetic drugs. Many patients suffer loss of short-term memory and become confused merely from being placed in the strange environment of a hospital. The addition of general anaesthesia and surgery further increases the confusion. Many people can supply anecdotal support to the notion that elderly patients are mentally affected after surgery, often pointing to a relative, patient or acquaintance who has 'never been the same' since the operation. Bedford (1955) reported in detail the cases of 18 normal elderly patients who, following general anaesthesia, showed the greatest degree of dementia. However, Simpson et al (1961) found no mental deterioration in their series of 250 patients following general anaesthesia for elective surgery.

Hole et al (1980) compared the use of epidural with general anaesthesia for total hip replacement in elderly patients. They found a significant reduction in $Pa\text{O}_2$ on days 1 and 3 postoperatively after general anaesthesia, and five patients in the general anaesthesia group suffered mental deterioration as evidenced by disorientation, confusion and restlessness. This reduced their quality of life several months later. None of these changes was found in the epidural group. These observations were not confirmed in a recent publication by Jones et al (1990). In their series of 146 patients over 60 years old, randomly allocated to receive regional or general anaesthesia for hip or knee replacement, they found that the anaesthetic technique did not influence the long-term mental function of the patients if scrupulous attention was paid to the avoidance of hypotension, hypoxia and hypocapnia.

Vertebrobasilar insufficiency may be present, therefore the head should be maintained in a neutral position. The autonomic nervous system responds less to stress in the elderly. For instance, Collins et al (1980) found that there is a decreased response to alteration in cardiac preload. There is also an enhanced response to agents such as adrenaline due to the reduced autonomic system output and increased receptor sensitivity. Bladder dysfunction is more likely, with a high incidence of urinary retention in elderly patients. A paralysed extremity secondary to a previous stroke is quite common, and care must be taken during anaesthesia to position the extremity in the neutral position.

Thermoregulation

The elderly patient is unable to control body temperature, particularly during major surgery in a cool theatre, thus body temperature should be monitored and maintained. Shivering on recovery from anaesthesia increases oxygen demands by as much as 300–800%. The elderly myocardium cannot cope with such a drastic increase as this. This is accentuated by the fact that a fall in temperature shifts the haemoglobin dissociation curve to the left and therefore reduces oxygen delivery to the tissues. Goldberg & Roe (1966) reviewed the problems of temperature regulation during surgery and showed that heat loss and a fall in temperature increased with age. Accidental perioperative hypothermia may be followed by deranged clotting, and prolongation of anaesthesia and muscle relaxation (MAC values fall with decreasing body temperature). Also, a fall in temperature may be accompanied by a fall in $Pa\text{CO}_2$, causing a reduction in cerebral perfusion. Vasoconstriction also occurs, causing a shift of fluid centrally, and hypovolaemia is masked until the patient warms up.

Endocrine function

Diabetes mellitus occurs in 15% of patients aged 65, and in 25% of 85-year-olds (Bennett 1976). This condition may not be detectable until routine preoperative urine screening and may, not uncommonly, become apparent postoperatively. These patients are usually non-insulin-dependent. The following acute problems may affect the patient's safety (see also Ch. 9):

- diabetic ketacidosis
- hyperosmolar nonketotic diabetes
- lactic acidosis
- hypoglycaemia.

The chronic problems include:

- delayed wound healing
- retinopathy
- nephropathy
- skin problems
- cardiovascular problems
- autonomic and peripheral neuropathy, which may affect the patient's suitability for spinal/epidural anaesthesia.

A significant number of elderly diabetic patients present for eye surgery, particularly for cataract. Poor eyesight and, perhaps, mental deterioration mean that self-administration of insulin may be inaccurate or impossible. Compliance with the oral hypoglycaemics and dietary control may also be problematical. Often these patients have significant cardiorespiratory and renal disease and, traditionally, many of these patients are operated on using local anaesthesia. Lang (1982) suggested that if a patient has a clear mind and he is likely to survive 6 months or more with an improved quality of life, then surgery with local anaesthesia is indicated. However, there is no statistical difference in survival between general and local anaesthesia.

Local anaesthetic, retrobulbar block in particular, has a number of life-threatening complications:

- vagal stimulation
- convulsions
- brainstem anaesthesia.

These complications may occur in about 5% of procedures, requiring anaesthetic personnel to be summoned.

Meyers (1986) suggests that anaesthetic personnel should always be present for local anaesthesia. Sedation can then be safely applied and the patient properly monitored. If the patient becomes uncooperative and in danger of coughing out the contents of his eye, conversion to general anaesthesia can take place.

Skeletal changes

Bone weakness is a common problem in the elderly and may be responsible for fractures of the vertebral body, femoral neck and distal end of the radius. These fractures may occur following trivial injury, or due to rough handling and poor positioning on the operating table. A fractured neck of the femur is associated with a high mortality. Severe arthritic changes, perhaps associated with vertebrobasilar insufficiency, makes endotracheal intubation particularly hazardous. The presence of osteophytes along the vertebral column tends to cause the intervertebral foramina to close off. This may be why epidural anaesthesia reaches a higher level. For this reason the volume of local anaesthetic solution administered needs to be reduced in the elderly.

Connective tissue

Many patients are edentulous. Endotracheal intubation may be easier, but gum margins may be abraided by inexperienced anaesthetists, resulting in dentures fitting poorly postoperatively. Floppy cheeks and edentulous gums make ventilation via a mask more difficult. The presence of loose, decaying teeth may cause problems during laryngoscopy and intubation. In the elderly the skin is thin and friable, so these patients are far more prone to developing pressure sores, particularly after a prolonged period on the operating table. The situation is often accentuated by poor nutrition in elderly patients with dental problems, systemic illness and poor financial status. Wound healing is poor and postoperative infections are more common. The skin should be protected with adequate padding and care must be taken in the use of sticky tape and ECG electrodes. Sheets and canvasses should be smooth, neither creased nor folded. Blood vessel fragility and atrophic skin make it difficult to cannulate veins, and bruising is more common. Sebaceous cysts may be present in large numbers, and large cysts may be responsible for difficulty at intubation (Fig. 13.2).

Altered sensitivity to drugs

A major problem facing the anaesthetist is that of drug interaction. Between 1977 and 1985 the Department of Health prescribing data showed a 27% increase in the average number of prescription items per person of pensionable age compared to a decrease of 6% in younger patients (Elderly people: their medicines and their doctors 1990). The data were obtained from a structured sample of people aged 65 and over. Of those interviewed 70% had been prescribed medication, 60% within the previous 24 hours. On average 2.8 drugs had been prescribed per patient. Apart from a significant number of inappropriate medications and dosages and lack of compliance, there was a 4% incidence of duplication, e.g. propanolol and inderal, and in 17% of cases a potential for harmful interactions. The most common drugs prescribed to this age group are diuretics, potassium supplements, analgesics, digitalis and psychotropic drugs. One important drug interaction is that associated with ecothiopate eyedrops which are still prescribed for the treatment of glaucoma. These prolong the activity of succinylcholine. The elimination half-life and peak blood levels of the anaesthetic agents used are increased in elderly patients and requirements are generally reduced. The reasons for this are:

1. Reduced renal excretion. There is a 50% reduction in renal blood flow by the age of 70. The reduction in muscle mass means that serum creatinine does not accurately reflect renal function (Friedman et al 1972).
2. Reduction in serum albumin. This results in a higher proportion of free drug.
3. The sensitivity of tissue receptors to drugs is increased.
4. Liver function is reduced, therefore drug metabolism is reduced.

Several studies have demonstrated the effect of age on the handling of anaesthetic agents. Sear et

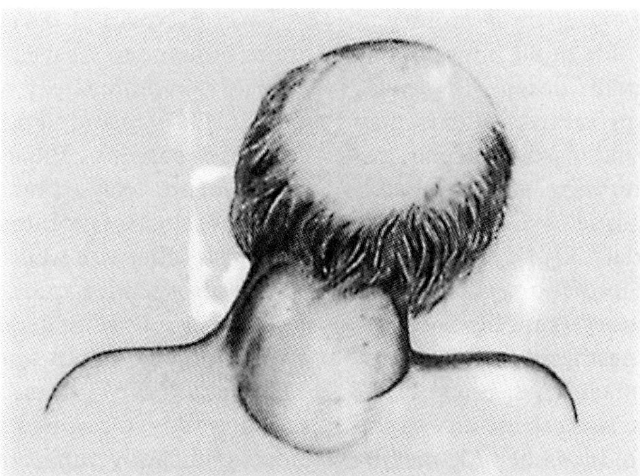

Fig. 13.2 Sebaceous cyst of the neck in a 75-year-old man causing difficulty at intubation (from the Association of Anaesthetists of Great Britain and Ireland: © 1983).

al (1983), using the postbox test, showed that patients over 50 years old had a longer recovery time with thiopentone. Christensen et al (1983) concluded that elderly patients were far more sensitive to thiopentone and suggested midazolam given as 1–2 mg boluses to be a preferable induction agent. MAC values of inhalational agents are reduced with age. For example, halothane MAC of 0.75% at 40 yrs reduces to 0.64% at 80, and isoflurane in N_2O 70% has a MAC value of 0.5% at 40 yrs but this becomes 0.37% at 80.

The cardiovascular stability of pancuronium is usually offset by its tendency to cause tachycardia which may embarrass the elderly myocardium, and by the prolongation of recovery (Marsh et al 1980) which may be as much as 30 min. Atracurium and vecuronium may be preferable muscle relaxants. The use of glycopyrrolate, instead of atropine with neostigmine, has been found preferable for two reasons:

1. There are fewer arrhythmias, especially with halothane (Muravchicks et al 1979).
2. Simpson et al (1985) demonstrated a reduction of cognitive function after atropine but not with glycopyrrolate.

Alfentanil is a useful perioperative opioid because of its short duration of action, which reduces the likelihood of postoperative respiratory depression. Klotz et al (1975) demonstrated that the half-life of diazepam is prolonged from 20 hours in 20-year-olds to 90 hours in 80-year-olds. Even with small doses of benzodiazepines in the elderly, protective reflexes may be lost, and respiratory and cardiovascular depression may occur. Monitoring of the sedated patient should include pulse oximetry, blood pressure, ECG and end tidal CO_2.

The use of regional anaesthetic techniques in order to avert the respiratory complications associated with general anaesthesia may lead to high blood levels of local anaesthetic. Blood levels are more likely to be in the toxic range due to the slow circulation time and reduced hepatic metabolism. Additionally, less than adequate local anaesthesia necessitates the administration of sedatives, many of which have prolonged effects.

Problems related to specific surgery for the elderly

Transurethral resection of prostate

In Desmond's series (1970), about 90% of the patients having transurethral transection of prostate (TURP) were over 60 years old. The particular problems related to this form of surgery are covered in Chapter 17 (p. 256). Lange et al (1988) concluded that regional anaesthesia is, at present, the most appropriate technique for this form of prostate surgery. Absorption of irrigating fluid may occur not only during TURP, but also during transanal resection of rectal tumours.

Fractured neck of femur

Patients presenting with fractured neck of femur (FNF) have a 40% incidence of arrhythmias detected on preoperative continuous ECG monitoring, 30% incidence of Parkinsonism and 23% incidence of hypoxia, with $P\text{aO}_2$ preoperatively less than 60 mmHg (Covert & Fox 1989). The optimum timing of surgery and the most appropriate technique for this operation has been the subject of much debate. Anderson (1971) summarized his doctrine for patients with FNF stating: 'Unless moribund the indication for internal fixation of the patient's hip is inversely proportional to the general condition of the patient, in fact, internal fixation may offer the only hope of survival.'

Lyon & Nevin (1984) have suggested that it is more humane to treat nursing home patients previously non-ambulatory without surgery. Kenzora et al (1984) recommends 24 hours stabilization prior to surgery. Villar et al (1986) do not recommend delay in operating for FNF because of suboptimal laboratory investigations if the patient is otherwise well.

In a prospective multicentre trial of mortality, at 4 weeks following general or spinal anaesthesia for nonprosthetic hip fracture in elderly patients, Davis et al (1987) found that out of 538 patients the mortality for spinal anaesthesia (6.6%) was not significantly different from that for general anaesthesia (5.9%). However, mortality was increased by a delay of more than 24 hours from admission to surgery.

Covert & Fox (1989) reported that postoperative confusion was not dependent on anaesthetic techniques for FNF. There was, however, higher $Pa\text{O}_2$ postoperatively in the regional group and a reduction in the incidence of DVT from 70% after general anaesthesia to 40% for regional anaesthesia. A confused patient who cannot be positioned adequately and who may be receiving low-dose heparin, may not be an ideal candidate for regional anaesthesia.

FNF was the subject of a recent report by the Royal College of Physicians (Summary and Recommendations 1989). The report showed that in England and Wales in 1983, FNF was responsible for the occupancy of 3500 beds per day with a high perioperative and later mortality. The estimated cost per year was £160 million. The report's recommendations included the following:

- Each Health District develops a strategy for FNF which is annually audited and reviewed.
- Patients with FNF spend no longer than 1 hour in Casualty, and should be assessed not only by an orthopaedic surgeon, but geriatricians should be involved.
- Operative intervention should occur during the day by senior orthopaedic and anaesthetic staff within 24 hours of admission.
- Postoperative care and rehabilitation should take place under the combined care of orthopaedic surgeons and geriatricians.

Total hip replacement

Total hip replacement has been a major advance in the treatment of chronic arthritis of the hip, and provides patients with relief from pain and increased mobility. To try to reduce the incidence of hypotension and cardiac arrest following insertion of the methyl methacrylate cement, it is usual to use a catheter to act as a medullary cavity vent. Insertion of cement is delayed for 2 min after mixing to reduce the amount of free monomer present (Gray et al 1980). About 60% of patients presenting for THR are more than 65 years of age. About 25% have rheumatoid arthritis with multiple joint involvement, including atlantoaxial and temporomandibular joints. Approximately 10% had problems with intubation, primarily due to rheumatiod arthritis and ankylosing spondylitis (Koide et al 1974). Covert & Fox (1989) reported a 4-week mortality of 1% following THR, mostly due to pulmonary embolism. It has been claimed that the incidence of DVT and intraoperative blood loss may be reduced by the use of regional anaesthetic techniques.

SUMMARY

In the elderly, surgery needs to be rapid, but not at the expense of unnecessary blood loss. The idea that modern anaesthesia permits hours of unhurried surgery may be true in the young, but is less so in the elderly. The reduced organ function in old people not only decreases the margin of error permissible to the anaesthetist, but also increases the penalties for even minor shortcomings in patient care. It is no longer acceptable to ascribe perioperative death to the patient's age and general decrepit state. The only justification for embarking on surgery and anaesthesia in any patient, young or old, is the expectation of improvement in their physical status and life expectancy. Like any other group of patients the elderly have their own constellation of problems, and ignorance of or indifference towards them is as culpable as it would be in a neonate. If you can't help people, you should leave them alone.

The following ideas may be of help to us in improving the service we give as anaesthetists to elderly patients:

1. Where possible patients should not be operated on outside normal working hours by the most junior anaesthetists and surgeons.
2. A 24-hour anaesthetic and surgical consultant input should be available.
3. There should be adequate high dependency and intensive care back-up

4. Minimally invasive surgery should be encouraged.
5. Geriatricians, cardiologists, respiratory physicians should more often be involved in perioperative management.
6. More day care surgery should be employed where possible. The patient must have a telephone at home.
7. Consider the appropriateness of major surgery in the individual about to be anaesthetised. For instance it may be illogical to perform aortobifemoral graft procedures for claudication in patients with untreated angina. If the angina is adequately treated, the claudication may improve.
8. A regular review of anaesthetic practice in the elderly should take place looking at morbidity and mortality. Surgery should not be undertaken unless there is a reasonable chance that the patient's quality of life can be improved. If there is no such assurance the patient may prefer to take his or her chance at home rather than risk dying in theatre or the intensive care unit.

REFERENCES

Anderson L D 1971 Fractures. In: Crenshaw A H (ed) Campbells's operative orthopaedics. C V Mosby, St Louis, pp 471–691

Atkinson R S, Rushman G B, Lee A J 1977 A synopsis of anaesthesia, 9th edn. Wright, Bristol, p 515

Balin A K, Allen R G 1989 Molecular basis of biologic aging. Clin Geriatr Med 1(1): 21

Barlow A, Crumplin M, Zarisag et al 1989 Surgery in a geriatric population. Ann R Coll Surg Eng 71: 110–114

Bedford P P 1955 Adverse cerebral effects of anaesthesia on old people. Lancet 2: 259–263

Bennett P M 1976 Report of work group on epidemiology. National Commission of Diabetes 3, US Department of Health Education and Welfare, 76–1021, part 2, pp 65–135

Casey W F 1984 Respiratory failure following intercostal nerve blockade. Anaesthesia 39: 351–354

Christensen J H, Andreasen F, Jansen J A 1983 Thiopentone sensitivity in young and elderly women. Br J Anaesth 55: 33–40

Collins K J, Exton-Smith A N, James M H et al 1980 Functional changes in the autonomic nervous system with aging. Age Aging 9: 17–24

Cooperman M, Pflug B, Martin E W, Evans W E 1978 Cardiovascular risk factors in patients with peripheral vascular disease. Surgery 84: 505–508

Covert C R, Fox G S, 1989 Anaesthesia for hip surgery in the elderly. Can J Anaesth 36(3): 311–319

Currie I C, Robson A K, Scott J A, Horrocks M 1992 Quality of life of octogenarians after aneurysm surgery. Ann R Coll Surg 74: 269–273

Davenport H T 1983 Anaesthesia for the geriatric patient. Can Anaesth Soc J 30(3): S51–S55

Davis F M, Wooner D F, Frampton C, Wilkinson A, Grant A, Harrison R T, Roberts M T, Thadaka R 1987 Prospective multicentre trial of mortality following general or spinal anaesthesia for hip fracture surgery in elderly patients. Br J Anaesth 59: 1080–1088

Davidson K 1986 Anaesthesia for major vascular procedures in the elderly. In: Anaesthesia for the geriatric patient. Clinics in Anesthesiology 4(4): 935

De Busk F L 1972 The Hutchinson-Gilford progeria syndrome. J Paed 80: 697

Desmond J 1970 Complications of transurethral prostatic surgery. Can Anaesth Soc J 17(1): 25–36

Dodson M E 1987 Aspects of anaesthesia in the elderly. Br J Hosp Med 37(2): 114–120

Elderly people: Their medicines and their doctors 1990 Drugs and Therapeutics Bulletin 28(20): 77–79

Farrow S C, Fawkes F G R, Lunn J N, Robertson I B, Samuel P 1982 Epidemiology in anaesthesia II: Factors affecting mortality in hospital. Br J Anaesth 54: 811–817

Friedman S A, Raizner A E, Roson H, Solomon N A, Sy W 1972 Functional defects in the ageing kidney. Ann Intern Med 76(1): 41–45

Gallo J A 1986 Anaesthesia and the elderly patient. Clinics in Anesthesiology 4(4): 824

Goldberg M J, Roe C F 1966 Temperature changes during anaesthesia and operation. Arch Surg 93: 365–369

Goldman L, Caldera D, Nussbaum R et al 1977 Multifactorial index of cardiac risk in non-cardiac surgical procedures. N Engl J Med 297(16): 845–50

Gray T C, Nunn J F, Utting J E 1980 General anaesthesia, 4th edn. Butterworths, London, vol 2, pp 1175–1176

Growing older 1981 HMSO, London

Hole V, Terjesen T, Breivik H 1980 Epidural versus general anaesthesia for total hip arthroplasty in elderly patients. Acta Anaesthesiol Scand 24: 279–287

Jones M J T, Piggott S E, Vaughan R S et al 1990 Cognitive and functional competence after anaesthesia in patients aged over 60: controlled trial of general and regional anaesthesia for elective hip or knee replacement. Br Med J 300: 1683–1687

Jones R M 1989 Anaesthesia in old age. Anaesthesia 44: 377–378

Kaplan M, List J, Stenmiar E, Connoly J 1972 Surgical management of peptic ulcer disease in the aged patient. Arch Surg 104: 667–671

Kenzora F E, McCarthy R E, Lowell F D, Sledge C B 1984 Hip fracture mortality. Clin Orthop Relat Res 186: 45–56

Kitamura H, Sava T, Kezono E 1972 Postoperative hypoxaemia: the contribution of age to the maldistribution of ventilation. Anesthesiology 36: 244–252

Klotz V, Avant G R, Hoyumpa A et al 1975 The effects of age and liver disease on the disposition and elimination of diazepam in adult man. J Clin Invest 55: 347–359
Knight P R, Hantler C B 1980 Anaesthesia and the geriatric patient: hypertension in the elderly. Clinics in Anesthesiology 4(4): 1003–1023
Koide M, Pilone R N, Vandam L D, Lowell J D 1974 Anaesthetic experience with total hip replacement. Clin Orthop Surg 99: 78–85
Lang D W 1982 Morbidity and mortality in ophthalmology. In: Bruce R A, McGoldrick K E, Oppenheimer P (eds) Anaesthesia for ophthalmology. Birmingham Aesocolapius pp 195–204
Lange R, Rupieper N, Ringert R H 1988 Anaesthesia in transurethral surgery. Urol Augs A 27: 86–88
Lehot J J, Muchada R, George M, Ferrier C, Winnock S, Mercier M, Renard A, Estauve S 1989 Dobutamine during anaesthesia of patients at risk for heart failure: a controlled prospective multicenter study of 93 surgical patients over 64 years of age. CAH Anaesthesiol 37: 319–326
Leppo J A, 1989 Dipyridamole-thallium imaging: the lazy man's stress test. J Nucl Med 30(3): 281–287
Levy D M 1990 Letter to editor. Anaesthesia 45: 488–489
Lunn J N, Mushin W W 1982 Mortality associated with anaesthesia. Nuffield Provincial Hospitals Trust
Lyon L F, Nevin M A 1984 Management of hip fractures in nursing home patients. J Am Geriatr Soc 32: 391–395
Marsh R H K, Chimielewski A T, Goat V A 1980 Recovery from pancuronium: a comparison between old and young people. Anaesthesia 35: 1193–1196
Meyers E F 1986 Anaesthesia for ophthalmologic surgery in the aged. In: Anaesthesia and the geriatric patient. Clinics in Anesthesiology 4(4): 979–1002
Muravchicks S, Owens W D, Ifelts J A, 1979 Glycopyrrolate and cardiac dysrhythmias in geriatric patients after reversal of neuromuscular blockade. Can Anaesth Soc J 20: 22–25
Nascher I R 1914 Geriatrics: the diseases of old age and their treatment. Blakistons Son, Philadephia
O'Donnell T F, Darling R C, Linton R R 1976 Is 80 years too old for aneurysmectomy? Arch Surg 3: 1250–1257
Palmer C A, Reece Smith H, Tayler I 1986 Personal communication
Pontoppidan H, Beecher H K 1960 Progressive loss of protective reflexes in the airways with the advance of age. J Am Med Assoc 174: 2209–2213
Saklad M 1941 The grading of patients for surgical procedures. Anesthesiology 2: 281–284
Sear J W, Cooper G M, Kumar V 1983 The effects of old age on recovery: a comparison of the kinetics of thiopentone and althesin. Anaesthesia 38: 1158–1161
Seymour D G, Pringle R 1983 Postoperative complications in the elderly surgical patients. Gerontology 29: 262–270
Shoemaker W C, Appel P L, Kram H B 1988 Prospective trial of supranormal values of survivors as therapeutic goals in high risk surgical patients. Chest 94: 1176–1186
Simpson B R, Williams M, Scott J F, Crampton-Smith A 1961 The effects of anaesthesia and elective surgery on old people. Lancet 2: 888–893
Simpson K H, Smith R J, Davies L F 1985 Comparison of the effects of atropine and glycopyrrolate on cognitive function following general anaesthesia. Br J Anaesth 57: 821
Summary and Recommendations of a Report of the Royal College of Physicians 1989. J R Coll Physicians 23: 8–12
Smith R 1990 The church on aging. Br Med J 301: 829–830
Veterans Administration Co-operative Study Group on Antihypertensive Agents 1972 Effects of treatment on morbidity in hypertension III: influence of age, diastolic pressure and prior cardiovascular disease: further analysis of side effects. Circulation 45: 991–1004
Villar R N, Allen S M, Barnes S J 1986 Hip fractures in healthy patients: operative delay v prognosis. Br Med J 293: 1203–1204
Wolf P A, Kannel W B, Sorlie P, McNamara P 1981 Asymptomatic carotid bruit and risk of stroke. The Framlingham Study. J Am Med Assoc 245(14): 1442–1445

14

Obesity and the safety of anaesthesia

T. H. Taylor

INTRODUCTION

Despite a constant stream of advice on the dangers of obesity, many individuals in the western world are overweight, in some cases grossly so. It has been estimated that 26% of North Americans are obese according to published life insurance tables. Rosenbaum et al (1985) estimated that about 15% of adults are overweight in the UK, and this figure is in close agreement with Van Itallie (1985) in the USA. Although the condition is not uncommon in the elderly, the risks of obesity are much greater in those under the age of 45. Kral (1985) related the incidence and severity of diseases thought to be associated with obesity in early life to the degree of overweight and found them to be exponentially related. The disease entities incriminated in this excess morbidity and mortality are diabetes mellitus, ischaemic heart disease, cancer and hypertension. Furthermore, in addition to making the tasks of the surgeon and anaesthetist technically more difficult, there seems little doubt that obesity increases the morbidity and the mortality of operative procedures, thus making them more hazardous for the obese than the normal population (Andres 1980, Pasulka et al 1986). It is also likely that these people take less regular physical exercise, and are therefore less physically fit, in the commonly understood meaning, than the slimmer individual.

Definitions

The term obesity is used casually by doctors and others, but such is the need for a precise definition that much time and effort have been expended in enunciating one. The use of definite mathematical language is helpful and also aids clinical research. There are two commonly used methods of defining obesity, described below.

The first is the Ideal Body Weight tables so beloved of the insurance companies. Many people are not infrequently aggrieved by the apparently low weights set as normal for a given height by these tables. Ideal body weight can be roughly determined by subtracting 100 from the height in centimetres and expressing the result as kilogrammes. For females, 105 should be deducted. A person 20% or more over the ideal body weight can be considered to be obese. If the excess is greater than 60% the associated disorders, as reported by Kral (1985), reach exponential proportions. At 100% above the desirable weight individuals are deemed to have 'morbid obesity', which carries very serious implications for anaesthesia and, indeed, for life itself. Between 1% and 2% of the population are affected by morbid obesity. This proportion is obviously higher if the more rigorous definition of 'ideal body weight plus 45 kilos' is used, as advocated by some experts in the field.

The second method is more frequently employed in the USA. This is the calculation of the Body Mass Index. The index can be calculated for an individual by dividing the weight in kilogrammes by the square of the height in metres. According to Bray (1976), if the index is under 25 there is no obesity, those between 25 and 30 are overweight, an all over 30 are, by definition, obese. The morbidly obese have an index greater than 35. As mentioned earlier, obesity is of added importance in those younger than 45 years.

In clinical practice it may be easier to use a simple calculation of the ratio of the waist measurement to the hip measurement as a measure of obesity. Obese patients may have the fat distributed primarily to the abdomen (android) or the hip, buttocks and thigh (gynaecoid). In males the waist/hip ratio should not exceed unity, but in females it is somewhat lower, that is the buttocks are larger than the waist (Buckley 1989). There is evidence that fat distributed to the abdomen carries a higher mortality from heart disease than similar weight gain distributed over the buttocks and thighs, as is more commonly seen in women.

Patients in all these categories have a positive calorie intake and, in theory (although rarely in practice), could reduce their weight by dieting before routine surgery. Perhaps by spelling out the inherent dangers of obesity in anaesthesia, patients could be better motivated in seeking a preoperative weight loss before undergoing elective surgery.

PHYSIOLOGICAL CHANGES IN OBESITY

In discussing the anaesthetic problems presented by the obese patient, it is important to comprehend the alterations in normal physiology that progressively occur as the weight of the individual increases (Fisher et al 1975). All systems of the body are involved to a greater or lesser degree, and this involvement is more profound in those whose weight greatly exceeds their ideal. Thus not all individuals over the age of 45 and only moderately obese are at particularly great risk, although logically it would be expected that a threshold could be found where the risks markedly increased. Most of the physiological data presently used have been extrapolated from the morbidly obese patient.

Respiratory reserves

The presence of a large mass of adipose tissue within and on the chest wall and abdomen reduces chest wall compliance. This in turn increases respiratory work and the increased oxygen cost of breathing reduces respiratory muscle efficiency. Lung volume is reduced and the diaphragm assumes a higher position in the chest. Functional residual capacity (FRC) decreases, but residual volume is unchanged. As a result of decreased FRC, airway closure occurs during normal tidal respiration with a consequent reduction in arterial oxygen saturation. Certain postures required for surgery, for example lithotomy, Trendelenberg, prone and even supine positions further reduce FRC and oxygen saturation. Because posture also has a profound effect on extrapulmonary compliance, the component of the compliance that is grossly abnormal in the obese, the untoward effects of these positions required during surgery may be further enhanced.

The extra body mass of the obese patient demands increased oxygen supply and there is an increased output of carbon dioxide. This requires increased alveolar ventilation. Taking this into account and the factors mentioned immediately above, it is obvious that there is a significant increase in the work of breathing at rest. During exercise, oxygen consumption is greatly increased over the normal.

As a result of the reduced oxygen saturation and diminished expiratory reserve volume, obese patients are unable to tolerate even short periods of apnoea without serious hypoxia. Since their anatomical configuration may lead to difficulty in passing an endotracheal tube, constant watch should be kept on the oxygen saturation in the periphery at this stage of an anaesthetic and provision made by the anaesthetist to forestall the rapidly increasing hypoxia which can accompany a slow intubation.

It is notable that most fat patients compensate well for the respiratory disability; the few that do not are the morbidly obese who are clearly at severe risk. The majority of obese patients therefore have a normal arterial carbon dioxide level, but a small proportion suffer from obesity-hypoventilation syndrome (OHS). In this condition, also known as the Pickwickian syndrome, patients are both hypoxic and hypercarbic.

Cardiovascular reserves

In those patients with a considerable degree of obesity, the work of the heart is increased since both the blood volume and the cardiac output are found to be raised, probably in response to the increased total body need for oxygen. The increased flow is predominantly to the splanchnic area and the adipose tissues. Various estimates of the actual rise in these values have been made, and it is probable that it amounts to 0.1 l/min of cardiac output for every kilogramme of excess adipose tissue. The heart rate is usually normal, although it may be slow, so this increase in output is achieved by an increase in stroke volume, thus eventually producing left ventricular hypertrophy. Many observers have directly related a rise in blood pressure to weight gain, and this hypertension is, in the early stages, reversed by a corresponding weight loss. The increased stroke volume and cardiac output in obese patients adds to the total body oxygen consumption and, since total systemic vascular resistance is unaltered, these factors contribute to the increase in systolic and diastolic blood pressure seen in obesity.

Alteration in posture not only changes respiratory parameters, but also affects the cardiovascular system. Moving from the sitting to the supine position is associated with increased cardiac output and pulmonary artery pressure, and because of the added work of respiration is accompanied by a simultaneous increase in oxygen consumption. Alveolar-arterial oxygen difference may remain unchanged if the increased cardiac output is sufficient to mask the effects of increased shunting, but in those patients unable to increase their cardiac output, hypoxia may rapidly develop. Reduction in cardiac output by anaesthesia in the supine position with spontaneous respiration may have an even greater effect.

Pulmonary hypertension is more common than in the normal population, and the rate of myocardial infarction is doubled.

Metabolic reserves

In common with all other organs in the body, the liver of obese subjects is infiltrated by fat. Biochemical tests of liver function may be abnormal, but the degree of fatty infiltration can only be accurately established by liver biopsy, since morphological changes are often more extensive than the biochemical abnormality. It is therefore reasonable to assume that all morbidly obese patients have abnormal liver function and that any decrease in liver blood-flow or oxygen delivery should be avoided. It is reasonable to extrapolate this information to the somewhat less obese, although quantification is less well-documented.

The choice of anaesthetic technique is therefore important in these patients, since it can be seen from the preceding discussion that both patient posture and anaesthetic agents conspire to reduce arterial oxygen tension. It is now clearly established that almost all volatile anaesthetic agents undergo biotransformation in the liver and the toxic effect of free fluoride ion on the kidney is well established. Young et al (1975) demonstrated that the fluoride levels in obese patients may be well within the toxic range after only 3 hours exposure to methoxyflurane. This may partly reflect the large quantities of the highly lipid-soluble substance retained in the fat deposits and consequently available to be metabolised. Vaughan (1982) found that serum fluoride levels were higher in the morbidly obese than in patients of normal weight, following anaesthesia with methoxyflurane, halothane and enflurane.

Young et al (1975) have also demonstrated a small but significant rise in free fluoride levels in obese patients during halothane anaesthesia. While the increases were not to a level considered to be toxic to the kidney, the changes demonstrate that reductive metabolism of halothane is occurring in the obese subject and this might be related to the incidence of unexplained jaundice following anaesthesia. Several studies have suggested that obesity may increase the incidence of 'halothane hepatitis', but the evidence is by no means conclusive since it is now known that obese patients may demonstrate postoperative increases in liver enzymes whatever the anaesthetic technique employed. Tinker et al (1976) have shown that free bromine levels in plasma may also be abnormal following halothane anaesthesia. The degree of elevation of bromine levels was directly related to the inspired concentration and duration of exposure (i.e. MAC hours). Although peak concentrations were not achieved for 2–3 days postoperatively, they remained elevated for up to 22 days. It is conceivable, although not yet proved, that plasma bromine levels would be further elevated in the obese patient as a result of the increased amount of the agent contained in the fatty tissue. Such elevation of bromide concentration, if present, might be expected to produce some additional sedative effect, thus enhancing the action of other depressant drugs on these patients.

The metabolism of enflurane is also enhanced in the obese subject, with a consequent increase in the level of free fluoride ions in the blood. In the absence of further data it would be prudent to be cautious with this drug, especially during a prolonged administration. From the evidence so far available, isoflurane would be the drug of choice because of the relatively low level of biotransformation.

Statistically there is a greater incidence of maturity onset diabetes in obese patients, and many others are resistant to insulin and have a mildly abnormal glucose tolerance curve. They also have high blood levels of cholesterol and triglycerides, and this may be reflected in the degree of atheroma some patients exhibit. There is also a three-fold increase in the incidence of diseases of the biliary tract and the gallbladder.

Pharmacokinetics

The diagnosis of obesity means, by definition, that the individual's body has a smaller proportion of muscle mass and water, and a greater proportion of fat than a normal individual. Thus the distribution of drugs may be different in the obese when compared with those of normal weight, and this may be further modified by poor hepatic and renal function. Diabetes mellitus is more common and may also have an effect, and hyperlipidaemia may affect the protein binding of some drugs. In theory there should be a marked difference in behaviour of the drugs in the hydrophyllic and fat soluble groups.

When a drug is injected intravenously it is initially distributed throughout the central compartment. The overall volume of this compartment appears to increase in obesity, but when expressed in litres per kilogramme its volume is similar in both lean and obese individuals. It is therefore theoretically reasonable to administer the same dose of induction agent per kilogram body weight in both lean and fat patients. In contrast to the central compartment the volume of distribution at steady state (Vdss) is markedly increased in obesity. This may be best defined as that volume of plasma that would be required to contain all the administered drug at the concentration present in the plasma. In the case of thiopentone the Vdss exceeds the total body volume (1.4–2.3 l/kg), so it represents a notional volume only. It may be increased by increased protein binding and for highly lipid-soluble drugs. It is also increased by the presence of extra body fat. Intravenous infusion anaesthesia with thiopentone would be particularly difficult in the obese subject. Very large doses would be required to saturate the increased distribution volume and, although clearance of the drug, adjusted for body weight, is unchanged, terminal elimination half-life is prolonged due to the large body store of the drug. Recovery should therefore be prolonged. Any anaesthetic technique employing repeated intravenous doses of highly fat-soluble drugs in obese patients would lead to a similar situation, that is a prolonged elimination time and therefore delayed recovery.

Hydrophylic drugs have similar volumes of distribution, elimination half-life and metabolic clearance rates in the obese and the normal.

The range of drugs used in anaesthesia includes many that are highly fat-soluble. These include the benzodiazepines and thiopentone, as well as the volatile agents and the opioids, fentanyl and alfentanil. Theoretically, volatile agents, which are distributed eventually to the body fat, and are administered in large doses over time, show disadvantages compared with intravenous agents, the absolute dosage of which can be better controlled. Volatile agents have an increased volume of distribution, with a more select distribution to the fat stores of the body which do not enjoy a rich blood supply. This should mean a longer elimination half-life and should lead to a considerable increase in the time required for recovery in obese individuals. However, Cork et al (1981) compared fentanyl, enflurane and halothane during gastric stapling in the grossly obese. They showed that, used in a normal way for operations of moderate duration, there was no delayed awakening or prolongation of recovery with lipid-soluble volatile agents or with fentanyl. Bentley et al (1981) showed that fentanyl has a similar distribution in the body in the obese and the non-obese patient, with a similar elimination half-time. They suggest that fentanyl should be given on a basis of lean body mass rather than total body weight. In the case of halothane (and other volatile agents) it is probable that a time of exposure of around 24 hours would be required before any delay in recovery time became apparent (Landergaard-Pederson 1981).

HAZARDS OF OBESITY IN ANAESTHETIC PRACTICE

The decision to abandon a projected operation because of the dangers of severe obesity is clearly one to be taken by the surgeon and anaesthetist together, weighing the benefits of the surgery to the patient against the manifest extra dangers of the obesity. The urgency of the procedure must also be taken into account. The morbidly obese are now being subjected to various weight-reducing surgical procedures, commonly to limit their calorie intake, and these provide a special problem of anaesthetic assessment. The anaesthetist must be prepared to emphasize those dangers that arise from the physiological matters outlined above, and explain, if necessary, how the surgery contemplated may add to those dangers.

Preoperative assessment

Simple observation may be sufficient to alert the anaesthetist to the problem of obesity. However some indication of the severity of the obesity may be obtained from a detailed history before any specific tests are undertaken. Thus the importance of taking an adequate history cannot be overemphasized. The previous experience of anaesthesia is important, and direct questions should be asked about dyspnoea and the degree of activity, orthopnea, and snoring. In severe cases there may be a history of daytime sleeping. It is also worth asking the patient about the effect of posture on his breathing.

Clinical examination of an obese patient is more difficult than in a normal subject. Unless care is exercised, vital signs may be missed. In view of this, and the probability of cardiorespiratory abnormalities, the importance of testing lung function and obtaining an adequate chest X-ray cannot be overstressed. A recent ECG is also required. When this evidence is available, an assessment should be made of the potential difficulty on intubation and the technique to be employed should be decided. Soft-tissue X-rays or CT scans of the upper airway may assist in evaluating the degree of difficulty in intubation.

General problems

The difficulties posed by the obese patient are obvious in some respects from the start, for they present formidable problems to the nursing and portering staff responsible for the patient's general care. The difficulty of clinical examination has been mentioned above. X-ray examination may not be so clear, and access to the veins for blood sampling is more difficult, as is induction of anaesthesia and the setting up of intravenous infusions. In some cases it may be wise to insert an arterial cannula for direct pressure measurement and blood-gas sampling. The radial artery at the wrist is often accessible for this purpose, and is easier to enter than the veins. Cuffs for measuring blood pressure do not function well and tourniquets may be too short. Positioning obese patients on the operating table, as well as their subsequent removal, calls for a deal of thought and muscle. Some postures on the operating table, such as the lithotomy position and Trendelenberg position, enhance many of the physiological difficulties of obesity, as mentioned previously.

Premedication

A suitable premedication should usually be given, but the dose may be somewhat less than the gross body weight would suggest, and it should be administered in such a way as to ensure absorption by the time of induction. A subcutaneous injection into body fat is notoriously slow in reaching maximum concentration, presumably because of the relatively poor blood supply of this tissue. This may mean altering the usual time interval, ensuring a deep intramuscular injection, or giving the drugs intravenously. The dose of respiratory depressant drugs must be carefully controlled.

Induction of anaesthesia

There are a number of hazards in the induction phase of anaesthesia, the most important of which are listed below:

1. Vascular access may be so difficult that cannulation of a central vein or a peripheral cutdown may be advisable before induction.
2. Stringent precautions should be taken to prevent aspiration of gastric contents. This is more likely in the obese because the volume of the resting gastric juice is raised and the intragastric pressure is high. The lower oesophageal sphincter is more likely to be incompetent, and the incidence of hiatus hernia, diagnosed or not, may increase this risk. A preoperative antacid regime should be used, for example as recommended in the Appendix 1 (p. 735).
3. Upper airway obstruction during anaesthesia is likely in the grossly obese, and all patients should probably be intubated, except for the most trivial procedures.
4. Difficulty in intubating obese patients is common. The dangers of hypoxia are great and all these patients should be preoxygenated for a suitable period. Inflation via a face mask is undesirable because it increases the dangers of aspirating gastric contents. All available aids to intubation should be on hand, especially a full range of laryngoscopes. If severe difficulty is experienced in a non-urgent case there should be no hesitation in abandoning the procedure until more information or help is available. The required dose of suxamethonium for intubation may be greater than normal, as there is greater activity of pseudocholinesterase in these patients (Bentley et al 1982). Eventually, intubation in an awake patient with local anaesthetic, or even preliminary tracheostomy, may be the only safe course.
5. Cyanosis develops rapidly during apnoea or in the course of respiratory obstruction. Preoxygenation will delay the onset and is mandatory. A pulse oximeter should be in place at all times, although it should be remembered that this device only gives a late warning of hypoxaemia. An end-tidal carbon dioxide analyser is useful, especially in the few patients allowed to breathe spontaneously. It will, of course, also confirm the correct placement of the endotracheal tube.
6. Non-invasive blood-pressure measuring techniques may be unreliable because of the circumference of the patient's arm. The inflatable cuff should occupy at least 75% of the circumference. If monitoring of blood pressure becomes difficult with a non-invasive technique, or for the more major procedures, it is justifiable to insert an arterial cannula. This may also be required to monitor the blood gases. A continuous ECG monitor should also be employed. If a peripheral nerve stimulator is used it may be

necessary to use needle electrodes to apply an appreciable stimulus to obtain a satisfactory endpoint.

Maintenance of anaesthesia

No consensus exists on the ideal anaesthetic sequence for the obese patient. Personal preference must predominate but, whichever technique is chosen, due note must be taken of the alterations in respiratory, cardiovascular and liver functions discussed on pages 214–217. The nearest to a generally accepted technique is a 'balanced anaesthetic' where reflex suppression, analgesia and hypnosis are provided by a combination of drugs, including a muscle relaxant, all given by the intravenous route. The drugs chosen should either have a short duration of action or be easily reversed, so that no postoperative respiratory depression is produced. Large doses of highly lipid-soluble drugs should be avoided and ventilation should be controlled. The advantages of such an anaesthetic sequence would include control of arterial carbon dioxide tension, improved ventilation-perfusion ratios and minimal cardiovascular depression from inhalational agents, and consequently a rapid recovery of consciousness.

The posture of the patient is of utmost importance. It would seem that obese patients are more at risk from nerve palsies occurring during anaesthesia, possibly from increased pressure on the superficial nerves. In particular, ulnar nerve paralysis may occur in obese patients where the elbows are flexed and the hand rests on the chest, especially if this flexion is forced to enable injections into an indwelling needle in the back of the hand.

Recovery from anaesthesia

At the conclusion of the surgical procedure, muscle relaxants should be fully reversed and respiratory depression from opioids minimal. Tidal volumes should have returned to near preoperative levels, and the patient should be awake and responding before the endotracheal tube is removed. This advice is the same for the safe recovery of any patient, but the obese require closer attention to detail if all the many hazards are to be avoided. If any doubt exists over the ability of the patient to breathe adequately, a period of controlled ventilation is mandatory to allow time for the elimination of depressant drugs. There is no margin for any error in this respect in obese subjects. As soon as the general condition permits, the patient should be sat up to assist normal respiration, for the extrapulmonary compliance is improved by relatively reducing the weight of the abdominal wall fat and contents in that position.

Mortality and morbidity

In the longer term the evidence suggests that the obese suffer a higher mortality and morbidity from operations than those of normal weight. Operation wounds tend to break down more easily, and the incidence of both wound and chest infection is higher. Long-term immobilization easily leads to pressure sores, and this is not aided by the difficulty in nursing care mentioned on page 217. Deep-vein thrombosis is common, and this in turn leads to a greater incidence of pulmonary embolism. Obesity of itself is, in the opinion of many, an indication for preoperative and postoperative therapy with subcutaneous heparin, as well as the use of all other prophylactic measures.

Local anaesthesia

From the foregoing paragraphs it would seem that local anaesthetic techniques are indicated for many procedures in the obese patient. However, regional blocks are difficult to perform in these subjects, when even the bony landmarks may be impossible to find. The patients, if awake, often find the postures required of them during surgery difficult to sustain and, as has been previously mentioned, heavy sedation leading to respiratory depression is contraindicated.

When surgery on a limb is contemplated it would seem sensible to avoid general anaesthesia and all sedative drugs, provided that the posture required is tolerable for the awake patient.

Spinal and epidural analgesia are unpredictable in the obese, and hypotension may be profound and require prompt treatment. As a result of increased intra-abdominal pressure in obese patients the epidural veins may be dilated, rendering this technique particularly difficult, reducing the volume of the space and extending the effect of the injected drugs. Dosage may therefore need to be reduced. Continuous observation will be required to prevent hypoventilation and to reduce the discomfort of the postures required for operation. In some cases undergoing abdominal surgery, the addition of a light general anaesthetic consisting mainly of muscle relaxant, to allow controlled ventilation, and nitrous oxide sedation, together with a spinal or epidural anaesthetic, may prove to be a most effective technique.

OBESITY HYPOVENTILATION SYNDROME

The practical comments above all refer to the simple obese subject, although much of the research and physiological data on which it is based is derived from the morbidly obese, that is those patients with a body mass index in excess of 35. The true morbidly obese constitute between 1% and 2% of the population, but about 8% of overweight people have such poor respiratory reserves that constant underventilation ensues, leading to a chronic elevation of the blood carbon dioxide level. In the extreme case they represent the so-called 'Pickwickian Syndrome'. They characteristically show hypoventilation, somnolence during the day, hypoxia and terminally cor pulmonale. These patients present a very real anaesthetic hazard, and should be identified and treated before any surgery is contemplated. It is as a result of problems arising in the surgical treatment of the gross obesity in these subjects that the dangers are now fully realized. The patients have major changes in their cardiovascular and respiratory systems, and only the most urgent procedures should be undertaken in the absence of proper facilities for their postoperative care, which will inevitably mean management in an Intensive Care Unit.

REFERENCES

Andres R 1980 Effect of obesity on total mortality. Int J Obes 4: 381

Bentley J B, Borel J D, Gillespie T S, Vaughan R W, Gondolfi A J 1981 Fentanyl pharmacokinetics in obese and non-obese patients. Anesthesiology 55: A177

Bentley J B, Bond J B, Vaughan R W, Gondolfi A J 1982 Weight, pseudocholinesterase activity and succinylcholine requirements. Anesthesiology 57: 48–49

Bray G A 1976 Who are the obese? In: The obese patient. W B Saunders, Philadelphia, pp 5–43

Buckley F P 1989 Anaesthetic management of the obese. In: Nimmo W S, Smith G (eds) Anaesthesia. Blackwell Scientific, Oxford, vol 1, p 805

Cork R C, Vaughan R W, Bentley J B 1981 General anaesthesia for morbidly obese patients: an examination of post-operative outcomes. Anesthesiology 54: 310–314

Fisher A, Waterhouse T D, Adams A P 1975 Obesity: its relation to anaesthesia. Anaesthesia 30: 633–647

Kral J G 1985 Morbid obesity and related health risks. Ann Intern Med 103: 1043–1047

Landergaard-Pederson M J 1981 Recovery from general anesthesia in obese patients. Anesthesiology 55: 720

Pasulka P S, Bistman B R, Benotti P N, Blackburn G L 1986 The risk of surgery in obese patients. Ann Intern Med 104: 540

Rosenbaum S, Skinner R F, Knight A B, Garrow J S 1985 A survey of height and weight in Great Britain 1980. Ann Hum Biol 12: 115–127

Tinker J H, Gondolfi A J, Van Dyke R A 1976 Elevation of plasma bromide levels in patients following halothane anesthesia: time correlation with total halothane dosage. Anesthesiology 44: 195–196

Van Itallie T B 1985 Health implications of overweight and obesity in the United States. Ann Intern Med 103: 983–988

Vaughan R W 1982 Biochemical and biotransformation alterations in obesity. In: Brown B R (ed) Anesthesia and the obese patient. Contemporary Anesthetic Practice Series. F A Davis, Philadelphia, pp 55–77

Young S R, Stoelting R K, Peterson C, Madura J A 1975 Anesthetic biotransformation and renal function in obese patients during and after methoxyflurane or halothane anaesthesia. Anesthesiology 42: 451–457

FURTHER READING

Adams A P 1982 Nutritional disorders. In: Vickers M D (ed) Medicine for anaesthetists, 2nd edn. Blackwell Scientific, Oxford, ch 12, p 401

Brown B R (ed) 1982 Anaesthesia and the obese patient. G A Davis, Philadelphia

Papers on several aspects of obesity. Br J Hosp Med 1973 10: 8–44

Hazards related to surgical factors

15

Hazards of postoperative pain and its management

M. Morgan

INTRODUCTION

Pain following surgery is probably the most common form of acute, severe pain suffered by man. In recent years there has been an increasing number of publications concerned with its relief, interest in the topic being, no doubt, stimulated by editorial remarks in leading journals, castigating the efforts of the profession in dealing with such an apparently simple problem. Even the Royal College of Surgeons and the College of Anaesthetists have entered the debate with their own report, critical of postoperative pain relief in the UK (1990).

But is it necessary to relieve pain after surgery? The pain, after all, is self-limiting and will eventually go away. Apart from purely humanitarian grounds, however, there are very good reasons why pain relief will result in an improvement in physiological function. The effects of severe pain emanating from thoracic and abdominal incisions on respiration can easily be seen, but the effects of pain resulting in alterations in hormone levels, on metabolic and cardiac function are more subtle and not so immediately obvious. Although there would be little disagreement that postoperative pain should be relieved, it must be remembered that the methods used to achieve this, particularly the more sophisticated techniques, can have serious, and indeed lethal, consequences. It is therefore essential that the potential dangers of the analgesic technique are balanced against the problems that arise from not providing optimum pain relief.

It is not the purpose of this chapter to evaluate the various methods of postoperative analgesia, but rather to consider the complications that may arise from not relieving severe pain after surgery, and those of the various methods used to relieve such pain. There are also a number of non-surgical causes of postoperative discomfort that are usually labelled minor which will be discussed.

HAZARDS OF POSTOPERATIVE PAIN

Although a significant number of the population are so called 'placebo reactors', most anaesthetists would not agree with the use of a placebo in studies on the management of postoperative pain. As a result, controlled trials, in which the hazards of severe pain can be ascertained by withholding treatment in one group of patients, are not possible. Rather the hazards have to be inferred or gleaned from the effects of inadequate analgesia which, unfortunately, is all too common.

Physiological effects

Whether the experience of postoperative pain has a permanent effect on the mental state of patients such that it affects their everyday life is not known. Parbrooke et al (1973) have shown that patients who are unduly apprehensive preoperatively do experience more pain postoperatively. There is also a close correlation between the preoperative neuroticism score and the reduction in vital capacity seen after upper abdominal surgery; this in turn is related to the chest complication rate (Boyle & Parbrooke 1977). Identification of these patients before surgery will indicate the use of more sophisticated methods of pain relief postoperatively, thereby reducing the incidence of complications. Such methods of identification, however, are time-consuming and hardly feasible in most busy hospitals.

That pain after surgery does dwell on the mind is indicated by opinions expressed in the lay and medical press. Thus MacInnes (1976) wrote of his experience of pain after major surgery as 'the grave defect in English public hospital treatment which ... is a cruel and callous disgrace' and condemned 'the nonchalant attitude of the medical profession to quite unnecessary suffering'. Eminent members of the medical profession have also felt moved to record their experiences of major surgery. Following open-heart surgery, Donald (1976) stated, 'I would be a liar if I did not straightaway admit that the pain defies description', while Rhodes (1983) commented on his experiences of being moved after a total hip replacement: 'I shrieked and cursed with pain and was ticked off for doing so'.

Such experiences must be shared by a considerable number of patients who are not in a position to communicate their experiences to the medical profession at large. Every anaesthetist has met patients on their preoperative visit whose main anxiety has been of postoperative pain. On purely humanitarian grounds, therefore, efforts must be made to produce satisfactory analgesia after surgery.

Respiratory effects

The most obvious effects of postoperative pain are on respiration, while the most important single factor determining the severity of such pain is the site of the incision, it being at its worst following thoracic and abdominal surgery.

The response to such pain has been summarized by Bromage (1978). Respiration is markedly inhibited and breathing adopts a grunting nature with tightened muscles in an attempt to prevent further aggravation of the pain. Vital capacity and peak expiratory flow are considerably reduced, and there is a reduction in functional residual capacity and compliance. Respiration is shallow and the lung is ventilated below functional residual capacity so that there are varying degrees of airway closure. Due to the tenseness of the muscles, intrathoracic end-expiratory pressure rises and hence central venous pressure increases. There is a marked impairment of the ability to cough so that secretions may be retained, with resultant areas of collapse, increased shunting and hypoxaemia. Such effects are particularly serious in the presence of pre-existing lung disease. These changes occur to a lesser extent following lower abdominal operations. Surgery on the limbs has virtually no effect on respiration.

The result of abolishing pain after upper abdominal surgery has been accurately described by Simpson et al (1961): 'The patient becomes completely unaware of the existence of an upper abdominal wound; his face loses its expression of anxiety and strain and it is an exciting experience to see a patient, a few hours after gastrectomy, taking deep breaths, coughing vigorously and reaching enthusiastically for his dressing gown.'

Metabolic, endocrine and cardiovascular effects (see also Ch. 8)

The cause-and-effect relationship between pain and hormonal levels, and consequent metabolic and cardiovascular changes in the postoperative period are not as clear-cut as the effects on respiration. Surgical trauma leads to a response characterized by increased adrenergic activity, substrate mobilization and energy consumption. These changes are also pronounced in the post-operative period when there are no direct surgical stimuli; hence Kehlet (1982) has suggested that pain might be a factor contributing to the stress response. Kehlet et al (1980) have pointed out that, following completely uneventful surgery, unexpected complications occur, such as thromboembolism, stress ulcers, myocardial and pulmonary insufficiency, impaired immunocompetence and prolonged convalescence. They proposed that these events are probably precipitated by the endocrine-metabolic response to injury. They summarized existing data in this field and showed that neurogenic blockade plays a major part in inhibiting the stress response to surgery and therefore may result in less postoperative demands on total body function. They therefore suggest that inhibition of the response may lower postoperative morbidity in high-risk patients.

It should be stated that definitive evidence for such a statement does not exist. Again, because it would be quite unethical to withhold analgesia postoperatively, a controlled trial cannot be performed to confirm or refute this hypothesis. Evidence will only eventually come from studying a large number of patients over a prolonged period of time. It can, however, be stated that complete removal of pain inhibits the endocrine-metabolic response to surgery only partially. This response can only be totally prevented during surgery of the lower limb or pelvis. During abdominal hysterectomy a sensory block must extend from S5 to T4 to block the cortisol response. Sensory blockade from S5 to T8 does not affect the cortisol response, even though the patients are pain-free postoperatively (Engquist et al 1977), thus it is essential to block all the sympathetic afferents involved. During upper abdominal surgery, extensive epidural blockade will not inhibit the cortisol response even when combined with vagal blockade (Traynor et al 1982).

There have been few measurements of plasma catecholamine levels during surgery and the postoperative period. Halter et al (1977) showed that both adrenaline and noradrenaline levels were raised during surgery and remained elevated at comparable levels for at least 2 hours postoperatively. The mean arterial blood pressure in these patients showed a positive correlation with the change in plasma catecholamines. More recently, Rutberg et al (1984) measured plasma catecholamines for 24 hours after upper abdominal surgery, pain relief being supplied by epidural bupivacaine, epidural morphine or intravenous morphine. They found that epidural analgesia with bupivacaine suppressed the increase in catecholamines postoperatively and it was noteworthy that the patients who experienced the greatest pain (intravenous morphine group) had the highest catecholamine levels. Experimental work in patients suggests that it is the increase in adrenaline that causes the metabolic and cardiovascular effects, as the levels of noradrenaline attained pre- and postoperatively are insufficient to produce such changes (Silverberg et al 1978, Clutter et al 1980).

It would thus be reasonable to assume that severe postoperative pain plays a predominant part in the increases in arterial blood pressure and cardiac arrhythmias frequently seen postoperatively and mediated by the accompanying increase in circulating catecholamines. Complete relief of pain therefore plays an important part in preventing potentially dangerous cardiovascular changes postoperatively.

Other effects

Following surgery energy expenditure is increased. That pain plays an important role in this effect is illustrated by the fact that the increased oxygen uptake after surgery can be reduced to almost preoperative levels by regional block or narcotic analgesics (Wiklund 1975). Pain also limits movement, thereby contributing to muscle wasting and the possible development of bedsores, which add to the general debility that can occur postoperatively.

Although it was once thought that early mobilization after surgery reduced the incidence of thromboembolic disease, this is now in some doubt. Nevertheless, epidural analgesia extended into the postoperative period markedly reduces the incidence of deep-vein thrombosis and pulmonary embolism (Modig et al 1981). Neurogenic blockade produced by an epidural does not influence the coagulation and fibrinolytic response to surgery (Rem et al 1981). This effect is probably due to the accelerated blood flow produced by the sympathetic block, aided by the patient's ability to move because of his pain-free state.

HAZARDS OF POSTOPERATIVE ANALGESIA

From the above discussion there would be little disagreement about the suggestion that pain contributes substantially to postoperative morbidity, and indeed mortality, and that attempts must be made to relieve pain. However, it must be remembered that the drugs and techniques used to produce analgesia are potent instruments, and complications resulting from their incorrect use can add significantly to postoperative morbidity and even mortality. This particularly applies when sophisticated methods are being used, especially when such methods are not properly controlled due to a lack of adequate facilities to monitor their effects.

By far the most common drugs used to relieve severe pain are the opioids, which may be given by a variety of routes. Less frequently used, although producing superior analgesia, are local anaesthetic agents. Potentially lethal complications are associated with both types of drug.

Complications of opioid analgesia

All opioid analgesics, be they pure or partial agonists, will provide adequate pain relief if given in sufficient amounts. There are some differences between the pure agonists with regard to the incidence and severity of side effects and their pharmacokinetic profiles. The partial agonists share many of the side effects of the pure agonists, but differ in some of their adverse reactions, namely psychotomimetic effects and the much smaller incidence of addiction, although the latter is hardly a problem in the management of postoperative pain.

Varying degrees of sedation will always accompany the administration of opioid drugs. Although this might be desirable from the point of view of the patient, it can have adverse effects by making the patient drowsy and uncooperative so that adequate physiotherapy cannot be carried out. The other basic actions of these drugs, such as inhibition of ciliary activity and of the cough reflex, will also add to the possibility of retention of secretions and consequent pulmonary complications. However, by far the most serious complication associated with the use of opioid analgesics is respiratory depression.

Respiratory effects

Patients differ considerably in the amount of opioids they require to relieve pain after surgery. Mather (1983) has suggested two main reasons for this variability. Firstly, pharmacokinetic variability, which relates to rates of absorption, distribution and elimination of drugs. Secondly, pharmacodynamic variability, which concerns the differences in responses that occur when the tissues of different individuals are presented with the same concentration of a drug. It follows that these two factors also apply to the appearance of complications, such as respiratory depression.

It has been stated that it is a feature of opioids that levels necessary to provide adequate analgesia are always associated with respiratory depression (Bennett & Adams 1983). Indeed it has been noticed that during infusion of pethidine, significant ventilatory depression occurs at pethidine levels below that necessary for analgesia (Rigg et al 1981). Jennett (1977), however, has pointed out that a drug that decreases ventilation does not necessarily cause respiratory depression. Pain might contribute to respiratory drive, and the drug itself may cause metabolic depression, thereby reducing the requirements for ventilation so that a decrease in the latter is appropriate. Jennett has also pointed out that all opioid analgesics that have been compared at approximately equianalgesic doses show very similar respiratory depressant effects, and that they differ only in the timing of the peak effect after administration and in the dose–response relationship.

The respiratory depressant effects of opioids used intraoperatively can extend for some time into the postoperative period, especially when large doses have been used. Particularly disturbing is the fact that prolonged respiratory depression may follow intraoperative use of so-called short-acting narcotics, such as fentanyl. Thus Becker et al (1976) showed a biphasic response of respiration to carbon dioxide challenge postoperatively, which had not returned to normal 4 hours after the last dose of fentanyl. The clinical relevance of this finding was confirmed by Adams & Pybus (1978), who described severe narcosis in two patients 2–4 hours following administration of low to moderate doses of fentanyl. There are also other causes of respiratory depression in the early postoperative period, such as the residual effects of neuromuscular blocking drugs. All of these factors must be taken into account before commencing treatment of postoperative pain with narcotic analgesics.

Another important factor is to eliminate hypoxia as a cause of restlessness after surgery before giving opioids. Administration of these drugs under these circumstances, particularly to dark-skinned patients, can have disastrous consequences, as is documented in several of the reports on confidential enquiries into maternal mortality. Age, too, is an important factor in the appearance of respiratory depression after narcotics. Arunasalam et al (1983) showed that, when given morphine intravenously, more patients in the over-65 age group had periods of apnoea and periodic breathing than those aged between 28 and 37 years. Arunasalam et al concluded that the older patients were in much more danger of becoming hypoxic and that extra care should be taken in monitoring them for evidence of respiratory depression.

There is a large amount of evidence in the literature that suggests the conventional method of postoperative analgesia, namely an intramuscular injection of an opioid given at the discretion of a nurse, is quite inadequate for the vast majority of patients. Sublingual and oral administration of appropriate preparations will also result in inadequate analgesia if prescribed in the same manner, although, given on a regular basis, they might provide adequate pain relief (Derbyshire et al 1984). The reason for the inadequate analgesia is obviously insufficient dosage given at too infrequent intervals. As a result, of course, clinically significant respiratory depression is virtually never reported following conventional postoperative analgesia. Of much more importance are the potential consequences following intravenous use.

Intravenous infusion of opioids

The most rapid way of achieving adequate analgesia with narcotics is to give the drug intravenously. Titration of small doses against the patient's needs has been used for many years. A logical consequence of this is to utilize a continuous infusion, thereby eliminating fluctuations in blood levels achieved with bolus injections. It has also been pointed out that, should any complication occur during an intravenous infusion, stopping the infusion will result in an immediate fall in the blood level, as opposed to the relentless absorption that will occur following intramuscular injection.

Administration of the drug intravenously, however, will result in the agent rapidly reaching the vital centres in the medulla, hence it is not surprising that respiratory depressant effects will be seen more frequently and be more severe than with other routes of administration. All opioids decrease the sensitivity of the respiratory centre to carbon dioxide and the rate of respiration is affected rather than the depth. Thus, with increasing dosage, respiration becomes slower until eventually complete apnoea results.

Catling et al (1980) investigated the breathing pattern of patients receiving a continuous intravenous infusion of papaveretum after cholecystectomy. Satisfactory pain relief was associated with respiratory depression indicated by a rise in arterial carbon dioxide tension, slow respiratory rate and periods of apnoea of up to 40 s. There was no correlation with dose, indicating a large individual variation. Further work by Catley et al (1982a) revealed that an oxygen saturation of less than 80% associated with periods of paradoxical respiration occurred in patients receiving a morphine infusion after surgery. This evidence of respiratory depression occurs much less frequently when a regional block is used to provide postoperative analgesia (Catley et al 1982b).

In the obstructive sleep apnoea syndromes, profound hypoxia has been shown to occur. This in turn may have caused the deaths that have been reported in several such patients due to arrhythmias. It is quite possible that a similar sequence of events might result during continuous infusions of narcotics in the postoperative period. Here there is already a fall in arterial oxygen tension due to impaired gas exchange that occurs following surgery. This would be compounded by the respiratory depression produced by the narcotic which, together with the periods of apnoea, could lead to profound hypoxia and possible cardiac arrhythmias.

The available evidence indicates that even modest doses of narcotics used postoperatively may produce periodic breathing, which in some patients may cause life-threatening hypoxaemia. Patients receiving continuous intravenous infusions of narcotics must therefore be closely monitored.

Patient-controlled analgesia

As the patient is the only judge of the amount of pain experienced, the technique of patient-controlled anaesthesia (PCA) is being used increasingly and undoubtedly provides better analgesia than conventional methods. Sophisticated machinery is required, however, and thus there is always the potential for complications to occur with the development of profound respiratory depression.

White (1987) has highlighted three main areas where things can go wrong with PCA. The most common is operator errors, with mistakes in programming, failure to clamp or unclamp tubes, improper filling of syringes, failure to respond to safety alarms and misplacing the PCA pump key. Patient errors result from failure to understand the method and the device, and possibly intentional analgesic abuse. Mechanical problems can also occur with the machine failing to deliver on demand, defective valves and cracked syringes. Notcutt & Morgan (1990) also reported equipment malfunction as the most common problem with PCA, but noted that inadequate monitoring on the ward was also common.

Partial agonists

Partial agonists, such as pentazocine, butorphanol, buprenorphine and nalbuphine will have a lower maximum effect than pure agonists, and this will apply to respiratory depression as well as to analgesia. The presence of a 'ceiling effect', that is a point at which no further respiratory depression will occur despite an increase in dose, has been shown for these drugs. Animal experiments indicate that, with regard to buprenorphine, autoantagonism might occur producing a bell-shaped dose–response curve (Cowan et al 1977). This does not mean that these drugs can be used with immunity, as severe respiratory depression and hypoxaemia do occur. It is not known whether autoantagonism occurs in man, but doses of up to 7 mg of buprenorphine have been given intravenously for postoperative pain with no adverse effect (Budd 1981).

Epidural and intrathecal opioids

The discovery of opiate receptors in the spinal cord soon led to the demonstration in animals, then man, of prolonged and effective analgesia following injection of small doses of opioids epidurally and intrathecally. At last it was hoped that it would be possible to divorce analgesia from respiratory depression with these drugs. However, this was not to be, and reports soon appeared of profound respiratory depression following both intrathecal and epidural administration, but particularly the former. Even more sinister was the fact that respiratory depression could be delayed for several hours after injection, particularly following morphine, when the patient might have been transferred back to an ordinary ward. The respiratory depression is readily reversed by naloxone.

The incidence of respiratory depression can only be gleaned from reports of large series, although numerous case reports can be found in the literature. Such series have only been reported after epidural morphine (Table 15.1), where respiratory depression can be delayed for as long as 16 hours and can also recur after treatment with naloxone. With the more fat-soluble drugs, the complication can occur soon after injection due to systemic absorption. Nevertheless, occasional cases of profound, delayed respiratory depression have been reported (Table

Table 15.1 Respiratory depression following epidural opioids (references from Morgan 1989)

Morphine	n	Dose	Respiratory depression Number	Incidence	Fat soluble opioids	Dose	Respiratory depression Time after injection
Stenseth et al 1985	1085	4–6 mg	10	1:109 (0.9%)	Diamorphine	2–10 mg	20 min–4.5 h
Ready et al 1988	623	4–5 mg	4	1:156 (0.6%)	Pethidine	50–100 mg	5–30 min
Writer et al 1985	128	5 mg	4	1:32 (3.1%)	Methadone	4–6 mg	20 min–4 h
					Hydromorphone	1 mg	4.5 h
					Sufentanil	50 μg	5–15 min
					Fentanyl	100 μg	100 min

15.1). Particularly disturbing is the report of such a case in a fit, healthy, young woman, given 100 μg fentanyl, who had received no other central depressant drugs (Brockway et al 1990). Previously there had been no authenticated reports following this very fat-soluble opioid.

Wheatley et al (1990) investigated the incidence of postoperative hypoxaemia in healthy patients who had received PCA with diamorphine, epidural diamorphine or intramuscular morphine for postoperative analgesia. They found that hypoxaemia occurred in all groups, but tended to last for longer periods in those given epidural diamorphine. The periods of hypoxaemia usually occurred at night.

Certain factors appear to predispose to the appearance of respiratory depression (Cousins & Mather 1984). These include advanced age, high dose, intrathecal injection, thoracic epidurals, grunting respiration, concomitant use of central depressant drugs by other routes, intolerance to opioids and the use of hydrophilic drugs such as morphine. A fat-soluble drug, for example diamorphine, pethidine or fentanyl, will be rapidly absorbed into the circulation and some degree of early respiratory depression might be expected (Table 15.1). That entering the cerebrospinal fluid (CSF) would be 'leached' into the spinal cord with its high fat content and only very little would remain in the CSF. Morphine is very poorly fat soluble and would enter the spinal cord only slowly. Much more drug would linger in the CSF and be available for rostral spread. The higher incidence of delayed respiratory depression with this agent is borne out in clinical practice. Cousins & Mather have also pointed out that, given parenterally, only about 0.1% of morphine is taken up into the brain. Thus of 100 mg morphine given intravenously, only 100 μg would penetrate the CNS, whereas a typical intrathecal dose would be 250–500 μg.

'Minor' complications are also common after spinal (especially intrathecal) opioids, and are again more common after morphine. Incidences of pruritus, nausea and vomiting, and urinary retention of 40–60% are frequently reported. The latter is probably the most problematical complication.

The nature and incidence of the complications following spinal opioids have important implications for postoperative management. These patients cannot be looked after on an ordinary ward. Surveillance has to be continuous, and monitoring simple and applicable to several patients at once. The constant presence of a properly trained nurse provides the best monitor. It has been shown that a slow respiratory rate is an unreliable and late sign of ventilatory depression and is poorly correlated to hypoxaemia (Catley et al 1985). The reduction in minute volume after epidural morphine is largely due to a reduction in tidal volume. Selection of monitoring is therefore important. Apnoea alarms are of no use as this is the very complication that should have been prevented. Continuous capnography would be an excellent monitor but such machines are not readily available for postoperative use. Oximetry has the disadvantage of a delay in response and there would be many false alarms when the oxygen mask slipped off the face. Instructions must be left as to the treatment of both major and minor complications, and naloxone must be immediately available.

Spinal opioids have now been in use for over 10 years in the treatment of postoperative pain, and a number of conclusions can be drawn:

1. Although there are a number of factors that make the appearance of delayed respiratory depression more likely, its occurrence is largely unpredictable.
2. Morphine, because of its high incidence of complications, is not a suitable drug for postoperative pain relief by the spinal route.
3. Delayed respiratory depression is much more rare after the fat-soluble drugs, but can still appear after 4–5 hours. Early depression within 30 min is more likely.
4. All opioid drugs have the propensity to cause respiratory depression when injected epidurally. Although clinical reports are lacking after some opioids, they have nevertheless been shown experimentally to possess this action.
5. Because of all the known facts concerning spinal opioids it would be insouciant to nurse such patients on an ordinary ward postoperatively.

Reversal of respiratory depression

As a competitive antagonist is available in the form of naloxone, it can be argued that respiratory depression is not a problem following agonist drugs since it can be reversed instantly. However, naloxone reverses all the actions of narcotics including analgesia, and indeed can cause hyperalgesia, resulting in unacceptable discomfort for the patient. The necessary use of naloxone has been described as a failure of narcotic management (Bennett & Adams 1983). Although naloxone is generally regarded as being a very safe drug, sudden death has been reported immediately following its use (Andree 1980). Furthermore, naloxone will satisfactorily reverse the respiratory depression of a partial agonist such as pentazocine, but is usually ineffective in restoring ventilation in the case of buprenorphine, which is tightly bound to the receptors.

Naloxone is also a short-acting drug. Doxapram, a non-specific antagonist acting via the chemoreceptors, is as effective as naloxone in reversing narcotic-induced respiratory depression and has no effect on the analgesic action. It is the recommended drug for the reversal of ventilatory depression due to buprenorphine. However, doxapram is also relatively short-acting and can produce unpleasant central effects.

Pharmacokinetics

It is now possible to measure small amounts of drugs in plasma due to improved assay techniques. This has led to suggested schemes of achieving a constant plasma level of a drug by continuous infusion preceded by a bolus or loading infusion dose. The use of such schemes for infusions of narcotics in the postoperative period is potentially dangerous. Such methods rely on computer programs, which may be inaccurate, and on the plasma assay of drugs. Mather (1983) has emphasized the need for critical evaluation of the methods of drug assay. The infusion regimens are usually suggested following measurements in a few fit and healthy patients or volunteers, and therefore cannot be applied to all patients, who will have varying degrees of hydration, and of hepatic and renal function. The effects of other drugs must also be borne in mind.

There is an enormous variation in response to narcotics, and it is generally agreed that a relationship between plasma concentration and analgesia does not exist for many drugs. Reilly et al (1985) reviewed all the data then available on the pharmacokinetic parameters of fentanyl and found a wide discrepancy in the reported results. They questioned the clinical application of current pharmacokinetic data for this drug. Thus it must be emphasized that infusion rates of analgesics postoperatively must be regulated to each individual patient's needs.

Cardiovascular effects

In normal man the potent narcotic agonists have little effect on arterial blood pressure. Some slight fall might be expected due to a combination of sedation, pain relief, vasomotor centre depression and histamine release. This fall would be accentuated by adoption of the upright posture, hypovolaemia and the presence of other drugs, such as phenothiazines. Occasionally, pethidine can be accompanied by a considerable reduction in arterial pressure, and experimentally it produces 100–200 times greater myocardial depression than morphine (Strauer 1972). Pentazocine causes a slight rise in blood pressure and heart rate following intravenous use, associated with a rise in circulating catecholamines. Buprenorphine causes little circulatory disturbance.

Other effects

There are several other unpleasant side effects associated with all opioid analgesics, the incidence varying according to the particular agent. Nausea and vomiting can be particularly distressing, although there are many other causes of this in the postoperative period. Nausea and vomiting are more common when patients move postoperatively, indicating an increased sensitivity of the vestibular apparatus. The problem is also more frequent when blood opioid concentrations change rapidly, as with an intravenous bolus injection, than if the same concentration were reached slowly (Mather 1983). The study of Andersen & Krogh (1976), however, showed that relief of pain by opioids resulted in a reduction in the incidence of nausea and vomiting, while these were unabated if pain relief was inadequate. Opioid analgesics markedly delay gastric emptying and retard the return of normal gastrointestinal function postoperatively.

Physical dependence (addiction) is not a complication that need be feared in the treatment of postoperative pain. It is interesting to note, however, that a survey of nursing and junior medical staff reported that quite a number thought this might be a problem in a significant number of patients (Weiss et al 1983).

COMPLICATIONS OF REGIONAL ANAESTHESIA (see also Ch. 38)

The use of local anaesthetics to relieve pain after surgery has the advantage that analgesia is complete with no central depression. Nevertheless, serious complications can occur and might be related to the toxic effects of the drug or to the physiological changes produced by the nerve block. Any nerve can be blocked after surgery provided it is accessible, but the only two techniques that are really feasible are intercostal and epidural blocks.

Intercostal block

Intercostal block can provide complete somatic analgesia after thoracic and upper abdominal surgery. As the block is frequently performed bilaterally and therefore involves a relatively large volume of local anaesthetic solution at multiple sites, it is not surprising that plasma concentrations are high. The same applies when the nerves are blocked using the interpleural technique. Signs of systemic toxicity must therefore always be sought, but reports of such occurrences are extremely rare. This might be related to the increase in alpha acid glycoprotein which occurs in the plasma postoperatively and provides the binding sites for bupivacaine (Wulf et al 1988). Thus increased plasma bupivacaine levels can occur without an increase in the free level of drug, which is responsible for systemic toxicity.

The production of a pneumothorax is always possible following intercostal block. This would be particularly serious in patients with chronic pulmonary disease who would be most likely to benefit from this form of pain relief. However, the complication is very rare. Moore (1975) reported an incidence of 0.07% in over 10 000 blocks, and this only rises to 0.4% when routine X-rays are taken afterwards (Thompson 1980). Figures following interpleural block are not available as large series have yet to be reported.

Although the limiting effects of pain on ventilation are well known and are particularly serious in patients with pre-existing chest disease, paralysis of intercostal and abdominal muscles by an intercostal block in these patients can have serious consequences. Following studies in patients with chronic lung disease, Sharp et al (1977) concluded that such patients are liable to have abnormal diaphragmatic function and that ventilation depends to a greater extent than normal on the rib-cage musculature. Carey & Mulroy (1981) and Casey (1984) have described patients with the condition who developed respiratory failure following bilateral intercostal block for postoperative pain relief. Engberg (1978) reported that bilateral intercostal block after surgery was associated with a higher incidence of pulmonary complications than unilateral block, this figure being 50% in those over 60 years of age. It is interesting to note that most studies of lung function that compare complete pain relief with epidural block and narcotic analgesia have specifically excluded those with lung disease. When using local anaesthetics, therefore, it is important to choose a concentration that produces minimal interference with motor function, particularly in the elderly and those with chronic lung disease.

Epidural analgesia (see also pp. 600–604)

There would be no disagreement that epidural block provides the best pain relief after surgery. However, the technique is sophisticated and associated with a number of complications, some of which are potentially lethal. Thus continuous monitoring is mandatory for patients receiving this type of analgesia postoperatively.

Any of the technical problems associated with epidural analgesia may be seen. A dural puncture rate of around 0.5% can be expected, with all its consequences that might add to patient discomfort. There is also a small incidence of failure to locate and/or cannulate the epidural space. Occasional cases of nerve damage, sometimes paraplegia, are reported. These result either from direct needle damage or following the physiological effects of extensive sympathetic blockade. By far the most common and potentially dangerous complication is hypotension. It is essential that, before any local anaesthetic solution is injected, the circulating volume must be adequate, and a vasopressor and atropine must be available for immediate use. Conacher et al (1983) reported that 62% of their patients developed hypotension during an epidural infusion of bupivacaine into the thoracic region after pulmonary surgery. In 36% this was described as being moderate or severe. Urinary retention occurred in 31% of patients, while possible toxicity to the local anaesthetic occurred in 3%. Because of the complications, the technique was abandoned in 3% of patients. Griffiths et al (1975) also found that hypotension was troublesome during thoracic epidural analgesia, but the blood pressure was more stable when the local anaesthetic was given by continuous infusion rather than by intermittent injection, although the incidence of urinary retention was higher.

Prolonged use of local anaesthetics via the epidural route might also lead to tachyphylaxis. A careful watch must therefore be kept for evidence of drug toxicity.

Other methods of analgesia

The use of a cryoprobe has been described for pain relief after surgery and complete analgesia lasting several weeks can result. However, the loss of sensation may result in damage occurring to the appropriate area of skin without the patient's knowledge.

Nitrous oxide can be extremely useful in providing pain relief in the immediate postoperative period, particularly in patients requiring artificial ventilation. It is now well established that nitrous oxide interferes with the metabolism of vitamin B_{12} and that prolonged exposure is not necessary to produce an effect. The clinical relevance of this in man is dubious, although it should not be used in patients with known disorders of vitamin B_{12} metabolism. Prolonged use of nitrous oxide results in bone marrow depression.

MINOR SEQUELAE

There are a number of minor sequelae that occur postoperatively and are so called because they are presumably not life-threatening. They may, however, be in no way regarded as minor by the patient, and can adopt a significance that is far greater than the discomfort produced by the surgical wound.

Traumatic sequelae

Damage to the lips and gums during tracheal intubation can produce considerable discomfort postoperatively, as can dental trauma which has been reported in 1.2% of 513 patients interviewed by Edmonds-Seal & Eve (1962). Multiple attempts at venepuncture can result in painful bruising. This can last for several days and may be quite incapacitating if situated on the dorsum of the hand. It is important to protect a patient's eyes, particularly when in the prone and lateral positions, and when the head is covered by towels. Corneal abrasions are extremely painful and occurred in 0.6% of patients in the above series. Permanent damage with scarring is possible.

Backache

Edmonds-Seal & Eve (1962) reported that some 11% of patients developed symptoms post-operatively that were associated with lifting and moving them while anaesthetized. In particular, 24% of patients placed in the lithotomy position were troubled by backache postoperatively. A number of patients also complained of pain in the heels, around the knee and in the elbow.

As a large-diameter needle is used to perform an epidural block, it might be expected that there would be a high incidence of backache, but this is certainly not so after an atraumatic epidural. The incidence of backache is much higher in obstetric patients, but is more or less the same whether an epidural is used or not (Moir & Davidson 1972).

Headache can also be a problem post-operatively, but this is a common everyday problem and certainly a tendency to headaches is the most important factor determining its occurrence after surgery. It is more common in women, and unrelated to the severity of surgery and duration of anaesthesia, but halothane may be a causative factor (Tyrell & Feldman 1968).

Suxamethonium pains

Muscle pains and stiffness in the early post-operative period may occur as a result of suxamethonium administration, the reported incidence varying from virtually zero to almost 100%. These pains are usually located in the neck, shoulders, anterior chest-wall and upper abdomen, and are rare in the limbs. The pains usually occur within 24 hours, but occasionally may be more delayed and can last for as long as 5–6 days. They can be severe enough to limit activity. The factors determining the appearance of these pains have been summarized by Craig (1964). They are more common following early ambulation and less common in children. There is no relationship between their severity, and the degree of physical fitness and muscle development, nor is there any correlation with the severity of visible muscle fasciculations.

Waters & Mapleson (1971) attributed the pain to damage in muscle caused by incoordinate contractions preceding the paralysis. They therefore predicted, and indeed confirmed, that the incidence of pains would decrease if large single doses were used, as the degree of synchrony of contraction would be greater. Also, multiple doses, each being given following full recovery from the previous dose, will increase the probability of pain. It is noteworthy that Crawford (1971) reported a very low incidence of pains (1.5%) in pregnant patients in whom paralysis was induced with suxamethonium (100 mg) and maintained with a continuous infusion.

A number of pharmacological approaches have been used to reduce the incidence of these pains, but the only easily applied methods involve the administration of a small 'taming' dose of suxamethonium (Strom & Jansen 1984) or of a small dose of a competitive relaxant. Use of the latter, however, although effective, does antagonize the action of suxamethonium so that larger amounts have to be used. Suxamethonium pains can be so disabling postoperatively that serious consideration must be given to this drug's use in patients who will be ambulatory soon after surgery.

Sore throat (see also p. 498)

Sore throat is another complaint that can be extremely distressing to a patient in the post-operative period. The reported incidence again varies widely. In a large series, Wolfson (1958) reported a frequency of 16%, with the condition being severe in 2.5% of cases. A hoarse voice occurred in 3%. Symptoms lasted from 3 hours to 7 days, lasting longer than 2 days in 10% of patients. As with other reports, the incidence was more common in women and following surgery in the prone position.

There are several factors that determine the appearance of sore throats. A sore throat can occur in patients who are not intubated and the presence of a cuff on the tracheal tube has little effect on the number of affected patients (Loeser et al 1980). Loeser et al have shown that, surprisingly, lubrication of the tube provides no advantage in terms of sore throat, and that the incidence may even be increased by use of local anaesthetic jelly or ointment on the tube. Intubation time, age and intracuff pressure do not appear to be causative factors, but sore throat is highly correlated with the length of the tracheal tube cuff. The area of contact between the cuff and the trachea has been confirmed by others to be related to the incidence of sore throat (Jensen et al 1982). Other causative factors include drying of secretions with anticholinergics, use of throat packs and administration of suxamethonium.

CONCLUSIONS

Apart from the almost indescribable distress caused by severe postoperative pain, the restriction on all movement and physiological changes occasioned by the presence of this pain can result in serious disturbances of normal function, particularly in those patients with pre-existing respiratory and cardiovascular disease. Every effort should therefore be made to treat this pain.

In 1944, Waters commented: 'Relief of pain is purchased always at a price. The price in both morbidity and mortality does not greatly differ whatever the agent or agents used.' This statement remains largely true today. All methods of pain relief are attended by complications, some of which are potentially lethal. The latter particularly applies to those sophisticated methods necessary to bring about the most effective pain relief and especially so in those patients who would most benefit from it, that is those with pre-existing cardiorespiratory disease. It must therefore be stressed not only that any method of pain relief must be effective, but also that it must be safe and feasible within the context of the staff and facilities that are available in any particular environment. With the constraints that apply within the UK today, it is regrettable that the superior methods of pain relief cannot be applied to the majority of patients because of the lack of staff and facilities to provide the constant supervision necessary to deal with any complications. The choice of patients for such treatment should lie with the individual anaesthetist.

At the moment it seems that postoperative pain will continue to be treated in the majority of patients with opioid drugs. The advent of many new agents in this field has not proved to be an advance. It remains to be seen whether modifications to the molecules of the endogenous opioids will result in the production of better analgesia without the attendant complications. Another approach might be the inhibition of the breakdown of these substances by enkephalinase inhibitors. Both types of agent have been used experimentally.

The so-called minor complications of anaesthesia can cause considerable patient discomfort. As Riding (1975) pointed out, the frequency of these complications is such that 'attention to refinements in the management of anaesthesia would be advantageous to the patients'.

REFERENCES

Adams A P, Pybus D A 1978 Delayed respiratory depression after use of fentanyl during anaesthesia. Br Med J 1: 278–279

Andersen R, Krogh K 1976 Pain as a major cause of post-operative nausea. Can Anaesth Soc J 23: 366–369

Andree R A 1980 Sudden death following naloxone administration. Anesth Analg 58: 524–525

Arunasalam K, Davenport H T, Painter S, Jones J G 1983 Ventilatory response to morphine in young and old subjects. Anaesthesia 38: 529–533

Becker L D, Paulson B S, Miller R D, Severinghaus J W, Eger E I 1976 Biphasic respiratory depression after fentanyl-droperidol or fentanyl alone used to supplement nitrous oxide anaesthesia. Anesthesiology 44: 291–296

Bennett M R D, Adams A P 1983 Postoperative respiratory complications of opiates. In: Bullingham R E S (ed) Opiate analgesia. Saunders, London pp 41–56

Boyle P, Parbrooke G D 1977 The interrelation of personality and postoperative factors. Br J Anaesth 49: 259–264

Brockway M S, Noble D W, Sharwood-Smith G H, McLure J H 1990 Profound respiratory depression after extradural fentanyl. Br J Anaesth 64: 243–245

Bromage P R 1978 Epidural analgesia. Saunders, Philadelphia.

Budd K 1981 High dose buprenorphine for postoperative analgesia. Anaesthesia 36: 900–903

Carey P C, Mulroy M 1981 Postoperative respiratory failure following intercostal block. Anesthesiology 54: 418–419

Casey W F 1984 Respiratory failure following intercostal nerve blockade. Anaesthesia 39: 351–354

Catley D M, Thornton C, Jordan C, Royston D, Lehane J R, Jones J G 1982a Postoperative respiratory depression with continuous morphine infusion. Br J Anaesth 54: 235P

Catley D M, Thornton C, Jordan C, Royston D, Lehane J R, Jones J G 1982b. Continuous postoperative monitoring reveals oxygen desaturation associated with paradoxical respiration. Am Rev Respir Dis 125: 105

Catley D M, Thornton C, Jordan C, Lehane J R, Jones J G 1985 Pronounced episodic oxygen desaturation in the postoperative period: its association with ventilatory pattern and analgesic regimen. Anesthesiology 63: 20–28

Catling J A, Pinto D M, Jordan C, Jones J G 1980 Respiratory effects of analgesia after cholecystectomy: comparison of continuous and intermittent papaveretum. Br Med J 281: 478–480

Clutter W E, Bier D M, Shah S D, Cryer P E 1980 Epinephrine plasma metabolic clearance rates and physiological thresholds for metabolic and hemodynamic actions in man. J Clin Invest 66: 94–101

Conacher I D, Paes M L, Jacobson I, Phillips P D, Heaviside D W 1983 Epidural analgesia following thoracic surgery: a review of two years' experience. Anaesthesia 38: 546–551

Cousins M J, Mather L E 1984 Intrathecal and epidural administration of opioids. Anesthesiology 61: 276–310

Cowan A, Lewis J W, MacFarlane I 1977 Agonist and antagonist properties of buprenorphine, a new antinociceptive agent. Br J Pharmacol 60: 537–545

Craig H J L 1964 The protective effect of thiopentone against muscle pain and stiffness which follows the use of suxamethonium chloride. Br J Anaesth 56: 612–619

Crawford J S 1971 Suxamethonium muscle pains and pregnancy. Br J Anaesth 43: 677–680

Derbyshire D R, Vater M, Maille C I D, Larsson I M, Aitkenhead A R, Smith G 1984 Non-parental postoperative analgesia: a comparison of sublingual buprenorphine and morphine sulphate (slow release) tablets. Anaesthesia 39: 324–328

Donald I 1976 At the receiving end: a doctor's personal recollection of second-time valve replacement. Scott Med J 21: 49–57

Edmonds-Seal J, Eve N H 1962 Minor sequelae of anaesthesia: a pilot study. Br J Anaesth 34: 44–48

Engberg G 1978 Relief of postoperative pain with intercostal blockade compared with the use of narcotic drugs. Acta Anaesthesiol Scand Supplement 70: 36–38

Engquist A, Brandt M, Fernandes A, Kehlet H 1977 The blocking effect of epidural analgesia on the adrenocortical and hyperglycaemic response to surgery. Acta Anaesthesiol Scand 21: 330–335

Griffiths D P G, Diamond A W, Cameron J D 1975 Postoperative epidural analgesia following thoracic surgery: a feasibility study. Br J Anaesth 47: 48–55

Halter J B, Plug A E, Porte D 1977 Mechanism of plasma catecholamine increase during surgical stress in man. J Clin Endocrinol Metab 45: 936–944

Jennett S 1977 Respiratory effects of strong analgesics. In: Harcus A W, Smith R, Whittle B (eds) Pain: new perspectives in measurement and management. Churchill Livingstone, Edinburgh, pp 34–40

Jensen P E, Hommelgaard P, Søndergaard P, Eriksen S 1982 Sore throat after operation: influence of tracheal intubation, intracuff pressure and type of cuff. Br J Anaesth 54: 453–457

Kehlet H 1982 The endocrine-metabolic response to post-operative pain. Acta Anaesthesiol Scand Supplement 74: 173–175

Kehlet H, Brandt M R, Rem J 1980 Role of neurogenic stimuli in mediating endocrine-metabolic response to surgery. J Parenter Enteral Nutr 4: 152–156

Loeser E A, Stanley T H, Jordan W, Machin R 1980 Post-operative sore throat: influence of tracheal tube lubrication versus cuff design. Can Anaesth Soc J 27: 156–158

MacInnes C 1976 Cancer ward. New Society 36: 232–234

Mather L E 1983 Pharmacokinetic and pharmacodynamic factors influencing the choice, dose and route of administration of opiates for acute pain. In: Bullingham R E S (ed) Opiate analgesia. Saunders, London, pp 17–40

Modig J, Hjelmstedt A, Shalstedt B, Maripuu E 1981 Comparative influences of epidural and general anaesthesia on deep vein thrombosis and pulmonary embolism after total hip replacement. Acta Chir Scand 147: 125–130

Moir D D, Davidson S 1972 Postpartum complications of forceps delivery performed under epidural and pudendal nerve block. Br J Anaesth 44: 1197–1199

Moore D C 1975 Intercostal block for postoperative somatic pain following surgery of thorax and upper abdomen. Br J Anaesth 47: 284–286

Morgan M 1989 The rational use of intrathecal and extradural opioids. Br J Anaesth 63: 165–188

Notcutt W G, Morgan R J M 1990 Introducing patient

controlled analgesia for postoperative pain control into a district general hospital. Anaesthesia 45: 401–406
Parbrooke G D, Steel D F, Dalrymple D G 1973 Factors predisposing to postoperative pain and pulmonary complications. Br J Anaesth 45: 21–23
Reilly C S, Wood A J J, Wood M 1985 Variability of fentanyl pharmacokinetics in man: computer predicted plasma concentrations for three intravenous dosage regimens. Anaesthesia 40: 837–843
Rem J, Feddersen C, Brandt M, Kehlet H 1981 Postoperative changes in coagulation and fibrinolysis independent of neurogenic stimuli and adrenal hormones. Br J Surg 68: 229–233
Rhodes P 1983 Getting a new hip joint. Br Med J 287: 747–748
Riding J E 1975 Minor complications of anaesthesia. Br J Anaesth 47: 91–101
Rigg J R A, Ilsley A H, Vedig E 1981 Relationships of ventilatory depression to steady state blood pethidine concentrations. Br J Anaesth 53: 613–619
Royal College of Surgeons of England and the College of Anaesthetists 1990 Commission on the Provision of Surgical Services. Report of Working Party on Pain after Surgery.
Rutberg H, Hakanson E, Anderberg B, Jorfeldt L, Martensson J, Schuldt B 1984 Effects of extradural administration of morphine, or bupivacaine, on the endocrine response to upper abdominal surgery. Br J Anaesth 56: 233–238
Sharp J C, Goldberg N B, Druz W S, Fishman H C, Danon J 1977 Thoracoabdominal motion in chronic obstructive pulmonary disease. Am Rev Respir Dis 115: 47–56
Silverberg A B, Shah S D, Haymond M W, Cryer P E 1978 Norepinephrine hormone and neurotransmitter in man. Am J Physiol 234: E252–256
Simpson B R, Parkhouse J, Marshall R, Lambrechts W 1961 Extradural analgesia and the prevention of post-operative respiratory complications. Br J Anaesth 33: 628–641
Strauer B E 1972 Contractile responses to morphine, piritramide, meperidine and fentanyl: a comparative study of effects on the isolated ventricular myocardium. Anesthesiology 37: 304–310
Strom J, Jansen E C 1984 Pain-reducing effect of self-taming suxamethonium. Acta Anaesthesiol Scand 28: 40–43
Thompson G E 1980 Celiac plexus, intercostal and minor peripheral blockade. In: Cousins M J, Bridenbaugh P O (eds) Neural blockade in clinical anesthesia and management of pain. Lippincott, Philadelphia pp 384–404
Traynor C, Paterson J L, Ward I D, Morgan M, Hall G M 1982 Effects of extradural analgesia and vagal blockade on the metabolic and endocrine response to upper abdominal surgery. Br J Anaesth 54: 319–323
Tyrrell F M, Feldman S A 1968 Headache following halothane anaesthesia. Br J Anaesth 40: 99–102
Waters R M 1944 Anesthesia and breathing. Minn Med 207: 909–912
Waters D J, Mapleson W W 1971 Suxamethonium pains: hypothesis and observation. Anaesthesia 26: 127–141
Weiss O F, Sriwatanakul K, Alloza J L, Weintraub M, Lasagna L 1983 Attitudes of patients, housestaff and nurses towards postoperative analgesic care. Anesth Analg 62: 70–74
Wheatley R G, Somerville I D, Sapsford D J, Jones J G 1990 Postoperative hypoxaemia: comparison of extradural, I. M. and patient controlled opioid analgesia. Br J Anaesth 64: 267–275
White P F 1987 Mishaps with patient controlled analgesia. Anesthesiology 66: 81–83
Wiklund L 1975 Splanchnic oxygen uptake in relation to systemic oxygen uptake during postoperative splanchnic blockade and postoperative fentanyl analgesia. Acta Anaesthesiol Scand Supplement 58: 29–40
Wolfson B 1958 Minor laryngeal sequelae of endotracheal intubation. Br J Anaesth 30: 326–332
Wulf H, Winckler K, Maier C, Henzow B 1988 Pharmacokinetics and protein binding of bupivacaine in postoperative epidural analgesia. Acta Anaesthesiol Scand 32: 530–534

16

Postoperative respiratory problems

A. G. Marshall

INTRODUCTION

Deaths associated with anaesthesia are responsible for about 2% of surgical mortality (Harrison 1978), and of these nearly 62% occur during the immediate recovery phase (Edwards et al 1956, Bodlander 1975). Pulmonary complications are the most common cause of this morbidity and mortality after surgical operations (Bartlett 1980), with a frequency of some 20% in healthy individuals, an incidence difficult to reduce despite many advances in anaesthesia (Garibaldi et al 1981).

In an attempt to protect the patient during this critical postsurgical phase, recovery areas have developed for supervision and observation of patients by specially trained nurses. The common problems seen during this recovery phase are described in Chapter 27.

Hypoxaemia remains one of the most common postoperative problems. It is often difficult to detect, but potentially lethal, especially in combination with other complications. Cyanosis is not clearly visible until oxygen saturation is below 80% (equivalent to an oxygen tension of 7.6 kPa [50 mmHg]). At this level there are generally some signs of respiratory insufficiency: rapid shallow respiration may be followed by periodic breathing, cardiovascular depression and restlessness. Carboxyhaemoglobin and pigmented skin may mask the development of cyanosis. Cyanosis is best seen inside the mouth, both in white and dark-skinned people, as 'blue fingers' may merely reflect poor peripheral perfusion, cold, or bad lighting. The use of pulse oximetry in recovery has become an essential monitor, a fall in saturation being treated by increasing ventilation or inspired oxygen, provided cardiac output has remained stable.

The cause of postoperative hypoxaemia may be divided into early (which reflects preoperative, perioperative and immediate postoperative factors) and late (which although related to perioperative factors are usually the result of progression of pulmonary mechanical factors).

Early postoperative hypoxaemia is described in detail in Chapter 27 and summarized in Table 27.3.

PATHOPHYSIOLOGY

Hendenstierna et al (1987) described the cause for abnormal gas exchange during anaesthesia, demonstrating dependent lung alterations by computed tomography. This supported Craig's (1981) traditional view that the early postoperative hypoxaemia is an extension of the disorders in gas exchanges that occur during anaesthesia. This lung alteration is reversed only partially by lung inflation. The reduction in functional residual capacity (FRC) is more likely related to changes in chest wall muscle tone and thoracoabdominal blood volumes. These mechanisms have been reviewed by Jones et al (1990).

The importance of upper airway obstruction must be emphasized, and the transient effect of the early elimination of nitrous oxide diluting alveolar gas must be avoided by allowing the patient to breathe 100% oxygen for a few minutes.

Some of the early-phase respiratory depression may also be explained by the depression of the normal hypoxic drive to respiration by concentrations of halothane and enflurane as low as 0.1 minimum alveolar concentration (MAC). Such concentrations are not improbable in the early postoperative phase (Knill & Gelb 1978).

The effects of narcotics, including fentanyl, may depress respiration for some hours after surgery and indeed may cause disturbances of respiratory control leading to obstructive sleep apnoea. This is rarely associated with the slow respiratory rate characteristic of narcotics, but may be dependent on the mode of administration of the opioid analgesic, that is intramuscular, intravenous or extradural. Obstructive apnoea may occur whenever the patient falls asleep, night or day. If this is related to a reduced central drive then a respiratory stimulant, for example doxapram or almitrine, may be useful. Doxapram increases both tidal volume and arterial oxygen tension in fit patients after abdominal surgery, and has been advocated for use over the first postsurgical day (Jansen et al 1990). Short-term improvements in ventilation may be achieved at the cost of excessive breathlessness. Usually, central drive is appropriate. Attempts should be made to reduce load by improving respiratory muscle force and to optimize capacity and pressure generation.

The problems of early respiratory depression are probably less hazardous to the patient than those of the later phase because the level of observation is usually high immediately after anaesthesia. These later phases, which may last up to a week, are more likely after thoracic and upper abdominal surgery in the immobile, the aged, smokers, the obese and those with pre-existing cardiorespiratory disease. These late changes have also been characterized by a decrease in FRC related to changes in the chest wall, mucous plugs, collapse of perfused alveoli and blood-volume shifts.

Sudden oxygen desaturation in the late postoperative period may be due to a disturbed sleep pattern (Knill et al 1987) or the effects of opioids on ventilatory control (Catley et al 1985). Such hypoxaemia may put patients with cardiovascular disease at considerable risk (Rosenburg et al 1990).

Early postoperative hypoxaemia

Early respiratory problems should be sought in at-risk patients to prevent serious complications developing later. The site and duration of surgery, the type of anaesthesia and the degree of postoperative immobilization may also affect respiratory function(Jansen et al 1990).

Obesity

Obese patients provide significant difficulties both during and after surgery (Schwartz 1955). Airway maintenance may be difficult, as can be intubation, causing trauma to teeth or larynx with subsequent stridor. Associated cardiovascular disease and chronic hypoxaemia caused by restricted diaphragm and chest movements are common, and reduced functional residual capacity and vital capacity (Barrera et al 1967) may be exaggerated postoperatively (Carture et al 1970, Marshall & Melvill 1972) by airway closure (Alexander et al 1973) and muscle fatigue. Postoperative pneumonia is more common in the obese (Garibaldi et al 1981). Management during the recovery and immediate postoperative days needs constant patient encouragement with attention to airway and breathing. A change in position from supine to sitting may not necessarily improve diaphragmatic movement, and patients weighing over 100 kg should be considered for elective ventilation and intensive-care management postoperatively. Narcotics and atropine should be used cautiously because of their depressant and drying effects, respectively.

Age

Due to increasing airway closure and musculoskeletal changes with age, the normal Pa_{O_2} declines to about 8.4 kPa by the age of 70 years (Marshall & Millar 1965, Jones 1982). There may also be associated cardiorespiratory disease predisposing to pneumonia or pulmonary oedema.

Reaction to drugs, particularly opiates, may be unpredictable and an increased incidence of apnoeic spells has been reported (Arunasalam et al 1983).

Smoking

The increased incidence of postoperative pulmonary complications in smokers has long been recognized (Morton 1944). Measurable changes in lung function, airflow, closing volume, FVC and maximum midexpiratory flow rate (Burrows et al 1977, Beck et al 1981, Buist et al 1981) are seen in smokers, and their severity is related to the duration of the addiction and the quantity of tobacco used. Cessation of smoking should be encouraged preoperatively, although return towards normal function is slow. Bronchorrhoea often occurs for 2–3 days after stopping smoking and thereafter the productive cough is reduced. However, improvement in lung function takes at least 2 months.

Cardiorespiratory disease

A predisposition to postoperative chest infection exists with chronic obstructive airway disease (Garibaldi et al 1981). Physiotherapy with controlled bronchodilator therapy, together with mucolytic agents and steroids, should be used during the preoperative period to obtain optimum chest conditions.

The profuse secretions of chronic bronchitis may compromise the airway lumen allowing resorption atelectasis to occur. The continuation of physiotherapy, together with the therapeutic measures outlined above, will minimize the complication.

Pulmonary heart disease (cor pulmonale) may be secondary to chronic respiratory disease such as chronic bronchitis and emphysema, obesity or recurrent emboli, and, rarely, pectus excavatum. As a result of hypoxia, pulmonary vasoconstriction may increase pulmonary artery pressure (Fishman 1966). Further increases in pulmonary vascular resistance may be minimized by oxygen therapy, avoiding acidosis, and by using vasodilators such as isoprenaline, nitroprusside and nitroglycerine. Digitalis and diuretics should be used in the presence of congestive heart failure.

Elective surgery should be postponed in the presence of upper respiratory tract infection as it is reported to increase the risk of postoperative chest infection. The acutely inflamed pharynx and larynx may also be rendered more sensitive to developing laryngospasm.

The usual defence mechanisms of nasal filtration, airway reflexes, alveolar macrophage system and mucociliary clearance may be modified during anaesthesia, allowing access to the usually clean lower airways. Mucociliary action is also altered by dehydration, atropine and high concentrations of oxygen (see Ch. 4).

Chronic respiratory infections should be treated with early preoperative hospital admission and vigorous chest physiotherapy until optimum conditions are reached. In many circumstances it may not be possible to clear the lung of disease completely, but broad-spectrum antibiotic cover, with careful attention to the anaesthetic and postoperative recovery period, will reduce morbidity.

Careful preoperative assessment is important (Brindley et al 1982, Gothard & Branthwaite 1982). Generally, arterial oxygen levels are probably not as significant as an elevated arterial carbon dioxide, particularly during thoracic surgery, as shunting through the abnormal lung will improve when the diseased part is removed.

Various parameters of lung function are shown in Table 16.1. Patients whose lung function exceeds these limits should be free of untoward postoperative respiratory complications. These factors should always be measured preoperatively in the patients most at risk.

Table 16.1 Parameters of lung function

Factor	Limit
FVC	>50% predicted
FEV	>50% predicted
FVC^1/TLC	<50%
Diffusion capacity	>50% predicted
FEV_1/fractional perfusion	>0.8
Mean pulmonary artery pressure	<35 mmHg
PaO_2	>6.0 kPa

Late postoperative hypoxaemia

The pathophysiology of late hypoxaemia has been described above and includes central changes in chemosensitivity, reduced airway patency, decreased respiratory muscle activity, and persisting intrapulmonary shunting and ventilation/perfusion (V/Q) mismatch. If V/Q abnormalities already exist from pre-existing lung disease the V/Q ratio will be further reduced.

The pulmonary circulation can adjust itself to varying V/Q situations tending to direct blood from poorly ventilated areas to better-ventilated zones, but clinical intervention is often necessary. Fibrotic lung disease and oedema may produce low oxygen tension due to diffusion block between alveolar gas and pulmonary capillary blood. Hypoxaemia may also be exaggerated by a persisting low haemoglobin, increased oxygen demand, decreased cardiac output or changes in acid-base state.

All these mechanisms may be present to some degree after major surgery. In the absence of signs of decreased cardiac output or increased oxygen consumption, a mixed venous blood sample should be obtained by pulmonary artery catheter to determine the arteriovenous oxygen content difference and hence the pathology.

The most important causes of late postoperative hypoxaemia are discussed in detail below. These are:

- chest infection
- aspiration
- atelectasis
- pneumothorax
- fat embolism
- pulmonary embolism
- amniotic fluid embolism
- bypass lung.

Postoperative chest infection

The common 'postoperative chest' with segmental atelectasis, hypoxaemia, pyrexia and purulent sputum may complicate about 5% of all operations. The incidence is highest following abdominal operations (at least 10%), and Saady (1974) reported figures as high as 80%.

The condition may be initiated by trauma to the tracheobronchial tree or by contamination of respiratory equipment. Depressed mucociliary clearance due to drugs and oxygen or gas irritation are also factors. During thoracic procedures contamination of the good lung by secretions from the pathological areas may occur. Many factors predispose to the development of chest infection. These include age, obesity, smoking, pre-existing lung disease, emergency surgery, abdominal pain and sepsis, and the inability to cough. Debility, malnutrition and alcoholism are additional factors.

The site of surgery and its duration will alter the incidence of postoperative infection even in the absence of chronic respiratory disease. Chronic obstructive respiratory disease does, however, increase the risk of pneumonia after all surgery by 19% and after upper abdominal surgery by 25% (Gracey et al 1974). Following thoracotomy, severe respiratory insufficiency may develop as a result of segmental pneumonia on top of an already diminished reserve after resection. The clinical features of pyrexia and purulent sputum may be accompanied by localized auscultatory signs. The chest X-ray may not be distinctive unless segmental collapse has occurred, when tachycardia and tachypnoea will also be present. The lower lobes are most often involved, and if infection is allowed to progress bronchopneumonia will develop. This can progress to lung abscess. The arterial oxygen tension may decrease even when respiratory function appears to be normal initially. Persisting lung pathology will lead to tachypnoea, tachycardia, cyanosis, restlessness, confusion and delayed recovery. It should be remembered however that oxygen tension may decrease significantly before respiratory function appears abnormal. Respiratory muscle function, particularly the onset of respiratory fatigue, may be exacerbated by sepsis and critical illness, hastening the onset of respiratory failure (Rochester & Esau 1988).

Treatment is essentially preventive, but once infection is established physiotherapy, intelligent use of analgesics, antibiotics and tracheal intubation and/or bronchoscopy may be needed.

Patients with chronic respiratory disease, and those undergoing cardiac surgery or thoracotomy, should receive antibiotics preoperatively and for 3 days postoperatively, accompanied by frequent physiotherapy.

Effective analgesia may allow the patient to breathe deeply and cough effectively. Regional techniques with local anaesthetics can be used and Entonox during physiotherapy may relieve discomfort. Chest locks and abdominal belts have been recommended by some, but they further restrict respiratory movement and increase the risk of atelectasis.

Aspiration of gastric contents (including acid aspiration syndrome)

Despite preoperative preparation to ensure an empty stomach, the use of special precautions in susceptible patients, and the avoidance of agents likely to cause vomiting, regurgitation of gastric contents and their subsequent aspiration remains a major cause of postanaesthetic morbidity and mortality. The incidence is difficult to assess as silent regurgitation has been reported in 7.8% of patients in one series, and of these, 8.6% aspirated the material. In a recent UK study (Lunn & Mushin 1982) 11 of 58 anaesthetic deaths were thought to be due to aspiration. The sequelae of aspiration depend on the nature and volume of the aspirated fluid. Gastric pH below 3 is said to be associated with severe pulmonary damage (Banister & Sattilaro 1962). Aspiration may go unnoticed by the anaesthetist until pulmonary symptoms occur, particularly if actual vomiting has not been observed. The aspiration of larger food particles may lead to obstruction of the airway and suffocation. Incomplete obstruction results in cyanosis, tachypnoea, dyspnoea and the X-ray changes of pulmonary collapse. With an acid liquid aspirate, intense bronchospasm, hypoxia, dyspnoea and pneumonitis may rapidly develop, and this is worse if small food particles are also inhaled.

Histologically, pulmonary mucosal oedema, congestion, and haemorrhages with extensive exudate and bronchial epithelial degeneration can be demonstrated. Within 36 hours a polymorphonuclear infiltration begins with necrosis and sloughing off of mucosal lining cells, and alveolar consolidation (Wynne & Modell 1977).

Late consequences may be adult respiratory distress syndrome (ARDS) (Fein et al 1982), lung abscess and pulmonary fibrosis. The differential diagnosis should include: leaky lung, often associated with fat embolism and septicaemia; high-pressure pulmonary oedema of left-sided heart failure and fluid overload; hypoproteinaemia of nephrotic syndrome; and malnutrition. Abnormal capillary membrane permeability should be suspected in the presence of radiographic pulmonary oedema with a normal pulmonary wedge pressure and normal colloid osmotic pressure.

While particularly likely to occur in obstetric patients it is important to remember that acid aspiration may occur before, during or after anaesthesia, particularly during the first few postoperative days in sick patients.

The training of anaesthetists to recognize susceptible patients, to prevent or minimize the effect and to treat the established condition is essential to decreased morbidity and mortality from aspiration. The factors increasing the risk of regurgitation of gastric contents are:

1. full stomach
    - pyloric obstruction
    - peritonitis
    - blood in stomach
    - abdominal distension
    - oesophageal pouch or obstruction
2. intestinal obstruction
3. delayed emptying
    - labour
    - emotional stress
    - pain
    - serious illness
    - drugs
4. hiatus hernia
5. indwelling nasogastric tube
6. pregnancy
7. obesity.

Treatment of acid aspiration syndrome

While all would agree that aggressive therapy is essential for the patient with signs of respiratory distress, the patient with a suspected aspiration and no signs poses a particular dilemma. If there is a strong suspicion of gastric aspiration, my own practice is to institute therapy immediately rather than wait for evidence of respiratory dysfunction, particularly if a sample of gastric juice proves to have a low pH. Management consists of oxygenation, intubation, endotracheal suction, mechanical ventilation overnight with 5 cmH_2O positive end-expiratory pressure and the administration of steroids and antibiotics. If, by the following morning, no signs of respiratory dysfunction have developed, controlled ventilation can be discontinued.

The difficulty, of course, is knowing whether the therapy has been effective or grossly overenthusiastic. The potential consequences of acid aspiration are, however, so disastrous that I am content to be overcautious. Thus far I have had no cause to regret this policy.

Tracheal suction should only be performed after preoxygenation, and if solid aspirate is seen or suspected, bronchoscopy should be performed. Bronchial lavage in connection with suction has been recommended, but is likely to increase the area of involvement, disperse surfactant and cause an initial increase in airways resistance followed by a prolonged fall in compliance and arterial oxygenation. It is therefore not recommended.

Positive end-expiratory pressure (PEEP) is of value in conditions of alveolar instability and closure, but will not relieve the hypoxia of obstructed airways and pneumonitis. Circulating blood volume must be maintained, as the increase in intrathoracic pressure may cause a fall in cardiac output and increase the intrapulmonary shunt, thus exaggerating the hypoxaemia. Reduced cardiac output may also be related to developing pulmonary oedema in established cases. Fluid replacement with colloid, such as salt-free albumin, may reduce oedema formation. However, if capillary damage is severe, protein may also leak into the alveoli making subsequent removal of the oedema even more difficult. Metabolic acidosis is a frequent complication at this stage.

The use of steroids is controversial, but I consider that they have an important place given as a short course (24 hours maximum) of high-dose methylprednisolone (30 mg/kg). Prophylactic antibiotics have not led to improved prognosis, although broad-spectrum antibiotics are still generally prescribed. There is perhaps more logic in the use of antibiotics specifically aimed at anaerobic organisms. Bronchodilators such a salbutamol, isoprenaline and adrenaline may help to alleviate the bronchospasm, but can exaggerate the ventilation-perfusion mismatch.

Atelectasis

Atelectasis may account for as much as 42% (Wightman 1969) of the observed pulmonary complications following abdominal surgery, and is even more common after thoracic and cardiac surgery. It is also the most common respiratory finding on chest X-ray during the first 48 postoperative hours (Hamilton 1961). The pain and trauma of the surgical procedure, particularly upper abdominal or thoracic surgery, leads to splinting of the ribs and diaphragm, causing a reduced vital capacity. Tidal volume falls but respiratory rate rises and spontaneous sigh is reduced in both depth and frequency. These lead to a fall in functional residual capacity (see Ch. 4). This may be further reduced by small airway closure. Secondary to the limited inspiratory capacity and impairment of cough mechanisms, changes in surfactant production and accumulation of secretions may reduce lung compliance with the inevitable reduction of lung volume and the creation of a focus for infection.

Atelectasis may present on X-ray of the chest or as a low-grade postoperative fever with cough and a widening alveolar-arterial oxygen gradient. Radiographically it may appear as plate-like bands, patchy infiltration, lobar shadowing or a change in density of parts of the cardiac shadow. Lobar collapse implies a proximal obstruction and occurs frequently after thoracic and upper abdominal surgery, typically involving the lower lobes. A large heart may also directly compress the left lower lobe in a supine patient.

Total lung atelectasis is less common, and implies obstruction to a major bronchus. Total lung collapse may occur with mechanical obstruction, mucus secretions, foreign bodies, poorly placed endotracheal tubes and tooth aspiration. Removal of the obstruction by bronchoscopy, positive pressure reinflation and postoperative deep breathing with physiotherapy is necessary treatment. All degrees of atelectasis contribute to postoperative hypoxaemia, and may cause hypercapnia and lead to ventilatory failure in patients with underlying lung disease.

Patients must be encouraged to inspire deeply postoperatively. Thoracic epidurals for control of post-thoracotomy and upper abdominal pain have led to easier ambulation while avoiding the depressive effects of analgesics and sedatives. The role of intercostal nerve blocks is controversial. Special techniques, such as transcutaneous electrical nerve stimulation, have also been used effectively (Ali 1979). However, the mainstay of postoperative respiratory care is physiotherapy. The techniques and devices used by the physiotherapist that encourage a large and sustained increase in transpulmonary pressure will expand collapsed lung units. These include intermittent positive pressure breathing ('bird' therapy) and positive end-expiratory pressure breathing, together with percussion, postural drainage and coughing. Early and periodic ambulation will also encourage better distribution of air in the lungs.

Bypass lung

Exposure of blood to the unphysiological events of cardiopulmonary bypass and the formation of heparin/protamine complexes initiates a systemic inflammatory response, probably via the release of complement $C3_a$ and $C5_a$. Blood levels of these anaphylatoxins and interleukin 1 may be related to postoperative sequelae, particularly the post perfusion syndrome (Haeffner-Caraillon et al 1989). The mechanisms of damage are exposure of blood to various abnormal events and altered flow patterns. The damage is manifested after bypass by a tendency to bleed, a diffuse whole-body inflammatory reaction characterized by increased capillary permeability and increased interstitial fluid, leucocytosis and fever, peripheral and central vasoconstriction, and breakdown of red blood cells resulting in haematuria and anaemia. These lead to dysfunction in various organs. One manifestation of this may be varying degrees of pulmonary oedema with or without an elevated left atrial pressure.

Plasma proteins, albumin, lipoprotein and immunoglobulins are damaged by exposure to non-biological surfaces leading to fat microemboli. The humoral amplification system, both complement and fibrinolytic cascades, is activated. Complement activation leads to the release of glycoproteins active in cell lysis and phagocytosis, increased vascular permeability, smooth muscle contraction and leucocyte chemotaxis. These cause pulmonary sequestration of polymorphonuclear leucocytes and pulmonary dysfunction. Leucocyte-mediated pulmonary endothelial damage is one of the mediators of the adverse effect of cardiopulmonary bypass on pulmonary function. The damaged leucocytes release lysosomes against the pulmonary basement membrane and endothelial cells causing damage. Platelets are reduced in number and function. Red blood cells may fragment or have damaged cell membranes.

The sheer stress of pump suction, and acceleration and deceleration of blood in the cannulae also cause cell damage. The damaged platelets then aggregate in the lungs, causing a pulmonary reaction which may lead to a raised pulmonary artery pressure. This, together with the relative pulmonary ischaemia during bypass, may result in a decrease of the pulmonary surfactant and a strong tendency to atelectasis.

Contact activation also initiates the kallikrein-bradykinin system causing increased vascular permeability, dilated arterioles and smooth muscle contraction.

The net result of the damage during bypass is the 'postperfusion' or postpump syndrome (Kirklin 1989). Although mild degrees of this syndrome will follow most bypass surgery, failure to compensate will lead to severe physiological disturbances. The syndrome is manifest by pulmonary dysfunction, particularly pulmonary oedema, without an elevated left-atrial pressure. Increased capillary permeability, with consequent transcapillary plasma loss and increased interstitial fluid, is partly responsible. An abnormal bleeding tendency may be associated with red cell breakdown resulting in haemoglobinuria and anaemia.

This may lead to renal failure. Peripheral and central vasoconstriction, which usually persist for a variable time after bypass, may result in both haemodynamic and metabolic problems. Fever and leucocytosis also occur.

Prevention lies largely in the choice and management of the bypass equipment, although steroids may have a role in reducing compliment levels. A skilful operation, choice of patients not affected by advanced heart disease, and attention to perioperative and postoperative care, will help to limit the damaging effects of bypass, but even under these circumstances unexplained dysfunction can occur.

Pneumothorax

Air may remain in the chest cavity following any intrathoracic procedure, accidental opening of the pleura by fractured ribs or following extrathoracic surgical procedures, such as cervical sympathectomy. Anaesthetic procedures, such as intercostal nerve blocks, brachial plexus blocks and insertion of central venous cannulae are known to cause this complication. Barotrauma from controlled ventilation as a result of high positive pressures may cause pneumothorax, but positive pressure ventilation will accentuate any leak of air from the lung or tracheobronchial tree into the pleural cavity. Pleural drains are usually inserted after thoracotomy with an underwater seal bottle to maintain a closed pleural space. If drains are not to be inserted, air can be expressed by maintaining a positive pressure on the lungs during wound closure.

A chest radiograph should be taken in the recovery room if there is a possibility of pneumothorax following any of the above procedures. Interpretation of the chest X-ray may be difficult in the presence of diseased lungs, abnormal soft-tissue shadows, hyperinflation emphysema and thoracic tubes, which may loculate along the pleura or mediastinum. Suspicion should be roused by the presence of fractured ribs, surgical emphysema or a small collection of pleural fluid.

A pneumothorax of less than 20% may not be clinically detectable, but the presence of chest pain (worse with inspiration), cyanosis, a fall in pulmonary compliance, rapidly deteriorating vital signs and diminished or absent breath sounds, with tracheal deviation, should warn of tension pneumothorax, especially if associated with positive pressure ventilation. Immediate drainage is necessary. A dramatic change in compliance during anaesthesia may be the first obvious sign, preceding deteriorating vital signs and impairment of normal blood gas levels. Nitrous oxide should be discontinued if pneumothorax is suspected. Chest X-ray may show total lung collapse, ipsilateral rib spread and depressed diaphragm.

Treatment for pneumothorax of more than 10% is by pleural drainage; less than this will absorb over a few days. Progress should be followed by regular chest X-ray. The site of drain insertion should depend on localizing signs and chest X-ray, although in the supine and semierect positions air usually collects anterosuperiorly and therefore the drain should be anterosuperior. Common insertion sites are:

- posterior to the pectoralis major in the anterior axillary line through the fifth interspace
- anteriorly in the midclavicular line through the second interspace
- posteriorly through the first intercostal space.

Argyle-type thoracic catheters with an introducer or Tudor-Edwards trocar and a malecot catheter are most frequently used. To avoid damage to other organs I prefer a small transverse incision at the insertion site, with blunt dissection to puncture the parietal pleura and insertion of a gloved finger to clear a path for the drain. The procedure should be sterile and painless. Drains should remain for 24–48 hours postoperatively or until drainage of blood, fluid or air stops.

Thoracotomy drains should only be inserted by doctors experienced in the dangers of the procedure. The lung, liver, spleen, stomach, colon and kidney may be lacerated. The tube may not be accurately placed, and leaking around the drainage site can cause alarming surgical emphysema. Damage may also occur to the intercostal arteries, veins and the ribs themselves. A chest radiograph should confirm the position of the drain and reduction of the pneumothorax. The drainage tubes should not be permanently clamped in case air or fluid accumulate in the chest. Should it be necessary to elevate the drainage bottle above the chest, brief clamping to prevent siphoning of fluid from the bottle is permissible.

Suction on the drain is not usually necessary as long as the tube remains patent. Breaking the tube to measure fluid loss or to move the patient may contaminate the system or cause recurrent pneumothorax. On removal of the tube the patient should take a deep breath and perform a Valsalva manoeuvre to prevent air entrainment and pneumothorax.

In an emergency a 20 ml syringe filled with saline and connected to a needle can be inserted into the pneumothorax space. The plunger is removed and an effective water-seal drain results.

Fat embolism

'Fat embolism syndrome' should be distinguished from the presence of embolic fat in the circulation. While embolization of fat is relatively common the full syndrome is fortunately rare. Fat droplets may frequently be demonstrated in sputum, blood or urine following injury, but these are not diagnostic of 'fat embolism syndrome'. The syndrome has the radiological features of an interstitial pneumonitis, with dyspnoea, hypoxaemia, tachycardia and respiratory failure in its most serious form. Cerebral involvement may show the features of confusion, restlessness, and ultimately cerebral oedema and coma. Petechia confined to the anterior chest, neck, axillae and conjunctivae are present in 50–60% of cases (Sevitt 1962).

Pathophysiologically, microaggregates of fat droplets, platelets, red and white blood cells, and thrombin impair small-vessel perfusion and cause endothelial damage in the pulmonary capillaries by liberation of toxic free-fatty-acids and vasoactive peptides. This leads to V/Q mismatch, vascular congestion, interstitial haemorrhage, alveolar wall damage and collapse. Mortality in the full-blown syndrome approaches 10–45% (Peltier 1969).

Management of these patients requires early stabilization of the fracture, and cardiovascular and respiratory support, including mechanical ventilation with added oxygen and PEEP. There is no definitive treatment. Ethanol infusion, high-dose heparin, low molecular weight dextran, hypertonic glucose, clofibrate, phynoxybenzamine and steroids have all been tried, but none has been proved effective. Ventilatory assistance and expedient fracture management are acceptable cornerstones of management.

Pulmonary embolism

Pulmonary embolism is a significant cause of death during the postoperative and postpartum periods. More than 90% of emboli originate in the deep veins of the pelvis and the legs, the separated portion of thrombus lodging in one of the pulmonary arteries (see Ch. 18).

The classical triad of sudden pleuritic pain, dyspnoea and haemoptysis occurs in less than 20%, and, generally, tachypnoea, fever, anxiety, pleural rub, wheeze, cough and signs of right ventricular strain should raise suspicion.

If the embolism is large, cardiovascular collapse usually occurs, and death will result if embolectomy is not performed. ECG changes are transient and non-specific, leading to difficulty in the differential diagnosis from myocardial ischaemia.

Chest X-ray is usually unhelpful, although small pleural effusions may develop. Elevation of the hemidiaphragm is not uncommon. Selective pulmonary angiography is the most accurate method of diagnosis, although pulmonary perfusion scans (technetium-labelled albumin microspheres) and combined ventilation-perfusion scanning are used.

Amniotic fluid embolism

A rare complication of both vaginal and caesarean delivery is the escape of amniotic fluid from the amniotic sac to the uterine venous sinus, particularly during contractions. This may cause a sudden massive pulmonary microvascular obstruction leading to 'shock' and death. The emboli may be the solid particles in the amniotic fluid or the fibrin emboli of the disseminated intravascular coagulation that follows. Pulmonary hypertension and oedema occur and cardiovascular collapse may follow. Treatment with oxygen and cardiopulmonary support may be necessary and heparin therapy has been advocated.

SUMMARY

The diagnosis and management of postoperative hypoxaemia require answers to three questions:

1. What is happening in the lungs?
2. How good is the central control system?
3. Is oxygen delivery and utilization adequate?

The most appropriate monitor postoperatively is the pulse oximeter. Its use should be extended with continuous oxygen therapy into the third and fourth postoperative days for patients at risk, especially when high-dependency units are unavailable.

Some benefit may be gained from using drugs acting on the chemoreceptor mechanisms and by choosing effective pain relief methods.

Marshall B E, Millar R A 1965 Some factors influencing 10

REFERENCES

Alexander J I, Spence A A, Parikh R K, Stuart B 1973 The role of airway closure in postoperative hypoxaemia. Br J Anaesth 43: 34

Ali J 1979 The effects of intermittent positive pressure breathing on postoperative pulmonary function. Ann Coll Physicians Surg Can 12: 36

Arunasalam K, Davenport H T, Painter S, Jones J G 1983 Ventilatory response to morphine in young and old subjects. Anaesthesia 38: 529–533

Banister W K, Sattlaro A J 1962 Vomiting and aspiration during anaesthesia. Anesthesiology 23: 251–264

Barrera F, Reidenberg M M, Winters W L 1967 Pulmonary function in the obese patient. Am J Med Sci 254: 785–796

Bartlett R H 1980 Pulmonary pathophysiology in surgical patients. Surg Clin North Am 60: 1323

Bartlett R H, Bazzaniga A B, Geraghty T R 1973 Respiratory maneuvers to prevent postoperative pulmonary complication. J Am Med Assoc 22: 1017–1021

Beck G J, Doyle C A, Schachter E N 1981 Smoking and lung function. Am Rev Respir Dis 123: 149–155

Bodlander F M S 1975 Deaths associated with anaesthesia. Br J Anaesth 47: 36

Brindley G V, Walsh R E, Scnarr W T, Allen G W, Mendenhall M K, Ahlgran E W 1982 Pulmonary resection in patients with impaired pulmonary function. Surg Clin North Am 62: 192–214

Buist A S, Seton G V, Nagy J M et al. 1981 The effects of smoking cessation and modification on lung function. Am J Respir Dis 114: 115–122

Burrows B, Knudson R J, Cune N G et al. 1977 Quantitative relationships between cigarette smoking and ventilatory function. Am Rev Respir Dis 115: 195–205

Catley D M, Thornton D, Jordan D, Lehane J R, Royston D, Jones J G 1985 Pronounced episodic oxygen desaturation in the postoperative period: its association with ventilatory pattern and analgesia regimen. Anesthesiology 63: 20–28

Couture J, Picken J, Trop D et al 1970 Airway closure in normal obese and anaesthetised supine subjects. Fed Proc 29: 269

Craig D B 1981 Post op recovery of pulmonary function. Anesth Analg 60: 48–52

Edwards G, Morton H J V, Pask E A, Wylie W D 1956 Deaths associated with anaesthesia. Anaesthesia 11: 194

Fein A M, Goldberg S K, Uppman M L, Fisher R, Morgan L 1982 Adult Respiratory distress syndrome. Br J Anaesth 54: 723–726

Fishman A P 1966 Chronic cor pulmonale: state of the art. Am Rev Respir Dis 355–374

Garibaldi R A, Britt M R, Coleman M L, Reading J E, Pace N L 1981 Risk factors for postoperative pneumonia. Am J Med 70: 677–680

Gothard J W W, Branthwaite M A (eds) 1982 In: Anaesthesia for thoracic surgery. Blackwell, Oxford, pp 8–22

Gracey D R, Divertie M B, Didier E P 1974 Preoperative pulmonary preparation of patients with chronic obstructive pulmonary disease. Chest 76: 123–129

Haeffner-Cavaillon N, Roussellier N, Ponzio O et al 1989 Induction of interleukins production in patients undergoing cardiopulmonary bypass. J Thor Cardiovasc Surg 98: 1100–1106

Hamilton W K 1961 Atelectasis, pneumothorax and aspiration as postoperative complications. Anesthesiology 22: 708–722

Harrison G G 1978 Death attributable to anaesthesia. Br J Anaesth 50: 1041–1046

Hendenstierna G, Tokies L, Strandberg A, Lundquist H, Brismar B 1987 Correlation of gas exchange impairment to development of atelectasis during anaesthesia and muscle paralysis. Acta Anaesthesiol Scand 57: 949–953

Jansen J E, Sorensen A I, Naesh O, Erichsen C J, Pedersen A 1990 Effects of doxapram on post op complications after upper abdominal surgery in high risk patients. Lancet 335: 936

Jones J G 1982 Closing volume. In: Kaufman L (ed) Anaesthesia, revised edn. Churchill Livingstone, Edinburgh pp 43–54

Jones J G, Sapsford D J, Wheatley R G 1990 Postoperative hypoxaemia: mechanisms and time course. Analg 45: 566–573

Kirklin J K 1989 The postperfusion syndrome. In: Tinker J H (ed) Cardiopulmonary bypass: current concepts and controversies. W B Saunders, Philadelphia, pp 131–146

Knill R L, Gelb A W 1978 Ventilatory response to hypoxia and hypercapnia during halothane sedation and anaesthesia in man. Anesthesiology 49: 244–257

Knill R L, Moote C A, Rose E A, Skinner M I 1987 Masked hypoxaemia after gastroplasty due to disorders of breathing in REM sleep. Anesthesiology 67: A552

Lunn J N, Mushin W W 1982 Mortality associated with anaesthesia. Nuffield Provincial Hospital Trust, London

Marshall B E, Millar R A 1965 Some factors influencing postop hypoxaemia. Anaesthesia 20: 488

Marshall B E, Melville Q W 1972 Hypoxaemia during and after anaesthesia. Anesthesiology 37: 178–209

Morton H J V 1944 Tobacco smoking and pulmonary complications after operation. Lancet 1: 368–370
Peltier L F 1969 Fat embolism: a current concept. Clin Orthop Relat Res 66: 241
Rochester D F, Esau S A 1988 Critical illness, infection and the respiratory muscles. Am Rev Respir Dis 138: 258–9
Rosenberg J, Rasmussen V, Von Jenssen F, Ullstad T, Kehlet H 1990 Late postoperative episode and constant hypoxaemia and accounted ECG abnormalities. Br J Anaesth 65: 684–691
Saady A 1974 Pulmonary consequences of upper abdominal surgery: therapeutic considerations. Anaesthetics and Internal Chemistry 2: 221
Schwartz H 1955 The problem of obesity in anaesthesia. N Y State J Med 55: 3257
Sevitt S 1962 Fat embolism. Butterworths, London
Wightman J A K 1969 A prospective survey of the incidence of postoperative pulmonary complications. Br J Surg 55: 85–91
Wynne J W, Modell J H 1977 Respiratory aspiration of stomach contents. Ann Intern Med 87: 466–476

17

Complications of fluid therapy

D. R. Bevan

INTRODUCTION

The early prevertebrates on earth lived in an environment similar in composition to the fluid surrounding their cells. As evolution progressed, species learned to live under more hostile conditions: in fresh water and on land. Survival, then, was only possible with the development of sophisticated processes to preserve consistency of the milieu interieur (Smith 1959). In particular, the vascular tuft, or glomerulus, allowed filtration of blood, and the composition of the filtrate could be modified by the nephron.

The maintenance of the individual's body water content and its distribution between intra- and extracellular regions is important for the continued function of all tissues. If the overall volume status decreases, tissue perfusion may fail and any increase may cause oedema. The constancy of solute concentration is equally important because the body cannot tolerate osmotic gradients, except at a few sites. Thus volume and osmotic factors are both concerned in the control of the volume and composition of body fluid. Disorders of fluid volume will be associated with alteration of solute content and vice versa. Small changes (1–2%) in plasma osmolality produce considerable alteration in thirst, antidiuretic hormone (ADH) secretion and water excretion in an attempt to restore the status quo.

Major surgery offers a series of challenges to the delicate control of salt and water homeostasis. Intake may be modified by either the patient or his medical attendants, and the hormonal environment of surgery, mainly in response to cardiovascular threats, may limit any additional reactions that may be necessary to counteract fluid loss from the circulation, gut, lungs and skin. In particular, the development of surgical complications, especially sepsis, leads to additional insensible loss and continued secretion of stress hormones.

METABOLIC RESPONSE TO TRAUMA

Major surgery is accompanied by powerful adaptive responses to preserve the milieu interieur. Although the sources and sites of action of the stimuli inducing the changes are largely unknown, the efferent limb of the response results in a massive outpouring of hormones resulting in changes in metabolism and fluid balance. Similar reactions occur in many acute disorders. The qualitative reactions to severe trauma, major surgery, burns, sepsis and acute myocardial infarction are similar, so that the common response is known as 'the metabolic response to trauma' (see also Ch. 8).

Major surgery is followed by conservation of water and salt by the kidney. The response may be less intense during deep anaesthesia, or in the presence of high narcotic doses or regional anaesthesia. Paradoxically, sodium retention is associated with hyponatraemia: serum sodium concentrations between 130 and 135 mmol/l are common in the early postoperative period. During surgery, renal perfusion is reduced following sympathetic stimulation, the vasoconstrictive action of catecholamines and ADH, and activation of the renin-angiotensin system. In particular, angiotensin II seems to have an important role. Generalized stress hormone activation is reinforced by perioperative starvation, dehydration and third-space extracellular fluid (ECF) losses. Consequently, urine produced during surgery is of small volume and low concentration.

In the postoperative period, several of the surgical initiating factors persist so that the patient remains relatively intolerant of salt and water loads. Hyponatraemia, although common, appears to be unimportant and seldom requires treatment as long as sodium-containing fluids are given to replace losses. Probably the most common perioperative fluid and electrolyte disorders are iatrogenic, resulting from fluids that have been administered without regard to the needs of the patient.

PERIOPERATIVE FLUID THERAPY

In the perioperative period, patients require fluid for daily maintenance of water and electrolytes and to replace losses of blood, ECF or other fluid, including that from the gut, lungs and skin.

Maintenance

The minimal water requirement per day is the sum of that required to excrete the solute load and that needed to replace insensible losses, less that available from endogenous production. The normal urinary solute excretion in the perioperative period is approximately 10 mOsm/kg/day (Zideman et al 1978, Read & Manners 1983). The urine volume depends on the urine concentration, which is usually between 500 and 1000 mOsm/kg. Thus, for a 70 kg man, the excretion of 700 mOsm will require between 700 and 1400 ml/day. Insensible losses from the skin and lungs are about 40ml/m^2/hour at 20–25°C and a relative humidity of 20–60%. This amounts to a daily loss of about 1400 ml, from which should be subtracted 300–400 ml of endogenous water. Insensible losses increase by about 12% for each 1°C increase in temperature.

Thus the total daily fluid requirement for the maintenance of body fluids is about 30–40 ml/kg. The requirements for sodium and potassium are about 1 mmol/kg/day, although potassium is often omitted until renal function is well established on the second postoperative day. The fluids may be administered in any combination of water (5% dextrose) or salt, so long as isotonic fluids are given. This regimen is quite suitable for the previously healthy patient following hysterectomy or cholecystectomy. Preoperative deficiencies or abnormal losses should be measured or estimated in terms of the volume and composition that should be replaced.

ECF replacement

Extracellular fluid accumulates in traumatized tissue, peritonitis, burns, crush injuries and ascites (Shires et al 1961). The fluid is 'lost' to the circulation and third space, and with massive trauma or major surgery may result in hypovolaemia. The extent of this reduction of 'functional' ECF volume is difficult to estimate. During major abdominal surgery 5 ml/kg/hour Ringer's lactate can be given in addition to the replacement of blood and maintenance fluid. Replacement in more extensive surgery, or in the patient who has suffered prolonged complications, should be guided by maintaining adequate cardiac filling pressures for the determination of which pulmonary artery catheters should be more frequently used. Therapy titrated according to filling pressures is more likely to maintain haemodynamic stability than arbitrary infusion rates based on anticipated third-space fluid accumulation.

Blood and colloid replacement

Most anaesthetists recommend blood transfusion to replace blood loss when the haemoglobin concentration is less than 8–10 g/dl. This arbitrary limit assumes that the tissue demands for oxygen can be met without difficulty at this level. However, transfusion may be advisable earlier in patients with a fixed or limited cardiac output, and in those with pulmonary disease which limits arterial oxygenation. It should also be remembered that the shift to the left of the haemoglobin dissociation curve in stored blood limits its ability to transfer oxygen for about 24 hours (see Ch. 10). Increased awareness of the roles of transfusion, particularly the transmission of diseases such as hepatitis and AIDS, has encouraged the more conservative use of blood products.

There are three choices of fluid for blood replacement: stored blood, colloids (plasma or plasma substitutes) and crystalloids (saline or Ringer's lactate). If crystalloids are chosen they will be distributed throughout the ECF, so the blood volume will be maintained only if three times the volume of blood loss is given. Several colloid solutions are available: blood derivatives: plasma protein, albumen; dextrans: dextran 40 and 70; hydroxyethyl starch; gelatins: haemaccel. All have some disadvantages. Blood derivatives are expensive and have the potential for disease transmission, but have a very low incidence of severe reactions. Dextrans have a low incidence of anaphylactoid reactions. Their use is limited to 1–2 l/day due to their interference with haemostasis (Isbister & Fisher 1980). The amount of hydroxyethyl starch infused is limited, but there remains a small (1:200) incidence of anaphylactoid reaction (Ring & Messmer 1977). However, hydroxyethyl starch is not associated with the histamine release of the gelatins (Lorenz et al 1976).

The use of colloids (oncotic therapy) is controversial. According to Starling's law:

$$V = Kf[(Pc - Pif) - (\pi p - \pi if)]$$

the transcapillary rate of fluid movement (V) is related to the capillary filtration coefficient (Kf), the hydrostatic pressure in the capillaries (Pc) and interstitial fluid (Pif), and the oncotic pressures of the plasma (πp) and interstitial fluid (πif). The net effect is to produce a small gradient across the capillary membrane to encourage movement of fluid into the interstitial space to be returned via the lymphatic system. Unfortunately, only two of the terms from Starling's equation can be measured clinically (Pc and πp). Replacement of plasma losses with colloid to limit oedema formation, particularly as infusion of only 1 l of crystalloid in normal subjects may affect pulmonary function (Collins et al 1973), is an attractive hypothesis, but clinical studies have been unable to support this hope. Colloids do not offer any advantage over crystalloids in preventing pulmonary dysfunction after transfusion. When non-cardiac oedema is present, oncotic therapy is of little benefit in removing it. In cardiogenic pulmonary oedema oncotic therapy is indicated only after digitalis, diuretics, oxygen and narcotics have been ineffective, and when colloid pressure (πp) is known to be low (Bevan 1980). Nevertheless, the debate between crystalloid and colloid administration continues (Twigley & Hillman 1985). The theoretical advantage of using colloids with oxygen-carrying capacity (fluosol-DA) has not met with the anticipated benefits (Tremper et al 1982), even in hypoxic conditions.

Hypertonic saline

Recently, hypertonic saline (7.5%) has been used in place of isotonic crystalloids and colloids in fluid resuscitation (Velasco et al 1980). It was hoped that the fluid would be inexpensive and avoid both oedema formation and anaphylactoid reactions. However, the beneficial haemodynamic effects are brief (Prough et al 1988) and, except in burn resuscitation (Monafo et al 1986), appear to offer no benefit over existing solutions.

Glucose solutions

Glucose solution of 5% strength is an isotonic fluid used only in modest amounts to replace body water losses. It is inappropriate for fluid resuscitation: its effect on increasing plasma volume is small because it is distributed throughout the body, both intracellularly and extracellularly. Recently there have been several disturbing reports, both clinical (Longstreth et al 1984) and laboratory (Lanier et al 1987), that have demonstrated that the extent of cerebral damage following cardiac arrest is related to blood-glucose concentration. The reason for the increased dysfunction is unclear, but may result from lactic acid accumulation in the absence of aerobic metabolism. As a consequence the use of dextrose-containing solutions during surgery has almost ceased (Sieber et al 1987).

Hypertonic glucose solutions may be used with insulin in the management of the diabetic patient or to control hyperkalaemia. Unless the blood-sugar concentration is carefully controlled by frequent monitoring, this may result in polyuria and hypovolaemia. Also, hypertonic glucose solutions may be part of a parenteral nutrition regimen. This may increase carbon dioxide production so that, to maintain normocapania, ventilation will need to be increased (Askanazi et al 1980). This could be of particular importance in the patient with chronic lung disease, in whom the institution of parenteral nutrition may induce respiratory failure.

Renal failure

The principles of fluid therapy are no different in the absence of renal function. Fluids are still required in the same volume and composition for the maintenance and replacement of losses, although urinary losses will be reduced. Problems may be encountered in renal failure when sympathetic blockade with its accompanying hypotension is produced by spinal or extradural analgesia. Fluids to restore ECF volume may produce an overload when the block wanes. Consequently, vasoconstrictor agents may be more appropriate to counteract the vasodilatation.

Ascites and liver disease

It is still disputed whether ascites results primarily from obstruction to hepatic venous outflow or from salt and water retention by the kidney. Therapeutically the difference is important. In the former the ascites is associated with hypovolaemia, and tapping of the ascites would cause severe and rapid hypotension. Peritoneovenous shunting would be more appropriate to induce natriuresis following an increase in intravascular volume (Epstein 1980). Interestingly, when up to 5 l of ascitic fluid is drained before insertion of the shunt, hypotension is seldom observed. This suggests that for many patients the ascites exists without hypovolaemia and that the renal disturbance is secondary to hepatic cirrhosis (Levy & Allotey 1978). Nevertheless, rapid drainage of ascitic fluid in the cirrhotic patient needs careful observation to avoid the consequences of rapid hypovolaemia. The principles of replacement are similar for all losses: if in doubt, volume and electrolyte content should be measured and replaced appropriately.

Neonates and infants

The total body water of a 3 kg neonate is only 2 l, of which 40% is extracellular. The major problem of fluid replacement in the very small patient is assessing the size of losses and deficits. Losses that would be innocuous in the older child and adult are life-threatening to the neonate. Particular attention should be paid to recognize dehydration and to replace losses from fasting. In situations where major losses are anticipated, an aterial line and central venous or pulmonary artery catheter may be indicated.

Replacement of blood and extracellular fluid losses is similar in principle to the adult. Water turnover is more rapid in the very young so that maintenance requirements for the neonate are increased to a volume of 100 ml/kg/day and 2.5 mmol/kg/day for sodium and potassium. The requirements decrease to adult values at 7–8 years of age (see Ch. 12).

COMMON DISORDERS OF FLUID AND ELECTROLYTE BALANCE

Osmotic disturbances

Intracellular processes are exquisitely sensitive to rapid changes in extracellular osmolality. In particular, the central nervous system demonstrates similar clinical manifestations during hyper- or hypoosmolar states as a result of swelling or shrinking of brain cells. Osmolar changes may follow alteration in the amount of solvent (water) or solute (mainly salt). Osmoreceptors respond to an increase in ECF osmolality by stimulating thirst and encouraging ADH secretion so that water retention is increased. Indeed, there are close correlations between serum osmolality, serum antidiuretic activity (arginine vasopressin concentration) and urine concentration (Fig. 17.1). Non-osmotic ADH secretion may be stimulated by hypotension, pain, emotional stress and various drugs, including opiates, general anaesthetic agents and beta sympathomimetics. Thus, surgery provides an environment that encourages water retention and an intolerance to fluid loads.

Hyperosmolar syndromes

Hyperosmolality is usually the result of fluid loss with the loss of water exceeding that of salt, so that hypernatraemia is the rule. There are several predisposing factors (Table 17.1). In the surgical patient alimentary losses, hyperosmolar diets and hypertonic intravenous therapy are the principal precipitating causes. Polyuric renal failure associated with fluoride toxicity is a relic of prolonged methoxyflurane anaesthesia. Extracellular fluid volume may be high, normal or low depending on the aetiology. Clinical features will be mainly cerebral with cardiovascular effects depending upon the ECF volume. Water deficits should be corrected slowly (over 48–72 hours) by the administration of oral or intravenous hypotonic fluids. Too rapid correction may induce convulsions. Volumes for replacement can be calculated from the serum osmolality and by assuming that the deficits exist throughout the total body water.

Hypoosmolar syndromes

All hypoosmolar patients are also hyponatraemic, although the converse may not be true: hyperglycaemia or mannitol encourage fluid transport from within cells to dilute extracellular sodium to maintain normal osmolality. Of the many causes of hypotonic hyponatraemia, third-space losses and the sick-cell syndrome are the most common in the postoperative patient. In addition, ADH

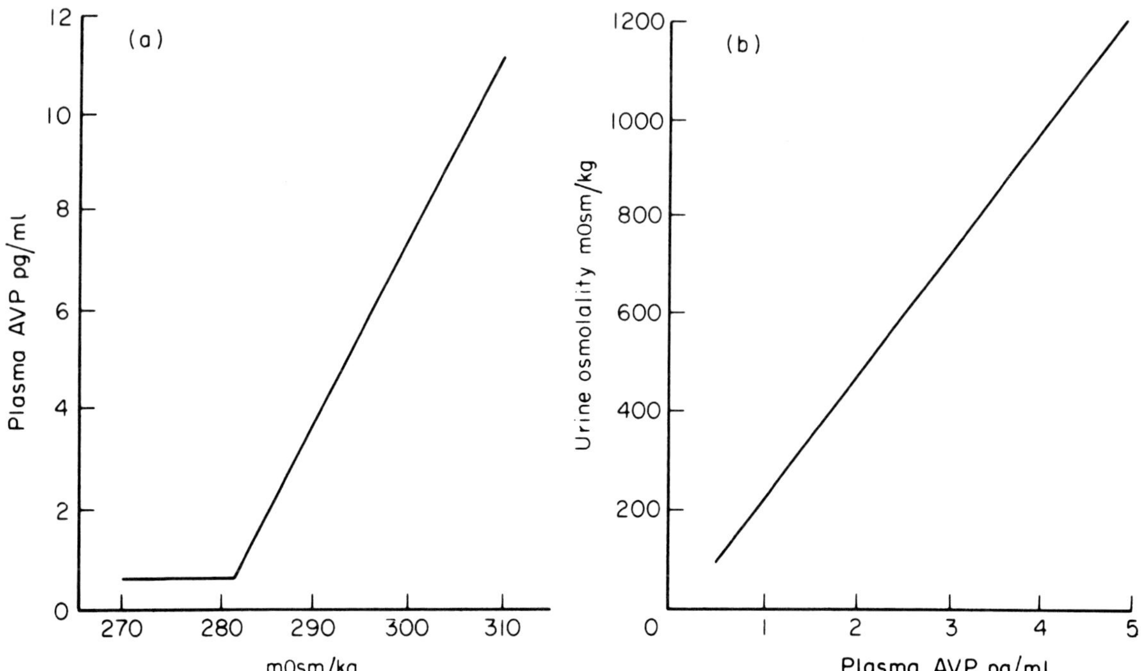

Fig. 17.1 Correlation between plasma AVP concentration and (a) plasma osmolality, (b) urine osmolality (modified from Robertson et al 1976).

Table 17.1 Causes of hypernatraemic hyperosmolality

HYPERNATRAEMIA

HYPEROSMOLALITY (>295 mmol/l)

Salt loss with larger water loss		Water loss	Water gain with larger salt gain
Renal	*Extra renal*		
diuretics	adrenal deficiency	diabetes insipidus	iatrogenic (8.4% $NaHCO_3$)
glycosuria	alimentary losses	reset osmostat	infant feeding
renal failure	respiratory losses	skin losses	hypertonic fluids
ureteric obstruction	skin losses	fluoride toxicity	mineralocorticoid excess
ECF volume LOW		NORMAL	HIGH

secretion, following either non-osmotic or pharmacological stimulation, and the TURP syndrome are common causes of water excess (Table 17.2).

Clinical evaluation of ECF volume and measurement of urine sodium concentration are helpful to differentiate the cause, and as a basis for therapy. When ECF volume and urine sodium concentration are low, intravenous saline is appropriate therapy. Hypertonic saline is only necessary when the serum sodium concentration is less than 120 mmol/l. Cardiovascular signs are only present in the water-deficient group.

TURP syndrome. The occurrence of cardiovascular and cerebral disturbances during transurethral resection of the prostate (TURP) is well described (Marx & Orkin 1962, Desmond 1970, Osborn et al 1980). The symptoms are the result of absorption of bladder-irrigating fluid (usually 1.5% glycine), causing hypervolaemia and hypotonicity. Fluid is absorbed during the resection in considerable amounts (10–30 ml/min) via open prostatic venous sinuses, and also into extravascular sites through small perforations of the bladder or through defects in the prostatic capsule (Oester & Madsen 1969, Aashein 1973). Sometimes, evidence of water intoxication is seen very quickly (within 15 min; Hulbert & Wingard 1979).

Glycine at a strength of 1.5% is hypotonic (osmolality approximately 200 mOsm/kg), so that its absorption leads to plasma hypotonicity associated with extracellular to intracellular shifts of water and glycine and dilutional hyponatraemia. The relationship between plasma osmolality, and plasma concentrations of glycine and sodium, are variable. It depends on the rate of fluid and solute shifts, and the composition of intravenous fluid therapy. Glycine absorption is also associated with hypervolaemia, but its extent is variable depending on blood losses and fluid replacement (Zucker & Bull 1984). In addition, glycine itself may demonstrate cardiac and cerebral toxicity, either directly or by its metabolism to ammonia and glyoxylic acid.

The symptomatology and plasma osmolar changes are modified by several factors. In particular the amount of glycine absorbed will depend on the duration and extent of surgery, the surgeon's skill, the hydrostatic pressure of the irrigant (which should never exceed 100 cmH_2O) and the presence of sepsis. Hypervolaemia may result in a small increase in systolic blood pressure and elevation of central venous pressure (CVP). In the presence of hypoosmolality, pulmonary and peripheral oedema are encouraged. Cardiovascular disturbances are particularly common in elderly men who may have underlying coronary and carotid artery disease, and who are receiving multiple therapy.

The syndrome is easier to recognize when the patient is awake, so regional, especially spinal anaesthesia, may be preferable to general anaes-

Table 17.2 Hyponatraemic hypoosmolar syndromes (modified from Schrier & Berl 1976, Narins et al 1982)

HYPONATRAEMIA

HYPERTONIC >285 mmol/kg
1. hyperglycaemia
2. hypertonic infusions
   - mannitol
   - glycine
   - glucose

ISOTONIC 280–285 mmol/kg
1. pseudohyponatraemia
   - hyperlipidaemia
   - hyperproteinaemia
2. isotonic infusions
   - mannitol
   - glycine
   - glucose

HYPOTONIC <280 mmol/kg

Total body water deficit with larger sodium deficit		Excess body water	Excess total body sodium with larger water excess
Renal losses diuretics renal tubular acidosis salt-losing nephritis hypoadrenalism urinary tract obstruction	*Extra renal losses* vomiting diarrhoea 'third space' 'sick cell syndrome' skin losses lung losses pancreatitis	Pain emotion drugs (e.g. chlorpropamide) SIADH TURP syndrome reset osmostat water intoxication hypokalaemia	Cardiac failure cirrhosis nephrotic syndrome
ECF volume: LOW		NORMAL-HIGH	HIGH
Urine sodium concentration >20 mmol/l	<10 mmol/l	>20 mmol/l	<10 mmol/l

thesia. Careful cardiovascular monitoring, including blood pressure and ECG is important, and CVP monitoring should be used more frequently. All patients for TURP should have a postoperative urine flow exceeding 0.5 ml/kg/hour. Dilution is recognized early with decreased concentrations of sodium, haemoglobin and urea. The decreases in concentration are greater than expected by the moderate decrease of serum osmolality. If in doubt postoperatively, the serum sodium concentration should be measured after TURP.

Mild degress of haemodilution will be corrected by spontaneous diuresis. However, the presence of cerebral and cardiovascular symptoms needs treatment with hypertonic saline (5%) and diuretics (frusemide 40–80 mg). Resolution is usually rapid, although acute cardiovascular collapse may necessitate inotropic agents, including calcium chloride (Charlton 1980).

Potassium balance

Hyperkalaemia

In the perioperative period, hyperkalaemia may have several causes:

1. increased input
   - diet
   - cellular damage, haemolysis
   - insulin deficiency
2. acidaemia
   - metabolic and respiratory
3. impaired excretion
   - renal failure
   - impaired renin-angiotensin-aldosterone axis
   - drugs: spironolactone, amiloride, digitalis.

The most important are those associated with renal failure, intracellular release after tissue damage and metabolic acidosis. Alimentary symptoms of irritation include vomiting and diarrhoea which lead to fluid losses. When the serum potassium concentration exceeds 7 mmol/l, arrhythmias are common, and these may be induced following administration of suxamethonium, particularly in the burned or injured patient. Rapid reduction of serum potassium concentration can be achieved with an infusion of 100 ml 50% dextrose containing 24 units of insulin, and 10 ml 10% calcium chloride (see Ch. 5).

Hypokalaemia

Gastrointestinal and diuretic-induced renal losses are the most common causes of hypokalaemia in the surgical patient (Table 17.3). In addition, stress responses induce potassium loss which the surgeon is reluctant to replace until adequacy of renal function is assured.

Symptoms are uncommon unless the serum potassium concentration is less than 2.5 mmol/l. This is associated with generalized muscle weakness including cardiac muscle. Hypotension unresponsive to catecholamines is common. During anaesthesia, hypokalaemia is associated with increased sensitivity to non-depolarizing neuromuscular blocking drugs (Waud et al 1982).

Restoration of potassium losses should, if possible, be completed before surgery. Oral replacement can be given up to a total of about 15 g (195 mmol) per day. Doses above that are irritant and nauseating. Intravenous replacement should not exceed a concentration of 40 mmol/l and should not be given at a rate greater than 0.5 l/hour.

Table 17.3 Aetiology of hypokalaemia

Factor	Cause
Decreased input	Diet
Alkalosis	–
Increased losses	Diuretics, saline loading, diabetes mellitus, hyperaldosteronism, 'stress' response, alkalosis

Calcium

Postoperative hypocalcaemia

Acute hypocalcaemia may occur after parathyroidectomy, radical neck surgery or thyroidectomy (see Ch. 9). Cardiovascular and neuromuscular symptoms are common. Hypotension is frequent and, rarely, is associated with congestive cardiac failure. The electrocardiogram demonstrates characteristic prolongation of the Q–T interval. Tetany is the hallmark of neuromuscular instability. Latent tetany may be detected by tapping over the facial nerve to elicit a twitch in the facial muscles (Chvostek's sign). Carpal spasm (Trousseau's sign) can be induced by inflating a blood pressure cuff around the arm above systolic pressure for 3 min. Carpal spasm is the direct effect of ischaemia potentiating nerve irritability.

Initial treatment is with 20–30 ml 10% calcium gluconate intravenously and, if symptoms persist, an infusion of calcium should be started. Long-term therapy, after total parathyroid ablation, includes oral calcium supplements, phosphorus restriction and vitamin D preparations.

Chronic hypocalcaemia is often seen in chronic renal failure. It produces a chronic parathyroid stimulation so that after successful transplantation hypercalcaemia may follow (Agus et al 1982). This may necessitate parathyroidectomy to control the serum calcium concentration.

Magnesium

Magnesium is the second most abundant intracellular cation, but little importance has been attached to disturbances of magnesium balance until recently. Half is present in bone and most of the remainder is found in soft tissue. Less than 1% is present in ECF. A normal diet contains about 12–15 mmol magnesium/day, of which 25–60% is absorbed. Regulation of the serum magnesium concentration is under the control of the kidney, although the mechanisms involved are uncertain. In general, the kidney offers a better defence against hypermagnesaemia than hypomagnesaemia.

Hypermagnesaemia

Hypermagnesaemia is usually iatrogenic and results from excess magnesium administration, antacids, enemas and dialysis fluids to patients in renal failure. Less commonly it follows the treatment of toxaemia of pregnancy with magnesium sulphate. When the serum magnesium concentration exceeds 2 mmol/l, muscle weakness is detectable and sensitivity to curare-like drugs can be demonstrated. When levels exceed 5 mmol/l, flaccid paralysis, respiratory failure and apnoea may follow. Hypotension with a characteristic increase in PR interval of the ECG occurs at high levels. This progresses to complete heart block at concentrations greater than 7.5 mmol/l. Treatment is by stopping magnesium therapy, administration of 10 ml 10% calcium glyconate and peritoneal dialysis should be considered.

Hypomagnesaemia

Hypomagnesaemia is common. Usually it has an alimentary aetiology; either decreased intake, including parenteral nutrition, or increased loss from enteritis or malabsorption. Renal losses may be increased with a variety of tubular magnesium-wasting disorders, but particularly in combination with diuretics or aminoglycoside administration (Dirks 1983). Potassium-wasting and hypokalaemia are common accompaniments of magnesium deficiency. Presenting features occur when the serum magnesium concentration is less than 0.5 mmol/l. They include personality change, tremor, fasciculation, carpopedal spasm and generalized spasticity. Treatment is by the resumption of a normal diet, supplemented, if necessary, with magnesium oxide. Magnesium sulphate is available for parenteral use.

CONCLUSION

The management of fluid and electrolyte balance in the surgical patient should follow a logical plan. Preoperative losses should be assessed and replaced before anaesthesia. During surgery all patients require fluid for maintenance and to replace losses. In the postoperative period, inadequate replacement is more common than excessive administration. When losses are abnormal their volume and electrolyte content should be measured for accurate replacement. The goals of therapy are to maintain cardiovascular integrity and osmolar equilibrium.

REFERENCES

Aashein G M 1973 Hyponatraemia during transurethral surgery. Can Anaesth Soc J 20: 274–280

Agus Z S, Wasserstein A, Goldfarb S 1982 Disorders of calcium and magnesium homeostasis. Am J Med 72: 473–488

Askanazi J, Rosenbaum S H, Hyman A I 1980 Respiratory changes induced by the large glucose loads of TPN. J Am Med Assoc 243: 1444–1447

Bevan D R 1980 Colloid osmotic pressure. Anaesthesia 35: 263–270

Charlton A J 1980 Cardiac arrest during transurethral prostatectomy after absorption of 1.5% glycine. Anaesthesia 35: 804–806

Collins J V, Cochrane G M, Davis J, Benetar S R, Clark J H 1973 Some aspects of pulmonary function after rapid saline infusion in healthy subjects. Clin Sci Mol Med 45: 407–410

Desmond J 1970 Complications of transurethral prostatic surgery. Can Anaesth Soc J 17: 25–36

Dirks J H 1983 The kidney and magnesium regulation. Kidney Int 23: 771–777

Epstein M 1980 The Le Veen shunt for ascites and the hepatorenal syndrome. N Engl J Med 302: 628–632

Hulbert B J, Wingard D W 1979 Water intoxication after 15 minutes of transurethral resection of the prostate. Anesthesiology 50: 355–356

Isbister J P, Fisher M McD 1980 Adverse effects of plasma volume expanders. Anaesth Intensive Care 8: 145–151

Lanier W L, Stangland K J, Scheithauer B W, Milde J H, Michenfelder J D 1987 The effects of dextrose infusion and head position on neurologic outcome after complete cerebral ischemia in primates: examination of a model. Anesthesiology 66: 39–48

Levy M, Allotey J B K 1978 Temporal relationship between urinary salt retention and altered systemic hemodynamics in dogs with experimental cirrhosis. J Lab Clin Med 92: 560–565

Longstreth W T, Inui T S 1984 High blood glucose level on hospital admission and poor neurological recovery after cardiac arrest. Ann Neurol 15: 59–63

Lorenz W, Doenicke A, Messmer K, Reiman H-J, Therman N, Lahn W, Berr J, Schmal A, Dorman P, Egenfuss P, Hamelmann H 1976 Histamine release in human subjects by modified gelatin (Haemaccel) and dextran: an

explanation for anaphylatoid reactions observed under clinical conditions. Br J Anaesth 48: 151–165
Marx G F, Orkin L R 1962 Complications associated with transurethral surgery. Anesthesiology 23: 802–813
Monafo W W, Chuntrasakul C, Ayvazian V H 1973 Hypertonic sodium solutions in the treatment of burn shock. Am J Surg 126: 778–783
Narins R G, Jones E R, Stom M C, Rudnick M R, Basti C P 1982 Diagnostic strategies in disorders of fluid, electrolyte and acid-base homeostasis. Am J Med 72: 496–520
Oester A, Madsen P O 1969 Determination of absorption of irrigating fluid during transurethral resection of the prostate by means of radioisotopes. J Urol 102: 714–719
Osborn D E, Rao P V, Greene M J, Barnard R J 1980 Fluid absorption during transurethral resection. Br Med J 281: 1549–1550
Prough D S, Johnson J C, Stump D A, Stallken E A, Poole G V Jr, Howard G 1986 Effects of hypertonic saline versus lactated Ringers solution on cerebral oxygen transport during resuscitation from hemorrhagic shock. J Neurosurg 64: 627–632
Read D H, Manners J M 1983 Osmolal excretion after open heart surgery. Anaesthesia 38: 1053–1061
Ring J, Messmer K 1977 Incidence and severity of anaphylactoid reactions to colloid volume substitutes. Lancet 1: 466–470
Roberson G L, Shelton R L, Athar S 1976 The osmoregulation of vasopressin. Kidney Int 10: 23–37
Schrier R W, Berl T 1976 Disorders of water metabolism. In: Schrier R W (ed) Renal and electrolyte disorders. Little Brown, Boston, p 39
Shires T, Williams J, Brown F 1961 Acute changes in extracellular fluids associated with major surgical procedures. Ann Surg 154: 803–810
Sieber F E, Smith D S, Traystman R J, Wollman H 1987 Glucose: a re-evaluation of its intraoperative use. Anesthesiology 67: 72–81
Smith H W 1959 From fish to philosopher: the story of our internal environment. Ciba, Summit, New Jersey
Tremper K K, Friedman A E, Levine A M, Lapin R, Camarillo D 1982 The preoperative treatment of severely anemic patients with perfluoro-chemical oxygen-transport fluid, Fluosol DA. N Engl J Med 303: 291– 292
Twigley A J, Hillman K M 1985 The end of the crystalloid era? Anaesthesia 40: 860–871
Velasco I T, Pontiem V, Rocha C, Silva M R Jr, Lopes O U 1980 Hyperosmotic NaCl and severe hemorrhagic shock. Am J Physiol 239: H664–H673
Waud B E, Mookerjee A, Waud D R 1982 Chronic potassium depletion and sensitivity to tubocurarine. Anesthesiology 57: 111–115
Zideman D A, Dudley H A F, Bevan D R 1978 Osmolar output in the peri-operative period. Anaesthesia 33: 788–793
Zucker J R, Bull A P 1984 Independent plasma levels of sodium and glycine during transurethral resection of the prostate. Can Anaesth Soc J 31: 307–313

18

Postoperative thrombosis and embolism

D. Goldhill

INTRODUCTION

The incidence and hazards of venous thrombosis in patients subjected to prolonged bed rest or in the perioperative period are such that vigorous preventative efforts should be taken with patients at risk. Pulmonary emboli (PE) are the most important and potentially fatal complication, however the serious long-term nature of postphlebitic disease should not be forgotten. Diagnosis of deep-vein thrombosis (DVT) is difficult as clinical signs and symptoms are often absent or non-specific. PE often occur without warning, and here again clinical diagnosis is made difficult by the lack of specific indicators.

AETIOLOGY OF VENOUS THROMBOSIS

In the mid-nineteenth century, Virchow described the triad of factors associated with the development of venous thrombosis. These are hypercoagulation, damage to the vessel wall and stasis. The last factor is probably the most common cause for venous thrombosis in the perioperative period and also in those patients confined to bed for any length of time. Most cases of venous thrombosis originate in areas of stasis around the valve cusps in the lower limb. In this region of sluggish circulation the activated factors causing the thrombosis are protected from blood-borne inhibitors, from clearance by the liver and from dissolution by fibrinolysis. Thrombin generated in these areas causes fibrin formation and platelet aggregation. The resulting nidus increases in size by forward propagation and retrograde extension, and may eventually fill the entire lumen of large veins.

THE INCIDENCE OF DEEP-VEIN THROMBOSIS

Venous thrombosis affects both medical and surgical patients, but the incidence is greater in patients with severe trauma or undergoing major surgery. Many seriously ill patients are at risk, and a proximal DVT is found at necropsy in about 25% of patients who die in hospital (Lindblad et al 1991). Postoperatively the incidence depends not only on the surgery undertaken, but on other risk factors that the patient may possess. The incidence varies from some 0.4% in women after childbirth to 12–15% in patients with soft-tissue injury of the lower limbs and 50% or more in elderly patients with major orthopaedic trauma. Table 18.1 shows the incidence of DVT and PE in various groups at risk.

Surgical patients can be classified as high, moderate or low-risk for developing thromboembolism depending primarily on the nature of the surgical procedure to be performed (Table 18.2; Hull et al 1986). High-risk patients are those having major orthopaedic lower-limb surgery, or extensive pelvic or abdominal surgery for malignant disease (NIH 1986). Also included are older patients with a history of DVT or PE. Patients at moderate risk are older people undergoing surgery

Table 18.1 Incidence of DVT and fatal PE in various groups

At-risk group	DVT	Fatal PE
General surgery	19–25%	1%
Orthopaedic surgery (hip or knee)	45–70%	1–3%
Urological surgery	25%	—
Gynaecological surgery	7–45%	1%
Neurosurgery	9–50%	1.5–3%
Major trauma	20–40%	1–4%
Critically ill	30%	—

of longer than 30 min. There is a low risk in younger healthy patients undergoing uncomplicated surgery or in fit adults older than 40 years of age for minor surgery of short duration. In all three groups the risk will be increased by additional factors (Goucke 1989). These are:

- surgery and other trauma
- previous history of venous thromboembolism
- increasing age
- malignancy
- obesity
- varicose veins
- prolonged immobilization
- oestrogen containing oral contraceptives
- pregnancy and the puerperium
- cardiac disease (especially myocardial infarction and congestive cardiac failure)
- hypercoagulation.

Although DVT are classically described as occurring at about 5 days after surgery and causing a PE on perhaps the tenth postoperative day, they can occur as early as the first day after surgery. Patients may be at increased risk of developing a DVT for as long as 6 weeks after surgery, well after they are ambulant and have been discharged from hospital.

Immobilization, causing venous stasis, is the most common factor preceding DVT and may be due to disabling problems such as lower limb fractures, paralysis, debilitating cardiopulmonary disease or extended best rest. Under this category will also come anaesthesia and the immediate post-operative recovery period, when the patient may have limited mobility because of pain or sedation. Congestive cardiac failure, recent myocardial infarction, cardiomyopathy and constrictive pericarditis increase the possibility of venous stasis and thus DVT. No significant difference in the frequency of DVT has been identified between males or females, although in women the oestrogen-containing oral contraceptives are a significant risk factor. Studies in the 1970s with the higher-dose oestrogen pills, no longer commonly in use, found that there was a two- to eight-fold increase in the relative risk of venous thrombosis. An increased risk of DVT remains even if women use oral contraceptives containing low doses of oestrogen (Helmrich et al 1987). Although there is an increased incidence of DVT in women taking the oral contraceptive, but not having perioperative prophylaxis, it is still not high. This is almost certainly because these women possess few other risk factors. During pregnancy, platelet levels and many coagulation factors are increased and this may be the cause of the higher incidence of thrombosis found in women, especially multiparae, during the postpartum period and also in the third trimester of pregnancy.

Older patients are more likely to have a DVT and there is a peak incidence between 50 and 65 years of age, although this also reflects the increased incidence of disease in the elderly. The hazard of DVT is multiplied with all neoplasms, being greatest with cancer of the lung, pancreas, and alimentary and genitourinary tracts. It has been suggested that in malignancy, mucin-producing cells are associated with thrombus formation and that abnormal haemostatic control may also play a part. In addition, neoplastic cells sometimes produce a variety of substances capable of activating the coagulation system (Bell & Simon 1982). Thromboembolism is also more common in a small number of patients with specific haematological diseases. These include those with reduced protein C levels or antithrombin III deficiency. Other conditions

Table 18.2 Classification of the risk of postoperative thromboembolism

Level of risk	Calf vein thrombosis	Proximal vein thrombosis	Fatal PE
High	40–80%	10–20%	1–5%
Moderate	10–40%	2–10%	0.1–0.7%
Low	<10%	<1%	<0.01%

associated with DVT formation include polycythaemia rubra vera, myeloproliferative diseases, splenectomy and blood group A. An increaed incidence has been found in the nephrotic syndrome, inflammatory bowel disease, lupus anticoagulant and metabolic conditions such as diabetes mellitus, homocystinuria and Behçet syndrome.

The incidence of pulmonary emboli

PE are the most serious and commonly fatal complication of DVT. It has been estimated that, in the USA, DVT and PE are associated with 300 000–600 000 hospital admissions per year, and that some 50 000 individuals die each year as a result of PE (NIH 1986). In the UK, PE may account for some 10% of all hospital deaths (Sandler & Martin 1989). Nearly 25% of surgical patients who die have been shown to have a PE which, in about half the cases, either caused or contributed to death (Bergqvist & Lindblad 1985). Without prophylaxis against DVT, between 0.1% and 1% of patients undergoing major operative surgery would die from a PE (Dismuke & Wagner 1986). PE are often rapidly fatal, and after a symptomatic PE about 10% of patients die within one hour, with up to a further 20% dying subsequently (Bell & Simon 1982). Although, as expected, most postoperative patients who die of their PE do so within the first few days of surgery, the problem can present some time after surgery with some 15% dying more than 30 days after the operation (Bergqvist & Lindblad 1985). An estimated 15–20% of DVT embolize, with about two-thirds of the fatal PE that result originating from proximal DVT in the ileofemoral segments of the leg veins (Bell & Simon 1982). Postmortem studies indicate that 65–85% of PE are associated with DVT (Sandler & Martin 1989, Lindblad et al 1991). Although DVT do not account for all PE, they are thought to be the cause in about 80% of fatal cases. Other sources of PE include thrombi in the right atrium, septic foci, tumours without evidence of intravascular thrombosis, amniotic fluid, bone marrow, fat and air (Bell & Simon 1982).

THE DIAGNOSIS OF DEEP-VEIN THROMBOSIS

The clinical diagnosis of DVT is based on the presence of calf tenderness, ankle oedema, an increase in skin temperature overlying the suspected DVT and changes in the circumference of the lower limb. Clinical signs result either from obstruction of venous outflow or from inflammation of the vessel wall or perivascular tissues. Unfortunately these do not occur with many potentially dangerous DVT, and up to two-thirds of venous thrombi are silent and are never clinically suspected. Even when clinical signs and symptoms are present they typically appear at least 24–36 hours after the DVT is detectable by other means (Kakkar et al 1970). Furthermore there are many other causes of a hot, painful, swollen leg, and thrombi are present only half the time that signs and symptoms suggest their existence (Salzman 1986). Therefore many postoperative patients will have a DVT that remains unsuspected and undiagnosed, and the use of objective diagnostic tests is essential before a patient thought to have a DVT is subjected to a prolonged course of anticoagulant treatment.

It is regrettable that the objective tests for DVT tend to be non-specific, inconvenient, technically demanding or expensive (Salzman 1986). The sensitivity and specificity of some methods of detecting DVT are shown in Table 18.3. The gold standard is venography, even though the deep femoral vein, and the common femoral and iliac veins are sometimes difficult to visualize adequately. Venography is a difficult technique and requires considerable experience to execute and interpret accurately. It is also expensive, causes local discomfort and allergic reactions, and may itself predispose to venous thrombosis in a small percentage

Table 18.3 Investigations for DVT

Method	Sensitivity	Specificity
Venography	98%	95%
^{125}I fibrinogen	94%	92%
Doppler	45–95%	41–96%
Plethysmography	90–95%	85–95%
Thermography	93%	98%

of patients. In addition, patients are exposed to radiation and this makes repeat studies undesirable. Venography is therefore not acceptable as a screening test for DVT and should be used only when one is suspected on other grounds. Blood tests for identifying the products of coagulation or accompanying fibrinolysis lack specificity and are of limited clinical value. Radioactive ^{125}I-labelled fibrinogen uptake has been used extensively as a screening test in patients at risk. A scintillation detector is used to make daily counts of isotope activity over several sites on the lower limbs. It detects distal (calf) thrombi but is of little use for detecting the thrombi above mid-thigh, which are the ones most likely to embolise. This test is insensitive to a clot that is not actually extending, takes at least 24 hours to obtain a result, and is invasive, requiring exposure of the patient to ionizing radiation. Because of the risk of infection from blood products it is likely that this test will not be available in the future. Plethysmography is one practical method that shows great promise as a screening test for occlusive proximal thrombi. With this technique a cuff is placed around the thigh and inflated to cause venous occlusion. As arterial inflow continues the calf increases in volume with the retained venous blood. At the end of the inflation period the thigh cuff is rapidly deflated and venous outflow is estimated by measuring the rate of change in the circumference of the calf. Reduced venous outflow is suggestive of occlusion of one of the main limb veins by a DVT. The calf circumference is usually measured with a strain gauge or by impedance. This test is simple to perform, non-invasive and repeatable. If consistent results are to be obtained the technique must be carefully applied. Non-occlusive DVT and those in the calf will be missed, and measurements in patients with reduced venous outflow, especially those who have suffered a DVT in the past, may give rise to false positive readings. Doppler ultrasound can also be used to detect DVT by examining flow through the venous system. However this test is subjective, and requires considerable skill and experience to be performed reliably and interpreted accurately. Duplex ultrasound imaging promises to be a satisfactory method of identifying DVT. Particular vessels can be imaged and the flow within the lumen studied. More advanced machines allow colour flow mapping where the colour on the screen is related to the velocity of blood flow. This method is non-invasive, repeatable and poses no hazard to the patient. It is likely to become the gold standard of the future for detecting DVT. There are as yet few published studies comparing this technique to venography. It is relatively poor in the detection of DVT from calf veins and in the iliac veins of patients who are obese or have had recent abdominal surgery. At present the necessary equipment is expensive. Other techniques, including thermography (Aronen 1981), have been explored but appear at present to be of little clinical use.

The diagnosis of pulmonary emboli

PE, just like DVT, are difficult to diagnose clinically (Dehring & Arens 1990). The vascular obstruction of the PE, and the release of chemical mediators from poorly perfused areas of lung, cause vasoconstriction and bronchoconstriction, and these give rise to ventilation/perfusion abnormalities. The pulmonary vasoconstriction may cause a decline in systemic blood pressure, a rise in pulmonary artery pressure and right-sided cardiac pressures. Clinically a PE can present as anything from a fever of unknown origin or chronic cardiopulmonary problem, to an overwhelming catastrophic disaster. The classic picture is described as hypotension, raised jugular venous pressure, right ventricular failure, chest pain, haemoptysis and fever. Unfortunately the patient with a PE rarely conforms to this ideal (Table 18.4; Bell & Simon 1982). Presentation often suggests congestive cardiac failure, pneumonia or other pulmonary disease, myocardial

Table 18.4 Symptoms and signs in patients with PE

Symptoms	%	Signs	%
Chest pain	88	Tachypnoea	92
Dyspnoea	85	Rales	58
Apprehension	59	Tachycardia	44
Cough	53	Pyrexia	43
Syncope	13	Gallop rhythm	34
		Haemoptysis	30

infarction, angina or even lung cancer. Symptoms may include apprehension, difficulty in breathing and pleuritic pain. Physical signs, such as tachypnoea, wheeze and fever are non-specific, and are present in a wide variety of diseases. The patient's heart rate is commonly normal and severe hypotension only occurs with about 10% of PE, almost always associated with a massive embolus. Although the signs and symptoms are often non-specific they provide the clinical suspicion on which further investigations are based.

The arterial blood gas will often show hypoxia and less frequently a low $P\text{aCO}_2$. A chest X-ray and ECG may exclude other acute diseases from the differential diagnosis, but they will often not prove a PE has occurred as changes may be absent, non-specific, transient or delayed. In approximately 80% of patients with suspected PE the ECG is of no value, although right-axis shift, T wave changes and abnormal S–T segments are common with massive PE. Invasive haemodynamic monitoring or echocardiography only are able to confirm the presence of a massive PE. A normal perfusion scan will exclude a PE but may have an incidence of false positive results as high as 50%. Ventilation/perfusion (V/Q) scans will correctly diagnose about 85% of PE where there are segmental or large areas of V/Q mismatch, but they are unreliable with subsegmental V/Q mismatch and in the presence of other lung pathology such as pulmonary oedema. The definitive diagnosis of a PE is made with angiography, an invasive procedure with an associated mortality. In urgent cases it may be possible to obtain a diagnosis by echocardiography or by injecting contrast dye into central venous or pulmonary artery catheters. Diagnosis of a DVT will support the suspicion that a PE has occurred and may decrease the necessity to perform angiography.

PROPHYLAXIS OF DVT

DVT are common in postoperative patients, difficult to diagnose, and the major cause of PE. DVT prophylaxis is therefore the best method to prevent PE. Prophylactic measures to guard against DVT should be taken in all surgical patients who fall into high- and moderate-risk categories (Table 18.2) (NIH 1986, Goucke 1989). This strategy not only decreases the incidence of DVT, but is also cost effective (Bergqvist et al 1988a). Although the prevention of PE is the main aim of prophylaxis, it should not be forgotten that swelling of the legs, varicose veins and ulceration are additional undesirable sequelae of extensive DVT and these will also be prevented.

Before subjecting a patient to surgery and the attendant risk of a DVT and PE, preoperative risk factors, such as cardiac failure, should be minimized. When time allows, consideration is necessary as to whether women taking oestrogen-containing oral contraceptives should change their form of contraception. Although women taking these contraceptives have an increased chance of developing a DVT, opinion is divided as to how they should be managed. Advice ranges from discontinuing the oral contraceptive four weeks before major elective surgery with heparin prophylaxis when discontinuation is not possible (Guillebaud 1985), to continuing the pill and not using prophylaxis, which is thought unnecessary (Sue-Ling & Hughes 1988). It should be noted that manufacturers generally advise stopping the oral contraceptive for 6 weeks before an operation, and this may impose a medico-legal constraint on the clinician.

Methods of prophylaxis can be divided into pharmacological and mechanical techniques (Goucke 1989) as listed below:

1. pharmacological
   - heparin: low dose subcutaneous
adjusted dose subcutaneous
ultralow dose
low molecular weight
   - oral anticoagulants: warfarin
   - antiplatelet therapy: aspirin (of dubious benefit)
   - dextran: dextran 40 or 70
   - dihydroergotamine
2. mechanical
   - pneumatic leg compression
   - electrical calf stimulation
   - graduated compression stockings
   - early ambulation
   - regional anaesthesia: spinal and epidural.

In some groups of patients more than one prophylactic regime may be effective, and the best prophylaxis often consists of a combination of techniques. In addition, the method of anaesthesia employed may also affect the likelihood of developing a DVT. Many researchers have examined the efficacy of prophylactic regimens to prevent DVT in the postoperative period. The practical difficulty of identifying patients with DVT means that studies are often on a small scale, using a variety of methods on a range of different patient groups. Unsurprisingly this often produces conflicting results. Although the efficacy of a particular method of prophylaxis in a specific situation is not always unqualified, it is clear that the incidence of DVT and PE can be significantly reduced in patients at risk. Suggestions for prophylaxis are given in the list below:

- all patients: early postoperative ambulation
- low risk: graduated compression stockings
- moderate risk: heparin subcutaneous 5000 i.u. 12-hourly
  - or low molecular weight heparin subcutaneous 2500 i.u. daily
  - or dextran 500ml intraoperatively and daily for 3–4 days
  - intermittent pneumatic leg compression (recommended for intracranial neurosurgery)
  - graduated compression stockings
  - regional anaesthesia
  - antithrombotic therapies should be avoided as even minor haemorrhage is potentially dangerous
- high risk: as for moderate risk but also consider adjusted dose heparin or low dose warfarin.

These suggestions may need to be modified for individual patients and particular surgical procedures (Bell & Simon 1982, NIH 1986, Goucke 1989, Dehring & Arens 1990).

As venous thrombosis is to a great extent the result of venous stasis, an aggressive approach should be adopted in the pre-, peri- and postoperative periods to maintain venous flow in the veins of the lower limbs. Preservation of an adequate cardiac output is important and increased blood viscosity should be prevented, where necessary by the administration of intravenous fluid. Care must be taken to avoid undue calf compression, and pressure points must be protected by padding. A 15° head-down tilt will also increase the blood flow rate in the veins of the legs.

Heparin is the most widely used drug in the prophylaxis of DVT. It acts by potentiating the activity of antithrombin III on Factor Xa inhibition, its antithrombotic effect, and it inhibits Factor IIA, its anticoagulant effect. A meta-analysis of heparin prophylaxis trials shows that heparin is effective in reducing DVT in a range of situations (Collins et al 1988). Overall, heparin reduced the incidence of DVT by about 60% and the number of fatal PE to one third for a reduction in mortality of about 20%. There was a small increase in the number of wound haematoma but no significant increase in deaths from bleeding. If subcutaneous heparin is used this should be started 2 hours before surgery and continued at least until the patient is fully mobile. Administering 12-hourly doses is as effective as an 8-hourly regime but is less likely to cause wound haematoma. Various refinements on the use of heparin have been described. These include adjusted-dose subcutaneous heparin, where the dose is adjusted to keep the activated partial thromboplastin time (APTT) between 31.5 and 36 s, and ultra low-dose heparin as a continuous infusion of 1.0 i.u./kg/hour. More recently, trials have been performed with low molecular weight fractionated heparin. This consists of short heparin fragments, about 18 monosaccharide units long, with an average molecular weight of 4000–6000 Da. Compared with standard heparin, this preparation has more antithrombotic potency with less risk of bleeding complications. Furthermore it has a long half-life so that it need only be administered once a day (Bergqvist et al 1988b). Oral anticoagulation with warfarin is widely used in the treatment of DVT and PE. Although it has been employed in the prophylaxis of DVT, the increased risk of haemorrhage and the need for close monitoring of prothrombin time make this method unsuitable for most patients. Antiplatelet therapy, particularly aspirin, has undergone several randomized trials for prophylaxis of DVT and opinions remain divided on the benefit of this therapy. Intravenous dextran is effective in decreasing the incidence of DVT in high-risk patients by causing a relative haemodilution, thus decreasing blood viscosity, and by alterating platelet function and the ability of fibrin to polymerize. Both dextran 40 and dextran 70 appear to be equally effective in the prevention of DVT. An anaphylactoid reaction and fluid overload are possibilities when using dextran, and prophylaxis with this technique is more expensive than with heparin. Dihydroergotamine causes an increase in venous smooth-muscle tone, reducing peripheral venous pooling and increasing femoral vein blood flow velocity. It is usually used in combination with heparin. A side effect is arterial spasm which has, on occasion, resulted in gangrene.

Several mechanical devices decrease the risk of DVT by increasing venous return through the deep veins of the lower limb. Pneumatic devices intermittently compress the calf, sometimes in a sequential or wave-like manner. These mechanical devices are probably more effective than electrical calf stimulation. Elastic graduated compression stockings, when properly applied, are of benefit in low-risk general surgical patients and may be useful in combination with other techniques. Regional anaesthesia will help minimize the incidence of DVT in elective and emergency hip surgery, and this should be considered when selecting an anaesthetic technique for these procedures.

TREATMENT OF DVT AND PE

If a patient has a confirmed DVT the aim of therapy is to minimize thrombus extension, minimize damage to the deep venous system of the leg, and prevent a PE. Because of its immediate action, heparin is the anticoagulant of choice for initial treatment. Although it will not dissolve formed thrombus, it will prevent extension of the thrombus and may stimulate fibrinolysis. Heparin should be given as an intravenous infusion to maintain the activated partial thromboplastin time (e.g. kaolin cephalin clotting time [KCTT]) at 1.5–2.5 times control value (Fennerty et al 1988). A loading dose of heparin (5000 i.u.) is given over 5 min and an infusion started at 1400 i.u./hour. The KCTT is checked after 6 hours and the dose of heparin adjusted accordingly (Fennerty et al 1988). Oral anticoagulation with warfarin is typically started after 3 days of heparin treatment. The effectiveness of the warfarin is measured using the international normalized ratio (INR), which expresses the prothrombin time using a world standard for thromboplastin reagents. The heparin is discontinued when a therapeutic INR of 2.0–2.5 is achieved. Recommendations on the optimum duration of oral anticoagulation range from 3 weeks to 6 months. Warfarin can cause major life-threatening haemorrhage and the risk of this occurring increases with the duration of treatment. It has been suggested that a maximum of 4 weeks' warfarin therapy may provide the best compromise when treating a first episode of thromboembolism (Fennerty et al 1988). Patients with repeat thromboembolic events will require longer treatment.

Initial management of a PE is supportive to prevent hypoxia and cardiovascular collapse. Therapy includes administration of oxygen, mechanical ventilation, intravenous fluid resuscitation, and the use of vasopressors, inotropes and antiarrhythmics. At present, no selective pulmonary vasodilators are available, and systemic and venous dilatation are potentially harmful to a patient with a major PE. Limited data suggest that hydrallazine may be better than other vasodilators in relieving pulmonary hypertension (Dehring & Arens 1990). Further treatment of a massive PE lie between thrombolytic therapy, surgical pulmonary embolectomy, transvenous catheter embolectomy, and inferior vena cava (IVC) filter. Management algorithms for the treatment of PE are given below (Dehring & Arens 1990):

1. no contraindication to anticoagulation:
   give heparin bolus

- if stable: confirm with V/Q scan, pulmonary angiography, DVT studies treat with heparin and warfarin
- if unstable: confirm with pulmonary angiogram
- central PE: treat with fem-fem bypass, embolectomy, IVC filter or thrombolysis
- peripheral PE: treat with IVC filter or thrombolysis

continue with heparin and warfarin

2. contraindication to anticoagulation and thrombolysis:
   - central PE: treat with catheter embolectomy and IVC filter
   - peripheral PE: treat with IVC filter

3. contraindication to thrombolysis: give heparin bolus
   - unstable central PE: treat with fem-fem bypass, embolectomy, IVC filter
   - peripheral PE: treat with IVC filter

   continue with heparin and warfarin.

Thrombolytic therapy with streptokinase or urokinase will dissolve thromboemboli, a treatment that has been suggested for both DVT and PE (Bailey & Spielman 1985). These drugs activate the body's natural fibrinolytic system by converting plasminogen to plasmin. Streptokinase activates fibrinolysis by combining with and changing the conformation of plasminogen, whereas urokinase is a direct activator of the plasminogen-plasmin system. Tissue plasminogen activator (t-PA) has also been used for thrombolysis. Lysis of thrombus must be followed by conventional anticoagulation to prevent rethrombosis and embolization. Because thrombolytic therapy also lyses other tissue blood clots, treatment is relatively contraindicated within 7–10 days of surgery. Major bleeding complications affect about 10% of patients and thrombolysis is probably best reserved for patients with an acute massive embolism where embolectomy is not advisable.

Surgical pulmonary embolectomy carries a mortality of 50% or greater, although there is some evidence that improved survival rates can be achieved with the use of cardiopulmonary bypass before embolectomy (Dehring & Arens 1990). Proponents of thrombolytic therapy believe embolectomy should only be performed when thrombolysis is contraindicated or ineffective. Transvenous catheter embolectomy can be performed under local anaesthesia with a steerable catheter designed to remove central PE. The reported mortality in unstable patients is 27%.

Vena caval interruption to prevent thrombi reaching the lungs should be considered if anticoagulation or thombolysis is contraindicated or fails, after embolectomy, or with chronic embolization. Ligation or plication of the inferior vena cava has a mortality of 10–15%. Transvenous placement of intracaval devices, such as umbrella filters, have largely replaced surgical methods.

ANAESTHESIA AND THROMBOEMBOLISM

Several studies, primarily examining hip or knee surgery, have demonstrated a decrease of about 50% in the incidence of postoperative DVT in patients anaesthetized with a regional technique (spinal or epidural), compared with general anaesthesia (McKenzie 1991). General anaesthesia has a detrimental effect on lower limb blood flow which is reduced by about 50%. This is exacerbated by positive pressure ventilation. Before a spinal or lumbar epidural block it is common to give a fluid load to counteract the sympathetic effects of the local anaesthetic. The resulting decrease in blood viscosity, the lower intravascular hydrostatic pressure from vasodilatation, and the improved deformability of red and white cells after a subarachnoid block may all contribute to this advantage of regional over general anaesthesia.

Regional anaesthesia and anticoagulation

Many anaesthetists apparently consider that low-dose heparin DVT prophylaxis is a contraindication to epidural block because of concern that an epidural haematoma is made more likely. This problem is rare and may occur spontaneously in patients who have neither a coagulation disorder nor a regional anaesthetic. Definitive studies on the safety of epidural or spinal anaesthesia in patients on low-dose heparin have not been performed and would be difficult to conduct (Owens et al 1986, Wille-Jørgensen et al 1991, Wildsmith & McClure 1991). Opinion has been expressed that this combination is safe (Wille-Jørgensen et al 1991), whereas others have added the proviso that the block should not be performed within 4–6 hours of the administration of heparin, or alternatively that giving heparin should be delayed until after the block is performed (Wildsmith & McClure 1991). The safest time to remove an epidural catheter from a patient on low-dose heparin is about an hour before a dose is due.

There is general agreement that central nerve blockade is contraindicated if the patient is fully anticoagulated or has recently received thrombolytic therapy. Administration of heparin after performing an epidural or spinal block appears to be safe as long as sufficient time is allowed for any bleeding caused at the time of the block to stop. If possible, epidural catheters should be removed when the anticoagulation has worn off or been reversed.

The effect on platelet aggregation caused by aspirin lasts for 7–10 days, and the concerns that apply to heparin and regional anaesthesia arise with patients on aspirin. There is, as yet, little information on the risk of haematoma in this situation. A bleeding time of 10 min has been suggested as the level above which an epidural catheter should not be inserted, but this is probably a test that is not widely applied to patients at risk. To avoid the potential hazard posed by aspirin therapy, medication would have to be stopped for at least 72 hours, perhaps longer, before an extradural block (Macdonald 1991).

REFERENCES

Aronen A J 1981 Thermography in deep venous thrombosis of the leg. Am J Roentgenol 137: 1179–1182

Bailey A, Spielman F J 1985 Thrombolytic therapy. Can Anaesth Soc J 32: 385–389

Bell W R, Simon T L 1982 Current status of pulmonary thromboembolic disease: pathophysiology, diagnosis, prevention, and treatment. Am Heart J 103: 239–261

Bergqvist D, Lindblad B 1985 A 30 year survey of pulmonary embolism verified at autopsy: an analysis of 1,274 surgical patients. Br J Surg 72: 105–108

Bergqvist D, Jendteg S, Lindgren B, Mätzsch T, Persson U 1988a The economics of general thromboembolic prophylaxis. World J Surg 12: 349–355

Bergqvist D, Mätzsch T, Burmark U S, Frisell J, Guilbaud O, Hallböök T, Horn A, Lindhagen A, Ljungnér H, Ljungström K-G, Onarheim H, Risberg B, Törngren S, Örtenwall P 1988b Low molecular weight heparin given the evening before surgery compared with conventional low-dose heparin in prevention of thrombosis. Br J Surg 75: 888–891

Collins R, Scrimgeour A, Yusuf S, Peto R 1988 Reduction in fatal pulmonary embolism and venous thrombosis. N Engl J Med 318: 1162–1173

Dehring D J, Arens J F 1990 Pulmonary thromboembolism: disease recognition and patient management. Anesthesiology 73: 146–164

Dismuke S E, Wagner E H 1986 Pulmonary embolism as a cause of death: the changing mortality in hospitalized patients. J Am Med Assoc 255: 2039–2042

Fennerty A, Campbell I A, Routledge P A 1988 Anticoagulants in venous thromboembolism: guidelines for optimum treatment. Br Med J 297: 1285–1288

Goucke C R 1989 Prophylaxis against venous thromboembolism. Anaesth Intensive Care 17: 458–465

Guillebaud J 1985 Surgery and the pill. Br Med J 291: 498–499

Helmrich S P, Rosenberg L, Kaufman D W, Strom B, Shapiro S 1987 Venous thromboembolism in relation to oral contraceptive use. Obstet Gynecol 69: 91–95

Hull R D, Raskob G E, Hirsh J 1986 Prophylaxis of venous thromboembolism: an overview. Chest 89: 374S–383S

Kakkar V V, Howe C T, Nicolaides A N, Renney J T G, Clarke M B. 1970 Deep vein thrombosis of the leg: Is there a 'high risk' group? Am J Surg 120: 527–530

Lindblad B, Sternby N H, Berqvist D 1991 Incidence of venous thromboembolism verified by necropsy over 30 years. Br Med J 302: 709–711

Macdonald R 1991 Aspirin and extradural blocks. Br J Anaesth 66: 1–3

McKenzie P J 1991 Deep venous thrombosis and anaesthesia (Editorial). Br J Anaesth 66: 4–7

NIH 1986 Consenus Conference: Prevention of venous thrombosis and pulmonary embolism. J Am Med Assoc 256: 744–749

Owens E L, Kasten G W, Hessel E A 1986 Spinal subarachnoid hematoma after lumbar puncture and heparinization: a case report, review of the literature, and discussion of anaesthetic implication. Anesth Analg 65: 1201–1207

Salzman E D 1986 Venous thrombosis made easy (Editorial). N Engl J Med 314: 847–848

Sandler D A, Martin J F 1989 Autopsy proven pulmonary embolism in hospital patients: are we detecting enough deep vein thrombosis? J R Soc Med 82: 203–205

Sue-Ling H, Hughes L E 1988 Should the pill be stopped preoperatively? Br Med J 296: 447–448

Wildsmith J A W, McClure J H 1991 Anticoagulant drugs and central nerve blockade. Anaesthesia 46: 613–614

Wille-Jørgensen P, Jørgensen N, Rasmussen L S 1991 Lumbar regional anaesthesia and prophylactic anticoagulant therapy: is the combination safe? Anaesthesia 46: 623–627

SECTION 4

Hazards related to anaesthetic drugs

19

Adverse effects of drugs given by injection

J. W. Sear

INTRODUCTION

Adverse, unwanted or unexpected side effects are seen with all drugs. If a drug is administered directly into the circulation, the onset of these effects will often be rapid. For intravenously and intramuscularly delivered anaesthetic agents, adverse reactions can be divided into those that are predictable and hence potentially avoidable, and those that occur at random and are usually the result of some form of idiosyncrasy or hypersensitivity. In addition to these true adverse reactions there are other unwanted side effects which may influence a drug's usefulness or efficacy. In the case of the intravenous hypnotic induction agents, examples of the latter include spontaneous movement during induction, hypertonus, pain on injection, and venous sequelae such as phlebitis and thrombosis. These adverse effects generally have a high incidence and are dose dependent, but are associated with a low mortality (e.g. the overall incidence of thrombophlebitis after i.v. induction of anaesthesia may be as high as 40%, and the overall incidence of postoperative vomiting 30%).

Among the adverse reactions that may be considered as predictable are the prolongation of the effects of suxamethonium in patients receiving propanidid, procainamide, procaine, lignocaine or certain of the chemotherapeutic cytotoxic agents (e.g. methotrexate and cyclophosphamide), and the cardiotoxicity of bupivacaine associated with the release of the tourniquet after intravenous regional anaesthesia.

Overall, there is little doubt that the incidence of adverse reactions to drugs is on the increase. This may relate to the high percentage of patients receiving intercurrent medication. If such individuals present for anaesthesia and surgery, the possibility of drug–drug interactions is more likely. A report by Levy et al (1979) indicated that about 4% of all hospital admissions were the result of adverse responses to therapeutic doses of drugs. However, to put the incidence of these adverse reactions in perspective, they range from 1:5000–1:20 000 for anaphylaxis, to 1:150 000 for hepatic necrosis following halothane, and 1:20 000–1:200 000 for malignant hyperpyrexia. The overall mortality of adverse reactions in two large series was 4% (Clarke et al 1975, Fisher & More 1981).

In this chapter, various aspects of the problems of adverse drug reactions will be discussed: what are the mechanisms involved? what are the clinical features? what are the predictors of or predisposing factors to a reaction? how should the reactions be treated when they occur? how can the affected patient be studied in order to prevent re-exposure to the causative agent?

Before examining these immunological mechanisms, other adverse drug responses will be considered (those predictable responses already mentioned).

WHAT FACTORS MAY BE RESPONSIBLE FOR PREDICTABLE DRUG REACTIONS?

Overdose

There are two types of overdose:

1. Absolute overdose due to acute excess administration, or to accumulation as a result of reduced elimination or metabolism.
2. Relative overdose due to patient factors, such as hypovolaemia, extremes of age, intercurrent disease (especially cardiac, renal or hepatic impairment) and drug–drug interactions.

Bacterial contamination

This may occur due to the use of non-aseptic techniques when handling the hypnotic agent, propofol. This drug is made up in egg phosphatide emulsion which contains no antimicrobial preservatives and may support the growth of microorganisms.

Incompatible drug mixtures

The precipitation reaction that occurs when thiopentone and d-tubocurarine are administered in the same syringe, or via the same intravenous cannula, is an example of an incompatible drug mixture. This interaction is also seen with some of the other non-depolarizing muscle relaxants (e.g. alcuronium, pancuronium and atracurium). Excess dilution of lipophilic drugs formulated in solubilizing agents may result in the solution becoming unstable. Similarly, changes in the pH of the blood or tissues may lead to precipitation of drugs from solution, for example thiopentone and methohexitone in acidic environments.

Side effects

Examples of side effects are excessive hypotension or bradycardia, which are seen following the administration of large doses of the intravenous hypnotic agents and opioids, respectively. Also, methaemoglobin formation is associated with the metabolism of prilocaine (an amide local anaesthetic) to o-toluidine. This occurs when large doses of prilocaine (>600 mg) are used as part of a plexus or intravenous regional technique.

Secondary effects

Secondary effects include competition for the same metabolic degradation pathway, as can be seen with propanidid and suxamethonium (see Appendix 2 for important drug–drug interactions).

Idiosyncratic effects

Idiosyncratic effects occur under circumstances, or in conditions, where the administration of a specific drug or group of drugs is contraindicated. This is often due to the presence of a genetic or inherited abnormality (e.g. porphyria, malignant hyperpyrexia, plasma pseudocholinesterase deficiency, glucose-6-phosphate dehydrogenase deficiency and the genetic polymorphism of drug metabolism: fast and slow acetylators of hydralazine, slow and fast hydroxylators of desbrisoquin or propranolol). The incidence of these predictable drug responses is higher than that of the true allergic or immunological reactions. In addition, there are the other pharmacological effects of drugs apart from those for which they are principally used. Some examples of these unwanted pharmacological effects are given below.

Opioid agents

Unwanted effects of opioid agents include: respiratory depression; euphoria or dysphoria; postoperative nausea and vomiting; miosis; decreased intestinal peristalsis and sphincteric constriction; vasodilatation in high dosage.

Hypnotic agents

Unwanted effects of hypnotic agents include: respiratory and myocardial depression; laryngospasm; postoperative disorientation, vertigo and euphoria; venous sequelae; antanalgesia (barbiturates); decreased cerebral metabolism (barbiturates, etomidate, Althesin and propofol); anticonvulsant effects; hallucinations (ketamine); adrenal cortex suppression (etomidate); hypothalmopituitary modulation of the neuroendocrine responses to surgery or trauma (midazolam).

Benzodiazepines

Unwanted effects of benzodiazepines include: central nervous system (CNS) depression and drowsiness; muscle weakness; ataxia; dysarthria; interactions with alcohol.

Local anaesthetics

Unwanted effects of local anaesthetics include: neurocytotoxicity; CNS excitement, euphoria and convulsions; respiratory and cardiovascular depression (bupivacaine); membrane stabilization (lignocaine and mepivacaine); mydriasis; tachyphylaxis; locally mediated adverse effects such as spinal cord ischaemia, arachnoiditis and radiculitis.

Muscle relaxants

Unwanted effects of muscle relaxants include: blockade of sympathetic ganglia to produce hypotension (d-tubocurarine), or of vagal postganglionic fibres to cause tachycardia and arterial hypertension (gallamine, pancuronium). Contraindications to succinylcholine are listed in Appendix 3. For further discussion of the predictable side effects of these agents, the interested reader is referred to any standard text book of pharmacology and Fisher (1984).

With the increasing number of agents available to the anaesthetist, it is important that he chooses his drugs carefully and logically according to the particular patient and the specific clinical situation.

WHAT ARE THE MECHANISMS INVOLVED IN IMMUNOLOGICAL REACTIONS?

Adverse immunological responses to foreign proteins or other substances normally require either antibody formation or an alternative humoral mechanism leading to a hypersensitivity reaction. The occurrence of a reaction depends upon two separate events: recognition of the protein or foreign substance (in this case a drug) and a secondary response.

Under normal conditions the primary exposure of an individual to a foreign substance will result in antibody production. Following antigen exposure, B lymphoctye transformation occurs with the subsequent synthesis of antibodies by plasma cells and other lymphocyte populations. A second or subsequent exposure to the same foreign substance usually results in only a localized response with antigen and antibody interaction. However, in the case of an allergic reaction to repeat exposure to a particular chemical or drug, a systemic response to the formation of the antigen–antibody complex occurs.

Antibodies

The immune system consists of a variety of molecules and cells of which the immunoglobulins and lymphocytes are the most important. There are two types of lymphocytes: T and B cells. The former are involved in cellular immunity, whereas the B cells are of importance for humoral immunity. After exposure to an antigen, B cells differentiate into plasma cells which can synthesize antibodies to interact with the antigen.

Antibodies are immunoglobulins, part of the larger group of molecules termed glycoproteins, which contain 82–96% protein and 4–18% carbohydrate. Each immunoglobulin is made up of two identical heavy chains and two identical light side chains linked by disulphide bonds. Most human immunoglobulins have a flexible region between the N-terminal F_{ab} arms and the C-terminal F_c fragments. The F_{ab} fragments contain the antigen binding sites, while the F_c fragments have effector function sites (e.g. binding of complement [IgG binding to Cl_q]; binding to protein A or G [ex. *Staphylococcus aureus* and *streptococcus* sp., respectively]; binding to F_c receptors on leucocytes, which are responsible for promoting cell phagocytosis, clearance of immune complexes, antibody cell-mediated cytotoxicity, release of chemical mediators and superoxide production).

There are nine immunoglobulin heavy chain isotypes (IgM, IgD, IgE, IgG_{1-4} and IgA_{1-2}). IgE is the main immunoglobulin involved in drug reactions. It is able to bind avidly to the surface membrane of mast cells and basophils through the F_c portion. For anaphylaxis to occur the antigen must be polyvalent (binding two or more IgE molecules). This binding results in stereochemical changes within the cells, and hence cellular disruption and the release of primary or secondary mediators (histamine, heparin, eosinophil and neutrophil chemotactic factors [primary or preformed mediators], leukotrienes B–E_4 [slow releasing substance of anaphylaxis: SRSA], prostaglandins, platelet-activating factor and kinins [secondary or formed mediators]). The release of both types of mediators is dependent on the presence of calcium ions.

In addition to cell degranulation, there is oxidative metabolism of arachidonic acid to leukotrienes, thromboxanes and platelet aggregating factors. The onset of a reaction is usually immediate, but it may occur up to about 20 min after parenteral drug administration (so-called 'hypersensitivity reactions' to drugs).

The mechanisms involved in these hypersensitivity reactions have been classified into four main types; each of which is discussed below.

Type I hypersensitivity

In Type I (immediate) hypersensitivity the antigens interact with specific IgE reaginic antibodies. These antibodies are often bound to the surface of mast cells and basophils, which, following antigen–antibody interaction, become degranulated and release histamine and other vasoactive amines.

Type II hypersensitivity

In Type II (cytotoxic-like) hypersensitivity, IgA, IgG or IgM antibodies bind to an antigen located on the cell surface and initiate phagocytosis through either opsonization, or NK-cell mediated non-phagocytic extracellular cytotoxicity. The antibody–antigen interaction then activates the classical complement pathway, leading to cell lysis and death. The antigens involved may be integral components of the cell membrane (e.g. blood-group antigens) or molecules (haptens) which adhere to the cell membrane (e.g. penicillin).

Type III hypersensitivity

In Type III (immune-complex-mediated) hypersensitivity the interaction of antibody and antigen results in immune complex formation with the resulting activation of the classical complement pathway. If the antibody is present in excess there occurs a localized (Arthus) response; if antigen is in excess, a diffuse systemic reaction (serum sickness type) occurs.

Type IV hypersensitivity

In Type IV (cell-mediated or delayed) hypersensitivity, T lymphocytes with specific surface receptors are stimulated through antigen contact and release lymphokines which mediate the hypersensitivity reaction.

Thus, both type II and III hypersensitivity reactions can result in activation of the classical complement pathway. IgG or IgM antibodies must be involved, as IgE antibodies do not bind to complement.

MECHANISMS OF ANAPHYLAXIS

Most drugs administered during anaesthesia are of low molecular weight (≤1000 daltons) and as such are not capable *on their own* of initiating an immune response with the production of specific antibodies. However, many drugs are able to combine in vivo with a carrier protein (hapten) to form an antigenic moiety. The extent of basophil and mast cell degranulation will depend on the amount of drug injected, the affinity of the drug for the antibodies and the amount of cell-bound antibodies produced.

A number of vasoactive compounds have already been described as undergoing release following mast cell and basophil degranulation. Each of these has different pharmacological effects (Table 19.1). There is little doubt, however, that histamine is the most important vasoactive compound released by degranulation, and is the only substance proven to be essential for anaphylaxis to occur.

Table 19.1 Chemical mediators released by degranulation of mast cells and basophils (from Altman 1981)

Mediators	Pharmacological effects
Preformed	
Histamine	Increased capillary permeability, bronchoconstriction
Eosinophil chemotactic factor of anaphylaxis (ECF-A)	Attraction of eosinophils
Neutrophil chemotactic factor of anaphylaxis (NCF-A)	Attraction of neutrophils
Heparin	Anticoagulant, inhibition of complement system activation
Newly synthesized	
Arachidonic acid metabolites	
Slow-reacting substance of anaphylaxis (SRS-A; leukotrienes C_4, D_4, E_4)	Bronchoconstriction, increased capillary permeability, coronary vasoconstriction, pulmonary vasoconstriction (D_4), altered inotropy
Prostaglandins	Bronchoconstriction (PGD_2, PGF_{2a}), bronchodilatation (PGE_1, PGE_2), pulmonary hypertension, peripheral vasodilatation
Thromboxane A_2 (TA_2)	Platelet aggregation, bronchoconstriction, vasoconstriction
Prostacyclin	Increased capillary permeability, antagonism of effects of TA_2
Platelet activating factor	Platelet aggregation and degranulation, increased capillary permeability
Kinins (prekallikrein and bradykinin)	Increased capillary permeability, vasodilatation

Anaphylactoid reactions

Anaphylactoid reactions occur as a result of either a direct pharmacological effect or another non-immune response by which the drug causes the release of histamine. For some drugs, particularly those with basic properties (e.g. d-tubocurarine, suxamethonium, morphine, thiobarbiturates and trimetaphan), there is direct competitive displacement of histamine (another basic molecule) from the mast cell.

As will be discussed later, there are, in addition, predisposing factors that may also play a role in the genesis of these anaphylactoid responses.

The main aetiologies of these anaphylactoid hypersensitivity reactions to drugs can be subdivided into: alternate complement pathway activation and direct pharmacological effects.

Complement pathway

There are more than 22 complement proteins which are synthesized as acute phase proteins in the liver. Their concentrations vary greatly from 3.0 μg/ml to 1.2 mg/ml. Activation of the complement pathway can be achieved via two separate pathways. These are termed classical complement activation and alternate pathway activation. Normally the complement proteins exist in an inactive form due to the presence of inhibitor proteins and the spontaneous breakdown of activated enzymes. The complement system has various functions:

1. Opsonization. This involves the coating of foreign particles to increase their attractiveness to phagocytes.
2. Lysis of foreign proteins. This is probably of little relevance in vivo.
3. Augmentation of the inflammatory response. This may occur by:
   - increasing the chemotaxis of neutrophils
   - increasing white cell mobilization from the bone marrow
   - activating macrophages
   - increasing the permeability of capillary vessels.

The interaction of the various components of the two complement pathways is shown in Figure 19.1.

Classical complement pathway

The activation of the classical complement pathway can be achieved by several initiators:

- immune complexes containing IgG or IgM antibodies
- aggregated IgG

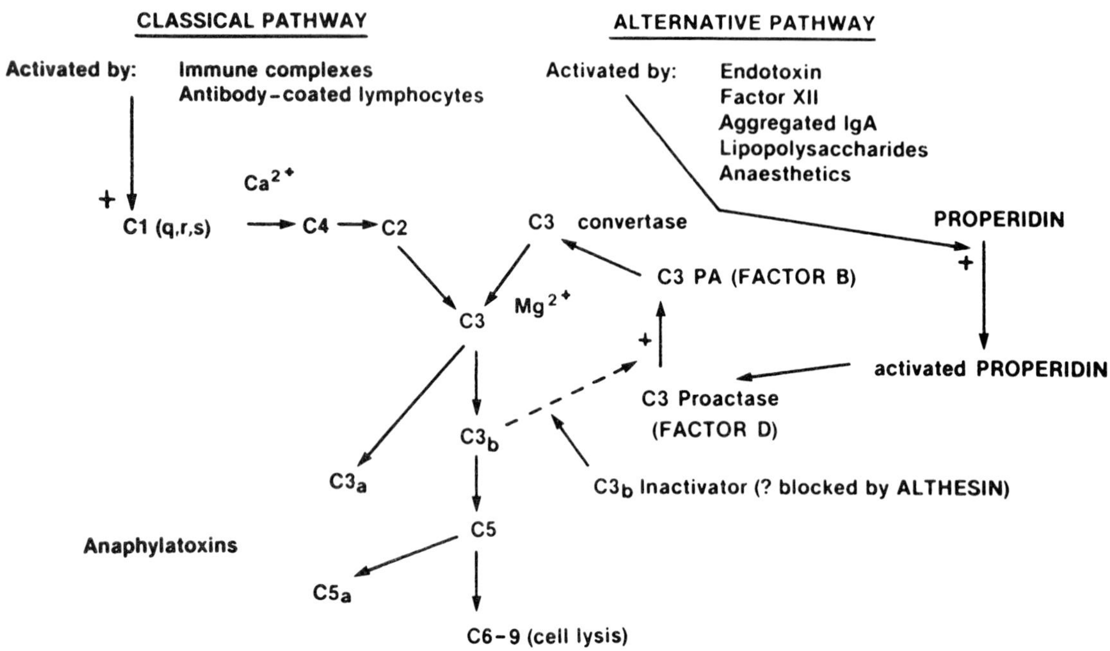

Fig. 19.1 Component proteins and activation cascades of the classical and alternative complement pathways.

- C-reactive protein
- polyamines, polynucleotides or polyvalent cations
- proteolytic enzymes
- gram-negative bacteria, parasites and mitochondrial membranes
- the lipid A moiety of endotoxin
- some RNA viruses.

For an adverse drug reaction to be mediated via the classical pathway there must be interaction between the antigen (drug) and the antibody (i.e. previous exposure to the drug or the presence of a cross-reacting antibody). The interaction results in comformation changes in the protein structure of the antibody, leading to the exposure of the complement binding sites. Once binding of the antigen–antibody to complement protein Cl_q has occurred, activation of the cascade occurs via the complement proteins Cl_r, C4 and C2. The resulting activation of C3 to $C3_a$ then triggers the activation of the remaining proteins, C5–C9, which have lytic or phagocytic functions, or result in the release of anaphylotoxins. These lead to antigen destruction. The formation of the anaphylotoxins $C3_a$ and $C5_a$ are responsible for mast cell disruption and the release of histamine. It is also these active protein fragments that produce the increased vascular permeability, and so allow the passage of phagocytes from extravascular sites to enter the bloodstream and break down the antigens. These activated proteins also bring about the contraction of smooth muscle.

In addition, $C5_a$ interacts with specific high-affinity receptors on granulocytes and platelets to initiate cell aggregation by increased cell adherence and positive chemotaxis. The activated neutrophils liberate arachidonic acid metabolites, oxygen-free radicals and lysosomal enzymes.

$C5_a$ is inactivated by carboxypeptidase B and C5 convertase to form $C5_a$ des Arg, which is not anaphylatoxic but still has chemotactic and lysosomal disruptive properties. Other activated fragments include $C5_b$ (which is cytotoxic), plus $C3_b$ and $C4_b$ which increase immune adherence and opsonization.

Alternative complement pathway

Unlike the classical pathway, preformed antibodies to a particular antigen are not necessary for alternative pathway activation. Hence prior exposure to the drug or endotoxin is not necessary. There are a number of activators of the alternative pathway:

- bacterial cell-wall carbohydrates
- zymogen from yeast cells
- endotoxin
- aggregated IgA
- contrast media
- renal dialysis membranes and membranes of some other artificial organs.

The activity of the two pathways may be further modulated by other factors. Lewis et al (1982) have shown a significant reduction in overall classical pathway activity in patients undergoing anaesthesia and surgery, with C3 concentrations being diminished to a greater extent than other complement proteins. In addition, drugs such as Althesin were capable of activating the alternate complement pathway via the protein Properdin and inhibition of $C3_b$ inactivator. The conversion of C3 to $C3_a$ and $C3_b$, and the subsequent release of $C5_a$, resulted in histamine release with bronchospasm, vasodilation, hypotension and tachycardia. In the absence of persistence of the antigen, or if it was present in a low titre, the majority of these reactions tended to be milder in nature than those that occurred as a result of classical pathway activation (Radford et al 1982).

As well as occurring in response to the specific pathway activators listed above, it has been suggested that direct complement activation may be more likely in conditions associated with complement abnormalities, for example pregnancy and disseminated carcinoma. In these conditions the plasma levels of the normal inhibitory proteins may be reduced. Because IgE has no binding potential to any of the complement proteins, it is probably inappropriate to attempt a correlation of the occurrence of an adverse reaction with the presence of high circulating IgE levels, as are found in the atopic or allergic patient.

Direct pharmacological effects of drugs

Although adverse drug reactions may involve activation of one or other of the complement pathways, the majority are better described as anaphylactoid in nature and occur as a result of a dose-related direct effect of the drug on mast cells and basophils. Such reactions may be manifest as either local cutaneous signs or the more severe systemic signs and symptoms of histamine release. With drugs such as thiopentone and some of the neuromuscular blocking agents, a flush-and-wheal reaction is often seen following their intravenous injection. The systemic features of the reactions are usually mild (e.g. hypotension and tachycardia) and without the other stigmata of histamine release. Why some of these cases (for which no immunological basis will be found on subsequent testing) progress to produce more generalized systemic symptoms is uncertain.

WHAT ARE THE PREDISPOSING FACTORS TO THE DEVELOPMENT OF ADVERSE REACTIONS?

These factors may be considered in three groups: patient factors, possible pharmacological factors and potential at-risk groups.

Patient factors

Age

In general, adverse reactions in children are rarer than in the adult population. However, it has been suggested that there is a steady increase in hypersensitivity reactions occurring in the young (Radford et al 1982).

Sex

When adverse reactions are analysed on the basis of actual numbers of operations in male and female patients, there is probably no difference in incidence. However, the apparently high incidence of reaction reported in gynaecological patients may not just be the result of the frequency of such operations, but due to the large number of patients who are coincidentally pregnant (see below).

Pregnancy

There is no doubt that pregnancy alters the activity of activators and inhibitors of the complement cascade system. Thus the high incidence of adverse reactions on first or subsequent exposure to certain intravenous anaesthetics in the pregnant patient may be the result of two influences. Firstly, there is the choice of drugs suitable for short gynaecological procedures, such as vaginal termination of pregnancy and evacuation of retained products of conception. Secondly, the altered immune status of these patients must be considered. The withdrawal of Propanidid and the Cremphor containing hypnotic Althesin, and the reformulation of di-isopropyl phenol may be associated with the apparent decrease in the number of reported adverse reactions to intravenous agents in this group of patients.

Atopy

The incidence of hypersensitivity reactions to intravenous anaesthetic drugs is greater in atopic individuals than in the non-atopic normal population. However, this is in contradiction to the findings of Green & Rosenblum (1971) who found no correlation between atopy and the frequency of allergic reactions to penicillin.

Several studies have compared reactors and the non-reactors to intravenous anaesthetic agents. These show an increased incidence of atopy, asthma and allergy, and a previous history of drug reactions in the reacting patients (LaForest et al 1980, Watkins et al 1981). However, although Fee et al (1978) suggested that the same intravenous anaesthetic drugs should not be used in patients with a history of atopy or allergy undergoing repeat anaesthesia, this was not substantiated by the studies of LaForest et al (1980). Moreover, Watkins et al (1981) have postulated that a history of allergy or atopy in the presence of a high IgE level is a valuable predictor of the likelihood of a particular type of adverse reaction. If the patient has no history of allergy or atopy, or has a history of contact allergy or allergy to drugs other than penicillin, then he is more likely to show a delayed type hypersensitivity reaction (Type IV). However, if the patient suffers from extrinsic asthma, hay fever or penicillin allergy (and has elevated levels of IgE) he is more likely to show a Type I immediate hypersensitivity reaction on second exposure to thiopentone and other intravenous anaesthetic drugs.

This theory has not been supported by the findings of Fisher & Rolfe (1984). They examined the clinical details of 105 patients following reactions to intravenously administered drugs. They found it impossible to predict whether an adverse reaction would have been Type I or Type IV hypersensitivity on the basis of allergic history and IgE levels.

In general, the increased incidence of hypersensitivity reactions to first exposure in the atopic individual is small when compared with the higher incidence of hypersensitivity reactions seen in patients receiving repeat administration of the same anaesthetic agent.

Previous exposure to the anaesthetic agent

Case reports in the literature indicate that previous exposure to any intravenous agent is likely to predispose to hypersensitivity on a subsequent administration of either the same drug or another of similar constituents. Thus, in the case of the Cremophor formulated anaesthetics (Propanidid, Althesin and di-isopropyl phenol), there were many reports of cross-reactivity leading to hypersensitivity, often some years after the intial exposure to this solvent. Cross-reactivity has also been reported for reactions involving muscle relaxants and local anaesthetic agents (see pp. 290, 292).

When Radford et al (1982) studied the underlying mechanisms of reactions to second or subsequent exposure to Althesin, most cases implicated an antigen–antibody interaction leading to classical complement pathway activation. In many of the reactions, pronounced hypotension and bronchospasm were important features, particularly if the time interval between exposures was short.

Stress

There is an impression among anaesthetists that adverse reactions are more common in nervous, anxious patients and that appropriate heavy premedication is indicated in potentially susceptible individuals. Although adrenaline may initiate activation of the complement cascade, there are no good data to support the suggestion that stress is a definite aetiological factor in adverse reactions.

Possible pharmacological factors

Many of the intravenous drugs administered during anaesthesia are poorly water soluble. The addition of glycols, macrogols and non-ionic surfactants will increase the solubility of such agents.

Both propylene glycol and polyethylene glycol have been used as the solvent for etomidate and diazepam. When the latter was used as the solvent for etomidate, injection of the drug was accompanied by a significant reduction in the incidence of pain when compared with an aqueous etomidate solution. Similarly, the partial substitution of propylene glycol as the solvent for diazepam reduced the incidence of pain associated with intramuscular injection.

Of the non-ionic solvents, Cremophor EL was the most widely used. It consists of 83% lipophilic and 17% hydrophilic elements. Extraction of the hydrophilic part with n-butanol leaves Micellophor, the solvent for Propanidid.

Studies of the cardiovascular effects of Cremophor EL in fit, unpremedicated patients were reported by Savage et al (1973) and Kettler & Sonntag (1974). Lorenz et al (1972) and Doenicke et al (1973) studied the effects of Micellophor. Only doses in excess of 20 ml of Cremophor EL alone produced significant haemodynamic changes, despite the liberation of histamine that could be measured following clinical doses of either Propanidid and Althesin (<10 ml Cremophor EL).

Laxenaire et al (1977) showed that antihistamine premedication decreases histamine release in both normal and atopic individuals (Table 19.2). More important, premedication significantly reduced the occurrence of the systemic effects of histamine (6:25 in the non-treated group, 0:25 in the treated group; p<0.01).

Table 19.2 Efficacy of antihistamine premedication in decreasing the release of histamine during induction of anaesthesia with Althesin (from Laxenaire et al 1977)

	Mean (SD) histamine release (μg/ml) Preinduction	+5 min	+10 min
Unpremedicated			
Atopic (n=9)	193(51)	229(59)	214(34)
Normal (n=16)	134(37)*	163(52)*	153(41)*
Premedicated†			
Atopic (n=8)	126(50)	131(43)	128(34)
Normal (n=17)	103(31)	117(38)	121(30)

† Premedicated with tritoqualine, epsilon amino caproic acid and hydroxyzine.
*p<0.01.

There is no evidence to suggest that different doses or rates of administration of drugs influence the predisposition to 'pharmacological drug reactions'. Adverse reactions to Althesin were reported with 'test doses', bolus doses, repeated incremental administration and with infusions of the agent (Simpson et al 1985).

Potential at-risk groups

Apart from patients with a history of previous anaphylaxia or a proven sensitivity to one or more drugs, there are no other predictors of at-risk groups (Fisher et al 1987). Whether non-histamine-releasing drugs or drugs with a low propensity to histamine release should be the agents of choice in the atopic individual is a point of discussion; there is no evidence to favour either view.

WHAT ARE THE CLINICAL FEATURES OF AN ALLERGIC REACTION TO INTRAVENOUS AGENTS?

There is considerable variation in the severity and magnitude of the clinical features among different reactors. Factors that influence the severity of the symptomatology include the amount of drug injected, the reactivity of basophils and mast cells, the responsiveness of the bronchial and vascular smooth muscle and the activity of the autonomic nervous system. There has been some suggestion that chronically atopic individuals may have an imbalance between alpha and beta adrenergic activity, such that the injection or release of small amounts of histamine into the atopic patient will produce an exaggerated response. Control of peripheral autonomic nervous system activity is also regulated by higher centres. Thus the increased emotional activity of the asthmatic patient prior to anaesthesia and surgery may both enhance any existing symptomatology and exaggerate any adverse response to intravenous drug administration.

The various symptoms and signs that may occur during adverse reactions are listed below:

- skin: erythema, wheals, oedema (often periorbital or perioral), flare, pruritus and arthralgia (in awake patients)
- hypotension and tachycardia: with decreased systemic vascular resistance and pulmonary hypertension
- cough: a single cough on induction of anaesthesia may precede the development of a hypersensitivity reaction
- bronchospasm and arterial hypoxaemia: wheezing, laryngeal oedema, decreased pulmonary compliance, fulminant pulmonary oedema and acute respiratory distress
- hyperperistalsis
- cardiac arrest
- Other: ventricular conduction defects, atrioventricular block, clotting defects, leucopaenia, decrease in body temperature.

The maximum intensity of the symptoms often occurs rapidly, and usually within 30 min of intravenous drug administration. All of the clinical features can be attributed to mast cell and basophil degranulation. This knowledge has been made use of in some of the preoperative prophylactic methods advocated for patients with a history of drug allergy.

The usual order of clinical symptoms is: skin changes, hypotension with tachycardia, and bronchospasm with resulting arterial hypoxia.

Skin changes

Skin changes are characterized by the classic triple response, described by Lewis & Grant (1924) and given below:

1. *Erythema* occurs as a result of capillary dilatation, and is predominantly seen over the face, arms and necklace area of the upper chest.
2. *Wheal formation* occurs due to an increased vascular permeability, and secondary fluid transudation.
3. *Flares* are presumably due to an axon reflex response.

Although hypersensitivity to the intravenous barbiturates and many of the muscle relaxants is reflected solely by these three features at the site of administration, peri-orbital oedema may also be prominent. If the oedema extends to involve the upper airway tissues, bronchospasm and laryngospasm may occur.

Hypotension and tachycardia

Hypotension and tachycardia result from the transudation of fluid from the vascular to extravascular spaces. Histamine also causes vascular smooth muscle dilatation, and hence the venous pooling of blood may occur. The accompanying tachycardia is probably not a baroreflex response, but rather the chronotropic effect of increased circulating catecholamine levels following their release by histamine from the adrenal medulla.

Although several of the vasoactive mediators of anaphylaxis can affect animal hearts in vivo and human cardiac muscle in vitro, there is little evidence for allergic reactions resulting in *primary* cardiac dysfunction. Indeed, it has only been reported in two patients with pre-existing normal myocardia (Raper & Fisher 1988). Secondary cardiac dysfunction following anaphylaxis is, however, more common.

Bronchospasm

Bronchospasm is the most life-threatening of the symptoms and treatment must primarily be aimed at preventing severe arterial hypoxia.

THE LABORATORY DIAGNOSIS OF PATIENTS EXPERIENCING SUSPECTED ADVERSE ALLERGIC REACTIONS

There are several different tests available for adverse allergic reactions. These include:

1. Routine haematology, including haematocrit, should be measured. This will allow for correction of plasma protein concentrations to take account of the fluid changes brought about by the reaction or the administration of intravenous fluids during resuscitation. Changes in platelet and white cell numbers may be small, but of significance, as disappearance of basophils (expressed as a percentage of the total leucocyte count) are indicative of a Type I response (Theobald-Segalen et al 1982).
2. Serial measurements should be made of the plasma concentrations of total IgE antibodies and complement proteins (C3, C4 and breakdown products $C3_a$, $C3_b$ and C1 inhibitor) during the 72 hours after an adverse reaction. These samples should be taken into tubes containing EDTA as this affords better stability of frozen samples compared with those added to citrate or heparin. Poor storage may lead to in vitro activation. The absence of a true pre-operative control sample in most circumstances will, however, preclude the delineation of a clear profile of protein changes. Although Stoelting (1983) has suggested that a sample obtained 72 hours after a reaction may be used to determine the control 'normal values' of these proteins, work by the Department of Anaesthetics at Southmead Hospital, Bristol, has shown that it is better to wait until 6 or more weeks after the initial reaction to obtain a 'near-true' baseline sample (P Simpson, personal communication). Serial measurements of these proteins do not identify the causative drug, but rather suggest the occurrence of an allergic reaction. Again, the absolute IgE concentrations may be affected by fluid loss and replacement.

   Involvement of both C3 and C4 is indicative of an immune reaction which does not involve IgE antibodies, while C3 conversion alone is an indicator of a specific non-immune mechanism.
3. IgE levels: in contrast to the patients with increased levels (atopy), there are some individuals (10–20%) having very low levels. Such individuals appear to be prone to non-immune mediated clinical reactions and may produce positive intradermal tests to drugs having a high potential to histamine release (Lavery et al 1985). One hypothesis is that these patients respond to intravenous drug administration by histamine release because their mast cells lack sufficient endogenous IgE to mask those cell receptors responsible for histamine release following interaction with causative drugs (Watkins & Nimmo 1985).
4. Other in vivo or in vitro diagnostic tests may be useful for later assessment to establish the identity of the responsible drug:
   - intravenous challenge with putative drug: too dangerous for routine use
   - intradermal skin testing
   - IgE inhibition test
   - leucocyte histamine release test and basophil degranulation test
   - radioallergosorbent test (RAST)
   - delineation of specific antibodies.

Intradermal testing of acute adverse drug reactions

Intradermal testing has been suggested by Malcolm Fisher (1979, 1981) and Sage (1981). This approach involves the intradermal injection of a diluted solution of the suspected causative agent. Patients should not be taking medication such as glucocorticoids, sympathomimetics or antihistamines at the time of testing. A positive response is a characteristic wheal and flare with dilute solutions of the test agents. This occurs within 10 min of injection and persists for at least 30 min. The wheal diameter is usually greater than 10 mm for a 0.1 ml injectate. For induction agents the dilution used is 1:100; for relaxants, colloids, fentanyl and local anaesthetics 1:1000–1:10 000; and for other narcotics 1:100 000. The intradermal test has a 97% positivity for neuromuscular relaxants but is only rarely positive for thiopentone. In addition to the suspected drug, the possibility of an allergic reaction to the diluent or preservative must be excluded by separate intradermal testing.

In an assessment of the causative factor in 128 patients who had undergone acute anaphylactic reactions during anaesthesia, Fisher (1981) was able to make a positive confirmation of the aetiology in 100 patients. More recently, Galletly & Treuren (1985) reported the positive identification of the causative agent in 84% of patients suffering an intraoperative adverse reaction. Muscle relaxants were shown to be the responsible drug in 75% of the patients. Predisposing factors in those patients reacting to relaxant drugs were: being female, previous drug allergy and atopy.

The intradermal test does not appear to be of value in the diagnosis of reactions due to local anaesthetics or colloids.

A positive intradermal test suggests the presence of IgE or IgG antibodies. Nevertheless, the confirmation of these antibodies in reactions to anaesthetic agents has proved difficult. False positive intradermal tests may be induced by the local release of histamine due to mechanical trauma from the injection. This should be avoided by the simultaneous control intradermal injection of normal saline. Similarly, a false negative test may occur if conditions at the injection site do not permit the breakdown of the drug to an antigenic form, or the conjugation of the drug or its metabolites to a tissue protein carrier.

Although Fisher and his colleagues afford an enthusiastic approach to intradermal testing, this has not always been shared by other authorities (Watkins 1986).

A variation of the intradermal test is the Prausnitz–Kustner test. Here, 0.1 ml of plasma from a patient who has experienced a suspected allergic reaction is given intradermally to a non-allergic subject. After 24 hours the putative allergenic drug is injected at the same sites. If positive, there will be a wheal and flare reaction within 20 min due to local mast cell disruption following interaction of the tissue-fixed antibodies (IgG or IgE) with the allergen. IgE antibodies can be distinguished from IgG, as the former are heat labile and are destroyed by heating the plasma to 56°C for 2 h before injection.

Although easy to perform, the test subjects the non-allergenic subject to the risk of transmission of disease (hepatitis B, HIV, etc.), and the risks of a systemic adverse reaction. Apes can be used in place of human volunteers, but studies in lower primates appear less sensitive and less accurate.

IgE inhibition test

The IgE inhibition test is an in vitro model of what occurs when a patient experiences an anaphylactic reaction. The concentrations of IgE antibodies are measured before and after incubation of the patient's plasma with the suspected drug. If a specific antibody is present and an antigen–antibody interaction occurs, the level of IgE will decrease.

Leucocyte histamine release test and basophil degranulation test

Incubation of white cells from a patient who has suffered a drug-induced adverse reaction with the suspected drug (in drug concentrations ranging from 0.1 μg/ml to 1.0 mg/ml) provides another in vitro model of the anaphylactic reaction. The two tests only differ in the endpoints they measure: either an increased histamine concentration in the incubate (Hirshman et al 1982) or morphological evidence of basophil degranulation (>30% total cell numbers) due to histamine release (Shelley 1963). These tests are mainly useful to delineate anaphylactoid reactions where there is no other evidence of an immunological mechanism.

RAST and specific IgE antibodies

These techniques detect the presence of specific antibodies to a drug. Commercially prepared antigen is added in vitro to the plasma from a patient who has experienced an adverse reaction, so forming an antigen–antibody (IgE) complex.

After the further addition of radiolabelled anti-IgE and the precipitation of the antigen–antibody-anti-IgE complex, the radioactivity of the complex correlates the in vitro presence and concentration of specific IgE antibodies. However, at present there are only a few commercially available antigens so that the value of this test is limited (to succinylcholine, pethidine and thiopentone; Levy & Rockoff 1982, Dueck & O'Connor 1984, Harle et al 1984). The evidence from intradermal testing, passive transfer testing, basophil and leucocyte histamine release or degranulation and radioimmunoassay techniques suggest that IgE antibodies play an important role in a considerable number of reactions. However, such antibodies can be detected in less than 60% of all reactions.

PROPHYLACTIC MEASURES IN THE SUSCEPTIBLE PATIENT

Although the occurrence of a first exposure reaction of any drug is unpredictable, steps can be taken to prevent hypersensitivity reactions occurring on subsequent exposures. These steps are listed below:

1. Use of local rather than general anaesthesia. However, for some surgical procedures this may not be feasible or possible. In addition, hypersensitivity to the ester type of local anaesthetic has been reported (see p. 290).
2. In the patient needing general anaesthesia, the following guidelines may be useful:
   - Although there is little evidence to support the efficacy of such drugs, the use of adequate preoperative anxiolysis and premedication may reduce 'stress'.
   - Preoperative prophylaxis should be aimed at both reducing plasma histamine release and blocking its systemic effects:
     - sodium cromoglycate to stabilize mast cells, and so prevent degranulation and histamine release
     - salbutamol to prevent bronchospasm
     - hydrocortisone
     - antihistamines (H_1-receptor antagonists, e.g. chlorpheniramine in doses up to 0.3 mg/kg, or terfenadine)
     - H_2-receptor antagonists (e.g. cimetidine in doses up to 5 mg/kg, or ranitidine).

Histamine receptor antagonists do not inhibit histamine release, but rather compete at the receptors to attenuate the decreases in systemic vascular resistance.

- Avoid repeat exposure to any intravenous drug that the patient has received in the near past. However, as Radford et al (1982) found in patients reacting to repeat exposure to Althesin, the 'memory period' may be long.
- Use inhalational rather than intravenous agents whenever possible. However, the problems of hepatotoxicity to repeat administrations of the fluorinated hydrocarbons must not be forgotten.
- Avoid the use of plasma expanders such as Haemaccel and dextran.

DISCUSSION OF ALLERGIC RESPONSES TO INDIVIDUAL DRUGS

The Boston Collaborative Drug Surveillance Programme has determined the incidence of severe allergic reactions during general anaesthesia as 1:4395 general anaesthetics (Beard & Jick 1985).

Hypnotic and sedative drugs

Presently available hypnotic induction agents

Between 1964 and 1984 about 1000 reports of hypersensitivity reactions to intravenous anaesthetic agents were cited in the French and English language literatures. About 50% were due to neuromuscular relaxant drugs, 40% to the hypnotic agents and the remainder to opioids (3%), benzodiazepines (2%) and neuroleptic agents (<1%). Between 1985 and 1987 the Departments of Anaesthetics and Immunology in Sheffield investigated 241 cases of anaphylactoid responses during induction of anaesthesia (Watkins 1989).

Thiopentone. There are over 300 cases of allergic reactions to the barbiturates, most of which relate to thiopentone. The quoted incidences of adverse reactions to thiopentone and methohexitone are 1:14 000 and 1:7000, respectively. The classical features of the allergic response to thiopentone were first described by Hunter (1943). To date there have been over 250 reported cases of anaphylactic or anaphylactoid reactions to the drug. Cutaneous and cardiovascular manifestations predominate (65% and 56%, respectively) with respiratory side effects (laryngospasm or difficulty in ventilating the patient) being less common (35%). About 10 cases of death are recorded following thiopentone. Many patients will also give a history of atopy, allergy or a previous general anaesthetic (presumably one of the barbiturates). Unlike the increasing incidence of reactions to Althesin before its withdrawal, the rate of reactions to thiopentone appears fairly constant.

Laboratory testing after a suspected reaction usually shows a significant immediate decrease in the plasma levels of IgE with no significant change in the concentration of complement proteins C3 and C4. Lilly & Hoy (1980), in reporting an allergic reaction to thiopentone, found a 20% decrease in the IgE level within 4 hours of the reaction (Fig. 19.2). Thus these results suggest the involvement

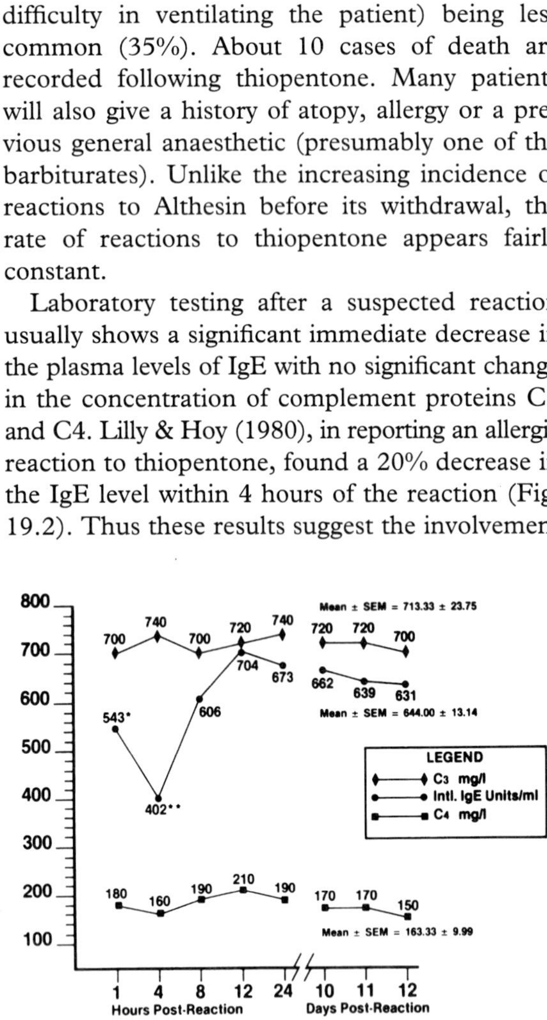

Fig. 19.2 Serially measured values of IgE and complement C3 and C4 after adverse reaction to thiopentone. Except where indicated (*, **), the difference of the value from its appropriate mean ± SEM was not significant (using Student's paired 't' test). The changes in IgE at 1 and 4 h postreaction were significantly different (* $p<0.05$, ** $p<0.002$, respectively; from Lilly & Hoy 1980).

of IgE without complement pathway activation, at least in a primary capacity. The incidence of IgE-mediated reactions to the thiobarbiturate has been estimated by Beamish & Brown (1981) to be about 1 in 23 000. In those rare cases in which both IgE and complement are involved, secondary complement activation probably occurs as a result of hypotension leading to metabolic derangement.

Frequent cutaneous manifestations of induction with thiopentone (histaminoid wheal and flaring) are seen in many patients. Whether these represent true reactions is uncertain. They may alternatively represent a local response to the extreme alkalinity of thiopentone in patients who are often nervous and peripherally vasoconstricted.

In the 75 adverse reactions to the thiobarbiturates reported to the Department of Anaesthetics at Sheffield University between 1974 and 1982, antibody (IgE) involvement was found in 20% of the cases, IgG and classical pathway activation in 12%, and alternate pathway activation in only 5% (Watkins 1984). Pharmacological, non-immune reactions constituted the remaining 63%. From 1985 to 1987 the same department investigated a further 191 cases in which thiopentone was a part of the anaesthetic induction technique (Watkins 1989). Three other cases of anaphylaxis to thiopentone (with positive detection of specific IgE antibodies supported by a positive intradermal test in two of the three) have been described by Fisher et al (1989). One interesting feature of this report was that all three patients had postoperative gastrointestinal symptoms. These are generally only observed in about 10% of patients experiencing anaphylaxis during anaesthesia. However, all three had received only short-duration anaesthesia (<10 min). It may be that involvement of the gastrointestinal system occurs more frequently than was previously realized, but that the symptoms are often masked by the continuation of anaesthesia during the resuscitation phase of adverse reactions.

More recently, Moneret-Vautrin et al (1990) reported two cases of simultaneous immune reactions to thiopentone and a neuromuscular blocking drug. The presence of specific IgE antibodies to thiopentone was demonstrated on the basis of positive passive cutaneous anaphylaxis, basophil degranulation, leucocyte histamine release and radioimmunoassay (Harle et al 1986).

Investigation. Apart from the measurement of serial IgE and complement protein levels, in vitro stimulation tests (basophil degranulation and leucocyte histamine release) are useful in categorizing the cause of a suspected reaction. The development of a RAST technique may prove useful in the study of these patients.

Methohexitone and other barbiturates. Clarke (1981) summarized 15 cases of suspected hypersensitivity to methohexitone, and two cases associated with thiamylal. Other cases may also have occurred, but the incidence is undoubtedly low and there have been no deaths reported. Most patients show periorbital and facial oedema, with no history of allergy. One of these recent cases of an adverse reaction to methohexitone presented with cutaneous signs of flushing and periorbital oedema, accompanied by severe hypotension. Laboratory testing showed significant decreases in the serum levels of C3 and C4 over the 24-hour period following the reaction, with a subsequent return of normal levels over the next 12–24 hours. Of relevance in deciding the aetiology of this reaction was the previous use of thiopentone for the induction of anaesthesia. The clinical signs and confirmatory laboratory tests indicated an anaphylactic response due to a Type I hypersensitivity reaction. The probable cause of the response was a passive sensitization to the barbiturates following a previous anaesthetic (i.e. cross-sensitivity may exist between the two barbiturates).

Hirshman et al (1982, 1985) have investigated dose-related histamine release from human cutaneous mast cells and leucocytes by intravenous barbiturates. At equimolar concentrations, release was greatest after thiopentone and thiamylal, with significant responses seen at the clinical concentration range (10^{-5}–10^{-3} M).

Etomidate. There were five reports between 1978 and 1982 of possible adverse reactions to the etomidate (Watkins 1983). All involved widespread cutaneous flushing or urticaria and postoperative vomiting. None of the patients showed complement activation. A further two cases reported to Watkins in 1982 both exhibited anaphylactoid responses with signs of cyanosis, marked hypotension and, in one case, oedema. Whether these were due to etomidate is difficult to decide, as the drug was administered concurrently with suxamethonium or alcuronium. Nevertheless, complement C3 activation was shown in one of the cases.

Krumholz et al (1984) have described a further reaction to etomidate, with generalized erythema, urticaria, tachycardia and hypotension. Sold & Rothhammer (1985) reported a similar picture in a patient scheduled for coronary artery surgery. Positive skin tests supported etomidate as the causative agent of this anaphylactoid reaction.

Fazackerley et al (1986) described a further case with urticaria and severe bronchospasm leading to hypoxic cardiac arrest following induction of anaesthesia with etomidate. There was no complement activation but the patient had a raised plasma IgE level, consistent with atopy. This is the first case of severe bronchospasm to etomidate but, unlike many of the other reports, a direct release of histamine or other immune mediators by the intravenous hypnotic agents seems the most likely explanation. In two other cases, etomidate was given at induction of anaesthesia with another intravenous drug, lignocaine or vecuronium (Bricker & Raitt 1987, Farrell et al 1988). Studies suggest these other drugs were the causative agents.

Whether or not these recent reports indicate an increase in the incidence of reactions to etomidate is uncertain, but from 1985 to 1987, Watkins and colleagues in Sheffield investigated 241 adverse reactions to intravenous agents. Etomidate was part of the anaesthetic in 19 of these cases (Watkins, 1989). However, the 12 case reports represent the only documented adverse reactions to a drug where over 4 million induction doses have been given. This is a very low incidence compared with those reported for the other intravenous hypnotic agents (Table 19.3).

Ketamine, a phencyclidine derivative, has been associated with only two reports of allergic reactions (Mathieu et al 1975, Laxenaire et al 1985), one probably having a non-immune basis, the other involving IgE.

Table 19.3 Incidence of adverse hypersensitivity reactions to intravenous hypnotic agents

Agent	Incidence
Thiopentone	1:14 000–1:20 000
Methohexitone	1:1600–1:7000
Propofol (as Cremophor formulation)	5 in 1131
Etomidate	1:50 000–1:450 000 (10+ cases)
Propofol as emulsion	1:80 000–1:100 000
for comparison:	
Althesin	1:400–1:11 000
Propanidid	1:500–1:17 000
Neuromuscular blocking drugs	1:5000
Penicillin	1:2500–1:10 000
Dextrans	1:3000
Gelatins	1:900
Hydroxyethyl starch	1:1200

Di-isopropyl phenol (propofol) was introduced for clinical trials in Belgium in 1977. This water-insoluble hypnotic agent was initially solubilized in Cremophor EL. At least five cases of hypersensitivity were reported among the 1131 patients receiving the agent. One of these (Briggs et al 1982) showed features of classical complement pathway activation with C3 conversion and C4 consumption. Because the patient had not received propofol previously, this must represent a reaction following exposure to some other Cremophor-containing substance.

The reformulation of propofol as a soybean oil emulsion (Cummins et al 1984, Glen & Hunter 1984) led to its reintroduction into clinical trials in 1983 and into general clinical practice in 1986. Data from the Committee on Safety of Medicines (to August 1991) indicate 22 cases of reports categorized as 'allergic, anaphylactoid or anaphylactic', with one associated death. Several of these cases have appeared in the literature as case reports (Jamieson and MacKenzie 1988, Laxenaire et al 1988, Dold & Konarzewski 1989, Kumar & McNeela 1989, de Leon-Casasola et al 1992, Laxenaire et al 1992, McHale & Konieczko 1992). Other side effects occurring with a high incidence (and which may be related to histamine or other mediator release) include erythematous rashes, bronchospasm, flushing and hypotension. Although the frequency of reports of allergic-type responses to propofol seems to be increasing, the concurrent administration of neuromuscular blocking drugs may be a significant causative factor.

Diazepam. There have been few reports of clinically overt adverse reactions to diazepam when formulated in propylene glycol (Valium; Roche) (Falk 1977). However, Schou Olesen & Huttel (1978) described five cases of reactions to a Cremophor formulation of the drug (Stesolid) in a total of 5200 administrations. Three patients suffered pronounced cardiovascular collapse, the other two had minor cutaneous sequelae. In a further case report of two more reactions to Stesolid, rash, bronchospasm and hypotension occurred in one patient, and erythema, facial oedema and cardiovascular collapse in the other. These reactions involved probable alternate pathway activation in one of the patients, with C3 consumption and conversion, and normal plasma C4 level (Huttel et al 1980). More recently, Brogger–Nielsen (1984) reported a 20-year-old woman who received Diazemuls (an emulsion formulation) for gastroscopy, and developed signs of flushing, urticaria and upper body oedema. This 'histaminoid' picture was not associated with activation of either complement pathway. Thus all three present formulations of this commonly prescribed benzodiazepine have been implicated in adverse reactions. To date there are no reports of allergic reactions to any other of the benzodiazepines commonly used in anaesthetic practice (midazolam, lorazepam and temazepam).

Evidence for involvement of Cremphor EL in immune reactions

When Cremophor EL is injected alone into the dog there is a high incidence (about 75%) of pulmonary distress with associated urticaria and marked hypotension. These reactions are often fatal. In cases where the solubilizing agent has been previously administered, there is evidence of complement activation. The liberation of $C3_a$, an anaphylatoxin, is usually promptly coupled with granulocyte margination. Thus, soon after a reaction, the peripheral white cell count will show a declining number of granulocytes. However, within 10–20 min the picture is reversed, with a 200–300% increase in blood granulocytes following their release from tissue pools.

Animal studies by Glen et al (1979) using the 'mini-pig' (Gottingen-derived strain) model showed that a second exposure to a Cremophor containing anaesthetic within 5–15 days of the first administration produced a high incidence of anaphylactic response: usually urticaria and hypotension. Between these times (i.e. before about 5 days after the initial exposure) the animal appeared tolerant to the Cremophor.

In man, administration of Althesin to a volunteer on two occasions 7 days apart resulted in the expected difference in blood white cell counts: an increase following the first exposure and a marked fall on the second occasion. A second exposure of a patient to Althesin, which resulted in a classical-complement-pathway-mediated adverse reaction, showed the same white cell picture. Although these white cell changes tend to be greatest where there is a short latent period, subclinical alterations have been reported when the exposures to Althesin have been more than 3 years apart.

Thus, in contrast to thiopentone, reactions to Althesin (and probably to other Cremophor formulated drugs) showed two distinct patterns. First exposure reactions tended to be mild and were mediated either via the alternative complement pathway or by a direct pharmacological effect on the mast cells and basophils. Repeat exposure adverse reactions led to classical complement pathway activation, with more severe symptomatology (Radford et al 1982). IgE antibodies were not detected in affected subjects, but Moneret-Vautrin et al (1983) found anti-Cremophor IgG antibodies.

The apparent clear distinction in aetiology of the reactions to Althesin depending on the existence or not of previous exposure (as proposed by Radford et al 1982) has been questioned by Watkins (1982).

In a further in vitro study, Tachon et al (1983) showed that Althesin (formulated in Cremophor) but not the individual steroids were allergenic. Thus, in contrast to Glen et al (1979) who demonstrated an effect in the mini-pig from Cremophor alone, the data of Tachon would imply that reactions require the combined presence of steroids and solvent.

Another feature seen in patients receiving Althesin was complement activation in the absence of clinical symptomatology (Simpson et al 1985). In a prospective study of 137 patients receiving a first exposure to Althesin, two had positive clinical signs of an adverse reaction in the absence of complement changes (i.e. probably anaphylactoid); six showed complement activation (C3 conversion) with no clinical signs (i.e. subclinical reaction); and a further two showed both clinical and immunological signs of an adverse reaction. There was no relationship between the dose of Althesin and the incidence of either clinical or subclinical changes. In contrast, no changes were seen in the control group of 46 patients receiving thiopentone. Of the 10 patients reacting to Althesin, eight were pregnant at the time of surgery. It may be, therefore, that the altered immunological status of the pregnant patient renders her more susceptible to Cremophor-associated reactions. This study suggested that the overall rate of reactions to Althesin in first time exposees might be as high as one in 14!

Whether these reactions to the Cremophor formulated drugs (Propanidid, Althesin, Diazepam [as Stesolid MR] and Di-isopropyl phenol) were due to the pharmacologically active components with the Cremophor acting as an adjuvant, or to the Cremophor itself, must now remain a matter of conjecture, as all three induction agent preparations have now been withdrawn from the British market.

However, it would appear that any further drugs solubilized in Cremophor EL are likely to possess allergenic potential, either in their own right or secondary to previous exposure to one of the other Cremophor containing compounds, such as miconazole (an antifungal agent), cyclosporine A, vitamin K and some proprietary hair shampoos. The reported reactions to cyclosporine include facial and upper thoracic flushing, acute respiratory distress with apnoea and wheezing, and blood pressure changes (Kahan et al 1984, Chapuis et al 1985, Friedman et al 1985, Leunissen et al 1985, Magalini et al 1986). The overall incidence of anaphylactoid reactions to intravenous cyclosporine is about 1 in 1000 administrations. An alternative intravenous formulation (made up of the enteral preparation dissolved in maize oil) has been shown to be non-allergenic in a one case. The patient showed erythematous changes, conjunctival oedema and tachycardia to both intravenous and oral formulations of the drug (van Hooff et al 1987). These formulations contain cyclosporine solubilized in Cremophor EL (i.v.) and polyoxyl-5-oleate, ethanol and olive oil, respectively.

Narcotics

Many of the narcotics, especially morphine, release histamine with the development of either local or systemic effects. Rosow et al (1982) showed a direct relationship between the plasma histamine concentration following morphine administration (1 mg/kg), and the associated decrease in systemic vascular resistance and mean arterial blood pressure (Figs 19.3 & 19.4). Although these responses are similar to those seen during anaphylactoid reactions, bronchospasm has not been observed in any patient. In contrast, fentanyl (50 μg/kg) caused no significant increase in plasma histamine and hence no related haemodynamic effects. Similarly, the newer fentanyl congeners, alfentanil and sufentanil, do not cause release of histamine in significant concentrations (Flacke et al 1987). The mechanism of morphine-induced hypotension is both a direct effect of the drug to increase venous capacitance as well as an indirect effect due to histamine release.

A single case of anaphylaxis to an opioid has been reported following the intravenous administration of pethidine (Levy & Rockoff 1982). The patient suffered urticaria, bronchospasm and profound hypotension but was successfully resuscitated. Subsequent RAST studies confirmed the presence of specific IgE antibodies to pethidine. Two further reports describe reactions to fentanyl and alfentanil. The former is confirmed on the basis of a positive skin test, the latter is suggestive of a non-immune histaminoid reaction (Pevny & Danhauser 1981, Coventry & Stone 1988).

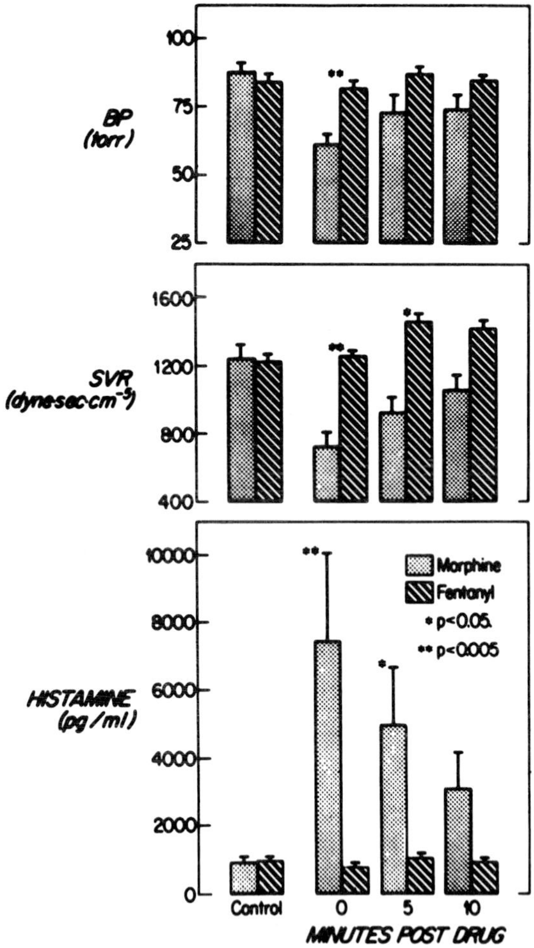

Fig. 19.3 Data (mean ± SEM) for plasma histamine, mean arterial pressure and systemic vascular resistance at the times indicated following morphine or fentanyl. Asterisks indicate significant differences (* p<0.05, ** p<0.005) (from Rosow et al 1982).

Local anaesthetic agents

True allergic or adverse responses to the local anaesthetic agents in current use are rare (constituting probably less than 1% of all reactions to the drugs; Schatz 1984). In most patients, other causes of drug reactions are responsible, for example systemic toxicity, simple fainting or reactions to added adrenaline. The recommended maximum dosage of these agents is shown in Table 19.4.

The ester group of local anaesthetics (cocaine, procaine, chloroprocaine and tetracaine) are more liable to provoke adverse reactions as they contain both a para-aminobenzoic acid grouping and methyl- or propylparaben as the added preservative. The systemic effects of adrenaline are undoubtedly the cause of some of these reported adverse reactions to local anaesthetics. Use of 1:800 000 adrenaline in dental anaesthesia is frequently accompanied by symptoms of tachycardia, palpitation and chest tightness. Verrill (1975) cited 21 deaths due to adrenaline administration over a 6-year period. By contrast, the occurrence of angina is rare.

Investigation of reactions to local anaesthetics

Some authorities have advocated the use of skin tests in investigating reactions to local anaesthetics. However, Aldrete & Johnson (1970) found positive skin tests in 25 out of 60 patients in the non-allergenic control group. This suggests that cross-sensitivity to other structurally related drugs may exist, hence the use of intradermal testing cannot be considered as reliable in eliciting the true cause of a suspected drug reaction. This cross-reactivity is thought only to occur among the esteric local anaesthetics, not the structurally dissimilar amides. However, this has been questioned by Incaudo et al (1978) and Fisher (1984).

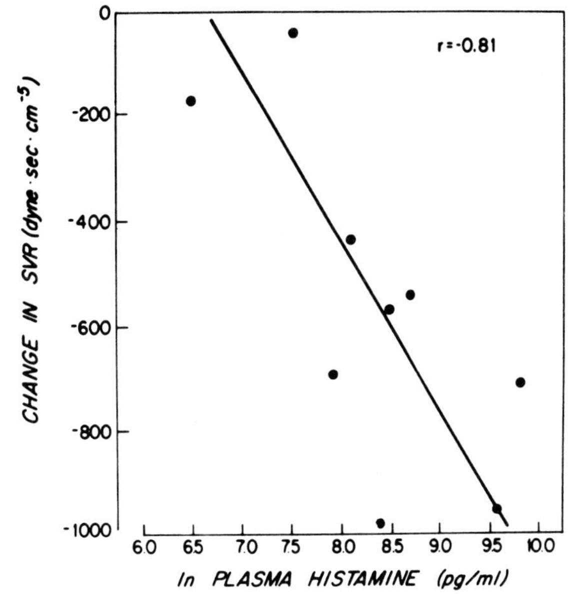

Fig. 19.4 Correlation plot of log plasma histamine concentration and peak change in systemic vascular resistance for patients given intravenous morphine (from Rosow et al 1982).

Table 19.4 Maximum doses and signs of toxicity for commonly used local anaesthetic agents

Agent	Maximum dose (mg) Plain	with Adr	Important toxic side effects
Amethocaine	100	—	Cardiac depression, may cause asystole and ventricular fibrillation
Bupivacaine	175	250	Cardiotoxicity, drowsiness and convulsions
Cinchocaine	50		
Chloroprocaine	800	1000	Neurotoxicity, prolongation of effect of suxamethonium
Cocaine	200		Sympathetic stimulation, excitement, restlessness, headache, vomiting, myocardial depression and cardiac arrhythmias
Etidocaine	300	400	Less toxic than bupivacaine
Lignocaine	300	500	Convulsions, twitching and psychotic reactions
Mepivacaine	350	500	Less cardiotoxic than bupivacaine
Prilocaine	400	600	Methaemoglobinaemia
Procaine	500	700	CNS toxicity, may prolong the effect of suxamethonium, reduced procaine metabolism in patients with deficiency of pseudocholinesterase

Amide drugs (bupivacaine, cinchocaine, etidocaine, lignocaine, mepivacaine, prilocaine) have all been reported to precipitate malignant hyperpyrexia. Risk of hypersensitivity reactions to local anaesthetic agents is described in text.

Although rare, reports have shown patients to be sensitive to the amide drugs, for example lignocaine and prilocaine (Brown et al 1981, Ruiz et al 1987). Ruiz et al (1987) reported that two anaphylactoid responses to the use of prilocaine for intravenous regional anaesthesia were manifest as severe pain in the exsanguinated arm. The mechanism of these allergic responses probably involved IgE antibodies. Some authors have suggested that the cases of drug allergy to lignocaine may, in fact, be due to the preservative rather than the parent drug, or to the antioxidant, bisulphite or metabisulphite present in solutions of lignocaine containing vasoconstrictors. Of the three or so reports associated with adverse reaction unequivocally due to lignocaine itself, only that of Brown et al (1981) have indicated accompanying immunological changes involving alternate complement pathway activation.

Muscle relaxants

Anaphylactic reactions to muscle relaxants were also originally thought to be rare, with the majority of adverse reactions to these commonly used drugs being anaphylactoid in nature. However, Baldo & Fisher (1983b) have measured high titres of IgE drug-specific antibodies in the sera of subjects who have suffered life-threatening reactions to the muscle relaxants alcuronium and d-tubocurarine. Their findings also indicate that the IgE antibodies to one muscle relaxant may interact with other relaxants. The likely allergenic sites are the quaternary ammonium groups (Baldo & Fisher 1983a,b, Harle et al 1985, Baldo 1986).

Establishing the cause of a suspected adverse reaction involving muscle relaxants is difficult, as many of the drugs provoke histamine release. Even low drug concentrations (≤ 1 μg/ml) may elicit a positive wheal-and-flare response.

Succinylcholine

Although localized wheal-and-flare reactions at the site of injections are common after the administration of suxamethonium, there have been at least 250 cases of systemic reactions to the drug cited in the literature since the first report of anaphylaxis by Jerums et al (1967) and the first laboratory confirmed report of such a reaction by Royston & Wilkes (1978). In the majority of these patients, bronchospasm and hypotension, with or without generalized erythema, were the main clinical signs (Boileau et al 1985). True anaphylaxis is the aetiology in about 65% of the cases (Harle et al 1985, Vervloet et al 1983). Pre-existing factors in the affected patients included a history of allergy, asthma or chronic bronchitis. Interestingly, there appears to be a sex predominance with greater than 65% of the reported cases being in female patients. To date there have been few documented deaths due to the adverse reactions from succinylcholine (Assem & Ling 1988).

Because of the common structural similarities (quaternary ammonium groups) between the different relaxants, the potential for cross-reactivity has been suggested. This is thought to be the cause in as many as 80–90% of all cases (Moneret-Vautrin et al 1985).

The value of in vitro tests such as basophil histamine release in the investigation of succinylcholine reactions has been described (Assem et al 1981, Withington et al 1987). A further tool in the elucidation of the causative drug may be detection of IgE specific antibodies by RAST (Assem & Ling 1988). Serial measurements on serum samples stored from an adverse reaction occurring in a 7-year-old child in 1973, and re-examined 14 years later together with a further blood sample, confirm the apparent in vitro stability of the allergen-specific IgE antibodies and the in vivo persistence of immunological memory (Assem & Symons 1989).

D-Tubocurarine

Allergic responses to d-tubocurarine have typically been described after the first exposure to the drug. It is probably the most potent histamine releaser of the current relaxant drugs (Galletly 1986), with the first case report of bronchospasm, presumed due to histamine release, by West (1936). Most adverse responses result in only mild and insignificant changes in airway resistance, although severe reactions may occur, particularly in patients with pre-existing obstructive airway disease. Other features may include urticaria and cardiovascular collapse. The literature contains no unequivocal reports of true anaphylaxis to the relaxant, and to date there have been no fatalities to the drug following adverse reactions.

Other relaxants

The histamine-releasing potential of gallamine is less than that of d-tubocurarine, but 65 or more reactions have been described in the literature. Watt (1973) described a reaction in a patient who had had previous exposure to gallamine, suggesting the possibility of an anaphylactic reaction. However, no confirmatory immunological tests were carried out. Fisher (1978) described three cases of anaphylaxis and cited details of three others occurring in the absence of previous exposure to the muscle relaxant (i.e. suggesting a cross-reactivity to an unknown allergen). More recently, anaphylaxis to a pre-curarizing dose of gallamine has been reported (Harrison & Bird 1986).

Following the early reports of Buckland & Avery (1973) and Heath (1973), 12 cases of anaphylactoid reactions to pancuronium (bronchospasm being the main feature) have been cited in the literature. These are of interest as histamine release by the drug has not been demonstrated in animals or man. Skin testing may prove useful in the investigation of suspected reactions to pancuronium (Patriarca et al 1989).

Alcuronium releases only minimal amounts of histamine and, although originally thought of as being of low incidence, cases of anaphylaxis have been reported (Chan & Young 1972, Fisher et al 1978). To date, over 80 reactions to the drug (mainly circulatory collapse) have been described (Fisher & Baldo 1983, Pusey et al 1987). Immunological testing has shown the cause to be anaphylaxis in over 90% of cases. This high incidence of adverse reactions may result from a presensitizing of patients to the quaternary ammonium group (which is present in many shampoos, drugs and soaps).

Newer drugs

Vecuronium is said not to cause significant release of histamine. The ability of atracurium to release histamine is approximately 50% that of dimethyl-tubocurarine and one third that of tubocurarine when compared at equipotent neuromuscular blocking doses.

Atracurium. There are many reports of cutaneous reactions to the administration of atracurium, with an incidence of 25–47%, and two cases of marked hypotension following histamine release (Mirakhur et al 1983, Philbin et al 1983). In further reports, Mercer (1984) described a case with bronchospasm and hypotension as the major symptoms and immunological evidence of an anaphylaxis; Aldrete (1985) a case presenting with diffuse upper thoracoabdominal and facial erythema, increased inspiratory resistance and hypotension; and Cohen & Frank (1987) an anaphylactoid reaction with periorbital and conjunctival oedema. However, Barnes et al (1986) showed no correlation between the incidence of cutaneous reactions to atracurium and plasma histamine levels.

Vecuronium. Although vecuronium is said to be free of histamine-releasing properties, four case reports have described release together with the onset of bronchospasm following administration of this drug (Clayton & Watkins 1984, Lavery et al 1985, O'Callaghan et al 1986, Farrell et al 1988). The mechanism differs between the four cases: one having raised IgE levels but no evidence of complement activation; two showing positive intradermal tests to vecuronium, and cross-reactivities to tubocurarine, atracurium and pancuronium; the fourth case had shown a previous reaction to tubocurarine, and exposure to vecuronium resulted in hypotension, wheezing and facial swelling and erythema. The laboratory tests revealed a low IgE, and no complement activation. Negative skin-testing would suggest this to be a case of non-immune histamine release (i.e. anaphylactoid). A similar case of cross-reactivity to vecuronium has been described by Moneret-Vautrin et al (1984). More recently, Durrani & O'Hara (1987) have reported a similar case of a histaminoid reaction to vecuronium

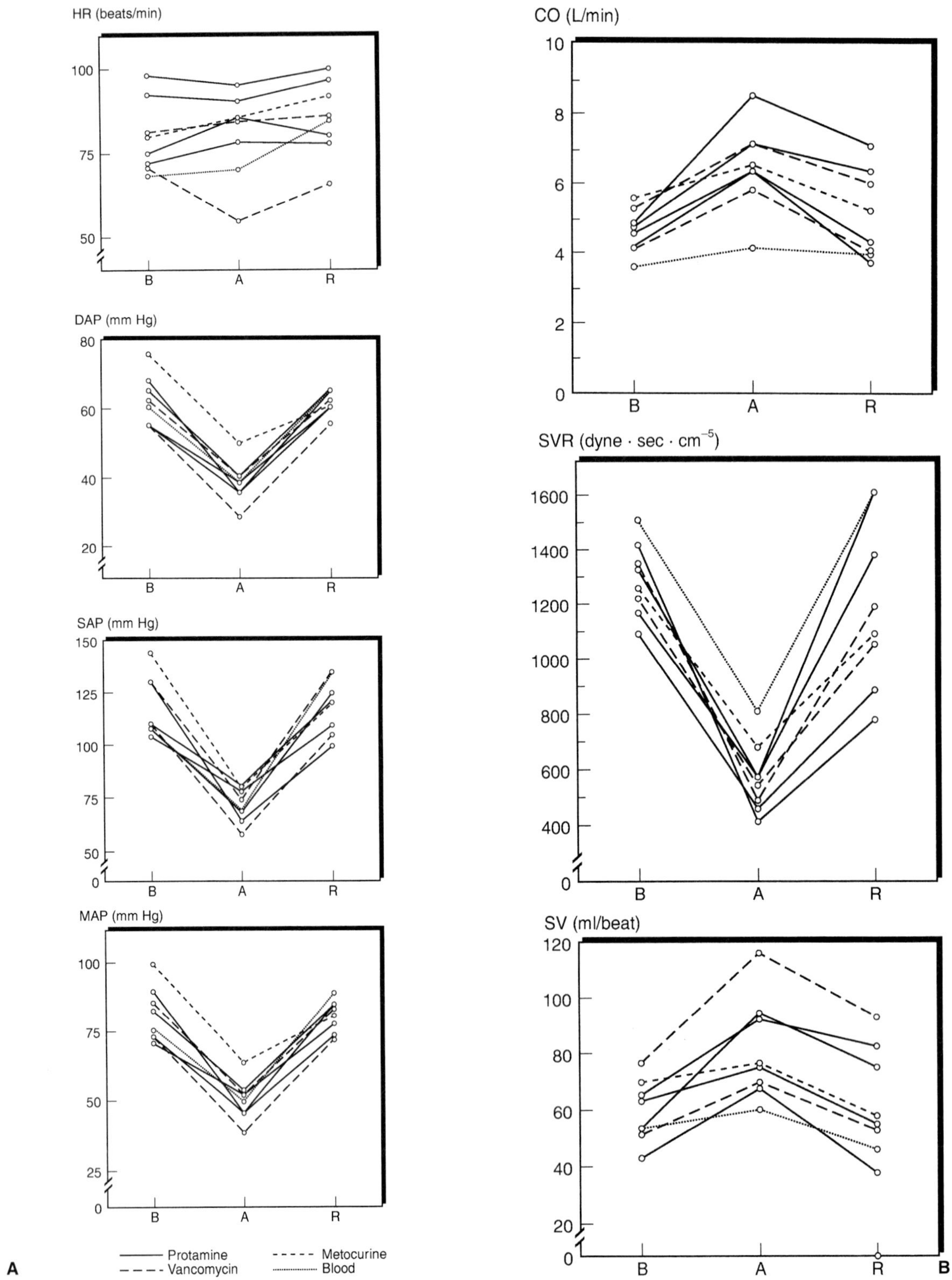
HR (beats/min)
DAP (mm Hg)
SAP (mm Hg)
MAP (mm Hg)
CO (L/min)
SVR (dyne · sec · cm^{-5})
SV (ml/beat)
B
A
R
Protamine
Vancomycin
Metocurine
Blood
A
B

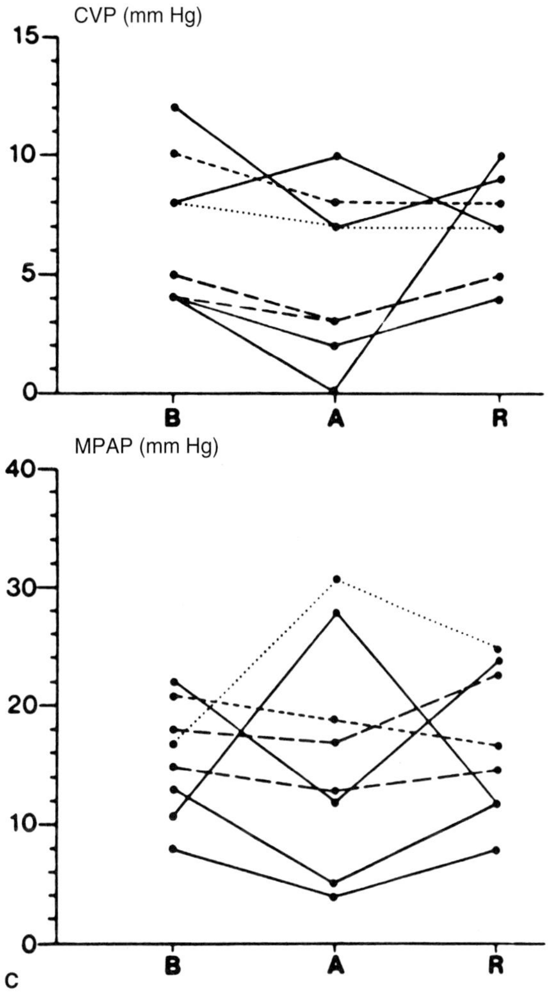

Fig. 19.5 (A to C) Cardiovascular changes during anaphylaxis. a: individual values of heart rate (HR), systolic blood pressure (SAP), diastolic blood pressure (DAP) and mean arterial blood pressure (MAP) at baseline (B), during anaphylactic reaction (A) and during recovery (R) in eight patients. b: individual values of cardiac output (CO), systemic vascular resistance (SVR) and stroke volume (SV). c: individual values of central venous pressure (CVP) and mean pulmonary artery pressure (MPAP). = protamine, — — - vancomycin, - - - - - - = metocurine, and . . . . = blood (from Levy 1986).

with an upper torso macular erythema and difficulty in breathing following a 'priming dose' (17 ug/kg) of the drug. Their suggestion that such a dose may be a useful predictive test for histamine release is ill-conceived, as even a small dose may trigger a full-blown anaphylactic reaction (Brinquin 1985, Conil et al 1985, Farrell et al 1988, Treuren & Buckley 1990). Because of its monoquaternary structure, vecuronium is still likely to be the least allergenic of the relaxants and the least likely to cross-reactivity.

HAEMODYNAMIC RESPONSES DURING ANAPHYLAXIS

There are few reports of the detailed cardiovascular changes occurring during anaphylactic or anaphylactoid reactions (Beaupre et al 1984). Levy (1989) has recently described eight such cases from a population of 1743 cardiac surgical patients over a 1-year period. The causative drug was protamine in four cases, vancomycin in two and a blood transfusion or metocurine in the others. All showed significant falls in blood pressure and systemic vascular resistance, while both stroke volume and cardiac output increased (Fig. 19.5). Associated clinical features were cutaneous wheals or flushing, and bronchospasm. Recovery to pre-allergy haemodynamic values occurred within 14 min (mean) following administration of intravenous catecholamines (ephedrine [two patients] or adrenaline). Previous reports have suggested that the decrease in blood pressure was due to a decrease in cardiac output (Enjeti et al 1983). However, in Levy's anaesthetized subjects, vasodilatation *not* decreased output was the cause of the hypotension. Increased stroke volume (and cardiac output) may occur secondary to the acute reduction in afterload, or to the inotropic effects of histamine on the heart (Bristow et al 1982).

TREATMENT OF ALLERGIC REACTIONS TO DRUGS

Various authors have reviewed the management of severe histamine release reactions (Fisher 1975, Stoelting 1983, Simpson 1984, Fisher, 1986, Levy 1986). As listed by Stoelting, the aims of treatment must be to correct arterial hypoxia, inhibit further release of chemical mediators and restore the vascular fluid volume (preferably with colloids). If the combination of adrenaline and adequate volume replacement do not produce clinical improvement, use of noradrenaline may be considered and prove life-saving. The following list details a management approach to allergic reactions:

1. Aims
   - correct arterial hypoxaemia
   - restore intravascular fluid volume
   - inhibition of further release of chemical mediators
2. Routine
   - stop administration of antigen
   - airway
   - added inspired oxygen
   - adrenaline: i.v., i.m. or via the endotracheal tube (depending on the severity of the reaction); 4–8 μg i.v. for hypotension, 0.5 ml of 1:1000 (0.5 mg) for cardiovascular collapse
   - fluids: both crystalloids and colloids, although the former may be ineffective in some cases
   - bronchodilators: if there is bronchospasm, give aminophylline or adrenaline; if during anaesthesia, consider use of halothene, diethyl ether, ketamine or isoflurane for relief of bronchoconstriction
   - positive pressure ventilation: especially in cases of pulmonary oedema
   - inotropes: to support circulation; adrenaline 2–4 μg/min, noradrenaline 2–4 μg/min, isoprenaline 0.5–1.0 μg/min
   - antiarrhythmics
   - cerebral resuscitation: consider if prolonged period of cardiac arrest, low output or arterial hypoxaemia; useful drugs include mannitol, dexamethasone, frusemide and IPPV with mild hypocapnia
   - correct acidosis.

Note: No benefit is gained from steroids in the acute phase, but methylprednisolone may be helpful in cases thought to be complement-mediated. No agent affects gastrointestinal symptoms. Isoprenaline increases the dead space and may increase arterial hypoxaemia. Antihistamines are only useful in angioneurotic oedema.

There is considerable controversy as to whether steroids should be given routinely. Cortisol has no effect on inhibiting the allergen–antibody interaction, nor on the release of vasoactive amine from mast cells and basophils. Thus steroids are probably only indicated for the treatment of severe bronchospasm. Other stimulant drugs, such as isoprenaline, should only be given cau-tiously in the presence of cardiac arrhythmias or hypovolaemia. Vasoconstrictors should also be used with care as they can provoke acute pulmonary oedema when coupled with rapid fluid infusion. Anticholinergic drugs such as atropine may attenuate the release of histamine by decreasing the intracellular concentrations of the second messenger, cyclic guanosine monophosphate. However, there is only limited data from which to draw conclusions. In cases of severe or intractable bronchospasm there is need for drugs other than aminophylline (e.g. glucocorticoids, adrenaline, isoprenaline, salbutamol, and even general anaesthetic agents with bronchodilator properties: diethyl ether, halothane, ketamine and isoflurane). For persistent vasodilatation, dopamine, dobutamine, ephedrine or adrenaline, given by repeat bolus doses or infusion, are the drugs of choice. There is no evidence of any acute value in the administration of H_1 and H_2 blocking drugs; however, these drugs may have a role in prophylaxis.

The postrecovery management of these patients must include adequate laboratory investigation to allow the establishment of a diagnosis, counselling of the patient and an explanation of the significance of hypersensitivity, reassurance as to future anaesthesia, and registration of the patient with Medic Alert or other organizations. In addition, a clear summary of the reaction should be placed in the patient's notes and sent to the general practitioner.

OTHER ADVERSE EFFECTS OF INTRAVENOUS ANAESTHETIC AGENTS

Hypnotic agents

Effects on endocrine glands

Normally, stress and surgery result in an increase in the activity of the neuroendocrine axis. Clarke et al (1970) have shown the magnitude of this response to be proportional to the severity of the trauma or surgical procedure.

There are few studies investigating the effects of intravenous anaesthetic agents on neuroendocrine activity in the absence of surgery. Engelhardt et al (1984) compared the influence of thiopentone (4 mg/kg) and etomidate (0.3 mg/kg) on plasma ACTH and serum cortisol concentrations in groups of male volunteers. The cortisol levels fell in both groups: by 30% in the thiopentone group and by 62% in those volunteers receiving etomidate. Following thiopentone, the plasma ACTH concentration showed an initial decline and then returned to the basal preanaesthetic level. In contrast there was a 100% increase in ACTH in those volunteers who received etomidate.

When given by either bolus dose or continuous infusion for the maintenance of anaesthesia in the surgical patient, etomidate obtunds the normal increases in both cortisol and aldosterone (Fragen et al 1984, Wagner & White 1984, Moore et al 1985). The decreased concentrations of cortisol and aldosterone were coupled with increases in 11-deoxycortisol and 11-desoxycorticosterone (DOC) (Duthie et al 1985, Moore et al 1985, Sear et al 1988). The increase in plasma ACTH in the surgical patient was similar in patients receiving either thiopentone or etomidate for the induction and/or maintenance of anaesthesia (Fragen et al 1984, Wagner & White 1984, Moore et al 1985).

Fry & Griffiths (1984) and Wagner & White (1984) studied the effects of administration of $ACTH^{1-24}$ (Synacthen) in patients receiving thiopentone or etomidate for induction (and maintenance) of anaesthesia. In those patients receiving thiopentone, ACTH caused marked increase in both cortisol and aldosterone. However, in the patients receiving etomidate the cortisol and aldosterone responses were blunted. In a separate study of four patients undergoing cardiac or vascular surgery, the effect of ACTH stimulation was assessed 4 and 24 hours after the last dose of etomidate (Wagner et al 1984). At the time of the first test there was a flattened response in the increases in cortisol and aldosterone, but by 24 hours the responses to ACTH had returned to normal.

Several reports have described the mechanisms of this interaction. In vitro studies in the rat indicated an inhibitory effect on the hypothalamus as well as the adrenal gland, but studies in man have all shown the effects of the drug to be limited to the adrenal cortex. Enzyme inhibition occurs in the pathways of both glucocorticoid and mineralocorticoid synthesis through high-affinity binding of etomidate to cytochrome(s) P-450, resulting in the inhibition of steroid metabolism (Vanden Bossche et al 1984, Horai et al 1985). Inhibition of steroid synthesis occurs at drug concentrations lower than those associated with hypnosis and anaesthesia. If the estimated drug concentration 1 min after a single induction dose of thiopentone, etomidate or propofol is calculated, and then compared with the in vitro concentration of the drug needed to 50% inhibit ACTH-stimulated cortisol synthesis in isolated bovine or guinea pig adrenal cells, the magnitude of the cortisol inhibition will be 10%, 100% and 40% respectively (Kenyon et al 1985, Lambert et al 1985).

There are several probable sites of adrenocortical action of etomidate. Bolus doses (0.3 mg/kg) and infusions up to 1.2 mg/kg total dose inhibit the 11 beta hydroxylase enzyme. This leads to the decreased levels of cortisol and aldosterone, and the increased plasma concentrations of their precursors, 11-deoxycortisol and DOC. However, Sear et al (1988) showed that the increase in DOC was greater in patients receiving a bolus dose of etomidate than in those receiving an infusion of the drug. This suggests, therefore, a second dose-related inhibition of DOC synthesis through an early pathway effect. Further evidence for a second inhibitory site between cholesterol and progesterone has been obtained through measurements of plasma concentrations of progesterone and 17-alpha hydroxyprogesterone (Moore et al 1985, Sear 1987). Although there was a dose-related inhibition of cortisol and aldosterone secretion, the effect of etomidate on the synthesis of progesterone appears to be an all-or-none response.

What is the significance of these effects of etomidate on the adrenal gland with respect to the clinical use of the drug? Watt & Ledingham (1984) reported an increased mortality when etomidate by infusion was used for sedation of the critically ill patient in the intensive care unit. Our own studies and those of other authors investigating the biochemistry of the adrenal cortical inhibition have all failed to detect clinical signs of acute adrenal insufficiency in the perioperative period (Fragen et al 1984, Wagner & White 1984, Moore et al 1985, Duthie et al 1985, Sear et al 1988). However, Van Lambalgan et al (1982) demonstrated cardiovascular depression in the dog when etomidate (4 mg/kg/hour) was infused for 4 hours 30 min. There is also limited evidence from the Cleveland Clinic suggesting a higher incidence of postoperative pulmonary complications in cardiac surgical patients induced with etomidate and fentanyl than in those induced with fentanyl alone (Zurick et al 1986). However, the study has apparently not been completed, hence the value of their preliminary account must be considered with due caution.

We have been searching for several years for methods of inhibiting the stress response to surgery, and in some respects etomidate may represent the ideal agent. However, it has also been clearly demonstrated that the patient receiving etomidate is unable to respond by an increase in cortisol secretion to a stressful event in the perioperative period (Fragen et al 1984, Wagner et al 1984a,b).

Some authorities have doubted the significance of this inhibition of cortisol synthesis and the associated low plasma cortisol levels in the perioperative patient.

As a result of these findings with etomidate, other intravenous agents have also been investigated for their effects on the neuroendocine responses to surgery. Studies with propofol showed no inhibition of the increase in plasma cortisol and aldosterone concentrations associated with surgery (Sear et al 1985, Fragen et al 1987, Herregods et al 1987). The response to injury or trauma is also not obtunded when propofol has been used by continuous infusion for sedation in the intensive care unit (Newman et al 1987, Aitkenhead et al 1989, Harris et al 1990).

There are also data to confirm that both methohexitone and ketamine given by continuous infusion have no effect on the neuroendocrine responses to surgery (Lacoumenta et al 1984, Mehta et al 1985, Crozier et al 1987). However midazolam (an imidazobenzodiazepine) has been shown to affect the hormonal response to surgery, but in a different manner to that described for etomidate. Crozier studied patients undergoing orthopaedic body-surface surgery in whom anaesthesia was induced with methohexitone, midazolam or etomidate (Crozier et al 1987). The midazolam group showed a blunting of the pituitary responses to surgical stress, with an absence of the expected increase in ACTH and beta endorphin concentrations (both being increased in the other two groups), and hence no increase in the plasma cortisol concentration. Thus, although both etomidate and midazolam may prevent the rise in cortisol concentrations, the mechanism is different. Midazolam causes a central inhibition of ACTH release from the anterior pituitary. Glisson (1987) has shown a similar effect in a canine model subjected to hypovolaemic hypotension under midazolam hypnosis, where there was an accompanying decrease in adrenergic output as well as ACTH and cortisol. There is no evidence, to date, that this centrally mediated effect is associated with increased morbidity. However, in contrast to etomidate, the effect on ACTH release of midazolam can be overcome by greater magnitude surgical stresses (Dawson & Sear 1986, Nilsson et al 1988).

Other studies reported by Kapp (1988) show a similar decrease in both plasma ACTH and cortisol following oral and intravenous administration of morphine to volunteers. This opioid-mediated effect may be a highly relevant observation, as the intensive therapy unit (ITU) patients reported in the studies of Watt & Ledingham (1984) were sedated with an etomidate-morphine combination!

The adrenal–pituitary axis is not the only endocrine system affected by intravenous hypnotic drugs. Gottardis et al (1988) have shown a difference between propofol, and thiopentone and diazepam, on plasma growth hormone (HGH) and glucose concentrations. After 2 mg/kg propofol followed by 0.2 mg/kg/min for 10 min, 0.3 mg/kg diazepam or 5 mg/kg thiopentone, anaesthesia was maintained with halothane in nitrous-oxide-oxygen. In all three groups there were no significant changes in the blood glucose concentration. However, 15 and 30 min after induction HGH had risen in the thiopentone and diazepam groups, but not in those patients receiving propofol. The clinical significance and aetiology of these observations is uncertain at present.

Effects on blood chemistry, coagulation and fibrinolysis

The onset of anaesthesia with thiopentone was shown (Bond 1969) to cause a 5% decrease in haemoglobin concentrations within 15–30 min of induction. Similar decrements were found when Althesin, ketamine and propofol were given for induction and/or maintenance of anaesthesia (Lacoumenta et al 1984, Sear et al 1985). The mechanism of this haemodilution is uncertain, but it may represent either alterations in the capillary perfusion pressure vs. plasma oncotic pressure relationship, or a redistribution of blood rich in cells and blood poor in cells. Studies with bolus doses, and infusions of hypnotics and opioids have shown no significant changes in plasma electrolytes and urea concentrations during anaesthesia of 2–3 hours' duration (Sear 1987).

Most intravenous anaesthetic drugs have been shown to have little effect on routine liver function tests when used to supplement either nitrous oxide or opioids during body-surface or major abdominal surgery (Blunnie et al 1981, Kawar et al 1982, Sear et al 1983, 1984, Robinson et al 1985). However, large doses of thiopentone (>1.4 g) and infusions of methohexitone (both used as sole agents for anaesthesia) have been reported to increase urinary urobilinogen (Dundee 1955, Bittrich et al 1963), although subsequent studies with methohexitone as a supplement to nitrous-oxide-fentanyl anaesthesia have failed to support these findings (Prys-Roberts et al 1983).

The effects of ketamine on liver function tests are confusing. Dundee et al (1980) reported significant increases on day 3–4 postsurgery in aminotransferases, alkaline phosphatase and gammaglutamyl transpeptidase when ketamine was given by infusion. The magnitude of the increases in the measured enzyme activity was still within the normal quoted ranges. In addition, many of the studies to date have assayed enzymes that are not liver specific and may therefore reflect the effects of tissue damage elsewhere in the body (Sear et al 1983).

Viegas & Stoelting (1979) overcame this lack of specificity. They compared the changes in the plasma activity of the fifth isoenzyme of LDH (LDH_v) in patients receiving either halothane, enflurane or fentanyl to supplement 67% nitrous oxide in oxygen while undergoing cholecystectomy or abdominal hysterectomy. Changes in LDH_v (expressed as a percentage of total LDH) were comparable for all three anaesthetic techniques, but differed between groups based on the site of the surgery (Fig. 19.6). Cholecystectomy involves surgical manipulation of the liver and compression of its blood supply. The data of Viegas & Stoelting (1979) and the study of Thompson & Friday (1978) have demonstrated that the nearer the site of surgery is to the liver, the greater is the incidence of liver enzyme abnormalities. A further

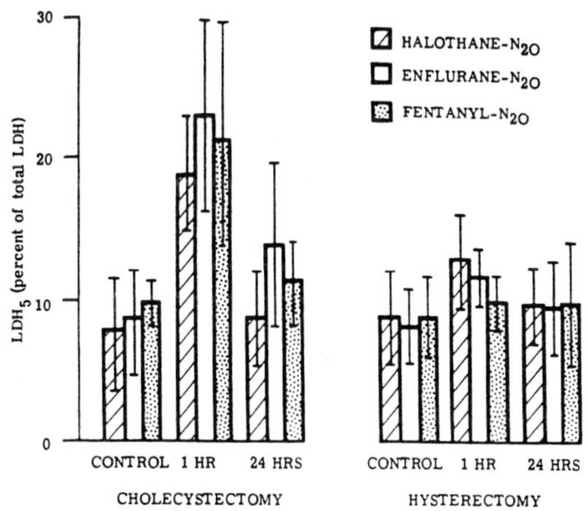

Fig. 19.6 LDH_v (as percentage of total LDH; mean ± SD) before and 24 h after elective cholecystectomy (30 patients) or abdominal hysterectomy (30 patients) in patients anaesthetized with 60% nitrous oxide in oxygen, supplemented with halothane, enflurane or fentanyl. Each group contained 10 patients. Normal LDH_v is 5–16% total LDH. LDH_v did not change following hysterectomy. By 1 h after cholecystectomy, values were significantly increased above control values in each group, and also above the corresponding values in those patients undergoing hysterectomy. By 24 h, there were no differences from the control values or in the levels seen in the two surgical groups, that is LDH_v changes did not appear to be influenced by the choice of anaesthetic technique (from Viegas & Stoelting 1979).

study in rats has shown that intraperitoneal dosing with fentanyl for 6 consecutive days may result in significant increases in alanine aminotransferase (Fassoulaki et al 1986).

Other functions of the liver include its synthetic properties relating to carbohydrate, lipid and protein metabolism. Recent work of de Sommer et al (1990) investigates the effects of infusions of propofol on lipid metabolism in patients undergoing arthroscopy. There were significant increases in serum triglyceride and free fatty acid concentrations during the infusion, with a return to baseline within 2 hours. There were also significant decreases in total serum cholesterol and apoprotein B. All fractions of very low density lipoproteins (VLDL) (except cholesterol and apoprotein C II) increased, while low density lipoproteins (LDL) and high density lipoproteins (HDL) fell. These data are in agreement with our own unpublished results which show a triglyceride clearance half-time of about 30 min after a 3-hour infusion of Intralipid (A Grant & J W Sear, unpublished). Surgery, trauma and fasting per se all promote lipolysis of triglycerides and increase free fatty acid concentrations. This may explain the differences between the data of de Sommer et al (1990) and that of Gottardis et al (1989). The latter found no significant changes in serum triglyceride, cholesterol and HDL-cholesterol when propofol was administered for prolonged sedation in the intensive care unit.

Other hypnotic agents used for sedation in the ITU have been reported to cause more significant biochemical and haematological changes. Gibbs et al (1984) investigated the effects of long-term continuous infusions of Althesin in 12 neurosurgical patients. The main changes were a decrease in serum albumin, an increase in triglycerides and an associated decrease in HDL. Haematological effects related to a 20% decrease in the haemoglobin level, and significant increases in plasma fibrinogen and plasma viscosity. Whether these changes were due to the sedative or its solvent remain uncertain, but clearly the latter is also present in intravenous cyclosporine formulations, and hence prolonged intravenous infusions for immunosuppression must be accompanied by monitoring of liver function. Other authors have described further biochemical changes following prolonged Althesin infusion: abnormal electrophoretic pre-beta band and an absence or decrease of the alpha band (Lawler et al 1983, Stewart et al 1983). Abnormalities in liver function tests were also seen when Althesin was used for prolonged ITU sedation (Ramsey et al 1974).

Lipid solutions and solvents in general may also affect the coagulation pathways. Gaszynski et al (1974) showed that both single doses and repeated increments of Althesin cause increased clot retraction, an increased platelet count and activation of plasma thromboplastins. More recent work, comparing the effects of Althesin and propofol to supplement nitrous oxide during body-surface surgery, showed no significant changes in platelet count, prothrombin ratio, thrombin time or partial thromboplastin time (Sear et al 1985). However, Amris et al (1964) reported in vivo acceleration of thrombin generation after infusion of Intralipid, while Reid & Ingram (1967) showed that lipid infusions possess weak antiplatelet activity.

Other work by Hulman et al (1982) suggests that fat emulsions may undergo in vitro agglutination or 'creaming' when added to the serum of patients with high levels of C-reactive and other acute phase proteins. Conditions most commonly associated with these high protein concentrations are neoplasia, sepsis, major surgery, trauma, and inflammatory disorders such as rheumatoid arthritis. If agglutination was to occur in vivo to a greater extent than can be rapidly cleared by the reticuloendothelial system, lipid microembolization might result. Indeed, there have been reports of tissue lipid deposition in some of the conditions listed above.

Opioid drugs

Many opioid drugs have effects on biochemical parameters. The influence of morphine on the plasma ACTH and cortisol levels of volunteers has already been mentioned (Kapp 1988). Use of parenteral opioids (and also opioids by the spinal route) has been shown effective in attenuating but not abolishing the neuroendocrine responses to anaesthesia and surgery (McQuay et al 1980, Child & Kaufman 1985, Kay et al 1985, Normandale et al 1985, Dowing et al 1986). The size of intravenous doses of opioid agonists (and partial agonists) needed to suppress the increases in catabolic hormones is considerable and can only be achieved at the expense of marked cardiorespiratory depression. Fentanyl, methadone, phenazocine, morphine and pethidine in normal doses have no significant effect. Buprenorphine, on the other hand, has been shown to attenuate the cortisol response in doses as low as 0.6 mg. Meptazinol (100 mg) had no effect on the postoperative catabolic hormonal responses to lower abdominal surgery. However its action (via the mu_1 receptor) to increase prolactin levels (Kay et al 1985) is of interest.

These negative findings of the opioids compare with the ability of spinally administered local anaesthetics to prevent the major part of the neuroendocrine response to surgery and trauma in lower abdominal surgery, although these drugs are also less effective in the management of patients undergoing upper abdominal or thoracic surgery (Kehlet 1982, Shirasaka et al 1986, Davis et al 1987). In contrast, extradural injections of local anaesthetic agents may block the glycoregulatory response to lower abdominal or peripheral body-surface surgery, but have little effect in upper abdominal and thoracic surgical procedures (Kehlet 1982, Hall 1985).

The value of properly controlled outcome studies investigating the efficacy of these different methods of hormonal modulation on morbidity and mortality are clearly needed. There are few data examining whether suppression of the cortisol response affects postoperative morbidity. Smith et al (1985) have reported an isoflurane-fentanyl combination to be associated with less intraoperative ischaemia than fentanyl alone in high-risk patients undergoing coronary artery bypass surgery. However, Benefiel et al (1986) have questioned this in a subsequent study showing less major morbidity following sufentanil anaesthesia when compared with isoflurane in a randomized study of patients undergoing aortic surgery. Thus improved efficacy in one area (e.g. cardiovascular stability or neuroendocrine effects) may be accompanied by other adverse side effects (e.g. convulsions, rigidity, immediate and delayed postoperative respiratory depression, nausea and vomiting, and delayed recovery; Janis 1972, Becker et al 1976, Rao et al 1982, Christian et al 1983, Chang & Fish 1985, Goldberg et al 1985, Mahla et al 1988, Jaffe & Coalson 1989, Krane et al 1990).

CONCLUSIONS

Despite the widespread recognition of the need to monitor the responses of patients to intravenous anaesthetic drugs, many unexpected observations go uncharted and unrecorded. The reporting of drug reactions to the Committee on Safety of Medicines probably represents about 10% of all cases that occur. Monitored release programmes for new drugs may go some way towards improving this figure, but the true incidence of allergic and other idiosyncratic reactions will only become apparent during the widespread usage of the drugs in clinical practice (rather than in the 'protected' environment of the clinical trial).

The anaesthetist gives most drugs by the intravenous route. The rapidity of onset of drug effects should improve the likelihood of his detecting adverse reactions. When such a reaction occurs, treatment must be prompt and aggressive, and subsequent investigation of the cause is the anaesthetist's responsibility.

Acknowledgment

I am grateful to the Committee on Safety of Medicines for some of the data in Table 19.3.

REFERENCES

Aitkenhead A R, Pepperman M L, Willatts S M, Coates D P, Park G R, Bodenham A R, Collins C H, Smith M B, Ledingham I McA, Wallace P G M 1989 Comparison of propofol and midazolam for sedation in critically ill patients. Lancet 2: 704–709

Aldrete J A 1985 Allergic reaction after atracurium. Br J

Anaesth 57: 929–930
Aldrete J A, Johnson D A 1970 Evaluation of intracutaneous testing for investigation of allergy to local anesthetic agents. Anesth Analg 49: 173–184
Altman L C 1981 Basic immune mechanisms in immediate hypersensitivity. Med Clin North Am 65: 941–957
Amris C J, Brockner J, Larsen V 1964 Changes in the coagulability of blood during the infusion of intralipid. Acta Chir Scand Suppl 325: 70–74
Assem E S K, Frost P G, Levis R D 1981 Anaphylactic-like reaction to suxamethonium. Anaesthesia 36: 405–410
Assem E S K, Ling Y B 1988 Fatal anaphylactic reaction to suxamethonium: a new screening test suggests possible prevention. Anaesthesia 43: 958–961
Assem E S K, Symons I E 1989 Anaphylaxis due to suxamethonium in a 7-year-old child: a 14 year follow-up with allergy testing. Anaesthesia 44: 121–124
Baldo B A 1986 Cross-reactions of neuromuscular blocking drugs and anaphylactoid reactions. Anaesthesia 41: 550–551
Baldo B A, Fisher M M 1983a Detection of serum IgE antibodies that react with alcuronium and tubocurarine after life threatening reactions to muscle-relaxant drugs. Anaesth Intensive Care 11: 194–197
Baldo B A, Fisher M M 1983b Anaphylaxis to muscle relaxant drugs: cross-reactivity and molecular basis of binding of IgE antibodies detected by radioimmunoassay. Molecular Immunology 20: 1393–1400
Barnes P K, de Renzy-Martin N, Thomas V J E, Watkins J 1986 Plasma histamine levels following atracurium. Anaesthesia 41: 821–824
Beamish D, Brown D T 1981 Adverse responses to iv. anaesthetics. Br J Anaesth 53: 55–58
Beard K, Jick H 1985 Cardiac arrest and anaphylaxis with anesthetic agents. JAMA 254: 2742
Beaupre P N, Roizen M F, Cahalan M K, Alpert R A, Cassorla L, Schiller N B 1984 Hemodynamic and two-dimensional transesophageal echocardiographic analysis of an anaphylactic reaction in man. Anesthesiology 60: 482–484
Becker L D, Paulson B A, Miller R D, Severinghaus J W, Eger E I 1976 Biphasic respiratory depression after fentanyl-droperidol or fentanyl alone used to supplement nitrous oxide anesthesia. Anesthesiology 44: 291–296
Benefiel D J, Roizen M F, Lampe G H, Sohn Y J, Fong K S, Irwin D H, Drusneck K, Smith J S, Stoney R J, Ehrenfeld W K, Goldstone J S, Reilly L M, Thisted R A, Eger E I 1986 Morbidity after aortic surgery with sufentanil versus isoflurane anesthesia. Anesthesiology 65: A516
Bittrich N M, Kane A V, Mosher R E 1963 Methohexital and its effects on liver function tests. Anesthesiology 24: 81–90
Blunnie W P, Zacharias M, Dundee J W, Doggart J R, McIlroy P D 1981 Liver enzyme studies with continuous intravenous anaesthesia. Anaesthesia 36: 152–156
Boileau S, Hummer-Sigiel M, Moeller R, Drouet N 1985 Reevaluation des resques respectifs d'anaphylaxie et d'histaminoliberation avec les substances anesthesiologiques. Annales francaises d'Anesthesie et de Reanimation 4: 195–204
Bond A G 1969 Determination of operative blood loss. Anaesthesia 24: 219–229
Bricker S R W, Raitt D G 1987 Angioneurotic oedema following etomidate/lignocaine. Anaesthesia 42: 323–324
Briggs L P, Clarke R S J, Watkins J 1982 An adverse reaction to the administration of disprofol (Diprivan). Anaesthesia 37: 1099–1101
Brinquin L 1985 Anaphylactic reaction to vecuronium. Annales francaises d'Anesthesie et de Reanimation 4:244
Bristow M R, Ginsburg R, Harrison D C 1982 Histamine and the human heart: the other receptor system. Am J Cardiol 49: 249–251
Brogger-Nielsen F 1984 Anaphylactoid reaction to Diazemuls. Br J Anaesth 56: 1179
Brown D T, Beamish D, Wildsmith J A W 1981 Allergic reaction to an amide local anaesthetic. Br J Anaesth 53: 435–437
Buckland R W, Avery A F 1973 Histamine release following pancuronium: a case report. Br J Anaesth 45: 518–521
Chan C S, Young M L 1972 Anaphylactic reaction to alcuronium. Br J Anaesth 44: 103–105
Chang J, Fish K J 1985 Acute respiratory arrest and rigidity after anesthesia with sufentanil: a case report. Anesthesiology 63: 710–711
Chapuis B, Helg C, Jeannet M, Zulian G, Huber P, Gumovski P 1985 Anaphylactic reaction to intravenous cyclosporin. N Engl J Med 312: 1259
Child C S, Kaufman L 1985 Effect of intrathecal diamorphine on the adrenocortical, hyperglycaemic and cardiovascular response to major colonic surgery. Br J Anaesth 57: 389–393
Christian C M, Waller J L, Moldenhauer C C 1983 Postoperative rigidity following fentanyl anesthesia. Anesthesiology 58: 275–277
Clarke R S J 1981 Adverse effects of intravenously administered drugs used in anaesthetic practice. Drugs 22: 26–41
Clarke R S J, Johnston H, Sheridan B 1970 The influence of anaesthesia and surgery on plasma cortisol, insulin and free fatty acids. Br J Anaesth 42: 295–299
Clarke R S J, Dundee J W, Garrett R T, McArdle G K, Sutton J A 1975 Adverse reactions to intravenous anaesthetics: a survey of 1000 reports. Br J Anaesth 47: 575–585
Clayton D G, Watkins J 1984 Histamine release with vecuronium. Anaesthesia 39: 1143–1144
Cohen A Y, Frank G 1987 Periorbital edema after atracurium administration. Anesthesiology 66: 431–432
Conil C, Bornet J L, Jean-Noel M, Conil J M, Brouchet A 1985 Choc anaphylactique au pancuronium et au vecuronium. Annales francaises d'Anesthesie et de Reanimation 4: 241–243
Coventry D M, Stone P 1988 Hypersensitivity reactions to alfentanil? Anaesthesia 43: 887–888
Crozier T A, Beck D, Wuttke W, Kettler D 1987 Endocrinological changes following etomidate, midazolam or methohexital for minor surgery. Anesthesiology 66: 628–635
Cummins C G, Dixon J, Kay N H, Windsor J P W, Major E, Morgan M, Sear J W, Spence A A, Stephenson D K 1984 Dose requirements of ICI 35868 (Propofol, 'Diprivan') in a new formulation for induction of anaesthesia. Anaesthesia 39: 1168–1171
Davis F M, Laurenson V G, Lewis J, Wells J E, Gillespie W J 1987 Metabolic response to total hip arthroplasty under hypobaric subarachnoid or general anaesthesia. Br J Anaesth 59: 725–729
Dawson D, Sear J W 1986 Influence of induction of anaesthesia with midazolam on the neuroendocrine

response to surgery. Anaesthesia 41: 268–271
de Leon-Casasola O A, Weiss A, Lema M J 1992 Anaphylaxis due to propofol. Anesthesiology 77: 384–386
de Sommer M R J, Driessen J H J, Willems C M E, Lust P C 1990 A comparative study of the effects of propofol in emulsion and Intralipid[R] on fat metabolism. Acta Anaesthesiol Belg 41: 133–138
Doenicke A, Lorenz W, Beigl R, Bezecny H, Uhlig G, Kalmar L, Praetorius B, Mann G 1973. Histamine release after intravenous application of short-acting hypnotics: a comparison of etomidate, Althesin (CT 1341), and propanidid. Br J Anaesth 45: 1097–1104
Dold M, Konarzewski W H 1989 Delayed allergic response to propofol. Anaesthesia 44: 533
Dowing R, Davis I, Black J, Winsor C W O 1986 Effect of intrathecal morphine on the adrenocortical and hyperglycaemic responses to upper abdominal surgery. Br J Anaesth 58: 858–861
Dueck R, O'Connor R D 1984 Thiopental: false positive RAST in patient with elevated serum IgE. Anesthesiology 61: 337–338
Dundee J W 1955 Thiopentone as a factor in the production of liver dysfunction. Br J Anaesth 27: 14–20
Dundee J W, Fee J P, Moore J, McIlroy P D, Wilson D B 1980 Changes in serum enzyme levels following ketamine infusions. Anaesthesia 35: 12–16
Durrani Z, O'Hara J 1987 Histaminoid reaction from vecuronium primimg: a case report. Anesthesiology 67: 130–132
Duthie D J R, Fraser R, Nimmo W S 1985 Effect of induction of anaesthesia with etomidate on corticosteroid synthesis in man. Br J Anaesth 57: 156–159
Engelhardt D, Doenicke A, Suttmann H, Kupper F J, Braun S, Muller C A 1984 Der einfluβ von etomidat und thiopental auf ACTH- und cortisolspiegel im serum. Der Anaesthesist 33: 583–587
Enjeti S, Bleecker E R, Smith P L et al 1983 Hemodynamic mechanisms in anaphylaxis. Circ Shock 11: 197–309
Falk R H 1977 Allergy to diazepam. Br Med J 1: 287
Farrell A M, Gowland G, McDowell J M, Simpson K H, Watkins J 1988 Anaphylactoid reaction to vecuronium followed by systemic reaction to skin testing. Anaesthesia 43: 207–209
Fassoulaki A, Andreopoulou K, Williams G, Pateras C 1986 The effect of single and repeated doses of thiopentone and fentanyl on liver function in the rat. Anaesth Intensive Care 14: 145–147
Fazackerley E J, Martin A J, Tolhurst-Cleaver C L, Watkins J 1988 Anaphylactoid reaction following the use of etomidate. Anaesthesia 43: 953–954
Fee J P H, McDonald J R, Clarke R S J, Dundee J W, Pal P K 1978 The incidence of atopy and allergy in 10 000 preanaesthetic patients. Br J Anaesth 50: 74–78
Fisher M McD 1975 Severe histamine mediated reactions to intravenous drugs used in anaesthesia. Anaesth Intensive Care 3: 180–197
Fisher M McD 1978 Anaphylactic reactions to gallamine. Anaesth Intensive Care 6: 62–65
Fisher M McD 1979 Intradermal testing in the diagnosis of acute anaphylaxis during anaesthesia: results of five years experience. Anaesth Intensive Care 7: 58–61
Fisher M McD 1981 The diagnosis of acute anaphylactoid reactions to anaesthetic drugs. Anaesth Intensive Care 9: 235–241
Fisher M McD (ed) 1984 Adverse reactions. Clinics in Anaesthesiology 2(3): 447–697. W B Saunders, London
Fisher M McD 1986 Clinical observations on the pathophysiology and treatment of anaphylactic cardiovascular collapse. Anaesth Intensive Care 14: 17–21
Fisher M McD, Hallowes R C, Wilson R M 1978 Anaphylaxis to alcuronium. Anaesth Intensive Care 6: 125–128
Fisher M McD, More D G 1981 The epidemiology and clinical features of anaphylactic reactions in anaesthesia. Anaesth Intensive Care 9: 226–234
Fisher M McD, Baldo B 1983 Adverse reactions to alcuronium: an Australian disease? Medical Journal of Australia 1: 630–632
Fisher M McD, Rolfe D J 1984 Allergy, atopy and IgE. Anaesthesia 39: 213–217
Fisher M McD, Outherd A, Bowey C J 1987 Can clinical anaphylaxis to anaesthetic drugs be predicted from allergic history? Br J Anaesth 59: 690–692
Fisher M McD, Ross J D, Harle D A, Baldo B 1989 Anaphylaxis to thiopentone: an unusual outbreak in a single hospital. Anaesth Intensive Care 17: 361–365
Flacke J W, Flacke W E, Bloor B C, Van Etten A P, Kripke B J 1987 Histamine release by four narcotics: a double-blind study in humans. Anesth Analg 66: 723–730
Fragen R J, Shanks C A, Molteni A, Avram M J 1984 Effects of etomidate on hormonal responses to surgical stress. Anesthesiology 60: 652–656
Fragen R J, Weiss H W, Molteni A 1987 The effect of propofol on adrenocortical steroidogenesis: a comparative study with etomidate and thiopental. Anesthesiology 66: 839–842
Friedman L S, Dienstag J L, Nelson P W, Russell P S, Cosimi A B 1985 Anaphylactic reaction and cardiopulmonary arrest following intravenous cyclosporine. Am J Med 78: 343–345
Fry D E, Griffiths H 1984 The inhibition by etomidate of 11ß hydroxylation of cortisol. Clin Endocrinol 20: 625–629
Galletly D C 1986 Comparative cutaneous histamine release by neuromuscular blocking agents. Anaesth Intensive Care 14: 365–369
Galletly D C, Treuren B C 1985 Anaphylactoid reactions during anaesthesia: seven years' experience of intradermal testing. Anaesthesia 40: 329–333
Gaszynski W, Winiarski T, Orzechowski S, Sokot-Kobielska E 1974 Studies of blood clotting system during intravenous general anaesthesia with Althesin. Anaesth Resusc Intensive Ther 2: 345–350
Gibbs N, Cameron P D, Thompson W R, Purser C, Oh T E 1984 Effect of long term continuous infusion of Alfathesin on clinical biochemical and haematological parameters. Anaesth Intensive Care 12: 108–112
Glen J B, Davies G E, Thomson D S, Scarth S C, Thompson A V 1979 An animal model for the investigation of adverse responses to iv. anaesthetic agents and their solvents. Br J Anaesth 51: 819–827
Glen J B, Hunter S C 1984 Pharmacology of an emulsion formulation of ICI 35868. Br J Anaesth 56: 617–626
Glisson S N 1987 Investigation of midazolam's influence on physiological and hormonal responses to hypotension. J Cardiovasc Pharmacol 9: 45–50
Goldberg M, Ishak S, Garcia C, McKenna J 1985 Postoperative rigidity following sufentanil administration. Anesthesiology 65: 199–201

Gottardis M, Fessler R, Luger Th J, Mutz N, Kornberger R 1988 Das verhalten des menschlichen wachstumhormons (hGH) nach anaesthesieeinleitung mit propofol. Der Anaesthesist 37: 690–693
Gottardis M, Khuenl-Brady K S, Koller W, Sigl G, Hackl J M 1989 Effect of prolonged sedation with propofol on serum triglyceride and cholesterol concentrations. Br J Anaesth 62: 393–396
Grant A, Sear J W 1982 Personal communication.
Green G R, Rosenblum A 1971 Report of the penicillin study group, American Academy of Allergy. J Allergy Clin Immunol 48: 331–343
Hall G M 1985 The anaesthetic modification of the endocrine and metabolic response to surgery. Ann R Coll Surg Engl 67: 25–29
Hall G M, Young C, Holdcroft A, Alaghband-Zadeh J 1978 Substrate mobilisation during surgery: a comparison between halothane and fentanyl. Anaesthesia 22: 924–930
Harle D G, Baldo B A, Fisher M M 1984 Detection of IgE antibodies to suxamethonium after anaphylactoid reactions during anaesthesia. Lancet 2: 930–932
Harle D G, Baldo B A, Fisher M M 1985 Assays for, and cross reactivities of, IgE antibodies to the muscle relaxants gallamine, decamethonium and succinylcholine (suxamethonium). J Immunol Methods 78: 293–305
Harle D G, Baldo B A, Smal M A, Wajon P, Fisher M M 1986 Detection of thiopentone reactive IgE antibodies following anaphylactoid reactions during anaesthesia. Clinical Allergy 16: 493–498
Harris C E, Grounds R M, Murray A M, Lumley J, Royston D, Morgan M 1990 Propofol for long-term sedation in the intensive care unit: a comparison with papaveretum and midazolam. Anaesthesia 45: 366–372
Harrison J F, Bird A G 1986 Anaphylaxis to precurarising doses of gallamine triethiodide. Anaesthesia 41: 600–604
Heath M L 1973 Bronchospasm in an asthmatic patient following pancuronium. Anaesthesia 28: 437–440
Herregods L, Rolly G, Versichelen L, Rosseel M T 1987 Propofol combined with nitrous oxide-oxygen for induction and maintenance of anaesthesia. Anaesthesia 42: 360–365
Hirshman C A, Peters J, Cartwright-Lee I 1982 Leukocyte histamine release to thiopental. Anesthesiology 56: 64–67
Hirshman C A, Edelstein R A, Eastman C L 1985 Histamine release by barbiturates in human mast cells. Anesthesiology 63: 353–356
Horai Y, White P F, Trevor A J 1985 The effect of etomidate on liver: rabbit liver microsomal drug metabolism in vitro. Drug Metab Dispos 13: 364–367
Hulman G, Pearson H J, Fraser I, Bell P R F 1982 Agglutination of Intralipid by sera of acutely ill patients. Lancet 2: 1426–1427
Hunter A R 1943 Dangers of pentothal sodium anaesthesia. Lancet 1: 46–48
Huttel M S, Schou Olesen A, Stofferson E 1980 Complement mediated reactions to diazepam with Cremophor as solvent (Stesolid MR). Br J Anaesth 52: 77–79
Incauto G, Schatz M, Patterson R, Rosenberg M, Yamamoto F, Hamburger R N 1978 Administration of local anesthetics to patients with a history of prior adverse reaction. J Allergy Clin Immunol 62: 339–345
Jaffe R S, Coalson D 1989 Recurrent respiratory depression after alfentanil administration. Anesthesiology 70: 151–153
Jamieson V, Mackenzie J 1988 Allergy to propofol? Anaesthesia 43: 80
Janis K M 1972 Acute rigidity with small intravenous doses of innovar: a case report. Anesthesia and Analgesia: Current Researches (Cleveland) 51: 375–376
Jerums G, Whittingham S, Wilson P 1967 Anaphylaxis to suxamethonium: a case report. Br J Anaesth 39: 73–76
Kahan B D, Wideman C A, Flechner S, van Buren C T 1984 Anaphylactic reaction to intravenous cyclosporin. Lancet 1: 52
Kapp W 1988 Opioids in anaesthesia. Acta Anaesthesiol Scand Suppl 32 (87): 33–37
Kawar P, Briggs L P, Behar M, McIlroy P D, Dundee J W, Merrett J D, Nesbitt G S 1982 Liver enzyme studies with disoprofol ('Diprivan') and midazolam. Anaesthesia 37: 305–308
Kay N H, Allen M C, Bullingham R E S, Baldwin D, McQuay H J, Moore R A, Price R K, Sear J W 1985 Influence of meptazinol on metabolic and hormonal responses following major surgery. Anaesthesia 40: 223–228
Kehlet H 1982 The modifying effect of general and regional anaesthesia on the endocrine metabolic response to surgery. Reg Anaesth 7: s38–s48
Kenyon C J, McNeill L M, Fraser R 1985 Comparison of the effects of etomidate, thiopentone and propofol on cortisol synthesis. Br J Anaesth 57: 509–511
Kettler D, Sonntag H 1974 Intravenous anesthetics: coronary blood flow and myocardial oxygen consumption (with special reference to Althesine). Acta Anaesthesiol Belg 3: 386–401
Krane B D, Kreutz J M, Johnson D L, Mazuzan J E 1990 Alfentanil and delayed respiratory depression: case studies and review. Anesth Analg 70: 557–561
Krumholz W, Muller H, Gerlach H, Russ W, Hempelmann G 1984 Ein fall von anaphylaktoider reaktion nach gabe von etomidat. Der Anaesthesist 33: 161–162
Kumar C M, McNeela B J 1989 Ocular manifestation of propofol allergy. Anaesthesia 44: 266
Lacoumenta S, Walsh E S, Waterman A E, Ward I, Paterson J L, Hall G M 1984 Effects of ketamine on the metabolic response to pelvic surgery. Br J Anaesth 56: 493–497
LaForest M, More D, Fisher M M 1980 Predisposing factors in anaphylactoid reactions to anaesthetic drugs in an Australian population: the role of allergy, atopy and previous anaesthesia. Anaesth Intensive Care 8: 454–459
Lambert A, Mitchell R, Robertson W R 1985 Effect of propofol, thiopentone and etomidate on adrenal steroidogenesis in vitro. Br J Anaesth 57: 505–508
Lavery G G, Hewitt, Kenny N T 1985 Possible histamine release after vecuronium. Anaesthesia 40: 389–390
Lawler P G P, McHutcheon A, Bamber P A 1983 Potential hazards of prolonged steroid anaesthesia. Lancet 1: 1270
Laxenaire M C, Chastel A, Borgo J, Kim K M, Medot J M, Fossard J M, Barlier J 1977 Prevention des accidents d'histaminoliberation survenant apres administration d'agents anesthetiques et adjuvants. Annales Anesthesie Francaise XVIII: 711–719
Laxenaire M C, Moneret-Vautrin D, Vervloet D 1985 The French experience of anaphylactoid reactions. Int Anesthesiol Clin 23: 145–160
Laxenaire M C, Gueant J L, Bermejo E, Mouton C, Navez M T 1988 Anaphylactic shock due to propofol. Lancet 2: 739–740
Laxenaire M-C, Mata-Bermejo E, Moneret-Vautrin D A,

Gueant J-L 1992 Life-threatening anaphylactoid reactions to propofol ('Diprivan'). Anesthesiology 77: 275–280
Leunissen K M L, Wateral P W G, van Hooff J P 1985 Anaphylactic reaction to intravenous cyclosporine. Lancet 1: 636
Levy J H 1986 A therapeutic protocol for the management of acute anaphylaxis. In: Anaphylactic reactions in anesthesia and intensive care. Butterworths, Boston, Ch 9, p. 103–111
Levy J H 1989 Anaphylactic/anaphylactoid reactions during cardiac surgery. J Clin Anesth 1: 426–430
Levy M, Lipshitz M, Eliakim M 1979 Hospital admissions due to adverse drug reactions. Am J Med Sci 277: 49–56
Levy J H, Rockoff M R 1982 Anaphylaxis to meperidine. Anesth Analg 61: 301–303
Lewis T, Grant R T 1927 Vascular reactions of the skin to injury. Heart 11: 209–265
Lewis R E, Cruse J M, Richey J V 1982 Effects of anesthesia and operation on the classical pathway of complement activation. Clin Immunol Immunopathol 23: 666–671
Lilly J, Hoy R H 1980 Thiopental anaphylaxis and reagin involvement. Anesthesiology 53: 335–337
Lorenz W, Doenicke A, Meyer R, Reimann H-J, Kusche J, Barth H, Geesing H, Hutzel M, Weissenbacher B 1972 Histamine release in man by propanidid and thiopentone: pharmacological effects and clinical consequences. Br J Anaesth 44: 355–369
McHale S P, Konieczko K 1992 Anaphylactoid reaction to propofol. Anaesthesia 47: 864–865
McQuay H J, Bullingham R E S, Paterson G M C, Moore R A 1980 Clinical effects of buprenorphine during and after operation. Br J Anaesth 52: 1013–1019
Magalini S C, Nanni G, Agnes S, Citterio F, Castagneto M 1986 Anaphylactic reaction to first exposure to cyclosporine. Transplantation 42: 443–444
Mahla M E, White S E, Moneta M D 1988 Delayed respiratory depression after alfentanil. Anesthesiology 69: 593–595
Mathieu A, Goudsouzian N, Snider M T 1975 Reaction to ketamine: anaphylactoid or anaphylactic. Br J Anaesth 47: 624
Mehta M F, Dillman J B, Sherman B M, Ghoneim M M, Lemke J H 1985 Etomidate anesthesia inhibits the cortisol response to surgical stress. Acta Anaesthesiol Scand 29: 486–489
Mercer J D 1984 A severe anaphylactic reaction to atracurium. Anaesth Intensive Care 12: 262–263
Mirakhur R K, Lyons S M, Carson I W, Clarke R S J, Ferres C, Dundee J W 1983 Cutaneous reaction after vecuronium. Anaesthesia 38: 818–819
Moneret-Vautrin D A, Laxenaire M C, Viry-Babel F 1983 Anaphylaxis caused by anti-Cremophor EL IgG STS antibodies in a case of reaction to Althesin. Br J Anaesth 55: 469–471
Moneret-Vautrin D A, Laxenaire M C, Mouton C 1984 Anaphylaxie croisee avec le vecuronium. Annals francaise d'Anesthesie et de Reanimation 3: 467
Moneret-Vautrin D A, Mouton C, Widmer S 1985 Anaphylaxie aux myorelaxants. Valeur predictive des intradermoreactions et recherche de l'anaphylaxies croisee. Annales francaises d'Anesthesie et de Reanimation 4: 186–191
Moneret-Vautrin D A, Widmer S, Gueant J-L, Kamel L, Laxenaire M C, Mouton C, Gerard H 1990 Simultaneous anaphylaxis to thiopentone and a neuromuscular blocker: a study of two cases. Br J Anaesth 64: 743–745
Moore R A, Allen M C, Wood P J, Rees L H, Sear J W 1985 Perioperative endocrine effects of etomidate. Anaesthesia 40: 124–130
Newman L H, McDonald J C, Wallace P G M, Ledingham I McA 1987 Propofol infusion for sedation in intensive care. Anaesthesia 42: 929–937
Nilsson A, Persson M P, Hartvig P, Wide L 1988 Effect of total intravenous anaesthesia with midazolam/alfentanil on the adrenocortical and hyperglycaemic response to abdominal surgery. Acta Anaesthesiol Scand 32: 379–382
Normandale J P, Schmulian C, Paterson J L, Burrin J, Morgan M, Hall G M 1985 Epidural diamorphine and the metabolic response to upper abdominal surgery. Anaesthesia 40: 748–753
O'Callaghan A C, Scadding G, Watkins J 1986 Bronchospasm following the use of vecuronium. Anaesthesia 41: 940–942
Patriarca G, Nucera E, Schiavino D, Romano A, Di Rienzo V, Pellegrino S, Fais G 1989 Pancuronium allergy: a case report. Br J Anaesth 62: 210–212
Pevny I, Danhauser I 1981 Anaphylaktischer shock wahrend der narkose mit positivem hauttest auf fentanyl und alloferin. Der Anaesthesist 30: 400–404
Philbin D M, Machaj V R, Tomichek R C, Schneider R C, Alban J C, Lowenstein E, Lineberry C C 1983 Haemodynamic effects of bolus injections of atracurium in patients with coronary artery disease. Br J Anaesth 55: 131s–134s
Prys-Roberts C, Sear J W, Low J M, Phillips K C, Dagnino J 1983 Hemodynamic and hepatic effects of methohexital infusions during nitrous oxide anesthesia in humans. Anesth Analg 62: 317–323
Pusey J M, Charlton S M, Skinner J B, Assem E S K 1987 Anaphylactoid reaction to alcuronium. Anaesthesia 42: 164–167
Radford S G, Lockyer J A, Simpson P J 1982 Immunological aspects of adverse reactions to Althesin. Br J Anaesth 54: 859–863
Ramsey M A R, Savage T M, Simpson B R J, Goodwin R 1974 Controlled sedation with alphaxalone/alphadolone. Br Med J 2: 656–659
Rao T L K, Mummaneni N, El-Etr A A 1982 Convulsions: an unusual response to intravenous fentanyl administration. Anesth Analg 61: 1020–1021
Raper R F, Fisher M M 1988 Profound reversible myocardial depression after anaphylaxis. Lancet 1: 386–387
Reid D J, Ingram G I C 1967 Changes in blood coagulation during infusion of Intralipid. Clin Sci 33: 399–407
Robinson F P, Patterson C C 1985 Changes in liver function tests after propofol ('Diprivan'). Postgrad Med J Suppl 61 (3): 160–161
Rosow C E, Moss J, Philbin D M, Savarese J J 1982 Histamine release during morphine and fentanyl anesthesia. Anesthesiology 56: 93–96
Royston D, Wilkes R G 1978 True anaphylaxis to suxamethonium chloride. Br J Anaesth 50: 611–615
Ruiz K, Stevens J D, Train J J A, Watkins J 1987 Anaphylactoid reactions to prilocaine. Anaesthesia 42: 1078–1080
Rutberg H, Hakansson E, Anderberg B, Jorfeldt L, Mortensson J, Schildt B 1984 Effects of extradural administration of morphine or bupivacaine on the endocrine response to upper abdominal surgery. Br J

Anaesth 56: 233–238
Sage D 1981 Intradermal drug testing following anaphylactoid reactions during anaesthesia. Anaesth Intensive Care 9: 381–386
Savage T M, Foley E I, Simpson B R 1973 Some cardiorespiratory effects of Cremophor EL in man. Br J Anaesth 45: 515–517
Schatz M 1984 Skin testing and incremental challenge in the evaluation of adverse reactions to local anaesthetics. J Allergy Clin Immunol 74: 606–616
Schou Olesen A, Huttel M S 1978 Circulatory collapse following intravenous administration of Stesolid MR. Ugeskr Laeg 140: 2644
Sear J W 1987 Toxicity of iv. anaesthetics. Br J Anaesth 59: 24–45
Sear J W, Prys-Roberts C, Dye A 1983 Hepatic function after major vascular reconstructive surgery. A comparison of four anaesthetic techniques. Br J Anaesth 55: 603–609
Sear J W, Walters F J, Wilkins D G, Willatts S M 1984 Etomidate by infusion for neuroanaesthesia: kinetic and dynamic interaction with nitrous oxide. Anaesthesia 39: 12–18
Sear J W, Uppington J, Kay N H 1985 Haematological and biochemical changes during anaesthesia with propofol ('Diprivan'). Postgrad Med J Suppl 61(3): 165–168
Sear J W, Edwards C R W, Atherden S 1988 Dual effect of etomidate on mineralocorticoid biosynthesis. Acta Anaesthesiol Belg 39: 87–94
Shelley W B 1963 Indirect basophil degranulation test for allergy to penicillin and other drugs. J Am Med Assoc 184: 171–178
Shirasaka C, Tsuji H, Asoh T, Yakeuchi Y 1986 Role of the splanchnic nerves in endocrine and metabolic response to abdominal surgery. Br J Surg 73: 142–145
Simpson P J 1982 Personal communication.
Simpson P J 1984 Adverse reactions to intravenous anaesthetic agents. Clinics in Anaesthesiology (ed. J W Sear) 2(3): 185–201. W B Saunders, London
Simpson P J, Radford S G, Lockyer J A, Sear J W, Cooper G M 1985 Some predisposing factors to hypersensitivity reactions following first exposure to Althesin. Anaesthesia 40: 420–423
Smith J S, Cahalan M K, Benefiel D J, Lurz F W, Lampe G H, Byrd B J, Schiller N B, Yee E S, Turley K, Ullyot D J, Hamilton W K 1985 Fentanyl versus fentanyl and isoflurane in patients with impaired left ventricular function. Anesthesiology 63: A 18
Sold M, Rothhammer A 1985 Lebensbedrohliche anaphylaktoide reaktion nach etomidat. Der Anaesthesist 34: 208–210
Stewart G O, Dobb J G, Craig I A 1983 Clinical trial of continuous infusion of alphaxalone/alphadolone in intensive care patients. Anaesth Intensive Care 11: 107
Stoelting R K 1983 Allergic reactions during anesthesia. Anesth Analg 62: 341–356
Tachon P, Descotes J, Laschi-Loquerie A, Guillot J P, Evreux J C 1983 Assessment of the allergenic potential of Althesin and its constituents. Br J Anaesth 55: 715–717
Theobald-Segalen C, Sainte-Laudy J, Pons A, Benveniste J 1982 Interet de l'exploration des basophiles humains dans le diagnostic de l'allergie medicamenteuse. Annales francaises d'Anesthesie et de Reanimation 1: 285
Thompson D S, Friday C D 1978 Changes in liver enzyme values after halothane and enflurane for surgical anesthesia. South Med J 71: 779–782
Treuren B C, Buckley D H F 1990 Anaphylactoid reaction to vecuronium. Br J Anaesth 64: 125–126
Vanden Bossche H, Willemsens G, Cools W, Bellens D 1984 Effects of etomidate on steroid synthesis in subcellular fractions of bovine adrenals. Biochem Pharmacol 33: 3861–3868
van Hooff J P, Bessems P, Beuman G H, Leunissen K M L 1987 Absence of allergic reaction to cyclosporin capsules in patient allergic to standard oral and intravenous solution of cyclosporin. Lancet 2: 1456
Van Lambalgan A A, Bronsveld W, van den Bos G C, Thijs L G, Teule G J J 1982 Cardiovascular and biochemical changes in dogs during etomidate-nitrous oxide anaesthesia. Cardiovasc Res 16: 599–606
Verrill P J 1975 Adverse reactions to local anaesthetics and vasoconstrictor drugs. Practitioner 214: 380–387
Vervloet D, Nizankowska X, Arnaud A, Senft M, Alazi M, Charpin J 1983 Adverse reactions to suxamethonium and other muscle relaxants under general anesthesia. J Allergy Clin Immunol 71: 552–558
Viegas O, Stoelting P K 1979 LDH_5 changes after cholecystectomy or hysterectomy in patients receiving halothane, enflurane or fentanyl. Anesthesiology 51: 556–558
Wagner R L, White P F 1984 Etomidate inhibits adrenocortical function in surgical patients. Anesthesiology 61: 647–651
Wagner R L, White P F, Kan P B, Rosenthal M H, Feldman D 1984 Inhibition of adrenal steroidogenesis by the anesthetic etomidate. N Engl J Med 310: 1415–1421
Watkins J 1982 Hypersensitivity reactions to drugs and other substances. In: Scurr C F, Feldman S (eds) Scientific foundations of anaesthesia, 3rd edn. Heinemann, London, pp 516–523
Watkins J A 1983. Etomidate: an 'immunologically safe' anaesthetic agent. Anaesthesia Suppl 38: 34–38
Watkins J 1984 Immunological effects of anaesthetic drugs. Clinics in Anaesthesiology 2(3): 463–483
Watkins J 1986 Antibody involvement in reactions to neuromuscular blocking drugs. Anaesthesia 41: 655
Watkins J 1987 Investigation of allergic and hypersensitivity reactions to anaesthetic agents. Br J Anaesth 59: 104–111
Watkins J 1989 Second report from an anaesthetic reactions advisory service. Anaesthesia 44: 157–159
Watkins J, Clarke R S J, Fee J P H 1981 The relationship between reported atopy or allergy and immunoglobulins: a preliminary report. Anaesthesia 36: 582–586
Watkins J, Nimmo W S 1985 'Allergic' drug reactions during anaesthesia. Anaesthesia 40: 813–814
Watt H K 1973 Anaphylactic shock from gallamine. New Zealand Society of Anaesthetists Newsletter 20: 21
Watt I, Ledingham I McA 1984 Mortality amongst multiple trauma patients admitted to an intensive therapy unit. Anaesthesia 39: 973–981
West R 1936 Intravenous curarine in the treatment of tetanus. Lancet 1: 12
Withington D E, Leung K B P, Bromley L, Scadding G K, Pearce F L 1987 Basophil histamine release: a study in allergy to suxamethonium. Anaesthesia 42: 850–854
Zurick A M, Sigurdsson H, Koehler L S, Ghattas M A, Dhun H S, Roberts M M, Estafanous F G 1986 Increased postoperative respiratory morbidity with a single dose of etomidate. Crit Care Med 14: 322

20

Adverse effects of drugs given by inhalation

D. E. R. Burt

INTRODUCTION

One hundred and forty years after their introduction, anaesthesia with inhalational anaesthetic agents is still the most widely practised form of the art. That this should be so at a time when there has been much concern about the adverse effects of atmospheric pollution on operating theatre staff, and a strong interest in total intravenous anaesthesia, attests to their popularity.

It is the ease of use, facility of control, and safety that are the most attractive features of these agents. The success of isoflurane has encouraged the search for volatile agents ever more close to the goal of the ideal anaesthetic agent. The very limited marketing of sevoflurane (restricted at present to Japan) would suggest that it offers few new advantages. However, the new decade has seen reports of the first clinical trials of desflurane, an agent of interest if for no other reason than that its high cost of production and low boiling point will necessitate the use of closed-circle systems and modified vaporizers.

This is not to say that inhalational agents are totally free from undesirable attributes, but that their adverse effects are well known and predictable, and have been reduced as newer agents have been developed. In this brief review we shall consider the effects of volatile agents and anaesthetic gases on the major systems of the body, and make mention of particular hazards of individual agents.

THE RESPIRATORY SYSTEM

Inhalational anaesthetics in general have a depressant effect on respiration, producing a reduction in alveolar ventilation and an increase in the dead space–tidal volume ratio with subsequent change in the acid-base state of the patient. In addition they tend to reduce, by differing amounts, the ventilatory response to increases in CO_2 concentration and to hypoxia.

Anaesthesia produces a reduction in the functional residual capacity (FRC) with increase in airway resistance and deterioration in gas exchange. Upper airway obstruction is a common feature following induction of anaesthesia, and the response to obstruction, either of the airway or the breathing circuit, is blunted.

These features have been recognized for some considerable time, but only recently has research begun to suggest mechanisms by which they may occur. A review of this work has been prepared by Jones (1987). He suggests that the underlying mechanism is a reduction in phasic and tonic activity of respiratory muscles.

Phasic drive

Phasic drive is directed by chemoreceptor stimulation responding to a rise in arterial $P\text{CO}_2$, fall in $P\text{aO}_2$ or pH, and by increased surgical stimulation. Volatile anaesthetics depress phasic drive and reduce alveolar ventilation. Enflurane has the most depressant effect and ether the least.

Tonic drive

There is a reduction in tone in the muscles of the upper airway and rib cage, and to a lesser extent in the diaphragm, during general anaesthesia. In addition there is reduction of phasic activity in these muscles. This results in obstruction of the upper airway during anaesthesia. Upper airway patency requires adequate muscle tone to resist the negative forces generated during inspiration, and coordination of oropharyngeal muscles to dilate the airway and decrease its compliance to oppose airway closure (Rodenstein & Stanescu 1986). As long as this balance is maintained the oropharynx resists closure and flow can proceed. However, if the dilating forces are selectively decreased (during REM sleep, alcohol ingestion and anaesthesia) then oropharyngeal closure ensues.

Carbon dioxide drive

The ability to increase ventilatory effort in response to a rising CO_2 concentration is important in anaesthesia where obstruction to breathing from airway interference or increased resistance in breathing circuits may occur. Impairment of this response exposes the patient to the danger of hypoxia. This increase in ventilation is a result of activity in the rib-cage musculature rather than the diaphragm. However, anaesthesia impairs muscle tone and movement of the rib cage much more than that of the diaphragm (Jones 1977). Thus the response of the anaesthetized patient to a CO_2 challenge is much diminished because the rib cage contribution is reduced by about 90%.

Functional residual capacity

Reduction in FRC of about 500 ml and an increase in the alveolar–arterial $P\text{O}_2$ gradient are constant features of anaesthesia, requiring increase of inspired oxygen from 21% to at least 33% in order to maintain normal oxygen saturation.

It had been suspected that atelectasis in dependent parts of the lung was responsible for this, and Strandberg et al have demonstrated this using computerized tomography (Strandberg et al 1986). They have shown that dependent lung atelectasis commenced within 5–10 min after induction of anaesthesia, in 50% of patients persisted for more than 24 h, and that the mode of ventilation, whether spontaneous or mechanical, had no influence. This atelectasis was seen both with and without volatile agents, and the extent of the atelectasis correlated with the magnitude of the shunt produced and impairment of arterial $P\text{O}_2$ (Hedenstierna et al 1986).

It has been postulated that the reduction in FRC would produce closure of basal airways as the FRC fell below the closing volume. It now appears that as the closing volume (the lung volume at which airway closure begins) is itself reduced during anaesthesia, this may not be a common event (Jones 1987).

Reduction in FRC occurs when the reduced tone in the diaphragm during anaesthesia no longer resists the pressure of the abdominal contents, and the diaphragm moves cranially. In the awake patient maintenance of FRC in the face of increasing hydrostatic pressure in the abdomen requires outward movement of the rib cage. The reduced rib-cage tone during anaesthesia prevents this happening. As the lung volume is reduced the airways narrow, and this effect is greatest in the dependent areas. It would be expected that inward movement of the abdominal wall would accompany the cranial shift of the diaphragm and abdominal contents, but this has been shown not to occur (Hedenstierna et al 1985). There is therefore speculation that the fall in FRC must be accompanied by a shift of blood from the thorax to the abdomen. The splanchnic vessel dilating effects of volatile anaesthetics may well have an important part to play in this mechanism.

Hypoxic vasoconstriction

Inhaled anaesthetics can be demonstrated to reduce the pulmonary vascular response to alveolar hypoxia. This is known as hypoxic vasoconstriction (HPV). It is a protective mechanism to divert blood away from areas of underventilated lung, and to reduce the V/Q mismatch and pulmonary shunt. Although reduction of HPV produced by volatile agents might be considered to be detrimental, in clinical practice the changes are subtle, and influenced by the response of pulmonary vasculature to reduction in cardiac output and mixed venous saturation. In clinical concentrations it is unlikely that volatile agents will have any other than minor effects (Augustine & Benumof 1984).

Both carbon dioxide production and oxygen consumption are reduced during anaesthesia as a result of diminished activity, and in the case of oxygen consumption by the action of inhalational anaesthetics as general metabolic depressants. Depression of respiration may be a desirable feature in an anaesthetic agent if controlled ventilation is anticipated, but is undesirable if the patient is breathing spontaneously and normal levels of PaO_2, $PaCO_2$ and pH are required. The stimulus provided by surgery and the use of nitrous oxide as a carrier gas will reduce the overall respiratory depressant effect.

Nitrous oxide

Nitrous oxide does not produce respiratory depression in clinical use. This may be demonstrated by the absence of any rise in the $PaCO_2$ of volunteers during spontaneous respiration breathing concentrations of 1.0–1.5 MAC (minimum alveolar concentration) nitrous oxide in a pressure chamber (1.0 MAC nitrous oxide = 110% atm). If nitrous oxide is used as the carrier gas then the concentrations of volatile agents required to maintain anaesthesia can be reduced. For example, the isoflurane requirement decreases by slightly less than 1% of MAC for each per cent of nitrous oxide used. This means that the respiratory depression produced by a nitrous oxide–oxygen-agent mixture will be less than that produced if the equivalent depth of anaesthesia were achieved by an oxygen-agent mixture alone. It should be noted, however, that nitrous oxide markedly reduces the CO_2-ventilatory response curve.

Cyclopropane

Cyclopropane produces a decrease in tidal volume and an increase in respiratory rate. The overall effect is a progressive reduction in alveolar ventilation as anaesthesia deepens and a rise in $PaCO_2$. The increased respiratory rate may be due to sensitization of pulmonary stretch receptors or may be mediated by the respiratory centre in response to a rise in $PaCO_2$. Hypercapnia, with concomitant stimulation of the sympathetic nervous system, is particularly undesirable with this agent in view of the serious cardiac dysrhythmias that occur in conjunction with catecholamines and cyclopropane (Price et al 1958). Opiate premedication abolishes the increase in respiratory rate and leads to a greater rise in $PaCO_2$ during induction than in the unpremedicated patient, and apnoea may occur at a lighter plane of anaesthesia. Cyclopropane is irritating to the respiratory tract in concentrations above 40%, and high inspired concentrations may provoke laryngeal spasm. Bronchoconstriction has been shown to occur in animals during cyclopropane anaesthesia, and although this is not commonly seen in clinical practice its possibility should be borne in mind when anaesthetizing patients with reactive airways.

Trichloroethylene

Trichloroethylene is non-irritant to the respiratory tract, although too rapid a rate of increase in concentration during induction may lead to coughing and breathholding as the agent has a strong odour. This, coupled with the length of time that induction takes compared to more recently introduced agents, may make induction of anaesthesia with this agent a taxing experience for the tyro.

Trichloroethylene produces a reduction in tidal volume, but its most striking feature is the pronounced tachypnoea that is produced. Respiratory rates in excess of 40 breaths/min are not uncommon. Previously it was considered that this tachypnoea was due to sensitization of the pulmonary stretch receptors in the alveoli and small bronchioles, and subsequent initiation of the inflation and deflation reflexes known as the Hering–Breuer reflexes (Whitteridge & Bulbing 1944). However, this original work was performed in animals, and it is known that the Hering–Breuer reflexes are very weak in man. Additional animal experimentation has shown that bilateral section of the vagi carrying the afferent impulses from the pulmonary stretch receptors does not prevent trichloroethylene tachypnoea in cats (Ngai et al 1961). It is more likely, therefore, that this effect of trichloroethylene, which is an extreme manifestation of the tendency of all inhalational agents to increase the respiratory rate, has a central origin. It was customary to control the tachypnoea by the administration of small intravenous doses of opiates, a practice which can only further increase the already elevated $Pa\text{CO}_2$. Trichloroethylene has been largely supplanted by newer agents for the spontaneously breathing patient, but its potent analgesic effects and relative lack of cardiovascular effects still make it a useful adjuvant to a nitrous oxide/oxygen/relaxant technique.

The manufacture of trichloroethylene was discontinued in the United Kingdom by ICI in 1988, due to falling demand. Supplies in the UK were due to expire by late 1989, and reference to it was removed from the British National Formulary at the end of 1989.

Ether

Ether differs from other inhalational anaesthetic agents in that, initially, respiratory stimulation is marked and $Pa\text{CO}_2$ may be maintained at normal or even reduced levels. This effect lasts until deep levels of anaesthesia (alveolar concentration of 6%) are reached at which point carbon dioxide levels start to rise. The reason for the overall stimulation of respiration is unclear, but depression of the respiratory centre occurs at deeper levels of anaesthesia and the CO_2–ventilatory response curve is flattened. Ether vapour is highly irritating to the respiratory tract and induction may be stormy. Increase in inspiratory concentration must be carried out carefully to avoid breath-holding and laryngospasm. The high blood/gas coefficient of ether means that changes in alveolar ventilation during induction are reflected in rapid changes in blood and brain concentrations, and fluctuating depths of anaesthesia may be produced. Antisialogogues are necessary to control excessive salivation. Ether produces relaxation of the bronchial musculature and has been used for the relief of bronchospasm in asthmatics.

Halothane

Halothane produces a rise in respiratory rate accompanied by a fall in tidal volume leading to an overall reduction of alveolar ventilation and a rise in $Pa\text{CO}_2$. At light levels of anaesthesia this rise in carbon dioxide is modest, and unstimulated volunteers breathing halothane in oxygen at 1 MAC show $Pa\text{CO}_2$ levels of 6 kPa, a level which the addition of surgical stimulation and nitrous oxide would reduce. The ventilatory response to hypoxia is also diminished by some 80% of the awake values at 0.5 MAC, and is completely abolished by 1.1 MAC halothane (Knill & Gleb 1978). Halothane is, however, a less potent respiratory depressant than either isoflurane or enflurane. Halothane vapour is not irritating to the respiratory tract and produces a smooth induction of anaesthesia. Laryngeal and pharyngeal reflexes are obtunded at light planes of anaesthesia and oral or nasopharyngeal airways may be inserted early. Halothane blocks both direct and reflex-mediated bronchoconstriction and is a suitable agent for patients with reactive airways. It has been used to treat bronchospasm in asthmatics.

Enflurane

Enflurane is a profound respiratory depressant producing a fall in tidal volume and a slight rise in respiratory rate accompanied by occasional sighing respirations. The net effect is to reduce the alveolar ventilation and elevate the arterial carbon dioxide tension. Enflurane is a more potent respiratory depressant than either halothane or isoflurane. 1 MAC enflurane in oxygen results in $Pa\text{CO}_2$ levels of 8 kPa in the unstimulated patient, and apnoea is produced at 2 MAC (Calverly et al 1978a). Addition of surgical stimulation and nitrous oxide will reduce these levels, but respiration should be assisted during deep anaesthesia. Enflurane is not irritating to the respiratory tract and secretions are not stimulated. Enflurane does not normally produce any change in airway conductance and is suitable for patients with chronic obstructive airways disease. There are a few case reports that suggest that there are occasional patients in whom enflurane anaesthesia may provoke bronchoconstriction, which may be relieved by substitution with halothane or isoflurane (Lowry & Fielden 1976).

Isoflurane

Isoflurane produces a dose-related depression of the respiratory system leading to a rise in $P\text{aCO}_2$. Its effect is greater than halothane but less than enflurane (Fourcade et al 1971). It is not irritating to the respiratory tract and does not provoke secretions. It has a pungent smell, and a rapid increase in concentration during induction may lead to breath-holding. Its respiratory depressant effect is reduced by surgical stimulation and the use of nitrous oxide as a carrier gas. Isoflurane is suitable for use in patients with reactive airways, and may be preferable to halothane when bronchoconstriction occurs since the arrhythmia potential of aminophylline with isoflurane is considerably less than with halothane (Stirt et al 1983). Isoflurane has been used in the management of status asthmaticus (Bierman et al 1986).

THE CARDIOVASCULAR SYSTEM

Haemodynamic effects

Nitrous oxide

Nitrous oxide has a direct depressant effect on the heart, producing a reduction in cardiac output caused by diminished myocardial contractility and a slowing of the heart rate. It also has a stimulatory effect on the sympathetic nervous system due to brainstem activity and causes a modest rise in circulating noradrenaline. This increases the systemic vascular resistance, and the net effect is to maintain blood pressure at awake levels. Such cardiovascular depression as does occur has only a slight effect in healthy individuals. In patients with severe cardiac decompensation even such a small degree of reduction in cardiac performance may be unacceptable, although a recent report (Mitchell 1989) suggests that, even in patients with coronary artery disease and poor left ventricular function (left ventricular ejection fraction <40%), nitrous oxide did not induce clinically detectable myocardial ischaemia. As with its effects on the respiratory system, the lesser degree of cardiovascular depression produced by nitrous oxide in comparison with more potent anaesthetic agents may be put to good use. By reducing the amount of potent agents required to maintain anaesthesia when nitrous oxide is introduced (which is often as much as a 50% reduction for a 50% concentration of nitrous oxide) the overall cardiovascular depressant effect of the anaesthetic is reduced (Stevens et al 1975).

Ether

Ether is a direct myocardial depressant. However, during light ether anaesthesia remarkably little change in blood pressure, heart rate or cardiac output will be seen. This is due in part to a vagal depressant action, and also to considerable stimulation of the sympathetic nervous system and release of noradrenaline. Plasma levels of noradrenaline are seen to rise in relation to increasing concentrations of ether. In deep ether anaesthesia the myocardial depressant effect will predominate and blood pressure and cardiac output will fall. Peripheral vasodilatation occurs initially due to a direct effect on the smooth muscle of the vessel walls, followed at deeper levels of anaesthesia by central depression of the vasomotor centre. This greatly reduces the ability of the peripheral vascular system to compensate for hypovolaemia and produces a reduced tolerance to haemorrhage.

Cyclopropane

Cyclopropane has a direct depressant effect on the myocardium. In light anaesthesia, however, sympathetic stimulation and a release of catecholamines result in an increase in cardiac output. This is due mainly to an enhancement of stroke work and a rise in right ventricular stroke volume. The blood pressure is usually well maintained and a falling blood pressure is often indicative of an overdosage of cyclopropane or the effect of bradycardia produced by vagal stimulation. As the depth of anaesthesia increases so cardiac output falls to normal or reduced levels.

It was the increased cardiac output during light to moderate levels of anaesthesia that made cyclopropane such a popular agent when surgery was required in patients with a generally poor clinical condition.

Cyclopropane shock is a condition where circulatory collapse occurs soon after the return of a patient from the operating theatre to the ward (Dripps 1947). It is accompanied by a slow pulse. The exact mechanism is uncertain, however it is most probably related to the high circulating levels of catecholamines resulting from the sympathetic stimulation caused by cyclopropane and enhanced by hypercarbia. This leads to vasoconstriction during surgery and an increase in systemic blood pressure, and tends to mask the effects of blood loss. When anaesthesia ceases, an undertransfused patient is suddenly deprived of the support of a stimulated sympathetic nervous system and the hypovolaemia becomes apparent. This condition should not occur if the patient is adequately ventilated during the operation and careful replacement of blood loss is carried out.

Halothane

Halothane is a potent depressant of the cardiovascular system, and in excess dosage may produce peripheral vascular collapse and cardiac arrest. This cardiovascular depression is the result of a number of factors. Halothane produces direct depression of the myocardium and vascular smooth muscle, a reduction in sympathetic nervous system activity by depression of medullary centres (and possibly by reducing their afferent input) and blockade of the sympathetic ganglia. The net result is a progressive fall in systemic blood pressure as the depth of anaesthesia increases. This effect may be compounded by a bradycardia. Concentrations of 1–2 MAC halothane will depress the I–J wave of the ballistocardiogram (a measure of cardiac contractility) by 30–60% of awake values (Eger et al 1970). Recently more consideration has been given to the principle of reducing myocardial oxygen demand and maintaining coronary flow in patients with ischaemic heart disease. In these circumstances the negative inotropic effects of halothane may be of particular advantage, although the same does not apply to patients with congestive cardiac failure where positive inotropic support may be required.

Enflurane

Enflurane produces a dose-dependent depression of the cardiovascular system which is due to a combination of direct myocardial depression (Calverly et al 1978b) and a reduction in sympathetic activity (Gothert & Wendt 1977). Its effects are similar to those of halothane.

Isoflurane

Isoflurane produces a dose-dependent depressant effect on myocardial contractility. This is compensated to some extent by a greater decrease in systemic vascular resistance than seen with other anaesthetics, the net effect of this reduction in afterload being to maintain the stroke volume. In younger patients (less than 45 years) there is often an increase in heart rate of 5% which will tend to maintain cardiac output (Forrest et al 1982). Elderly patients do not show the same degree of rise in heart rate as younger patients, and a greater degree of dose-related hypotension might be anticipated (Table 20.1).

Isoflurane and the coronary steal syndrome

Coronary vasodilatation occurs with all volatile anaesthetics. The effect is most pronounced with isoflurane, which led to the suggestion by Reiz et al (1983) that redistribution of coronary blood

Table 20.1 Effects on the cardiovascular system of light to moderate levels of anaesthesia

Effect	Agent
Stimulation	Cyclopropane
Little Effect	Nitrous oxide Trichloroethylene Isoflurane
Equivocal	Ether
Depression	Chloroform Methoxyflurane Halothane Enflurane

flow during isoflurane anaesthesia may divert blood away from ischaemic areas of the myocardium. This luxury perfusion of non-ischaemic myocardium at the expense of those ischaemic areas dependant on collateral circulation has been termed the 'coronary steal syndrome'.

If this situation did, in fact, exist, then the use of isoflurane in patients with ischaemic heart disease would be questionable. There has been much investigation of this subject in recent years, and the complex interrelated factors such as the preoperative therapy (beta blockers and calcium channel blockers), preoperative myocardial function, type of anaesthetic technique used (MAC and nitrous oxide) and the relevance of animal models has made interpretation difficult. It would appear, however, that in many studies purporting to demonstrate coronary steal the inspired concentrations of isoflurane were higher than normally used in clinical practice and that coronary perfusion pressure (mean arterial pressure) was substantially reduced.

At present the consensus is that isoflurane may safely be used in patients with ischaemic heart disease as part of a balanced anaesthetic technique in concentrations below 1%, provided mean arterial pressure is not reduced.

Some benefit in the use of isoflurane to control hypertension during anaesthesia has been demonstrated by Brusset (Brusset et al 1986) in comparison with halothane, where isoflurane increased the cardiac index and ejection fraction.

Production of arrhythmias

The following inhalational anaesthetics predispose to dysrhythmias:

- halothane
- chloroform
- cyclopropane
- trichloroethylene

while the following do not:

- nitrous oxide
- ether
- methoxyflurane
- enflurane
- isoflurane.

Nitrous oxide

Nitrous oxide does not induce arrhythmias and is safe to use when catecholamines are being administered.

Ether

Ether produces an initial tachycardia due to sympathetic stimulation and the release of endogenous catecholamine coupled to vagal depression. Arrhythmias are rare and the use of adrenaline containing solutions is relatively safe.

Cyclopropane

With cyclopropane there is little change in the heart rate of unpremedicated patients. In patients who have received a narcotic premedication a bradycardia may be produced, and if atropine is subsequently given a very considerable increase in heart rate may be seen, with arrhythmias and the possibility of ventricular fibrillation.

Arrhythmias. Two types of arrhythmia may occur:

1. Bradycardia. A nodal rhythm may occur as a result of vagotonic stimulation. As with other nodal rhythms, unless accompanied by hypotension no action need be taken.
2. Ventricular ectopic beats. These may occur singly, as coupled beats, or as runs of ventricular tachycardia. They tend to be related to the level of $P\text{aCO}_2$ and may occur:
    - at concentrations of cyclopropane greater than 20% with normal $P\text{aCO}_2$
    - during infusion or infiltration of adrenaline or noradrenaline
    - after the injection of atropine
    - as a result of hypercarbia.

Plasma catecholamine levels during hypercarbia may only be a tenth as great as during adrenaline infusions, but a similar incidence of arrhythmias will be produced. As the concentration of cyclopropane rises, so the level of $P\text{aCO}_2$ at which arrhythmias occur is lowered.

Adrenaline. A subcutaneous injection of 1:60 000 adrenaline during cyclopropane anaesthesia with normal levels of $Pa\text{CO}_2$ has been shown to induce ventricular arrhythmias in 30% of patients. Adrenaline injection should therefore be avoided during cyclopropane anaesthesia.

Trichloroethylene

Arrhythmias are common with trichloroethylene. Sinus tachycardia and nodal rhythm occur during light anaesthesia and ventricular extrasystoles during deep anaesthesia. Since trichloroethylene is now nearly always used to supplement a nitrous oxide-oxygen-relaxant technique in low concentrations, few problems are likely to be encountered.

Adrenaline increases the incidence of ventricular extrasystoles and may lead to ventricular fibrillation.

Halothane

Halothane may produce a nodal bradycardia which, when accompanied by hypotension, should be treated with intravenous atropine. It may also produce bigeminy and ventricular extrasystoles.

Adrenaline. Halothane sensitizes the myocardium to the effects of catecholamines. At 1.25 MAC, submucosal infiltration with 2.1 μg/kg of adrenaline will produce ventricular extrasystoles in 50% of patients (Johnston et al 1976); (see Table 20.2). If adrenaline is given in lignocaine instead of saline, the infusion threshold is raised to 3.7 μg/kg. Translated into clinical practice this suggests that rates of infiltration of adrenaline should be:

1.0–1.5 μg/kg/10 min (10 ml of 1:100 000 adrenaline for 70 kg adult)

Table 20.2 Production of ventricular extrasystoles with submucosal adrenaline

Agent	ED50 at 1.25 MAC
Halothane	2.1 μg/kg
Isoflurane	6.7 μg/kg
Enflurane	10.9 μg/kg*

*Note the different dose-response curve of enflurane allows occasional extrasystoles to occur at concentrations of 4μg/kg and below.

and

less than 4 μg/kg total dose in any 1 h period (30 ml of 1:100 000 adrenaline; Katz et al 1962).

Enflurane

Arrhythmias are less common with enflurane than with halothane.

Adrenaline may be infiltrated at up to three times the dose permissible with halothane. This is therefore 4 μg/kg (30 ml of 1:100 000 adrenaline) per 10 min for a 70 kg adult. Note that one effect of the difference in dose–response curve between enflurane and halothane is that occasional extrasystoles may be seen in some patients at less than 4 μg/kg of adrenaline infiltration (Johnston et al 1976).

Isoflurane

Isoflurane produces a rise in heart rate which may not be seen in elderly patients. Arrhythmias with isoflurane are uncommon, but where they occur they tend to be associated with intraoperative rises in blood pressure (Levy 1982).

Adrenaline. Isoflurane does not sensitize the heart to the effects of catecholamines. There is a three- to five-fold increase in the dose of adrenaline required to produce arrhythmias as compared to halothane. The amount of adrenaline needed to produce arrhythmias in dogs anaesthetized with isoflurane did not differ significantly from that required in awake animals. Thiopentone can precipitate adrenaline-induced arrhythmias. Plasma levels of adrenaline required to produce four or more premature ventricular contractions in 15 s with isoflurane were four times higher than the level required to produce the same effect with enflurane (Atlee & Roberts 1986).

When used in conjunction with aminophylline, isoflurane has less potential for arrhythmia production than halothane and may be more suitable in situations where bronchospasm has occurred (Stirt et al 1983).

Effects of beta blockade

Many patients present for surgery while being treated with beta-receptor antagonists for antihypertensive therapy, the control of symptoms of ischaemic heart disease or as part of the treatment of hyperthyroidism. There has been considerable discussion about the advisability of discontinuing beta-blocker therapy prior to anaesthesia, on the grounds that synergism between the negative inotropic effects of anaesthetic agent and beta blocker would lead to undue depression of the cardiovascular system to the detriment of the patient. However, studies have shown that there is little or no interaction of beta blocker and volatile agent at the sinoatrial node. Clinical practice has not shown this to be a problem provided the anaesthetist is aware that alterations in heart rate in response to blood loss will be attenuated, and should inotropic support be required an increased dosage will be necessary.

There are positive advantages for the hypertensive patient being treated with beta blockers to continue therapy up to the time of surgery, as less lability of blood pressure is seen than in hypertensive patients whose therapy has been stopped. Sudden withdrawal of propranolol in patients with coronary artery insufficiency has been associated with a rebound phenomenon leading to crescendo angina and sudden death.

Effects of calcium channel blockers

Calcium channel blockers (verapamil, diltiazem and nifedipine) have been introduced over the past decade for the treatment of angina and hypertension, and more recently (nimodipine) the treatment of subarachnoid haemorrhage. These drugs bind with high affinity to receptor sites on one of the postulated types of calcium channel, the long-lasting large current receptor-operated L-channel, and inhibit the entry of Ca^{2+} ions into the cell or mobilization from intracellular stores.

The effect of individual calcium channel blockers on AV node conduction or SA rate appears to depend, in part, on whether the agent delays recovery of activation of the slow (Ca^{2+}) channel.

Calcium channel blockers influence myocardial contractility, systemic and coronary vascular resistance and AV node conductance in varying degrees, and have a spectrum of actions similar to the volatile anaesthetics halothane, enflurane and isoflurane, which are themselves blockers of the calcium channel.

As was the case in the early days of beta blockade, so the introduction of calcium channel blockers into clinical practice was accompanied by reports of deleterious interactions with volatile anaesthetics. These events (of which I have uncomfortable personal experience) consisted of sustained bradycardia (<30 beats/min) accompanied by hypotension, amenable only to discontinuation of the anaesthetic.

To consider the types of interaction that may occur it is helpful to classify the calcium channel blockers according to their effect on contractility, conduction and systemic vascular resistance, and to compare these to similar effects produced by volatile anaesthetics (Fig. 20.1).

Verapamil

Verapamil significantly reduces contractility and conductance, and produces considerably more depression in ventricular function in patients whose existing ventricular function is already compromised by disease (Chew et al 1981). The use of halothane, with a similar profile, in such patients would have additive detrimental effects, and the risk of producing first- or second-degree block. A recent study (Marijic et al 1988) suggests that while the effects of isoflurane and halothane on the AV conduction time and atrial rate in the presence of verapamil are additive, the effect of verapamil and enflurane are synergistic.

Diltiazem

Diltiazem has less effect on contractility and AV conductance than verapamil, limited effect on systemic vascular resistance, and shares similar properties with enflurane.

Nifedipine

The dihydroperidine calcium channel blockers (nifedipine and nicardipine) are used primarily for the treatment of angina and hypertension.

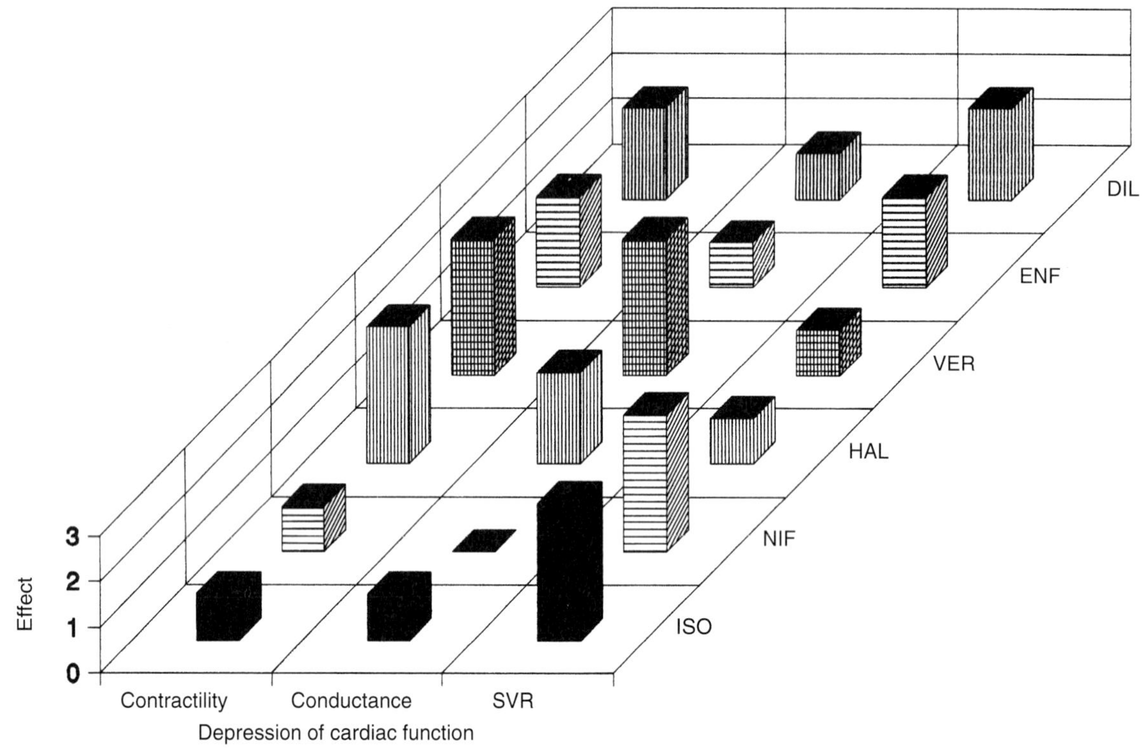

Fig. 20.1 Comparative effect of volatile agents and calcium blockers. Representation of cardiovascular effects (using arbitrary scale) of diltiazem (DIL), enflurane (ENF), halothane (HAL), Isoflurane (ISO) nifedipine (NIF) and verapamil (VER). SVR: systemic vascular resistance.

They cause a reduction in systemic and coronary vascular resistance with little effect on contractility and conductance. Their effects are thus very similar to those of isoflurane.

Evidence of interaction between volatile anaesthetics and calcium channel blockers requires careful interpretation in view of the different experimental models used. In closed-chest animals, using both acute and chronic models, only at high doses of anaesthetics (>1.5 MAC) and/or high plasma levels of calcium channel blockers were clinically significant haemodynamic interactions observed. The most serious finding was atrioventricular (AV) conduction deficit and sinus arrest resulting in sustained bradycardia. However, in open-chest models marked depression of ventricular function following calcium channel blocker administration and volatile agents has been reported, although these effects are considerably less marked with nifedipine and nicardipine.

In routine clinical practice the use of calcium channel blockers at therapeutic plasma levels and volatile anaesthetics at clinical concentrations produces little untoward effect, and in view of the rationale of calcium channel blockade their use during anaesthesia is probably beneficial to the patients (Merin 1987).

Amiodorone

Amiodorone prolongs action potential duration and refractory period in all cardiac tissues, and is used to treat both ventricular and supraventricular arrhythmias. It also causes peripheral vasodilatation, myocardial depression, atropine-resistant bradycardia and sinus arrest. Amiodorone alters digoxin pharmacology and may be responsible for sinus arrest and asystole in patients receiving digoxin. Caution should be exercised when anaesthetizing patients that are being treated with amiodorone.

THE CENTRAL NERVOUS SYSTEM

All the inhalational anaesthetic agents share the common property of causing cerebral vasodilatation with an increase in cerebral blood flow (CBF), and producing a decrease in the cerebral metabolic rate (CMR) as shown by a rise in cerebral venous oxygen saturation. It is unclear whether the increase in $CBF/CMRO_2$ ratio that inhalational anaesthetics produce exerts any protective effect on the brain during anaesthesia, however there appears to be an approximately linear relationship between increase in this ratio and depth of anaesthesia. Those agents, such as halothane, that produce a large increase in CBF (20–25% increase in CBF at 1 MAC) produce a proportionally smaller reduction in $CMRO_2$ than, for example, enflurane which produces a 25–30% reduction in $CMRO_2$ at 1 MAC (Smith & Wollman 1972).

The increase in cerebral blood flow produced by this cerebral vasodilatation will lead to an increase in the intracranial pressure (ICP). This may be considerable in the case of patients with cerebral oedema or space-occupying lesions. The effect that the use of an inhalational agent will have on the cerebral circulation will depend on a number of factors including: the presence or absence of a space-occupying lesion, the integrity of cerebral autoregulation, the baseline level of ICP, the arterial $P\text{CO}_2$ and the systemic blood pressure.

Intracranial pressure

The pressure–volume curve relating the ICP to the size of a space-occupying lesion shows that initially there is an ability to compensate for the increased volume of the lesion without a rise in pressure. This is achieved by a translocation of cerebral spinal fluid and a reduction in cerebral blood volume. However when this compensating ability is exhausted, further increase in the size of the lesion is accompanied by a rapid rise in ICP. On this non-compliant part of the pressure–volume curve an increase in cerebral blood volume, as may be caused by inhalational agents, will also cause rapid rise in ICP. Thus the effect that an inhalational agent will have on the ICP depends upon the preoperative level of ICP (which may be monitored by an intracranial pressure transducer) and whether specific measures to reduce the ICP, such as hyperventilation or the use of osmotic diuretics, have been taken. In patients with reduced compliance it may be wise to withhold volatile agents until the dura has been opened. The rise in ICP caused by nitrous oxide is in general small, and its use is rarely contraindicated.

Cerebral blood flow

Cerebral autoregulation will maintain the CBF in normotensive individuals between mean systemic blood pressures of 60 and 120 mmHg. Cerebral autoregulation is impaired by cerebral damage and following surgery and anaesthesia. It can be demonstrated that autoregulation is abolished at concentrations of 1 MAC of enflurane and halothane, although the response of the cerebral vessels to changes in $P\text{aCO}_2$ is maintained (Miletich et al 1976). Cerebral perfusion during and immediately after surgery will therefore be directly related to systemic blood pressure. Local regional perfusion may also be impaired. It has been suggested that cerebral steal, the diversion of blood by the vasodilatation of vessels in normal areas of brain at the expense of damaged areas whose vessels are already maximally dilated, may be produced by inhalational agents, but the evidence for this taking place is inconclusive.

Despite the problems associated with their use, inhalational anaesthetic agents are widely and successfully employed in neuroanaesthetic practice.

Nitrous oxide

The replacement of nitrogen by nitrous oxide in gas-filled cavities and the subsequent expansion in size of these cavities as a result of the differing rates of diffusion of the two gases has implications in three areas of neuroanaesthesia:

1. The air encephalogram, the radiological identification of the ventricles by subarachnoid injection of air, has largely been replaced as a diagnostic tool by

computerized tomography. However, if it is performed on a patient with suspected raised ICP, nitrous oxide should not be used.

2. Air embolism, arising from opened veins in which there is a negative pressure, is a hazard of both neurosurgical operations and surgical operations in the area of the neck. To limit the size of the embolism, nitrous oxide should be discontinued whenever air embolism is diagnosed or suspected.
3. There will be some air remaining in the cranial cavity for 2–3 weeks following craniotomy, and it has been suggested that in the event of reoperation during that time nitrous oxide should be avoided during induction.

Hearing loss after general anaesthesia

A small number of cases of hearing loss following general anaesthesia in non-otological surgery have been reported (Hochermann & Reimer 1987). If those following cardiac surgery are excluded (where the mechanism is assumed to be microembolic in nature), then the remainder have all had, or been assumed to have had, an anaesthetic using nitrous oxide. Changes in middle ear pressure during nitrous oxide anaesthesia have been recorded, with an increase in pressure (of up to 450 mmH_2O) during surgery. During recovery, subatmospheric pressures may be produced. Pressure changes in the middle ear are normally equalized by swallowing, utilizing the Eustachian tube. Patients with Eustachian tube dysfunction may be vulnerable to middle ear pressure changes during anaesthesia, particularly during manual ventilation. In a number of cases, rupture of the round window has been shown to be the cause of the hearing loss.

Electrical activity

Although the appearance of seizures may be demonstrated on the EEG at concentrations of ether (4 MAC) and cyclopropane above those in clinical use, enflurane alone has the property of inducing epileptic-like seizure activity in the EEG of patients receiving normal anaesthetic concentrations. This effect is influenced by both concentration of enflurane and the $Pa\text{CO}_2$. At normal $Pa\text{CO}_2$ spiking is maximal at inspired concentrations of 2–3% and is reduced with increase in CO_2. The minimum epileptogenic enflurane concentration is reduced by 1% when the $Pa\text{CO}_2$ is less than 2.6 kPa, and raised by 1% when the $Pa\text{CO}_2$ is more than 8.0 kPa.

The electrical activity may be accompanied by abnormal twitching of individual muscle groups or occasionally tonic-clonic activity. A history of convulsive disorders does not appear to increase this convulsive activity, and there is no evidence that permanent CNS dysfunction is produced. If twitching occurs during anaesthesia, isoflurane or halothane should be substituted for enflurane.

Convulsions during anaesthesia

Convulsions occurring during the course of anaesthesia have been reported most frequently with ether, but may occur with any inhalational agent. They occur characteristically in feverish children or young adults in hot and humid operating conditions, particularly after atropine premedication. As with all types of convulsion the aim of treatment is to prevent hypoxia and terminate the convulsive episode. The inhalational agent should be withdrawn and the patient treated with intravenous diazepam or thiopentone. In refractory cases suxamethonium should be given. Cooling should be instituted and adequate oxygenation ensured.

Evoked potentials

Brainstem

A neurophysiological indicator to measure depth of anaesthesia would be of considerable benefit to anaesthetists and their patients. The measurement of evoked potentials for such an indicator has been suggested. Somatosensory evoked potentials (auditory and visual) recorded in the brainstem are depressed in a dose-dependent fashion by halothane, enflurane and isoflurane, while nitrous oxide has no effect when used alone (Sebel et al 1986).

Extradural

Assessment of spinal cord function during operations such as scoliosis correction has traditionally been achieved by 'wake up' tests. These have significant disadvantages and alternative methods have been sought, for example recording motor evoked potentials from the extradural space. In contrast to brainstem evoked potentials it appears that anaesthetic agents, at least halothane, do not have any significant effect on the amplitude or latency of the motor evoked potential (Loughnan & Hall 1989).

RENAL EFFECTS

Inhalational anaesthetic agents produce a mild depression of renal function during anaesthesia as shown by reduced glomerular filtration rate, renal plasma flow and urine output. These effects are, in general, secondary to the haemodynamic changes of diminished cardiac output and blood pressure produced by general anaesthesia.

Renal vascular tone may be altered by sympathetic activity, particularly with ether and cyclopropane, and halothane is known to stimulate the release of antidiuretic hormone. Autoregulation of the renal circulation may be impaired during anaesthesia. These effects are short lived and a return to normal function will usually occur within 2–3 h after anaesthesia ceases, although recovery may be delayed following prolonged operations.

The fact that inhalational agents are not excreted by the kidneys makes their use particularly appropriate for patients with diminished renal function, although care should be taken to avoid hypotension and ensure adequate oxygenation.

The biotransformation of halogenated hydrocarbons with the release of inorganic fluoride ions has been a matter of some concern (Mazze et al 1971). There is considerable evidence that inorganic fluoride causes damage to the distal tubule, resulting in the retention of uric acid and the production of renal failure associated with a diuresis and increased levels of serum osmolarity and urea.

This was brought to light by the discovery of cases of high output renal failure in patients following the use of methoxyflurane. A number of fatalities ensued and post mortem examination revealed the presence of oxalate crystals in the renal tubules. Damage to the renal tubule is associated with a serum fluoride level in excess of 50 μmol/l (Cousins & Mazze 1973). All the halogenated hydrocarbons will release inorganic fluoride, but to a lesser extent than methoxyflurane. After 2.7 MAC h of enflurane anaesthesia in human volunteers, peak serum fluoride levels of 20 μmol/l were found. For halothane and isoflurane 4 MAC h produced levels of less than 5 μmol/l (Mazze et al 1974). Although the incidence of renal toxicity with methoxyflurane was low (0.03% in 17 000 administrations), its occurrence largely contributed to the disuse of this agent.

Obesity, enzyme induction and prolonged anaesthesia enhance biotransformation. Although halothane and isoflurane do not produce high free-fluoride levels even under these circumstances, enflurane may provoke renal toxicity if given to very obese patients for prolonged periods.

Isoniazid specifically induces biotransformation of enflurane to fluoride ion (Mazze et al 1982), hence should be avoided in patients receiving antituberculous therapy with isoniazid.

The use of oral fluoride therapy (1 mg/day) in dental patients receiving enflurane anaesthesia has been studied (Oikkonen et al 1987). Maximum levels of serum fluoride of 10 μmol/l were produced following enflurane administration, well below the threshold for renal toxicity. However, the authors caution that if patients are using topically applied fluoride gel much higher free-fluoride levels will be produced and enflurane should be avoided.

EFFECTS IN PREGNANCY

A number of inhalational agents have used in the past to provide analgesia during labour. Trichloroethylene and methoxyflurane, when administered from specially designed draw-over vaporizers delivering fixed percentages of agent in air (Emotril and Tecota MK 6 deliver 0.35% and 0.5% trichloroethylene in air; the Cardiff Penthrane Inhaler delivers 0.35% methoxyflurane in air) were approved for use by the Central Midwives Board (CMB). Apart from drowsiness occurring in the patient after prolonged use, they were used successfully in obstetric practice for many years. The use of volatile agents in this field has now been largely supplanted by the inhalation of premixed nitrous oxide in oxygen (Entonox) and by epidural analgesia.

With the exception of nitrous oxide, all the inhalational agents produce a dose-related reduction in uterine contractility. In the case of trichloroethylene and cyclopropane, concentrations in excess of normal requirements are necessary before this effect is clinically noticeable. Halothane, enflurane and isoflurane all depress uterine contractility, frequency of contraction and maximum tension developed in the myometrium. At 0.5 MAC the effect is minimal, contraction being diminished by about 20%, but as the concentration rises to 1.5 MAC the reduction in contraction is greater than 70% (Munson & Embro 1977). Uterine tone may be restored and excessive blood loss prevented by the administration of oxytocics, although, as the uterine response to these is diminished by inhalational anaesthetics, repeated doses or an infusion of oxytocin may be required. In vitro experiments with isoflurane demonstrate adequate reversal of the inhibitory effects on uterine contractility by oxytocics with concentrations up to 1.5%. This suggests that isoflurane would be a useful agent for manual removal of the placenta and other agents when transient uterine relaxation coupled with rapid recovery of contractility are desirable (Abadir et al 1987).

During pregnancy there is an increase in the minute volume of ventilation and a decrease in FRC. This results in an increase in the rate of rise of alveolar concentrations of inhalational anaesthetics. There is also a decrease in MAC requirements during pregnancy. It has been shown in sheep that pregnancy decreases the MAC for isoflurane by 40%, for halaothane by 25% and for methoxyflurane by 32% (Palahniuk et al 1974). Administration of normal concentrations of inhalational anaesthetics will result in deeper levels of anaesthesia being achieved more rapidly in the pregnant patient.

Inhalational agents readily cross the placental barrier and uterine blood levels will reflect levels in maternal blood. The level of anaesthetic concentration in foetal blood is determined by two factors: the rate of rise in alveolar concentration in the mother and induction–delivery time. By the same token the more soluble agents will be eliminated more rapidly by the neonate after delivery. In common with adults, neonates show respiratory depression following exposure to an anaesthetic agent, although they are more tolerant to halogenated hydrocarbons. It is unlikely that the concentrations of volatile anaesthetics used during delivery will have significant deleterious effects on the neonate. The advantage of using 50% oxygen with a rapidly acting agent like halothane, enflurane or isoflurane can be demonstrated in the improved clinical condition of the neonate (Moir 1970) while providing a measure of protection against maternal awareness. Isoflurane (0.75%), halothane (0.5%) and enflurane (1%), each with 50% nitrous oxide, have been shown to produce no difference in Apgar scores or neurobehavioural scale scores in the neonate when compared to anaesthetic techniques employing just nitrous oxide in oxygen. There were, however, instances of awareness in the group not receiving volatile supplements (Warren et al 1983). Recent reports of maternal awareness during caesarean section emphasize the need to provide adequate anaesthesia for the mother.

THE IMMUNOLOGICAL DEFENCE SYSTEM

As early as 1896 it was recognized that anaesthetic agents could affect the immunological responses of patients when it was shown that anaesthesia with diethyl ether produced a leucocytosis appearing within a few hours of induction and lasting for several days.

The immunological defence system of the body may be considered as consisting of two parts. The non-specific or resistance mechanisms exist to create a climate inimical to bacteria and viruses. Included among these mechanisms are the cilia of the respiratory tract, bactericidal secretions contained in tears and saliva, mucous secretions, and the effect of lactic acid and fatty acids in sweat. The second part of the immune system consists of the cellular response of lymphocytes and macrophages responsible for the identification and destruction of invading organisms.

Anaesthetics may act directly on the immune systems of the body, or their effects may be mediated by the hormones that they cause to be released during the course of anaesthesia. In considering these effects it is always difficult to separate what is caused by anaesthetics themselves, from the hormonal effects produced as a result of the 'stress' of surgery and anaesthesia. This is particularly so as the hormone release produced by the stress response is much greater than that caused by anaesthetic agents. It is difficult to evaluate experimental work performed on human subjects as anaesthesia unaccompanied by surgery is rarely conducted. Animal experiments where anaesthesia is performed alone are not always helpful as there is considerable interspecies variability and direct extrapolation of animal results to man is not always feasible.

Hormone release during anaesthesia

When catecholamines are released (by either anaesthesia or stress) there are increases in both the neutrophil and leucocyte counts, and alteration in their distribution and mobilization. Steroids reduce the synthesis of both DNA and RNA, and depress the mitotic phase of cell division. ACTH depresses phagocytosis and is accompanied by a neutrophilia. Ether increases ACTH release, raises plasma corticosteroid levels and increases plasma catecholamines. These factors explain the leucocytosis originally noted to accompany the use of ether. Cyclopropane has a similar stimulatory effect on the sympathetic nervous system. Enflurane anaesthesia may depress plasma catecholamines and in the absence of surgery decreases plasma corticosteroids, however it will not prevent a marked increase in corticosteroid levels when surgery commences. Similar effects are seen with isoflurane (Oyama et al 1975), however halothane does depress the stress response although altering catecholamine and corticosteroid levels little.

Effects on the non-specific mechanisms

During anaesthesia the upward sweeping motion of the cilia in the respiratory tract is disorganized, thus impairing the removal of particles of foreign material from the lungs (Forbes 1976). This is the result of depression of microtubule activity in the cilia and it can be demonstrated that several anaesthetics, including halothane, cyclopropane, chloroform and ether, are capable of producing reversible depression of microtubular activity. This effect is made worse by the action of atropine and increased inspired concentrations of oxygen. Reduction of microtubule activity is also thought to explain the reduction in phagocyte and lymphocyte migration out of the blood vessels towards areas of foreign material. Leucocytes are attracted to areas of infection by the process of chemotaxis, but this does not appear to be diminished by anaesthesia. Reduced phagocytic activity by fixed macrophages within the reticulo-endothelial system has been demonstrated in man (Lofstrom & Schildt 1974), but these effects appear to be minimal. The total effects seen with anaesthesia are small in comparison to those caused by the stress response.

Cell division and leucopaenia

Lassen et al (1956) reported that patients being treated for tetanus had developed signs of acute bone marrow aplasia and megaloblastic red blood cell production after 5–7 days treatment. The treatment included curarization and ventilation with a 50% nitrous oxide in oxygen mixture. Although in the majority of cases this effect on the bone marrow was reversible, there were two fatalities. Lassen et al were able to demonstrate that the leucopaenia was due to the prolonged administration of nitrous oxide.

Further reports have demonstrated a condition resembling subacute combined degeneration of the cord in subjects chronically exposed to high concentrations of nitrous oxide (Layzer 1978).

Animal experiments have demonstrated inactivation of vitamin B_{12} by nitrous oxide. This results in inactivation of the enzyme methionine synthase, subsequent disruption of methionine metabolism and depletion of its two products, methionine and tetrahydrofolate. This leads to a failure of myelination, the production of subacute combined degeneration of the cord and a depression of DNA synthesis, leading to megaloblastic changes and agranulocytosis.

Megaloblastic changes in bone marrow are consistently found in patients that have been exposed to more than 24 h of nitrous oxide, and an abnormal deoxyuridine suppression test can be demonstrated (Skacel et al 1983). It is clear that exposure to nitrous oxide for periods longer than 24 h is now unacceptable. It is, however, considerably less clear whether the changes in hepatic methionine synthetase activity, which can be demonstrated after exposure to nitrous oxide of periods as short as 2 h, are of any consequence. This subject is comprehensively reviewed by Nunn (1987). He concludes that those who feel nitrous oxide is an agent that has usefully served its historical purpose and should be retired gracefully will accept this as evidence for their cause, while others will point to the absence of demonstrable deleterious effect in normal clinical practice of a gas used successfully by generations of anaesthetists.

Leucopaenia (in animals) has also been reported following long-term exposure to halothane (Bruce & Koepke 1966), nitrous oxide, hydrocarbons and inert gases. Short-term leucopaenia has been seen in some species during anaesthesia with ether, chloroform and halothane. The effect in animals varies from species to species. Halothane has been seen to arrest cell division at the metaphase (c-mitosis) DNA-synthetic and post-synthetic phases. Leucopaenia seen after prolonged exposure to anaesthetic agents may result from adverse effects at many different stages of the cell cycle as part of the overall depression of cellular metabolism. The effect of prolonged anaesthesia may be of importance in patients with pre-existing bone marrow depression.

Lymphocytes

The activity of both thymus-dependent T-lymphocytes responsible for cell mediated immunity and bursa-dependent B-lymphocytes responsible for the synthesis of circulating antibody is depressed after surgery and anaesthesia. A reduction in the number of splenic antibody-producing cells and antibody production may result following prolonged exposure to a variety of different anaesthetics. Transient decreases in the level of IgG have been reported following anaesthesia but, in general, levels of preformed antibodies are not altered. The T-cell population decreases during anaesthesia and surgery. The responsiveness of lymphocytes is decreased following induction of anaesthesia, but recent evidence suggests that preoperative stress in the absence of adequate premedication may itself produce depression of lymphocyte activity and tend to overemphasize the effects of anaesthetic agents (Walton 1979).

Anaesthesia and infection

Although postoperative infections produce a high morbidity in hospital patients and increase the length of hospital stay by over 1 million days/year (3% of total acute hospital bed occupancy), there is little evidence to allow us to compare the effects of different anaesthetic techniques with postoperative rates of infection. Studies early in the twentieth century produced conflicting results with anaesthesia appearing to enhance an infection in some species while offering protection against specific bacteria in others. More recently, halothane has been shown to reduce the survival time in mice with salmonella peritonitis (Bruce & Koepke 1966), while cyclopropane and methoxyflurane reduce pulmonary bactericidal activity in the same species. Although bacterial growth is inhibited by inhalational agents, as might be expected from the effects of anaesthesia on dividing cells, the overwhelming effect of steroid release would tend to favour the bacteria rather than the host.

Anaesthesia and malignancy

A close relationship exists between a fully functioning immunological system and resistance to malignant disease. Malignancy itself will tend to depress the immune function in the host. It is as yet unclear to what extent anaesthesia will alter this balance as animal experiments have yielded conflicting results. However, the recurrence of tumour metastases following minor surgery in patients that had had a primary tumour successfully treated a number of years previously has been documented. Once again the effects of surgical stress as a whole are likely to be greater than any particular component of anaesthetic technique. The contribution of inhalational anaesthetic agents to the depression of immunological defences is probably slight when compared to the effects of the stress response to surgery.

Although these effects are in general of little detriment to the majority of patients, there are individuals with abnormal immune systems, or who are suffering from a malignancy, in whom anaesthesia and surgery may have an adverse effect, especially if anaesthesia is prolonged. In these patients stress-free anaesthesia, based on high-dose opiate regimens or techniques of regional analgesia, may be more appropriate.

DIFFUSION EFFECTS OF NITROUS OXIDE

Nitrous oxide is 36 times more soluble in blood than is nitrogen, the relevant blood–gas partition coefficients being 0.470 and 0.013. This means that dissolved nitrous oxide will diffuse from blood into a gas-filled space more rapidly than nitrogen can diffuse out. This leads to an increase in volume if the space is able to expand or to an increase in pressure in a confined cavity. This has important implications during anaesthesia.

Expanding lesions

Pneumothorax, pneumoperitoneum and pneumopericardium will expand rapidly in the presence of nitrous oxide with subsequent adverse effects. Air embolism occurring during cardiac surgery or neurosurgical operations will expand and may form a serious obstruction to the circulation. The extent of the expansion is related to the inspired concentration of nitrous oxide (Munson 1974; Table 20.3). Air contained in the gut will also expand.

Pressure increases

Those gas-filled cavities where expansion cannot occur will respond to nitrous oxide administration with a rise in pressure within the cavity. In a brain with reduced compliance, nitrous oxide should be avoided during air encephalography and for anaesthesia occurring up to 3 weeks following a craniotomy. Nitrous oxide will raise the pressure in the middle ear and may make placing the graft during an overlay myringoplasty difficult. It has also been implicated in postoperative hearing losses and eardrum rupture (Owen et al 1978).

Diffusion hypoxia

The rapid diffusion of nitrous oxide from the bloodstream into the alveoli at the end of anaesthesia may reduce the alveolar oxygen tension and lead to the diffusion hypoxia described by Fink (1955). The extent of this effect is dependent on the length of nitrous oxide administration, and is of particular importance in the elderly and

Table 20.3 Volume expansion following nitrous oxide

% inspired nitrous oxide	% increase in volume of air space
33	150
50	200
75	400
80	500

in those patients with reduced respiratory reserves or diminished cardiac output. The problem may be avoided by the provision of increased concentrations of inspired oxygen postoperatively during the phase of nitrous oxide excretion.

ENTONOX

Self-administration of nitrous oxide for analgesia by women in labour under the supervision of midwives has been available since 1936. The original gas and air apparatus was first described in 1933 by Minnitt (1949), and in various commercial forms was available until withdrawal of approval by the CMB in 1970. Minnitt's apparatus delivered a 50% mixture of nitrous oxide in air, which supplied a 10.4% concentration of oxygen to the mother. Although the apparatus was used successfully for over a generation, concern was raised in the early 1960s that the hypoxic mixture might have an adverse effect on the fetus. Cole & Nainby-Luxmoore (1962) demonstrated reductions in maternal arterial oxygen saturation to 92% in the first stage of labour, falling to 88% during the latter part of the second stage. In addition, Nainby-Luxmoore (1964) showed that there was considerable variation in the composition of the mixture at different gas flows, and at minute volumes below 6 l/min some machines were delivering less than 5% of oxygen.

The advent of premixed cylinders of nitrous oxide and oxygen, produced by the British Oxygen Company after the suggestion of Tunstall (1961), made the provision of hypoxic mixtures of gas and air obsolete. A cylinder containing a 50% nitrous oxide in oxygen mixture, fitted with the Entonox patient demand valve, has been approved by the CMB for use in obstetric analgesia. Such a mixture has the considerable advantage of supplying the mother with an increased inspired oxygen concentration to the advantage of the fetus. The physical properties behind the manufacture of this premixed gas led to its one important hazard. Entonox is manufactured by bubbling oxygen through liquid nitrous oxide. The liquid nitrous oxide and the gaseous oxygen dissolve in one another to form a homogeneous gas mixture. The stability of this mixture is dependent on temperature, and a 50% nitrous oxide in oxygen mixture will show separation of liquid nitrous oxide at a temperature of –7°C (a 60% nitrous oxide mixture will separate at 1°C). If the cylinder is used in the vertical position after separation has occurred, the first gas to be issued will contain an increased concentration of oxygen and will supply inadequate analgesia, while that gas issued as the cylinder becomes exhausted will contain a hypoxic mixture.

Recent winters in this country have shown that night time temperatures as low as –7°C are not that uncommon, and Entonox cylinders stored outdoors or in the boot of a midwife's car are vulnerable. The separated mixture may easily be restored to its gaseous form by rewarming, either by placing the cylinder horizontally in an ambient temperature of at least 10°C for a period of 2 h, or by placing it in a bath of water at 52°C for 5 min, and inverting the cylinder three times to ensure adequate mixing (Cole 1964). Some protection is offered by the fact that the Entonox patient demand valve ensures that no flow occurs once the pressure in the cylinder has fallen to below 13 kPa × 100. This means that the final 10% of the contents are wasted, but if cooling and separation has occured that would be the fraction with the lowest oxygen content.

TRICHLOROETHYLENE AND SODA-LIME

In the presence of heat and alkali, trichloroethylene will decompose to form dichloroacetylene and hydrochloric acid. Dichloroacetylene is toxic and inflammable and may itself decompose further into phosgene and carbon monoxide. Dichloroacetylene will produce cranial nerve palsy, and cases of neurological damage and death have been reported following the use of trichloroethylene in a closed circuit.

Characteristically it is the trigeminal nerve that is involved, but lesions of all cranial nerves except the olfactory, glossopharyngeal and accessory have been reported. The onset usually begins with numbness or coldness around the lips starting 24–48 h following anaesthesia, and areas of sensory loss may then spread. Recovery in milder cases begins 5–10 days later and may be complete after 2 weeks.

The rate of decomposition of trichloroethylene is slow below 10°C, is significant at 40°C and rapidly increases as the temperature rises above 60°C. Lumley & Morgan (1976) investigated the temperature reached inside modern carbon dioxide absorbers and confirmed that under 'normal' operating conditions the temperature inside a circle absorber reached 40°C, and inside a 'to and fro' cannister some 5°C higher. These temperatures are dependent on the rate of carbon dioxide production by the patient, the environmental temperature and, particularly with a Waters' cannister, accidental insulation of the absorber. It is possible to raise the temperature inside a Waters' cannister to 104°C if sufficient carbon dioxide is added.

There is no safety interlock on modern anaesthetic machines to prevent the accidental inclusion of a trichloroethylene vaporizer in a closed circuit. Particular care must be taken to avoid using trichloroethylene in the presence of soda-lime, especially since its decreased use has reduced the awareness of anaesthetic staff to this hazard. Closed-circuit anaesthesia is almost certain once again to become a significant technique in anaesthesia in the UK as the high cost of inhalational agents encourages the use of low-flow techniques in budget-conscious times. The availability of inspired gas and vapour concentration monitors has made this technique much safer, and although trichloroethylene tends to be used by enthusiasts, this almost historical interaction is worth emphasizing.

EFFECTS ON THE LIVER

Since the introduction of chloroform, occasional cases of jaundice or liver failure have been described following anaesthesia. Although most inhalational agents transiently depress liver function it has been the potential hepatotoxic effects of anaesthetics that has caused most concern. The 'halothane hepatitis' controversy, with its attendant medico–legal implications, has focused attention on the previously unexpected extent to which volatile anaesthetics undergo metabolism in the liver. Some of these metabolites, particularly those formed by reductive biotransformation, have the potential for causing tissue damage. Recent investigations have suggested that the influence of perioperative hypoxaemia and poor nutritional state of the patient may be as important as the production of specific metabolites in the aetiology of liver damage following anaesthesia.

Chloroform

As early as 1850 an association between liver damage and chloroform anaesthesia was noted. A central hepatic necrosis was produced, the effects becoming apparent some 2–3 days following anaesthesia. The incidence of this complication was greater in malnourished patients, and where hypercarbia or hypoxia were noted to have occurred. A preoperative diet rich in carbohydrates, and the use of oxygen rather than air as the carrier gas, reduced the incidence of this effect. Repeated short administrations were thought to sensitize the liver and damage was potentiated by enzyme-inducing agents. During metabolism of chloroform the free radicals $^{\bullet}CCl_2$ and $^{\bullet}CCl_3$ are formed. These are highly reactive and may be responsible for the hepatic damage.

Ether and trichloroethylene

Ether and trichloroethylene transiently decrease liver function and, although rare, hepatic toxicity has been reported following their administration.

Cyclopropane

Cyclopropane has a specific vasoconstrictor effect on the splanchnic vasculature and reduces hepatic blood flow. It should be avoided in patients with hepatic dysfunction.

Enflurane

Only about 2.5% of the absorbed dose of enflurane is biotransformed. Enzyme induction secondary to enflurane administration occurs, but there is little evidence that repeated exposure increases the metabolism of enflurane itself. Isolated cases of clinically evident hepatic dysfunction have been reported, but their incidence is very small.

Eight years after the introduction of enflurane to the USA, Lewis et al (1983) published a series of 24 cases of jaundice 'possibly' associated with enflurane, and concluded that enflurane caused damage in some, but not all, of these instances. It was suggested that patients seemingly injured by enflurane had signs and symptoms reminiscent of halothane-induced hepatitis (chills, fever, nausea, anorexia and eosinophilia) and history of previous exposure to halogenated anaesthetics. It was also suggested that cross-sensitivity between halothane and enflurane existed.

In 1986, Eger et al (1986) reviewed the 88 reports of hepatic injury available since the release of enflurane in the USA in 1972. During this time some 20 million enflurane anaesthetics had been administered. Fifteen cases remained 'possible' after evaluation of other causes of hepatic injury, but no consistent pathology was detected. Eger et al concluded that the data did not demonstrate a causal relationship between enflurane anaesthesia and subsequent liver damage, and that if severe injury is caused by enflurane it is an extremely rare event (1 in 800 000 administrations). This incidence is less than that of viral hepatitis. No contraindications to the use and subsequent use of enflurane exist at this time.

Isoflurane

Isoflurane is metabolized to the least extent of all the inhalational agents in clinical use, only some 0.2% of the absorbed dose being oxidatively biotransformed. Clinical experience has not demonstrated any hepatotoxic effect. The US Food and Drug Administration have analysed 45 reports of unexplained hepatic dysfunction following isoflurane (Stoelting et al 1987). They concluded that a causal relationship between isoflurane and postoperative hepatic dysfunction could not be demonstrated.

If liver oxygen deprivation is the most common reason for perioperative liver damage (Gelman 1986), then the fact that total hepatic blood flow is better maintained with isoflurane than halothane as a result of increase in hepatic artery flow (Gelman et al 1985), and that hepatic tissue blood flow was less reduced (Kosaka et al 1986), would suggest that isoflurane would be less likely to produce hepatic damage. This is confirmed by studies (Gelman & Dillard 1985) demonstrating better maintenance of the ratio of hepatic oxygen delivery to hepatic oxygen demand with isoflurane.

Halothane

There has been a controversy about the alleged hepatotoxic effects of halothane since the early 1960s, by which time there had been numerous reports suggesting there was a causal relationship between the administration of halothane and postoperative hepatitis. Following small-scale retrospective studies the US National Halothane Study was undertaken (1969). This massive epidemiological survey reviewed over 850 000 anaesthetics, but was unable to provide conclusive results. However, reports of hepatic damage following halothane administration continued, and it is generally accepted that, although small, there is an incidence of hepatic dysfunction associated with halothane which may be of the order of 1 per 10 000 administrations. These reports have been reviewed by Stock & Strunin (1985).

Multiple exposures to halothane, often with a relatively short interval between exposures, has been a feature of these reports. Although halothane undergoes considerable biodegradation (20% of the absorbed dose), a form of liver damage specific to halothane has not been found. The discovery of the reductive pathway of metabolism for halothane and the isolation of two reductive metabolites, difluorochloroethylene and trifluorochloroethylene, excited interest because this might prove to be the mechanism of hepatocellular damage. Although this pathway does fit animal models (Widger et al 1976), there is as yet no evidence that the presence of the metabolites is correlated with the clinical syndrome of halothane hepatitis (Mazze 1984). The possible mechanisms of toxicity have been reviewed by Brown & Gandolfi (1987).

The balance of evidence would suggest that, although uncommon, two types of liver damage secondary to halothane administration may be detected. The first is fulminating hepatic failure associated with a hypersensitivity reaction. This less common manifestation is thought to occur when oxidative biotransformation of halothane leads to conjugation of an intermediate, trifluoroacetylchloride, with liver macromolecules, which in turn form a hapten (Callis et al 1986). This produces an immune response in certain individuals. The antibodies can be detected in immunological assays, but there is still debate as to whether the presence of antibodies is the cause or result of tissue injury. This is a slow reaction developing over 6–14 days into progressive and often fatal hepatotoxicity.

The second type of liver damage is a lesser form of hepatocellular jaundice which may be associated with hypoxia. It involves the quantitative enhancement of the reductive biotransformation of halothane by a variety of factors producing a biochemical insult to the liver from reactive intermediates. The onset of liver damage is rapid (1–3 days), but the disease is mild and remits.

Some of the factors that have been suggested to be of importance in the aetiology of post-halothane hepatic dysfunction are:

1. repeated administrations of halothane, particularly less than 6 weeks apart (about 80% of reported cases have had more than one exposure)
2. previous unexplained pyrexia or unidentified liver damage following halothane
3. obesity
4. gender (women have twice the risk of men)
5. age (middle-aged 40–50 years old patients are more susceptible)
6. patients (particularly women) with a tendency to organ-specific autoimmune disease
7. hypoxaemia
8. poor nutritional state.

The occurrence of hepatic dysfunction in children following halothane anaesthesia is considerably less than in adults, although a number of cases have been reported (Walton 1986). The value of halothane in paediatric anaesthesia is such that its continued use has not been challenged by these reports.

In recent years the dilemma facing anaesthetists when confronted with a patient requiring anaesthesia following a previous halothane anaesthetic has been resolved by the availability of first enflurane and latterly isoflurane. It follows that prudence would dictate that, in the light of strong circumstantial evidence, repeat halothane anaesthetics should be avoided within at least a 6-week period and probably 3 months between administrations would provide the greatest margin of safety.

REFERENCES

Abadir A R, Humayun S G, Calvello D, Gintautas J 1987 Effects of isoflurane and oxytocin on gravid human uterus in vivo. Anesth Analg 66: S1

Atlee J L, Roberts F L 1986 Thiopental and epinephrine-induced dysrhythmias in dogs anaesthetised with enflurane or isoflurane. Anesth Analg 65: 437–443

Augustine S D, Benumof J L 1984 Halothane and isoflurane do not impair arterial oxygenation during one-lung ventilation in patients undergoing thoracotomy. Anesthesiology 61: A484

Bierman M I, Brown M, Muren O et al 1986 Prolonged isoflurane anaesthesia in status asthmaticus. Crit Care Med 14: 832–833

Brown B R, Gandolfi A J 1987 Adverse effects of volatile anaesthetics. Br J Anaesth 59: 14–23

Bruce D L, Koepke J A 1966 Changes in granulopoeisis in the rat associated with prolonged halothane anaesthesia. Anesthesiology 27: 811–816

Brusset A, Coriat P, Pazvanska E, Froucht S, Mouquet C, Viars P 1986 Isoflurane versus halothane in the control of intra-operative hypertension: effects on left ventricular function. Anesthesiology 65: A2

Callis A H, Brooks S D, Waters S J et al 1986 Evidence for a role of the immune system in the pathogenisis of halothane hepatitis. In Roth S H, Miller K W (eds) Molecular and cellular mechanisms of anaesthetics. Plenum, New York

Calverly R K, Smith N T, Jones C W, Prys-Roberts C, Eger E I 1978a Ventilatory and cardiovascular effects of enflurane anaesthesia during spontaneous ventilation in man. Anesth Analg 57: 610–618

Calverly R K, Smith N T, Prys-Roberts C, Eger E I, Jones C W 1978b Cardiovascular effects of enflurane during controlled ventilation in man. Anesth Analg 57: 619–628

Chew C Y C, Hecht H S, Collett J T, McAllister R G, Singh B H 1981 Influence of severity of ventricular dysfunction on haemodynamic responses to intravenously

administered verapamil in ischaemic heart disease. Am J Cardiol 47: 917–922
Cole P V 1964 Nitrous oxide and oxygen from a single cylinder. Anaesthesia 19: 3–11
Cole P V, Nainby-Luxmoore R C 1962 The hazards of gas and air in obstetrics. Anaesthesia 17: 505–518
Cousins M J, Mazze R I 1973 Methoxyflurane nephrotoxicity: a study of dose response in man. J Am Med Assoc 225: 1611–1616
Dripps R D 1947 The immediate decrease in blood pressure seen at the conclusion of cyclopropane anesthesia, 'Cyclopropane shock'. Anesthesiology 8: 15–35
Eger E I, Smith N T, Stoelting R K, Cullen D J, Kadis L B, Whitcher C E 1970 Cardiovascular effects of halothane in man. Anesthesiology 32: 396–409
Eger E I, Smuckler E A, Ferrell L D, Goldsmith C H, Johnson B H 1986 Is enflurane hepatotoxic? Anesth Analg 65: 21–30
Fink B R 1955 Diffusion anoxia. Anesthesiology 16: 511–519
Forbes A R 1976 Halothane depresses mucociliary flow in the trachea. Anesthesiology 45: 59–63
Forrest J B, Buffington C, Cahalan M K et al 1982 A multicentre clinical evaluation of isoflurane. Can Anaesth Soc J 29: S1–S32
Fourcade H E, Stevens W C, Larson C P et al 1971 The ventilatory effects of Forane, a new inhaled anaesthetic. Anesthesiology 35: 26–31
Gelman S 1986 Halothane hepatotoxicity: again? Anesth Analg 65: 831–834
Gelman S, Dillard E 1985 Hepatic oxygen supply-demand relationship during anaesthesia in the dog. Anesthesiology 63: A540
Gelman S, Fowler K C, Smith L R 1985 Liver circulation and function during isoflurane and halothane anaesthesia. Anesthesiology 61: 726–730
Gothert M, Wendt J 1977 Inhibition of adrenal medullary catecholamine secretion by enflurane. I. Investigations in vivo. Anesthesiology 46:400–403
Hedenstierna G, Strandberg A, Brismar B, Lundquist H, Svensson L, Tokics L 1985 Functional residual capacity, thoracoabdominal dimensions and central blood volume during general anaesthesia with muscle paralysis and mechanical ventilation. Anesthesiology 62: 247
Hedenstierna G, Tokics L, Strandberg A, Lundquist H, Brismar B 1986 Correlation of gas exchange impairment to development of atelectasis during anaesthesia and muscle paralysis. Acta Anaesthesiol Scand 30: 183–191
Hochermann M, Reimer A 1987 Hearing loss after general anaesthesia. J Laryngol Otol 101: 1079–1082
Johnston R R, Eger E I, Wilson C 1976 A comparative interaction of epinephrine with enflurane, isoflurane and halothane in man. Anesth Analg 55: 709–712
Jones J G 1977 The chest wall-tone and movement. Anesthesiology 47: 325–326
Jones J G 1987 Mechanism of some pulmonary effects of general anaesthesia. Br J Hosp Med 38: 472–476
Katz R L, Matteo R S, Papper E M 1962 Anesthesiology 23: 597–600
Knill R L, Gleb A W 1978 Ventilatory responses to hypoxia and hypercapnia during halothane sedation and anaesthesia in man. Anesthesiology 49: 244–251
Kosaka F, Yamada T, Taniguchi M et al 1986 Alterations in hepatic blood flow during halothane, enflurane and isoflurane inhalation in dogs. Anesthesiology 65: A566
Lassen H C A, Henriksen E, Neukirch F, Kristensen H S 1956 Severe bone marrow depression after prolonged nitrous oxide anaesthesia. Lancet 1: 527–530
Layzer R B 1978 Myeloneuropathy after prolonged exposure to nitrous oxide. Lancet 2: 1227–1230
Levy W 1982 Cardiac arrhythmias: clinical evaluation of isoflurane. Can Anaesth Soc J 29: S28–S32
Lewis J H, Zimmerman H J, Ishak K G, Mullick F G 1983 Enflurane hepatotoxicity: a clinico-pathologic study of 24 cases. Ann Intern Med 98: 984–992
Lofstrom B, Schildt B 1974 Reticuloendothelial function under general anaesthesia. Acta Anaesth Scand 18: 34–40
Loughnan B A, Hall G M 1989 Spinal cord monitoring 1989. Br J Anaesth 63: 587–594
Lowry C J, Fielden B P 1976 Bronchospasm associated with enflurane anaesthesia: three case reports. Anaesth Intensive Care 4: 254–258
Lumley J, Morgan M 1976 The temperature inside carbon dioxide absorbers. Anaesthesia 31: 63–68
Marijic J, Bosnjak Z, Stowe D, Kampine J 1988 Effects and interaction of verapamil and volatile anaesthetics on the isolated perfused guinea pig heart. Anesthesiology 69: 914–922
Mazze R I 1984 Metabolism of the inhaled anaesthetics: implications of enzyme induction. Br J Anaesth 56: 27S
Mazze R I, Trudell J R, Cousins M J 1971 Methoxyflurane metabolism and renal dysfunction: clinical correlations in man. Anesthesiology 35: 247–252
Mazze R I, Cousins M J, Barr G A 1974 Renal effects and metabolism of isoflurane in man. Anesthesiology 40: 536–542
Mazze R I, Woodruff R E, Heerdt M E 1982 Isoniazid induced enflurane defluoridation in humans. Anesthesiology 57: 5–8
Merin R E 1987 Calcium channel blocking drugs and anaesthetics: is the drug interaction beneficial or detrimental? Anesthesiology 66: 111–113
Miletich J D, Ivankovitch A D, Albrecht R F, Reimann C R, Rosenberg R, McKissie E D 1976 Absence of autoregulation of cerebral blood flow during halothane and enflurane analgesia. Anesth Analg 55: 100–106
Minnitt R J 1949 Gas and air analgesia, 4th edn. Balliere Tindall, London
Mitchell M M, Prakash O, Rulf E N R, van Daele M E R M, Cahalan M K, Roeland J R T C 1989 Nitrous oxide does not induce myocardial ischaemia in patients with ischaemic heart disease and poor ventricular function. Anesthesiology 71: 526–534
Moir D D 1970 Anaesthesia for caesarian section: an evaluation of a method of using low concentrations of halothane and 50% oxygen. Br J Anaesth 42: 136–142
Munson E S 1974 Transfer of nitrous oxide into body air cavities. Br J Anaesth 46: 202–209
Munson E S, Embro W J 1977 Enflurane, isoflurane and halothane and isolated human uterine muscle. Anesthesiology 46: 11–14
Nainby-Luxmoore R C 1964 Further hazards of gas and air in obstetrics. Anaesthesia 19: 421–423
National Halothane Study 1969 Possible association between halothane anaesthesia and postoperative hepatic necrosis. J Am Med Assoc 197: 775–788
Ngai S H, Farhie S E, Brody D C 1961 Effects of trichloroethylene, halopropane and methoxyflurane on

respiratory regulatory mechanisms. J Pharmacol Exp Ther 131: 91
Nunn J F 1987 Clinical aspects of the interaction between nitrous oxide and vitamin B_{12}. Br J Anaesth 59: 3–13
Oikkonen M, Haavio M L, Rosenberg P, Kari K 1987 Serum and dental fluoride concentrations in patients on fluoride prophylaxis and anaesthetised with enflurane. Proc Finn Dent Soc 83: 43–46
Owen W D, Gustave F, Sclaroff A 1978 Tympanic membrane rupture with nitrous oxide anaesthesia. Anesth Analg 57: 283
Oyama T, Latto P, Holaday D A 1975 Effect of isoflurane anaesthesia and surgery on carbohydrate metabolism and plasma cortisol levels in man. Can Anaesth Soc J 22: 696–702
Palahnuik R J, Shnider S M, Eger E I 1974 Pregnancy decreases the requirement for inhaled anaesthetic agents. Anesthesiology 41: 82–83
Price H L, Lurie A A, Jones R E, Price M L, Linde H W 1958 Cyclopropane anaesthesia. II. Epinephrine and norepinephrine in initiation of ventricular arrhythmias by carbon dioxide. Anesthesiology 19: 619–630
Reiz S, Balfors E, Sorensen M T, Ariola S, Friedman A, Truedsson H 1983 Isoflurane: a powerful coronary vasodilator in patients with coronary artery disease. Anesthesiology 59: 91–97
Rodenstein D O, Stanescu D C 1986 The soft palate and breathing. Am Rev Respir Dis 134: 311–325
Sebel P S, Ingram D A, Flynn P J, Rutherford C F, Rogers H 1986 Evoked potentials during isoflurane anaesthesia. Br J Anaesth 58: 580–585
Skacel P O, Hewlett A M, Lewis J D, Lumb M, Nunn J F, Chanarin I 1983 Studies on the haemopoeitic toxicity of nitrous oxide in man. Br J Haematol 53: 189–200
Smith A L, Wollman H 1972 Cerebral blood flow and metabolism: effects of anesthetic drugs and techniques. Anesthesiology 36: 378–400
Stevens W C, Dolan W M, Gibbons R T et al 1975 Minimum alveolar concentration (MAC) of isoflurane with and without nitrous oxide in patients of various ages. Anesthesiology 42: 197–200
Stirt J A, Berger J M, Sullivan S F 1983 Lack of arrhythmogenicity of isoflurane following administration of aminophylline in dogs. Anesth Analg 62: 568–571
Stock J G L, Strunin L 1985 Unexplained hepatitis following halothane. Anesthesiology 63: 424–439
Stoelting R K, Blitt C D, Cohen P J, Merin R J 1987 Hepatic dysfunction after isoflurane anaesthesia. Anesth Analg 66: 147–153
Strandberg A, Tokics L, Brismar B, Lundquist H, Hedenstierna G 1986 Atelectasis during anaesthesia and in the postoperative period. Acta Anaesthesiol Scand 30: 154–158
Tunstall M E 1961 Obstetric analgesia: the use of a fixed nitrous oxide and oxygen mixture from one cylinder. Lancet 2: 964
Walton B 1979 Effects of anaesthesia and surgery on immune status. Br J Anaesth 51: 37–43
Walton B 1986 Halothane hepatitis in children. Anaesthesia 41: 575–578
Warren T M, Datta S, Ostheimer G W, Naulty J S, Weiss J B, Morrison J A 1983 Comparison of the maternal and neonatal effects of halothane, enflurane and isoflurane for caesarean delivery. Anesth Analg 62: 516–520
Whitteridge D, Bulbing E 1944 Changes in activity of pulmonary receptors in anaesthesia and their influence on respiratory behaviour. J Pharmacol Exp Ther 81: 340
Widger L A, Gandolfi A J, van Dyke R A 1976 Hypoxia and halothane metabolism in vivo: release of inorganic fluoride and halothane metabolite binding to cellular constituents. Anesthesiology 44: 197–201

21

Malignant hyperthermia

F. R. Ellis

INTRODUCTION

Malignant hyperthermia (MH) has been recognized as a clinical entity for 30 years, since Denborough & Lovell (1960) reported briefly an Australian family in which there had been multiple anaesthetic deaths. Hyperthermia, even in 1960, was recognized as a potential hazard of anaesthesia as it had been reported sporadically from 1900 (Gibson 1900, Moschowitz 1916). Most pre-1960 authors interpreted the hyperthermia as a type of 'heat stroke' and clearly did not appreciate the crucial hypermetabolic element.

It is interesting to note that another complication of ether anaesthesia also associated with hyperthermia was first described in 1922, namely ether convulsions. The similarities between ether convulsions and MH are marked and include abnormal muscle activity, high body temperature, severe acidosis, developing cyanosis and a high mortality. An important difference is the epileptiform type of muscle activity and the later observation that many of those who develop ether convulsions can be shown to have 'spike and dome' electroencephalogram (EEG) activity indicating an epileptic predisposition.

A third variety of hypermetabolism seen during anaesthesia is thyroid crisis, which also carries a high mortality. The most dangerous feature of thyroid crisis is the effect on cardiac function, so it differs from ether convulsion which causes death by hypoxaemia, and MH in which often the most dangerous feature is the hyperthermia. While MH has never been reported in association with overt hyperthyroidism, abnormal thyroid function was detected in MH susceptible pigs, but the reverse has also been shown (Gronert 1980).

MH has passed through various phases over the last 30 years. Initially the condition was infrequently recognized and, perhaps as a consequence, was usually fatal. From the early 1970s when the abnormality in muscle was increasingly observed, MH grew in complexity, and the literature of that decade contains many unsubstantiated cases and spurious associations between MH and many other diseases. There should be no excuse for this type of lax reporting today as MH can so easily be confirmed using the well-described screening procedures (see p. 334).

A third phase has been entered with the specific genetic studies showing that the MH gene is on human chromosome 19. In due course this will lead to a simplification of the recognition of MH susceptibles (MHS) and hopefully will allow a much wider screen to be applied to patients being prepared for anaesthesia.

THE CLINICAL SYNDROME

There are various types of clinical presentation that can be either recognized or deduced, namely:

- fulminant/classical
- mild
- aborted
- missed

- masseter spasm
- atypical.

Fulminant reaction

The early clinical descriptions of MH illustrate the gross derangement of metabolism that occurs if the reaction proceeds untreated for more than an hour. The signs can be most easily considered in two groups, namely hypermetabolism and muscular signs.

Hypermetabolism

The hypermetabolism is characterized by a rapid progressive and uncontrolled rise of body temperature of around 5–6°C/h typically, with developing cyanosis, and a mixed respiratory and metabolic acidosis. Increased oxygen demand by the hypermetabolic tissue causes a tachycardia and tachypnoea which reflect the body's attempt to deliver more oxygen to the tissues. The increased production of CO_2 may be the first sign and is recognized by an increasing $P_{ET}CO_2$ ($P_{ET}CO_2$ = partial pressure at CO_2 in the end-tidal gas). The metabolic acidosis may reflect only the degree of anaerobic metabolism.

Muscular

The majority of patients develop muscle rigidity (spasm and contracture) with suxamethonium and/or with inhalational anaesthetics. The spasm results in muscle damage which can be extreme. The evidence for muscle damage includes release from the muscle of K^+, creatine kinase (CK), myoglobin and other muscle enzymes. A sudden rise in serum K^+ has potentially damaging effects on the cardiac muscle and may cause early cardiac arrest. Intense myoglobinaemia results in myoglobinuria and renal tubular obstruction producing renal failure.

Mild and aborted reactions

The severity of an MH reaction depends at least in part on the length of time it has been allowed to develop and on the amount of trigger agent administered. Mild reactions are often seen with shorter duration anaesthesia. Under these conditions the signs of MH may be poorly developed or not apparent. With suxamethonium-induced muscle spasm, many anaesthetists would consider terminating the procedure pending further investigation. Many of these aborted cases prove to be normal and suxamethonium myotonia must be considered to occur in normal individuals (Van de Spek et al 1987, Leary & Ellis 1990).

Missed reaction

A previous MH reaction may only be suspected after MH has been confirmed in another family member. Also, a preanaesthetic personal or family history may arouse suspicion. Unfortunately, clinical records of previous reactions may be inadequate or lost.

Masseter spasm

Masseter spasm following suxamethonium is becoming more of a problem. Roughly 50% of patients investigated for MH have had suxamethonium spasm (Ellis & Halsall 1984) and roughly 50% of patients presenting with muscle spasm can be shown to be MHS. Thus masseter spasm and MH are associated, but in view of the work of Van de Spek et al (1987) and Leary & Ellis (1990) mentioned above, which indicates that suxamethonium spasm occurs in apparently normal subjects, the muscle spasm cannot be considered to be the causation of an MH response. It may be that MHS individuals have a muscle condition that responds in a myotonic fashion to a variety of stressors, including depolarizing relaxants and inhalational anaesthetic vapours. This may relate to the intracellular calcium lability suggested by the findings of Lopez et al (1987).

At present it would be dangerous to interpret suxamethonium-induced masseter spasm as anything other than an early sign of MH until research elucidates the problem. The main difficulty is the clinical recognition of masseter spasm. When masseter spasm occurs with either hypermetabolic signs, or signs of muscle disruption, there is a significantly raised probability of an MH reaction occurring.

Atypical reaction

MH may present in other ways. It may be the underlying or unappreciated cause of a peroperative cardiac arrest, a postoperative renal failure or perioperative brain damage. With better monitoring it is difficult to see how this type of situation arises, though it must be admitted that, until comparatively recently, MH was unrecognized as a clinical entity. The vast majority of postoperative pyrexias are found to be unrelated to MH (personal observation).

DIFFERENTIAL DIAGNOSIS

An important feature of MH is the relative non-specificity of the MH signs. There are many causes of all of the signs taken individually, but the more that occur concurrently the greater the probability of an MH aetiology.

Raised body temperature

Causes of a rise in body core temperature unrelated to MH include infections, abnormal drug response, drug hypersensitivity and allergic reactions, blood transfusion reactions, cold stress, abnormal muscle activity (such as convulsions, shivering and myotonia), midbrain damage following a CVA or hypoxia.

Hyperkalaemia, raised creatine kinase and hypermyoglobinaemia

Causes of hyperkalaemia, raised CK and hypermyoglobinaemia unrelated to MH include the well-documented abnormal muscle responses to anaesthesia in patients with muscle disease such as myotonic dystrophy, Duchenne muscular dystrophy, glycogen storage and other metabolic diseases of muscle, crush syndrome and reaction to suxamethonium in apparently normal individuals.

TREATMENT

Treatment depends on how early the diagnosis is made.

Early

If an early provisional diagnosis is made, treatment consists simply of withdrawal of trigger agents and monitoring progress using electrocardiogram (ECG), blood pressure (BP), oximetry, capnography (if available), serum electrolytes, CK, blood gases, urinalysis and body core temperature. Management should be expectant and symptomatic. Warning signs include rising body temperature, falling pH, rising serum potassium and increase in muscle tone.

Later

If the diagnosis is made at a later stage when the metabolic status of the patient has been significantly compromised, a more active management is required:

1. Stop all trigger agents. Either terminate the procedure or continue anaesthesia with intravenous agents (and nitrous oxide) with short-acting non-depolarizing relaxants. Hyperventilate with at least 50% oxygen.
2. Infuse dextrose/saline to maintain central venous pressure (CVP). Force a diuresis. Catheterize the bladder.
3. Prepare and administer dantrolene (1 mg/kg^{-1}). Be prepared to repeat this dose several times until the musculature becomes flaccid and the metabolic status is returning to normal.
4. Control arrhythmias by reversing hyperkalaemia with procainamide or equivalent, beta adrenoblockers and possibly calcium antagonists. Verapamil and dantrolene should not be given concurrently.
5. Hyperkalaemia may persist and worsen progressively even with good metabolic control. Insulin/dextrose is helpful in the short term (rapidly reverse peaked T-waves on the ECG), but ion exchangers and even haemodialysis may be required later. I have personal knowledge of two teenage children who died of hyperkalaemia (13 and 15 mmol/1, respectively) around 12 h after the acute episode.

6. Cooling is often unnecessary if good control is achieved with the above measures. If, however, the temperature reaches 41°C, it would be a brave anaesthetist that would reject cooling as part of the management. Surface cooling is comparatively easy but not very effective, except in children. Cooled intravenous fluids can be used and nasogastric cooling has also been advocated. With an open chest or abdomen, cavity cooling could be considered.
7. Other supportive measures, such as intravenous sodium bicarbonate (1–2 mmol/kg) for persistent acidosis and calcium gluconate for a failing heart, should be given as necessary. Clotting mechanisms should be tested and treated if a coagulopathy develops.

Late

All patients who have had a likely MH episode should be nursed postoperatively in an ICU where serum potassium, calcium, pH, $P\text{CO}_2$ and $P\text{O}_2$ can be closely followed. Renal failure due to tubular obstruction by myoglobin is rare nowadays but can be prevented by forced diuresis during the acute episode. If it occurs, however, haemodialysis may be necessary for several weeks. It usually resolves completely. Hypoxic damage to the brain is rare and usually only follows frank cardiac arrest during the acute episode. A diagnostic conundrum may arise from the difficulty of resolving whether hyperthermia is due to brain damage or vice versa. Recrudescence of MH can occur and require further active dantrolene treatment.

Finally

The family history should be evaluated and the patient referred for confirmatory screening using the muscle contracture tests described later. It is quite surprising that sometimes obvious clinical 'MH' cases are shown to be normal on muscle testing and another cause must be sought.

TESTING FOR MHS

Many tests for susceptibility to MH have been devised. These include serum CK, serum pyrophosphate, red cell osmotic fragility, white blood cell calcium release, chemiluminescence and red cell membrane fluidity. The only tests that have consistently differentiated MHS from normals (MHN) are the in vitro contracture tests of living muscle.

The contracture tests used at present are derived from the original caffeine (Kalow et al 1970) and halothane (Ellis et al 1971) contracture tests. The few laboratories offering screening services in the 1970s all adopted different methods, particularly in North America. In 1983 the European MH Group (EMHG) was formed. One of their primary aims was to agree a test protocol for the laboratory screening procedures (EMHG 1984, 1985). The tests are now combined and the results expressed as:

- MHS, when a sustained halothane contracture occurs with 2% halothane (0.44 mmol/1) or less *and* a sustained caffeine contracture occurs with 2 mmol/1 caffeine or less
- MHN, when neither of the above tests is positive
- MHE, when only one of the above tests is positive.

The MHE (equivocal) diagnosis can be used to differentiate an abnormal, or positive, halothane result (MHE_h) and an abnormal caffeine result (MHE_c).

The discrimination of the EMHG test can best be demonstrated by confirming that controls, that is patients with no personal or family MH history, fall into the MHN group and fulminant/classical cases fall into the MHS group. Within the European MH Group over 70 of the former and 10 of the latter have been confirmed.

At present there is great optimism that MHS screening will become much simplified using biogenetic techniques. In some families the MH gene resides on the long arm of chromosome 19 and the most likely candidate gene is the Human Ryanodine Receptor (RYR) gene (MacLennan et al 1990). Even if the MH gene and the RYR gene are the same, the problems of screening are not yet over. The RYR gene is 150 000 amino acids in length. To develop a specific test for MH it is necessary to identify the MH abnormality in the RYR gene and then to develop a suitable, quick and cheap biochemical test for it.

Some of the imponderables include the possibility that MH occurs with a variety of different RYR abnormalities, that the disease may involve another, perhaps recessive, gene as well, and that the RYR gene may not be the MH gene but just close to it. These are exciting times for geneticists but they are entirely dependent on the current screening tests and even more basically on the clinical recognition of MH in the operating theatre.

ARE THERE ANY OTHER DISEASES RELEVANT TO MH?

Various causes of hypermetabolism during anaesthesia have been linked with MH. Any cause of increased metabolic activity will result in a rise in body temperature above normal unless the increase is itself triggered by a lowering of body temperature. None of these causes has been shown to be related to MH.

It is now accepted that MH is a metabolic disease of muscle. It is therefore natural to suspect that other muscle disease may be causally associated with MH. Both Harriman (1988) and Mortier (1990) have reviewed this subject and neither has provided substantiated evidence that MH occurs with any other muscle disease consistently. Mortier (1990) and Lehmann-Horn & Iaizzo (In press) have tested the muscle from many patients with a rich variety of neuromuscular conditions. They have shown some muscle to be MHE and some even MHS. In interpreting these results it is thought likely that in some muscle diseases there could be a defect similar to the MH defect (such as intracellular calcium flux lability) that causes the muscle to develop contracture in vitro with either caffeine or halothane, or both. However the defect need not be, and almost certainly is not, the same as in MH. Brownell (1988) carefully assessed the muscle diseases in relation to MH and concluded that the only one likely to be associated was central core disease (CCD). Ranklev-Twetman (unpublished) and Ellis & Halsall (unpublished) have investigated CCD families and found MHS and CCD to be imperfectly correlated.

It is important not to diagnose MH simply from an in vitro test but to apply preconditions to the test including a good reason for performing it.

ANAESTHESIA FOR MHS

As more MHS individuals and families are identified, anaesthesia is becoming a bigger problem. MH trigger agents, which include depolarizing muscle relaxants and all inhalational anaesthetic vapours, should be avoided. As MH and the neuroleptic malignant syndrome (NMS) are separate entities (Hermesh et al 1988) the neuroleptics and phenothiazines need not be avoided. Heavy premedication may help to reduce stress which may be harmful for MHS. Similarly, deeper levels of anaesthesia should be maintained during surgery.

Monitoring should include body temperature, BP, ECG, capnography and oximetry if possible. There should be no need for blood gases or serum biochemistry if the anaesthesia is properly conducted. If trigger agents are avoided there is no need to use dantrolene as a preventative. If a potentially dangerous drug is to be used, dantrolene (1 mg/kg *q.d.s.* for 24 h) can be administered orally. Cooled intravenous solutions and dantrolene should be immediately available. Anaesthetic machinery should be equipped with clean tubing, and vaporizers should have been removed from the circuit. The anaesthetic machine should be flushed for an hour or so after this.

The following agents are probably completely safe:

1. premedication:
   - benzodiazepines
   - opioids
   - atropine
2. induction:
   - thiopentone
   - propofol
   - etomidate
3. maintenance:
   - nitrous oxide
   - atracurium

- vecuronium
- pancuronium
- opioids

4. reversal:
   - neostigmine
   - atropine
   - naloxone
5. Postoperative:
   - opioids
   - metoclopramide.

All local anaesthetics seem to have been used on MHS safely.

MOLECULAR BASIS OF MH

It is now widely accepted that MH is a muscle disease with a disordered intracellular calcium ion regulation (Ellis & Heffron 1985). Muscular rigidity is one of the earliest and most consistent signs of MH. This is not blocked by conventional non-depolarizing muscle relaxants, therefore the lesion is neither neurological nor at the neuromuscular synapse. It is now recognized that dantrolene will arrest and reverse the muscular rigidity. As dantrolene acts on the excitation–contraction coupling mechanism, this is likely to be the site of the MH defect.

Mitochondria from MHS swine have been investigated extensively and no consistent abnormality has been found. In particular, uncoupling of oxidative phosphorylation, thought to be a likely source of the heat generation in MH, does not occur with halothane.

The sarcolemma is slightly less stable in MH muscle compared with normal, with reduced K^+ and mechanical thresholds to stimulation. However, an important recent study by Iaizzo et al (1989) demonstrated that the sarcolemma is essentially normal.

The only other source of intracellular calcium is the sarcoplasmic reticulum (SR) which is mainly responsible for controlling intracellular ionic calcium concentrations. Recent studies of the interaction of the T-tubular system and the SR, at what are known as triadic junctions or triads, has demonstrated the presence of ionic channels specific for calcium which bridge the two structures. The T-tubule contains the slow calcium channel and the hydroxypyridine-sensitive channel. The adjacent SR contains a calcium channel which is partially blocked by the vegetable toxin ryanodine, hence the term 'ryanodine receptor-controlled channel'.

It is likely that the molecular abnormality responsible for MH lies in the protein controlling the ryanodine receptor. The gene controlling the formation of this protein is 150 000 amino acids in length. There may be several defects that could result in MH, a particular defect, or series of defects, occurring in a particular pedigree. Elucidation of the amino acid sequence for the MH and normal human HRYR gene is awaited. The rabbit HRYR gene has been sequenced. Even when the HRYR abnormality has been identified it will still be necessary to define the abnormal reaction that occurs when halothane and other inhalational anaesthetic vapours interact with the proteins.

If the study of the molecular mechanism of cystic fibrosis is taken as the model, it could be some years before the mechanisms involved in MH are fully understood.

SOCIAL CONCERNS

Possession of the MH gene rendering the individual MHS has social implications. Some types of employment that carry either a greater risk of trauma with the subsequent need for anaesthesia (such as the armed services) or a chemical pollution risk (such as the dry-cleaning industry) are inadvisable. The need to warn anaesthetists of the MHS state may become a problem after severe trauma and unconsciousness, and when travelling in foreign countries. In the UK the MHS subject may receive valuable support from the British MH Association which supplies suitable documentation in all European languages.

REFERENCES

Brownell, A K W 1988 Malignant hyperpyrexia: relationship to other diseases. Br J Anaesth 60: 303–308

Denborough M A, Lovell R R H 1960 Anaesthetic deaths in a family. Lancet 2: 45

Ellis, F R, Halsall P J unpublished observation

Ellis F R, Halsall P J 1984 Suxamethonium spasm: a diagnostic conundrum. Br J Anaesth 56: 381–383

Ellis F R, Harriman D G F, Keaney N P, Kyei-Mensah K, Tyrrell J H 1971 Halothane induced muscle contracture as a cause of hyperpyrexia. Br J Anaesth 43: 721–722

Ellis F R, Heffron J J A 1985 Clinical and biochemical aspects of malignant hyperpyrexia. Recent Advances in Anaesthesia and Analgesia 15: 173–207

European M H Group 1984 A protocol for the investigation of malignant hyperpyrexia susceptibility. Br J Anaesth 56: 1267–1269

European M H Group 1985 Laboratory diagnosis of malignant hyperpyrexia susceptibility (MHS). Br J Anaesth 57: 1038

Gibson C 1900 J Am Med Assoc 35: 1685

Gronert G A 1980 Malignant hyperthermia. Anesthesiology 53: 395–423

Hermesh H, Aizenberg D, Lapidot M, Munitz H 1988 Risk of malignant hyperthermia among patients with neuroleptic malignant syndrome and their families. Am J Psychiatry 145: 1431–1434

Harriman D G F 1988 Malignant hyperthermia myopathy: a critical review. Br J Anaesth 60: 309–316

Iaizzo P, Lehmann-Horn F, Taylor S R, Gallant E M 1989 Malignant hyperpyrexia: effects of halothane on the surface of the membrane. Muscle & Nerve 12: 178–183

Kalow W, Britt B A, Terreau M E, Haist C 1970 Metabolic error of muscle metabolism after recovery from malignant hyperthermia. Lancet 2: 895–898

Leary N P, Ellis F R 1990 Masseteric muscle spasm as a normal response to suxamethonium. Br J Anaesth 64: 488–492

Lehmann-Horn F, Iaizzo P in press Are myotonias and periodic paralyses associated with susceptibility to malignant hyperthermia. Br J Anaesth

Lopez J R, Medina P, Alamo L 1987 Dantrolene sodium is able to reduce the resting ionic [Ca^{2}+]: in muscle from humans with malignant hyperthermia. Muscle & Nerve 10: 77–80

MacLennan D H, Duff C, Zorato F et al 1990 Ryanodine receptor gene is a candidate for predisposition to malignant hyperthermia. Nature 343: 559–561

Mortier W 1990 Malignant hyperpyrexia: a relation to other diseases. Acta Anaesthesiol Belg 41: 55–62

Moschowitz A 1916 Postoperative heatstroke. Surg Gynecol & Obstet 23: 443–451

Ranklev-Twetman E unpublished observation

Van de Spek A F L, Fang W B, Ashton-Miller J A, Stohler C S, Carlson D S, Schork M A 1987 The effect of succinylcholine on mouth opening. Anesthesiology 67: 459–465

22

Medical conditions with specific drug contraindications

R. A. Mason

INTRODUCTION

This chapter discusses a variety of unrelated medical conditions in which certain anaesthetic drugs are said to be contraindicated. Sometimes recommendations have been made on sound clinical, scientific or theoretical bases. In other cases the evidence on which the claim has been based is more tenuous. Information may be handed down uncritically from one textbook to another and thereby achieves a historic respectability. Thus for many years it was accepted that thiopentone caused bronchoconstriction in asthmatics. However, it is now known that the bronchospasm is most frequently a reflex response to tracheal intubation under light anaesthesia. The induction agent itself had simply failed to prevent this response, rather than necessarily being the direct cause of it. Thiopentone in high dosages may actually have a protective effect against bronchospasm.

Evidence that a drug has undesirable effects in a particular disease can originate from a variety of sources: from individual or multiple case reports; by extrapolation, relating the known pharmacology of a drug to the physiology of the condition; from collection of data by an agency, such as the Committee on Safety of Medicines (CSM), involved in voluntary reporting of complications; from controlled clinical trials; from in vitro human tissue tests; and occasionally from research involving animal or tissue models.

The contraindication may be absolute because of the serious nature of the reaction, as in the use of inhalational agents or suxamethonium in malignant hyperthermia. Sometimes the interaction may be quantitative, in the sense that the pathology of the condition results in undue sensitivity to the normal clinical dosage of the drug. This is seen in the use of non-depolarizing neuromuscular blockers in myasthenia gravis. In other cases the advice is cautionary and based on general physiological principles, as in the use of vasoactive drugs or myocardial depressants in Riley Day syndrome.

Three of the most important conditions–malignant hyperthermia, plasma cholinesterase deficiency and myotonic dystrophy–will not be discussed further as they are described in detail elsewhere. Particular consideration will be given to the use of anaesthetic agents in the following conditions:

- asthma
- epilepsy
- muscular dystrophy (Duchenne)
- myasthenia gravis
- Eaton–Lambert syndrome or myasthenic syndrome
- porphyria.

ASTHMA

Asthma is an inflammatory condition of the tracheobronchial tree that is associated with hyperreactivity of the airways. The importance of the inflammatory element has only recently been recognized. There are pathological changes within the submucosa of the airways. These include infiltration by inflammatory cells (especially eosinophils and lymphocytes), oedema of the bronchial mucosa, secretion of mucus and epithelial desquamation. The presence of inflammation results in the airways being hyperresponsive to a variety of exogenous and endogenous stimuli.

Histamine, the leukotrienes and platelet-activating factor are thought to be the most active chemical mediators, while neural mechanisms may also contribute to the bronchial responses. As obstruction worsens, smaller airways are affected. Expiration is prolonged, residual volume and functional residual capacity are increased, while vital capacity, inspiratory capacity and expiratory reserve volume are reduced. Widespread ventilation perfusion inequalities may occur to produce hypoxia, at a time when the work of breathing is considerably increased. The airway obstruction is usually reversible, but in the later stages of asthma it may become irreversible.

The inflammatory component is particularly significant for the patient needing anaesthesia. The effect of reflex increases in airway tone depends on the initial calibre of the airway. If inflammation is present, causing mucosal oedema and secretion of mucus, then reflex bronchospasm may have profound effects on airway resistance. An apparently asymptomatic patient that has inflamed airways may thus develop complete airway closure after tracheal intubation.

Intercurrent drug treatment of asthma

Therapy in asthma can be aimed at blocking airway reflexes, relaxing smooth muscle, inhibiting the release of inflammatory mediators and increasing beta adrenergic tone.

An increasing appreciation of the role of the inflammatory component has led to a change of emphasis in drug therapy for long-term treatment (Barnes 1989, British Thoracic Society 1990a,b). Bronchodilators are primarily indicated for short-term relief of bronchospasm, acute asthma attacks and the prevention of exercise-induced asthma. The main bronchodilators are, in decreasing order of effectiveness: beta 2 agonists, theophylline derivatives and anticholinergics.

For the chronic state, emphasis is now placed on the early introduction of regular inhaled anti-inflammatory drugs such as corticosteroids (beclomethasone dipropionate or budesonide), sodium cromoglycate and nedocromil sodium. As their onset of action is slow, long-term therapy is required. The use of the aerosol forms of bronchoactive drugs reduces systemic side effects. In addition, bronchodilators given by inhalation act more rapidly than oral, and equally as fast as intravenous preparations.

Anaesthetic management of the asthmatic patient

Elective surgery should not take place in the presence of infection or untreated bronchospasm. Preoperative preparation may include physiotherapy, bronchodilators, antibiotics and corticosteroid cover if these drugs have been used within the previous 12 months. A short course of steroids is also indicated before surgery if inflammation is present (Hirshman & Bergman 1990). In severe cases it is important to assess the likelihood of the need for intermittent positive pressure ventilation (IPPV) after operation. An FEV1 of less than 1 l, or an FEV1/VC ratio of less than 40% and a raised $P\text{aCO}_2$, may all indicate the need for postoperative IPPV. A PEFR of less than 120 l/min and an MVV of less than 50% of the predicted level also indicate severe obstruction. If, however, IPPV is required it carries a high risk of complications such as pneumothorax, cardiac arrhythmias, pneumonia and heart failure.

Anxiety may be a significant feature in the asthmatic patient. Care and understanding should be shown at the preoperative visit and a sedative premedication, such as an antihistamine, is advantageous. The potential seriousness of this disease must not be underestimated.

Despite having a drying effect on secretions, atropine may be desirable for a smooth induction. It can also improve dilatation of the larger bronchi by blocking vagal bronchoconstrictor effects. Although pethidine has been promoted as a bronchodilator, it has recently been shown to be a more common cause of histamine release than morphine. There is, however, no evidence that opiates in normal doses cause bronchoconstriction.

Even in the absence of bronchospasm, some form of preoperative bronchodilator therapy is advisable. Beta blockers are contraindicated because even those with a primarily cardiac action can aggravate airway obstruction.

The choice of induction agent in asthma is controversial. Bronchoconstriction can arise from the drug itself or directly from tracheal intubation. It is difficult to separate these potential causes. Even when asthmatic attacks are infrequent, tracheal intubation is one of the most common causes of bronchospasm in patients that have any history of asthma. In a computer-aided incidence study of 136 929 anaesthetics it was found that bronchospasm was usually triggered by mechanical stimuli, not drugs (Olsson 1987). The carina is particularly sensitive to stimulation.

Thiopentone may affect the airways in a variable, dose-related, manner. There is evidence that airway reflexes are depressed at high, but not at low doses. If used, a larger than normal dose should be given. There are no particular contraindications to the use of benzodiazepines, etomidate or propofol. However, since none of these depresses airway reflexes, premature intubation must be avoided. Sufficient depth of anaesthesia should be attained before airway stimulation. Rapid sequence induction can be difficult in asthmatics.

Ketamine is the one induction agent known to have bronchodilator properties. It has a protective effect against bronchospasm in dogs when compared with thiopentone. This effect is abolished by beta adrenergic blockers. Ketamine has been suggested as a suitable induction agent for emergency anaesthesia in asthmatics, when a rapid sequence induction is required (Kingston & Hirshman 1984). It has also been used to treat status asthmaticus. The use of intravenous lignocaine prior to induction has also been recommended. There is evidence that this prevents the reflex bronchospasm caused by intubation, but not that due to the release of allergic mediators. Topical lignocaine is not effective and may actually induce bronchoconstriction in asthmatic patients (McAlpine & Thomson 1989).

Halothane, enflurane and isoflurane are all effective at reversing antigen-induced bronchospasm (Hirshman et al 1982). However, halothane sensitizes the heart to the effect of exogenous and endogenous catecholamines. In addition, it can interact with aminophylline to produce serious ventricular arrhythmias, even when theophylline levels are within the therapeutic range. The choice of isoflurane or enflurane may therefore be more appropriate. By reducing hypoxic pulmonary vasoconstriction, inhalational agents may worsen ventilation perfusion inequalities and increase hypoxia.

Despite traditional teaching to the contrary, there is no evidence of significant differences between the modern neuromuscular blockers with respect to histamine-related side effects. Nor is there evidence that patients with asthma are more likely to develop anaphylactic reactions to anaesthetic drugs. Although anticholinesterases may produce bronchoconstriction by parasympathetic effects, this effect should be blocked by muscarinic receptor antagonists.

Regional analgesia may be used for surgery or during labour. A retrospective study of asthmatic parturients showed that epidural analgesia could be safely administered, even during acute exacerbations of asthma (Ramanathan et al 1990).

Should acute bronchospasm occur following tracheal intubation, the easiest initial manoeuvre is to attempt to deepen the anaesthetic by the use of an inhalation agent. Residual bronchospasm can be treated with 5 mg/kg aminophylline over a period of 10–15 min. If necessary, an infusion of 0.5 mg/kg/h is started. During anaesthesia, however, there is decreased inactivation of aminophylline by the liver, so caution is required. In addition, plasma theophylline levels must be estimated if treatment is prolonged for more than 24 h. The therapeutic range is 10–20 mg/l, but toxic effects such as fits, arrhythmias and cardiac arrest have been described with plasma levels as low as 25 mg/l. If the patient has already been taking sustained release theophylline preparations, extreme caution will be necessary. Alternatively, bronchodilatation can be achieved with either salbutamol or terbutaline. Salbutamol is given as 200 μg over 10 min or by a salbutamol infusion (3–20 μg/min; 5 ml of 1mg/ml solution added to 500 ml 0.9% saline to give a final concentration of 100 μg/ml). 250 μg terbutaline can be given over 10 min or by an infusion of 3–20 μg/min (British Thoracic Society 1990a,b).

EPILEPSY

A seizure is an abnormal paroxysmal discharge from a group of neurones, resulting in a clinical manifestation or a sensory perception. It may occur with or without loss of consciousness. Epilepsy is a clinical diagnosis based on the occurrence of at least two seizures. Elucidation of the type of epilepsy is usually made on the pattern of the fit, the age at onset, the timing and electroencephalogram (EEG) changes. The international classification of seizure types and epileptic syndromes is complex, and detailed discussion is beyond the scope of this chapter. However, seizures can be broadly divided into 'partial' (which include the former terms Jacksonian, temporal lobe and psychomotor epilepsy) and 'generalized' (previously described as grand mal or major convulsions). Partial seizures begin locally in the cortex and have an aura reflective of the origin of the discharge. This type of seizure can be further subdivided into simple, complex, and those that have become secondarily generalized. Generalized seizures are characterized by a sudden loss of consciousness without an aura, and bilateral manifestations. Further subdivisions include tonic-clonic, absence and myoclonic seizures.

It is unusual to obtain an EEG during a fit, but the interictal EEG usually shows abnormal features which may further assist diagnosis. However, if the epilepsy is mild the EEG can be normal between fits. In addition, if the neuronal discharge originates from a medial temporal focus a specialized lead may be required to record an abnormality, even during a fit.

The incidence of epilepsy is 0.5–1.0%. As many as 5% of the population will have a seizure at some stage of life. It may be a symptom of an underlying pathology, in which case there is a focal cerebral lesion. Alternatively it may be idiopathic. In the latter there is a constitutional and sometimes hereditary disposition to seizures, and a focal lesion is not necessarily demonstrated. However, with the increasing use of magnetic resonance imaging, focal lesions may be found even in apparent idiopathic epilepsy. Below the age of 10 and above the age of 60 the incidence of epilepsy increases. The age at onset may give a guide to the aetiology.

Every individual has the potential to have a seizure if the stimulus applied is great enough. It is important to remember this if an isolated seizure occurs in an apparently non-epileptic patient during the perioperative period. There are normal fluctuations in seizure threshold. In most people this threshold is considerably above the baseline and seizures never occur. An acute traumatic, metabolic or toxic event can thus precipitate a seizure even in a normal individual. Head injury, hypoxia, hypoglycaemia, hyponatraemia, or sudden withdrawal of benzodiazepines, alcohol or barbiturates in a chronic abuser can act as a provocative stimulus. Periodically, 'seizures' have been reported in association with anaesthesia, sometimes during induction with a drug that has excitatory effects, and sometimes during the recovery period.

In an epileptic patient, an individual in whom the threshold for seizures is already reduced, the application of an appropriate stimulus may increase the chance of a seizure occurring. Anticonvulsant therapy might also have been inadvertently omitted during the perioperative period. Sudden withdrawal of drugs can increase the likelihood of convulsions.

The controversies

In epileptic patients, perioperative seizures are occasionally reported. Their occurrence leads to speculation about the immediate cause, the role of anaesthetic drugs with pro- and anticonvulsant effects, and their possible relationship to epilepsy or other pre-existing but undiagnosed cerebral pathology. Considerable confusion has arisen in the terminology used for perioperative excitatory events because a number of anaesthetic drugs, such as the opioids, propofol and etomidate, have been reported to cause rigidity or myoclonus in subjects that do not have a history of epilepsy. These reactions should not be classed as seizures. Perioperative drug-induced excitatory events and their probable neurophysiological basis are discussed in more detail in Chapter 28.

Diagnosis of a seizure

If an overt epileptiform event occurs in an epileptic during the perioperative period, it is important to try to establish whether it was a genuine seizure resulting from cortical epileptiform activity or simply a form of drug-induced rigidity or myoclonus. Clinical observations may be critical. If sudden loss of consciousness was followed by a typical grand mal tonic-clonic convulsion, a seizure is likely to have occurred. Occasionally, simultaneous EEG recording will have confirmed seizure activity. However, the subsequent recording of a normal EEG does not mean that a seizure did not take place. In any case, subcortical or temporal lobe events will not be recorded using only the conventional placement of scalp electrodes.

Potential epileptogenic anaesthetic agents

Evidence for or against a direct relationship between an anaesthetic agent and an epileptic fit may be gathered in a variety of ways. Initially there may be isolated clinical reports of perioperative epileptiform events, usually without, but occasionally with, concurrent EEG monitoring. Studies, with EEG control, of the drug in question may be undertaken in normal or epileptic patients. Subsequent examination of the traces is undertaken for evidence of excitatory effects such as spikes, spike-wave formation or actual seizure activity. Effects of a drug on seizure duration in electroconvulsive therapy (ECT) may be explored. There may be animal experiments, either using EEG recording or with metabolic studies, to determine regional increases in cerebral metabolic rate for oxygen and cerebral blood flow. Alternatively, the capacity of a drug to alter the threshold in artificially induced convulsions may be measured.

The evidence implicating some drugs may be paradoxical. The pro- and anticonvulsant effects of anaesthetic drugs have been reviewed in detail (Modica et al 1990a,b). Some appear to possess both properties in that they have been linked with events thought to be epileptiform on the one hand and yet used in the treatment of status epilepticus on the other. Neurones are subjected to both excitatory and inhibitory influences and anaesthetic agents can produce, at different times or in different neuronal populations, either excitation or depression. This observation is thus not as contradictory as may have appeared at first glance. In cases where the EEG has been recorded during administration of a drug, a spectrum of effects may be observed ranging from depression of EEG activity to excitation, and occasionally to EEG seizures. Only rarely do actual tonic-clonic convulsions occur.

The onset of unexpected, unmonitored seizures is of interest. They may occur soon after administration of the drug or drug combination, but sometimes their appearance is delayed until the recovery period. Recovery of different regions of the brain may possibly occur sequentially during emergence from anaesthesia, such that removal of inhibition from one group of neurones may enhance activity in others, especially when excitation has already been produced by a particular agent. This may be similar to the convulsions that may occur during withdrawal from central nervous system (CNS) depressants such as alcohol, benzodiazepines or other addictive drugs. The effect of a drug on brain cells may be dose related, as suggested by the dose of methohexitone used to localize focal epilepsy being much lower than that used for anaesthesia. Isolated seizures occurring several hours, or occasionally several days, after an anaesthetic are more difficult to explain.

If, as is frequently the case, more than one agent has been used, it is difficult to identify positively the one drug responsible for the seizure. A combined effect is possible.

Adverse effects of a seizure

During a seizure, there are marked systemic changes such as hypertension, tachycardia, respiratory and metabolic acidosis, hypoxia and hyperthermia. Traumatic injury may occur. At a cellular level, focal increases in metabolism may cause local hypoxia or ischaemia. Sometimes postoperative fits are recurrent and status epilepticus carries significant morbidity and occasional mortality.

Genuine epileptic seizures have social and legal implications. Should a perioperative seizure occur it is important that anaesthesia is recognized as the cause (Fariello 1980) and stated in the notes, for if it is not a controlled epileptic might lose his eligibility to drive, or a non-epileptic might be accidentally misdiagnosed as having epilepsy. A seizure must count as a highly undesirable event during anaesthesia and recovery.

If it can be established that a particular drug is able to produce epileptiform activity on EEG in a normal patient, is it more likely to precipitate a seizure in an epileptic? If so, is its use contraindicated when anaesthetizing a known epileptic patient? There is no satisfactory answer to these questions since the literature contains conflicting advice.

Methohexitone, etomidate and enflurane have all been used to provoke focal discharges in epileptics undergoing surgery for focal epilepsy. Many authors therefore advocate their avoidance in epilepsy except under these particular circumstances. Others have argued that this effect only applies to focal epilepsy and that not all paroxysmal discharges demonstrated on EEG result in an overt seizure. However, it does seem that methohexitone is more likely to produce a clinical seizure in an epileptic whose medication has been withdrawn. Clinical reports of perioperative seizures are also relatively more common in patients with a previous history of epilepsy than those without. In epileptics, as there are well-recognized stress factors that increase seizure frequency, it would seem logical to avoid using anaesthetic drugs that are known to activate the EEG. However, it must not be forgotten that, provided the anticonvulsant medication is continued, the risk of a seizure occurring in an individual epileptic is very low.

Anaesthetic drugs and epileptiform events

Induction agents

Thiopentone is an effective anticonvulsant although at low doses spike waves may be seen on EEG. In higher doses, brain metabolism and oxygen consumption are reduced.

Methohexitone is particularly interesting. The importance of structure–activity relationships in determining the actions of the different barbiturates has long been recognized. A methyl group introduced into position 1 gives a high incidence of excitatory phenomena. Varying extents of excitatory activity also result from pharmacological differences between the isomeric forms of methohexitone. The early unfractionated preparations produced convulsions in both epileptic and non-epileptic patients and the present formulation retains some excitatory effects. There is therefore still the potential to induce seizure activity in epileptic patients classified as having partial seizures. Several isolated reports of fits have occurred. In one study, 48 epileptics had their anticonvulsant medication withheld. Methohexitone-activated EEG analysis was undertaken using incremental doses followed by an infusion (Male & Allen 1977). Two developed grand mal fits during induction and three others had status epilepticus (two of the petit mal type and one of the myoclonic type) after the infusion was stopped.

In much lower doses than those required for anaesthesia, methohexitone can be used to provoke epileptic foci on EEG during surgical treatment of focal cortical epilepsy. Certain premedicant drugs may also alter the response to barbiturates. Promethazine and hyoscine premedication increases the incidence of excitatory effects especially with methohexitone, whereas opiates cause a reduction.

Benzodiazepines are effective anticonvulsants and increase beta activity on EEG. Diazepam, midazolam and lorazepam have all been used to treat status epilepticus.

Etomidate may produce marked myoclonic movements on induction of anaesthesia (Ghonheim & Yamada 1977). These are reputed not to be associated with epileptiform discharge on EEG. However, in some epileptics, increased epileptiform discharges on EEG have been seen (Opitz et al 1983, Ebrahim et al 1986). Generalized seizures have been reported with etomidate, often when given with fentanyl (Kreiger & Koerner 1987). As with methohexitone, etomidate has been used to activate epileptic foci. Both generalized and focal seizures have occasionally occurred after etomidate infusions (Grant & Hutchinson 1983), and in rats, myoclonic movements have been accompanied by increases in brain glucose utilization. There is powerful activation of beta activity on EEG and recording from scalp electrodes may be obscured. Several authors have suggested the avoidance of etomidate in epilepsy. However, it has been used successfully as an anticonvulsant.

The use of propofol has been associated with a number of CNS effects, more than 30 of which have been recorded in the literature. These include convulsions, opisthotonos, myoclonus and prolonged unconsciousness. Prior to October 1989, 101 similar events had been reported to the Committee on Safety of Medicines (CSM) (Shearer 1990). Nearly one-third of 37 patients who had seizures were epileptics (CSM 1989). In some cases, repeated fits have occurred, and in one patient these continued for 7 days (Bredahl 1990). Conversely, a decreased duration of fits during ECT has been documented (Simpson et al 1988) and propofol has been used for treatment of status epilepticus.

Ketamine given to both epileptics and non-epileptics did not show cortical or clinical seizure activity on EEG studies (Corssen et al 1974, Celesia et al 1975). However, ketamine is known to be excitatory to the thalamus and limbic system, in which it produces a seizure pattern that does not extend to the cerebral cortex (Ferrer-Allado et al 1973). Thus cortical electrodes do not reflect seizure activity. Increases in cerebral blood flow and oxygen consumption have been shown and activation of experimentally induced corticoreticular epilepsy in cats has been reported. However, ketamine also possesses anticonvulsant properties and has been used to treat status epilepticus.

Inhalation agents

Halothane has been shown to reduce the incidence of epileptic abnormalities in children with generalized or focal epilepsy. Studies in 12 epileptic children given halothane anaesthesia showed a decrease in EEG abnormalities which increased during recovery (Mecarelli et al 1981). Halothane reduces the clearance of pethidine, norpethidine and phenytoin. Phenytoin toxicity has been reported after halothane anaesthesia.

During enflurane anaesthesia, EEG studies have shown that an increase in depth of anaesthesia is accompanied by the appearance of high-voltage spikes and spike waves with burst suppression. A reduction in $P\text{aCO}_2$ increases the occurrence of these abnormalities (Neigh et al 1971). Enflurane has been used to activate epileptic foci during surgery for epilepsy. Convulsions have been reported at times varying from minutes to several hours, and in one case several days (Grant 1986), after such anaesthesia. On another occasion, status epilepticus occurred (Nicoll 1986). In all cases, enflurane was not the sole agent used and, in the main, no seizures had occurred previously. Cerebral glucose utilization studies in rats suggested activation of intercortical and corticothalamic pathways (Nakakimura et al 1988). However, in one study when enflurane was given to 21 epileptics, EEG recordings could not demonstrate provocation of epileptic foci (Opitz et al 1977). Inhibition of seizure activity during enflurane anaesthesia has also been reported (Opitz et al 1983).

Isoflurane has anticonvulsant properties and has been used to treat status epilepticus refractory to treatment (Kofke et al 1989). Again there have been isolated reports of fits noted during induction of anaesthesia.

Opioids

A number of reports have described rigidity and epileptiform or myoclonic movements after high-dose opioids. In several, simultaneous cortical EEG recordings have shown no abnormal activity in man although animal studies have shown accompanying seizure activity on the EEG and activation of subcortical brain metabolism. High-dose pentazocine, used for cardiac surgery, has been associated with seizures. Grand mal convulsions have occurred during induction with fentanyl, but not necessarily at high dosage. In those in which EEG recording was available no cortical seizure activity was seen. During a study of alfentanil-induced rigidity in 10 patients the EEG showed no evidence of seizure activity and a neurochemical mechanism has been suggested (Benthuysen et al 1986). A subsequent study of 127 patients with high-dose opioids produced similar conclusions (Ty Smith et al 1989).

Pethidine has been associated with seizures, particularly when used over a long period or in patients with renal failure. Norpethidine, one of the metabolites, was probably responsible.

Potential problems with anticonvulsant drugs

Most anticonvulsants cause enzyme induction and can interfere with the metabolism of other drugs. The folate deficiency and megaloblastic anaemia that are sometimes seen in patients on long-term therapy with phenytoin, phenobarbitone or primidone are probably due to this.

Sodium valproate may interfere with haemostasis. Thrombocytopenia is the most common defect. Its incidence is dose related and is more common in children than in adults. Platelet dysfunction, prolonged bleeding time and hypofibrinogenaemia have been reported. Caution is needed if anticoagulants or antiplatelet drugs are given.

Phenytoin has a narrow therapeutic range and certain drugs (including sulphonamides, cimetidine and halothane) have been known to precipitate acute phenytoin toxicity. Ataxia, nystagmus and repiratory depression are clinical signs of this.

Fentanyl requirements are increased in those patients requiring prolonged treatment with anticonvulsants. The underlying mechanism remains unclear (Tempelhoff et al 1990). Interactions between neuromuscular blocking agents and anticonvulsants have also been reported.

As might be expected, there is an increased likelihood of convulsions when epilepsy is poorly controlled (Modica & Tempelhoff 1989).

Conclusions

The incidence of perioperative seizures is unknown but must be very low. However, certain anaesthetic agents have sometimes been associated with EEG epileptiform activity and occasionally even seizures. This risk would appear to be increased in epileptics, especially if anticonvulsant medication has been withdrawn.

Methohexitone, etomidate, enflurane, ketamine and propofol are agents particularly implicated in the production of clinical excitatory events. The first three have also been associated with EEG excitation. While in an individual patient the chance of seizures is low, if they do occur there is significant morbidity. It would thus seem prudent to avoid these drugs in epileptics, if at all possible. However, should the use of any one of these drugs be particularly indicated, then provided adequate anticonvulsant therapy is given in the perioperative period, the risk of precipitating seizures must be slight.

MUSCULAR DYSTROPHY

An X-linked recessive, severe muscle dystrophy (Duchenne) usually presents with proximal lower limb and pelvic muscle weakness. The weakness, which is progressive and varies between muscles, is caused by a decrease in the total number of muscle fibres. Pseudohypertrophy of the calf muscles occurs secondary to infiltration with fatty tissue. Scoliosis develops and is progressive. There may be disease of the cardiac muscle with characteristic ECG changes and a hypertrophic cardiomyopathy. The condition steadily progresses to involve other muscles. Vital capacity falls and diaphragmatic weakness may result in hypoventilation and hypoxia in the later stages. Death, usually from respiratory failure (75% of cases) occurs between the ages of 10 and 20. The creatine kinase (CK) may be grossly raised, the highest levels often occurring early in the disease.

Anaesthetic complications

Although many apparently uneventful anaesthetics have been given to patients with Duchenne muscular dystrophy (DMD), a substantial number of individual cases has been reported in which serious complications have occurred. Some have resulted in death. Attempts have been made to quantify the risks of anaesthesia in DMD (Worthen et al 1987, Sethna et al 1988, Larsen et al 1989). Most studies have been retrospective. Problems were reported with 16–27% of patients having general anaesthesia for a variety of procedures. Those operations performed under local anaesthesia were uneventful. Complications were usually associated with halothane and suxamethonium. Isoflurane has also recently been implicated (Chalkiadis & Branch 1990). Although the precise aetiology of the anaesthetic complications has not always been clear, they can be broadly divided into respiratory problems, abnormal metabolic responses and cardiac events. The metabolic complications may resemble those seen in malignant hyperthermia (MH) and it had been thought that DMD was associated with an increased incidence of this condition. This seems to be unlikely. Occasionally the two conditions have been noted to coexist, but both traits may occur independently (Brownell 1988).

Respiratory problems

Respiratory problems tend to occur with advanced disease. They are associated with the residual effects of anaesthetic agents on patients with poor respiratory reserve, and impairment of the reflexes involved in airway protection and swallowing. Several cases have been reported in which delayed respiratory insufficiency occurred after 'uneventful' anaesthetics. In several instances difficulty in breathing, swallowing and clearing secretions necessitated tracheal reintubation and IPPV. In spite of respiratory support a number of these children later had fatal cardiac arrests (Smith & Bush 1985). Major surgery has resulted in the need for prolonged artificial ventilation. The response to non-depolarizing agents may be abnormal, and in the presence of hypoventilation there may be sensitivity to sedatives, hypnotics and opiate analgesics.

Abnormal metabolic responses

Suxamethonium, halothane and isoflurane have all been reported to be triggering agents for a variety of non-specific complications. These include pyrexia, tachycardia, acidosis, hyperkalaemia, asystole, ventricular fibrillation, muscle spasm, acute rhabdomyolysis, myoglobinuria and renal failure. Unlike the respiratory events, these metabolic problems can occur in the early stages of the disease. In some cases, cardiac arrest during anaesthesia was the first indication that the child had a muscle dystrophy.

When biochemical evidence was available, the acute cardiac events seemed mostly to be associated with hyperkalaemia. Cardiac arrest has usually occurred immediately after administration of suxamethonium but has been reported at any stage, even during the recovery period. Presumably this is because suxamethonium-induced hyperkalaemia persists longer in patients with DMD. In normal individuals given suxamethonium the rise in plasma potassium usually lasts for less than 10 min, whereas in DMD it may be significantly prolonged. Hyperkalaemia may also be precipitated by inhalation agents alone. In one particular case in which cardiac arrest occurred during recovery from anaesthesia with isoflurane, the serum potassium did not return to normal levels until 5 h after the initial event, despite active treatment (Chalkiadis & Branch 1990).

The other metabolic events, primarily rhabdomyolysis, myoglobinuria and renal failure, can also be attributed to sudden loss of the integrity of the muscle membrane and subsequent muscle breakdown. Myoglobinuria after adenoidectomy was the first indication of DMD in a 5-year-old boy (Rubiano et al 1987).

Cardiac problems

It is difficult to separate cardiac events secondary to hyperkalaemia from those associated with a cardiomyopathy. Early cardiac arrest and ventricular fibrillation unassociated with suxamethonium have been reported, as has cardiac failure. Should cardiac arrest occur the cardiomyopathic heart may be resistant to resuscitative measures.

Management

If advanced disease is present, the wisdom and possible benefits of surgery should be weighed against the risks. Elective surgery has resulted in the need for prolonged IPPV and sometimes death. Respiratory function should be carefully assessed if the child is old enough to cooperate. Diaphragmatic involvement occurs in advanced disease. It is indicated by a difference in vital capacity of more than 25% between the erect and supine positions. It has been suggested that for major surgery, such as correction of scoliosis, a vital capacity of at least 20 ml/kg or 30% of predicted is required (Milne & Rosales 1982).

Suxamethonium should not be used in patients with DMD as many of the major complications are associated with its use. Non-depolarizing neuromuscular blocking agents may be used cautiously but, in view of the variability of response, the effects of incremental doses should be monitored. Although many patients have been safely anaesthetized with halothane, the use of this agent has been challenged, particularly when the CK is markedly elevated (Roizen 1987).

Observation in a high-dependency area for the first 24–48 h after anaesthesia will assist in the early detection of pulmonary insufficiency. If doubt arises it is much safer to support ventilation until all drugs have been eliminated.

MYASTHENIA GRAVIS

Myasthenia gravis is an autoimmune disease of the neuromuscular junction involving the post junctional acetylcholine receptors. Specific antibodies against these receptors have been identified in 80–90% cases of myasthenia gravis and microscopic changes in the membrane demonstrated. Not only is there a reduction in the number of acetylcholine receptors at the postjunctional membrane, but there also appears to be a variation in the functional ability of the antibodies to block the receptors (Drachman 1987). The condition is characterized by muscle weakness and fatigue on repeated use of that muscle. There is a 2:1 predominance of females and an association with thymic enlargement and thymomata, both benign and malignant.

Symptoms are primarily those of increasing muscle weakness and neuromuscular fatigue which improve after resting. Muscles of the eye and face are affected early in the disease and result in ptosis and diplopia. Bulbar palsy may produce swallowing and speech difficulties, and neck muscles may be affected. Sometimes there is early involvement of respiratory muscles. Variable progression or remission may occur. The involvement of particular muscle groups is inconstant, but proximal muscles of the upper limbs are affected more frequently than the lower limbs. The diagnosis may be confirmed by EMG or by demonstrating an improvement within 10–30 s of giving 2–10 mg intravenous edrophonium. This improvement lasts for about 5 min.

The current first line of treatment is immunological suppression to eliminate the antibody. Azathioprine or steroids are used and benefit 90% of cases. Immunosuppression may lead to neutropenia and serious infection. Thymectomy may be indicated, and surgery is now more frequently performed via the transcervical rather than the transsternal approach. Symptomatic relief is obtained with anticholinesterase preparations which act by potentiating the effects of acetylcholine. Pyridostigmine and neostigmine are most commonly employed. Concurrent use of atropine or propantheline may be required to block muscarinic effects, such as intestinal colic. Plasma exchange may be used for short-term treatment, particularly in a crisis, and its use before thymic surgery in severely affected patients may reduce the duration of postoperative IPPV (d'Empaire et al 1985).

Myasthenic crises may occur due either to the disease itself or to excessive amounts of an anticholinesterase. Cholinergic and myasthenic crises may be confused. Experimentally an excess of anticholinesterase has been shown to reduce the number of functioning receptors. Patients in a cholinergic crisis may need artificial ventilation.

Anaesthetic implications

Anaesthesia may be required for thymectomy or for other incidental surgery. Thymectomy is performed either via a median sternotomy or a transcervical approach. The former produces the greater anaesthetic difficulties.

In any type of surgery the main problem is the management of three variables: the muscle weakness produced by the patient's disease, his preoperative anticholinesterase medication and the surgeon's requirement for muscle relaxation. Respiratory function must be maintained in the pre- and postoperative period, and yet adequate intraoperative muscle relaxation should be provided for surgical access.

Neuromuscular blocking agents and anticholinesterases

The response to suxamethonium is unpredictable. Some resistance to normal doses has been reported, but recovery can sometimes be prolonged and incomplete due to a phase II block (Wainwright & Brodick 1987, Eisenkraft et al 1988). Suxamethonium can be used for rapid sequence induction of anaesthesia, provided its effect is monitored. Myasthenics may or may not have an increased sensitivity to non-depolarizing neuromuscular blockers. The blockade of the acetylcholine receptors by antibody resembles partial curarization, therefore the amount of a drug required to produce effective paralysis is often reduced. There is, however, wide variation in patient response to these drugs. The actual dose needed will depend on factors such as the stage of the disease, the presence or absence of a remission, the muscles being tested and whether or not anticholinesterase medication has been given preoperatively.

The method of management depends on the severity of the myasthenia, the type of operation and the anaesthetist's personal preference. In a series of 100 cases of transcervical thymectomy (Girnar & Weinreich 1976), those patients with mild myasthenia were given half their normal dose of pyridostigmine, while those with severe disease received their full dose. Anaesthesia and tracheal intubation were achieved with thiopentone, nitrous oxide, oxygen and either halothane or ethrane. IPPV was maintained without neuromuscular blocking agents and 92 patients were extubated successfully within 2 h of operation. Other authors have advocated inhalation induction with isoflurane, which produced sufficient muscle relaxation for transsternal thymectomy (Rowbottom 1989).

Upper abdominal surgery requires a greater degree of muscle relaxation than can be produced by inhalation agents alone. With the advent of clinical neuromuscular monitors, good control can be achieved using only small doses of non-depolarizing agents. The satisfactory use of atracurium in incremental doses has been reported (MacDonald et al 1984, Ward & Wright 1984). While the final doses required to produce 90–95% blockade varied from 0.05 to 0.33 mg/kg, it was agreed that with atracurium a relatively rapid rate of spontaneous recovery took place when compared with other neuromuscular blockers. Sensitivity to vecuronium has been shown and incremental dosages of 0.02–0.05 mg/kg are recommended (Hunter et al 1985, Eisenkraft et al 1990).

At the end of surgery, either reversal of neuromuscular blockade or restoration of respiration in the myasthenic may be achieved by the routine use of neostigmine and atropine. However, care must be taken not to give a dose in excess of the patient's normal requirements, otherwise a cholinergic crisis may occur (Eisencraft & Papatestas 1988). The patient's usual anticholinesterases may have to be given intravenously until oral medication can be taken. Approximately equivalent doses are:

neostigmine: 1 mg intravenously = 30 mg orally
pyridostigmine: 4 mg intravenously = 120 mg orally.

Postoperative complications

All patients will initially require high-dependency facilities and some patients will need postoperative IPPV. Attempts have been made to devise a scoring system to predict the need for postoperative IPPV (Leventhal et al 1980), but it has proved to be of limited value because of surgical variables (Grant & Jenkins 1982, Eisenkraft et al 1986). Appropriate surgical approaches to the thymus are still debated, although the transcervical approach is being increasingly used rather than the more traumatic transsternal route. The cervical approach is associated with a reduced requirement for prolonged postoperative IPPV. Thoracic epidural analgesia with light general anaesthesia has been described for transsternal thymectomy (Burgess & Wilcosky 1989).

It should be remembered that respiratory failure in myasthenic patients may be secondary to either a myasthenic or a cholinergic crisis. If there is doubt, IPPV should be instituted, anticholinesterase therapy stopped, and then only cautiously reintroduced after testing with intravenous edrophonium. An improvement suggests a myasthenic cause, while deterioration indicates a cholinergic crisis. Facilities should always be available for the rapid reinstitution of IPPV.

In advanced disease, respiratory muscle or bulbar weakness may occur perioperatively and can predispose the patient to pulmonary aspiration, chest infection or respiratory failure. Tracheostomy may occasionally be required, but only if artificial ventilation is prolonged and excess secretions are a problem.

EATON–LAMBERT SYNDROME

The Eaton–Lambert (Lambert–Eaton or myasthenic) syndrome is a myasthenia-like disorder due to an abnormality of neuromuscular transmission. It was originally described in association with carcinoma of the lung, but cases were subsequently reported in which no carcinoma was found. There is now evidence that both types of Eaton–Lambert syndrome are autoimmune in origin. There is a presynaptic abnormality that results in a decrease in the quanta of acetylcholine released by the passage of a nerve impulse. This contrasts with myasthenia gravis in which the abnormality involves the postganglionic receptors. The tumour-associated cases are almost exclusively found in association with small cell carcinoma of the lung, and the syndrome sometimes precedes the tumour by as much as 2 years. Tumour therapy may result in improvement of the neurological problems.

In a review of 50 cases, half of the patients had a malignancy (O'Neill et al 1988). The main neurological features were proximal lower limb weakness (100%), reduced or absent tendon reflexes (92%), posttetanic facilitation (78%), autonomic dysfunction (in particular dryness of the mouth; 74%) and mild to moderate ptosis (54%). The patients tended to be older than those with myasthenia gravis.

Electrophysiological criteria for diagnosis include a decrease in amplitude of EMG muscle potentials and further decline at low rates of stimulation. In contrast, there is an increase in amplitude of the action potential in response to stimulation at high rates or following muscle contraction.

Some symptomatic improvement has been reported with guanidine and 4-aminopyridine. The latter enhances the release of acetylcholine but the dose that can be given is limited by CNS excitation. More recently, 3,4-diaminopyridine, an oral preparation with fewer CNS effects, has been used (McEvoy et al 1989).

Anaesthetic implications

Neuromuscular problems

Prolonged paralysis can occur after the use of non-depolarizing neuromuscular blockers. Respiratory failure following anaesthesia may be a presenting feature (O'Neill et al 1988) and reversal with anticholinesterases may be incomplete (Telford & Hollway 1990). Neuromuscular blockers should therefore, if possible, be avoided. If essential, the effects of small doses should be monitored carefully with a nerve stimulator.

Improvements in evoked action potential have been reported after treatment with intravenous 4-aminopyridine (Agoston et al 1978) and oral 3,4-diaminopyridine (Telford & Hollway 1990). Where possible a local anaesthetic technique may be appropriate. Respiratory insuffiency should be treated promptly with IPPV.

Autonomic disturbances

Autonomic dysfunction may be a prominent feature (Mamdani et al 1985). Symptoms can include constipation, urinary retention and mouth dryness. Orthostatic hypotension and decreased R–R intervals on the ECG may be noted. In such patients there may be impairment of cardiovascular responses to hypotension, so drugs producing myocardial depression or peripheral vasodilatation should be used with caution.

PORPHYRIA

Porphyria is a rare group of disorders of porphyrin metabolism due to defects in certain enzymes involved in the synthesis of haem. They may be inherited or acquired. Haem, which is synthesized in the liver, bone marrow and erythrocytes, is required for the manufacture of haemoglobin, myoglobin and a number of other respiratory pigments, such as the cytochrome enzymes. In the hepatic porphyrias only the liver is involved in the abnormality of haem synthesis. It is this group of porphyrias that is of particular concern to the anaesthetist, and only these are discussed.

Biochemistry

In the hepatic porphyrias there is a relative deficiency of one of a number of enzymes involved in the hepatic synthesis of haem. The majority of haem manufactured by the liver is used in the biosynthesis of the cytochrome P-450 enzyme system. This system is important for drug metabolism.

The administration of certain drugs to patients with porphyria can, on occasion, result in severe neurological defects. Most of the drugs that are potentially dangerous in porphyria can increase delta-aminolaevulinic acid (ALA) synthase activity. This is the first enzyme required to initiate the sequence that results in the manufacture of haem. These drugs are usually lipid soluble. To assist their excretion by the kidneys they require transformation into water-soluble compounds by the cytochrome P-450 enzyme system. The presence of any of these drugs can increase the activity of this system. In other words, they have the potential to induce the cytochrome P-450 system. A demand for haem secondary to this induction of cytochrome P-450 results in a feedback mechanism stimulating further production of ALA synthase. The hepatic haem metabolic pathway is thus stimulated, but because the underlying enzyme deficiencies cannot fully cope with this extra activity there is an accumulation of certain porphyrins or their precursors at specific levels in the metabolic chain. These levels will vary according to the particular relevant enzyme deficiency. However, the evidence for this mechanism has been difficult to produce for a number of drugs, and some other explanation for their porphyrinogenicity must be sought.

Clinical features

The exact relationship between the biochemistry, the clinical features of porphyric crises and the neurological deficits is not known. However, there are characteristic pathological lesions in the brain, the spinal cord and the autonomic ganglia. Axon degeneration and demyelination are particular features. It has been suggested that the signs and symptoms of porphyria can be entirely attributed to neurological damage (Laiwah et al 1987). However, porphyrin precursors do not seem to be the main cause of the neurotoxicity, as has been previously postulated. Existing evidence suggests that the nervous system lesions are primarily secondary to a deficiency of haem, while neurotoxicity due to increased levels of ALA and porphobilinogen (PGB) may be an additional factor in their evolution.

Clinical and biochemical features of the hepatic porphyrias rarely appear before puberty, and, inexplicably, many patients remain permanently asymptomatic. Symptoms, which depend on the particular type of porphyria, may involve the gastrointestinal tract, the nervous system and the skin. Intermittent acute crises which may result in severe neurological deficits and occasionally death, may be precipitated by a variety of drugs. Crises may also be associated with menstruation, acute infection and pregnancy. The length of an attack, which may feature tachycardia and hypertension, can vary from hours to days. Acute abdominal crises with abdominal pain and vomiting can result in undiagnosed porphyrics being subjected to surgery. Specific tests to discover the exact type of porphyria exist for different precursors and/or porphyrins. Haematin, which suppresses ALA synthase activity, has been used to relieve the symptoms of porphyria.

Acute intermittent porphyria

Acute intermittent porphyria (AIP) is an autosomal dominant condition in which there is a reduction in porphyrobilinogen deaminase. During an attack there are increased amounts of ALA produced and excreted. AIP often presents with episodes of acute abdominal pain, vomiting, constipation and pyrexia in adult life. Motor, sensory and autonomic deficits may occur. There may be severe neuropsychiatric manifestations and the incidence in psychiatric populations is still much greater than in the normal population. Recently, family studies have shown that a high proportion of the individuals that are deficient in the enzyme never develop clinical symptoms of porphyria.

Hereditary coproporphyria

Hereditary coproporphyria (HC) is a rare condition with predominantly neural and visceral symptoms, similar to, but often milder than, AIP. Cutaneous photosensitivity may occur. There is a deficiency of coproporphyrinogen oxidase so that coproporphyrin levels may be elevated, in addition to those of ALA and porphobilinogen.

Variegate porphyria

Variegate porphyria (VP) results from a deficiency of protoporphyrinogen oxidase; the enzymatic block is therefore one step further on. The main symptoms are once again neural and visceral. Cutaneous lesions are present, commonly on the hands and face. Photosensitivity is due to the presence of certain porphyrins in the skin. In South Africa the incidence of VP is 0.3%.

Anaesthetic implications

A wide range of drugs, including anaesthetic agents, possess a potential for increasing the production of porphyrins or their precursors. Thus they may precipitate an acute porphyric attack. The use of any of these drugs may result in severe neurological deficits, including paraplegia or quadriplegia.

Since the overall number of porphyrics presenting for anaesthesia is small, experience with any individual anaesthetic drug is limited. In addition, a patient's response to a particular drug will vary according to the state of his porphyria. A retrospective analysis of 78 anaesthetics given to 47 patients suggested that, if the patient was in a latent period, the risks of using thiopentone were small. In contrast, seven in 10 patients given thiopentone during an acute episode had a worsening of porphyric symptoms (Mustajoki & Heinonen 1980). However, with such potentially devastating complications, the scope for prospective human 'studies' is limited.

For this reason, experimental models are used to assess the porphyrinogenicity of certain anaesthetic drugs. Various drugs have been tested for their ability to increase hepatic ALA synthase activity and produce intermediate porphyrins using such systems (Blekkenhorst et al 1980, Harrison et al 1985). While animal studies cannot necessarily be extrapolated to man, additional testing with known safe and unsafe drugs has provided some measure of control.

A simple method of drug classification has been suggested as a clinical guide to therapy in porphyria (Disler et al 1982):

- Category A drugs are those that have, in terms of clinical experience, been reported as dangerous or safe by three or more authorities.
- Category B drugs have been reported as being dangerous or safe by only two or fewer authorities. (Category A and B are usually associated with corroborated experimental animal data.)
- Category C drugs have been evaluated only in the experimental rat model.
- Category D drugs have been evaluated in chick embryo liver cell culture or in ovo. (Neither Category C nor Category D have corroborative reports of human cases.)

As is to be expected, the available data about some drugs is conflicting. For detailed general prescribing, reference to the work of Disler et al 1982 and Moore & Disler (1988) is recommended.

Potentially dangerous drugs of anaesthetic interest include: alcuronium, barbiturates, carbamazepine, carbromal, chloramphenicol, chlordiazepoxide, cimetidine, enflurane, ergot alkaloids, erythromycin, etomidate, flunitrazepam, frusemide, glutethimide, griseofulvin, hydantoins, imipramine, lignocaine, meprobamate, methyl dopa, metoclopramide, nalidixic acid, nikethimide, nitrazepam, pancuronium, pargyline, pentazocine, phenoxybenzamine, prilocaine, steroids, sulphonamides, sulphonylurea antidiabetic agents, theophylline, tranylcypromine and valproic acid.

Other drugs exist that have been used often, without complication, but single case reports or experimental data have implicated them as being porphyrogenic. This group includes: corticosteroids, diazepam, halothane, hydralazine, ketamine, pancuronium, pethidine, paraldehyde, and the sex hormones.

Although a single dose of etomidate produced equivocal results using a rat model, a continuous infusion of etomidate caused an increase in ALA synthase, coproporphyrin and protoporphyrin levels. It was therefore suggested that it should be considered as Category C and thus potentially porphyrinogenic (Harrison et al 1985). In this same study, ketamine did not produce any change but another single case report has implicated ketamine as porphyrinogenic. Other clinical and experimental evidence, however, suggests that it is safe (Rizk et al 1977, Blekkenhorst et al 1980, Capouet et al 1987).

Halothane, fentanyl, pethidine and pancuronium have been implicated in single case reports only, and have been used on other occasions without complication (Disler et al 1982).

Several recent clinical and experimental reports have suggested that propofol may be safe as an induction agent, although there have been two reports of asymptomatic increases in urinary porphyrins (Weir & Hodkinson 1988). The safety of atracurium and vecuronium is not yet known.

Anaesthetic management

General measures

A careful history and examination must be made to document existing neurological deficits. If a patient is admitted in a porphyric crisis, correction of fluid and electrolyte balance may be required. After this, and if necessary, tachycardia and hypertension can be treated with beta blockers. Autonomic neuropathy may be prominent during acute porphyria, but undergoes remission when the attack resolves.

Glucose administration inhibits enzyme induction and fasting increases it. Administration of dextrose should therefore begin before a period of starvation. Haematin has been reported to be effective in aborting clinical episodes of porphyria by decreasing ALA synthase activity.

Anaesthetic agents

All drugs known definitely to precipitate acute crises should be avoided. Individual clinical judgements must be made about the controversial ones, taking into account the presence or absence of an acute attack. Further advice can be obtained from the Porphyria Research Unit, Western Infirmary, Glasgow G11 6NT; Tel. 041 339 8822.

Drugs that are reported to be safe in porphyrics (Disler et al 1982, Moore & Disler 1988) include: adrenaline, aminoglycosides, aspirin, atropine, beta blockers, biguanides, bupivacaine, buprenorphine, cephalosporins, chlorpheniramine, chlorpromazine, codeine, coumarins, cyclopropane, diazoxide, digitalis, droperidol, d-tubocurarine, erythromycin, ether, fentanyl, heparin, hyoscine, insulin, labetolol, lorazepam, morphine, neostigmine, nitroglycerin, nitrous oxide, paracetamol, penicillins, procaine, prochlorperazine, promazine, promethazine, propranolol, sodium nitroprusside, suxamethonium, thyroxine and trifluoperazine.

The uneventful use of regional techniques with bupivacaine for childbirth has been reported (Brennan et al 1990, Mc Neill & Bennet 1990). Fears have sometimes been expressed about its inadvisability for medico–legal reasons lest subsequent neurological deterioration due to the disease itself might be attributed to the procedure.

REFERENCES

Agoston S, van Weerden T, Westra P, Broekert A 1978 Effects of 4-aminopyridine in Eaton Lambert syndrome. Br J Anaesth 50: 383–385

Barnes P J 1989 A new approach to the treatment of asthma. N Engl J Med 321: 1517–1527

Benthuysen J L, Ty Smith N, Sanford T J, Head N, Dec-Silver H 1986 Physiology of alfentanil-induced rigidity. Anesthesiology 64: 440–446

Blekkenhorst G H, Harrison G G, Cook E S, Eales L 1980 Screening of certain anaesthetic agents for their ability to elicit acute porphyric phases in susceptible patients. Br J Anaesth 52: 759–762

Bredahl C 1990 Krampeanfald og opitotonus efter propofol-anaestesi. (Seizures and opisthotonos after propofol anesthesia: a possible connection.) Ugeskr Laeg 152: 748–749

Brennan L, Halfacre J A, Woods S D 1990 Regional anaesthesia in porphyria. Br J Anaesth 65: 594–597

British Thoracic Society 1990a Guidelines for management of asthma in adults. I. Chronic persistent asthma in adults.

Br Med J 301: 651–653
British Thoracic Society 1990b Guidelines for management of asthma in adults. II. Acute severe asthma in adults. Br Med J 301: 797–800
Brownell A K W 1988 Malignant hyperthermia: relationship to other diseases. Br J Anaesth 60: 303–308
Burgess F W, Wilcosky B Jr 1989 Thoracic epidural anesthesia for transsternal thymectomy in myasthenia gravis. Anesth Analg 69: 529–531
Capouet V, Dernovoi B, Azagra J S 1987 Induction of anaesthesia with ketamine during an acute crisis of hereditary coproporphryia. Can J Anaesth 34: 388–390
Celesia C, Chen R, Bamforth B 1975 Effects of ketamine in epilepsy. Neurology 25: 169
Chalkiadis G A, Branch K G 1990 Cardiac arrest after isoflurane anaesthesia in a patient with Duchenne's muscular dystrophy. Anaesthesia 45: 22–25
CSM May 1989 Current problems 26
Corssen G, Little S, Tavakoli M 1974 Ketamine and epilepsy. Anesth Analg 53: 319
d'Empaire G, Hoaglin D C, Perlo V P, Pontoppidan H 1985 Effect of prethymectomy plasma exchange on postoperative respiratory function in myasthenia gravis. J Thor Cardiovasc Surg 89: 592–596
Disler P B, Blekkenhorst G H, Eales L, Moore M R, Straughan J 1982 Guidelines for drug prescription in patients with the acute porphyrias. S Afr Med J 61: 656–660
Drachman D B 1987 Present and future treatment of myasthenia gravis. N Engl J Med 316: 743–745
Ebrahim Z Y, DeBoer G E, Luders H, Hahn J F, Lesser R P 1986 Effect of etomidate on the electroencephalogram of patients with epilepsy. Anesth Analg 65: 1004–1006
Eisencraft J B, Papatestas A E, Kahn C H, Mora C T, Fagerstrom R, Genkins G 1986 Predicitng the need for postoperative mechanical ventilation in myasthenia gravis. Anesthesiology 65: 79–82
Eisenkraft J B, Book W J, Mann S M, Papatestas A E, Hubbard M 1988 Resistance to succinylcholine in myasthenia gravis: a dose response study. Anesthesiology 69: 760–763
Eisenkraft J B, Papatestas A E 1988 Anaesthesia for trans-sternal thymectomy in myasthenia gravis. Ann Coll Surg Engl 70: 257–258
Eisenkraft J B, Book W J, Papatestas A E 1990 Sensitivity to vecuronium in myasthenia gravis: a dose-response study. Can J Anaesth 37: 301–306
Fariello R G 1980 Epileptogenic properties of enflurane and their clincial interpretation. Electroencephalogr Clin Neurophysiol 48: 595–598
Ferrer-Allado T, Brechner V L, Dymond A, Cozen H, Crandall P 1973 Ketamine-induced electroconvulsive phenomena in the human limbic and thalamic region. Anesthesiology 38: 333–344
Ghoneim M, Yamada T 1977 Etomidate: a clinical and encephalographic comparison with thiopental. Anesth Analg 56: 479
Girnar D S, Weinreich A I 1976 Anesthesia for transcervical thymectomy in myasthenia gravis. Anesth Analg 55: 13–17
Grant I S 1986 Delayed convulsions following enflurane anaesthesia. Anaesthesia 41: 1024–1025
Grant I S, Hutchinson G 1983 Epileptiform seizures during prolonged etomidate sedation. Lancet 2: 511–512
Grant R P, Jenkins L C 1982 Prediction of the need for postoperative mechanical ventilation in myasthenia gravis: thymectomy compared with other surgical procedures. Can Anaesth Soc J 29: 112–116
Harrison G G, Moore M R, Meissner P N 1985 Porphyrinogenicity of etomidate and ketamine as continuous infusions. Br J Anaesth 57: 420–423
Hirshman C A, Bergman N A 1990 Factors influencing intrapulmonary airway calibre during anaesthesia. Br J Anaesth 65: 30–42
Hirshman C, Edelstein G, Peetz S, Wayne R, Downes H 1982 Mechanisms of action of inhalational agents on airways. Anesthesiology 56: 107–111
Hunter J M, Bell C F, Florence A M, Jones R S, Utting J E 1985 Vecuronium in the myasthenic patient. Anaesthesia 40: 848–853
Kingston H G G, Hirshman C A 1984 Perioperative management of the patient with asthma. Anesth Analg 63: 844–855
Kofke W A, Young R S K, Davis P et al 1989 Isoflurane for refractory status epilepticus: a clinical series. Anesthesiology 71: 653–659
Kreiger W, Koerner M 1987 Generalized grand mal seizure after recovery from uncomplicated fentanyl-etomidate anesthesia. Anesth Analg 66: 284–285
Laiwah A C Y, Moore M R, Goldberg A 1987 Pathogenesis of acute porphyria. Q J Med 241: 377–392
Larsen U T, Juhl B, Hein-Sorensen O, Olivarius B de F 1989 Complications during anaesthesia in patients with Duchenne's muscular dystrophy (a retrospective study). Can J Anaesth 36: 418–422
Leventhal S R, Orkin F K, Hirsch R A 1980 Prediction of the need for postoperative mechanical ventilation in myasthenia gravis. Anesthesiology 53: 26–30
McAlpine L G, Thomson N C 1989 Lidocaine-induced bronchoconstriction in asthmatic patients: relation to histamine airway responsiveness and effect of preservatives. Chest 96: 1012–1015.
MacDonald A M, Keen R I, Pugh N D 1984 Myasthenia gravis and atracurium. Br J Anaesth 56: 651–654
McEvoy K M, Windebank A J, Daube J R, Low P A 1989 3,4-Diaminopyridine in the treatment of Lambert-Eaton myasthenic syndrome. N Engl J Med 321: 1567–1571
McNeill M J, Bennet A 1990 Use of regional anaesthesia in a patient with acute porphyria. Br J Anaesth 64: 371–373
Male C G, Allen E M 1977 Methohexitone-induced convulsions in epileptics. Anaesth Intensive Care 5: 226–230
Mamdani M B, Walsh R L, Rubino F A, Brannegan R T, Hwang M H 1985 Autonomic dysfunction and Eaton Lambert syndrome. J Auton Nerv Syst 12: 315–320
Mecarelli O, De Feo M R, Romanini L, Calvisi V, D'Andrea E 1981 EEG and clinical features in epileptic children during halothane anaesthesia. Electroencephalogr Clin Neurophysiol 52: 486–489
Milne B, Rosales J K 1982 Anaesthetic considerations in patients with muscular dystrophy undergoing spinal fusion and Harrington rod insertion. Can Anaesth Soc J 29: 250–254
Modica P A, Tempelhoff R 1989 Seizures during emergence from anesthesia. Anesthesiology 71: 296–300
Modica P A, Tempelhoff R, White P F 1990a Pro- and anticonvulsant effects of anesthetics. Part I. Anesth Analg 70: 303–315

Modica P A, Tempelhoff R, White P F 1990b Pro- and anticonvulsant effects of anesthetics. Part II. Anesth Analg 70; 433–444
Moore M R, Disler P B 1988 Drug-sensitive diseases. I. Acute porphyrias. Adverse Drug React Bull 129: 484–487
Mustajoki P, Heinonen J 1980 General anaesthesia in 'inducible' porphyrias. Anesthesiology 53: 15–20
Nakakimura K, Sakabe T, Funatsu N, Maekawa T, Takeshita H 1988 Metabolic activation of intercortical and corticothalamic pathways during enflurane anesthesia in rats. Anesthesiology 68: 777–782
Neigh J L, Garman J K, Harp J R 1971 The electroencephalographic pattern during anesthesia with Ethrane: effects of depth of anesthesia, Pa_{CO_2}, and nitrous oxide. Anesthesiology 35: 482–487
Nicoll J M V 1986 Status epilepticus following enflurane anaesthesia. Anaesthesia 41: 927–930
Olsson G L 1987 Bronchospasm during anaesthesia: a computer-aided incidence study of 136,929 patients. Acta Anaesthesiol Scand 31: 244–252
O'Neill J H, Murray N M, Newsom-Davies J 1988 The Lambert-Eaton myasthenic syndrome: a review of 50 cases. Brain 111: 577–596
Opitz A, Brecht S, Stenzel E 1977 Enfluran-Anaestheseien bei epileptikern. (Enflurane anaesthesia for epileptic patients.) Der Anaesthesist 26: 329–332
Opitz A, Marschall M, Degen R, Koch D 1983 General anaesthesia in patients with epilepsy and status epilepticus. Adv Neurol 34: 531–535
Ramanathan J, Osborne B, Sibai B 1990 Epidural anesthesia in asthmatic parturients. Anesth Analg 70: S317
Rizk S K, Jacobsen J H, Silvay G 1977 Ketamine as an induction agent for acute intermittent porphyria. Anesthesiology 46: 305–306.
Roizen M F 1987 Comment. Survey of Anesthesiology 31: 232–233
Rowbottom S J 1989 Isoflurane for thymectomy in myasthenia gravis. Anaesth Intensive Care 17: 444–447
Rubiano R, Chang J-L, Carroll J, Sonbolian N, Larson C E 1987 Acute rhabdomyolysis following halothane anesthesia without succinylcholine. Anesthesiology 67: 856–857
Sethna N F, Rockoff M A, Worthen H M, Rosnow J M 1988 Anesthesia-related complications in children with Duchenne muscular dystrophy. Anesthesiology 68: 462–465
Shearer E S 1990 Convulsion and propofol. Anaesthesia 45: 255–256
Simpson K H, Halsall P J, Carr C M E, Stewart K G 1988 Propofol reduces seizure duration in patients having anaesthesia for electroconvulsive therapy. Br J Anaesth 61: 343–344
Smith C L, Bush G H 1985 Anaesthesia and progressive muscular dystrophy. Br J Anaesth 57: 1113–1118
Telford R J, Hollway T E 1990 The myasthenic syndrome: anaesthesia in a patient treated with 3,4, diaminopyridine. Br J Anaesth 64: 363–366
Tempelhoff R, Modica P A, Spitznagel E L 1990 Anticonvulsant therapy increases fentanyl requirements during anaesthesia for craniotomy. Can J Anaesth 37: 327–332
Ty Smith N, Benthuysen J L, Bickford R G et al 1989 Seizures during opioid anaesthetic induction: are they opioid-induced rigidity? Anesthesiology 71: 852–862
Wainwright A P, Brodrick P M 1987 Suxamethonium in myasthenia gravis. Anaesthesia 42: 950–957
Ward S, Wright D J 1984 Neuromuscular blockade in myasthenia gravis with atracurium besylate. Anaesthesia 39: 51–53
Weir P M, Hodkinson B P 1988 Is propofol a safe agent in porphyria? Anaesthesia 43: 1022–1023
Worthen H M, Kuban K C K, Sullivan R N, Bresnan M D 1987 A national survey of anesthetic complications in children with Duchenne's muscular dystrophy. Anesth Analg 66: S190

23

Hazards of pseudocholinesterase deficiency

F. S. Jensen and J. Viby-Mogensen

INTRODUCTION

The depolarizing neuromuscular blocking agent, succinylcholine, is still commonly used to facilitate tracheal intubation due to its rapid onset and short duration of action. After an intravenous injection, succinylcholine is hydrolysed in plasma by plasma cholinesterase (pChe, pseudocholinesterase) in a few minutes and only 5–10% of the injected drug actually reaches the neuromuscular endplates. However, in patients with decreased plasma cholinesterase activity, a prolonged duration of action of succinylcholine is seen and some patients remain paralysed for hours (Viby-Mogensen 1983, Whittaker 1986, Pantuck & Pantuck 1987).

In this article the causes and the clinical significance of pChe deficiency are discussed. The main emphasis is placed on the significance of pChe for the hydrolysis of succinylcholine, but the relationship between abnormal pChe activity and the effect of the new non-depolarizing neuromuscular blocking drug, mivacurium, is also dealt with. Further, the recent developments in identification of pChe genotypes are presented.

THE NORMAL PLASMA CHOLINESTERASE ENZYME

Plasma cholinesterase (acylcholine-acylhydrolase E.C. 3.1.1.8) is a glycoprotein containing about 24% carbohydrate. It is primarily present as a tetramer of four identical subunits or peptide chains. The tetrameric subunits are held together by two interchain disulfide bridges and by hydrophobic, non-covalent forces (Lockridge et al 1979). Each subunit contains 574 amino acids and one active site, and has a molecular weight of approximately 85 000 Da. Each has two active sites, one negatively (anionic) charged binding to positively charged quaternary ammonium groups at the substrate, the other an esteratic site breaking ester bonds (Muensch et al 1976).

Plasma cholinesterase is synthesized in the liver and immediately released into the plasma. The concentration here is a reflection of the rate of hydrolysis (Whittaker 1986). The enzyme is also found in both the central and peripheral nervous system of all animals as well as in cerebrospinal fluid (Kambam et al 1989). Since 1932 it has been recognized as an enzyme that hydrolyses choline esters (Stedman et al 1932). However, the physiological function of pChe is not known. The half-life has been estimated as about 12 days by measuring the decrease of enzyme activity following injection of purified pChe (Østergaard et al 1988).

DECREASED PLASMA CHOLINESTERASE ACTIVITY

Physiological variation

The pChe activity is known to vary with age, sex, body fat and with other parameters such as plasma lipids or lipoprotein fractions (Whittaker

1986). Females have lower activity than males (Propert & Brackenridge 1976). In the newborn the activity is about 50–60% of the healthy adult, but the activity increases gradually and by the age of 3–4 years the activity is approximately 30% higher than in adults. The cholinesterase activity decreases slowly to 75% during the years from puberty to 70–80 years of age.

In the first trimester of pregnancy the pChe activity decreases to 70–80% of prepregnant values. This is maintained until delivery, with a further decrease 2–4 days after delivery, after which time the activity returns to normal after 3–6 weeks. The low pChe activity during pregnancy is probably due to decreased synthesis by the liver.

Reduced activity due to disease

In 50–75% of patients with liver diseases such as hepatitis, liver abscess and cirrhosis, a decrease in pChe activity to about 50% or even lower is seen. In diseases with biliary obstruction, however, the activity of pChe is not affected unless there is damage to the liver cells as well (Jorge & Sanchez 1976, Singh et al 1976, Viby-Mogensen & Hanel 1978). In patients with acute or chronic renal disease the pChe may be reduced to a level of 30%, probably due to impaired liver synthesis. Following renal transplantation the activity initially decreases but returns to normal after about 4 weeks (Simon et al 1969, Zarday et al 1975, Whittaker 1986). Patients with malignant tumors often have a pChe activity 60–65% of healthy normal adult values. A more pronounced reduction in activity below 25% is seen in patients with gastrointestinal tumours or bronchogenic carcinomata (Kaniaris et al 1979). A decrease in activity to 20% of normal is seen in patients with severe burns a few days after the trauma. There is a correlation between the degree of injury and the pChe activity (Viby-Mogensen et al 1975).

Iatrogenic changes

Many different drugs reduce pChe activity, either by inhibition of the enzyme in the plasma or by a reduced synthesis of the enzyme in the liver. Inhibitors are usually classified as reversible or irreversible. A great variety of drugs is known to cause a reversible reduction in pChe activity, that is anaesthetic agents, neuromuscular blocking drugs and reversal agents, antibiotics, cytotoxic drugs and several hormones. Clinically, the most important drugs are ecothiopate eyedrops, pesticides and the new bronchodilator drug, bambuterol (see p. 364). Ecothiopate eyedrops used in the treatment of glaucoma inhibit the activity by 70–100% (Cavallaro et al 1968). The most potent irreversible pChe inhibitors are organophosphates such as pesticides, which may reduce the pChe activity by 100%.

The inherited variants

The biosynthesis and the structural quality of pChe is controlled by at least four autosomal allelic genes at locus E_1, which is located on the long arm of chromosome 3 (Yang et al 1984, Soreq et al 1987). The four allelic genes are the E_1^u (usual), responsible for the normal or usual form, the E_1^a (atypical), the E_1^f (fluoride resistant) and the E_1^s (silent) gene with no detectable enzymatic activity. Combination of these genes can give anyone of ten genotypes, that is homozygous for two normal genes (E_1^u E_1^u), heterozygous for one normal and one abnormal gene (E_1^a E_1^u, E_1^u E_1^f, E_1^u E_1^s), heterozygous for two abnormal genes (E_1^a E_1^f, E_1^f E_1^s, E_1^a E_1^s), and homozygous for two abnormal genes (E_1^a E_1^a, E_1^f E_1^f, E_1^s E_1^s). During the last decade, several additional variants have been discovered: E_1^j (Garry et al 1976), E_1^k (Rubinstein et al 1978) and E_1^h (Whittaker & Britten 1987).

The frequency of the different cholinesterase variants varies in different populations (Whittaker 1986). In Caucasians, 95–97% have normal pChe phenotype (E_1^u E_1^u) and only 2.5–4.0% (1:25) will be heterozygous for the usual and the atypical gene (E_1^u E_1^a). The incidence of other heterozygous genotypes is lower: E_1^u E_1^f in 0.4% of the population (1:250) and E_1^u E_1^s in 0.5% of the population (1:200). Clinically, the most important variant is the homozygous atypical genotype (E_1^a E_1^a), with an incidence of 0.04% (1:2500). This is connected with long-lasting neuromuscular blockade following a normal dose of succinylcholine. In other ethnic groups the gene frequencies vary. In certain Eskimo groups, for example, the E_1^s variant is common and the E_1^a variant is very rare.

DETERMINATION OF PLASMA CHOLINESTERASE ACTIVITY AND PHENOTYPES

Until recently the determination of the different pChe variants has been done on the basis of biochemical studies, clinical information available and comprehensive family studies, often necessary for a correct determination of phenotypes.

Plasma cholinesterase activity is determined by measuring the rate of hydrolysis of a substrate (an ester) catalyzed by pChe. Most commonly used today is ultraviolet spectrophotometry using benzoylcholine or propionylthiocholine as a substrate (Kalow & Lindsay 1955, Whittaker 1986). It is not possible to differentiate the various genotypes of pChe by measuring the enzyme activity alone because the activity of different phenotypes overlaps. Furthermore, the enzyme from the various phenotypes differs quantitatively. The atypical (dibucaine-resistant) form of human pChe, with reduced affinity for choline ester substrates, was first described by Kalow & Genest (1957). They classified the types of esterases as usual, intermediate or atypical according to differences in sensitivity to inhibition by the local anaesthetic dibucaine hydrochloride. From the percentage inhibition of cholinesterase by a 10^{-5} molar concentration of dibucaine (DN or dibucaine number) under specific experimental conditions, the usual esterase was inhibited about 80% and the atypical esterase was inhibited about 20%. Heterozygous carriers for the normal and the atypical gene showed inhibition values of about 60%.

It is not possible to differentiate all phenotypes solely by the DN, therefore other inhibitors, that is fluoride and urea, have been used to identify the pChe variants (Harris & Whittaker 1961, Hanel & Viby-Mogensen 1977).

By combining the dibucaine, fluoride and urea numbers it is usually possible to determine the patient's phenotype. However, patients homozygous for the usual gene cannot be distinguished biochemically with certainty from patients heterozygous for the silent and the usual gene, and patients homozygous for the atypical gene cannot be distinguished from patients heterozygous for the atypical and the silent gene. In these cases family studies are of decisive significance. In patients homozygous for the silent gene no, or very little, pChe activity is found (Liddell et al 1962). Recent studies indicate that the silent variant in fact represents two, or possibly even several, different genes. So far two types have been recognized: Type I with no activity and Type II with about 2% of the usual activity (Viby-Mogensen 1983). The relationship between pChe activity and the dibucaine, fluoride and urea numbers of the various well-established pChe variants at locus E_1 is given in Table 23.1.

To detect the new alleles, j, k, and h (Evans & Wardell 1984, Whittaker & Britten 1987), another inhibiting substance, trimethylammonium bromide

Table 23.1 The biochemical characteristics of the various cholinesterase variants (locus E_1; from the Danish Cholinesterase Research Unit, Viby-Mogensen 1983)

Genotype	No. of patients	pChe activity (U/l)	Dibucaine number	Fluoride number	Urea number
$E_1^u E_1^u$ *	970	690–1560	79–87	55–66	41–53
$E_1^u E_1^a$ *	745	433–1197	55–72	40–53	54–69
$E_1^a E_1^a$ *	207	190–732	14–27	16–30	86–100
$E_1^u E_1^s$ *	78	329–870	78–86	56–66	42–52
$E_1^a E_1^s$ *	33	146–450	16–27	19–30	86–100
$E_1^s E_1^s$	9	0–48	—	—	—
$E_1^u E_1^f$ †	21	514–1150	74–80	44–53	61–71
$E_1^a E_1^f$ †	12	318–777	45–52	25–33	75–100
$E_1^f E_1^s$ †	2	351–509	63–64	26–38	90–91

*indicates that 2.5 and 97.5 percentiles are given.
†indicates that ranges are given.

(Ro2-0683, the dimethylcarbamate of 2-hydroxy-5-phenylbenzyl), is used. The k and j genes can only be identified with certainty when they occur together with the atypical variant. The two phenotype combinations, $E_1^a\ E_1^k$ and $E_1^a\ E_1^j$, give rise to characteristic Ro2-inhibitor numbers. A reduction in pChe activity by 33% and 66% is seen due to the k and j genes, respectively.

The new h-variant is a quantitative variant and, when segregating with the atypical gene, it reduces the enzymatic activity by approximately 90%. The activity can be as low as that found in some patients homozygous for the silent genes (Whittaker & Britten 1987).

NEW DEVELOPMENTS IN IDENTIFICATION OF GENOTYPES:

Structural analysis of variants at DNA level

The increasing number of possible phenotypes has complicated the identification of phenotypes using only biochemical analysis. A DNA structural basis for cholinesterase phenotyping would be valuable, as well as being a logical frame of reference for developing future diagnostic methods to distinguish the important new genotypes.

Molecular biological studies are the basis for new, specific, diagnostic methods to identify pChe variants. The complete amino acid sequence of the normal enzyme was determined by Lockridge et al (1987). Each of the four subunits was found to contain 574 amino acids and the active site serine was found to be the 198th residue from the amino terminus. The DNA sequence coding for the usual form of pChe could then be compared to the analogous coding for other variants of the enzyme, hence it was possible to deduce the amino acid alterations in the protein (Table 23.2 & Fig. 23.1).

New specific diagnostic methods are now being developed using DNA from peripheral blood cells, the polymerase chain reaction (PCR) amplification, allele-specific oligonucleotide probes and colorimetric (non-radioactive) detection methods. There is no doubt that future studies using gene technology will increase our understanding of the physiological and clinical significance of pChe and its variants.

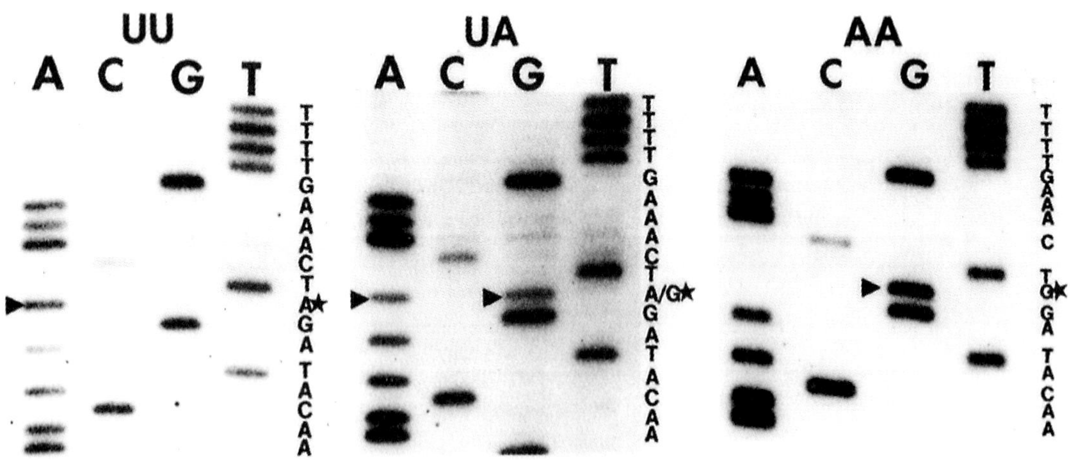

Fig. 23.1 DNA sequence of usual ($E_1^u\ E_1^u$), heterozygous ($E_1^u\ E_1^a$), and atypical ($E_1^a\ E_1^a$) cholinesterases showing the nucleotide substitution in atypical cholinesterase. Total genomic DNA from three individuals was amplified by the polymerase chain reaction with oligonucleotides corresponding to the coding region of the cholinesterase gene. Both strands of the double-stranded, amplified DNA were sequenced simultaneously. The sequences are identical except for the nucleotide marked with a star. Codon 70 is GAT in $E_1^u\ E_1^u$, GAT and GGT in $E_1^u\ E_1^a$, and GGT in $E_1^a\ E_1^a$. (From McGuire et al 1989.)

Table 23.2 Current status of identification of human pChe variants at DNA level

Common name	Amino acid change	DNA change
Usual	None	None
Atypical	70 Asp → Gly	nt 209 (GAT → GGT) (Lockridge et al 1979)
Silent	117 Gly → frameshift	nt 351 (GGT → GGAG) (Nogueira et al 1990)
Fluoride 1	243 Thr → Met	nt 728 (ACG → ATG) (Bartels et al 1990)
Fluoride 2	390 Gly → Val	nt 1169 (GGT → GTT) (Bartels et al 1990)
K-variant	539 Ala → Thr	nt 1615 (GCA → ACA) (Bartels et al 1992a)
H-variant	142 Val → Met	nt 424 (GTG → ATG) (Jensen et al 1992b)
J-variant	497 Glu → Val	nt 1490 (GAA → GTA) (Bartels et al 1992)

DNA bases: A, adenine; C, cytosine; G, guanine; T, thymine. Amino acids: Asp, aspartate; Glu, glutamine; Gly, glycine; Met, methionine; Thr, threonine; Val, valine.

RELATION BETWEEN PLASMA CHOLINESTERASE ACTIVITY AND REACTION TO SUCCINYLCHOLINE

After intravenous injection, succinylcholine (or succinyldicholine) is first hydrolyzed to the monocholine ester of succinic acid and choline. Succinylmonocholine, which has almost no neuromuscular blocking activity, is later hydrolyzed to succinic acid and choline. The dicholine is hydrolyzed at a rate approximately six times as fast as the monocholine (Whittaker 1986). According to this, a larger proportion of succinylcholine reaches the neuromuscular endplate if the pChe activity is decreased, and this may cause a prolonged neuromuscular block.

When discussing the correlation between phenotypes and recovery of neuromuscular function following succinylcholine the phenotypes can conveniently be divided into four groups, that is those homozygous for the usual gene, those heterozygous for the usual and one of the abnormal genes, those heterozygous for two abnormal genes and finally those patients homozygous for two abnormal genes.

Phenotypically normal patients

In phenotypically normal patients (E_1^u E_1^u) the first neuromuscular response to peripheral nerve stimulation is seen 5–10 min after an intubation dose of succinylcholine (1 mg/kg) and the time to 90% twitch height recovery is 6–13 min (Viby-Mogensen 1980; Table 23.3). A good correlation exists between pChe activity and the time to first evoked response in patients with normal genotype (Fig. 23.2). However, within the reference values of normal pChe activity, time to first evoked response is practically independent of the enzyme activity, and even pChe activities as low as 400 U/1 cause only a moderate prolongation of the block. Only when the activity is severely depressed will the time to first evoked response be significantly prolonged. In patients with normal pChe activity and phenotype a typically depolarizing block with equal inhibition of all four responses in the train-of-four (TOF) (Ali et al 1970) is seen following succinylcholine injection. However, prolonged administration of succinylcholine, as repeated injection or infusion, alters the reaction to nerve stimulation. The original depolarizing block, or Phase I block, changes to a non-depolarizing-like block or a Phase II block, characterized by fade in the TOF response. There are large individual variations as to how easily a Phase II block develops. In some patients it is seen following relatively small doses of 2–3 mg/kg, whereas others might receive large doses of succinylcholine and not show a Phase II block.

Table 23.3 Time to response to train-of-four nerve stimulation and to 90% twitch height recovery following 1 mg/kg succinylcholine (Viby-Mogensen 1980, 1981a, b). Means and ranges are given

Genotype	No. of patients	First evoked response (min)	90% twitch height recovery (min)
$E_1^u E_1^u$	41	5.6 (4.0–8.0)	9.3 (6.0–13.0)
$E_1^u E_1^a$, $E_1^u E_1^s$, $E_1^u E_1^f$	39	8.6 (4.0–15.0)	13.0 (7.5–22.0)
$E_1^a E_1^f$, $E_1^f E_1^s$	4	24.5 (22.5–25.0)	29.5 (29.0–30.0)
$E_1^a E_1^a$	12	38.0 (35.0–40.0)	160.0 (120.0–180.0)

The development of a Phase II block depends on the amount of succinylcholine that reaches the neuromuscular endplate, and this, of course, depends on both the pChe activity and the dose of succinylcholine.

Patients heterozygous for the usual and one of the abnormal genes

Patients heterozygous for the usual and one of the abnormal genes, (E_1^u E_1^a, E_1^u E_1^s and E_1^u E_1^f) normally show a depolarizing block following a single dose of succinylcholine and the duration of action may be normal or slightly prolonged (Table 23.3; Viby-Mogensen 1981a). However, if the patient is precurarized with a small dose of a non-depolarizing relaxant, that is pancuronium, and given an increased dose of succinylcholine (e.g. 1.5 mg/kg) to facilitate tracheal intubation, a Phase II block and prolonged respiratory insuf-

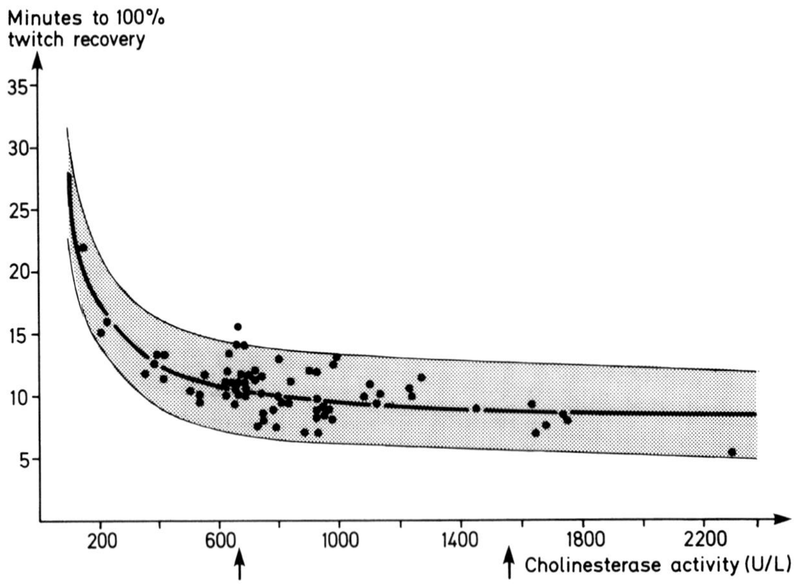

Fig. 23.2 Correlation between cholinesterase activity and time to recovery of 100% twitch height following administration of succinylcholine 1 mg kg^{-1} i.v. to 70 phenotypically normal patients anaesthetized with thiopental, N_2O/O_2, halothane. The fitted regression line and 95% prediction region are given. Arrows indicate the normal range of cholinesterase activity in phenotypically normal patients. (From Viby-Mogensen 1980.)

ficiency might be seen. This may also occur if the pChe activity is low because of pregnancy, disease or the administration of a drug that depresses the enzyme activity (i.e. bambuterol, see p. 365).

Patients heterozygous for the fluoride-resistant and the silent gene or atypical and fluoride-resistant gene

Patients heterozygous for the fluoride-resistant and the silent gene (E_1^f E_1^s) or atypical and fluoride-resistant gene (E_1^a E_1^f) do not have normal enzyme activity and the hydrolysis of succinylcholine is slower. A Phase II block is seen following succinylcholine (1 mg/kg) and the time to 90% twitch height recovery is slightly prolonged (Table 23.3; Viby-Mogensen 1981a).

Patients homozygous for the atypical gene or heterozygous for the atypical and silent gene

In patients homozygous for the atypical gene (E_1^a E_1^a) and patients heterozygous for the atypical and the silent gene (E_1^a E_1^s) a Phase II block is always seen following 1 mg/kg succinylcholine. The mean duration of apnea (or time to first response to nerve stimulation) is 50–60 min following this dose. Time to adequate clinical recovery is 140–150 min (Table 23.3 & Fig. 23.3; Viby-Mogensen 1981b).

Patients homozygous for the silent gene

No controlled study using a nerve stimulator in patients with genotype E_1^s E_1^s (homozygous for the silent gene) has been published. Because of the lack of enzyme activity, these patients will probably react like patients homozygous for the atypical gene.

Patients homozygous for the fluoride-resistant gene

In patients homozygous for the fluoride-resistant gene (E_1^f E_1^f) no controlled study has been published using a nerve stimulator, but normal or slightly prolonged apnea has been reported following normal doses of succinylcholine.

DIAGNOSIS AND TREATMENT OF PROLONGED RESPONSE TO SUCCINYLCHOLINE

If prolonged apnoea is suspected to be caused by succinylcholine, the first part of treatment is patience on the part of the anaesthetist. While the patient is kept anaesthetized and ventilated, a nerve stimulator is applied to determine whether or not the prolonged apnoea is, in fact, caused by succinylcholine. If a normal reaction to nerve stimulation is seen, the prolonged apnoea is not caused by the neuromuscular blocking drug. An abnormal reaction to nerve stimulation indicates that the prolonged apnoea may be due to an overdose of succinylcholine, an abnormal pChe activity and/or an abnormal phenotype. In a Danish survey it was found that 60% of patients with prolonged response to a normal dose of succinylcholine had inherited deficiency of pChe, 10% had normal phenotype but low activity and 30% had normal phenotype and normal activity indicating that

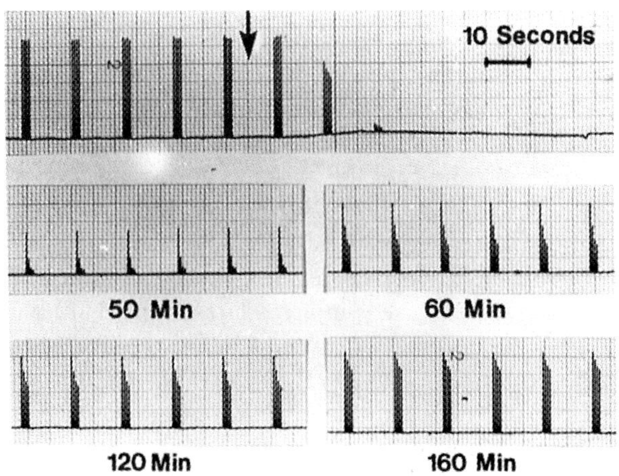

Fig. 23.3 The reaction to train-of-four (TOF) nerve stimulation after intravenous administration of succinylcholine 1 mg kg^{-1} (arrow) in a patient homozygous for the atypical gene (E_1^a E_1^a). Anaesthesia: thiopental, N_2O/O_2, halothane. The neuromuscular blockade is markedly prolonged compared with that seen in normal patients and there is pronounced fade in the TOF response (phase II block). (From Viby-Mogensen 1983.)

other causes of prolonged apnoea are common, for instance respiratory depression or hyperventilation (Viby-Mogensen & Hanel 1978).

The treatment of patients with prolonged apnoea following succinylcholine depends on the cholinesterase activity and genotype. If the patient has a normal genotype, only succinylcholine bound to the receptors persists after a short time (minutes). There is a 'pure' Phase II block which is reversible by anticholinesterases (Viby-Mogensen 1983, Donati & Bevan 1985).

In patients with abnormal phenotypes the presence of a Phase II block does not indicate that reversion of a block can be produced by a cholinesterase inhibitor. The effect of the anticholinesterase drug is unpredictable and depends on the phenotype, the dose of the inhibitor and the dose of succinylcholine.

In patients homozygous for the atypical enzyme a mixed block with both a depolarizing and a non-depolarizing element is often seen. This is due to the fact that succinylcholine persists for a longer time both in plasma and at the neuromuscular junction. Immediately after administration of succinylcholine the depolarizing block dominates; later the non-depolarizing part of the block becomes more important (Viby-Mogensen 1981b). These two kinds of block have to be treated separately. The depolarizing block can be treated with human cholinesterase and the non-depolarizing part with anticholinesterase. If purified human cholinesterase is administered within 30 min after the injection of succinylcholine, it will hydrolyze the persisting free succinylcholine and a faster recovery is seen. The remaining part of the block may be restored by neostigmine. If the cholinesterase is injected later than 35–40 min after the injection of succinylcholine, recovery will be prolonged (Fig. 23.4). If the TOF ratio is low (<0.70), neostigmine or edrophonium may be administered to treat the remaining non-depolarizing part of the block.

In daily clinical practice the patient's cholinesterase activity and phenotype are normally not known when a prolonged response to succinylcholine is seen.

Hence the most important action is to keep the patient anaesthetized and ventilated. If an abnormal pChe phenotype cannot be excluded the block should not be treated solely with an anticholinesterase drug; this may prolong the block. To avoid the complications of succinylcholine the initial dose should not exceed 1.0–1.5 mg/kg, and no other relaxant drug should be administered until there are at least signs of recovery of neuromuscular function. Furthermore, monitoring the neuromuscular function with a peripheral nerve stimulator is recommended.

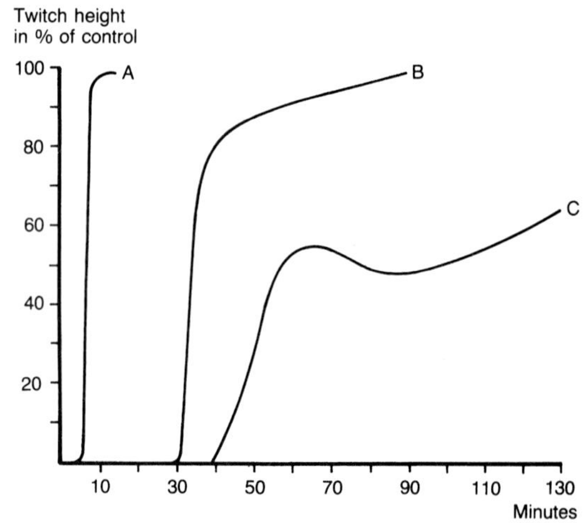

Fig. 23.4 Recovery of thumb twitch (% of control) following intravenous administration of 1 mg/kg succinylcholine. **A**: spontaneous recovery in genotypically normal patients. **B and C**: recovery in patients homozygous for the atypical enzyme following intravenous administration of human plasma cholinesterase 30 and 90 min following succinylcholine, respectively. See text for further explanation. (From Østergaard & Viby-Mogensen 1989.)

NEW ASPECTS OF PLASMA CHOLINESTERASE

Bambuterol

Most drugs that inhibit pChe activity prolong the duration of action of succinylcholine only moderately (20–25 min). However, the new bronchodilator prodrug of terbutaline, bambuterol, causes a clinically significant prolongation of the duration of action of succinylcholine due to its very pronounced pChe inhibiting effect (Fisher et al 1988, Bang et al 1990a). Bambuterol is an inactive prodrug formed by linking two carbamate groups to terbutaline. The drug has no $beta_2$ agonistic activity itself, and is broken down to terbutaline by a combination of oxidative metabolism and esterase-catalyzed hydrolysis by pChe. However, as the carbamates are strong inhibitors of pChe, bambuterol slows down its own hydrolysis by the inhibition of pChe. The effect of bambuterol on the pChe activity has been found to be maximal 2–3 h after oral administration and to remain for about 8 h. Bang et al 1990a found that in patients with the normal phenotype the median inhibition of enzyme activity 2 h after bambuterol (30 mg orally) was 90%. Following an injection of succinylcholine (1 mg/kg) at that time the neuromuscular recovery was 3–4 times prolonged. In some patients with very low pChe activity a Phase II block developed, resulting in a clinically very significant prolonged neuromuscular blockade.

In patients heterozygous for the usual and the atypical gene, bambuterol (20 mg) causes a two- to three-fold prolongation of the duration of action of succinylcholine. In some patients a clinically very significant prolonged neuromuscular blockade may be seen and a respiratory insufficiency of 2–3 h duration may follow (Bang et al 1990b).

Mivacurium

Mivacurium is a new short-acting non-depolarizing relaxant that has been designed to undergo hydrolysis by pChe. In vitro, the hydrolysis rate of mivacurium by purified human pChe is about 70–80% of the rate of hydrolysis of succinylcholine (Savarese et al 1988). Other routes of metabolism and excretion of mivacurium do exist, but the clinical significance of these is not known.

Clinical studies in patients with the normal phenotype and a low or normal pChe activity have shown an inverse correlation between pChe activity and the duration of action of mivacurium (Østergaard et al 1992).

In phenotypically abnormal patients the duration of action of mivacurium is prolonged. In patients heterozygous for the usual and the atypical gene the time to neuromuscular recovery is prolonged by about 30% compared to normal patients (Østergaard et al submitted). So far, only very few patients homozygous for the atypical gene have been given mivacurium. Initial studies indicate that the patients are extremely sensitive. One patient given a very small dose of mivacurium, equivalent to ED_{10}, was totally paralysed for more than 2 h. Two other patients showed a somewhat lesser sensitivity.

Prolonged respiratory insufficiency after succinylcholine is comparatively rare. It is, however, a very unpleasant and straining experience for both the patient and the anaesthetist. The introduction of bambuterol and mivacurium into clinical practice will increase the frequency with which an anaesthetist will face a patient with a prolonged neuromuscular response caused by an abnormal pChe activity. Knowledge of pChe is therefore still essential for the anaesthetist.

REFERENCES

Ali H H, Utting J E, Gray C 1970 Stimulus frequency in the detection of neuromuscular block in humans. Br J Anaesth 42: 967–977

Bang U, Viby-Mogensen J, Wirén J E, Skovgaard L T 1990a The effect of bambuterol (carbamylated terbutaline) on plasma cholinesterase activity and suxamethonium-induced neuromuscular blockade in genotypically normal patients. Acta Anaesthesiol Scand 34: 596–599

Bang U, Viby-Mogensen J, Wirén J E 1990b The effect of bambuterol on plasma cholinesterase activity and suxamethonium induced neuromuscular blockade in subjects heterozygous for abnormal plasma cholinesterase. Acta Anaesth Scand 37: 600–607

Bartels C F, Nogueira C P, McGuire M C, Adkins S, Rubinstein H M, Lubrano T, Van der Spek A F L, Lightstone H, Lockridge O, La Du B N 1990 Identification of two different mutations associated with human butyrylcholinesterase fluoride resistance in serum. Third International Meeting on Cholinesterases (Abstract). La Grande-Motte, France, p 103

Bartels C F, Jensen F S, Lockridge O et al 1992a DNA mutation associated with the human butyrylcholinesterase K-variant and its linkage to the atypical variant mutation and other polymorphic sites. Am J Hum Genet 50: 1086–1103

Bartels C F, James K, La Du B N 1992b DNA mutations associated with the human butyrylcholinesterase J-variant. Am J Hum Genet 50: 1104–1114

Cavallaro R J, Krumperman L W, Kugler F 1968 Effect of echothiopate therapy on the metabolism of succinylcholine in man. Anesth Analg 47: 570

Donati F, Bevan D R 1985 Antagonism of phase II succinylcholine block by neostigmine. Anesth Analg 64: 773–776

Evans R T, Wardell J 1984 On the identification and frequency of the j and k cholinesterase phenotypes in a Caucasian population. J Med Genet 21: 99–102

Fisher D M, Caldwell J E, Sharma M, Wirén J E 1988 The influence of bambuterol (carbamylated terbutaline) on the duration of action of succinylcholine-induced paralysis in humans. Anesthesiology 69: 757–759

Garry P J, Dietz A A, Lubrano T, Forde P C, James K, Rubinstein H M 1976 New allele at cholinesterase locus 1. J Med Genet 13: 38–42

Hanel H K, Viby-Mogensen J 1977 The inhibition of serum cholinesterase by urea. Br J Anaesth 49: 1251–1257

Harris H, Whittaker M 1961 Differential inhibition of human serum cholinesterase with fluoride: recognition of two new phenotypes. Nature 191: 496–498

Jensen F S, Bartels C F, La Du B N 1992 Structural basis of the butyrylcholinesterase H-variant segregating in two Danish families. Pharmacogenetics (accepted)

Jorge A D, Sanchez D 1976 Serum levels of C3 and cholinesterase in various diseases of the liver. Acta Hepato-Gastroenterol 23: 19–25

Kalow W, Genest K 1957 A method for the detection of atypical forms of human serum cholinesterase: determination of dibucaine numbers. Can J Biochem 35: 339–346

Kalow W, Lindsay H A 1955 A comparison of optical and manometric methods for the assay of human serum cholinesterase. Can J Biochem Physiol 33: 568–574

Kambam J R, Horton B, Parris W C V, Hyman S A, Berman M L, Sastry B V R 1989 Pseudocholinesterase activity in human CNS. Anesth Analg 69: 486–488

Kaniaris P, Fassoulaki A, Liarmakopoulou K, Dermitzakis E 1979 Serum cholinesterase levels in patients with cancer. Anesth Analg 58: 82–84

Liddell J, Lehmann H, Silk E 1962 A 'silent' pseudocholinesterase gene. Nature 193: 561–562

Lockridge O, Eckerson H W, La Du B N 1979 Interchain disulfide bands and subunit organization in human serum cholinesterase. J Biol Chem 254: 8324–8330

Lockridge O, Bartels C F, Caughan T A, Wong C K, Norton S E, Johnson L L 1987 Complete amino acid sequence of human serum cholinesterase. J Biol Chem 262: 549–557

McGuire M C, Nogueira C P, Bartels C F, Lightstone H, Hajra A, van der Spek A F L, Lockridge O, La Du B N 1989 Identification of the structural mutation responsible for the dibucaine-resistant (atypical) variant form of human serum cholinesterase. Proc Natl Acad Sci USA 86: 953–957

Muensch H, Goedde H W, Yoshida A 1976 Human serum cholinesterase subunits and number of active sites of the major compartment. Eur J Biochem 70: 218–223

Nogueira C P, McGuire M C, Graeser C et al 1990 Identification of a frameshift mutation responsible for the silent phenotype of human serum cholinesterase Gly 117 (GGT->GGAG). Am J Hum Genet 46: 934–942

Østergaard D, Viby-Mogensen J 1989 Prolonged apnea after succinylcholine. Problems in Anesthesia 3: 455–464

Østergaard D, Viby-Mogensen J, Hanel H K, Skovgaard L T 1988 Half-life of plasma cholinesterase. Acta Anaesthesiol Scand 32: 266–269

Østergaard D, Jensen F S, Jensen E, Viby-Mogensen J 1989 Influence of plasma cholinesterase activity on recovery from mivacurium induced neuromuscular blockade in phenotypically normal patients. Acta Anaesthesiol Scand 1992: 36: 702–706

Østergaard D, Jensen F S, Jensen E, Viby-Mogensen J Mivacurium-induced neuromuscular blockade (NMB) in patients heterozygous for the atypical gene for plasma cholinesterase. Acta Anaesthesiol Scand (submitted)

Pantuck E J, Pantuck C B 1987 Prolonged apnea following succinylcholine administration, side effects and rational approach to relaxation. Azar, I (ed) Dekker, New York, p 205–209

Propert D N, Brackenridge C J 1976 The relation of sex, age, smoking, status, birth rank and parental ages to pseudocholinesterase activity and phenotypes in a sample of Australian Caucasian adults. Hum Genet 32: 181–188

Rubinstein H M, Dietz A A, Lubrano T 1978 E_1^k, another quantitative variant at cholinesterase locus 1. J Med Genet 15: 27–29

Savarese J J, Ali H H, Basta S J, Embree P B, Scott R P F, Sunder N, Weakly J N, Wastila W B, El-Sayad H A 1988 The clinical neuromuscular pharmacology of mivacurium chloride (BW B1090U). Anesthesiology 68: 723–732

Simon N M, Greco F D, Dietz A A, Rubinstein H M 1969 Serum cholinesterase deficiency in renal failure. Trans Am Soc Artif Intern Organs 15: 328–332

Singh D S, Shukla P K, Gupta J P, Dube B 1976 Serum cholinesterase in hepatic disorders. J Indian Med Assoc 66: 49–51

Soreq H, Zamir R, Zevin-Sonkin D, Zakut H 1987 Human cholinesterase genes localized by hybridization to chromosomes 3 and 16. Hum Genet 77: 325–328

Stedman E, Stedman E, Easson L H 1932 Cholinesterase: an enzyme present in the blood of the horse. Biochem J 26: 2056–2066

Viby-Mogensen J 1980 Correlation of succinylcholine duration of action with plasma cholinesterase activity in subjects with genotypically normal enzyme. Anesthesiology 53: 517–520

Viby-Mogensen J 1981a Succinylcholine neuromuscular blockade in subjects heterozygous for atypical plasma cholinesterase. Anesthesiology 55: 231–235

Viby-Mogensen J 1981b Succinylcholine neuromuscular blockade in subjects homozygous for atypical plasma cholinesterase. Anesthesiology 55: 429–434

Viby-Mogensen J 1983 Cholinesterase and succinylcholine. Dan Med Bull 30: 129–149

Viby-Mogensen J, Hanel H K 1978 Prolonged apnoea after suxamethonium: an analysis of the first 225 cases reported to the Danish Cholinesterase Research Unit. Acta Anaesthesiol Scand 22: 371–380

Viby-Mogensen J, Hanel H K, Hansen E, Sørensen B, Graae J 1975 Serum cholinesterase activity in burned patients. I: Biochemical findings. Acta Anaesth Scand 19: 159–168

Whittaker M 1986 Cholinesterase. Beckman, L (ed) Karger, Exeter

Whittaker M, Britten J 1987 A new allele at cholinesterase locus 1. Hum Hered 37: 54–58

Yang F, Lum J B, McGill J R, Moore C M, Naylor S L, van Bragt P H, Baldwin W D, Bowman B H 1984 Human transferrin: cDNA characterization and chromosomal localization. Proc Natl Acad Sci USA 81: 2752–2756

Zarday Z, Deery A, Tellis I, Soberman R, Foldes F F 1975 Plasma and red cell cholinesterase activity in uremic patients (effects of hemodialysis and renal transplantation). J Med 6: 337–349

24

Hazards of reversal of neuromuscular blockade

N. O. Boheimer

INTRODUCTION

Ever since the introduction of curare into clinical practice by Griffith in 1942, there has been a need for reversal of the actions of non-depolarizing neuromuscular blockers by anticholinesterase drugs. Anticholinesterases bind to and inactivate acetylcholinesterase and pseudocholinesterase, increasing the local concentration of the neurotransmitter, acetylcholine (ACh), at the neuromuscular junction, autonomic ganglia and postganglionic parasympathetic synapses. Unchecked stimulation of the parasympathetic nervous system leads to bradyarrhythmias, hypotension, bronchospasm, excessive salivation and contraction of the gut. To counteract these effects it is neccessary to administer an anticholinergic drug with the anticholinesterase. The commonly used anticholinesterases in anaesthetic practice are neostigmine and edrophonium, in combination with either atropine or glycopyrrolate. Pyridostigmine has also been used. 4-aminopyridine is not an anticholinesterase. It enhances the release of ACh from the motor nerve terminal, though its clinical usefulness is limited by a tendency to cause convulsions.

Problems at reversal fall into two main categories: failure of the anticholinesterases to reverse the neuromuscular block and specific side effects of the reversal agents. Failure to breathe following successful antagonism of neuromuscular blockade may be due to other factors, including overdose of perioperative opiates, volatile agents or as a consequence of an intraoperative incident (e.g. hypoxia or cerebral vascular accident), but discussion of these is beyond the scope of this chapter.

Complication-free reversal requires a thorough knowledge of the currently available muscle relaxants, particularly of their differing durations of action and recovery profiles (Fig. 24.1). Awareness of the influence of other drugs, disease processes, electrolyte disturbances, body temperature and age on neuromuscular block is essential. Appreciation of the onset times and duration of action of neostigmine and edrophonium assists the choice of a suitable anticholinergic agent.

Intraoperative monitoring of the neuromuscular junction helps in assessing the need for supplementary doses or adjustment to infusion rates, especially with intermediate-duration muscle relaxants, but may not influence the incidence of postoperative pulmonary complications. Olsen et al (1988), in a study of 80 patients, noted that the use of the intermediate muscle relaxant vecuronium, rather than pancuronium, had more influence on improving postoperative train-of-four (TOF) ratios and reducing pulmonary complications than the use of perioperative TOF monitoring.

THE NEUROMUSCULAR JUNCTION

The neuromuscular junction is composed of a prejunctional nerve terminal, separated by a synaptic cleft from the folded postjunctional membrane of the endplate of skeletal muscle. Acetylcholine, the neurotransmitter, is stored in vesicles in the nerve terminal. Nicotinic cholinergic receptors are sited on the pre- and postjunctional membranes. The postjunctional receptor consists of five protein subunits (two α, β, γ and δ) arranged in a circular fashion to form an ion channel.

Acetylcholine is released into the synaptic cleft following the arrival of an impulse at the nerve terminal and the associated influx of calcium. Simultaneous binding of an acetylcholine molecule to each of the alpha subunits of the postjunctional receptor causes conformational changes in the receptor. These open the ion channel resulting in a net efflux of K^+ and influx of Na^+, producing a miniature endplate potential (MEPP). If enough receptors are simultaneously stimulated, the MEPPs summate to depolarize the postjunctional membrane from its resting potential of –90 mV to the threshold potential of –45 mV. At this point an action potential is propagated over the surface of the muscle fibre, ultimately causing contraction. Bowman et al (1988) demonstrated that stimulation of the prejunctional receptor by ACh amplifies the process of neuromuscular transmission by causing an increased release of ACh from the motor nerve ending.

Acetylcholine survives long enough to bind to only one receptor. It is then hydrolyzed (within 15 ms) by acetylcholinesterase which is located in the junctional folds of the synaptic cleft within. This leads to the restoration of the membrane potential. Neuromuscular blockers may bind at pre- and postjunctional receptors. Individual agents have different affinities for each site. Prejunctional binding inhibits positive feedback of neuromuscular transmission. Binding to one or both alpha units of the postjunctional receptor prevents ion channel opening and MEPP production. At least 70% of receptors must be blocked before a clinically useful paralysis is apparent. Anticholinesterases inactivate acetylcholinesterase located at the junctional folds, thereby lengthening ACh survival time.

Table 24.1 Comparable recovery data of various neuromuscular blockers following bolus intravenous injection

Duration of action	Recovery index (min)	Reversal time (min)	(min)
Atracurium ED 95 (Basta et al 1982)	44.0	12.0	10.5
Pancuronium 1.2 × ED95	73.0	31.0	17.0
Vecuronium 1.2 × ED95 (Engbaek et al 1983)	32.0	10.0	8.0
Mivacurium 1.2 × ED95 (Savarese et al 1988)	24.5	7.0	6.0
Doxacurium ED95 (Basta et al 1988)	128.4	51.0	15.0

MONITORING RECOVERY

Recovery and depth of paralysis can be monitored by assessing visually, mechanically, electrically or simply by feel the evoked muscle response to electrical stimulation of a peripheral nerve. The response in adductor pollicis brevis to stimulation of the ulnar nerve at the wrist or elbow by a TOF, is widely used. The TOF consists of four supramaximal single stimuli of 0.1–0.2 ms duration, applied to the nerve at a frequency of 2 Hz for 2 s, and repeated every 12–20 s. If, as is usual in a clinical setting, the response of the stimulated muscle is assessed visually or by feel, it is only possible to quantify the number of responses to stimulation. This is defined as the train-of-four count. The degree of block can be estimated from the number of twitches noted. At least two twitches should be present before reversal is considered.

It is possible to analyse the results if the response is recorded graphically. T1 is the height of the first twitch, T4 the height of the fourth twitch and T0, the magnitude of the first twitch prior to drug administration, acts as a control. Depression of the ratio T1:T0 reflects the postjunctional activity of a neuromuscular blocking drug, while reduction in the ratio T4:T1, sometimes referred to as the TOF ratio, mirrors prejunctional action or fade.

Recovery

Recovery from neuromuscular block occurs when the local concentration of ACh is sufficient to displace the muscle relaxant. As a consequence of redistribution and metabolism, a concentration

Table 24.2 Comparison of clinical tests for detecting residual paralysis

Test	Sensitivity	Remarks	Cooperation needed?
Tidal volume	Poor		Yes
Vital capacity	Poor		Yes
Inspiratory force	Moderate	Specialized equipment	Yes
Train of four	Moderate	Uncomfortable	No
Head lift	Moderate	Easy to perform	Yes
Tetanic fade	Good	Very painful	No
Expiratory force	Good	Specialized equipment	Yes
Hand grip	Good	Specialized equipment	Yes
Residual diplopia	Good	Simple equipment	Yes

gradient develops between neuromuscular junction and plasma. This results in a net flow of drug away from its site of action. Eventually, spontaneous recovery from any muscle relaxant will occur, but this process may be prolonged, particularly when a long-acting neuromuscular blocking drug is used (Fig. 24.1). It is usual in clinical practice to accelerate recovery by administering reversal agents.

To achieve safe reversal at least 10% of spontaneous recovery (T1 >10% T0) must have taken place, especially if a long-acting agent has

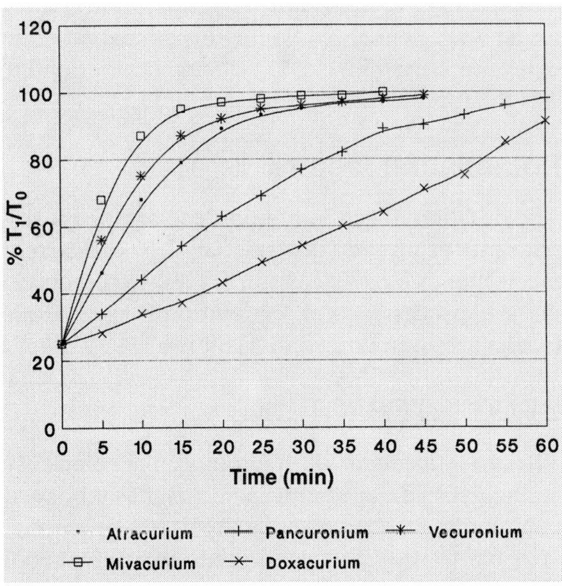

Fig. 24.1 Spontaneous recovery from neuromuscular blockade plotted as T_1/T_0 percentage against time for five non-depolarizing muscle relaxants. Approximate ED 95, pooled data.

been used. Safe reversal is said to occur when T1 is 90% T0, or the TOF ratio is greater than 0.7. Recovery of the TOF ratio takes longer so it may be safer to take this as the yardstick of clinical recovery. Jones et al (1984) suggested that a TOF ratio of 0.5 was sufficient for safe recovery from atracurium paralysis, which reflects the more rapid recovery profile of the drug.

Reversal times for long-acting agents are longer than those of the intermediate-duration drugs. Goldhill et al (1988), investigating reversal of deep pancuronium paralysis (91–99% depression of T0) by neostigmine and glycopyrronium, suggested that the time to reversal to a TOF greater than 0.75 may be greater than 30 min. In another study, Caldwell et al (1987) noted reversal times to TOF 0.7 of 95% atracurium (0.15–0.2 mg/kg) or vecuronium (40–60 mcg/kg) paralysis by comparable doses of neostigmine and atropine (8.9 ± 3.7 and 7.10 ± 3.35 min, respectively; Fig. 24.2).

In the absence of neuromuscular monitoring, simple clinical tests have been used to assess reversal from neuromuscular blockade. The ability to lift the head for 5 s and take a deep breath have been accepted as markers of clinical recovery. However, Hutton et al (1988) demonstrated these to be insensitive tests compared to monitoring grip strength, expiratory force and detection of residual double vision. They noted diplopia up to 60 min, and failure of full recovery in grip strength and expiratory force up to 120 min after neostigmine reversal of pancuronium paralysis. The ability to lift the head is probably sufficient to return a patient to the ward, but does not guarantee street fitness. In view of Hutton et al's findings it would

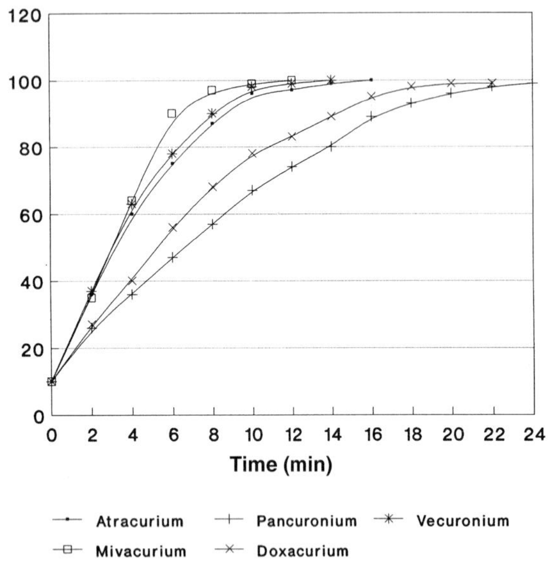

Fig. 24.2 Reversal times for five non-depolarizing muscle relaxants plotted as T_1/T_0 percentage against time following a standard dose of anticholinesterase. Approximate ED 95, pooled data.

be ill-advised to use pancuronium in out-patient anaesthesia.

Long-acting agents such as pancuronium or curare show slower recovery profiles than the intermediate duration drugs, atracurium and vecuronium. The character of recovery also differs for individual agents. Gallamine and vecuronium display similar degrees of fade during early spontaneous offset, but at 75% recovery of initial twitch height (T0) vecuronium shows more fade (Power et al 1988).

When comparing recovery from different relaxants it is important to use equipotent doses and similar anaesthetic techniques. The dose required to produce 95% depression of the twitch height (ED95) is frequently used. Sometimes workers refer to multiples of ED95 as it is common to administer two to three times the ED95 in clinical practice. It is usual to refer to the recovery index (T25%–T75%): the time taken to recover from 75% depression to 25% depression of T1. It may be more useful to measure a Spontaneous Recovery Time (T10%–T90%) as this may correlate better with clinical recovery and allow direct comparisons with reversal times (T10%–T90% following the administration of an anticholinesterase).

Increasing the administered dose of a muscle relaxant can prolong its duration of action and slow the rate of recovery. For example Fahey (1981) noted that changing the administered dose of vecuronium from 0.07 mg/kg to 0.28 mg/kg prolonged the recovery index from 8 to 38 min.

Failure to reverse

If overdosage of muscle relaxant is suspected, surgery finishes abruptly during profound block, or some other factor appears to be potentiating the block, the patient should remain anaesthetized and ventilated until early neuromuscular recovery can be detected, as immediate reversal is likely to be incomplete. Donati et al (1987) found that attempted reversal of 99% pancuronium paralysis by neostigmine (0.08 mg/kg) achieved only 83% recovery of T1 and 45% recovery of TOF after 10 min. Following edrophonium (1.15 mg/kg) recovery was even less satisfactory. Caldwell et al (1987) investigated the ability of equipotent doses of neostigmine and edrophonium to reverse profound unquantifiable block induced by vecuronium or atracurium. They found that neither could rapidly antagonize the neuromuscular blockade, though neostigmine was the more effective drug.

Potentiating factors

The duration of action of non-depolarizing muscle relaxants can be potentiated by concurrent medication, electrolyte disturbances, hypothermia, disease processes and extremes of age. These factors are summarized in Table 24.3.

DRUG INTERACTIONS (see Ch. 25)

The enhancement of neuromuscular block by aminoglycoside antibiotics and magnesium, used commonly in the USA to treat pre-eclampsia, appears to be associated with interference of calcium-mediated presynaptic release of ACh. An interesting study by Ramanathan et al (1988) demonstrated abnormal neuromuscular transmission in pre-eclamptic women receiving

Table 24.3 Diseases, drugs and physiological factors potentiating muscle relaxants

Potentiating factor	Muscle relaxant
Concurrent drug therapy	
Aminoglycoside antibiotics	All
Bambuterol	Mivacurium
Calcium channel blockers	All
Cardiac antiarrhythmics	All
Magnesium	All
Cimetidine	Vecuronium
Lithium carbonate	Pancuronium
Azathioprine	All
Cyclosporine	Pancuronium
Anaesthetic interactions	
Suxamethonium	Variable response
Volatile agents	All
Local anaesthetics	All
Pancuronium	Tubocurarine
Patient disease	
Renal failure	Gallamine Pancuronium Tubocurarine Vecuronium
Hepatocellular disease	Vecuronium
Biliary obstruction	Vecuronium Pancuronium Tubocurarine
Myasthenia gravis	All
Eaton–Lambert syndrome	All
Dystrophia myotonica	All, variable response
Miscellaneous	
Hypothermia	All, particularly atracurium
Acidosis	Tubocurarine Pancuronium Vecuronium Atracurium
Alkalosis	Gallamine
Hypokalaemia	All, variable response
Age:	
Neonates	All
Old age	All
Immediate postpartum period	Vecuronium

magnesium sulphate with serum magnesium levels within the normal range. The intensity of the transmission defect correlated significantly with increased magnesium levels and decreased calcium levels in serum.

Recently, Ulsamer (1988) demonstrated that vecuronium blockade was significantly prolonged by cimetidine but not by ranitidine. It would appear logical to use ranitidine if pretreatment with an H2 antagonist is needed when using vecuronium.

Bambuterol

Bambuterol, a bismethylcarbamate prodrug of terbutaline, is a new oral bronchodilator that is cleaved enzymatically to yield terbutaline and carbamate by plasma cholinesterase. The carbamate binds to and inhibits plasma cholinesterase. Viby-Mogensen (1989) reported that patients pretreated with bambuterol displayed prolonged apnoea following suxamethonium. The main metabolic pathway of the new non-depolarizing muscle relaxant, mivacurium, is hydrolysis by plasma cholinesterase. Neuromuscular blockade with mivacurium is prolonged in patients with plasma cholinesterase deficiencies and in those pre-treated with bambuterol (Viby-Mogensen 1989).

Procainamide

Procainamide, a potent antiarrhythmic drug, potentiates both depolarizing and non-depolarizing muscle relaxants. It inhibits the release of ACh at the neuromuscular junction. Reddy-Kambam et al (1987) demonstrated that, at therapeutic concentrations, procainamide inhibited plasma cholinesterase activity by 15-30%. It is possible that mivacurium will be potentiated by procainamide.

Calcium channel blockers

Potentiation of non-depolarizing muscle relaxants by the calcium channel blockers, verapamil and nifedipine, is well documented. Acute administration of verapamil for intraoperative tachyarrhythmias may prolong block but should not impede reversal, though reversal of residual block may be difficult in patients on long-term therapy. Wali et al (1987) demonstrated that edrophonium was more effective than neostigmine in reversing atracurium-verapamil induced blockade at the rat neuromuscular junction.

The potentiating effects of volatile agents are well known. The interaction between suxamethonium and non-depolarizing muscle relaxants appears confusing: some authorities cite a potentiating effect while others refute this. Prolonged depolarizing block after suxamethonium may occur in patients with absent, abnormal or inhibited plasma cholinesterase. Pancuronium priming of tubocurarine blockade causes synergism. Onset times are shortened in infants and children but not in adults, though the duration of action is prolonged in all groups.

Hepatic and renal disease

Atracurium is the relaxant of choice in renal failure. Recently, Lynam et al (1988) demonstrated a prolonged duration of action of vecuronium in patients with impaired renal function during isoflurane anaesthesia. Tubocurarine and pancuronium should be used with great caution in renal failure, and gallamine should be avoided. The action of vecuronium is prolonged by hepatocellular disease and biliary obstruction. Actracurium appears the relaxant of choice in hepatic disease. Changes in volumes of distribution prolong the onset times of most non-depolarizing muscle relaxants in chirrotic patients. With the exception of gallamine and atracurium, the duration of action is also increased.

Neuromuscular diseases

The sensitivity of patients suffering from myasthenia gravis or Eaton-Lambert syndrome to non-depolarizing muscle relaxants is well known. Monitoring the onset of block while small increments of drug are administered may avoid overdose. The response to non-depolarizing muscle relaxants appears to be normal in most patients with dystrophia myotonica and other myotonias, though some are sensitive. As the administration of anticholinesterases can precipitate myotonic contractions, a monitored spontaneous recovery from atracurium paralysis may be a useful alternative technique (Boheimer et al 1985).

Miscellaneous

Profound hypothermia, electrolyte disturbances including hypokalaemia and disorders of acid/base physiology can enhance non-depolarizing block. Patients suffering from these afflictions are often severely ill and require intermittent positive pressure ventilation as part of their treatment until physiological homeostasis is restored. Occasionally, hypokalaemia from chronic diuretic therapy potentiates muscle relaxation. The elderly and newborn are both sensitive to non-depolarizing muscle relaxants. In these patients they should be used with caution and in reduced dosage. The duration of action of atracurium appears to be least influenced by the patient's age. Postpartum women appear sensitive to vecuronium. Camp et al (1987) demonstrated a near two-fold increase in the duration of 0.1 mg/kg vecuronium in patients undergoing postpartum tubal ligation compared to controls.

CHOICE OF ANTICHOLINESTERASE

The calabar bean, source of the naturally occurring anticholinesterase physostigmine, was originally used by the Ibibio tribes of Nigeria as a weapon and ordeal poison. It comes as no surprise, therefore, that the routine use of this drug in anaesthesia may be associated with morbidity.

Neostigmine, a carbamate derivative, is the most extensively used anticholinesterase in UK anaesthetic practice. Pyridostigmine is used in the USA, but not commonly in the UK. Edrophonium, a phenyltrimethylammonium derivative, has the advantage of a more rapid onset than neostigmine and exerts fewer muscarinic side effects. Cronnelly et al (1982) noted that the duration of antagonism produced by edrophonium was similar to neostigmine, though there have been numerous recent reports questioning the reliability of edrophonium reversal.

Mirakhur (1987) compared the antagonism of the long-duration muscle relaxants, pancuronium and tubocurarine, with equipotent doses of neostigmine and edrophonium. Defining adequate recovery as a TOF ratio of 0.7, he found that, at approximately 30% spontaneous recovery of T1, attempted reversal by edrophonium was incomplete in 30% of patients receiving pancuronium, and in 40% of those receiving tubocurarine.

Donati et al (1989), comparing edrophonium and neostigmine as antagonists of moderate and profound atracurium blockade, concluded that the use of edrophonium as an antagonist of profound blockade should be avoided. Cashman et al (1989) determined that, following 0.3 mg/kg of intravenous atracurium and a halothane anaesthetic, safe reversal (TOF > 0.5) could only be rapidly and reliably achieved by 0.5 mg/kg edrophonium if more than 30 min had passed since the time of injection.

Neostigmine remains the anticholinesterase of choice. Edrophonium should only be used to reverse intermediate-duration muscle relaxants when at least 25% recovery of T1 has already occurred. Unlike neostigmine, edrophonium has no inhibitory effect on plasma cholinesterase. Although neostigmine has been used successfully, edrophonium may be a more appropriate agent to reverse residual mivacurium paralysis.

CHOICE OF ANTICHOLINERGIC AGENT

Atropine and glycopyrrolate are the anticholinergic agents used in anaesthetic practice to counteract the muscarinic side effects of anticholinesterases. The combination of neostigmine and atropine is not ideal, but has been used for many years. Glycopyrrolate with neostigmine is gaining popularity. Unlike atropine, glucopyrrolate and neostigmine are quaternary ammonium compounds and do not enter the central nervous system. Mirakhur (1985) has reviewed the advantages of glycopyrrolate over atropine when used with neostigmine. Atropine is normally used with edrophonium as a simultaneous injection. Glycopyrrolate may be used if administered 1 min earlier to compensate for its slower onset time with edrophonium (Dodd et al 1989).

COMPLICATIONS DUE TO REVERSAL AGENTS

Isolated cases of death following neostigmine were reported in the late 1940s. They appear to be related to the practice at that time of stimulating respiration with carbon dioxide prior to reversal. The clinically relevant complications of reversal are summarized in Table 24.4.

Cardiovascular complications

Changes in heart rate and rhythm are common at reversal. Atropine, a tertiary amine, has a more rapid onset and a shorter duration of action than neostigmine, leading to early increases in heart rate and late bradycardias. Glycopyrrolate and neostigmine have similar onset times and durations of action allowing greater cardiac stability and a lower incidence of dysrhythmias (Mirakhur 1983). Goldhill et al (1988), when comparing reversal of pancuronium by various doses of neostigmine (30, 60, 80 μg/kg) and glycopyrrolate (10 μg/kg), noted dysrhythmia in 17 of 51 patients. All but one were junctional and all settled spontaneously.

Satem at al (1985), when comparing glycopyrrolate and atropine in a mixture with neostigmine for reversal of neuromuscular blockade in cardiac patients, found that rate pressure product increases were significantly more marked following atropine. They also noted that concomitant beta

Table 24.4 Complications following reversal agents

Site	Anticholinesterase	Anticholinergic
Cardiovascular	Bradycardia, Arrhythmias	Tachycardia, Arrhythmias
Respiratory	Bronchoconstriction	
Gut	Contraction	Lower barrier Pressure
CNS	Vomiting	Slow arousal, confusion, short-term memory loss (atropine only)

adrenoreceptor blockade reduced these increases in both groups.

There have been isolated case reports of complete heart block and prolonged bradycardia with hypotension complicating reversal with neostigmine in patients receiving beta blockers. Lonsdale & Stuart (1988) reported a patient receiving 100 mg atenolol daily that developed complete heart block following the reversal of vecuronium paralysis with 2.5 mg neostigmine and 0.5 mg glycopyrrolate. Eldor et al (1987) reported prolonged bradycardia and hypotension after neostigmine and atropine administration in a patient receiving 50 mg atenolol daily.

Respiratory complications

Bronchospasm may occur after neostigmine, particularly when a low dose of anticholinergic agent is used. Pratt (1988) reported three patients that became wheezy following 2.5 mg neostigmine and 0.3-0.4 mg glycopyrrolate, one of whom was asthmatic.

Hammond et al (1983) measured changes in specific airway conductance at reversal with neostigmine (50 μg/kg) and either atropine (20 μg/kg) or glycopyrrolate (10 μg/kg). They showed significant reductions from baseline values with both anticholinergic agents, 10 min after reversal. There was an early increase in conductance in the atropine group reflecting the more rapid onset time of this drug.

The longer action of glycopyrrolate would make it a more logical choice of anticholinergic agent when reversing patients with asthma and other bronchospastic disorders.

Gastrointestinal tract complications

Neostigmine causes contraction of the gut which may disrupt recently fashioned intestinal anastomoses. In these circumstances an anaesthetic technique that avoids reversal could be considered. Reversal agents influence oesophageal barrier pressures and the incidence of postoperative vomiting. The physiological barrier to gastro-oesophageal reflux is the pressure differential (BrP) between the lower oesophageal sphincter (LOSP) and the stomach (GP). Anticholinergic agents tend to relax the lower oesophageal sphincter. Turner & Smith (1985) evaluated the combined effects of atropine and neostigmine on the lower oesophageal sphincter. Derrington et al (1987) evaluated the influence of glycopyrrolate and neostigmine. Following atropine there was an early transient decrease in LOSP which was negated after 3 min by the action of neostigmine. However, after glycopyrrolate there was significant reduction in LOSP throughout the 20 min studied. On the strength of this work, atropine and neostigmine are a more suitable reversal combination in cases where regurgitation is likely.

King et al (1988) compared reversal by neostigmine and atropine with spontaneous recovery from tubocurarine paralysis and noted that the incidence of postoperative vomiting and nausea was significantly reduced when no reversal agents were used.

Central nervous system complications

Atropine enters the central nervous system (CNS) and may cause anxiety, excitement, restlessness, confusion or cerebral depression. These complications are more likely in the elderly and may be treated by the centrally acting physostigmine. In a comparison of atropine and glycopyrrolate in combination with neostigmine, Simpson et al (1985) found that atropine caused a significant reduction in postoperative short-term memory.

SUMMARY

Complications due to inadequate reversal may be reduced by avoiding the use of long-acting neuromuscular blocking agents. Neostigmine remains the anticholinesterase of choice for elective anaesthesia, particularly when used in combination with glycopyrrolate. Atropine may be a more suitable anticholinergic drug when there is a high risk of aspiration.

Future prospects

The development of new monitoring patterns, post tetanic count and double burst stimulation and the new technique of accelerometry may increase the sensitivity of neuromuscular junction monitoring. The search for rapid onset, rapid offset nondepolarizing drugs may in the future make pharmacological reversal obselete.

REFERENCES

Basta S J, Ali H H, Savarese J J 1982 Clinical pharmacology of atracurium besylate (BW 33A): a new nondepolarising muscle relaxant. Anesth Analg 61: 723-729

Basta S J, Savarese J J, Ali H H, Embree P B, Schwartz A F, Rudd G D, Wastila W B 1988 Clinical pharmacology of doxacurium chloride. Anesthesiology 69: 478-486

Boheimer N, Harris J W, Ward S 1985 Neuromuscular blockade in dystrophia myotonica with atracurium besylate. Anaesthesia 40: 872-874

Bowman W C, Marshall I G, Gibb A J, Harborne A J 1988 Feedback control of transmitter release at the neuromuscular junction. Trends Pharmacol Sci 9: 16-20

Caldwell J E, Robertson E N, Baird W L M 1986 Antagonism of profound neuromuscular blockade induced by vecuronium or atracurium. Br J Anaesth 58: 1285-1289

Caldwell J E, Robertson E N, Baird W L M 1987 Antagonism of vecuronium and atracurium: comparison of neostigmine and edrophonium administered at 5% twitch height recovery. Br J Anaesth 59: 478-481

Camp C E, Tessem J, Adenwala J, Joyce T H 1987 Vecuronium and prolonged neuro-muscular blockade in post partum patients. Anesthesiology 67: 1006-1008

Cashman J N, Jones R M, Adams A P 1989 Atracurium recovery: prediction of safe reversal times with edrophonium. Anaesthesia 44: 805-807

Cronnelly R, Morris R B, Miller R D 1982 Edrophonium: duration of action and atropine requirements in humans during halothane anesthesia. Anesthesiology 57: 261-266

Derrington M C, Hindocha N, Smith G 1987 Evaluation of the combined effects of glycopyrrolate and neostigmine on the lower oesophageal sphincter. Br J Anaesth 59: 545-547

Dodd P, Day S J, Goldhill D R, Macleod D M, Withington P S, Yate P M 1989 Glycopyrronium requirements for antagonism of the muscarinic side effects of edrophonium. Br J Anaesth 62: 77-81

Donati F, Lahoud J, McCready D, Bevan D R 1987 Neostigmine, pyridostigmine and edrophonium as antagonists of deep pancuronium blockade. Can J Anaesth 34: 589-593

Donati F, Smith C E, Bevan D R 1989 Dose response relationships for edrophonium and neostigmine as antagonists of moderate and profound atracurium blockade. Anesth Analg 68: 13-19

Eldor J, Hoffnam B, Davidson J T 1987 Prolonged bradycardia and hypotension after neostigmine administration in a patient receiving atenolol. Anaesthesia 42: 1294-1297

Engbaek J, Ording H, Viby-Mogensen J 1983 Neuromuscular blocking effects of vecuronium and pancuronium during halothane anaesthesia. Br J Anaesth 55: 497-499

Fahey M R, Morris R B, Miller R D, Sohn Y J, Cronnelly R, Gencarelli P 1981 Clinical pharmacology of ORG NC45 (Norcuron TM). Anesthesiology 55: 6-11

Goldhill D R, Embree P B, Ali H H, Savarese J J 1988 Reversal of pancuronium. Anaesthesia 43: 443-446

Hammond J, Wright D, Sale J 1983 Pattern of change of bronchomotor tone following reversal of neuromuscular blockade: comparison between atropine and glycopyrrolate. Br J Anaesth 55: 955-959

Hutton P, Burchett K R, Madden A P 1988 Comparison of recovery after neuromuscular blockade by atracurium or pancuronium. Br J Anaesth 60: 36-42

Jones R M, Pearce A C, Williams J P 1984 Recovery characteristics following antagonism of atracurium with neostigmine of edrophonium. Br J Anaesth 56: 453-457

King M J, Milazkiewicz R, Carli F, Deacock A R 1988 Infuence of neostigmine on post operative vomiting. Br J Anaesth 61: 403-406

Lonsdale M, Stuart J 1988 Complete heart block following glycopyrronium/neostigmine mixture. Anaesthesia 43: 448-449

Lynam D P, Cronnelly R, Castagnoli K P 1988 The pharmacodynamics and pharmacokinetics of vecuronium in patients anesthetised with isoflurane with normal renal function or with renal failure. Anesthesiology 69: 227-231

Mirakhur R K 1987 Antagonism of pancuronium and tubocurarine blocks by edrophonium or neostigmine: a comparative study. Eur J Anaesthesiol 4: 411-419

Mirakhur R K, Dundee J N 1985 Glycopyrrolate: pharmacology and clinical use. Anaesthesia 38: 1195–1204

Olsen N V, Pederson T, Bang U, Jensen E, Viby-Mogensen J 1988 Perioperative use of a nerve stimulator: does it matter? 9th World Congress of Anesthesiologists A0536

Power S J, Pearce A C, Jones R M 1988 Fade profiles during spontaneous offset of neuromuscular blockade: vecuronium and gallamine compared. Br J Anaesth 60: 486-490

Pratt C I 1988 Bronchospasm after neostigmine. Anaesthesia 43: 248

Ramanathan J, Sibai P M, Pillai R, Angel J J 1988 Neuromuscular transmission studies in pre-eclamptic women receiving magnesium sulphate. Am J Obstet Gynecol 158: 40–46

Reddy-Kambam J, Franks J J, Naukam R, Sastry B V R 1987 Effect of quinidine on plasma cholinesterase activity and succinylcholine neuromuscular blockade. Anesthesiology 67: 858–860

Satem M G, Richardson J C, Meadows G A, Lamplugh G, Lai K M 1985 Comparison between glycopyrrolate and atropine in a mixture with neostigmine for reversal of neuromuscular blockade. Studies in patients following open heart surgery. Br J Anaesth 57: 184–187

Savarese J J, Ali H H, Basta S J 1988 The clinical neuromuscular pharmacology of mivacurium chloride (BW B1090U). Anesthesiology 68: 723-732

Simpson K H, Smith R J, Davies L F 1985 Comparison of the effects of atropine and glycopyrrolate on cognitive function following general anaesthesia. Br J Anaesth 57: 821P

Turner D A B, Smith G 1985 Evaluation of the combined effects of atropine and neostigmine on the lower oesophageal sphincter. Br J Anaesth 57: 956-959
Ulsamer B 1988 Effects of etomidate, ranitidine and cimetidine on pharmacodynamics of vecuronium bromide. Anaesthetist 37: 504-509
Viby-Mogensen J 1989 The clinical significance of plasma cholinesterase, new aspects. Critikon Lecture, Association of Anaesthetists of Great Britain and Ireland Scientific Meeting, Swansea
Wali F A, McAteer E, Suer A I L 1987 Interaction of verapamil with atracurium and reversal of combined block with edrophonium and neostigmine. I.J.M.S. July 215-218

25

Adverse drug interactions

N. E. Williams

INTRODUCTION

I was once approached by a somewhat disgruntled surgeon whose major case had been cancelled by a locum anaesthetist because the patient was taking promethazine for an allergic rhinitis. I was asked, 'How long before an elective surgical procedure should this drug be stopped?' The obvious answer seemed to be, 'about four hours if the drug is being taken orally'. After all, promethazine has useful sedative, antisialogogue and antiemetic properties, and many eminent anaesthetists have found it a most satisfactory premedicant drug.

Some years ago there was a vogue for stopping drugs for as long as possible before elective surgery. This approach was propagated by a natural fear of the consequences of polypharmacy, coupled with a relative lack of knowledge of drug kinetics and pharmacodynamics. With a greater awareness of the mechanisms of drug action and metabolism such an approach is no longer tenable. In many cases it is undesirable to interfere with existing drug therapy, provided it is beneficial to the patient, because there may be:

- an exacerbation of the underlying disease (e.g. hypertension, epilepsy, mental illness)
- difficulty in re-establishing active therapy (e.g. anticoagulants)
- intrinsic problems associated with sudden cessation of therapy (e.g. 'rebound phenomena' associated with withdrawal of clonidine, beta-adrenoceptor antagonists and antiepileptic drugs).

This is not to say that the problem of drug interaction associated with anaesthesia does not exist. Indeed, the overall potential for drug interactions is greater in anaesthesia than in other areas of medicine, because:

1. The patient who is being considered for anaesthesia may already be receiving several drugs. It has been stated that patients in one London hospital are concurrently taking five or six drugs, while one in 10 receives 10 drugs at the same time. In another hospital a patient was given 41 drugs during a single admission (Prescott 1973).
2. A patient may receive as many as 10 different drugs as part of his anaesthetic regimen.
3. The majority of responses that may occur due to drug interactions in anaesthetic practice are associated with acute depression of the nervous system and the inhibition of protective reflexes. Without any intervention the results may be catastrophic and long-term consequences may occur if the patient is not carefully monitored (Halsey 1987).

Thus it is imperative that, prior to any surgical procedure, a detailed history is taken from all patients regarding their current drug therapy, including any self-administered remedies. With such knowledge most ensuing drug interactions can be predicted, and either avoided or used to advantage by the anaesthetist.

DEFINITION

A drug interaction can be defined as the ability of one drug to alter the pharmacological effect of another drug that is administered concurrently. It should be understood that not all interactions are hazardous; many are actually advantageous and have become part of established therapeutics (Stockley 1974). Important examples of the former include the neutralization of heparin by protamine sulphate, and the inhibition of tubular transport of benzylpenicillin by probenecid. In anaesthetic practice the use of anticholinesterase drugs to antagonize the action of competitive neuromuscular blocking agents, and the administration of beta-adrenoceptor antagonists to prevent the reflex tachycardia which may occur when ganglion-blocking agents are used to induce deliberate hypotension, are instances of beneficial interactions.

Many drug interactions, once they are recognized and understood, can be allowed for by appropriate adjustment of drug dosage. However, in a significant number of cases the interaction between two drugs may render one of the agents therapeutically ineffective, or conversely enhance the likelihood of clinical toxicity. In a number of instances the pharmacological basis of drug interaction is obscure or poorly understood. The mechanism involved may be one of three types:

- pharmaceutical
- pharmacokinetic
- pharmacodynamic.

Pharmaceutical interactions

Pharmaceutical interactions occur prior to administration, that is outside the body, and usually relate to direct chemical combination between the drugs concerned. This may be responsible for the loss of activity of drugs and their precipitation or aggregation in solution. Such problems may be related to the mixing of solutions of different pH (e.g. thiopentone and suxamethonium) and the addition of drugs or electrolytes to fat emulsions (e.g. intralipid) or concentrated solutions (e.g. 20% mannitol; Grayson 1971).

Some drugs are unstable in solution with resultant loss of activity. A reducing agent, sodium metabisulphite, is added to local anaesthetic preparations to enhance the stability of the vasoconstrictor which may oxidize in solution. Other drugs (e.g. halothane and sodium nitroprusside) are decomposed by light or are sensitive to changes in temperature (e.g. isoflurane and enflurane). A classic example of a dangerous pharmaceutical interaction occurred when trichloroethylene was administered in anaesthetic circuits which incorporated soda-lime. This could lead to the production of the potentially neurotoxic vapour, dichloracetylene (Enderby 1944). Certain antibacterial drugs are rapidly inactivated in saline or dextrose solutions and the shelf life of methohexitone is considerably reduced when these solvents are used instead of water.

Physical properties may also account for interactions that may occur during the administration of drugs (Soni 1987). The concurrent infusion of blood with fluids of a different osmolarity (e.g. 5% dextrose and mannitol) may result in significant damage to the blood. Drugs may also interact with the administration sets through which they are given. Sorption refers to the lipophilicity and polarity of a solution, such as glyceryl trinitrate which is inactivated by binding if it is infused in bags or packs composed of polyvinyl chloride. Adsorption refers to the tendency of a drug to adhere to the surface of a container, as may occur with insulin in glass or plastic syringes. 'Salting out' may result when electrolytes are added to supersaturated solutions such as mannitol, and 'emulsion cracking' may ensue when calcium salts are added to fat emulsions.

Pharmaceutical interactions are not usually an important cause of complications in anaesthetic practice, but may be of particular import in the intensive therapy unit. Their occurrence can be minimized if drugs for continuous infusion are only added to crystalloid fluids; except in special circumstances, only one drug should be added to each unit of infusion fluid. Thorough mixing is necessary and whenever possible should be carried out in the pharmacy. The manufacturer's data sheet or the drug information pharmacist should be consulted in doubtful cases (Riley 1970).

Pharmacokinetic interactions

The kinetic disposition of any drug following administration is governed by the processes of absorption, distribution (which is itself considerably influenced by the degree of protein binding), biotransformation and excretion. It is clear that many drugs that may be administered concurrently can significantly modify one or more of these processes, thus influencing the concentration (and therefore the pharmacological effect) of the drug concerned at its site of action.

Absorption

Most drugs are administered by the oral route. Many factors are known to influence both the rate of absorption and the fraction of the drug that subsequently reaches the systemic circulation (bioavailability). These include the aqueous solubility of the drug (or its rate of dissolution if administered in soluble form), the rate of gastric emptying and subsequent transit time in the upper small intestine, the area of the absorbing surface and the local blood flow, and, not least, the dissociation constant (pKa) of the individual drug and the pH at the site of absorption. Drugs that alter the pH of the stomach (e.g. antacids and H_2 receptor antagonists) may influence the solubility of some basic drugs, such as the tetracyclines, which depend upon acid conditions. The rate of gastric emptying may be enhanced by metoclopramide or domperidone (which antagonize inhibitory dopamine receptors in the gut wall), or slowed by anticholinergic drugs or narcotic analgesics (Todd & Nimmo 1983). In clinical practice, such drugs are more likely to influence the rate of absorption, rather than the bioavailability, of concomitantly administered drugs. The timing of the peak effect of oral premedicants may thus be modified.

Drug interactions in the small intestine may decrease absorption due to the formation of insoluble complexes or chelates. The absorption of tetracyclines is reduced by the concurrent administration of calcium, magnesium or iron salts (Price et al 1957), and the absorption of chlordiazepoxide is slowed by the antacid mixture of aluminium and magnesium hydroxides ('Maalox'). The ion exchange resin cholestyramine may decrease the absorption of many other drugs, such as warfarin and aspirin.

Absorption from intramuscular sites is chiefly influenced by the aqueous solubility of the drug concerned and the regional blood flow. Absorption is delayed by formulating the drug as less soluble complexes (e.g. procaine penicillin, protamine zinc insulin), or as oily suspensions of esterized preparations composed of long-chain fatty acids (e.g. fluphenazine decanoate). Alternatively the rate of absorption may be diminished by the addition of a vasoconstrictor (catecholamine or synthetic derivative of posterior pituitary extract). The combination of these drugs with local anaesthetic agents will increase the duration of action and reduce the systemic toxicity of the latter. A number of drugs that may be administered systemically (e.g. sympathomimetic amines and beta blockers) can significantly modify skin and muscle blood flow. If tissue blood flow is decreased by such mechanisms, and extensive biotransformation of the parenterally administered drug occurs at tissue sites, its bioavailability will consequently be affected.

Distribution

When drugs are absorbed into the systemic circulation, they are present in plasma either in simple solution or bound to carrier proteins or erythrocytes, and are subsequently conveyed to their sites of action by the vascular system. The uptake and subsequent distribution of inhalational anaesthetic agents is primarily influenced by minute ventilation and cardiac output. The rate of rise of alveolar concentration, which correlates with the induction of anaesthesia, is largely determined by ventilatory activity. The onset of anaesthesia may thus be delayed by the presence of respiratory depressants (e.g. narcotic analgesics and barbiturates). Conversely, drugs that reduce cardiac output (e.g. intravenous induction agents and beta-adrenoceptor antagonists) will allow an increased rise of alveolar concentration and by reflex vasoconstrictor effects will lead to enhanced cerebral perfusion. The rate of induction of anaesthesia may therefore be increased.

Drugs bind to serum and to tissue proteins in a manner that has important implications on their subsequent distribution and elimination. Plasma protein binding influences the fate of drugs in that only the unbound fraction can diffuse through the capillary walls, reach the site of action and be subjected to the elimination processes. The pharmacodynamic response is considered to be proportional to free drug concentration. Most acidic drugs bind to serum albumin, while basic drugs bind to lipoproteins, gamma globulins and particularly $alpha_1$-acid glycoprotein which shows increased levels in certain disease states and stress (Piafsky 1980). Drugs that are extremely bound to plasma proteins, such as oral anticoagulants, may be displaced by certain anti-inflammatory analgesics and sulphonylureas. This interaction may significantly increase the free concentration of the anticoagulant concerned. However, it is unlikely that the displacement of drugs from plasma proteins is a prime factor in the causation of drug interactions. Any increase in the bound fraction of drug in plasma will be compensated by increased hepatic and renal clearance, so that a new steady state is established and drug distribution to the site of action is not significantly enhanced. Drugs that are involved in significant clinical interaction with warfarin, such as phenylbutazone, will also affect the metabolism of the anticoagulant. This is presumably due to competition at enzymatic sites, whose own protein configuration may be important in this context. The prior administration of certain sulphonamides (Csogor & Kerek 1970) and radio-opaque dyes is said to decrease the degree of protein binding of thiopentone; it is considered unlikely that this interaction is of any clinical significance.

Some drugs may be extensively bound to tissue proteins. The antimalarial agents pamaquin and mepacrine undergo significant binding to hepatic proteins, and interactions may occur between these two drugs because of competition for these sites. Many drugs used in anaesthetic practice (e.g. local anaesthetics and muscle relaxants) can be shown to sequester in various cellular reservoirs (lung, liver, kidney, muscle and cartilage), presumably due to protein binding at non-specific sites (Maclagan 1976). It is not known whether this phenomenon is associated with any significant drug interactions.

Biotransformation

Many drugs are extensively metabolized when they enter the systemic circulation. In some instances such biotransformation leads to the production of a more active substance, that is the drug administered can be regarded as a 'prodrug'. Examples include chloral hydrate, cyclophosphamide and certain steroids. In other cases the drug, though itself active, may be metabolized to a compound of similar pharmacological activity. Thiopentone is metabolized to pentobarbitone, a barbiturate with similar ability to induce central nervous system (CNS) depression, while the metabolites of diazepam possess their own intrinsic activity as minor tranquillizers. In the majority of cases, however, biotransformation leads to the production of more polar, less lipid-soluble compounds that are less able to penetrate cellular barriers but are more vulnerable to renal elimination, that is the administered drug is rendered inactive.

Drug interactions associated with biotransformation may evolve in two ways:

1. A number of drugs can increase the activity of enzymes concerned with their biotransformation (enzyme induction). In these circumstances autoinduction will occur and lead to tolerance when patients continue to receive the drug over a long period. Furthermore, this enzyme induction can also influence the degradation of other drugs which rely on similar metabolic pathways. The most familiar example of this is the propensity of barbiturates to reduce the pharmacological activity of oral anticoagulants when these drugs are administered concurrently (Goss &

Dickhaus 1965). Conversely, the sudden withdrawal of the barbiturate will increase the likelihood of toxicity with the existing dose of the anticoagulant.

2. Many drugs participate in the same enzymatic pathways. A drug that has the greater affinity for the enzyme system concerned can effectively delay the metabolic degradation of a second drug simultaneously administered (enzyme inhibition), and thus lead to a greater potency and likelihood of toxicity from the latter drug. Familiar examples to anaesthetists are the inhibition of pseudocholinesterase with prolongation of the action of suxamethonium by local anaesthetic esters, and the delayed metabolism (and increased toxicity) of pethidine in patients also receiving monoamine oxidase inhibitors.

Excretion

The elimination of drugs via the kidneys is effectively a balance between glomerular filtration, tubular secretion and tubular reabsorption. Glomerular filtration is directly related to renal perfusion, and drug removal may be decreased (and pharmacological activity thus enhanced) by other drugs which may reduce renal blood flow (e.g. catecholamines: drugs used to induce profound hypotension).

Both acid and basic drugs, and their metabolites, are also partially eliminated from plasma by secretion in the proximal renal tubule. Drug interaction may result from competition by two agents for the active transport sites. Benzylpenicillin is a weak acid whose active secretion can be suppressed by most diuretics and anti-inflammatory analgesics, as well as by probenecid.

Active transport is also involved in some aspects of tubular reabsorption (the principle of action of most uricosuric agents is to inhibit the enzyme responsible for the reuptake of the urate). However, in most instances reabsorption is a passive process, the extent of which is determined by the amount of unionized drug present in the renal tubules. Alkalization of the urine (with, e.g., sodium bicarbonate) will increase the ionization of acidic drugs such as barbiturates and salicylate, and thus facilitate their excretion. Similarly, acidification of the urine (with, e.g., ammonium chloride) will promote the removal of basic drugs such as narcotics and tricyclic antidepressants. Such beneficial interactions can be of value in the treatment of drug poisoning.

Liver blood flow is an important determinant of hepatic clearance and is of special significance when drugs, such as narcotic analgesics, have a high extraction ratio. Drugs that decrease liver blood flow (e.g. propranolol and phenothiazines) may increase the systemic bioavailability of morphine-related drugs and thus enhance their pharmacological profile. Similar effects on the hepatic clearance of a number of drugs may occur following the administration of general or regional anaesthetic techniques which result in a decrease in cardiac output or in systemic hypotension (Nies et al 1976).

Morphine is subjected to conjugation in the gut wall and liver, and is excreted into the upper small intestine as the glucuronide metabolite. Breakdown of this conjugate with subsequent release and reuptake of the parent compound occurs after exposure to the intestinal flora (enterohepatic recirculation). Antibacterial agents that inhibit the micro-organisms in the gut may prevent this breakdown and thus reduce the total bioavailability of morphine. A similar mechanism would appear to account for the attenuation of the effects of the contraceptive 'pill' when tetracyclines are administered concurrently.

Some highly basic and lipid-soluble narcotic analgesics (e.g. pethidine and fentanyl) may be excreted from the systemic circulation into the acidic environment of the stomach. Their subsequent reuptake from the small intestine may result in a 'secondary peak' effect. This gastroenteric recirculatory process may be modified by drugs that either influence splanchnic blood flow or produce changes in gastric pH (Calvey et al 1983).

Pharmacodynamic interactions

Pharmacodynamic interactions are due to interference with the effects of drugs at their sites of action in tissues. The resultant interaction may produce additive, synergistic, potentiating or antagonistic effects. Many antagonistic interactions are positively beneficial and form the basis of standard therapeutics. Examples include the use of protamine to reverse the anticoagulant effects of heparin, of naloxone to counteract the depressant effects of opiate analgesics, and the administration of chelating agents in the treatment of heavy metal poisoning. A much quoted example of pharmacodynamic antagonism producing an undesirable response is the inhibition of the active transport of guanethidine and related compounds into the adrenergic neurone by tricylic antidepressants and other drugs that block uptake mechanisms (Mitchell et al 1970).

More potentially harmful effects can occur when interactions are related to the additive effects of drugs at receptor or similar tissue sites. Such examples include the CNS (e.g. barbiturates, benzodiazepines and phenothiazines) and the autonomic nervous system (e.g. atropine-like drugs and tricyclic antidepressants). Instances of drug potentiation include the effect of chlorpromazine and other drugs which block alpha-adrenergic receptors in enhancing the hypotensive effects of other drugs (e.g. halothane and d-tubocurarine), and the increase in toxicity of cardiac glycosides in the presence of calcium salts or diuretic agents which effectively reduce serum potassium levels.

Receptor regulation

It can be demonstrated with the use of radioligands that the adrenergic receptor density is modified under certain conditions. In general, high catecholamine concentrations reduce the number and density of adrenergic receptors ('down regulation'; Harden 1983), while any fall in circulating adrenaline and noradrenaline, produced either by drugs or by denervation, increases the number of receptors. This adaptation process probably accounts for the phenomenon of supersensitivity, which may be exemplified by the exaggerated response to pressor agents that may occur in patients who are receiving adrenergic neurone-blocking drugs. It is postulated that similar receptor adaptation may occur in relation to other neurotransmitters and could help to explain the rebound phenomena which occur after the sudden withdrawal of drugs such as beta blockers, clonidine and anticonvulsants, and the adverse response to suxamethonium in patients with major neurological deficits.

DRUG INTERACTIONS IN ANAESTHETIC PRACTICE

The following text deals with interactions that may occur in anaesthetic practice and their possible avoidance or subsequent management. The interactions considered are those that may take place between pre-existing drug therapy and general/local anaesthetic agents, muscle relaxants, narcotic analgesics and drugs used in premedication. Interactions between anaesthetic drugs and their adjuvants are shown in Table 25.1.

Drugs affecting the cardiovascular system

Antihypertensive drugs

Many drugs used during an anaesthetic sequence can themselves lower the blood pressure by a number of different mechanisms, and interaction with coexistent antihypertensive therapy is therefore likely to occur. The original reports of complications of severe hypotension and bradycardia, or postural hypotension during recovery, were particularly associated with patients receiving reserpine therapy (Ominsky & Wollman 1969). At one time it was considered desirable that, whenever possible, antihypertensive drugs should be withdrawn for up to 14 days prior to anaesthesia and surgery. Various tests were also used to assess the magnitude of residual sympathetic activity. These included the measurement of blood pressure responses to the Valsalva manoeuvre or to postural changes, and the administration of indirectly acting sympathomimetic amines such as ephedrine or tyrosine (Crandell 1962). This view is no longer tenable: it is unjustified or even dangerous to stop antihypertensive therapy prior to anaesthesia. Rebound

Table 25.1 Interactions between drugs used during anaesthesia

Intravenous induction agents	Inhalational agents	Neuromuscular blockers	Analgesics	Local anaesthetics and sympathomimetic amines
Increased depressant effects on VMC and RC with inhalational agents	'Second gas' effects of N_2O will increase rate of uptake of other agents	d-tubocurarine can increase hypotensive effect of volatile agents	Effects on RC may influence uptake, distribution and elimination of inhalational agents	Increased risk of arrhythmias in presence of inhalational agents (H > E > I)
Increased depressant effects on RC with analgesics	Additive 'medullary' effects with intravenous induction agents and analgesics	Pancuronium may inhibit breakdown of suxamethonium	MAC value of inhalational agents may be reduced	Ester compounds may inhibit breakdown of suxamethonium
Increased likelihood of tachyarrhythmias with ketamine and anticholinergic premedication	Pharmacokinetics of neuromuscular blockers may be altered due to distribution factors	Increased likelihood of tachyarrhythmias if gallamine or pancuronium used with ketamine	Bradycardias more likely with inhalational agents	May potentiate neuromuscular block due to 'membrane stabilizing' effect
Diazepam decreases MAC value of H	Increased 'potency' of neuromuscular blockers due to central and peripheral effects (I > E > H)			
	'Dual' block more likely with repeated suxamethonium			
	Halothane anaesthesia may decrease clearance of analgesics			

E: enflurane, H: halothane, I: Isoflurane, RC: respiratory centre, VMC: vasomotor centre.

phenomena may occur due to sudden cessation of the drug therapy. Furthermore, hypertensive responses which can manifest during induction and endotracheal intubation may be exaggerated (Prys-Roberts et al 1971). It is recommended that treatment with beta-adrenoceptor antagonists is maintained up until the time of anaesthesia and the last dose given within a few hours of surgery (Foex 1983). It appears logical that a similar regime should be employed in patients receiving other antihypertensive agents.

Nevertheless, it can be anticipated that reflex autonomic responses may be obtunded during anaesthesia. Cardiovascular monitoring is essential, and particular attention should be paid to maintenance of blood volume, ventilatory parameters and positioning of the patient. Abnormal sympathetic responses may also be anticipated during the recovery period. The dose of intravenous induction agent should be reduced, particularly in those patients who are receiving antihypertensive agents that have a central sedative effect (e.g. methyldopa and reserpine). D-tubocurarine, which may produce additive effects because of its ganglion-blocking activity, is perhaps better avoided. Paradoxically, should pharmacological intervention be necessary to treat a profound fall in blood pressure, a test dose of vasopressor should be given initially to obviate the risk of supersensitivity.

Ganglion-blocking agents, which are used to induce hypotension during anaesthesia and occasionally in the management of hypertensive crises, may complicate neuromuscular block. They demonstrate affinity both for the acetylcholine receptor and for acetylcholine esterase. An anticurare effect has been observed, but in high doses these drugs will prolong competitive blockade (Blackman et al 1975). Trimetaphan also inhibits plasma cholinesterase and thus prolongs the effect of suxamethonium (Poulton et al 1979). Care is needed if muscle relaxants are administered at the same time as ganglion-blocking agents. There may be some reduction in dose requirements.

Antiarrhythmic agents

Many antiarrhythmic drugs have now become available. They have varying modes of action, including a slowing of the rate of depolarization of cardiac muscle due to suppression of Na^+ intake (e.g. procainamide and disopyramide) or Ca^{2+} antagonism (e.g. verapamil), a prolongation of the effective refractory period (amiodarone) and by antagonism of cardiac beta-adrenoceptors (e.g. propranolol). However, there is often some overlap in the modes of action of these various drugs, and the net result is the reduction of dysrhythmias whether they are due to enhanced automaticity of ectopic foci or to re-entrant phenomena. Sinus rhythm is often restored, the ventricular rate is usually slowed and the work of the heart reduced. New dysrhythmias not infrequently occur during therapy.

Interactions with antiarrhythmic agents may occur during anaesthesia when anaesthetic agents with intrinsic vagomimetic activity are used. Synergistic effects may lead to the development of a potentially dangerous bradycardia. The muscarinic effects of suxamethonium on the heart may be enhanced and the prior administration of atropine may be indicated when this relaxant is used. Bradycardia is not commonly associated with the use of enflurane and isoflurane, and these volatile agents are preferable to halothane in this context.

Some of these drugs have a significant 'membrane stabilizing' effect (e.g. quinidine and propranolol) and theoretically may inhibit depolarization at both pre- and postsynaptic sites. Prolongation of neuromuscular block by suxamethonium has occurred following the administration of intravenous quinidine (Grogono 1963).

Antianginal agents

Organic nitrates, beta blockers and calcium channel blocking agents are commonly used in the management of angina. This therapy should always be continued up to the immediate preoperative period as the risks of rebound phenomena (e.g. worsening of angina symptoms) outweigh those due to possible drug interaction. The percutaneous administration of glyceryl trinitrate is sometimes continued during anaesthesia to minimize the risks of anginal attacks in the perioperative period. There is a theoretical risk of potentiation of systemic hypotension or reflex tachycardia.

Calcium channel blockers

Calcium channel blockers are now widely used, as in the prophylaxis of angina pectoris. Dihydropyridine derivatives (e.g. nifedipine and nicardipine) are also well established as effective antihypertensive agents. Pharmacodynamic interactions between this group of drugs and those used during anaesthesia must be anticipated as there is considerable evidence that inhalational agents themselves can inhibit calcium fluxes across transcellular membranes (Bosjnak & Kampine 1986). Furthermore, verapamil has been shown in animal studies to reduce the minimum alveolar concentration (MAC) value for halothane by 25% (Maze & Mason 1983).

In consequence, a large number of studies have been undertaken, both in animals and in man, to assess the likelihood of drug interactions. It would appear that, under normal circumstances, clinical concentrations of volatile anaesthetic agents and therapeutic concentrations of calcium channel blocking drugs (preadministered by the oral route) do not produce significant additive effects (Merin 1987). However, experimental studies suggest that the administration of intravenous verapamil to dogs with depressed left ventricular function that were undergoing open-chest surgery and receiving volatile inhalational agents can lead to a further decrease in ventricular activity (Kates et al 1983). Furthermore, verapamil and related compounds may induce various degrees of heart block and these may be enhanced by volatile agents. Care in preoperative assessment and perioperative monitoring is especially important in patients receiving these drugs.

The effects of calcium channel blockers may be further enhanced by the concomitant administration of beta blockers, which will diminish the reflex responses to the depressant effects of the calcium channel blockers and augment their effects by reducing the availability of calcium channels (by lowering the intracellular levels of cyclic AMP; Lindemann et al 1982). Special vigilance is necessary in patients who are receiving combined therapy. Alternative techniques (e.g. regional blockade and high-dose fentanyl regimes) may be considered. If volatile anaesthetic agents are essential, evidence suggests that isoflurane is preferable to halothane or enflurane.

Calcium channel blockers may also be expected to potentiate neuromuscular blocking agents. Calcium is essential for the presynaptic release of acetylcholine and is important in the subsequent excitation–contraction coupling. Experimental evidence has confirmed the synergistic effects of muscle relaxants and calcium channel blockers. It is not clear whether dose requirements of relaxants are reduced in clinical practice in the presence of these drugs. However, monitoring of neuromuscular blockade is important in these circumstances and postoperative observations should be particularly vigilant to avoid the risk of unrecognized recurarization (Foex 1989).

Cardiac glycosides

The effect of digitalis and related drugs is partially mediated by the vagus. Suxamethonium may have additive effects and enhance digitalis toxicity (Avery 1973). The use of atropine may be necessary if there is evidence of a bradycardia or atrioventricular conduction defect. There is an increased risk of dysrhythmias when pancuronium is administered to digitalized patients. Toxic arrhythmias may be precipitated if calcium salts are being administered during anaesthesia (e.g. in association with major blood transfusion) in the presence of digitalis.

Autonomic drugs

Sympathomimetic amines

Drugs such as adrenaline, ephedrine and phenylpropanolamine may be encountered in 'over the counter' cough and cold remedies and in compound preparations used for nebulization therapy in obstructive airway disease. The relatively short half-life of these drugs makes it unlikely that any significant interaction can occur during anaesthesia, although they should not be administered prior to induction.

Aminophylline may have similar effects to catecholamines on cardiac receptors and may facilitate the release of noradrenaline from presynaptic sites. Ventricular tachycardia has been reported when halothane was administered to patients who had been given aminophylline shortly before induction or who were still receiving it by infusion (Roizen & Stevens 1978). Enflurane might be safer.

Fenfluramine is a sympathomimetic amine with mixed (direct and indirect) actions and is related to the amphetamines. It is used as an appetite-suppressant. Clinical and experimental studies suggest a significant interaction between fenfluramine and halothane. It is advised that fenfluramine should be discontinued a week before surgery if possible (Bennett & Eltrincham 1977).

Beta$_2$-adrenoceptor **stimulants** such as salbutamol and terbutaline are now extensively used, both as oral preparations and inhalants, in the treatment of asthma. Pretreatment with these agents would afford some protection from any hypersensitivity response that occurred during anaesthesia. However, these drugs may evince both central and peripheral effects of sympathetic stimulation. Tachyarrhythmias may occur and halogenated hydrocarbons should be used with caution. Theoretically, patients receiving these drugs may show an increased requirement of sedative and hypnotic drugs, and particular attention should be paid to the depth of anaesthesia.

Antagonists of sympathomimetic activity

Alpha-adrenoceptor antagonists (alpha blockers) such as tolazoline and phenoxybenzamine are used in the treatment of peripheral vascular disorders and to improve organ perfusion in the management of shock. Apart from prazosin (which is a useful antihypertensive agent), most drugs in this class affect both alpha$_1$ and alpha$_2$ receptors (Fig. 25.1). Thus, although peripheral resistance is reduced, noradrenaline output from the adrenergic neurone is actually increased and there may be significant 'overspill' on to the unblocked beta-receptors. Care is therefore necessary during the administration of halothane or with the use of adrenaline-containing solutions.

Beta-adrenoceptor antagonists (beta blockers) are chiefly used as antihypertensive and anti-arrhythmic agents but may be prescribed in a variety of other conditions, for example management of thyrotoxicosis, migrainous neuralgia and anxiety states. Beta blockers may enhance any bronchospasm that occurs during anaesthesia. Conversely they will exert a protective effect against dysrhythmias induced by exogenous or endogenous catecholamines.

Parasympathomimetic agents

Parasympathomimetic agents, including synthetic analogues of acetylcholine, naturally occurring alkaloids and anticholinesterases, are used as anti-arrhythmic agents, in the treatment of atony of bladder and gut and as miotics. Anticholinesterases are also used in the treatment of myasthenia gravis. In most instances the concurrent use of these drugs is unlikely to cause any interactions, although atropine may be indicated preoperatively. However, the anticholinesterase agents will inhibit plasma cholinesterase activity and prolong the action of suxamethonium. The concomitant use of the long-acting and relatively stable drug, distigmine, would theoretically have particular consequences.

Antagonists of parasympathomimetic activity

The chronic use of atropine, hyoscine and their analogues as antispasmodics, antiparkinsonian therapy or as mydriatics is unlikely to cause any

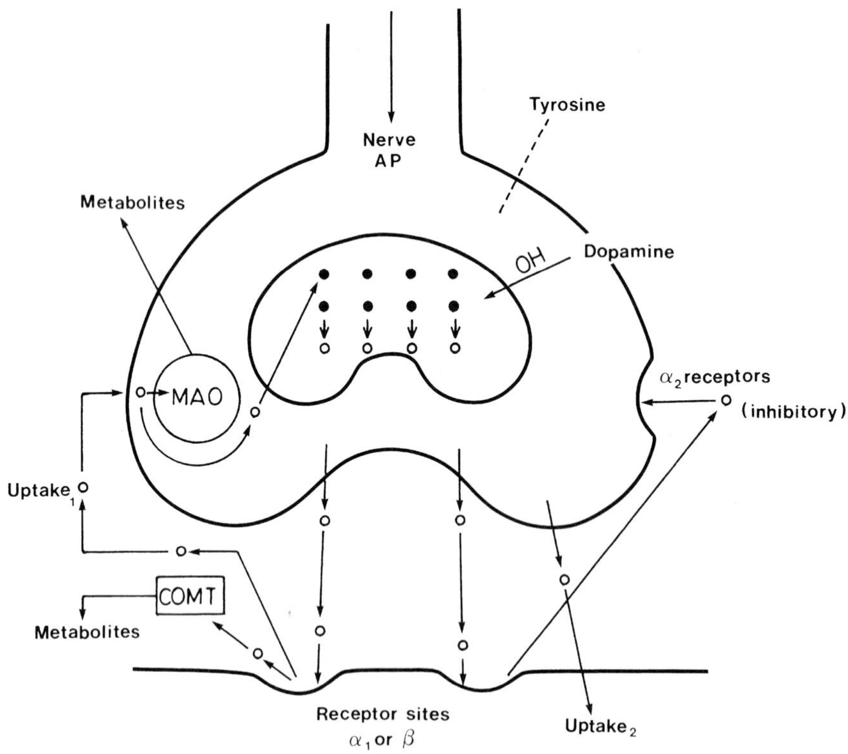

Fig. 25.1 The adrenergic nerve terminal showing the synthesis, release and reuptake of noradrenaline. AP: action potential, ●: Bound adrenaline, ○: unbound adrenaline, MAO: monoamine oxidase, COMT: Catechol-O-methyl transferase

significant drug interactions in anaesthesia. However, there is a possibility of tachyarrhythmias occurring if ketamine or gallamine is used in the anaesthetic sequence.

Miotics

Eye drops containing parasympathomimetic agents are used in the treatment of glaucoma. In most instances, interactions are unlikely, however the organophosphorous compound, ecothiopate, is a potentially irreversible inhibitor of cholinesterase enzymes and cases of suxamethonium apnoea have been reported in association with its use (Pantuck 1966). This interaction is now primarily of academic interest as this ophthalmic preparation is no longer available in the UK.

The beta-adrenoceptor antagonist, timolol, is used in the treatment of chronic simple glaucoma. Systemic absorption is known to occur following topical application. Marked bradycardia and hypotension have occurred during halothane anaesthesia in a patient who was using both timolol and pilocarpine eye drops. A significant plasma level of timolol was found (Mishra et al 1983).

Drugs acting on the central nervous system

Sedatives, hypnotics and minor tranquillizers

All general anaesthetic agents have a reversible depressant effect on the CNS. The prior administration of other drugs with similar actions will undoubtedly lead to additive effects. The MAC value of halothane has been shown to be reduced by about 35% in the presence of diazepam (Perisho et al 1971). Serious problems are unlikely but a reduced anaesthetic requirement may be anticipated.

Antipsychotic drugs

Tricyclic antidepressants. The reuptake of endogenous catecholamines across the axonal membrane into the nerve terminal (Uptake$_1$, or the amine pump) is blocked by most tricyclic antidepressants (TCADs), which compete for the active transport mechanism (Fig. 25.1). In these conditions the effects of adrenaline on the circulation are potentiated by two or three times and the pressor response to exogenous noradrenaline is enhanced by four to nine times (Svedmyr 1968). In addition, circumstantial clinical evidence has suggested that significant drug interactions during dental surgery can occur when local anaesthetic solutions containing noradrenaline are administered to patients receiving TCADs (Boakes et al 1972). Such solutions are no longer commercially available in the UK, and present opinion suggests that provided proper attention is given to dosage and technique, the use of local anaesthetic solutions containing adrenaline in these circumstances will not lead to clinically significant drug interaction. Pancuronium and ketamine may also inhibit the neuronal reuptake of catecholamines. The administration of these drugs to patients who are receiving TCADs is not recommended as supra-additive effects may ensue (Dodson 1982). A number of these antidepressants may also produce drowsiness by central post-synaptic inhibitory mechanisms and general anaesthetic requirements may be reduced. The large number of antimuscarinic side effects that are associated with TCADs may theoretically be enhanced by atropine and related drugs which may be used for premedication.

Monoamine oxidase inhibitors. Following reuptake into the nerve terminal a significant amount of noradrenaline is metabolized by the enzyme monoamine oxidase located in the mitochondria. Inactivation of this enzyme by drugs will allow a greater fraction of noradrenaline to return to binding sites in the storage granules (Fig. 25.1). Increased amounts of noradrenaline will thus be available for release, either by the arrival of a nerve action potential or following the administration of indirectly acting sympathomimetic amines (e.g. ephedrine, amphetamines and various tyramine containing foodstuffs). Pressor responses will thus be accentuated. In contrast, monoamine oxidase inhibitors (MAOIs) themselves may exhibit antihypertensive effects, either by autonomic ganglionic blockade or by the production of 'false transmitters'.

Monoamine oxidase is also abundant in liver hepatocytes and probably plays an important role in the metabolism of other drugs and endogenous substances. In particular, the complex biotransformation of pethidine (and presumably analogues such as phenoperidine and fentanyl) is inhibited and significant amounts of one metabolite, norpethidine, which has convulsive properties, may accumulate (Clark 1967). Alternatively, the interaction between pethidine and MAOIs may relate to the production of critically high levels of 5-hydroxytryptamine within the CNS (Rogers & Thornton 1969).

Particular problems may be anticipated during anaesthesia for patients receiving such drugs, with regard both to levels of CNS activity and to peripheral autonomic control (Goldberg 1964). Manufacturer's recommendations still suggest that this medication should preferably be stopped 1–2 weeks before non-urgent procedures. However, this is by no means universal anaesthetic practice, and if a policy to withhold the drugs is enforced, effective alternative therapy must be provided in the interim period. If a decision to continue MAOI therapy is made, or more urgent surgery is contemplated, the use of pethidine and indirectly acting vasopressors is absolutely contraindicated. Pretreatment with drugs having significant alpha-blocking properties (e.g. phenothiazines) may be valuable. Hypotensive episodes should be managed with plasma expanders and hydrocortisone. Morphine may be used as an analgesic if a test dose (1–2 mg) produces no untoward effects.

Interactions between MAOIs and other drugs used during general anaesthetic procedures appear to be relatively uncommon. However, there is some evidence that phenelzine may decrease plasma cholinesterase levels. This may lead to prolongation of apnoea following the administration of suxamethonium during electroconvulsive therapy (Bodley et al 1969). Hepatotoxicity is an uncommon but serious side effect associated with the use of MAOIs; it would thus seem prudent to avoid the use of halothane with patients receiving these drugs (Stack et al 1988).

The use of local anaesthetic solutions containing adrenaline is not contraindicated in patients receiving MAOIs. Exogenous adrenaline is effectively destroyed by the enzyme catechol-O-methyl transferase, which is widely available at extraneuronal sites.

Major tranquillizers

Phenothiazines and related substances (butyrophenones and thioxanthenes) can have ubiquitous effects on peripheral receptors in addition to their central action on reticular pathways. It could thus be anticipated that they:

1. have additive effects on other CNS depressants (induction and inhalational agents)
2. potentiate narcotic analgesics by a central mechanism and by reducing the 'first pass' effect
3. enhance the hypotensive effect of some anaesthetic agents (e.g. halothane and enflurane)
4. increase the toxicity of exogenous catecholamines
5. prolong competitive neuromuscular blockade by a 'membrane-stabilizing' effect.

In spite of these possibilities, significant interactions associated with the use of these drugs have not been reported or experienced. However, a reduced requirement of general anaesthetic agents and narcotic analgesics, with a depression of autonomic reflex activity, could be anticipated. Some neuroleptic drugs, particularly chlorpromazine, can lower the seizure threshold and the concomitant use of anaesthetic agents with epileptogenic properties, for example ketamine and enflurane, would seem unwise.

Lithium is used in the treatment of manic depressive psychosis. Lithium inhibits depolarization at selective sites and can also modify the distribution of electrolytes such as sodium, magnesium and calcium. Animal studies have shown that lithium can prolong the effect of certain muscle relaxants (suxamethonium and pancuronium) and a similar effect has been observed in man (Borden et al 1974, Hill et al 1976). Lithium toxicity can occur if the surgery is associated with electrolyte imbalance or deteriorating renal function.

Anticonvulsants. Most antiepileptic agents have significant enzyme-inducing properties, but these are unlikely to be of any import during the course of a single anaesthetic. The general anaesthetic requirements may be lessened because of the sedative properties of the anticonvulsants. Conversely these drugs may not give adequate protection if agents with known convulsant properties (methohexitone, enflurane and analeptic agents) are used during the course of anaesthesia.

Drugs used in parkinsonism

In the treatment of parkinsonism, anticholinergic drugs have in the main been superseded by agents that effectively replenish dopamine stores in the basal ganglia system. Levodopa, the immediate precursor of dopamine, is commonly used. Both hypertensive and hypotensive episodes have been reported in association with anaesthesia (Bevan et al 1973). This may reflect the preponderance of either dopa or dopamine at peripheral adrenergic receptors and is presumably dose-related. The effects of antiemetic drugs with central dopaminergic blocking properties may be inhibited. Conversely the mutual antagonism of these drugs and levodopa may herald the reappearance of parkinsonism.

Diuretics

Diuretics can induce a metabolic alkalosis and may alter the plasma concentrations of potassium and magnesium. They may occasionally prolong the effects of competitive neuromuscular blocking agents (Feldman 1963).

Antibacterial agents

Sulphonamides produce a bacteriostatic effect by preventing para-aminobenzoic acid from being incorporated into the folic acid nucleus. Procaine and other local anaesthetic esters provide an excess of this substrate and thus antagonize the effect of sulphonamides (Pfeiffer & Grant 1944). The concomitant use of these two drugs is therefore undesirable.

Aminoglycosides and tetracyclines may inhibit neuromuscular transmission by preventing the presynaptic release of acetylcholine. Tetracyclines presumably produce this effect by chelating extraneuronal calcium. The mode of action of aminoglycosides at this site is less clear, but they are also considered to have postsynaptic effects. Neuromuscular function may become impaired in tuberculous patients on long-term streptomycin therapy, and neostigmine-resistant curarization has been reported following abdominal surgery in which large doses of intraperitoneal aminoglycosides were administered (Benz et al 1961, Pittinger et al 1970). However, in modern practice, gentamicin is frequently administered by intravenous injection just prior to, or during, surgery for gastrointestinal pathology. There is little clinical evidence of any significant prolongation of neuromuscular blockade or of difficulties encountered during reversal. Should any problem arise, calcium salts and 4-aminopyridine, which also induces the presynaptic release of acetylcholine, may be used to supplement anticholinesterase drugs.

The nephrotoxic effects of both aminoglycosides and tetracycline are potentiated by the now obsolete inhalational agent, methoxyflurane. This effect is related to the increased elimination of the main metabolite, inorganic fluoride. A limited increase in the urinary excretion of fluoride ions follows the administration of enflurane and there could be a slight risk of renal damage if potentially nephrotoxic antibiotics are being used concomitantly (Mazze 1984).

Rifampicin, an antituberculous drug, is a potent inducer of hepatic microsomal enzymes. A nearly fatal hepatotoxic reaction has been reported following the administration of halothane anaesthesia to a patient who was also receiving rifampicin (Most & Markle 1974).

Hormones

Hormonal preparations are administered in two main circumstances: replacement therapy and active therapy.

Replacement therapy

If replacement therapy in endocrinological disorders is adequate, it is illogical to think that drug interactions will occur. If replacement is inadequate or in excess, problems occurring during the administration of anaesthetic agents are more properly related to the underlying endocrine disorder and are dealt with elsewhere.

Active therapy

Steroids are prescribed in a wide number of conditions including asthma, the arthritides and various skin disorders. If the daily intake of steroids is in excess of the normal physiological secretion (equivalent to 30 mg hydrocortisone in 24 h), the hypothalamo–pituitary–adrenal axis is suppressed. Thus the ability of the adrenal gland to secrete increased amounts of hydrocortisone in response to surgical stress is obtunded or absent, and may contribute to severe hypotension and cardiovascular collapse which can occur in the postoperative period. Conversely, the administration of large doses of steroids in the perioperative period may lead to delayed wound healing, an increased risk of postoperative infection, fluid retention and problems with hyperglycaemia.

A balanced outlook is therefore necessary. Previous studies have shown that adrenal suppression is unlikely to occur in patients who have ceased steroid therapy more than 2 months prior to surgery. Furthermore, plasma cortisol levels were only slightly depressed in patients who were still receiving prednisolone at the time of operation (Plumpton et al 1969a). In patients in whom it is particularly desirable to avoid steroids, or those who will require repeated procedures, the adequacy of the response of the pituitary–adrenal axis to stress (e.g. the insulin hypoglycaemia test) may be usefully measured (Plumpton et al 1969b). Alternatively, the morning plasma cortisol (hydrocortisone) level may provide a useful guide.

Many regimes of replacement therapy have been described. Hydrocortisone is usually administered by the intramuscular route to allow for more sustained blood levels. A dose of 100 mg is frequently chosen and is given prior to anaesthesia for minor procedures such as endoscopy. For more extensive operations (e.g. herniorrhaphy) the dose is repeated 6-hourly for up to 24 h, while for major surgery (e.g. colectomy) this dose regime should be extended up to 72 h before tailing off gradually to reach the normal preoperative dose requirement.

Modern-day thinking has led to the search for 'stress free' anaesthesia. Perhaps this enlightened approach will result in a fresh outlook on steroid cover during surgery. It is probable that dose regimes could be significantly diminished provided the normal daily physiological requirement is at least replaced and that satisfactory postoperative surveillance is maintained.

Clinical impressions have suggested that preoperative steroids can antagonize the effect of competitive neuromuscular blocking agents. It is not known whether this is due to pharmacokinetic (e.g. changes in plasma volume influencing drug distribution) or pharmacodynamic (alteration of plasma pH and electrolyte levels or induction of the enzyme choline acetyltransferase) factors. Furthermore it has been suggested that steroids administered during anaesthesia may potentiate the effects of muscle relaxants (Argov & Mastaglia 1979). Further studies are necessary.

The chronic use of adrenocorticotrophic hormone (ACTH) and its analogue tetracosactrin will not lead to any suppression of the pituitary–adrenal axis, and no special precautions are necessary during anaesthesia in these circumstances.

Sex hormones

Oestrogen therapy is used in the treatment of carcinoma of the prostate and in some cases of carcinoma of the breast. Combined oestrogen–progestogen preparations have achieved widespread use as oral contraceptives. It was initially estimated that the incidence of thrombophlebitis in young women receiving the 'pill' was increased from six-fold to ten-fold (Vessey & Doll 1968). The more recently introduced low-dose oestrogen preparations reduce this risk but do not eliminate it (see Ch. 18).

Patients receiving oestrogens or combined oral contraceptives have been found to have accelerated blood clotting and raised plasma concentrations of some coagulation factors, as well as increased platelet aggregation. These effects may persist for weeks or months after discontinuing therapy. The risk of thromboembolism in the postoperative period is enhanced, although this is much more likely to be due to factors causing mechanical stasis than to any interaction with anaesthetic agents. It has generally been recommended that these drugs should be stopped at least 1 month prior to elective major surgery, although evidence suggests that up to 3 months may elapse before coagulation processes return to 'normal'. For minor surgery the risk would appear to be minimal. In emergency cases, and in all women who have not discontinued the pill for a month, other methods should be used to reduce the likelihood of thrombotic episodes. Low-dose heparin regimes with either aspirin or dipyridamole during the perioperative period (see Ch. 17) are valuable in this context. Physical aspects (e.g. the use of 'antiemboli' stockings and early mobilization) are of equal importance.

Posterior pituitary extracts

Posterior pituitary hormones and their synthetic analogues are used to induce labour. They can produce peripheral vasodilatation by an effect on vascular smooth muscle and may lead to hypotension if administered in high doses to the anaesthetized patient (Weis & Peak 1974). Reflex tachycardia may also be associated with these agents and arrhythmias have been reported with the concomitant use of cyclopropane anaesthesia.

Cytotoxic agents

Cytotoxic agents are widely used in a variety of malignant conditions and as immunosuppressive therapy during transplant surgery. It is often unclear whether problems encountered during the administration of anaesthesia to patients who are receiving such drugs are due to specific interactions or to the manifestations of the underlying disease. Certainly, many of these drugs can be hepatotoxic (e.g. alkylating agents) and can produce quantitative and qualitative effects on plasma proteins and enzymes. Others are neurotoxic (e.g. vinca alkaloids) and may accentuate the autonomic neuropathy that is often associated with the later stages of malignant disease. In such cases, abnormal responses may be anticipated when patients receive muscle relaxants or anaesthetic agents with significant autonomic effects. Certain alkylating agents (cyclophosphamide and thiotepa) are reported as potentiating the effects of suxamethonium (Zsigmond & Robins 1972).

Miscellaneous drugs

Magnesium sulphate

Large doses of magnesium sulphate are still occasionally administered by parenteral routes in the management of eclampsia. Mg^{2+} depresses the output of acetylcholine from presynaptic sites, and abnormal responses to the effects of simultaneously administered muscle relaxants have been reported. Calcium salts may be required in the reversal of neuromuscular blockade.

Cimetidine

Cimetidine, an H_2 antagonist, binds to Cytochrome P-450 and thus inhibits the activity of the microsomal mixed-function oxidase system. Cimetidine may potentiate the effect of certain benzodiazepines used in premedication (e.g. diazepam and nitrazepam) because of decreased hepatic metabolism. The biotransformation of propranolol, phenytoin and certain barbiturates is similarly inhibited (Sedman 1984). The clearance of lignocaine is diminished by both cimetidine and ranitidine due to their effect in reducing hepatic blood flow. An observation that cimetidine induced a marked prolongation of the action of suxamethonium has not been substantiated by subsequent clinical studies (Woodworth et al 1989).

Effects of anaesthesia on concomitant therapy

So far, consideration has been given to the possible undesirable effects of pre-existing drug therapy on the conduct of anaesthesia. It is also relevant to consider the converse problem, that is the effects of anaesthesia on coadministered drugs. Many agents used for premedication or anaesthesia, including thiopentone, diazepam, nitrous oxide and halothane, have been shown to induce the activity of hepatic drug-metabolizing enzymes. It is thus possible that the plasma concentration and therefore the pharmacological activity of certain other drugs (e.g. steroids, anticoagulants and anticonvulsants) could be reduced. Alternatively there may be a significant increase in the production of toxic metabolites of certain agents (e.g. isoniazid). The problem is complicated by the fact that the underlying disease and the associated surgical trauma may have a depressant effect on drug metabolism, and lead to higher plasma concentrations of drugs that are administered soon after surgery. Studies incorporating antipyrine as an index of the efficiency of hepatic drug metabolizing systems have been performed in the perioperative period. They have shown that short procedures are followed by increased enzyme activity, but in protracted operations the activity is decreased (Pessayre et al 1978).

SUMMARY

Drug interactions that occur during anaesthesia due to pre-existing therapy remain a potential hazard. However, in almost all cases serious problems should be avoidable or even used to advantage by the anaesthetist. Current opinion suggests that there are few, if any, indications for withdrawing active drug therapy prior to anaesthesia. In order to minimize the likelihood of complications the anaesthetist should:

- possess a sound knowledge of the underlying mechanisms involved in drug interaction
- take a careful drug history
- use the minimum amount of anaesthetic agent required to obtain the appropriate pharmacological response
- check equipment and institute appropriate monitoring
- have available a checklist describing the more unusual interactions (Grogono 1970).

In view of the multiplicity of interactions that have been described in the literature, some comfort can be taken from the relative rarity of mortality or permanent morbidity associated with anaesthesia (Attia & Grogono 1978). However, as we approach a more litigation-conscious era, attention must be paid to the fact that certain anaesthetic agents may occasionally produce side effects that are 'coincidental' or possibly 'unmask' those possessed by concomitant drug therapy (Mueller & Lundberg 1988). Examples include:

- the use of halothane in patients who are receiving potentially hepatotoxic drugs or drugs that have significant enzyme-inducing properties (e.g. MAOIs, dantrolene and rifampicin)
- the prolonged administration of nitrous oxide when drugs with a propensity to reduce bone marrow activity are also being given (e.g. chloramphenicol and fluorouracil)
- the administration of local anaesthetic agents by regional or spinal routes in the presence of drugs with neurotoxic properties (e.g. hydralazine and penicillamine).

In these circumstances a balanced view is essential. However, such problems should be minimized by the wide choice of agents now available for anaesthesia. Detailed examination of the CNS and the administration of Vitamin B_{12} or folinic acid in the perioperative period may be indicated.

REFERENCES

Argov Z, Mastaglia F L 1979 Disorders of neuromuscular transmission caused by drugs. N Engl J Med 301: 409–413

Attia R R, Grogono A W 1978 Drug and disease interactions. In: Attia R R, Grogono A W (eds) Practical anaesthetic pharmacology. Appleton Century Croft, New York, 15: 243–261

Avery G S 1973 Check list to potentially clinically important interactions. Drugs 5: 187–211

Bennett J A, Eltrincham R J 1977 Possible dangers in anaesthesia in patients receiving fenfluramine: results of animal studies following a case of human cardiac arrest. Anaesthesia 32: 8–13

Benz H G, Lunn J N, Foldes F F 1961 Recurarisation by intraperitoneal antibiotics. Br Med J 2: 241–242
Bevan D R, Monks P S, Calne D B 1973 Cardiovascular reaction to anaesthesia following treatment with levodopa. Anaesthesia 28: 29–31
Blackman J G, Gauldie R W, Milne R J 1975 Interaction of competitive antagonists: the anticurare action of hexamethonium and other antagonists at the skeletal neuromuscular junction. Br J Clin Pharmacol 54: 91–100
Boakes A J, Laurence D R, Lovel K W, O'Neil R, Veril P J 1972 Adverse reactions to local anaesthetic/vasoconstrictor preparations: a study of the cardiovascular responses to xylestesin and hostacain-with-noradrenaline. Br Dent J 133: 137–140
Bodley R P, Halwax K, Potts L 1969 Low serum cholinesterase levels complicating treatment with phenelzine. Br Med J 3: 510–512
Borden H, Clarke M T, Katz H 1974 The use of pancuronium bromide in patients receiving lithium carbonate. Can Anaesth Soc J 21: 79–82
Bosjnak Z J, Kampine J P 1986 Effects of halothane on transmembrane potentials, Ca^{2+} transients, and pupillary muscle tension in the cat. Am J Physiol 251: H374–H381
Calvey T N, Milne L A, Williams N E, Chan K, Murray G R 1983 Effect of antacids on the plasma concentration of phenoperidine. Br J Anaesth 55: 535–539
Clark B 1967 The in vitro inhibition of the n-demethylation of pethidine by phenelzine (phenylethylhydrazine). Biochem Pharmacol 16: 2369–2385
Crandell D LeR 1962 The anaesthetic hazards in patients on antihypertensive therapy. J Am Med Assoc 179: 495–500
Csogor S I, Kerek S F 1970 Enhancement of thiopentone anaesthesia by sulphafurazole. Br J Anaesth 42: 988–990
Dodson M E 1982 Drug interactions and anaesthesia. Hospital Update 8: 57–68
Enderby G E H 1944 The use and abuse of trichlorethylene. Br Med J 2: 300–302
Feldman S A 1963 Effects of changes in electrolytes, hydration and pH upon the reactions to muscle relaxants. Br J Anaesth 35: 546–551
Foex P 1983 Beta blockade in anaesthesia. Journal of Hospital and Clinical Pharmacy 8: 183–190
Foex P 1989 Calcium channel blockers. Curr Opin Anaesthesiol 2: 71–79
Goldberg L I 1964 Monoamine oxidase inhibitors: adverse reactions and possible mechanisms. J Am Med Assoc 190: 456–462
Goss J E, Dickhaus D W 1965 Increased bishydroxycoumarin requirements in patients receiving phenobarbital. N Engl J Med 273: 1094–1095
Grayson J G 1971 Incompatabilities of multiple additives to intravenous infusion fluids. Pharm J 206: 64–71
Grogono A W 1963 Anaesthesia for atrial defibrillation: effect of quinidine on muscular relaxation. Lancet 2: 1039–1040
Grogono A W 1970 Danger lists for the anaesthetist. Anaesthesia 25: 518–524
Halsey P J 1987 Drug interactions in anaesthesia. Br J Anaesth 59: 112–123
Harden T K 1983 Agonist-induced desensitisation of the b-adrenergic receptor-linked adenylate cyclase. Pharmacol Rev 35: 5–32
Hill G E, Wong K C, Hodges M R 1976 Potentiation of succinylcholine neuromuscular blockade by lithium bicarbonate. Anesthesiology 44: 439–442
Kates R A, Kaplan J A, Guyton R A, Dorsey L, Hug C C, Hatcher C R 1983 Haemodynamic interactions of verapamil and isoflurane. Anesthesiology 59: 132–138
Lindemann J P, Bailey J C, Watanabe A M 1982 Potential biochemical mechanisms for regulation of slow inward current: theoretical basis for drug action. Am Heart J 103: 746–756
Maclagan J 1976 Competitive neuromuscular blocking drugs. In: Zaimis E (ed) Handbook of experimental pharmacology: Neuromuscular Junction. Springer-Verlag, Heidelberg, vol 42, 593–660
Maze M, Mason D M 1983 Verapamil decreases the MAC for halothane in dogs. Anesth Analg 62: 274
Mazze R I 1984 Fluorinated anaesthetic nephrotoxicity: an update. Can Anaesth Soc J 31: S16–22
Merin R G 1987 Calcium channel blocking drugs and anaesthetics: is the drug interaction beneficial or detrimental? Anesthesiology 66: 111–113
Mishra P, Calvey T N, Williams N E 1983 Intraoperative bradycardia associated with timolol and pilocarpine eye-drops. Br J Anaesth 55: 897–899
Mitchell J R, Cavanaugh J H, Arias L, Oates J A 1970 Guanethidine and related agents. III. Antagonism by drugs which inhibit the norepinephrine pump in man. J Clin Invest 49: 1596–1604
Most J A, Markle G B IV 1974 A nearly fatal hepatotoxic reaction to rifampin after halothane anaesthesia. Am J Surg 127: 593–595
Mueller R A, Lundberg D B 1988 A manual of drug interactions for anaesthesiology. Churchill Livingstone, Edinburgh, p 1–336
Nies A S, Shand D G, Wilkinson G R 1976 Altered hepatic blood flow and drug disposition. Clin Pharmacokinet 1: 135–155
Ominsky A J, Wollman H 1969 Hazards of general anaesthesia in the reserpinised patient. Anesthesiology 30: 443–446
Pantuck E J 1966 Ecothiopate eye-drops and prolonged response to suxamethonium. Br J Anaesth 38: 406–407
Perisho J A, Buechel D R, Miller R D 1971 The effect of diazepam on minimal alveolar anaesthetic requirement (MAC) in man. Can Anaesth Soc J 18: 536–540
Pessayre D, Allemand H, Benoist C, Afifi F, Francois M, Benhamou J-P 1978 Effect of surgery under anaesthesia on antipyrine clearance. Br J Clin Pharmacol 6: 505–514
Pfeiffer C C, Grant C W 1944 The procaine-sulphonamide interaction: an evaluation of local anaesthetics for use with sulphonamide therapy. Anesthesiology 5: 605–614
Piafsky K M 1980 Disease-induced changes in the plasma binding of basic drugs. Clin Pharmacokinet 5: 246–262
Pittinger C B, Eryaza Y, Adamson R 1970 Antibiotic induced paralysis. Anesth Analg 49: 487–501
Plumpton F S, Besser G M, Cole P V 1969a Corticosteroid treatment and surgery. I. An investigation of the indications for steroid cover. Anaesthesia 24: 3–11
Plumpton F S, Besser G M, Cole P V 1969b Corticosteroid treatment and surgery. II. The management of steroid cover. Anaesthesia 24: 12–18
Poulton T J, James M F, Lockridge O 1979 Prolonged apnoea following trimetaphan and succinylcholine. Anesthesiology 50: 54–56
Prescott L F 1973 Clinically important drug interactions. Drugs 5: 161–186
Price K E, Zolli Z, Atkinson J C, Luther H G 1957 Antibiotic inhibitors. I. The effect of certain milk constituents. Antibiot Chemother 7: 672–688

Prys-Roberts C, Greene L T, Melroche R, Foex P 1971 Studies of anaesthesia in relation to hypertension. II. Haemodynamic consequences of induction and endotracheal intubation. Br J Anaesth 43: 531–547
Riley B B 1970 Incompatibilities in intravenous solutions. Journal of Hospital Pharmacy 28: 228–240
Rogers K J, Thornton J A 1969 The interaction between monoamine-oxidase inhibitors and narcotic analgesics in mice. Br J Pharmacol 36: 470–480
Roizen M F, Stevens W C 1 978 Multiform ventricular tachycardia due to the interaction of aminophylline and halothane. Anesth Analg 57: 738–741
Sedman A J 1984 Cimetidine-drug interactions. Am J Med 76: 109–114
Soni N 1987 Mechanisms of drug interactions (Appendix III). In: Feldman S, Scurr C F, Paton W (eds) Drugs in anaesthesia: mechanisms of action. Edward Arnold, London, p 408–427
Stack C G, Rogers P, Linter S P K 1988 Monoamine oxidase inhibitors and anaesthesia: a review. Br J Anaesth 60: 222–227
Stockley I 1974 Drug interactions and their mechanisms. Pharmaceutical Press, London P 1–78
Svedmyr N 1968 The influence of a tricyclic antidepressive agent (protriptylene) on some of the circulatory effects of noradrenaline and adrenaline in man. Life Sci 7: 77–84
Todd J G, Nimmo W S 1983 Effect of premedication on drug absorption and gastric emptying time. Br J Anaesth 55: 1189–1192
Vessey M P, Doll R 1968 Investigation of the relation between the use of oral contraceptives and thromboembolic disease. Br Med J 2: 199–205
Weis F R, Peak J 1974 Effects of oxytocin on blood pressure during anaesthesia. Anesthesiology 40: 189–190
Woodworth G E, Sears D H, Grove T M, Ruff R H, Kosek P S, Katz R L 1989 The effect of cimetidine and ranitidine on the duration of action of succinylcholine. Anesth Analg 68: 295–297
Zsigmond E K, Robins G 1972 The effects of a series of anti-cancer drugs on plasma cholinesterase activity. Can Anaesth Soc J 19: 75–82

26

Awareness during anaesthesia

A. R. Aitkenhead

INTRODUCTION

Awareness during anaesthesia has been recognized as a clinical entity for many years and gave rise to a modest number of law suits annually in the UK until 1985. In that year a patient who had experienced severe and prolonged pain during caesarean section (Ackers v Wigan Health Authority 1985) sued her anaesthetist and was awarded damages in excess of £13 000 amid a blaze of publicity. As a result the number of legal actions brought against health authorities for alleged medical negligence resulting in awareness escalated. However, it should not be forgotten that only a very small proportion of patients that have suffered from awareness during anaesthesia proceed with legal action. The principal reason for attempting to minimize its incidence should be humanitarian, not fear of litigation.

Awareness during anaesthesia has been defined (Brice et al 1970) as the 'ability to recall, with or without prompting, events which occurred during the period at which it was thought the patient was fully unconscious'. Subsequently, there has been considerable debate concerning the definition of the word 'unconscious' in relation to anaesthesia, and several demonstrations that patients may be able to recall, at least subconsciously, information perceived by some areas of the brain during otherwise adequate anaesthesia. Nevertheless, Brice's definition remains useful because it refers to the variety of awareness which is of most clinical relevance, and because it draws attention to the difficulties faced by the anaesthetist in determining the level of consciousness in the anaesthetized patient.

What is anaesthesia?

Prys-Roberts (1987) considers that anaesthesia is an all-or-none phenomenon and thus suggests that there can be no degrees or depths of anaesthesia. This is technically correct if the term anaesthesia is taken to mean lack of conscious recall of events or noxious stimuli, but is unhelpful in attempting to understand the functional mechanism of action of anaesthetic and analgesic agents. Much has been written about the meaning of 'consciousness' during anaesthesia (Pinsker 1986, Kissin & Gelman 1987, Vickers 1987, Russell 1989, Rupreht & Valkenburg 1990) and it is likely that no satisfactory solution to this philosophical argument will be found. The practising anaesthetist, who is, quite reasonably, content to equate clinical awareness with conscious recall of intra-operative events, seeks a more pragmatic approach that is consistent with the clinical signs that accompany anaesthesia and with the pattern of recall of patients who complain spontaneously of awareness.

White (1987) has described a continuum of anaesthesia (Fig. 26.1). Increasing 'depth of anaesthesia' results in a progression from full consciousness through a phase of intoxication to a 'level' at which conscious perception of pain is decreased. There follows a loss of conscious memory of the

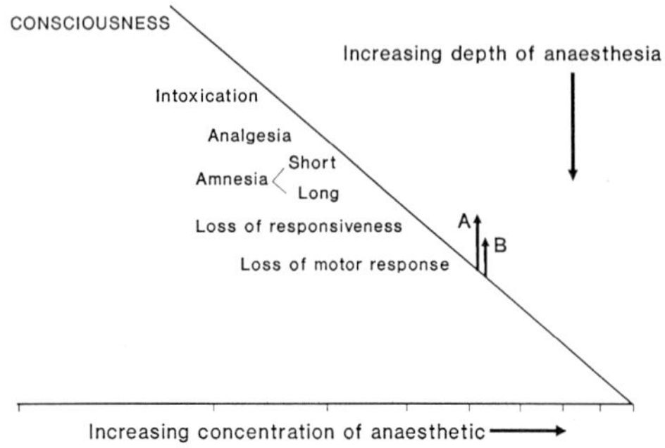

Fig. 26.1 Diagrammatic representation of the continuum of anaesthesia. Arrow A represents diagrammatically the response to a surgical stimulus, which tends to produce an effect opposite to that of the anaesthetic agents. Arrow B represents the influence of opioids on the response to surgical stimulation. See text for details (modified from White 1987).

various sensory modalities. Pain is the first modality to be affected, followed by tactile sensation and subsequently by auditory, visual and other senses. At this stage the patient may still respond to stimuli, including the spoken word, but retains no conscious memory of the event. Further movement down the continuum results in loss of responsiveness to command, and then to loss of the motor and autonomic responses to noxious stimuli.

It may be considered, simplistically, that increasing brain concentrations of anaesthetic agents result in movement down the continuum. However, clinical evidence suggests that noxious stimulation causes an increased 'level of consciousness', resulting in some 'upward' movement within the continuum (Fig. 26.1, arrow A). Although very large doses of opioids may produce an anaesthetic state, they appear to act in more conventional analgesic doses by reducing the 'upward' movement in response to a noxious stimulus from a point on the continuum determined by the concentration of anaesthetic agent in the brain (Fig. 26.1 arrow B). This effect is presumably a reflection of the action of opioids in reducing the transmission of noxious stimuli along the pain pathways to the brain. Thus the 'level of consciousness' is determined by the balance between the cerebral concentration of anaesthetic agent (determined by the anaesthetist) and the degree of cerebral arousal induced by surgical stimuli (which varies during the procedure and which may be modified by analgesic drugs). This concept is also of importance in considering methods of measuring 'depth of anaesthesia'.

What is awareness?

Jones & Konieczko (1986) have suggested that the effect of progressively increasing concentrations of anaesthetic drugs on the brain can be represented crudely by four stages:

- Stage 1: conscious awareness without amnesia
- Stage II: conscious awareness with amnesia
- Stage III: subconscious awareness with amnesia
- Stage IV: no awareness.

The majority of studies undertaken to investigate the incidence of awareness have depended on spontaneous recall upon questioning during the postoperative period (Stage I). This approach has been criticized (Millar & Watkinson 1983) on the basis that it relies not only on the patient's awareness of events, but also on his ability to remember them. A much higher incidence of awareness may be found using more sensitive tests of memory function, such as prompting under hypnosis and recognition testing (Stage III), or by using the isolated forearm technique to identify intraoperative response to command, but without conscious recall (Stage II). However, it remains unclear whether awareness without recall is of clinical importance. In contrast, recall of intraoperative events is distressing to the patient and may result in psychological sequelae that include insomnia, anxiety, irritability, repetitive nightmares and depression. A preoccupation with death may develop and there may be a morbid fear of hospitals, doctors and, in particular, of the need for future surgery. This 'post-traumatic stress syndrome' may persist for months or years, although it is often ameliorated or cured if the patient is able to discuss the memories openly and is assured that the memories are genuine. Following recent publicity, including newspaper reports, and radio and television programmes, there has been an increase in the number of patients seeking to sue their anaesthetist for negligence after an episode of alleged conscious recall of intraoperative events. The major part of the quantum of damages in successful actions relates to the psychological consequences rather than the experience of intraoperative pain. While those who pursue litigation represent only a small proportion of patients who remember intraoperative events, the fact that, to date, patients have sought recourse through the courts in respect only of 'conscious awareness without amnesia' suggests that this is the category of awareness that is of greatest clinical importance. It is also the category referred to by most anaesthetists who use the term 'awareness'. However, to differentiate between this category and other stages of awareness the term 'recall' will be used in the remainder of this chapter.

A distinction must be made between spontaneous recall of intraoperative events and dreams, illusions or hallucinations occurring during unconsciousness. An illusion has been defined by Garfield et al (1972) as 'a misinterpretation of a real sensory experience', and a hallucination as 'a false sensory perception in the absence of a sensory experience'. Wilson et al (1975) defined a dream as 'a train of thoughts or images passing through the mind, which the patient believes occurred between the induction of anaesthesia and the first moment of consciousness after the completion of the anaesthetic procedure'. Usually, spontaneous recall can be differentiated from dreams, illusions and hallucinations by the presence of verifiable conversation or events that occurred during operation. It is important also to differentiate between recall of experiences during anaesthesia and memories of events that occurred in the postoperative period.

INCIDENCE OF AWARENESS

Reported incidences of awareness vary widely. Part of this variation is due to differences in methods of detection.

Spontaneous recall

Studies of the ability of patients to recall spontaneously events that occurred during anaesthesia and surgery are reliable only if there has been a structured interview, consisting of questions such as:

- What is the last thing you remember before going to sleep for your operation?
- What is the first thing you remember on waking up after your operation?
- Do you remember anything in between?

The incidence of spontaneous recall after non-obstetric procedures in such studies is up to 1.6% (Hutchinson 1960, Harris et al 1971, McKenna & Wilton 1973, Wilson et al 1975), with up to 26% of patients reporting dreams (Table 26.1). One of the problems associated with studies of spontaneous recall is that anaesthetists may modify their normal technique if they know that such a study is in progress. This may result in an artificially low incidence of recall. Consequently, it is worth noting that the most recent investigation (Liu et al, 1991), in which 1000 patients were interviewed after surgery and in which the anaesthetists did not know of the existence of the study, found an overall incidence of spontaneous recall of 0.2% in patients

Table 26.1 Summary of incidences of awareness with recall and dreaming in studies using a structured interview, 1960–1990

Authors	Awareness (%)	Dreaming (%)	Sample size
Hutchinson (1960)	1.2	3.0	656
Harris et al (1971)	1.6	26.0	120
McKenna & Wilton (1973)	1.5	—	200
Wilson et al (1975)	0.8	7.7	490
Liu et al (1991)	0.2	0.9	1000

undergoing non-obstetric procedures. Both patients recalled events shortly after induction. It was the opinion of the investigators that anaesthesia had been inadequate because, in both cases, a low dose of intravenous agent had been given relative to the patient's weight, and in one the total concentrations of inhalational agents were inadequate before surgery started. No patient was aware during surgery. All patients received nitrous oxide supplemented by a volatile anaesthetic agent during the operative procedure.

The incidence of recall may be slightly higher during anaesthesia for obstetric operations (see below). However, it should be noted that recall during non-obstetric procedures was considerably more common in cases reported to the Medical Defence Union between 1982 and 1986 (Hargrove 1987; Table 26.2).

Hearing is the most common sensation recalled and is the last sense to disappear on losing consciousness. A more distressing complaint is recall of the sensation of pain during surgery. It has been estimated that about 10% of patients with spontaneous recall remember pain (Crawford 1984). Some patients are aware of being paralysed and of being unable to indicate to the anaesthetist that they are awake. These patients may not experience pain, but are usually distressed.

An alternative approach in the detection of recall has been to present the anaesthetized patient with a standardized auditory stimulus, usually tape-recorded words, sentences or music, and to test his ability to recall the stimulus during the post-operative period. The reported incidence of recall using this technique has ranged from 0 to 7% (McIntyre 1966, Terrell et al 1969, Brice et al 1970, Browne & Catton 1973, Eisele et al 1976). Up to 44% of patients have reported dreams.

Table 26.2 Types of operative procedure associated with cases of awareness with recall reported to the Medical Defence Union between 1982 and 1986 (from Hargrove 1987)

Type of procedure	Percentage of cases
General surgery	31
Obstetrics	28
Gynaecology	18
Orthopaedic surgery	11
Miscellaneous*	12

*Miscellaneous includes dental, ENT and ophthalmological procedures.

Conscious awareness with amnesia

The 'isolated forearm technique' (IFT) for demonstrating wakefulness during anaesthesia was described by Tunstall (1977). Prior to administration of a neuromuscular blocking drug, one forearm was isolated by inflation of a pneumatic tourniquet on the upper arm to a pressure exceeding arterial blood pressure. The patient was instructed at regular intervals to move the unparalysed arm, and a positive response was taken as an indication that wakefulness was present. 75% of patients undergoing caesarean section, with anaesthesia consisting of 33% nitrous oxide and 0.4% halothane in oxygen, appeared to respond correctly to command. None of the patients had recall of intraoperative events.

Breckenridge & Aitkenhead (1981) found no positive responders in general surgical patients anaesthetized with 66% nitrous oxide and fentanyl, despite clinical signs of light anaesthesia. In some patients the unparalysed arm responded purposefully to surgical stimulation. The IFT is unreliable after approximately 20 min as ischaemic paralysis occurs. Wilson (1981) has claimed that communication with the patient can be maintained by releasing the tourniquet after 20 min and re-inflating it prior to the administration of subsequent doses of neuromuscular blocking drugs. However, Clapham (1981) has demonstrated that blood concentrations of pancuronium are high enough 20 min after administration to cause significant paralysis.

Millar & Watkinson (1983) carried out a controlled study of the IFT in which one group of patients was instructed to move the paralysed hand while a control group was given no instructions. Approximately half of the patients in each group moved their hand intermittently at apparently random times, and the probability of a movement occurring at the time of a command was the same for patients who had received a command as for those in the control group, that is it could not be demonstrated that patients were responding directly to a command to move the hand.

Russell (1989) has demonstrated that up to 61% of patients may respond to command using the IFT if nitrous oxide/oxygen is used as the sole anaesthetic. 27% of these patients recalled being spoken to by the anaesthetist but had no other memory of intraoperative events.

The IFT may, if interpreted carefully, provide information that suggests that the patient is in Stage II of Jones & Konieczko's (1986) classification and may therefore be at risk of reaching Stage I (spontaneous recall) if anaesthesia is not supplemented. In the hands of its few enthusiasts the technique may be useful in routine use. However, it is probably of more value as an investigative tool.

Subconscious awareness with amnesia

Cued recall and recognition

Recognition of previously learned information is a simpler task for memory than recall, as the re-presentation of the stimulus may serve as a cue to its location in memory (Glucksberg 1962) and thus aid retrieval. This method of memory testing is likely to be much more sensitive than recall, particularly if the information is registered only weakly in memory, as may be the case if the stimulus is presented to the patient in a semiconscious state. Millar & Watkinson (1983) recorded lists each consisting of 10 words. They played repeatedly either a tape containing one of the lists or a tape of meaningless radio static to premedicated patients anaesthetized with 66% nitrous oxide and approximately 0.5% halothane. None of the patients had recall of events during anaesthesia. However, when presented with lists of words during the postoperative period, patients who had heard a list during anaesthesia were significantly more successful in recognizing words than patients who had heard meaningless noise. This suggested that awareness had occurred but recall was absent.

During normal sleep, learning can be demonstrated by subsequent recognition of word pairs presented to sleeping subjects (Evans 1972). The presentation of one word of the pair is used subsequently as a cue to recall of the other word. Although one attempt to reproduce this finding in anaesthetized subjects failed (Dubovsky & Trustman 1976), Millar & Watkinson (1983), using a more complex form of data analysis, showed that a significant degree of word recognition occurred in anaesthetized patients, although the total number of correct responses was extremely low. Eich et al (1985) and Stolzy et al (1987) were unable to replicate these results. There may be specific types of words that are recognized more easily than others, but on balance there is little evidence of any significant ability of patients to recognize auditory material presented during anaesthesia (Millar 1989).

Hypnosis

The induction of a hypnotic trance, with regression to the time of operation, has been used as a means of detection of awareness during anaesthesia (Levinson 1965). In a study that would now be considered unethical, 10 patients receiving deep anaesthesia with oxygen/nitrous oxide/ether were subjected to a 'crisis' in which the anaesthetist stopped the operation by announcing that the patient had turned blue and required oxygen. All of the patients were known to be susceptible to hypnotic techniques. One month later the patients were hypnotized and regressed to the time of operation. Four patients were able to repeat almost exactly the words of the anaesthetist. Another four remembered hearing something, and some were able to identify the speaker as being the anaesthetist. The latter patients all displayed marked anxiety. None of the patients had any conscious recall of intraoperative events. This is the only report that documents awareness during 'deep' anaesthesia. It suggests that, irrespective of the depth of anaesthesia, intraoperative auditory stimuli may be registered and retained by the brain. There have been other demonstrations of recall of *meaningful* sounds heard during surgical planes of anaesthesia when a hypnotic state was induced later (Cheek 1980). In addition, by coupling an auditory stimulus to an electric shock, animals can be conditioned during anaesthesia to respond later to the sound (Weinberger et al 1984). However, injection of adrenaline simultaneously with the stimulus during anaesthesia was necessary to obtain the postanaesthetic response. In clinical studies, hypnosis has failed to elicit recall of bland or innocuous words heard during anaesthesia, and it is possible that only words that cause arousal and stimulation of the sympathoadrenal system may be fixed in memory (Ewin 1990).

Unconscious perception

The term 'unconscious perception' has been used to describe the phenomenon of subconscious or unconscious retention in the brain of information presented during anaesthesia which may subsequently alter the patient's behaviour.

Several studies have demonstrated that patients may respond by changes in behaviour in the postoperative period to suggestions made during anaesthesia. Early reports (Wolfe & Millett 1960, Hutchings 1961) suggested that positive suggestions presented during anaesthesia regarding the quality of postoperative recovery reduced the incidences of postoperative pain, bronchospasm, nausea and vomiting, but there were no comparisons with control patients. However, two controlled trials (Pearson 1961, Bonke et al 1986) demonstrated that patients given positive therapeutic suggestions during anaesthesia recovered more rapidly, and left hospital sooner, than patients who heard music or blank tape recordings. However Bonke's group (Boeke et al 1988) were unable to reproduce this result in a later study. Evans & Richardson (1988) found a significant reduction in analgesic requirements, mobilization and time to discharge from hospital in a small group of patients who had undergone hysterectomy. Woo et al (1987) were unable to demonstrate any effect of positive suggestions on postoperative analgesic requirements, although McLintock et al (1990) found a significant reduction in analgesic requirement using the rather more precise technique of patient-controlled analgesia, but demonstrated no advantage in respect of time to discharge from hospital. Clearly, this is an area that requires further investigation to establish whether there are specific subgroups of patients who might benefit from hearing positive suggestions during anaesthesia.

Two studies appear to have demonstrated an ability of patients to respond to irrelevant suggestions heard during anaesthesia. Eleven patients who were told during anaesthesia to touch their ear during a postoperative interview with the investigator did so more frequently than control patients (Bennett et al 1985). This finding was confirmed in patients undergoing cardiac surgery (Goldmann et al 1987). However, there were no baseline data in either study, and subsequent investigations which have incorporated baseline observations (Eich et al 1985, Jansen et al 1990) have failed to confirm that behaviour may be altered by this type of suggestion.

The concept of subconscious awareness of auditory material with amnesia is consistent with the observation that anaesthetic agents do not abolish the transmission of auditory information to inner areas of the cerebral cortex, as has been demonstrated using evoked potentials (see p. 410). However, its implications are important. Although it has not been demonstrated, and indeed such experiments would be unethical, it seems reasonable to assume that, if it is confirmed that positive remarks may shorten hospitalization time, then pessimistic remarks heard during surgery may influence postoperative recovery adversely. Unconscious perception may be responsible also for psychological damage. Blacher (1975) reported a 'traumatic neurosis', consisting of repetitive nightmares, generalized irritability and anxiety, and a preoccupation with death, in six patients who had no specific recall of events during anaesthesia. Psychological aspects of anaesthesia are discussed more fully in Chapter 29.

CAUSES OF AWARENESS WITH RECALL

Spontaneous recall of intraoperative events is, by definition, due to delivery of inadequate concentrations of anaesthetic agents to the brain for the needs of the individual patient. The most common causes in cases reported to the Medical Defence Union between 1982 and 1986 (Hargrove 1987) are shown in Table 26.3. Although patients who pursue litigation are not necessarily typical of those who experience spontaneous recall, it is worthy of note that 70% of cases of recall were deemed to be caused by the use of an inappropriate anaesthetic technique. The specific details discussed in the following paragraphs do not relate specifically to the cases reported by Hargrove.

Faulty anaesthetic technique

Faulty anaesthetic technique is the most common single cause of awareness with recall. A faulty technique is one that could reasonably be predicted to result in recall of intraoperative events, or in which drug doses are not adjusted when clinical signs of inadequate anaesthesia become apparent. In general, the likelihood of recall is related inversely to the dose or concentration of anaesthetic drug administered (Fig. 26.1). However, high concentrations of most anaesthetic agents result in an increased incidence and severity of side effects, and delayed recovery. Consequently it became common, particularly in the UK, for anaesthetists to use paralysing doses of a muscle relaxant to prevent movement during surgery (in contrast to the smaller doses used in the USA) and to administer anaesthetic agents in concentrations of less than 1 MAC (minimum alveolar concentration which prevents movement in response to surgical stimulation in 50% of individuals). Awareness with recall occurs almost exclusively in patients who have received muscle relaxants.

Table 26.3 Causes of awareness with recall reported to the Medical Defence Union between 1982 and 1986 (from Hargrove 1987)

Causes	Percentage of cases
Faulty anaesthetic technique	70.0
Failure to check equipment	20.0
Genuine apparatus failure	5.0
Spurious claims	2.5
Justified risks/unknown cause	2.5

Inhalational anaesthetics

The alveolar concentration of inhaled anaesthetic agents required to produce loss of consciousness i.e. amnesia (MAC_{awake}) is about 0.6 MAC (Stoelting et al 1970). However, this is in the absence of surgical stimulation. A higher proportion of MAC is required to ensure amnesia during surgery. In addition there is individual variability in response; MAC and MAC_{awake} are average values, and the distribution of values among individuals conforms approximately to a normal distribution curve. Thus some patients require significantly higher alveolar concentrations of inhaled anaesthetics than others to ensure loss of consciousness.

Consequently, any technique that results in an alveolar concentration of inhaled anaesthetic which equates to 0.6–0.7 MAC will predictably result in awareness with recall in an unacceptably high proportion of patients. The use of unsupplemented nitrous oxide in concentrations of 60–70% provides about 0.65 MAC and is unsatisfactory. Utting (1987) reported definite or probable recall in 2.2.% of 500 patients anaesthetized with unsupplemented 70% nitrous oxide in oxygen. The addition of opioids may reduce the incidence of recall slightly but not significantly. Rosen (1959) demonstrated that auditory perception occurred in some patients breathing 60–75% nitrous oxide, despite an opioid premedication. Brown & Catton (1973) reported an incidence of recall of 5.3% in patients premedicated with pethidine or promethazine, and moderately hyperventilated using 60% nitrous oxide in oxygen.

The alveolar concentration of an inhalational agent is normally lower than the delivered concentration and 'overpressure' with volatile agents may be required initially to achieve the desired effect. Uptake is more rapid for agents with a low blood/gas solubility coefficient, and this may be of particular relevance to recall during tracheal intubation or at the start of surgery. The concentration of an inhalational agent delivered to a patient may be considerably less than the concentration set on the flowmeters or vaporizer if a circle system with vaporizer outside the circle (VOC) is used, especially with low fresh gas flow rates.

Intravenous anaesthetics

Anaesthetic drugs administered intravenously are less predictable than inhalational agents. Distribution volumes vary widely between individual patients. While distribution volume has some influence on the rate of uptake of inhalational drugs, its effect is relatively small because increased distribution is to a large extent compensated for by increased uptake from the lungs and the total dose of anaesthetic administered is increased. In contrast the total dose of an intravenous drug is selected by the anaesthetist, and the blood and brain concentrations are determined, at least in the short term, by redistribution to tissues that receive high blood flow. Recall may occur during tracheal intubation if a muscle relaxant has been given before clear signs of loss of consciousness have become apparent, or if inhalational anaesthetics are not given between induction and tracheal intubation. This risk is highest if a non-depolarizing relaxant has been used. In general, higher doses of intravenous anaesthetics are required to ensure lack of recall in unpremedicated out-patients in comparison to premedicated in-patients.

There may be a higher risk of recall in the paralysed patient if anaesthesia is maintained by an infusion of an intravenous agent than if inhalational anaesthetics are used. This is true particularly if the lungs are ventilated with oxygen-enriched air (total intravenous anaesthesia) rather than oxygen and nitrous oxide. An index of equipotency of anaesthetic effect comparable to MAC has been proposed for when intravenous anaesthetic agents are used by infusion to maintain anaesthesia (Sear 1983). When an intravenous agent is used the minimum infusion rate (MIR) preventing movement in response to surgical stimulation may be calculated. Both MIR and MAC are mean values and represent the ED_{50} for the agent under investigation. However, the distribution of values of MIR is log-normal, whereas that of MAC is Gaussian. In addition, the range of values is greater for MIR than MAC in populations studied (Eger et al 1965, Sear 1983). There is a relatively imprecise association between infusion rate of an intravenous agent and the resultant plasma concentration. During inhalational anaesthesia there is a predictable relationship between alveolar concentration and blood (or brain) concentration. However, blood concentration of an intravenous agent given by infusion is influenced by both the distribution volume (which varies widely among individuals) and the clearance, which may alter significantly with plasma concentration. For example, a five-fold increase in infusion rate of Althesin results in only a two-fold increase in plasma concentration, although this may not apply to all intravenous agents. However, even when sophisticated computerized apparatus is used in an attempt to attain a 'target' concentration, based on an algorithm derived from population kinetic data, there is wide variation in the plasma concentrations achieved (White & Kenny 1990). The difficulties inherent in predicting the pharmacological effects of intravenous anaesthetic agents may account for the 7.3% incidence of recall reported by Barclay et al (1980) in paralysed patients anaesthetized with flunitrazepam and ketamine. Many of the patients who reported recall had exhibited no outward signs of light anaesthesia. In a survey (Wright & Dundee 1982) of anaesthetists who had used total intravenous anaesthesia, 9% had abandoned its use because of difficulty in judging depth of anaesthesia. Although some anaesthetists have claimed never to have detected recall during total intravenous anaesthesia (Dundee & McMurray 1983), their methods of detection remain unknown.

Supplements of non-anaesthetic drugs

The use of opioids, butyrophenones or benzodiazepines to supplement nitrous oxide anaesthesia is common. In the doses usually employed these agents do not produce anaesthesia. Opioids may contribute to the prevention of recall, presumably by reducing transmission of nociceptive impulses. Lorazepam or diazepam have been used to contribute amnesia to an anaesthetic technique. They do not appear to offer reliable retrograde amnesia, as recall and unpleasant dreams still occur when either of these drugs is administered following delivery of the baby by caesarean section (Barr et al 1977). Their capacity to induce anterograde amnesia has also been questioned. Indeed, diazepam has been shown to improve the memory of anxious individuals (Desai et al 1983), and in normal individuals only certain aspects of memory are depressed (Jones et al 1979). Lorazepam appears to impair alertness and attention rather than memory per se (File & Lister 1982).

Caesarean section

The high incidences of recall of intraoperative events that have been reported over the years in obstetric patients who received general anaesthesia are attributable in part to a reluctance to use inhalational agents in adequate concentrations. This is because of fears of inducing depression of the fetus and of increasing haemorrhage from the uterus. There is no evidence that these fears are justified. The calculated dose of intravenous induction agent should not be reduced. If nitrous oxide is used in a concentration of only 50% before delivery, a higher concentration of volatile agent may be required than is necessary to supplement 67% nitrous oxide. In addition, the rate of uptake of the volatile agent is reduced because the influence of the concentration effect is less pronounced. Volatile anaesthetic agents with a low blood/gas solubility coefficient are preferable because there is usually a very short interval between induction of anaesthesia and the start of surgery. Methoxyflurane and trichloroethylene have been found to result in incidences of recall of 6% and 2%, respectively, at a concentration of 0.1% in 33% nitrous oxide during caesarean section (Crawford & Davies 1975). At a concentration of 0.2% these incidences were reduced to 0.7% and 0%, respectively, during emergency caesarean section, but were 3% and 6%, respectively, during elective section (Crawford et al 1976). Moir (1970) found an incidence of recall of 4% during caesarean section in patients receiving 70% nitrous oxide, but no recall in patients anaesthetized with 50% nitrous oxide supplemented by 0.5% halothane. However, the incidence of recall using this technique was 0.21% when the number of patients studied was extended to 1400 (Moir 1976), and 'under 1%' after 3000 patients had been interviewed (Moir & Thorburn 1986). 0.6% enflurane has been recommended as an alternative to 0.5% halothane (Moir & Thorburn 1986), but this is less than the 'MAC equivalent' concentration. 0.8% enflurane in 50% nitrous oxide before delivery and 1.5% thereafter, has been reported to produce no recall or dreaming when used for caesarean section (Farnsworth 1978), although the use of 1% enflurane in 50% nitrous oxide has been associated with recall of pain in 2% of patients (Bogod et al 1990). 0.75% isoflurane has been reported as effective in preventing awareness with recall in a small series of patients (Warren et al 1983). Most authors appear to agree that, while not eliminating the possibility of recall, supplementation of nitrous oxide anaesthesia with a volatile anaesthetic agent, particularly one of rapid onset (e.g. halothane, enflurane or isoflurane), substantially reduces the probability of its occurrence. There is normally no good reason to discontinue administration of the volatile agent after delivery of the baby. Lyons & Macdonald (1991) found that the incidence of spontaneous recall in patients who received general anaesthesia for caesarian section decreased from 1.3% to 0.4% when the practice in their maternity wait changed in 1986, and administration of a relative agent was.

The rationale for the use of a very high inspired oxygen concentration before delivery of the baby is based on work conducted 20 years ago. In these studies other factors, such as the induction-to-delivery interval, the uterine incision-to-delivery interval and the failure to use lateral tilt, may have influenced the condition of the fetus as much as, or more than, the maternal oxygen tension. A recent study (Lawes et al 1988), although not providing the definitive answer, suggests that an inspired oxygen concentration of 33% is adequate to ensure adequate fetal oxygenation, at least in the absence of fetal distress. There is no doubt that the adoption of a technique employing 67% nitrous oxide and a volatile anaesthetic supplement would reduce the incidence of recall substantially during the predelivery phase of caesarean section.

Difficult intubation

It is often desirable to discontinue the administration of nitrous oxide in order to maintain adequate oxygenation if tracheal intubation is difficult. This may lead to awareness with recall unless anaesthesia is maintained while attempts are made to intubate the trachea, either by administration of adequate concentrations of a volatile agent in oxygen between attempts or by further doses of an intravenous anaesthetic agent.

Premature discontinuation of anaesthesia

A desire to produce unnecessarily rapid recovery of consciousness after surgery may lead the anaesthetist to discontinue administration of a volatile anaesthetic agent or an intravenous infusion of anaesthetic drug several minutes before the end of the operation, or to switch off the nitrous oxide before reversal of the effects of neuromuscular blockers.

Failure to understand apparatus

Air is entrained by some mechanical ventilators if the supply of anaesthetic gases from the anaesthetic machine is less than the total minute volume delivered by the ventilator. Oxygen or air may dilute anaesthetic gases if tubing with an inadequate volume is used to connect a ventilator to a Bain system. Failure to understand the principles of the circle system may result in the delivery of inadequate concentrations of anaesthetic gases.

Failure to check apparatus

Apparatus must be checked before *and during* every anaesthetic. Common causes of recall include: failure to ensure that the anaesthetic gases are delivered to a mechanical ventilator of a type that does not depend upon the supply of fresh gas for its power; loose connections in the ventilator tubing or breathing system which result in loss of fresh gas and rebreathing or entrainment of air; failure to connect the vaporizer into the fresh gas supply at all or at least securely, or to lock the vaporizer on to a Selectatec block; failure to ensure that the vaporizer contains the anaesthetic agent; and failure to notice that a nitrous oxide cylinder has become empty. The emergency oxygen flush may be switched on accidentally, diluting the concentration of anaesthetic gases. An infusion of intravenous agent may become disconnected, leak or 'tissue', or the syringe in the infusion pump may become empty. A number of these events may occur during anaesthesia, even though a preanaesthetic check has been undertaken. There may also be misinterpretation of signs of light anaesthesia if electrocardiogram (ECG) monitors and automated blood pressure devices are not checked regularly. Recall may occur if an inaccurate inspired oxygen monitor or pulse oximeter causes the anaesthetist to increase the inspired concentration of oxygen inappropriately.

Genuine apparatus failure

In some circumstances, failure of apparatus could not reasonably have been predicted or detected by the anaesthetist. Flexible hoses connecting the supply of anaesthetic gases to the vaporizer may become perforated, resulting in a reduction in fresh gas flow rate. There may be a loss of fresh gas because of leaks in the back bar of the anaesthetic machine or a damaged flowmeter. Vaporizers may very occasionally deliver grossly inaccurate concentrations of volatile agent. Infusion pumps may malfunction without sounding an alarm. Ventilators may operate incorrectly despite appropriate external connections.

Spurious claims

Occasionally, patients complain of recall without foundation. Others may claim recall of intraoperative events that are found on detailed questioning to be memories of the early postoperative period, or a dream.

Justified risks

In a very small number of cases the patient is so seriously ill that there is a genuine risk to life if normally adequate doses or concentrations of anaesthetic drug are administered. The most common cause is profound hypotension caused by hypovolaemia when only surgery can effect a cure.

Unknown causes

Very occasionally there may be no identifiable factor to explain a genuine case of awareness with recall. It is possible that some of these cases are attributable to the variability in response to anaesthetic agents.

MONITORING DEPTH OF ANAESTHESIA

It is clear that the probability of recall is related to depth of anaesthesia. The major problem lies in detecting depth of anaestheia accurately and quantifying the relationship. A number of methods of monitoring depth has been described.

Clinical monitoring

During balanced anaesthesia involving the use of paralysing doses of muscle relaxants the clinical signs that are sought are predominantly those associated with stimulation of the autonomic nervous system. These may be affected by intercurrent disease or by the action of drugs.

Pupil size

In general the pupil size tends to decrease with increasing depth of anaesthesia, although the degree of constriction varies with different anaesthetic drugs and the pupil may dilate during very deep anaesthesia. The response to light may be present during inadequate anaesthesia. Opioids constrict the pupil and anticholinergics dilate it. Intense constriction or dilatation of the pupil may limit the ability to detect a light response.

Cardiovascular changes

Arterial pressure tends to decrease as anaesthesia deepens, except with ketamine. During ether or cyclopropane anaesthesia arterial pressure is well maintained until very deep planes of anaesthesia. Heart rate tends to decrease with increasing depth of anaesthesia. However, other drugs, for example muscle relaxants, may influence cardiovascular parameters without altering the conscious level. In addition, haemorrhage, drug reactions and body fluid abnormalities may affect the interpretation of arterial pressure and heart rate, as may drugs acting directly on the cardiovascular system, for example beta blockers, which may be administered by the anaesthetist or which the patient may have received preoperatively. Peripheral vasoconstriction may be associated with light anaesthesia, but is also influenced by body temperature and volaemic status.

Sweating and lacrimation

Sweating and lacrimation may be found during light anaesthesia or may be present when anaesthesia is adequate. lacrimation is a more sensitive index of light anaesthesia than sweating. Both may be reduced if anticholinergic drugs have been administered.

Clinical scoring system

A scoring system based on the clinical signs of anaesthesia has been described (Evans 1987). Based on arterial pressure, heart rate, sweating and tear formation, it has been termed the PRST score. Scores or 0–2 are allocated for each of the four components (Table 26.4). Initial studies suggest that a total score of 2–4 represents adequate anaesthesia. However, the system retains many of the disadvantages of conventional clinical monitoring in that the response to different anaesthetic agents varies and the scores may be influenced by the effect of other drugs.

Limitations

Clinical monitoring has always been, and remains, by far the most common method of attempting to gauge the depth of anaesthesia. There is no evidence that any instrument is more reliable. Clinical signs may be difficult to interpret in the presence of other drugs that act on the cardio-

Table 26.4 PRST scoring indices

Index	Condition	Score
Systolic arterial pressure (mmHg)	Less than control + 15	0
	Less than control + 30	1
	More than control + 30	2
Heart Rate (beats/min)	Less than control + 15	0
	Less than control + 30	1
	More than control + 30	2
Sweat	Nil	0
	Skin moist to touch	1
	Visible beads of sweat	2
Tears	No excess tears when eyelids open	0
	Excess tears visible when eyelids open	1
	Tears overflow from closed eyelids	2

vascular system and if hypovolaemia is present. Clinical signs of light anaesthesia are relatively common and usually are not associated with recall of intraoperative events. Conversely, awareness with recall may occur in the absence of clinical evidence of light anaesthesia if no confounding factors are persent. Consequently, evidence of inadequate anaesthesia. However, recall of intraoperative pain or distress is almost invariably associated with clinical evidence of light anaesthesia if no confounding factors are present. Consequently evidence of increased sympathoadrenal activity should be regarded as an indication to increase depth of anaesthesia immediately by administration of further doses or higher concentrations of anaesthetic agents. It may be appropriate to supplement, *but not to substitute*, the anaesthetic agent with an opioid analgesic and/or a muscle relaxant.

Response to verbal commands

The isolated forearm technique has been described above. It has significant disadvantages as a means of routine monitoring.

Instrumental monitoring

A number of instruments have been developed in an attempt to monitor depth of anaesthesia. Some of these are indirect monitors in that they record, in a peripheral tissue, activity that changes in a manner that may be related to alterations in the level of anaesthesia or in reflex neurological activity, while others are based on direct measurement of cerebral electrical activity.

Skin conductance

Measurement of alterations in skin conductance (the reciprocal of resistance) is in effect a quantification of sweat production and is more sensitive than clinical monitoring of sweating. The technique has been used in a number of contexts, including 'lie detection', because of the correlation between changes in skin conductance and activity in the sympathetic nervous system (SNS). Goddard (1982) reported the measurement of skin conductance in 67 anaesthetized patients. Conductance was low prior to induction of anaesthesia and increased as sleep ensued. In patients anaesthetized with oxygen/nitrous oxide/halothane, conductance remained high throughout surgery. However, in patients receiving a nitrous oxide/oxygen/relaxant anaesthetic supplemented by fentanyl, surgical incision and visceral traction reduced conductance (Fig. 26.2), which was increased by deepening the level of anaesthesia. A level of anaesthesia that maintained a high conductance often resulted in a prolonged recovery period, particularly in elderly patients. Clearly, factors that affect sweating, for example anticholinergic drugs or autonomic neuropathy, are likely to reduce substantially the accuracy of this type of monitoring.

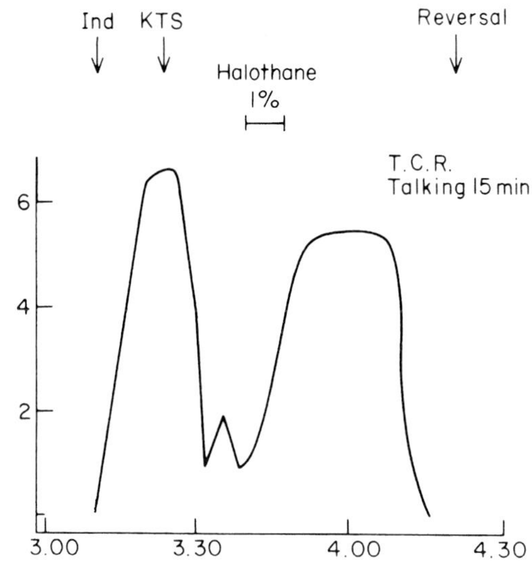

Fig. 26.2 Skin conductance changes at induction of anaesthesia (Ind), start of surgery (KTS) and in response to administration of 1% halothane in a 75-year-old patient undergoing vulvectomy (from Goddard 1982).

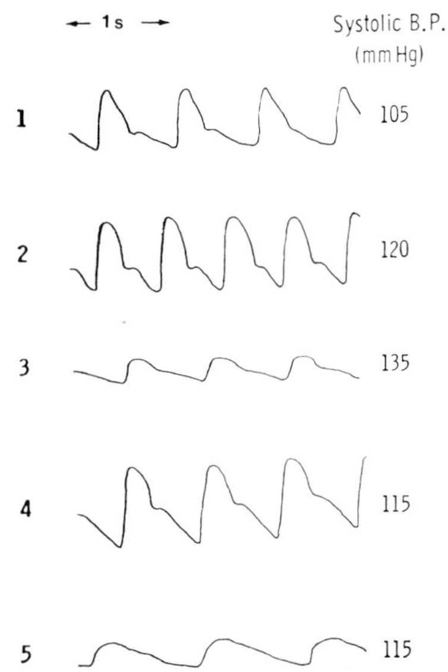

Fig. 26.3 Digital plethysmograph trace from a patient undergoing abdominal hysterectomy on arrival in the anaesthetic room (1), during nitrous-oxide-relaxant anaesthesia before surgery (2), during traction of the uterus (3), 5 min later after addition of halothane to the fresh gas mixture (4) and at the end of the procedure (5) (from Johnstone 1974).

Digital plethysmography

Vasoconstriction in the fingers is one of the earliest signs of SNS activity (Hertzman & Roth 1942). Digital plethysmography may be achieved by using a photoelectric or piezoelectric device, either of which produces a pulsatile trace on an oscilloscope or on paper, representing alterations in finger volume resulting from systolic blood flow. Vasoconstriction results in a decrease in amplitude of the trace, and vasodilatation in an increase (Fig. 26.3). Johnstone (1974) found that vasoconstriction was common during nitrous oxide/oxygen/relaxant anaesthesia, while supplementation with 0.5–1% halothane abolished the vasoconstrictor response to surgical stimulation. Supplementation with pethidine or fentanyl did not prevent vasoconstriction. However, this method of monitoring is subject to drift, and the signal is affected significantly by other causes of vasoconstriction such as hypovolaemia or hypothermia.

Lower oesophageal contractility

The musculature of the lower portion of the human oesophagus consists of smooth muscle fibres and is therefore unaffected by neuromuscular blocking drugs. Three types of oesophageal muscle activity are recognized. Primary and secondary activity are peristaltic in nature, and are responsible for propulsion of food along the oesophagus. Tertiary activity is non-propulsive and its function is obscure, but it is known to be increased by stress (Rubin et al 1962). Spontaneous tertiary activity measured with a balloon and pressure transducer produces contractions of the oesophagus of 2–5 s duration five or more times per minute during anaesthesia. It is suppressed, apparently in a dose-related manner, by most inhalational anaesthetic agents, intravenous anaesthetic drugs and opioids (Evans et al 1987). Spontaneous activity disappears at approximately 2 MAC or its equivalent. Lower oesophageal contractility (LOC) can also be provoked by inflation of a second balloon in the oesophagus. This results in a secondary peristaltic response with an amplitude that may be related inversely to the depth of anaesthesia. LOC is influenced by the type of surgical stimulus (Thomas & Aitkenhead 1990) but is altered by disease or drugs that affect smooth muscle or autonomic nervous system activity, and there is wide inter-individual variability. Its value in monitoring depth of anaesthesia is dubious (Cox & White 1987).

Ocular microtremor

Low-amplitude oscillations of the human eye at a frequency of approximately 100 Hz occur as a result of activity in extraocular muscle motor units and the normal 'hunting' effect of the brainstem gaze control mechanism. Coakley et al (1976) demonstrated that the frequency and amplitude of the resulting ocular microtremor, measured by a stylus on the sclera, were reduced by thiopentone or trichloroethylene anaesthesia (Fig. 26.4). However, the technique is unreliable in the presence of neuromuscular blocking drugs and requires exposure of the eye with the associated hazards to the cornea.

Electromyogram

Integrated electromyogram (EMG) recordings from the frontalis muscle have been used as a means of monitoring light anaesthesia (Harmel et al 1978). Electrodes are positioned on the forehead and mastoid process. The traces may be affected by ECG interference. In the absence of total muscle paralysis (the degree of neuromuscular blockade should also be monitored), lightening anaesthesia may result in subclinical frowning or grimacing which is detected as EMG activity. Although of limited use by itself, this system may have a place in monitoring the depth of anaesthesia in conjunction with information derived from the electroencephalogram (EEG).

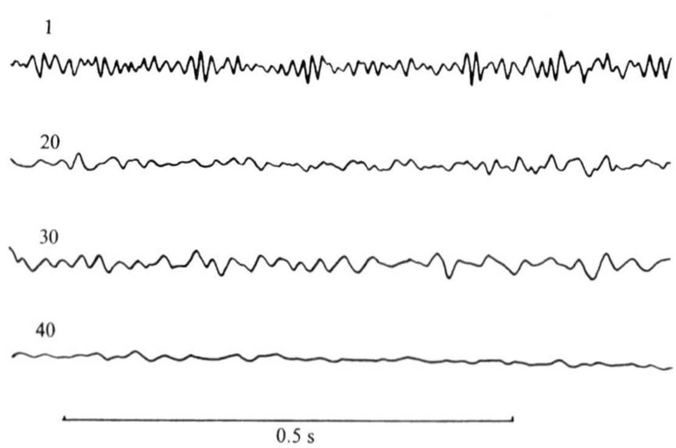

Fig. 26.4 Ocular microtremor 1, 20, 30 and 40 s after beginning injection of thiopentone (from Coakley et al 1976).

Electroencephalogram

Although it has been recognized for many years that the most logical method of monitoring depth of anaesthesia is to analyse cerebral function, success in this area has been elusive. The EEG is composed of a number of non-sinusoidal signals superimposed on low-amplitude random electrical activity. Limitations in its use as a monitor during anaesthesia are related in part to technical problems in analysing an extremely complex wave pattern, and partly to the difficulties inherent in interpretation of a two-dimensional signal from a three-dimensional organ. The major portion of the waveform emanates from superficial areas of the cerebral cortex. This may mask activity in deeper structures in the brain or changes in the function of such areas brought about by anaesthetic drugs. Nevertheless, a number of changes in EEG activity have been noted during anaesthesia, and several attempts have been made to process the EEG signal in such a way that any relationship between anaesthetic depth and EEG changes may be detected.

Raw EEG. The unprocessed EEG is an impractical tool for intraoperative monitoring. A large number of scalp electrodes is required and the equipment is bulky. Interpretation of the EEG trace obtained is unreliable.Volavka et al (1973) showed that the highest average correlation in interpretation of EEG traces by seven experienced readers was 56%. Although Courtin et al (1950) related seven different EEG patterns to levels of depth of anaesthesia, subsequent investigators (Galla et al 1958, Wolfson et al 1967) did not experience the same degree of success. While gross changes in the depth of anaesthesia may be detectable, more subtle changes, particularly during light anaesthesia, are inconsistent.

Processed EEG: pattern recognition. A sophisticated analysis of EEG traces has been designed (Gersch et al 1980) to recognize and compare patterns of activity of the patient being studied with 'control' EEGs from previous patients in whom, it was claimed, the depth of anaesthesia was known. While the technique has appeared successful during nitrous oxide and halothane anaesthesia it does not seem to have been investigated fully using other agents.

Total amplitude display. The overall amplitude of the EEG has been observed to increase during induction of anaesthesia and to decrease progressively as the depth of anaesthesia is increased (Bickford 1949). The cerebral function monitor (CFM) displays variations in overall amplitude of EEG activity from 2 to 20 Hz measured from two parietal scalp electrodes. Although a correlation was reported between CFM amplitude and depth of anaesthesia using intravenous agents (Dubois et al 1978, Prior et al 1978, Frank et al 1982), Sechzer & Ospina (1977) were unable to correlate CFM changes with depth of anaesthesia using a wide variety of inhalational and intravenous agents. The main uses of this device have been confined to the detection of adequate cerebral oxygenation, for example during neurosurgical or cardiothoracic operations, or during induced hypotension. It has been claimed that the ratio of the amplitude of delta waves to the amplitude of the entire EEG signal (augmented-delta quotient, ADQ) correlates well with the depth of anaesthesia, even using agents that produce markedly different EEG patterns (Volgyesi 1978).

Frequency/amplitude analysis. The use of Fourier analysis to identify the relative amplitudes of the component parts of a complex waveform has enabled EEG information to be displayed in a simpler form more amenable to interpretation. The most common method for display is compressed spectral array (CSA) (Fig. 26.5), producing a 'hills and valleys' appearance. Because 'hills' tend to obscure subsequent data an alternative method of display, density-modulated spectral array (DSA), has been suggested. Spectral arrays demonstrate changes in the frequency distribution of EEG activity in relation to increasing depth of anaesthesia

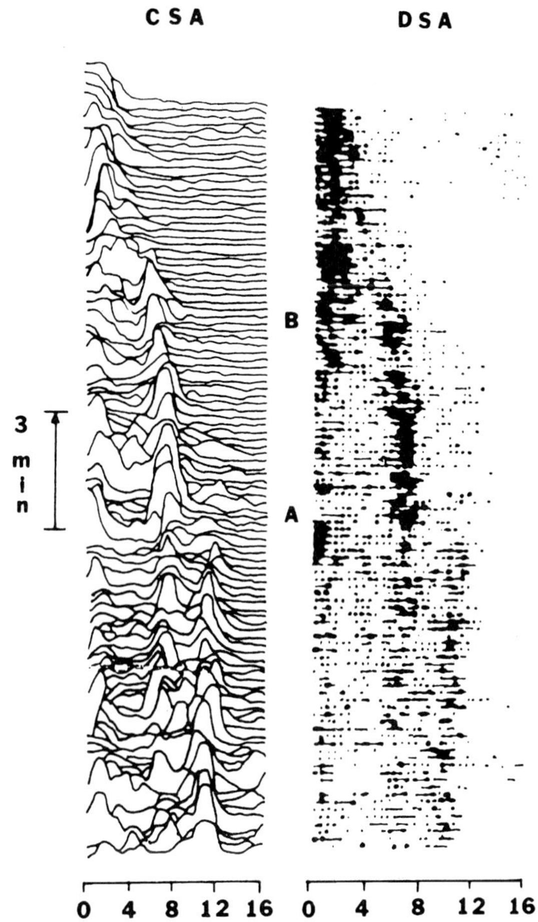

Fig. 26.5 A comparison of compressed spectral array (CSA) and density-modulated spectral array (DSA) in a patient undergoing gradually deepening halothane-nitrous oxide anaesthesia. The DSA is displayed in a dot-matrix form which retains information lost behind 'hills' in the CSA (from Levy et al 1980).

(Berezowskyj et al 1976, Levy et al 1980), but further investigation is required to define their role as intraoperative monitors.

Two derivatives of spectral analysis have been used to assess depth of anaesthesia. The median EEG frequency and the spectral edge (the frequency below which 95% of total EEG power is located) decrease with increasing doses of anaesthetic drug. It has been suggested that a median EEG frequency below 5 Hz is associated with non-responsiveness to verbal commands (Schwilden 1989).

The cerebral function analysing monitor (CFAM) is a development of the CFM. Rather than displaying the total EEG activity, the CFAM provides the mean and the 10th and 90th centiles of overall EEG amplitude distribution, together with a display of relative distribution of activity in the beta, alpha, theta and delta bands (Fig. 26.6). In addition, electrical activity from scalp muscle is monitored and evoked potentials (see below) may be obtained. Initial investigations (Maynard & Jenkinson 1984) suggest that alterations in beta activity reflect changes in conscious level during light anaesthesia. Data from the CFAM appear to be capable of detecting six levels of anaesthesia in baboons (Prior et al 1978), and a correlation has been established between plasma thiopentone concentrations and CFAM changes (Frank et al 1983). The frequency data enable the CFAM to be used for monitoring nitrous oxide and halothane anaesthesia (Sebel et al 1983), although Williams et al (1983) have found amplitude, but not frequency, to change predictably during inhalation of nitrous oxide.

Evoked potentials Auditory, visual and peripheral nerve (somatosensory) stimulation produce characteristic changes in the EEG. These are of very low amplitude and high frequency, and are obscured by other electrical activity in an EEG trace. However, by using repeated stimuli and computerized averaging techniques, it is possible to eliminate other EEG activity and obtain a display of the electrical changes produced as the impulse generated by the stimulus progresses up the brainstem and into the cortex.

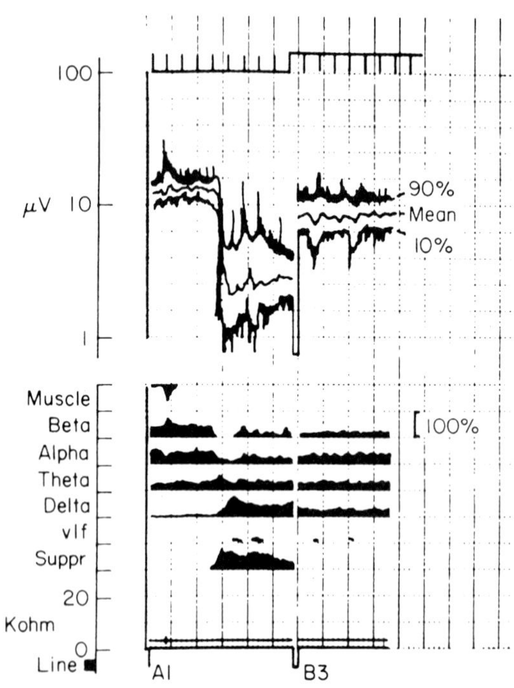

Fig. 26.6 A simulated CFAM trace (from Maynard & Jenkinson 1984).

Thornton et al (1984) found dose-related increases in latency and decreases in amplitude of some waves in the brainstem auditory evoked potential (EP) in patients anaesthetized with nitrous oxide and enflurane or halothane. However, intravenous anaesthetic agents had no effect on the brainstem EP (Thornton & Newton 1989). The later (more peripheral) waves of the cortical auditory EP are abolished by volatile anaesthetic agents. However, the earliest cortical waves remain relatively intact even during administration of inhalational anaesthetic agents in excess of MAC (Thornton & Newton 1989). This suggests that auditory stimuli may reach the inner areas of the cerebral cortex even during surgical anaesthesia. This may be related to the phenomenon of unconscious perception of auditory stimuli. The administration of inhalational anaesthetic agents is associated with a decrease in amplitude and an increase in latency of the waveform (Fig. 26.7). Similar changes accompany the administration of intravenous anaesthetic drugs. Of particular significance is the fact that the changes in the waveform are reversed in part by surgical stimulation, suggesting that EPs may indicate true depth of anaesthesia and are not acting only as bioassays of anaesthetic drug concentration in the brain.

Somatosensory EPs also show changes in latency and amplitude in response to the administration of anaesthetic and opioid drugs (Sebel et al 1987). However, the early cortical auditory EP appears at present to offer greater promise as a clinically useful index of depth of anaesthesia. Currently, investigations are in progress to evaluate a numerical 'AER index', based on the double differential of the waveform between 20 and 80 ms after each stimulus (Fig. 26.8). However, the apparatus used to generate EPs is expensive and is sensitive to interference from other equip-

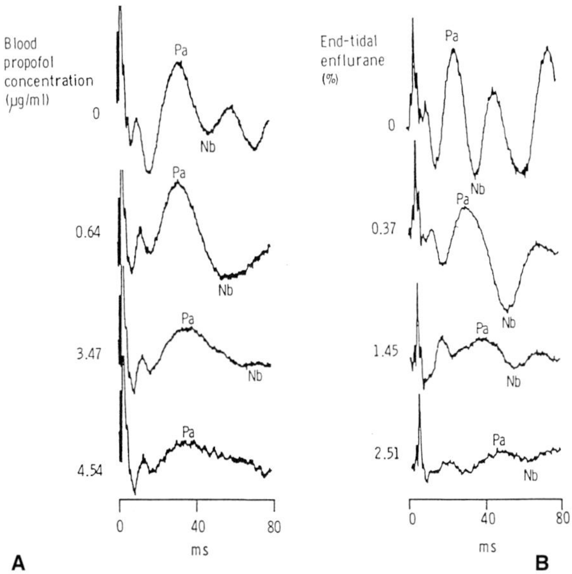

Fig. 26.7 Early cortical evoked potentials in patients given (A) propofol or (B) enflurane with 70% nitrous oxide. Note that the waves Pa and Nb are shifted to the right (increased latency) and their amplitudes decreased by increasing concentrations of anaesthetic (from Thornton & Newton 1989).

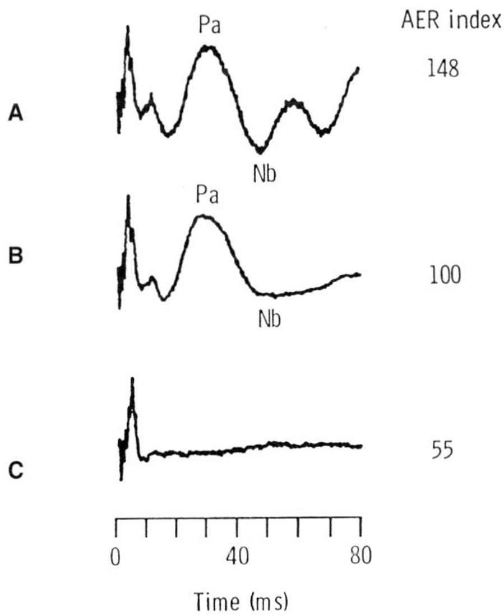

Fig. 26.8 Early cortical evoked response (AER) of a patient during (A) light, (B) moderate and (C) deep anaesthesia, with the AER index, which may relate to depth of anaesthesia, derived from the double differential of the waveform. See text (from Thornton & Newton 1989).

ment, particularly diathermy. In addition, changes occur with alterations in temperature and variations in arterial $P\text{CO}_2$.

PREVENTION OF AWARENESS WITH RECALL

Although it may not be possible to eliminate awareness with recall without administering doses or concentrations of anaesthetic drugs that will cause undesirable and potentially dangerous side effects in some patients (Blacher 1984), the risk of recall can be minimized by adherence to a small number of principles of clinical practice based on a knowledge of the potential causes:

1. All apparatus should be checked before every operating list, and the ventilator, vaporizer and breathing system before every new case. All apparatus must be serviced by qualified personnel at the recommended intervals and full records of servicing kept.
2. Patients should be resuscitated adequately whenever possible so that reduced concentrations of anaesthetic drugs are not required simply to prevent exaggerated cardiovascular side effects.
3. An adequate dose of intravenous induction agent should be administered. The 'sleep dose' should not be considered as the maximum, especially in young or unpremedicated patients. Consideration should be given to the duration of action of the agent.
4. The induction agent alone should not be relied upon to maintain unconsciousness during tracheal intubation if non-depolarizing neuromuscular blockers are used. Anaesthesia must be maintained while waiting for the relaxant to become effective.
5. If intubation is difficult and prolonged, anaesthesia must be maintained either by the use of an inhalational agent with oxygen between attempts or by supplementary doses of an intravenous drug.
6. Reliance should not be placed on nitrous-oxide-oxygen mixtures alone. A supplementary agent should be used. Volatile

agents are probably more predictable than intravenous agents in preventing recall in the paralysed patient.

7. Opioids in conventional doses are not effective anaesthetic agents. They form an important part of a balanced anaesthetic technique but must not be used as an alternative to adequate doses of anaesthetic agents.
8. Frequent checks of apparatus should be made during anaesthesia to ensure that all connections are intact and that reserves of anaesthetic agents in cylinders, vaporizers or infusion pumps are adequate. The patient's condition must be monitored continuously. The anaesthetist must never leave the patient unattended.
9. If nitrous oxide is used its administration should be continued until there is objective evidence of reversal of neuromuscular blockade. If other agents are employed their anticipated elimination profile should be considered carefully when determining the time at which their administration is discontinued. Volatile agents with a low blood/gas solubility coefficient are eliminated rapidly.
10. As hearing is the first sense to return it may be prudent to apply earplugs or earphones transmitting music or 'white noise' (Grant et al 1979). This precaution would also eliminate the risk of adverse postoperative effects from unconscious perception. It has been suggested that positive therapeutic suggestions might be given routinely during anaesthesia (Editorial 1986).

WHAT SHOULD THE PATIENT BE TOLD?

It is important that any patient who has experienced recall of intraoperative events should be identified. Ideally this would be accomplished by regular postoperative visits by all anaesthetists. However, this is not always achieved in practice and it is important that ward nurses and non-anaesthetic medical staff are educated about the subject in order that any complaint is dealt with appropriately. If informed of a patient who complains of recall, the anaesthetist should interview the patient in the presence of a witness and listen carefully to the complaint. If it is clear that intraoperative recall has occurred the anaesthetist should acknowledge the fact that he believes the account of events. The anaesthetist should apologize to the patient. He should explain that recall can occur without fault during anaesthesia in which muscle relaxants are employed because of the desire to avoid high and potentially toxic concentrations of anaesthetic drugs, and because of the difficulty in interpreting clinical signs. The patient should be reassured and informed that a note will be made in the hospital record so that other anaesthetists will know of the problem if anaesthesia and surgery are required in future. A full account of the interview should be recorded in the clinical notes. Junior anaesthetists should inform a consultant, who should be present when the patient is counselled.

It may be advisable to warn all 'high-risk' patients (e.g. the seriously ill and patients undergoing caesarean section under general anaesthesia) if low concentrations of anaesthetic are to be used, of the possibility of recall during anaesthesia (Aitkenhead 1990). Many patients are already anxious about the possibility of awareness because of recent publicity. In addition, the psychological stress resulting from awareness with recall may be reduced if a warning has been given. However, this should *not* be used as an excuse to omit the measures outlined above to reduce to a minimum the occurrence of this extremely distressing experience.

CONCLUSION

There is at present no definite evidence that the depth of anaesthesia affects the incidence of unconscious perception. However, the much more important problem of recall *is* related to depth of anaesthesia, and the most effective method of prevention is the administration of effective doses of anaesthetic agents. While a slight increase in time to recovery of consciousness may result, it is my view that in modern hospital practice this should be associated with a negligible risk. As yet there is no instrument, either mechanical or electrical, that has proved capable of assessing 'depth of anaesthesia' more reliably than simple clinical methods.

REFERENCES

Ackers v Wigan Health Authority 1985, referred to in Current Law, March 1986

Aitkenhead A R 1990 Awareness during anaesthesia: what should the patient be told? Anaesthesia 45: 351–352

Barclay A, Houlton P C, Downing J W 1980 Total intravenous anaesthesia: a technique using flunitrazepam, ketamine, muscle relaxants and controlled ventilation of the lung. Anaesthesia 35: 287–290

Barr A M, Moxon A, Woolam C H, Fryer M E 1977 Effect of diazepam and lorazepam on awareness during anaesthesia for Caesarean section. Anaesthesia 32: 873–878

Bennett H L, Davis H S, Giannini J A 1985 Non-verbal response to intraoperative conversation. Br J Anaesth 57: 174–179

Berezowskyj J L, McEwan J A, Anderson G B, Jenkins L C 1976 A study of anaesthesia depth by power spectral analysis of the electroencephalogram. Can Anaesth Soc J 23: 1–8

Bickford R G 1949 Neurophysiological applications of automatic anesthetic regulator controlled by brain potentials. Am J Physiol 159: 562–565

Blacher R S 1975 On awakening paralysed during surgery. J Am Med Assoc 234: 67–68

Blacher R S 1984 Awareness during surgery. Anesthesiology 61: 1–2

Boeke S, Bonke B, Bouwhuis-Hoogerwerf M L, Bovill J G, Zwaveling A 1988 Effects of sounds presented during general anaesthesia on postoperative course. Br J Anaesth 60: 697–702

Bogod D G, Orton J K, Yau H M, Oh T E 1990 Detecting awareness during general anaesthetic Caesarean section: an evaluation of two methods. Anaesthesia 45: 279–284

Bonke B, Schmitz P I M, Verhage F, Zwaveling A 1986 Clinical study of so-called unconscious perception during general anaesthesia. Br J Anaesth 58: 957–964

Breckenridge J, Aitkenhead A R 1981 Isolated forearm technique for detection of wakefulness during general anaesthesia. Br J Anaesth 53: 665–666

Brice D D, Hetherington R R, Utting J E 1970 A simple study of awareness and dreaming during anaesthesia. Br J Anaesth 42: 535–541

Browne R A, Catton D V 1973 Awareness during anaesthesia: a comparison of anaesthesia with nitrous oxide-oxygen and nitrous oxide-oxygen with Innovar. Can Anaesth Soc J 20: 763–768

Cheek D B 1980 Awareness of meaningful sounds under general anesthesia: considerations and a review of the literature 1959–1979. In: Wain H J (ed) Theoretical and clinical aspects of hypnosis. Symposia Specialists, Miami, p 87–106

Clapham M C 1981 Isolated forearm technique using pancuronium. Anaesthesia 36: 642–643

Coakley D, Thomas J G, Lunn J N 1976 The effect of anaesthesia on ocular microtremor. Br J Anaesth 48: 1122–1123

Courtin R F, Bickford R G, Faulconer A 1950 The classification and significance of electroencephalographic patterns produced by nitrous oxide-ether anesthesia during surgical operations. Proceedings of the Mayo Clinic 25: 197

Cox P N, White D C 1986 Do oesophageal contractions measure depth of anaesthesia? Br J Anaesth 57: 131P

Crawford J S 1984 Principles and practice of obstetric anaesthesia, 5th edn. Blackwell Scientific, Oxford, p 297

Crawford J S, Davies P 1975 A return of trichloroethylene for obstetric anaesthesia. Br J Anaesth 47: 482–490

Crawford J S, James F M, Davies P, Crawley M 1976 A further study of general anaesthesia for caesarian section. Br J Anaesth 48: 661–667

Davies W L, Evans J M, Fraser A C L, Barclay M 1982 Closed loop control of anaesthesia. In: Control systems, concepts and approaches in clinical medicine. Proceedings of the Institute of Measurement and Control Symposium, Brighton, p 87–90

Desai N, Taylor-Davies A, Barnett D B 1983 The effects of diazepam and oxprenolol on short term memory in individuals of high and low state anxiety. Br J Clin Pharmacol 15: 197–202

Dubois M, Savege T M, O'Carroll T M, Frank M 1978 General anaesthesia and changes in the cerebral function monitor. Anaesthesia 33: 157–164

Dubovsky S, Trustman R 1976 Absence of recall after general anesthesia: implications for theory and practice. Anesth Analg 55: 696–701

Dundee J W, McMurray T J 1983 Awareness during anaesthesia: a review. J R Coll Surg Engl 65: 330

Editorial 1986 Advertising during anaesthesia? Lancet 2: 1019–1020

Eger E I, Saidman L J, Brandstater B 1965 Minimum alveolar anesthetic concentration: a standard of anesthetic potency. Anesthesiology 26: 756–763

Eich E, Reeves J L, Katz R L 1985 Anesthesia, awareness and the memory/awareness distinction. Anesth Analg 64: 1143–1148

Eisele V, Weinreich A, Bartle S 1976 Perioperative awareness and recall. Anesth Analg 55: 513–518

Evans F J 1972 Hypnosis and sleep: techniques of exploring cognitive activity during sleep. In: Fromm E, Shor E (eds) Hypnosis: research developments and perspectives. Aldine-Atherton, Chicago, p 43–83

Evans J M 1987 Clinical signs and autonomic responses. In: Rosen M, Lunn J N (eds) Consciousness awareness and pain in general anaesthesia. Butterworths, London, p 18–33

Evans J M, Bithell J F, Vlachonikolis I G 1987 Relationship between lower oesophageal contractility, clinical signs and halothane concentration during general anaesthesia and surgery in man. Br J Anaesth 59: 1346–1355

Evans C, Richardson P H 1988 Improved recovery and

reduced postoperative stay after therapeutic suggestions during general anaesthesia. Lancet 1: 491–493
Ewin D M 1990 Hypnotic technique for recall of sounds heard under general anaesthesia. In: Bonke B, Fitch W, Millar K (eds) Memory and awareness in anaesthesia. Swetz & Zeitlinger, Amsterdam, p 226–232
Farnsworth G M 1978 Enflurane and the incidence of awareness in Caesarean section. Anaesthesia 33: 553
File S E, Lister R G 1982 Do lorazepam-induced deficits in learning result from impaired rehearsal, reduced motivation or increased sedation? Br J Clin Pharmacol 14: 545–550
Frank M, Savege T M, Leigh M, Greenwood J, Holly J M P 1982 Comparison of the cerebral function monitor and plasma concentrations of thiopentone and alphaxolone during total iv anaesthesia with repeated bolus doses of thiopentone and althesin. Br J Anaesth 54: 609–616
Frank M, Maynard D E, Major E, Coutinho P, Tsanaclis L M 1983 Comparison of plasma thiopentone concentrations and the cerebral function analysing monitor using repeated bolus injections of thiopentone. Br J Anaesth 55: 910
Galla S J, Rocco A G, Vandam L D 1958 Evaluation of the traditional signs and stages of anaesthesia: an EEG and clinical study. Anesthesiology 19: 328–338
Garfield J M, Garfield F B, Stone J G, Hopkins D 1972 A comparison of psychologic responses to ketamine and thiopental-nitrous oxide-halothane anesthesia. Anesthesiology 36: 329–338
Gersch W, Martinelli F, Yonemoto J et al 1980 A Kullback-Leibler nearest neighbour rule classification of EEGs. Comput Biomed Res 13: 283–286
Glucksberg S 1962 The influence of strength of drive on fixedness and perceptual recognition. J Exp Psychol 63: 36–41
Goddard G F 1982 A pilot study of changes in skin electrical conductance in patients undergoing general anaesthesia and surgery. Anaesthesia 37: 408–415
Goldmann L, Shah M, Hebden M 1987 Memory of cardiac anaesthesia: psychological sequelae of cardiac patients to intraoperative suggestions and operating theatre conversation. Anaesthesia 42: 596–603
Grant L J, Perkins M A, Babington P 1979 Prevention of hearing under anaesthesia. Anaesthesia 34: 921
Hargrove R L 1987 Awareness under anaesthesia. Journal of the Medical Defence Union (Spring) 9–11
Harmel M H, Klein F F, Davis D A 1978 The EEMG: a practical index of cortical activity and muscular relaxation. Acta Anaesthesiol Scand Suppl 70: 97–102
Harris T B J, Brice D D, Hetherington R R, Utting J E 1971 Dreaming associated with anaesthesia: the influence of morphine premedications and two volatile adjuvants. Br J Anaesth 43: 172–178
Hertzman A B, Roth L W 1942 The vasomotor components in the vascular reactions in the fingers to cold. Am J Physiol 136: 669
Hutchings D D 1961 The value of suggestion given under anesthesia: a report and evaluation of 200 consecutive cases. Am J Clin Hypn 4: 26–29
Hutchinson R 1960 Awareness during surgery. Br J Anaesth 33: 463–469
Jansen C K, Bonke B, Klein J, Bezstarosti-Van Eeden J, Tergau F, Custers W, van Dasselaar N 1990 Unconscious perception during balanced anaesthesia? In: Bonke B, Fitch W, Millar K (eds) Memory and awareness in anaesthesia. Swetz and Zeitlinger, Amsterdam, p 115–119
Johnstone M 1974 Digital vasodilatation: a sign of anaesthesia. Br J Anaesth 46: 414–419
Jones D M, Jones M E L, Lewis M J, Spriggs T L B 1979 Drugs and human memory: effects of low doses of nitrazepam and hyoscine on retention. Br J Clin Pharmacol 7: 479–483
Jones J G, Konieczko K 1986 Hearing and memory in anaesthetised patients. Br Med J 292: 1291–1293
Kissin I, Gelman S 1987 Three components of anesthesia: one more reason to accept the concept. Anesth Analg 66: 98
Lawes E C, Newman B, Campbell M J, Irwin M, Dolenska S, Thomas T A 1988 Maternal inspired oxygen concentration and neonatal status for Caesarean section under general anaesthesia: comparison of effects of 33% or 50% oxygen in nitrous oxide. Br J Anaesth 61: 250–254
Levinson B W 1965 States of awareness during general anaesthesia. Br J Anaesth 67: 544–546
Levy W J, Shapiro H M, Maruschak G, Meathe E 1980 Automated EEG processing for intraoperative monitoring. Anesthesiology 53: 223–236
Liu D, Thorp S, Graham S, Aitkenhead A R (in press) Incidence of recall of awareness during anaesthesia for non-obstetric surgery. Br J Anaesth
Lyons G, Macdonald R 1991 Awareness during caesarean section, Anaesthesia 46: 62–64
McIntyre J W R 1966 Awareness during general anaesthesia, preliminary observations. Can Anaesth Soc J 13: 495–499
McKenna J, Wilton T N P 1973 Awareness during endotracheal intubation. Anaesthesia 28: 599–602
McLintock T T C, Aitken H, Downie C, Kenny G N C 1990 The effect of intraoperative suggestions on postoperative analgesic requirements. In: Bonke B, Fitch W, Millar K (eds) Memory and awareness in anaesthesia. Swetz and Zeitlinger, Amsterdam, p 96–100
Maynard D E, Jenkinson J L 1984 The cerebral function analysing monitor: initial experience, application and further development. Anaesthesia 39: 678–690
Millar K 1989 Recall, recognition and implicit memory for intra-anaesthetic events. In: Jones J G (ed) Depth of anaesthesia. Baillière's clinical anaesthesiology: international practice and research 3: 487–510
Millar K, Watkinson N 1983 Recognition of words presented during general anaesthesia. Ergonomics 26: 585–594
Moir D D 1970 Anaesthesia for Caesarean section. Br J Anaesth 42: 136–142
Moir D D 1976 Obstetric anaesthesia and analgesia. Baillière Tindall, London, P 145
Moir D D, Thorburn J 1986 Obstetric anaesthesia and analgesia, 3rd edn. Baillière Tindall, London, p 193
Pearson R E 1961 Response to suggestions given under general anesthesia. Am J Clin Hypn 4: 106–114
Pinsker M C 1986 Anesthesia: a pragmatic construct. Anesth Analg 65: 819–820
Prior P F, Maynard D E, Brierly J B 1978 EEG monitoring for the control of anaesthesia produced by the infusion of Althesin in primates. Br J Anaesth 50: 993–1001
Prys-Roberts C 1987 Anaesthesia: a practical or impractical construct? Br J Anaesth 59: 1341–1345
Rosen J 1959 Hearing tests during anaesthesia with nitrous oxide and relaxants. Acta Anaesthesiol Scand 3: 1–8
Rubin J, Nagler R, Spiro M, Pilot M L 1962 Measuring the

effect of emotions on oesophageal motility. Psychosom Med 24: 1706
Rupreht J, Valkenburg M 1990 The anaesthetic state: evolution of a concept. In: Bonke B, Fitch W, Millar K (eds) Memory and awareness in anaesthesia. Swetz and Zeitlinger, Amsterdam, p 70–75
Russell I F 1989 Conscious awareness during general anaesthesia: relevance of autonomic signs and isolated arm movements as guides to depth of anaesthesia. In: Jones J G (ed) Depth of anaesthesia. Baillière's clinical anaesthesiology: international practice and research. 3: 511–532
Schwilden H 1989 Use of the median EEG frequency and pharmacokinetics in determining depth of anaesthesia. In: Jones J G (ed) Depth of anaesthesia. Baillire's clinical anaesthesiology: international practice and research. 3: 603–621
Sear J W 1983 General kinetic and dynamic principles and their application to continuous infusion anaesthesia. Anaesthesia Suppl 38: 10–25
Sebel P S, Maynard D E, Major E, Frank M 1983 The cerebral function analysing monitor (CFAM). Br J Anaesth 55: 1265–1270
Sebel P S, Glass P, Neville W K 1987 Do evoked potentials measure depth of anaesthesia? Int J Clin Monit Comput 5: 163–166
Sechzer P H, Ospina J 1977 Cerebral function monitor: evaluation in anesthesia/critical care. Curr Ther Res 22: 335–347
Stoelting R K, Longnecker D E, Eger E I 1970 Minimum alveolar concentrations in man on awakening from methoxyflurane, halothane, ether and fluroxene anesthesia: MAC awake. Anesthesiology 33: 5–9
Stolzy S, Couture L J, Edmonds H L 1987 A post-operative recognition test after balanced anesthesia. Anesth Analg 67: A377
Terrell R K, Sweet W O, Gladfelter J H, Stephen C R 1969 Study of recall during anesthesia. Anesth Analg 48: 86–90
Thomas D I, Aitkenhead A R 1990 Relationship between lower oesophageal contractility and type of surgical stimulation. Br J Anaesth 64: 306–310
Thornton C, Heneghan C P H, James M F M, Jones J G 1984 Effects of halothane or enflurane with controlled ventilation on auditory evoked potentials. Br J Anaesth 56: 315–323
Thornton C, Newton D E F 1989 The auditory evoked response: a measure of depth of anaesthesia. In: Jones J G (ed) Depth of anaesthesia. Baillière's clinical anaesthesiology: international practice and research. 3: 559–585
Tunstall M E 1977 Detecting wakefulness during general anaesthesia for Caesarean section. Br Med J 1: 1321
Utting J E 1987 Awareness: clinical aspects. In: Rosen M, Lunn J N (eds) Consciousness, awareness and pain in general anaesthesia. Butterworths, London, p 171–179
Vickers M D 1987 Detecting consciousness by clinical means. In: Rosen M, Lunn J N (eds) Consciousness awareness and pain in general anaesthesia. Butterworths, London, p 12–17
Volavka J, Matousek M, Feldstein S 1973 The reliability of electroencephalography assessment. Electroencephalography and Electromyography 4: 123
Volgyesi G A 1978 A brain function monitor for use during anaesthesia: preliminary report. Can Anaesth Soc J 25: 427–430
Warren T M, Datta S, Ostheimer G W, Naulty J S, Weiss J B, Morrison J A 1983 Comparison of the maternal and neonatal effects of halothane, enflurane, and isoflurane for cesarean delivery. Anesth Analg 62: 516–520
Weinberger N M, Gold P E, Sternberg D B 1984 Epinephrine enables Pavlovian fear conditioning under anesthesia. Science 223: 605–607
White D C 1987 Anaesthesia: a privation of the senses: an historical introduction and some definitions. In: Rosen M, Lunn J N (eds) Consciousness , awareness and pain in general anaesthesia. Butterworths, London, p 1–9
White M, Kenny G N C 1990 Intravenous propofol anaesthesia using a computerised infusion system. Anaesthesia 45: 204–209
Williams D J M, Morgan R J M, Sebel P S, Maynard D E 1983 Effect of nitrous oxide assessed by cerebral function analysing monitor (CFAM). Br J Anaesth 55: 908
Wilson M E 1981 Isolated forearm technique for detection of wakefulness during general anaesthesia. Br J Anaesth 53: 1234
Wilson S, Vaughan R, Stephen C 1975 Awareness, dreams and hallucinations associated with general anesthesia. Anesth Analg 54: 609–619
Wolfe L S, Millett J B 1960 Control of post-operative pain by suggestion under general anesthesia. Am J Clin Hypn 3: 109–112
Wolfson B, Siber E S, Ciccarrelli H E, Gray G H, Jones L 1967 The electroencephalogram as a monitor of arterial blood levels of methoxyflurane. Anesthesiology 28: 1003
Woo R, Seltzer J L, Marr A 1987 The lack of response to suggestion under controlled surgical anaesthesia. Acta Anaesthesiol Scand 32: 712–713
Wright P J, Dundee J W 1982 Attitudes to intravenous infusion anaesthesia. Anaesthesia 37: 1209–1213

27

Complications of recovery from anaesthesia

J. Cotter

INTRODUCTION

Recovery from anaesthesia is the process of reversal of the effects of the anaesthetic drugs used and of other effects due to anaesthetic techniques. It is not easy to define the exact point when the patient may be said to have recovered from the anaesthetic. It can be defined as the time when there are no residual effects from the anaesthetic drugs or the anaesthetic process. With general anaesthesia it is commonly taken as the point at which consciousness is regained, but there is no sharp endpoint to waking from coma, the ability to obey a command occurring before the ability to converse rationally. Even when this latter stage is reached the patient may have no recollection of the conversation the next day, indicating that he had not fully recovered from the effects of anaesthesia at the time of conversation. Other body systems may be affected by general anaesthetic drugs when recovery from cerebral effects has apparently taken place.

A patient with depressed consciousness preoperatively, or one who has suffered intraoperative brain damage due to anaesthetic or surgical mishap, may not regain consciousness when anaesthetic drugs have ceased to act.

It is rare for general anaesthesia to be used as a primary therapeutic measure, although it has been used as such in the treatment of status asthmaticus, status epilepticus and uterine tetany. Local anaesthesia is used in the treatment of pain. Anaesthesia is normally used to enable therapeutic or diagnostic procedures (both of which are included in the term 'operation' in this chapter) to be undertaken. Thus the patient recovering from anaesthesia will also be recovering from an operation, and both can produce complications postoperatively, singly or together. It can be difficult to differentiate the effects of anaesthesia from those of the operation, although it must be said that many of one's nursing and surgical colleagues seem to have no difficulty in ascribing a wide range of postoperative events solely to the anaesthetic.

Recovery from an anaesthetic is usually much quicker than recovery from the operation, but anaesthetic complications that have occurred intraoperatively or early in the recovery phase may be the cause of prolonged morbidity or late mortality.

RECOVERY OF CONSCIOUSNESS AFTER GENERAL ANAESTHESIA

Recovery of consciousness after operation is usually quite rapid. Farman (1978) reported an average waking time after entering the recovery room of 8.5 min. Various factors may affect the speed of recovery and some of the more important are listed below:

1. heavy premedication
2. delayed absorption of oral premedication
3. late premedication
4. long-acting anaesthetic agents
5. overdosage

6. delayed clearance of:
    - volatile agents due to:
        - respiratory depression
        - chronic respiratory disease
        - low cardiac output
    - intravenous agents due to:
        - low cardiac output
        - renal failure
        - liver failure
        - abnormal enzyme activity
7. age (the very young and very old)
8. obesity
9. poor physical status.

Clearly, speed of recovery will be affected by the type of anaesthetic drugs and techniques used, but it is often forgotten that one of the most common and easily remedied causes of slow recovery is low cardiac output. Volatile anaesthetic agents can only be excreted by the lungs if there is adequate pulmonary blood flow. If cardiac ouput is low, less anaesthetic will be cleared per unit time. Similarly, intravenous agents relying on liver or renal clearance will be metabolized and excreted much more quickly in the presence of adequate cardiac ouput. Frequently all that is required to speed up recovery is an infusion of fluid.

Cerebral depressant drugs, including sedatives, antidepressants and tranquillizers, taken prior to anaesthesia may summate with anaesthetic drugs and prolong the anaesthetic action. Where, however, the patient has taken cerebral depressant drugs for a considerable time, there may be resistance to the effects of cerebral depressants including general anaesthetics. Dundee & Wyant (1988) suggest that, although enzyme induction might play a part in resistance to intravenous anaesthetics shown by patients who have been receiving large doses of sedative and analgesic drugs, cross tolerance of the central nervous system to the drug is probably more important. Patients with a high alcohol intake form a group that is often resistant to general anaesthetic drugs.

Because of immaturity of metabolic pathways, neonates and infants metabolize or excrete some drugs more slowly than older patients. The elderly may be sensitive to the effects of anaesthetic drugs and may also have a decreased ability to metabolize and excrete them. Terminal elimination half-life of many drugs is prolonged in the elderly and dosage needs adjusting accordingly. A fuller description of hazards of anaesthesia in the elderly is given in Chapter 13.

Sick patients are particularly sensitive to anaesthetic drugs, as are patients hypovolaemic from any cause. Unless dosage is adjusted, recovery will be considerably prolonged. Diseases of systems involved in breakdown and excretion of drugs will also prolong anaesthesia. Metabolic disorders, particularly myxoedema, will also delay recovery.

In cases of unexpectedly prolonged recovery, cerebral causes of unconsciousness should be considered. Raised intracranial pressure (ICP) may have been present prior to anaesthesia and been made worse by anaesthetic factors. Embolism of blood components, air or fat may occur during certain forms of surgery, and the brain is sensitive to episodes of ischaemia and hypoxia. It should therefore not be assumed that if a patient fails to rouse following anaesthesia it is necessarily the fault of the anaesthetic. Unexplained unconsciousness requires investigation and an intracerebral cause needs to be excluded, if necessary with a brain scan. Fraser & Goat (1983) reported a case of prolonged unconsciousness following anaesthesia where the patient was found, some months later, to have a meningioma. Recovery may coincide with the postictal phase of an epileptic seizure. The tonic clonic phase of an epileptic seizure may not manifest itself in the presence of nondepolarizing muscle relaxants.

The Committee on Safety of Medicines (CSM 1989) drew attention to reports of eight patients that had either a delay of more than 1 h in regaining consciousness after propofol anaesthesia or who initially woke but subsequently lapsed into unconsciousness. They noted that these patients had undergone investigative procedures or minor surgery. Propofol is generally considered an ideal induction agent for day-case surgery, as in unpremedicated patients there is rapid recovery with clearheadedness. CSM advised that an adequate period of recovery must be allowed before discharging patients after day-case surgery.

The discharge of patients from day-case surgery normally adheres to strict guidelines. Saunders & Harris (1990) suggested that drug-induced decerebrate rigidity provides an explanation for the prolonged, fluctuating and relapsing unconsciousness observed in these patients. This is considered further in Chapter 28.

If recovery from anaesthesia is inexplicably delayed, contamination of the anaesthetic agents with impurities, or faulty anaesthetic equipment resulting in toxic doses of anaesthetic agents, must be considered. If necessary, any residual drug from broken ampoules or vaporizers used during the anaesthetic should be tested, as should vaporizers and anaesthetic machines used in the anaesthetic.

In considering complications of recovery in this chapter it is proposed to deal especially with complications presenting between the end of operation and the time at which the patient can safely be looked after with normal ward care. This period is referred to here as the primary recovery period. Events that occur at this time may persist or progress later.

THE RECOVERY ROOM AND THE CONDUCT OF POSTOPERATIVE AND POSTANAESTHETIC RECOVERY

The need for recovery rooms

It is accepted that a patient having a general anaesthetic, or a local anaesthetic technique which can cause major systemic effects, must be under the constant supervision of a trained individual whose sole commitment is to that patient, that is the anaesthetist.

As it is necessary for the anaesthetic to last at least until the end of operation and as current techniques do not allow instant cessation of the effects of anaesthetic drugs, there is a period after the end of operation during which the patient is still anaesthetized. Only when small doses of local anaesthetic have been used for minor surgery can the patient be regarded as past the primary recovery period at the end of surgery, although even in these cases analgesic tissue is still at risk of inadvertent damage. During the primary recovery period the patient is at risk of many of the complications that are a hazard to him during the operation and still requires the exclusive attention of a trained individual. This attention is required until the patient is conscious with functioning protective reflexes, and stable cardiovascular and respiratory systems, and may be required for minutes, hours or even days. Except where the patient is looked after in a specific high-dependency unit such as an intensive therapy unit, this care is best provided in a specially commissioned recovery room. The DHSS Building Note (1967) states that the function of a recovery room is 'to enable patients to be held under the care of appropriately skilled nursing staff with, when required, relatively easy access to a surgeon or anaesthetist during the immediate postoperative period'.

It would not be possible to conduct a trial allocating patients to undergo the primary recovery period in either a recovery room or an alternative site such as a corridor or ward! Patients in the recovery period need the best conditions that can be provided. Some of the basic requirements are listed below:

- adequate numbers of trained staff
- proximity to theatre
- good lighting to reflect natural flesh tints
- tipping trolleys or beds
- monitoring equipment
- oxygen
- suction
- power points
- full range of anaesthetic and resuscitation equipment, including a defibrillator
- resuscitation drugs
- analgesic and antiemetic drugs
- means of communication with theatres and other departments
- minor procedures equipment, for example a chest drain set and tracheostomy set.

It is necessary to make best use of staff and equipment and this can only be done in a dedicated area. Only if such an area is easily accessible to surgeons and anaesthetists can suitable medical help be rapidly provided in an emergency.

All anaesthetists with considerable experience will have been involved with situations in a recovery room where their intervention has been required to avoid disaster. Utting et al (1979), in considering cases reported to the Medical Defence Union of the UK, found failure of postoperative care to be the cause of 9.5% of deaths and cerebral damage. Life-threatening complications during the primary recovery period are usually related to the cardiovascular and respiratory systems. These complications may occur however careful the preparation of the patient, the administration of the anaesthetic and the performance of the operation. Anaesthetists must endeavour to minimize the incidence of complications and reduce their severity by early recognition and appropriate treatment.

A recovery room allows a surgical list to continue during a patient's recovery and thus makes the most efficient use of staff and equipment in the theatre suite.

Of course, a recovery room is only of use when it is staffed and open. Lunn & Mushin (1982) quote a DHSS estimate that 80% of acute hospitals have recovery rooms. Many hospitals do not provide recovery room facilities for surgery taking place outside normal working hours, thus many patients requiring emergency surgery and most in need of a recovery room do not have access to one.

In their survey on mortality associated with anaesthesia, Lunn & Mushin (1982) found that 18% of the patients surveyed did not go to a recovery room when the facility was available.

Site of the recovery room

The recovery room should be adjacent to the theatres it serves so that patients can be transferred rapidly and there is easy access for medical staff working in the theatres. It is best if entry can be made from both inside and outside the clean zone of theatres so that medical staff can easily see the patients if required.

Anaesthesia may be administered in departments that are remote from the main operating suite. In some hospitals the theatres are scattered. In such circumstances a decision must be made as to whether patients should remain at the site of anaesthesia or be transferred to a central recovery room for the primary recovery period. The advantages of a central recovery room have to be weighed against the inconvenience and potential dangers of transfer.

If recovery of the patient has to take place at a site other than a recovery room, the anaesthetist must supervise the recovery and ensure that it takes place in a suitably equipped area. This will usually be the place where anaesthesia was administered.

Size of the recovery room

The size of the recovery room should depend on the number of patient spaces required, which will in turn be dependent on the number of operating theatres, the speciality mix and the average duration of stay. Atkinson (1979) has recommended two to three bed spaces per operating theatre for the average district hospital. This is in excess of the number (1.5 per theatre) suggested in the DHSS Building Note (1967).

Each patient space should allow easy access around the bed; the DHSS Building Note (1967) specifies 100 sq. ft (9.3 m^2) per bed. In addition, considerable space is required for storage, administration, washing facilities and a sluice.

Staffing

The recovery room should be run by a sister or even a senior nursing officer with a staff of trained nurses. The recovery room nursing staff need to be trained in the management of the postoperative patient with emphasis on care of the unconscious patient. There is no special qualification in recovery room nursing in the UK; individual hospitals therefore have their own systems of selection and training for recovery room staff. If competent staff cannot be provided the patient is more safely 'recovered' under supervision of the anaesthetist in the operating theatre. Nominating a nurse as a 'recovery room nurse' without assessment or training is hazardous.

It would appear reasonable for the medical staff to assume that a nurse employed by a hospital to work in the recovery room is adequately trained to supervise the recovery of at least the uncomplicated postoperative patient. It must be remembered, however, that in some patients, problems such as management of the airway may tax the most experienced anaesthetist, and when such a problem exists the anaesthetist must be satisfied, before leaving the patient, that the nursing staff can cope.

Anaesthetists should be prepared to involve themselves in the training and assessment of recovery room nurses. It is also helpful if a named consultant takes responsibility for liaising with the recovery room staff over matters such as organization, policy, training and any problems that may arise. Responsibility for the individual patient must remain with the surgeon and anaesthetist who treated the patient.

The number of nurses required

The number of nurses required depends on the number of patients coming to the recovery room, their length of stay and the amount of nursing care they require. These factors depend on the type of surgery and anaesthesia, and on the patients' general condition. A patient who has had the exclusive attention of an anaesthetist in the operating theatre must have the exclusive attention of a trained individual until conscious with protective reflexes. Therefore the number of unconscious patients in the recovery room should not exceed the number of trained nurses and there should ideally be an extra person to act as a 'runner'. Later in the recovery period a one-to-one nurse:patient ratio is not usually necessary. The recovery room staff must have the authority to refuse to accept cases where space or staff constraints make it unsafe to take further patients, thus leaving the patient in the care of the anaesthetist.

Ideally, no nurse should be left alone with an unconscious patient, so a minimum of two people is always required in the recovery room. One of these, if acting as a 'runner', need not be qualified to supervise a patient's recovery.

The recovery room is a valuable training ground for student nurses, medical students and some other groups, but these should not be considered part of the basic recovery room complement.

Equipment

The list on page 419 details the essential requirements for the recovery room, including equipment. Much of the equipment is electrically powered. It is to be hoped that the recovery room will have emergency electrical power, but thought should be given to the provision of torches, suckers powered by rechargeable batteries or manually, and monitors with battery back up.

Developments in monitoring facilities available commercially and the rise in expectation of the quality of care needed have meant that the standard of monitoring required in operating theatres has undergone major improvements in recent years. Many hospitals have been unable or unwilling to make the financial commitment needed, and equipment in recovery rooms often comes a poor second to that in the operating theatres. I agree with the Recommendations for Standards of Monitoring During Anaesthesia and Recovery (Association of Anaesthetists 1988): 'The monitoring employed in the recovery area should be appropriate to the patient's condition and a full range of monitoring devices as employed during anaesthesia should be available.' Pulse oximetry shows desaturation of arterial blood before any clinical signs are apparent and is of particular use in coloured and anaemic patients. Automatic non-invasive machines to measure blood pressure allow readings to be obtained without the risk of neglecting airway management.

Selection of equipment should take into account the ability to work reliably on patients who shiver or move.

Conduct of primary recovery

Recovery from anaesthesia and surgery should take place in a safe and reassuring environment that is, as far as possible, quiet. The dignity of patients should be maintained: unnecessary nakedness should be avoided and an adult should normally be addressed by surname with the appropriate prefix.

Primary recovery starts in the operating theatre at the end of operation. At this time the theatre usually empties rapidly, and the remaining people are often concerned with clearing up after the case and preparing for the next operation. Help must be available to the anaesthetist at this dangerous time. If supports restraining the patient are removed the patient must be closely observed lest a limb fall from its support or the patient roll off the operating table. The patient may at this stage regain hearing, therefore discussion of the patient's pathology, prognosis, bodily habitus or personal peculiarities should be avoided in this period in theatre or in recovery room, as should discussion of other patients which may be interpreted by the patient as applying to him.

Transfer of the patient

At the end of the operation the patient must at some stage be transferred from the operating table to a bed or trolley. Transfer directly to the bed avoids a later transfer which may be painful for the patient. Transfer directly to the bed should be done only if the bed design allows rapid tipping of the patient. Space constraints in lifts, or staff shortages, may militate against bringing beds to the operating theatres. Transfer from the operating table to a bed or trolley should be safe, both for the patient and for those doing the transfer. When the patient is lifted on a canvas theatre stretcher the cervical spine can hyperextend if the head is not fully supported. An old or damaged canvas may tear and the patient fall. If a lifting pole is not in its channel in the canvas the patient can roll from the stretcher when lifting is attempted. A roller system risks the patient falling between operating table and bed or trolley if either can move during the transfer. When a patient is lifted without a stretcher there should be enough people to accomplish this without risk to the patient or to those lifting. The floor should be dry and unencumbered with equipment such as cables and suction tubing.

Transfer to the recovery room is a dangerous period because monitoring or treating a patient while moving is difficult, especially when corridors are long and poorly lit. The patient is between two well-equipped areas, the theatre and the recovery room.

Arterial oxygen saturation has been shown to fall in many patients breathing air during transfer from the operating theatre to the recovery room (Tyler et al 1985, Smith & Crul 1988). Even after breathing 100% oxygen for 5 min before transfer, the SaO_2 in some 30% of patients fell below 90% (Smith & Crul 1988). Portable suction and monitoring should accompany the patient if more than a short distance is to be covered or if there is a special indication in that patient. Transfer requires at least two people so that one can concentrate on the patient's well-being. The person thus in charge of the patient must be competent to supervise the transfer. There are great advantages if the transfer is supervised by either the anaesthetist or the nurse from the recovery room who is taking over the care of the patient as this allows direct communication between the anaesthetist and recovery room nurse. During the whole transfer from the operating table in theatre to the recovery room, care should be taken to avoid disconnection, displacement or breakage of monitoring leads, drainage tubes, etc. Nasogastric tubes with drainage bags attached seem to have a peculiar propensity to be withdrawn during transfer, and the tube is often best left spigoted until arrival in the recovery room.

Information

The nurse in charge of the patient's recovery should know:

1. what operation or investigation was performed
2. the drugs and fluids given intraoperatively
3. instructions as to further drug and fluid therapy
4. any procedures to be carried out, including removal of intravascular cannulae, and monitoring devices or packs
5. special observations required
6. any precautions concerning the airway, including liability to aspirate or abnormalities of dentition such as crowns, bridges or loose teeth

7. the presence of abnormalities of the cardiovascular or respiratory systems, for example dysrhythmias, hypertension or tachypnoea. It should be made clear within what limits these are acceptable in the patient.

The documentation of this information depends on local custom.

Observations in the recovery room

A patient arriving in the recovery room should immediately be assessed for colour of skin and mucous membranes, patency of the airway, and rate and depth of ventilation. Pulse and blood pressure should then be measured. Constant observation of colour and of airway patency should continue until the patient is conscious with functioning protective responses.

Responsibility of the anaesthetist during the primary recovery period

The anaesthetist must take responsibility for the effect of the drugs and techniques he has chosen to use on a patient. This responsibility extends into the primary recovery period because the effects of the drugs and techniques extend into this period. While the anaesthetist can quite properly delegate the care of the patient in the primary recovery period to a suitably qualified person, he cannot abrogate his responsibility.

The anaesthetist should therefore normally be available for consultation about a patient, or to provide help when requested by the recovery room staff, until the patient is conscious with functioning protective reflexes and no major impairment of the cardiovascular or respiratory systems due to the anaesthetic. If the anaesthetist is not available for this period a colleague should be asked to take over the responsibility for the specific patient. This colleague must be fully informed about the case.

Where patients are transferred to a high-dependency unit such as an intensive care unit it is proper for the anaesthetist to hand over his responsibility to the medical staff there.

There is a small group of patients where return of consciousness and protective reflexes may be very prolonged or may even never happen, for example after head injury or intraoperative cerebral damage. Similarly there can be prolonged abnormality of cardiovascular or respiratory function following trauma or certain other forms of organ damage. In these cases there is no clear end to the primary recovery period. The responsibility for the patient will have to be returned to the patient's medical team at some point when major effects of the anaesthetic drugs are judged to be no longer significant.

It must be remembered that the surgeons involved with the patient similarly have duties toward the patient during the primary recovery period.

COMPLICATIONS OCCURRING IN THE PRIMARY RECOVERY PERIOD

Complications seen in the primary recovery period may be a continuation of similar events occurring intraoperatively or may be new events in the recovery room. They may alternatively be associated with medical conditions existing preoperatively. Complications seen in the primary recovery period may contribute to prolonged morbidity or mortality at a later time. In considering complications it is not possible to delineate those solely due to anaesthetic causes and those due, at least in part, to surgical factors.

The type and incidence of complications seen in a recovery room will be influenced by the age and general health of the population being treated and the types of surgery performed. The criteria for selecting patients for treatment in a day surgery unit will rule out many less fit patients, who will thus undergo surgery in the main theatres of a major hospital. A paediatric hospital again deals with a different population.

Farman (1978) reviewed 29 583 patients going through the recovery rooms of a university-affiliated hospital. He found that 5349 complications (excluding pain) occurred, some patients having more than one complication, giving a complication rate of 1 in 5.5 patients. Zelcer &

Wells (1987) included pain as a complication when they did a prospective survey of 443 patients admitted in 1 month to the recovery room of a university-affiliated hospital. They found some form of complication in 30% of the patients, many patients having more than one complication.

Duncan & Cohen (1987) attempted to define what factors are important to the development of postanaesthetic complications. They found that more experienced anaesthetists had fewer postoperative complications. Patients experiencing complications in the operating theatre or those receiving pure spinal or narcotic techniques had a higher risk of postoperative complications. Preoperative conditions associatied with an increased risk of complications in the recovery room included cardiovascular, respiratory and renal disease. Increasing duration of anaesthesia was associated with a greater incidence of recovery room complications.

The patient regaining consciousness may complain of various symptoms including pain, nausea and feeling cold. Occasionally the patient complains of vivid dreams or hearing voices. This should alert staff to the possibility of the patient being awake during the procedure. In these circumstances it is important to treat the patient with considerable understanding since he may be too frightened to express fully his fear. A more detailed account of the effects of 'awareness' is given in Chapter 29, while the causes and methods of prevention are discussed in Chapter 26.

Disorders of tissue oxygenation

The overall aim of the recovery nurse must be to ensure adequate tissue oxygenation and carbon dioxide removal while the patient is allowed to recover consciousness as comfortably as possible. There are many factors that may make oxygen delivery to the tissues more difficult in the recovering patient. Some exist preoperatively (see Chs 3 & 4) and others occur during or after operation. Factors causing postoperative tissue hypoxia are:

- inadequate inspired oxygen concentration
- airway obstruction
- altered respiratory centre function
- altered nervous conduction in spinal cord or peripheral nerves
- prolonged neuromuscular blockade
- altered chest wall mechanics
- gas or fluid in pleural space
- altered lung mechanics
- low cardiac output
- pulmonary embolism
- low functioning haemoglobin due to anaemia, methamemoglobinaemia, etc.
- altered oxygen release by transfused stored blood
- increased oxygen demand.

Postoperatively, oxygenation of blood in the pulmonary capillaries is less than optimum. The postoperative patient may have a reduced oxygen-carrying capacity as a result of anaemia, or may be unable to release as much oxygen at tissue level because of blood transfusion with old stored blood. In addition the effect of many anaesthetic agents is to reduce cardiac output and hence blood flow to tissues. In recovering patients, tissue oxygen demands may be increased, particularly in response to shivering. Bay et al (1968) showed that in the early postoperative period oxygen consumption was 71–135% of basal in 14 non-shivering patients, but raised to the range 135–486% of basal in 10 shivering patients. The patient with good cardiovascular and respiratory function can usually meet this increased demand, but a patient where these systems are impaired for any reason may fail to do so.

With so many factors predisposing to postoperative hypoxaemia the use of oxygen therapy in the recovery period is mandatory. The reasons for relative hypoxaemia under anaesthesia are fully discussed in Chapter 4 and postoperative respiratory complications are dealt with in Chapter 16.

Postoperative respiratory complications

Patients with impaired respiratory function before operation are more susceptible to postoperative respiratory complications.

Airway obstruction

Airway obstruction seen in the recovery room is usually secondary to coma with loss of muscle tone and protective reflexes, but other causes must always be considered.

The tongue. In the unconscious patient the tongue/epiglottis tends to block the larynx, especially when the patient is supine. This needs to be excluded as the cause of obstruction before other causes are sought.

Pharyngeal wall collapse. When pharyngeal muscle tone is low the negative pressure produced during inspiration tends to cause pharyngeal collapse and obstruction. Obstruction by the tongue/epiglottis and pharyngeal wall collapse are the commonest causes of postoperative airway obstruction.

With the return of consciousness and muscle tone the patient usually maintains a clear airway. A patient who has regained a level of consciousness where specific commands are obeyed will usually maintain a patent airway. Some patients will maintain a clear airway when awake, but obstruct intermittently when they fall asleep or if sedated. Some of these have a mechanical abnormality of the airway such as a tumour, oedema or a tongue that is large relative to the mandible. Even people who have received no anaesthetic or other drugs may suffer episodes of obstruction and arterial desaturation, with snoring or with the obstructive sleep apnoea syndrome. Jennett (1984) has reviewed this problem and Hoffstein & Zamal (1990) have reviewed the role of the upper airway in sleep apnoea. Obese patients are particularly at risk of airway obstruction when sedated or asleep.The importance of snoring or intermittent obstruction in the postanaesthetic patient who has regained consciousness, but then falls asleep, is often difficult to assess. If there is any doubt, the patient should be kept under close observation, oxygen given and the arterial oxygen saturation measured if possible. A nasal airway is often of great help in such patients and will be tolerated when an oral airway will not.

Laryngospasm. Irritation of the larynx, even by small amounts of secretions, blood or gastric contents, can cause laryngospasm, especially in the lightly anaesthetized patient. Babies and small children are especially liable to laryngospasm, particularly at extubation. The incidence of laryngospasm can be minimized by extubating the patient either under deep anaesthesia or when nearly awake. In patients at risk of laryngospasm it is wise to extubate with the lungs held well expanded with a high percentage of oxygen to provide extra time before hypoxaemia ensues if laryngospasm occurs. Suxamethonium should be available to 'break' the laryngospasm and facilities for reintubation should be at hand.

Laryngeal oedema can be caused by various factors such as trauma (including an over-large endotracheal tube) or systemic allergic factors. Local allergic reactions to endotracheal tubes, lubricants or local anaesthetics are theoretically possible. Regurgitation of gastric acid may sufficiently irritate the larynx to cause oedema following extubation.

Laryngeal obstruction in obstetric cases has been described by Brock-Utne et al (1977) and by Mackenzie (1978). It is more common in patients with toxaemia of pregnancy. It need not cause respiratory embarrassment. Salt et al (1983) reported a case where laryngeal oedema developed 4 h after caesarean section and necessitated intubation. Any patient with generalized oedema is at risk of laryngeal oedema. In babies and small children even minimal laryngeal oedema can compromise the airway owing to its small diameter.

Tracheomalacia. Thyroid enlargement and subsequent surgery is occasionally associated with weakening of the tracheal wall. Vigorous inspiratory efforts are likely to cause narrowing of the lumen in such cases.

Compression of the larynx and trachea. Bleeding into the neck after surgery, classically after thyroidectomy, may compress the larynx or trachea and is often associated with oedema. Equipment to open both the skin and the deeper layers of the wound should be available after such operations. Opening the wound may not fully clear the obstruction as there may be oedema of the pharynx, larynx and trachea (Bexton & Radford 1982) which may necessitate intubation. Bleeding into the neck can also occur after carotid artery or internal jugular vein puncture. Tumours of the neck may cause compression, particularly in the unconscious patient lacking muscle tone.

Recurrent laryngeal nerve damage is mainly associated with surgery in the neck, especially thyroid surgery. Unilateral nerve damage usually gives voice changes without obstruction, but bilateral damage causes obstruction which may require intubation or tracheostomy.

Miscellaneous causes. Tumours can block the airway at various levels and aspiration of teeth, dental prostheses and other foreign bodies may cause sudden airway obstruction after extubation. Throat packs should obviously be removed prior to extubation and their removal recorded. The risk of a retained throat pack can be minimized by various means:

1. leaving part of the pack visible outside the mouth during surgery
2. ensuring that where more than one piece of packing is used they are fixed together
3. using a 'THROAT PACK' label on an easily visible part of the patient
4. including the throat pack in the swab count
5. ensuring that if a change of personnel takes place the new anaesthetist knows of the presence of the pack.

Central respiratory depression or altered sensitivity

Hypocarbia is usually due to hyperventilation during anaesthesia involving IPPV.

High inspired oxygen tension. In patients with a hypoxic respiratory drive due to chronic respiratory disease, uncontrolled oxygen therapy can induce apnoea. Patients exhibiting this condition are, however, rare, even among those suffering from chronic bronchitis.

Drugs. Many drugs used in anaesthesia, including inhalational agents, opioids, barbiturates and benzodiazepines, will depress the respiratory centre and their effects may summate. Some patients may show opioid-induced bradypnoea or apnoea after apparently waking and breathing satisfactorily. Possible mechanisms include a rise in blood level due to continued absorption of previously administered drug, the recirculation of the drug or reabsorption of the drug from the gut. Opioids given in the recovery room may summate with drugs previously administered. The use of intrathecal or epidural opioids can cause respiratory depression many hours after administration (Davies et al 1980). Morgan (1982) has discussed some aspects of this problem. Chapter 15 contains a detailed account of the problems of postoperative pain and its management.

Intracranial pathology The function of the respiratory centre may be affected by many pathological processes including infections, tumours, vascular disease and raised intracranial pressure.

Impaired spinal or peripheral nerve conduction

Pre-existing neurological disease. A variety of conditions (traumatic, degenerative, inflammatory and neoplastic) may affect the spinal cord. The impairment of respiratory function may be increased by surgical and anaesthetic factors. Respiratory problems associated with peripheral nerve damage are less common, but may occur with neuropathies, or damage to phrenic or intercostal nerves.

Regional blockade. High subarachnoid or epidural block causes ascending paralysis of the respiratory muscles. Weakness may present at the end of the operation performed under such a block, or may occur after 'top up' doses given in the recovery period. Total spinal block can occur after the injection of local anaesthetic into an epidural catheter which has previously been used without evidence of intrathecal administration. Patients must be carefully observed for 30–40 min after 'topping up' epidural blocks and trained staff with the necessary resuscitation equipment must be available during the period of observation.

Local anaesthesia. The phrenic nerve may be involved in brachial plexus or cervical blocks. Most patients tolerate paralysis of a hemidiaphragm without respiratory embarrassment, but when there are other respiratory problems respiratory inadequacy may result.

Damage to spinal cord or peripheral nerves. Where there is spinal instability due to trauma, inflammatory disease or other causes, ill-considered movement of the anaesthetized patient or manoeuvres such as extending the neck during intubation may cause permanent cord damage. The cord may also be damaged during spinal cord surgery and local damage to phrenic or intercostal nerves may occur at operation.

Abnormalities of neuromuscular transmission

Pre-existing disease. In conditions such as myasthenia gravis and the myasthenic syndromes, respiratory function may deteriorate sharply following an anaesthetic. This may require treatment for some days in an ITU. These patients are extremely sensitive to non-depolarizing neuromuscular blocking drugs (see Appendix 3).

Overdose of neuromuscular blocking drugs may be due to misjudgement or the operation proving to be unexpectedly short. There is also a wide patient variation to an otherwise normal dose and therefore a standard dose may be excessive for some susceptible patients. The problem must be treated if it occurs by prolonged intermittent positive pressure ventilation (IPPV), aided by monitoring neuromuscular blockade with a peripheral nerve stimulator.

Altered breakdown or excretion. Pseudocholinesterase deficiency or abnormality will prolong the action of suxamethonium. Renal or hepatic disease may prolong the duration of action of non-depolarizing drugs, as may pH and electrolyte abnormalities and altered plasma protein concentrations. These factors are fully discussed in Chapters 23 and 24.

Potentiation. Inhalational agents and certain antibiotics may potentiate the effects of non-depolarizing relaxants. Postoperative weakness due to neuromuscular blockade varies from mild weakness to complete paralysis. Complete paralysis can occur with pseudocholinesterase abnormality after administering suxamethonium, or after an overdose or abnormal response to non-depolarizing drugs. Many patients without full muscular power after non-depolarizing drugs are able to move but make small uncoordinated limb movements and wrinkle the forehead in trying to open the eyes. This must not be confused with other causes of abnormal muscle movements which are dealt with in Chapter 28. There may be secondary signs of hypoxia and this should, if required, be treated with IPPV.

Some partially paralysed patients may have sufficient respiratory exchange to maintain oxygenation, but will be unable to cough and clear secretions in a coordinated way. The weak and uncoordinated respiratory efforts and unsuccessful attempts to clear secretions can result in great distress in the conscious patient. The flaccid tongue and pharyngeal muscles may cause airway obstruction. Muscle power can be assessed by clinical testing of limb power or by getting the patient to hold his head clear of the pillows. The ability to sustain muscular effort by, for example, the ability to hold the head off the pillows for several seconds indicates good muscle power, but this test is usually not possible in the patient with an abdominal wound because of pain. A nerve stimulator can be used to indicate the type and degree of residual neuromuscular block. Single stimulus gives little information and tetanic or 'train of four' stimulation should be used. This will cause pain in the conscious patient. Patients who are incompletely reversed may maintain adequate ventilation for a short time after operation only to tire after a few minutes, especially if external stimuli are minimal. The potential danger of this situation cannot be overemphasized for it may lead to cardiorespiratory arrest.

Management of severe postoperative weakness

Severe weakness associated with hypoxia must be treated by manual ventilation with bag and mask prior to reintubation and ventilation. The patient with a milder degree of weakness can sometimes be managed with a high inspired oxygen concentration, careful observation and reassurance. The use of one further dose of anticholinesterase may help if a full dose has not already been given. Further doses are unlikely to help and may worsen the situation. Relieving any element of obstruction by use of an airway or intubation may enable a weak patient to breathe adequately.

Measurement of arterial oxygen saturation by pulse oximetry, arterial blood gases and pH, end-tidal carbon dioxide and plasma electrolytes may all be useful in assessing and treating a patient with postoperative weakness.

When there is doubt about respiratory adequacy, ventilation is mandatory. The conscious ventilated patient should be reassured and given adequate analgesia and sedation.

Pulmonary aspiration

Gastric contents, blood, pus, throat packs, or tissue displaced during surgery or intubation may be aspirated from the pharynx, as may the contents of a pharyngeal pouch. The need for careful suctioning prior to extubation is obvious. Oesophageal obstruction or a full stomach greatly increases the risk of aspiration in the unconscious patient. All unconscious patients are at risk both prior to intubation and after extubation in the recovery room. The effect of aspiration during anaesthesia, whether or not it is recognized, may not be apparent until the recovery period when withdrawal of ventilation, lowering of the inspired oxygen concentration or progression of the pathological consequences may cause symptoms and signs. Foreign bodies causing airway obstruction demand immediate relief, if necessary by bronchoscopy. Massive aspiration of gastric contents filling the tracheobronchial tree may cause rapid death from asphyxia, as may aspiration of anything that obstructs the larynx or trachea. Small amounts of gastric juice may, when aspirated, cause immediate bronchospasm or have little noticeable effect for some time (for discussion of the management of this problem see Ch. 16).

Pulmonary oedema

There are two main types of pulmonary oedema, namely cardiac and non-cardiac. High pressure or cardiac pulmonary oedema may be due to fluid overload, raised pulmonary artery and left atrial pressure due to excessive sympathetic activity and peripheral vasoconstriction, or simply due to left heart failure.

Non-cardiac oedema occurs as a result of altered pulmonary capillary permeability or reduced plasma oncotic pressure. Many factors can cause this including acid aspiration, septicaemia, fat embolism, amniotic fluid embolism and allergic reactions. Fortunately, inhalation of higher oxides of nitrogen from a contaminated nitrous oxide supply is less common (Clutton-Brock 1967, Greenbaum et al 1967), as is inhalation of ethylene oxide from anaesthetic equipment where, after sterilization with the gas, it has been improperly removed. The victims of accidents may have been exposed to hot air, smoke or blast injury, and lung damage from heat can occur with faulty hot-water humidifiers. Hypoproteinaemia predisposes to oedema formation, whether of cardiac or non-cardiac origin.

Bronchospasm

Bronchospasm may occur in the recovery period and be associated with pre-existing asthma, aspiration of irritant substances or drug therapy, whether as a pharmacological effect as with beta-sympathetic blockers or as part of an allergic reaction. Secretions from carcinoid tumours are a potent cause of bronchospasm and bronchospasm can also be a feature of pulmonary embolism.

Sputum retention

The irritant effects of some inhalational anaesthetic agents may increase sputum production. Copious sputum may cause coughing or laryngospasm. The effects of sputum retention are usually seen after the primary recovery period. Sputum retention is largely due to inadequate coughing in the postoperative period, but impaired mucociliary action due to anaesthetic drugs may also play a part.

Abnormalities of the pleural cavity

The presence of gas or fluid in the pleural cavity interferes with lung function. Severe mediastinal shift with tension pneumothorax can reduce venous return and cardiac output.

Pneumothorax may not be discovered until respiratory distress occurs in the recovery room on the cessation of controlled ventilation. It may have been present preoperatively as a result of trauma, or, more commonly, have arisen during operation, either from high inflation pressure during IPPV or as a result of the surgery. Supraclavicular brachial plexus block, and subclavian and internal jugular vein cannulation are common procedures during anaesthesia associated with a risk of pneumothorax.

Abdominal distension

Abdominal distension due to pregnancy, tumour, ascites or intestinal obstruction can interfere with respiration by 'splinting' the diaphragm.

Impaired hypoxic vasoconstriction

Anaesthetic agents may impair the normal pulmonary vasoconstrictive response to hypoxia and predispose to abnormal ventilation/perfusion ratios.

Diffusion hypoxia

Withdrawal of nitrous oxide at the end of anaesthesia has long been thought to contribute to postoperative hypoxaemia. The effect is due to displacement of oxygen from the alveolus by large quantities of the relatively insoluble nitrous oxide diffusing out. This was described by Fink (1955). Frumin & Edelist (1969), however, concluded that this does not exist as a clinically significant phenomenon in healthy patients who maintain normal ventilation. There are many other surgical and anaesthetic factors that can contribute to a fall in arterial oxygen saturation in the postoperative period and justify the use of oxygen in the primary recovery period.

Other miscellaneous causes of arterial desaturation in the immediate postoperative period include: anatomical shunting (especially in children with congenital heart disease), bronchopleural fistula and embolism.

Embolism

Pulmonary embolism, whether of blood clot, amniotic fluid or fat, is a rare cause of respiratory problems in the early postoperative period. A more detailed account of these complications is contained in Chapters 16 and 18.

Cardiovascular complications

Farman (1978) found the most common complications in the recovery room to be cardiovascular. The problems seen include hypertension and hypotension, dysrhythmias, heart failure and inadequate tissue perfusion.

Hypertension

Causes of early postoperative hypertension are listed below:

- pre-existing hypertension
- pain
- carbon dioxide retention
- cold vasoconstriction
- drugs
- endocrine disorders
- vascular and cardiac surgery
- raised intracranial pressure
- spinal cord trauma.

Preoperative hypertension of whatever cause is likely to persist in the recovery period. If therapy has been interrupted because of the surgery, controlled hypertension may become uncontrolled. Patients recovering from surgery on the aorta, the carotid or renal vessels, and those having open-heart surgery, are all likely to develop hypertension in the early postoperative period. Probably the most common cause of hypertension in the previously healthy patient, however, is severe pain. The cold, peripherally vasoconstricted patient may also be hypertensive. Carbon dioxide retention must always be excluded as a cause of hypertension before any treatment, particularly opioid analgesia, is instituted.

A variety of drugs may cause hypertension in the recovery period. These include ketamine, myocardial stimulants and vasoconstrictors. Endocrine causes include thyrotoxicosis, phaeochromocytoma and carcinoid tumours.

Postoperative hypertension increases the work of the myocardium and therefore the overall oxygen consumption, especially in the presence of tachycardia. Myocardial ischaemia may ensue in susceptible individuals with the risk of dysrhythmias, infarction and left ventricular failure. Hypertension encourages postoperative bleeding and there is a risk of disruption of vascular suture lines. In the presence of raised intracranial tension a rise in arterial blood pressure may cause a further rise in the tension.

Assessment and treatment of postoperative hypertension. The acceptable blood pressure in the individual patient must be considered in relation to age, coexisting pathology and preoperative blood pressure. Hypertension should be treated when there is a risk of any of the undesirable results listed above occurring. Where perfusion of certain organs is precarious, a high blood pressure may be necessary. When it is considered that the blood pressure should be lowered, any possible precipitating factors should be removed before hypotensive drugs are given.

Hypotension

Many factors may contribute to postoperative hypotension. These are listed below:

1. hypovolaemia
2. anaesthetic agents
3. hypotensive agents used preoperatively or intraoperatively
4. sudden posture changes
5. supine hypotensive syndrome:
   - pregnancy
   - large abdominal masses
6. cardiac dysrhythmias
7. myocardial ischaemia
8. tension pneumothorax
9. cardiac tamponade
10. hypoadrenalism
11. neurological causes:
    - intracranial pathology
    - spinal cord trauma.

Hypovolaemia is the most common cause of postoperative hypotension, either alone or with other factors.

When the legs are lowered from an elevated position, such as the lithotomy position, the increased venous filling of the limbs may cause hypotension if the patient is hypovolaemic. Drugs that can cause hypotension include induction and inhalational drugs, certain neuromuscular blocking drugs and opioids. Local anaesthetic may cause hypotension by a direct depressant action on the cardiovascular system as a result of systemic absorption or by inducing sympathetic blockade.

Assessment and treatment of postoperative hypotension. In defining the acceptable lower limit of blood pressure, the age of the patient and the preoperative blood pressure must be considered. The blood pressure recorded on hospital admission is often not representative of the patient's normal resting blood pressure. Evidence of circulatory impairment to vital organs, such as angina or a history of stroke, must be taken into account, and also the type of surgery. A fit adult, when asleep, may have a systolic blood pressure of under 80 mmHg (Richardson et al 1964), and such pressures may be quite acceptable in a sedated postoperative patient. A similar pressure in an elderly patient known to be hypertensive preoperatively may be associated with severe circulatory inadequacy leading to permanent sequelae.

The postoperative patient who is conscious and orientated with no signs or symptoms of myocardial ischaemia, and who has warm hands and feet and a satisfactory urine output, can usually be considered to have an adequate blood pressure.

All hypotensive patients must be given added inspired oxygen and the hypovolaemia corrected as soon as possible. Rapid infusion of 250–500 ml of intravenous fluid often raises the blood pressure by compensating for a relative hypovolaemia due to vasodilatation. If a bradycardia is present, hypoxia should first be excluded as a cause and then small increments of atropine or glycopyrrolate given to raise the pulse rate and thus the blood pressure. Any of the correctable factors in the previous list should be treated. If these attempts to raise the blood pressure fail, pharmacological methods may be indicated. Central venous pressure measurement should be used to help in the assessment and treatment of hypotension that does not readily respond to simple measures.

When the blood pressure is considered adequate although lower than expected, the possibility of bleeding must be excluded before the patient is discharged from the recovery room to the ward.

Dysrhythmias

Tachycardia. Some of the more common causes of postoperative tachycardia are listed below:

1. pain and anxiety
2. carbon dioxide retention
3. hypovolaemia
4. inadequate reversal of neuromuscular block
5. hypermetabolic states:
   - infection
   - non-infectious inflammatory conditions, for example, inflammatory bowel disease thyrotoxicosis, etc.
6. tachyarrhythmias
7. drugs, for example, atropine
8. acid-base abnormalities.

Tachycardias raise the workload of the heart and produce many of the deleterious effects seen with hypertension. When the rate is very fast there may be a decreased cardiac output and treatment then becomes urgent.

Bradycardia. Causes of postoperative bradycardia are listed below:

1. highly trained healthy individuals
2. hypoxia
3. drugs, for example:
   - neostigmine
   - local anaesthetics
   - inhalational agents
   - digoxin
   - opioids
   - beta blockers
4. high subarachnoid or epidural block
5. endotracheal suction or other vagal stimulation
6. heart block.

Bradycardia always accompanies terminal hypoxia preceding cardiac arrest, therefore hypoxia must always be eliminated before any other cause of a slow pulse is sought.

Bradycardia may be associated with arrhythmias, most commonly with breakthrough ventricular ectopics and with low cardiac output. The level at which bradycardia is of sinister import varies. If there is no arrhythmia, and blood pressure and cardiac output (as shown by tissue perfusion) are adequate, treatment is not usually required when the pulse rate is above 50/min and many anaesthetists find a lower rate acceptable. It would seem sensible that the anaesthetist should be informed of a pulse below 50/min before a patient is discharged from the recovery room.

Treatment of bradycardia should be undertaken when there are signs of inadequate cardiac output or blood pressure, or if arrhythmias occur. Use of small incremental doses of atropine or glycopyrrollate will often be successful when there is autonomic imbalance. Sympathomimetic agents are sometimes required and cardiac pacing may be indicated in heart block.

Arrhythmias may be caused by many factors, singly or in combination, some of which are listed below:

- pre-existing
- catecholamines
- inhalational anaesthetic agents
- hypercarbia
- hypoxia
- pH or electrolyte disturbance
- cardiac ischaemia or other disease
- intracardiac catheter
- cardiac or thoracic surgery
- cardiac tamponade
- pulmonary embolus.

Arrhythmias will often resolve when precipitating factors are removed. Thus excretion of inhalational agents, breakdown of catecholamines and correction of hypercarbia or hypoxia will frequently result in cessation of the arrhythmia. The combination of hypoxia, hypercarbia and an inhalational agent often results in an arrhythmia which can be corrected by a period of controlled ventilation.

When an arrhythmia causes no untoward effects, careful monitoring may be all that is required. It must be remembered that arrhythmias may progress to more hazardous forms that interfere with cardiac function. Under these circumstances pharmacological intervention is required.

Pain and other unpleasant sensations

Recovery of consciousness from general anaesthesia or cessation of action of local anaesthesia allows pain to be felt. The conscious patient will often experience other unpleasant sensations.

Postoperative pain, its deleterious effects and the hazards of its treatment are all considered in Chapter 15. Patients may not, however, only experience pain as a result of the surgery. The pressure of restraining equipment, or traction on limbs and malpositioning of joints, may cause pain that proves more of an inconvenience than the surgery. Back pain may also occur after surgery, and the pains attributable to suxamethonium fasciculations can be severe.

Pain associated with intubation and airway maintenance

Sore throat and the results of trauma to lips, mouth, pharynx and teeth may all present in the recovery period. Pressure on the mandible and face from the anaesthetist's fingers or from anaesthetic equipment can cause bruising and pain. These matters are considered more fully in Chapter 31.

Headache

Reported incidences of headache vary greatly. Edmonds-Seal & Eve (1962) found an incidence of 27% whereas Smith & Young (1976) reported an incidence of 81% in patients having dental operations as out-patients. Muir et al (1976) found no significant difference in the incidence of headache between patients having dental extraction under local analgesia and general anaesthesia.

Muscle pain

Muscle pain may occur after suxamethonium or vomiting, or as a result of surgical retraction and other manoeuvres.

Pain at injection site

There may be pain at intramuscular or subcutaneous injection sites or intravenous infusion sites.

Nausea, retching and vomiting

The incidence of nausea, retching and vomiting after anaesthesia and surgery is variable. Farman (1978) found some 2.5% of patients vomited in the recovery room. In some cases vomiting seems to be a consequence of anaesthetic drugs, but may be caused by other drugs including ergometrine and opioid analgesics. Late in the recovery period, vomiting is often due to the latter. It may also be related to the surgery, for example middle ear surgery. Gastrointestinal pathology, especially intestinal obstruction, and raised intracranial tension can cause vomiting.

Complications of nausea, retching and vomiting

The complications of nausea, retching and vomiting are as follows:

1. Nausea, retching and vomiting are unpleasant for the patient.
2. Dealing with vomit is unpleasant for staff.
3. Violent movements involved in retching or vomiting may be damaging to the surgery performed, for example microsurgery of the ear and ophthalmic surgery.
4. Soreness of the abdominal muscles may ensue.
5. Raised venous pressure can cause bleeding.
6. Rises in intraocular and intracranial tension can occur. After ophthalmic surgery or when intracranial tension is high these may be injurious.
7. Aspiration of vomit may occur if the patient's reflexes are depressed by coma or sedation,

or when the patient cannot expel the vomit because of the supine position or when the jaws are wired together.

Emptying a full stomach by nasogastric tube should reduce nausea and vomiting. Suggestion of the possibility of vomiting should be avoided. This can be difficult if the ward contains patients who are expert on the subject! Solicitous enquiries as to whether the patient 'feels sick' should be avoided in the recovery period.

Use of antiemetics if nausea occurs is of help, but the wide range of drugs available indicates none is fully effective. Prophylactic use of antiemetics is indicated if nausea or vomiting is especially likely or can have dangerous results. Unwanted effects of antiemetics include sedation and extrapyramidal effects. These are especially dangerous in the old and in children.

Other subjective sensations

After anaesthesia other subjective sensations can include inability to concentrate, dizziness, amnesia, drowsiness (which may, at least in part, be attributable to postoperative medication), dry mouth or unpleasant tastes and smells. There may be great anxiety or fear.

Temperature-associated complications

Temperature-associated complications can be caused by heat or cold and may be seen in the recovery period having arisen before, during or after operation.

Hypothermia

Patients entering recovery rooms following prolonged surgery are frequently cold. It is not uncommon to find central temperatures as low as 33°C, particularly if no attempt has been made to preserve body heat in the operating theatre. The combination of anaesthesia with its vasodilating effects, prolonged exposure and the use of cold fluids, together with the loss of heat in water vapour to the dry anaesthetic gases, is sufficient to cause this effect. Loss of heat from the operation site also contributes to cooling, particularly when major cavities are opened. A patient can be cold and vasoconstricted peripherally in spite of a normal core temperature.

In the paediatric patient the relatively higher body surface area and immature homeostatic mechanisms make maintenance of temperature intraoperatively even more difficult.

Being cold is not only unpleasant for the patient it is also positively harmful. Shivering as the patient recovers is almost inevitable. This increases the oxygen consumption considerably (Bay et al 1968) and oxygen should be given. Patients unable to increase their oxygen uptake because of respiratory or cardiac disease may well become hypoxic. Cold vasoconstriction makes assessment of peripheral tissue perfusion difficult and may contribute to severe postoperative hypertension. Dysrhythmias, including ventricular fibrillation, may occur without warning, and clearance of drugs will be modified. As the cold patient warms up postoperatively, vasodilation may cause hypotension due to hypovolaemia which has not been recognized in the vasoconstricted patient. There is little option for the recovery room staff but to gradually rewarm the patient, but the real solution lies in prevention of cooling during operation.

Pyrexia

The patient who is pyrexial in the recovery period may have developed the pyrexia before, during or after operation. Causes of pyrexia are listed below:

1. infection
   - preoperative
   - bacteraemia associated with:
     - instrumentation of the bladder
     - exploration of infected areas
2. overheating by warming device
3. inability of draped patient to lose heat
4. faulty heat exchange during cardiopulmonary bypass
5. certain forms of brain damage
6. malignant hyperpyrexia.

Burns

Burns caused during operation may present in the recovery period, and the unconscious patient in the recovery room is at risk from warming devices, etc. These matters are considered more fully in Chapter 43.

Haemorrhage in the recovery period

Haemorrhage usually occurs at the operation site, but may arise from other areas including injection and cannulation sites or areas traumatized at intubation. Disconnection of cannulae or lines associated with intravascular cannulae can cause bleeding.

Postoperative bleeding from the operation site is almost invariably from blood vessels divided at operation and may be due to inadequate haemostasis, a sudden rise in arterial or venous pressure dislodging clot, or vasodilatation of previously vasoconstricted blood vessels as injected vasoconstrictors wear off or cold areas warm up. Trauma to the operation site, as with over-enthusiastic use of a sucker following dental extracting or tonsillectomy, can cause bleeding.

Occasionally, haemorrhage is due to a bleeding disorder (See Ch. 10). This may be congenital, associated with the use of preoperative or intraoperative anticoagulants, due to dilution of clotting factors with massive transfusion or associated with a consumption coagulopathy, for example with incompatible blood transfusion. Where there is known to be a bleeding disorder the recovery room should be informed so as to avoid intramuscular and subcutaneous injection and any undue trauma.

The problems caused by haemorrhage are largely associated with hypovolaemia and pressure. A haematoma may become infected at a later stage.

Hypovolaemia

The classical signs associated with the cardiovascular effects of hypovolaemia are tachycardia and skin pallor (associated with catecholamine release), and hypotension (Baskett 1990). There may be cerebral signs such as confusion, tachypnoea and reduced urine output. The amount of blood loss a patient can tolerate must be considered as a percentage of the patient's normal blood volume, not an absolute amount. Many fit, unanaesthetized patients tolerate up to 15% loss of blood volume with little sign except a slight tachycardia, and may maintain their blood pressure up to a 30% loss (Baskett 1990). The effect of blood loss does, however, vary with the patient's age and general health, especially cardiovascular function. Many drugs, including anaesthetics, interfere with the body's compensatory mechanisms to hypovolaemia. The diagnosis of hypovolaemia can be confusing in the postoperative patient because of the variety of other causes of hypotension and tachycardia (see lists on pp 430–431). Cold vasoconstriction is common in postoperative patients. A trend in the results of cardiovascular measurements is often more informative than a single reading. Measurement of central venous pressure and its response to fluid therapy may be required.

Vasoconstricted patients may be sent back to the ward apparently stable, then suffer a drop in blood pressure some hours later when rewarming and vasodilatation reveal a degree of hypovolaemia.

Pressure effects

Pressure effects can have fatal consequences on respiratory and cardiovascular function. Compression of the airway, notably after neck surgery (see above) and haemothorax can affect respiratory function; haemopericardium can cause tamponade. Pressure from haematomata can interfere with the blood supply of organs or limbs.

Treatment of postoperative haemorrhage

Postoperative haemorrhage must be stopped. Observation of the patient and waiting for natural haemostatic mechanisms to work may be all that is required. Elevation of the operation site and/or pressure to the site may arrest the haemorrhage. If such measures do not suffice, surgical exploration may be required, but the patient must be adequately resuscitated before undergoing anaesthesia and operation. If a clotting defect is found this should be treated first. Help from a haematologist is often invaluable in this situation.

Hypovolaemia must be treated. The choice of fluid depends on the availability of fluids and the urgency for volume replenishment. Maintenance of circulating volume is generally more important than the haemoglobin level in the emergency situation, but the haemoglobin level must be monitored and is especially important in patients with a poor ability to raise their cardiac output to compensate for anaemia. Fluid replacement can itself cause complications such as haemodilution, change in pH and electrolyte levels and alteration in body temperature.

Problems of fluid and electrolyte balance

The problems and complications of fluid therapy are dealt with in Chapter 17. The state of hydration and electrolyte levels seen in the recovery period depend on the volumes and composition of fluid losses and fluid replacement that have occurred preoperatively, intraoperatively and postoperatively. Inappropriate volumes and types of replacement fluids can lead to over- or underhydration and abnormal electrolyte levels in the postoperative period. Fluid absorption leading to hyponatraemia during urological endoscopy is well recognized (Rao 1987) and similar problems can occur during laser photocoagulation of the endometrium (Morrison et al 1989).

Some special considerations regarding tissue damage

During recovery there is a considerable risk of damage to the teeth, lips and tongue. The patient recovering from anaesthesia may develop masseteric spasm, and any dental prostheses or loose or damaged teeth may be broken or displaced. Biting on an oral airway is particularly likely to cause breakage of crowns and bridges. Where there is a risk of the patient biting on crowns, or poor dentition, use of an oral airway should be avoided, a nasal airway usually being a satisfactory alternative. Where an oral airway is essential to maintain a clear airway it should be placed away from dental prostheses when possible, or some form of pack should be used to hold the teeth apart so that biting on the airway is impossible. Although the most careful anaesthetist may damage dental protheses or loose or bad teeth, this is hard to defend if the state of dentition has not been ascertained before anaesthesia.

The lips or tongue may be damaged by the teeth. A common cause is the careless insertion of an airway so that the lip lies between the teeth and airway. Cracked lips can occur in the unconscious patient. Sores at the corner of the mouth from an endotracheal tube or its fixation may be seen in the recovery room.

Urinary retention

In a large series of surgical patients, 4.7% of the males and 2.9% of the females developed total urinary retention postoperatively (Tammela et al 1986). Some 80% of the patients who developed retention gave an abnormal voiding history. Urinary retention can be distressing to the patient and makes assessment of urine output impossible. If the patient cannot micturate in response to simple measures such as change of position or use of non-opioid analgesics, catheterization eventually becomes necessary.

Psychological effects seen in the recovery period

It is in the recovery period, often in the recovery room, that patients may first become aware of the consequences of their surgery, whether mutilation or the fact that their condition is not curable by surgery. Thus anxiety and anguish are common and pain increases the distress. All this, together with the stress of illness, hospital admission, surgery and anaesthesia, can be confusing and disorientating. Patients need continual reassurance, reorientation and support postoperatively. This process can best be started with a calm and pain-free stay in the recovery ward.

REFERENCES

Association of Anaesthetists of Great Britain and Ireland 1988 Recommendations for standards of monitoring during anaesthesia and recovery. Association of Anaesthetists, London

Atkinson R S 1979 Postoperative care. In: Hewer C L, Atkinson R S (eds) Recent advances in anaesthesia and analgesia, 13. Churchill Livingstone, Edinburgh, Ch 9, p 185–197

Baskett P J F 1990 Management of hypovolaemic shock in ABC of major trauma. Br Med J 300: 1453–1457

Bay J, Nunn J F, Prys-Roberts C 1968 Factors influencing arterial PO_2 during recovery from anaesthesia. Br J Anaesth 40: 398–406

Bexton M D R, Radford R 1982 An unusual cause of respiratory obstruction after thyroidectomy. Anaesthesia 37: 596

Brock-Utne J G, Downing J W, Seedat F 1977 Laryngeal oedema associated with pre-eclamptic toxaemia. Anaesthesia 32: 556–558

Clutton-Brock J 1967 Two cases of poisoning by contamination of nitrous oxide with higher oxides of nitrogen during anaesthesia. Br J Anaesth 39: 388–392

CSM 1989 Current problems: propofol-convulsions, anaphylaxis and delayed recovery from anaesthesia. 26: 2

Davies G K, Tolhurst-Cleaver C L, James T L 1980 CNS depression from intrathecal morphine. Anesthesiology 52: 280

DHSS 1967 Hospital Building Note 26: operating department. HMSO, London

Duncan P G, Cohen M M 1987 Post-operative complications: factors of significance to anaesthetic practice. Can J Anaesth 34: 2–8

Dundee J W, Wyant G M 1988 Intravenous anaesthesia, 2nd edn. Churchill Livingstone, Edinburgh, ch 6, p 69–90

Edmonds-Seal J, Eve N M 1962 Minor sequelae of anaesthesia: a pilot study. Br J Anaesth 34: 44–48

Farman J V 1978 The work of the recovery room. Br J Hosp Med 19: 606–617

Fink B R 1955 Diffusion anoxia. Anesthesiology 16: 511–519

Fraser A C L, Goat V A 1983 Unrecognised presentation of a meningioma. Anaesthesia 38: 128–131

Frumin J M, Edelist G 1969 Diffusion anoxia: a critical reappraisal. Anesthesiology 31: 243–249

Greenbaum R, Bay J, Hargreaves M D et al 1967 Effects of higher oxides of nitrogen on the anaesthetised dog. Br J Anaesth 39: 393–404

Hoffstein V, Zamel N 1990 Sleep apnoea and the upper airway. Br J Anaesth 65: 139–150

Jennett S 1984 Snoring and its treatment. Br Med J 289: 335–336

Lunn J N, Mushin W W 1982 Mortality associated with anaesthesia. Nuffield Hospitals Trust, London

Mackenzie A I 1978 Laryngeal oedema complicating obstetric anaesthesia. Anaesthesia 33: 271

Morgan M 1982 Anaesthesia 37: 527–529

Morrison L M M, Davis J, Sumner D 1989 Absorption of irrigating fluid during laser photocoagulation of the endometrium in the treatment of menorrhagia. Br J Obstet Gynaecol 96: 346–352

Muir V M J, Leonard M, Haddaway E 1976 Morbidity following dental extraction: a comparative survey of local analgesia and general anaesthesia. Anaesthesia 31: 171–180

Rao P N 1987 Fluid absorption during urological endoscopy. Br J Urol 60: 93–99

Richardson D W, Honour H F, Fenton G W, Stott F H, Pickering G W 1964 Variation in arterial pressure throughout the day and night. Clin Sci 26: 445–460

Salt P J, Nutbourne P A, Park G R, Glazebrook C W 1983 Laryngeal oedema after caesarean section. Anaesthesia 38: 693–694

Saunders P R I, Harris M N E 1990 Opisthotonus and other unusual neurological sequelae after outpatient anaesthesia. Anaesthesia 45: 552–557

Smith B L, Young P N 1976 Day stay anaesthesia: a follow-up of day patients undergoing dental operations under general anaesthesia with tracheal intubation. Anaesthesia 31: 181–189

Smith D C, Crul J F 1988 Early post-operative hypoxia during transport. Br J Anaesth 61: 625–627

Tammela T, Kontturi M, Lukkarinen O 1986 Postoperative urinary retention. I. Incidence and predisposing factors. Scand J Urol Neprol 20: 197–201

Tyler I L, Tantisira B, Winter P M, Motoyama E K L 1985 Continuous monitoring of arterial oxygen saturation with pulse oximetry during transfer to the recovery room. Anesth Analg 64: 1108–1112

Utting J E, Gray T C, Shelley F C 1979 Human misadventure in anaesthesia. Can Anaesth Soc J 26: 472–478

Zelcer J, Wells D G 1987 Anaesthetic-related recovery room complications. Anaesth Intensive Care 15: 168–174

28

Adverse excitatory responses to anaesthetic agents

P. R. I. Saunders

INTRODUCTION

While some anaesthetic agents may increase the likelihood of convulsions in susceptible individuals, not all involuntary movements seen during induction and recovery from anaesthesia are epileptic in nature. This chapter discusses the adverse excitatory responses commonly seen at induction and recovery, and should be read in conjunction with Chapter 22 which specifically addresses the question of which anaesthetic agents might be contraindicated in patients with known epilepsy. There is, of course, considerable overlap since patients with diagnosed epilepsy may exhibit involuntary movements that are not true convulsions and, very occasionally, a previously 'normal' individual may suffer a grand mal convulsion in the perioperative period.

EXCITATORY PHENOMENA

There has been considerable confusion in the literature about the accurate definition of the neurophysiological basis of the variety of excitatory responses seen in patients during induction and recovery from anaesthesia. It is known that central nervous system (CNS) excitation occurs during induction of anaesthesia. Guedel (1937) developed his classic table of the signs of anaesthesia with divisions into stages and planes using open ether. The second stage was classified as excitement of uninhibited response and it represented a period of muscular activity associated with increased muscular tone. This is equally applicable to recovery from anaesthesia. Postanaesthetic shivering is common during recovery from anaesthesia and is undoubtedly a Stage II phenomenon in reverse. As with excitatory responses during induction of anaesthesia, shivering tends to occur in young muscular individuals who have had relatively short procedures. It can be minimized by adequate premedication, psychological reassurance and quiet surroundings. It is often associated with violent muscular activity. It can cause displacement of intravenous cannula, wound dehiscence, dental damage and disruption of delicate surgical repairs. There is an increase in metabolic rate of up to 400%. Hypoxaemia may result, placing patients with cardiopulmonary compromise at risk. Oxygen therapy is mandatory. In cases of severe masseteric spasm the airway may be compromised.

EXCITATORY CHANGE ON INDUCTION

Rosner & Clark (1973) showed that the origin of these excitatory effects within the neuroaxis depends on the excitatory and depressive effects of the anaesthetic agents on neurones located in the cortex, thalamus and reticular formation. However, it must be emphasized that they have a common path which results in disinhibition of spinal reflexes. Steen & Michenfelder (1979) and Meinck et al (1980) noted that excitatory effects, particularly in unpremedicated anxious patients, are observed frequently on induction of anaesthesia with well-established agents such as methohexitone and etomidate, and manifest as hypertonus, twitching and tremor. Although now withdrawn from anaesthetic practice, propanidid (Clarke & Dundee 1965) and Althesin (Samuel & Dundee 1973) produced a similar pattern. There are reports of generalized tonic clonic convulsions with all these agents on induction of anaesthesia (Uppington 1973, Barron 1974, Rees 1975). These convulsions have often been classified as epileptic in nature without confirmatory electroencephalogram (EEG) evidence. It is of interest that Savege et al (1971) noted apparent spontaneous limb movements occurring with burst suppression in Althesin anaesthesia. This kind of EEG pattern is generally taken to represent a considerable reduction in cortical activity and to be equivalent to a level of deep surgical anaesthesia. In other words the EEG implied that anaesthesia had become very profound but, in fact, clinically the patient was lightly anaesthetized.

EXCITATORY CHANGE ON RECOVERY

Weber (1979) reported generalized tonic clonic convulsions in the recovery phase with Althesin. There are similar reports by Cameron (1987) and Hopkins (1988) with propofol. This has not been a feature with other induction agents. Both Althesin and propofol have the ability to cause considerable reduction in cortical activity at light stages of anaesthesia. This facilitates more profound disinhibition of spinal reflexes and thus allows the more severe motor manifestations of hyperreflexia to present themselves in the recovery phase. Opisthotonus, the most severe manifestation of drug-induced decerebrate rigidity, has only been observed with propofol.

Laughlin & Newberg (1985), Goroszeniuk et al (1986) and Hansen & Drenck (1988) reported tonic clonic convulsions in the recovery phase following anaesthesia maintained by etomidate either as an infusion or as intermittent boluses. Grant & Hutchison (1983) reported several cases of generalized myoclonic activity during prolonged etomidate sedation in patients in intensive therapy units. In all these reports EEG recordings were either inappropriate or not recorded, thus there was no confirmation of epileptic discharge. Ebrahim et al (1986) reported the use of etomidate to activate the seizure focus in patients undergoing temporal lobectomy for the treatment of medically refractory complex partial seizures. This implies that etomidate, like methohexitone, lowers seizure threshold. However, there is no reason why these tonic clonic convulsions cannot be attributed to spinal disinhibition. Maintenance of anaesthesia with etomidate predisposes the patient to residual cortical anaesthesia with an activated reticular formation in the recovery phase resulting in disinhibition of spinal reflexes. This may be enhanced by a lowered threshold in excitatory neurones in the neuroaxis. Sloan et al (1988) showed that etomidate infusion produces a two- to twelve-fold increase in the amplitude of posterior tibial nerve somatosensory evoked potentials.

Opisthotonus and drug-induced decerebrate rigidity

The Committee on Safety of Medicines (CSM) drew attention in May 1989 to a total of 37 reports of 'seizures' during induction or recovery from anaesthesia induced by propofol. In addition, opisthotonus had occurred in 10 patients. It advised that care should be taken when this drug is used to anaesthetise epileptic patients. Recently, five of the reports of cases that involved opisthotonus have been published (Cameron 1987, Dingwall 1987, Hopkins 1988, Strowbridge 1989 and Saunders & Harris 1990). Each incident took place in the early recovery phase.

It has already been stated that hyperreflexia is a well documented and common neurological sequela after general anaesthesia and, although self-limiting in these circumstances, is likened to decerebrate rigidity. It is most commonly manifest as postanaesthetic shivering. Consequently it is not surprising that opisthotonus, a broadly facilitated state of muscle stretch reflexes, represents the most severe manifestation of decerebrate rigidity. This common physiological basis may well account for a wide range of unusual neurological sequelae of varying duration and intensity occurring during induction and recovery from anaesthesia. Excitatory effects, such as tremor and twitching, that arise on induction with etomidate and methohexitone are at the lower end of a spectrum of motor manifestations seen in drug-induced decerebrate rigidity. Decerebration resulting from brain injury is best considered a heterogeneous spectrum of motor manifestations and thus reinforces this concept. Bremer (1937) noted that section of the brainstem at the midcollicular level causes the EEG to become slow, synchronized and sleep-like. Thus the cortex 'sleeps' while the midbrain and spinal cord over-react.

Postanaesthetic shivering

Postanaesthetic shivering is frequently attributed to normal thermoregulatory shivering in response to intraoperative hypothermia. However, there is often a lack of correlation between perioperative hypothermia and the incidence of postanaesthetic shivering. Sessler et al (1988) showed that all patients experience inhibition of the normal thermoregulatory responses to cold during recovery from anaesthesia. Postanaesthetic shivering is tonic rigidity with generalized coarse phasic tremor. Piloerection, a characteristic feature of thermoregulatory shivering, is absent. Brichard & Johnstone (1970) likened postoperative rigidity to decerebrate rigidity, with clonus and exaggerated tendon reflexes. Soliman & Gillies (1972) drew attention to the appearance of muscle spasticity in nearly all postoperative patients. They noted that the spasticity occurred when the patient started to respond to painful stimuli and disappeared when the patient was responding to verbal command. Sessler et al (1988) analysed electromyogram (EMG) data from patients recovering from isoflurane anaesthesia. Two patterns were revealed: a tonic activity that did not resemble normal shivering, and 'clonic' activity similar to that produced by pathological clonus. In general, clonus occurs when descending cortical control fails to inhibit spinal reflex arcs. Rosenberg et al (1981) elicited abnormal reflexes such as clonus, nystagmus and Babinski's during recovery from anaesthesia. These findings suggest that postanaesthetic shivering is caused by spinal reflex hyperactivity which results when descending cortical control is inhibited by residual anaesthetic. Brichard & Johnstone (1970) showed that methylphenidate, a CNS stimulant, reliably abolished postanaesthetic shivering, and this reinforces the concept. Pathological clonus and flexion-induced clonus require both enhanced spinal cord reflexes and triggering by a mechanical stimulus, such as muscle stretching. Post-anaesthetic spontaneous EMG clonus and tonic EMG activity also may require enhanced reflexes and a trigger.

Sessler et al (1988) postulated that cutaneous receptors that sense skin coolness may play a significant role in postanaesthetic shivering as this symptom can be halted by localized skin warming. It is thus advisable to keep the patient warm in the recovery area and the ambient temperature high. Limb movement is a likely trigger as it often results in muscle stretching. This can occur during repositioning of the patient, maintaining an airway, recording blood pressure and securing the arm during intravenous administration of drugs.

CATALEPTOID CENTRAL NERVOUS SYSTEM EXCITATION

Winters (1972) stated that the implication that all anaesthetics induce CNS depression confuses our thinking about the anaesthetic state. The anaesthetic effects of diethyl ether refer specifically to Stage III anaesthesia. The anaesthetic properties of nitrous oxide refer to Stage II anaesthesia as this agent is not capable of inducing Stage III at 1 atm. However, Stage II induced either by diethyl ether or nitrous oxide is characterized by a state of hallucinosis and catalepsia. There is increased reticular formation neuronal activity. Thus there are two distinct types of agents capable of immobilizing patients for operation. Halothane, ultrashort acting barbiturates and diethyl ether at surgical levels act by CNS depression (Stage III). Agents of the second type, such as nitrous oxide, ketamine and enflurane, act by cataleptoid CNS excitation (Stage II). There is a tendency to assume that a reduction or lack of responsiveness is associated with depressed states only. The individual who is catatonic, hallucinatory or convulsing has a reduction in responsiveness to stimuli and a loss of memory but is in fact hyper-excited. Both types of anaesthesia can induce a state of unreponsiveness and amnesia. Drug-induced decerebrate rigidity conforms to this pattern. Drugs that induce CNS excitation to Stage II have the ability to change direction and cause CNS depression (Stage III diethy ether), to continue from Stage II to generalized convulsions (enflurane) or to induce Stage II catalepsia only (nitrous oxide and ketamine).

Ketamine

Ketamine is capable of causing convulsions with EEG changes consistent with epilepsy. Emergence delirium with nitrous oxide is short whereas that with ketamine is more prolonged. With ketamine there will be a tendency towards tonic clonic convulsions which have been observed experimentally in the absence of EEG changes. Although epileptic activity on EEG is observed only with higher doses of ketamine, Ferrer-Allado et al (1973) stated that grand mal seizures are still more likely to occur in epileptic patients using therapeutic doses. Ketamine is thus contraindicated in these patients. For most drugs used in anaesthesia subsequent EEG evaluation during their administration has helped to clarify whether or not a particular agent is truly epileptogenic. However, for certain anaesthetic agents, such as ketamine, the origin of epileptiform activity involves subcortical neuronal pathways and is detected only with implanted EEG depth electrodes, not by standard surface leads. In the recovery phase there will be increased muscle tone.

Smith et al (1980) postulated that ketamine may interact with opioid receptors in the basal ganglia and thus the increased muscle tone may have the features of narcotic-induced rigidity. Only accurate neurological assessment and investigation will confirm the exact nature of this muscle rigidity. Again, adequate premedication, particularly benzodiazepines, and quiet surroundings markedly reduce the unwanted effects of ketamine in the recovery phase.

Enflurane

Enflurane produces characteristic changes on EEG which are known to increase with depth of anaesthesia or change in $Pa\text{CO}_2$ and, as Burchiel et al (1977) showed, many persist for 30 days after administration. Opitz et al (1979) found that enflurane did not induce convulsions when given to a group of 45 epileptic patients receiving unspecified anticonvulsant drugs and the inspired concentrations of the anaesthetic agents were low. Since the introduction of enflurane there have been only 13 reports of convulsions on current CSM analysis. Convulsions in the recovery phase with enflurane are thus rare.

Most of the reports have been in non-epileptic patients using inspired concentrations unlikely to cause marked changes on EEG, and no EEG was taken immediately following the convulsion or even later. The nature of these tonic clonic convulsions is disputed. Drug-induced decerebrate rigidity is a most likely cause as hyperreflexia is common following enflurane anaesthesia. Experimentally, Darimont & Jenkins (1977) showed that enflurane causes CNS excitation at a subcortical level in concentrations normally used in anaesthetic practice and this would lend support to this explanation. Grant (1986) reported a patient who had fluctuating consciousness for 48 h immediately postoperatively. The patient remained hyper-reflexic and hypertonic for several days and as late as the 9th day postoperatively he had myoclonic convulsions with incomplete loss of consciousness. Repeat EEGs were normal. This is a classical picture of drug-induced decerebrate rigidity.

Nitrous oxide

The role of nitrous oxide is of particular interest. Tolerance is known to develop during inhalation of nitrous oxide and abrupt cessation is associated with a withdrawal syndrome or emergent delirium which may manifest itself in a variety of ways from confusion and restlessness to convulsions. Smith et al (1979) induced frank convulsive activity in mice after removal from 4–15 min exposure to 1.45 atm of nitrous oxide in air in a hyperbaric chamber. What contribution this has to excitatory effects observed in the recovery phase of anaesthesia is not clear.

Drug-induced decerebrate rigidity and epilepsy

Yanny & Christmas (1988) demonstrated that propofol causes marked cortical depression with an isoelectric EEG. Wood et al (1988) have used this agent successfully to treat status epilepticus. Mackenzie et al (1990) described two cases of unusual forms of status epilepticus that had not responded to conventional anticonvulsant therapy, but in which propofol successfully controlled the seizures as confirmed by EEG recordings before and after treatment. Dwyer et al (1988) and Rouse (1988) observed a reduction in seizure length in patients undergoing electroconvulsive therapy (ECT). This suggests that propofol is not an epileptogenic drug.

Myoclonic activity is known to occur at different levels of the neuroaxis. This activity can present as severe prolonged generalized tonic-clonic spasms and mimic a grand mal seizure, but the EEG is normal. It is a motor manifestation of drug-induced decerebrate rigidity. Clinically, a 'seizure' is usually considered epileptic in nature and this implies cortical disturbance detected as EEG changes. Thus without confirmatory EEG evidence of epileptic discharge the term 'seizure' commonly used in many reports may not be appropriate, and should probably be discontinued.

The CSM (1989) advised that care should be taken when propofol was used to anaesthetize epileptic patients as a significant number of the reports of 'seizures' involved epileptic patients. Postoperative grand mal seizures are a rare event with epileptic patients. Similar care was advised with Althesin before its withdrawal from anaesthetic practice. Both drugs cause marked reduction in cortical activity at light stages of anaesthesia and both have been used successfully in the treatment of status epilepticus. There is a strong association between opisthotonus in the postoperative period with the use of propofol and either a personal or family history of epilepsy. Propofol should be used with care in epileptic patients only because they are more susceptible to drug-induced decerebrate rigidity.

Hopkins (1988) stated that opisthotonus was followed by a grand mal seizure. Without confirmatory EEG evidence the latter may have been a generalized tonic clonic convulsion, part of the spectrum of neurological sequelae seen with drug-induced decerebrate rigidity. It is most likely that patients with a history of epilepsy or a family history that predisposed them to cortical dysrhythmia without EEG or clinical evidence, and those with a history of head injury, have modification of their supraspinal inhibitory pathways that makes them more prone to disinhibition of spinal reflexes in the presence of certain anaesthetic agents.

Shearer (1990) describes repeated grand mal seizures over 3 h in the recovery phase following propofol anaesthesia. The follow-up EEG was normal, although there was a history of head injury and investigations for petit mal epilepsy in childhood.

The term 'grand mal' should only be used when there is EEG evidence of seizure activity. The posture and the nature of movement during seizure activity should be accurately described to support the evidence of grand mal seizure. Otherwise the implications can be very serious for the patient. Unlike non-epileptic myoclonic activity, repeated grand mal seizure activity of this nature normally requires urgent attention.

Implications of drug-induced decerebrate rigidity in out-patient anaesthesia

Saunders & Harris (1990) described a case of a female patient with fluctuating consciousness associated with hyperreflexia lasting 36 h following propofol anaesthesia. The hyperreflexia manifested itself as episodic twitching and opisthotonus. EEG showed a sleep-like pattern, a feature of decerebrate rigidity. Hopkins (1988) reported a case of opisthotonus and tonic clonic convulsions associated with propofol anaesthesia with recurrent attacks up to 4 weeks post-operatively. An EEG at the onset of the attacks was consistent with sedation and this would rule out the possibility of a grand mal seizure.

There is no explanation at present of why the effects of drug-induced decerebrate rigidity can persist. It is likely that 30–40% of all surgery in the UK will be performed on an out-patient basis before the year 2000. Propofol is generally considered an ideal induction agent for day-case surgery. Milligan et al (1987) showed that propofol allows a more rapid return to 'street fitness'. Even though recovery is faster and better in the first hour, the patient should not be allowed home early. The CMS (1989) drew attention to reports of eight patients who had either a delay of more than an hour in regaining consciousness after propofol anaesthesia or who initially awoke but subsequently lapsed into unconsciousness. It advised that an adequate period of recovery must be allowed before discharging patients after day-case surgery. Their discharge normally adheres to strict guidelines.

Disturbances of CNS activity following day-care surgery are rare, but they are potentially hazardous after discharge from hospital. They may result in considerable anxiety to the patient. There are also medico–legal implications to consider. It is thus essential that the patient is escorted home and not left unattended for 24 h.

There is probably a critical residual CNS level of propofol that not only provides a background of cortical disinhibition, but also allows external stimuli to increase reticular formation activity. A spectrum of motor manifestations of drug-induced decerebrate rigidity can then follow. Thus a convulsing patient can be unresponsive and amnesic, but hyperexcited (Winters 1972). Biological variation in the individual patient's responsiveness to anaesthetic drugs could be a contributory factor. Weber (1979) reported two cases of convulsions occurring several hours after Althesin anaesthesia. A causal relationship was strongly suspected. Fahy (1987) reported a delayed convulsion in a discharged patient 6 h postoperatively after day-case anaesthesia with enflurane. There was no history of idiopathic epilepsy. Saunders & Harris (1990) observed hyperreflexia and twitching in the recovery phase following propofol-enflurane anaesthesia. The subject was unable to respond to verbal command or painful stimuli, but retrospectively there was patient awareness. Thus it is important to appreciate that an unresponsive patient with drug-induced decerebrate rigidity can be aware.

Narcotic-induced rigidity

Dose-dependent narcotic-induced rigidity has been observed with fentanyl and alfentanil. Benthuysen et al (1986) postulated that this phenomenon probably originates at a level above the spinal cord as tactile and auditory stimulation often markedly accentuate the rigidity. There has been no correlation with detectable EEG events. This observation is important because the rigidity occasionally resembled a tonic seizure in the suddenness of onset, and in the posture and general appearance of the patient, and could on occasion be misinterpreted as a seizure (Scott & Sarnquist 1985).

The final common pathway of narcotic rigidity may be shared by some of the motor abnormalities seen in Parkinson's disease and extra-pyramidal drug reactions. The cardinal features of Parkinsonism are hypokinesia, rigidity and tremor. Rigidity differs from that of corticospinal tract lesions by being characteristically present throughout the whole range of movement. Hypokinesia is characterized by difficulty in initiating and slowness in executing movement. Chest wall movement is reduced and restrictive ventilatory defect may occur. Christian et al (1983) showed that rigidity in the postoperative period after high dose fentanyl (up to 115 μg/kg) resulted in difficulty in ventilating the lungs of intubated patients. This effect has been described in doses as low as 150 μg and can be abolished with a dose of either 40 μg naloxone or 3 mg suxamethonium.

Extrapyramidal reactions

An adverse reaction to acute administration of neuroleptic drugs, including butyrphenones and phenothiazines, is the onset of extrapyramidal symptoms. These take the form of dyskinesia, including oculogyric crisis, torticollis, grimacing and other involuntary movements, and occurs in 12% of all patients given these drugs. It is most likely to occur in patients under the age of 20 years and in females. It may progress to more prolonged tonic contractions of the limb muscles leading to opisthotonus. This may be incorrectly diagnosed as hysteria, tetanus or epilepsy.

Another extrapyramidal disorder is drug-induced Parkinsonism or bradykinesia. This occurs more frequently in patients over the age of 65 years and presents with tremor, rigidity and facial masking. In fact the drug may unmask a latent form of idiopathic Parkinsonism.

These symptoms result from dopamine receptor antagonist activity. They are more likely to occur with prochlorperazine and perphenazine (commonly used antiemetics postoperatively) and less likely with premedicants such as cyclizine and promethazine. Droperidol is often used not only as an adjunct to anaesthesia, but also on induction of anaesthesia in those patients with a strong history of postoperative vomiting as it has powerful antiemetic properties.

In these reactions consciousness is typically not impaired, and symptoms are usually rapidly and completely reversed after the administration of agents with anticholinergic activity, including diphenhydramine. In contrast, cholinergic agonists such as physostigmine usually exacerbate the symptoms.

Postanaesthetic convulsions

Convulsions in the postoperative period are rare and their aetiology is often not clear. The following list indicates the differential diagnosis of convulsions in the postoperative period:

1. Structural
   - previous head injury
   - cerebral tumour, cerebral abscess, cerebral angioma
   - degenerative disorders (including cerebral atherosclerosis)
2. Congenital neuro-dysfunction (idiopathic epilepsy)
3. Vascular
   - cerebrovascular accident: haemorrhage, arterial or venous thrombosis or embolus
   - embolus: air, fat, amniotic fluid
   - hypertensive encephalopathy
4. Cerebral hypoxia
   - decreased cerebral blood flow
   - inadequate arterial oxygen tension
   - decreased oxygen availability due to alkalaemia
5. Metabolic
   - hyperpyrexia
   - hypoglycaemia
   - hypocalcaemia
   - uraemia
   - eclampsia
6. Iatrogenic
   - water intoxication and hyponatraemia
7. Drug-induced
   - deep ether anaesthesia
   - enflurane
   - methohexitone, ketamine, Althesin, propanidid, etomidate, propofol
   - fetanyl
   - bupivacaine, lignocaine
   - penicillin
   - intrathecal contrast media.

Incorrect diagnosis may result in patients being treated and labelled as 'epileptic' with wide-ranging implications.

Diagnosis of a causal relationship between an anaesthetic agent and an adverse CNS effect requires exclusion of idiopathic epilepsy, cerebral pathology and metabolic abnormality. Tonic clonic activity occurs throughout the neuroaxis and only confirmatory EEG evidence of epileptic foci can establish the diagnosis of grand mal seizure. Every grand mal seizure has the potential for status epilepticus. If diagnosed or strongly suspected it should not be dismissed lightly and requires vigorous treatment to prevent the complications.

The main systemic complications in tonic clonic (grand mal) status epilepticus are:

- hypoxia
- acidosis
- hyperthermia
- arterial hypotension
- hypoglycaemia.

The basic principles of resuscitation apply and, occasionally, it is even necessary to resort to general anaesthesia for control, otherwise repetitive seizures can result in irreversible cerebral oedema. The management of tonic clonic (grand mal status epilepticus) is described below:

1.
   - secure respiratory and cardiovascular function
   - intravenous routes for blood sampling and drug injection/infusion
   - intravenous diazepam, 10–20 mg (2–4 mg/min)
   - intravenous phenytoin, 20 mg/kg (i.e. 1000–1500 mg; 50 mg/min)
2. If seizures persist:
   - intravenous lignocaine test dose, 2–4 mg/kg in 30 s infusion, 6 mg/kg/h

   or
   - intravenous clomethiazole infusion, 0/8% solution (500 mg in 6 h)
3. If seizures persist:
   - general anaesthesia, intravenous thiopentone (EEG burst suppression)
4. Alternatives:
   - diazepam/clonazepam in larger doses
   - repeated intravenous injections/infusion
   - intravenous phenobarbitol
   - paraldehyde, valproate
   - propofol infusion.

CONCLUSION

A lack of knowledge of the neurophysiological basis of anaesthesia, together with a lack of awareness of the adverse CNS effects related to anaesthesia, may result in inappropriate classification and treatment. It may thus lead to misguided reporting or under-reporting to the CSM. An adverse CNS effect related to an anaesthetic agent may be attributed to pre-existing neurological disease rather than to the anaesthetic agent. Twitching may be mistaken for residual neuromuscular blockade. Adverse CNS effects that are brief or infrequent and associated with no subsequent morbidity may not be observed or reported, and there may be uncertainty as to which drug to report. The CSM Adverse Drug Analysis Information Service gives guidelines for all new drugs: 'Report all suspected reactions, that is, any adverse or untoward event, however minor, which could conceivably be attributed to the drug. Please report even if you are unsure of causal relationship or if the reaction is well recognized.' A number of reactions may occur in the same patient, for example twitching, opisthotonus and prolonged unconsciousness. It is obviously important to emphasize the correct primary reaction. In addition the adverse CNS effect may be misdiagnosed. For example opisthotonus may be confused with a grand mal seizure, or myoclonus with loss of consciousness may be interpreted as a grand mal seizure. In each case the implications are quite different. Posture and nature of muscle rigidity will help to differentiate between epileptic seizures, tonic clonic convulsions of drug-induced decerebrate rigidity and narcotic-induced extrapyramidal rigidity. Assessment by a neurologist, in conjunction with EEG evidence where appropriate, will provide a more accurate observation and definition of the adverse CNS effect. The following criteria can be used to describe convulsive activity following anaesthesia:

1. the patient's medical history, including negatives where appropriate
2. the patient's chronic preoperative medications, including antipyschotic medications and street drugs
3. a history of chemical dependency, including alcohol, with a description of the amount consumed and the date of the last consumption
4. the patient's emotional state on entering the operating room, including the presence or absence of hyperventilation
5. the presence or absence of fever
6. the alleged convulsive phenomenon, including rate of drug administration, time of onset in relation to the injection of the drug and the recovery period, speed of onset, parts of the body involved, duration and any indication of a postictal state
7. any cardiovascular changes
8. early postoperative neurological assessment and EEG. Ideally an independent EMG recording should also accompany the EEG.

Once an outline scheme such as this has been followed, appropriate treatment can be implemented.

The patient population (epileptic or non-epileptic), method of documentation (EEG or clinical observation) and method of EEG analysis (cortical or depth electrodes) must be used to analyse properly the preconvulsant and/or anti-convulsant properties of an anaesthetic or analgesic drug. As more information regarding the site and mechanism of action of drugs becomes available with advances in in vivo imaging techniques (magnetic resonance imaging and Positron emission tomography), our understanding of conditions responsible for producing excitatory responses to anaesthetic agents should improve. Further advances in neurophysiology and neurochemistry will lead to an improvement in the clinical use of anaesthetic and analgesic drugs with less adverse CNS effects during the peri-operative period.

REFERENCES

Barron D W 1974 Propanidid in epilepsy. Anaesthesia 29: 445–447

Benthuysen J L, Ty Smith N, Sanford T J, Head N, Dec-Silver H 1986 Physiology of alfentanil-induced rigidity. Anesthesiology 64: 440–446

Bremer F 1937 L'activite cerebrale au cours du sommeil et de la narcose, contribution a l'etude du mecanisme du sommeil. Bull Acad R Med Belg 2: 68–86

Brichard G, Johnstone M 1970 The effect of methylphenidate (ritalin) on post-halothane muscular spasticity. Br J Anaesth 42: 718–721

Burchiel K J, Stockard J J, Calverley R K, Ty Smith N 1977 Relationship of pre and postanaesthetic EEG abnormalities to enflurane-induced seizure activity. Anesth Analg 56: 509–514

Cameron A E 1987 Opisthotonus again. Anaesthesia 42: 1124

Christian C M, Waller J L, Moldenhauer C L 1983 Postoperative rigidity following fentanyl. Anesthesiology 58: 275–277

Clarke R S J, Dundee J W 1965 Clinical studies of induction agents XII: the influence of some premedicants on the course and sequelae of propanidid anaesthesia. Br J Anaesth 37: 51–56

Covino B G 1972 Local anaesthesia. N Engl J Med 286: 975–983

CSM 1989 Current problems: propofol-convulsions, anaphylaxis and delayed recovery from anaesthesia. 26: 2

Darimont P C, Jenkins L C 1977 The influence of intravenous anaesthetics on enflurane-induced central nervous system activity. Can Anaesth Soc J 24: 42–56

Dingwall A E 1987 Oculogyric crisis after day case anaesthesia. Anaesthesia 42: 565

Dwyer R, McLaughey W, Lavery J, McCarthy G, Dundee J W 1988 Comparison of propofol and methohexitone as anaesthetic agents for electroconvulsive therapy. Anaesthesia 43: 459–462

Ebrahim Z Y, DeBoer G E, Luders H, Hahn J F, Lesser R P 1986 Effect of etomidate on the electroencephalogram of patients with epilepsy. Anesth Analg 65: 1004–1006

Fahy L T 1987 Delayed convulsions after day case anaesthesia with enflurane. Anaesthesia 42: 1327–1339

Ferrer-Allado T, Brechner V L, Dymond A, Cozen H, Crandall P 1973 Ketamine-induced electroconvulsive phenomena in the human limbic and thalamic regions. 38: 333–344

Goroszeniuk T, Albin M, Jones R M 1986 Generalized grand mal seizure after recovery from uncomplicated fentanyl-etomidate anaesthesia. Anesth Analg 65: 979–981

Grant I S 1986 Delayed convulsions following enflurane anaesthesia. Anaesthesia 41: 1024–1025

Grant I S, Hutchison G 1983 Epileptiform seizures during prolonged etomidate sedation. Lancet 2: 511–512

Guedel A E 1937 Inhalation anesthesia: a fundamental guide. MacMillan, New York

Hansen H C, Drenck N E 1988 Generalized seizures after etomidate anaesthesia. Anaesthesia 43: 805–806

Hopkins C S 1988 Recurrent opisthotonus with anaesthesia. Anaesthesia 43: 904

Laughlin T P, Newberg L A 1985 Prolonged myoclonus after etomidate anesthesia. Anesth Analg 64: 80–82

Mackenzie S J, Kapadia F, Grant I S 1990 Propofol infusion for control of status epilepticus. Anaesthesia 45: 1043–1045

Meinck H M, Mohlenhof O, Kettler D. 1980 Neurophysiological effects of etomidate, a new short-acting hypnotic. Electroencephalogr Clin Neurophysiol 50: 515–522

Milligan K R, O'Toole D P, Howe J P, Cooper J C, Dundee J W 1987 Recovery from outpatient anaesthesia: a comparison of incremental propofol and propofol-isoflurane. Br J Anaesth 59: 1111–1114

Opitz A, Oberwetter W D 1979 Enflurane or halothane anaesthesia for patients with cerebral convulsive disorders. Acta Anaesthesiol Scand Suppl 71: 43–47

Rees L T 1975 Convulsions immediately following Althesin. Anaesthesia 30: 54–55

Rosenberg H, Clofine R, Bialik O 1981 Neurological changes during awakening from anaesthesia. Anesthesiology 54: 125–130

Rosner B S, Clark D L 1973 Neurophysiologic effects of general anaesthetics. II. Sequential regional actions in the brain. Anesthesiology 39: 59–81

Rouse E C 1988 Propofol for electroconvulsive therapy: a comparison with methohexitone: preliminary report. Anaesthesia Suppl 43: 61–64

Samuel I O, Dundee J W 1973 Clinical studies of induction agents XLII: influence of injection rate and dosage on the

induction complications with althesin. Br J Anaesth 45: 1215–1216
Saunders P R I, Harris M E 1990 Opisthotonus and other unusual neurological sequelae after out patient anaesthesia. Anaesthesia 45: 552–557
Savege T M, Foley E I, Coultas R J, Walton B, Strunin L, Simpson B R, Scott D F 1971 CT1341: some effects in man. Anaesthesia 26: 402–413
Scott J C, Sarnquist F H 1985 Seizure-like movements during a fentanyl infusion with absence of seizure activity in a simultaneous EEG recording. Anesthesiology 62: 812–814
Sessler D I, Israel D, Pozos R S, Pozos M, Rubinstein E H 1988 Spontaneous post-anaesthetic tremor does not resemble thermoregulatory shivering. Anesthesiology 68: 843–850
Shearer E S 1990 Convulsions and propofol. Anaesthesia 45: 255–256
Sloan T B, Ronai A K, Toleikis J R, Koht A 1988 Improvement of intraoperative somatosensory evoked potentials in humans. Anesthesiology 65: 584–589
Smith R A, Winter P M, Smith M, Eger E 1979 Tolerance to and dependence on inhalational anesthetics. Anesthesiology 50: 505–509
Smith D J, Rekoe G M, Martin L L, Coalgate B 1980 The interaction of ketamine with opiate receptor. Life Sci 26: 789–793
Soliman M G, Gillies D M M 1972 Muscular hyperactivity after general anaesthesia. Can Anaesth Soc J 19: 529–535
Steen P A, Michenfelder J D 1979 Neurotoxicity of anesthetics. Anesthesiology 50: 437–453
Strowbridge N F 1989 Postoperative opisthotonus following the use of propofol. Journal Royal Army Medical Corps 135: 79–80
Uppington J 1973 Epileptiform convulsion with Althesin. Anaesthesia 28: 546–550
Weber J 1979 Convulsions following althesin. Anaesthesia 34: 907–908
Weinberg S, Twersky R S 1983 Neuroleptic malignant syndrome. 62: 848–850
Winters W D 1972 Epilepsy or anaesthesia with ketamine. Anesthesiology 36: 309–312
Wood P R, Browne G P R, Pugh S 1988 Propofol infusion for the treatment of status epilepticus. Lancet 1: 480–481
Yanny H F, Christmas D 1988 Propofol infusions for status epilepticus. Anaesthesia 43: 514

29

Psychological responses to anaesthesia

G. M. Holt and P. M. Yate

INTRODUCTION

The continuing improvement in anaesthetic techniques, and a greater understanding of the physiological and pharmacological principles underlying anaesthesia, has enabled anaesthetists to look more carefully at the more subtle side of their practice. One effect of this has been a greater appreciation of the psychological complications of anaesthesia. There has been some change in medical practice in which patients seek a more holistic approach to their problems. Of special interest to the anaesthetist is the identification and reduction of patients' anxiety. This has led to a slight change in emphasis from pharmacological to psychological preparation. Of particular interest is the management of children and the elderly. With the increasing financial pressures on health care and the development of day-case surgery, greater consideration has to be given to psychological as well as physical recovery. At the other end of the spectrum the ability to perform increasingly major surgical procedures has led to a need to investigate the emotional and intellectual effects of these techniques.

THE PREOPERATIVE PATIENT

Anxiety can be subdivided into trait anxiety (the predisposition to react anxiously under stress) and state anxiety (the response to a specific circumstance). Anxiety is viewed as unpleasant by its sufferers, as demonstrated by Brice et al (1970). They reported on a series of postoperative interviews in which patients were asked what the most unpleasant feature of their visit to the operating theatre was. 46% volunteered the preoperative waiting and apprehension in contrast to 21% reporting postoperative pain.

The reported incidence of preoperative anxiety varies between studies, with figures of 60% or more being common. Ramsay (1972) found that 73% of patients admitted to fears when interviewed prior to operation. 62% of these had fears related to anaesthesia (of death, induction technique, waking up during the operation or feeling pain) and 15% to surgery. Norris & Baird (1967), however, in a similar study, found only 7% of their subjectively anxious patients related their state to anaesthesia. Studies cannot agree as to who is likely to be anxious. Ramsay found less fears at each end of the age spectrum (4–12 years and 62 years and over), but the sex of the patient and the severity of planned surgery was irrelevant in this respect, except that all the women with breast lumps feared cancer. Reynolds et al (1983) reported similar findings. In contrast, Norris & Baird (1967) and Lucente & Fleck (1972) found women to be more anxious than men.

Despite the difficulties in interpreting the research in this area it is clear that unpleasant preoperative anxiety is common. There is also evidence to suggest that it affects the pre- and postoperative course. Janis (1958) is largely responsible for the interest shown in this area. He reported on a study of pre- and postoperative interviews with 22 surgical patients and on a retrospective survey with 149 subjects. He suggested that a moderate amount of fear prior to surgery facilitated postoperative recovery, that such people prepared themselves for their ordeal (what Janis called the 'work of worrying') and that they showed less postoperative emotional disturbance, anger and criticism of hospital staff. Those with low fear presumably did not feel they needed such preparation, and those with high fear were too overwhelmed to do so. The curvilinear relationship between anxiety and response to stressful treatments has not been confirmed by more recent research (Cohen & Lazarus 1973). On the other hand, the importance of stress as a clinical variable has been repeatedly demonstrated. Kimball (1969) related preoperative anxiety to morbidity following open-heart surgery. The work of Chapman & Cox (1977) suggests that the context of the anxiety is important. They found that trait anxiety was related to postsurgical pain, anxiety and depression in general surgery and renal recipient patients, but not in kidney donors.

Others aspects of patients' mental states have been studied. Krantz et al (1982) found that preoperative measures of Type A behaviour (characterized by excessive competitive drive, impatience and hostility) were related to diastolic blood pressure increases and complications (mainly arrhythmias) in coronary bypass surgery. Kimball (1969), looking at open-heart surgery patients, found that those classified as depressed preoperatively had the highest mortality, those classified as anxious or as having a symbiotic relationship with their illness had the highest morbidity, while those characterized as adjusted did best. Boyle & Parbrook (1977) demonstrated that preoperative neuroticism in patients undergoing upper abdominal surgery was related to postoperative pain and limitation of vital capacity.

It is clear that the patient's mental state prior to surgery has important implications for his pre- and postoperative course. In particular the studies cited above demonstrate that high preoperative anxiety is associated with later complications. Egbert et al (1964) have shown the effectiveness of a reassuring, informative visit from an anaesthetist in producing a calm patient at the time of operation, reducing postoperative analgesia requirements and reducing length of hospital stay. The work of Leigh et al (1977) suggests that this role may also be filled by a non-anaesthetist (in this study a psychologist). They demonstrated that while an explanatory booklet reduced preoperative anxiety, it was not as effective as the psychologist providing the same information in an individualized and reassuring manner. There is high patient satisfaction with this approach (Reading 1981). Langer et al (1975) found that teaching patients how to cope with anxiety (e.g. by calming self-talk and by selective attention) is a potent method of reducing preoperative anxiety and postoperative requests for analgesia and sedation.

Whichever approach the anaesthetist adopts to the management of preoperative anxiety it must be tailored to the individual patient. Some patients may panic (Egbert et al 1964) if handled insensitively. Nevertheless, avoiding the frightened patient, exposes him not only to the discomfort of anxiety, but also to greater postoperative morbidity, as outlined above.

Premedication

Although premedication has been practised since the 1860s it was not until the early twentieth century that drugs were also used to allay preoperative anxiety. In 1908 McNaughton-Jones described the use of morphine and scopolamine to induce a 'calm, happy and hopeful state' before surgery. In modern anaesthetic practice, premedication has two objectives: first to minimize the risks of anaesthesia, for example giving atropine before cyclopropane; and second to produce a relaxed, calm patient in the anaesthetic room.

Despite the general use of premedication to reduce preoperative anxiety, studies have shown that a significant proportion of patients fail to benefit from these drugs, many of whose conditions are associated with physical and psychological complications. Egbert et al (1963) demonstrated that even a brief preoperative visit by an anaesthetist can be as effective as 2 mg/kg of pentobarbital in allaying preoperative anxiety. Eckenhoff & Helrich (1958), in a study of various premedicants, failed to demonstrate any lowering of the patient's apprehension when comparing narcotics with a placebo, and showed only a modest reduction after a barbiturate. This was reflected by the physiological findings, no difference being detected between the blood pressures of the premedicated and the placebo groups and, in addition, heart rate was significantly increased in those receiving narcotics. In another study, which compared two benzodiazepines with a placebo (Clark et al 1982), the anaesthetists in the induction room failed to differentiate between those patients receiving the active drugs and those receiving a placebo. A striking finding in a careful study by Forrest et al (1977) of five premedicants was that none of the drugs tested had any effect on preoperative apprehension relative to a placebo, as reported by the patient. In the opinion of the anaesthetists the placebo was a 'reasonably satisfactory premedicant'.

There is no general agreement as to the psychological requirements and indications for premedication. Most drugs in current use produce a degree of sedation that is not necessarily paralleled by a reduction in anxiety (Forrest et al 1977). Undoubtedly, in selected patients premedication produces a useful reduction of anxiety. The large number of agents used by anaesthetists indicates the wide divergence in views as to the ideal drug.

The mainstay of premedication over the past 50 years has been the narcotic analgesic. Several studies have, however, demonstrated the high incidence of physical and psychological side effects associated with its use (e.g. Eckenhoff & Helrich, 1958). Pethidine, in particular, has been implicated. One study even suggested that its use *increases* patients' anxiety (Feldman 1963). In the same report Feldman suggested that a combination of hyoscine and papaveretum produces fewer side effects, although it must be remembered that hyoscine may provoke confusion in the elderly. There are several reports of confusion related to atropine or hyoscine administration. In view of the fact that these drugs freely cross the blood–brain barrier, and cholinergic systems are important to central processing, this is hardly surprising. A recent study (Simpson et al 1987) demonstrated a greater memory defecit on the second postoperative day when atropine was used pre- and perioperatively compared to patients given glycopyrrolate which does not enter the brain. That elderly patients may be more susceptible to centrally acting anticholinergics may be due to a mild brain cholinergic deficiency which has been detected in the normal elderly brain (Perry 1986).

Recently there has been a move away from intramuscular administration, a technique hardly likely to improve a patient's mental state, to oral premedication. Droperidol was one of the drugs investigated. One study was abandoned because of the high number of patients suffering psychological sequelae, ranging from anxiety to bizarre behavioural disturbances. The work of Johnstone (1971) suggests that the use of nitrazepam with droperidol reduces these symptoms. The most suitable drugs are the benzodiazepines which, although not always successful in reducing anxiety, have few complications (Murray et al 1968). These, by nature of their amnesic and hypnotic activity, provide some prophylaxis against inadvertent perioperative awareness.

Children

Anaesthesia for small children has long been viewed as a special problem, both from the technical and psychological point of view. Sington (1926) discussed the importance of handling a child carefully, warning that frightening a child may lead to prolonged psychological consequences. It has been a common theme throughout the literature that hospitalization and surgery may be harmful for young children. Several studies have reported both immediate and long-term complications, and reports of acute distress in hospitalized children pepper the literature. Studies of the factors affecting the psychological responses of children to hospitalization, anaesthesia and surgery (it is often difficult to separate the three) agree with the importance of age (Levy 1945, Eckenhoff 1953, Prugh et al 1953). Korsch

(1975) describes how children of different ages relate to the world in different ways. The very small child is difficult to assess, but it has been suggested that separation may provoke behavioural difficulties, such as feeding and sleep disturbances, and if prolonged may interfere with parent–child relationships. Toddlers are beginning to develop a sense of mastery and independence. They find they can influence their environment by what they say and do. In contrast, when they arrive in hospital they may be physically restricted, experience pain and be forced into a passive role. The vivid imagination of the preschool child leads to fantasies of monsters and mutilation. They may interpret their illness and treatment as a form of punishment. As the child becomes older the problems are reduced. By school age, children are more accepting of new experiences, but may regress to earlier patterns of behaviour when confronted by stress. Adolescents, although now able to understand the need for surgery, have a fragile psyche and may be surprisingly vulnerable, but there is no doubt that in psychological terms the under-fives are the most vulnerable. If at all possible, surgery should be delayed until school age. The psychological disturbances following hospitalization have been divided into six types (Vernon et al 1966):

1. general anxiety and regression
2. separation anxiety
3. anxiety about sleep
4. eating disturbances
5. aggression towards authority
6. apathy and withdrawal.

Type 2 is particularly associated with younger children, Types 3, 4 and 5 with the longer-stay patient. A dramatic example was reported by Egerton & Kay (1964) of two children who became blind, mute and akinetic, and in whom no neurological deficit could be found. These children subsequently recovered and were found to have received no preoperative preparation. The specific place of anaesthesia and surgery in causing such problems is difficult to assess. Davenport & Werry (1970) in a well-controlled study of children over a wide age range were unable to show any postoperative behavioural upset. They pointed out that much of the work in this area is anecdotal and uncontrolled. Most studies relate to minor surgery and short hospital stays, as did their own.

Great strides have been made in the care of children in hospital with the development of a child-centred environment in the modern children's ward. The most important feature is the easy access of the child to a parent, especially at the stressful moments, despite the deterioration in the child's behaviour this may cause. The higher incidence of problems in the preschool child is mainly due to separation, therefore anaesthetists should encourage the presence of a parent both in the induction room (or until the onset of premedication-induced sleep) and in the recovery room. Even junior anaesthetists, if encouraged, do not find the parent's presence in the anesthetic room a problem (Hannallah et al 1984).

There have been many suggestions for minimizing psychological stress. It is important that whatever method is used the child's intellectual and emotional development is considered. The simplest technique is preoperative verbal preparation. This can be used prior to admission by the parents, and later continued by the hospital staff. Advice and information should also be given to the parents, as anxious parents produce anxious children. When talking to children one must realize that they are concrete thinkers, and explanation by analogy is unlikely to succeed. They may have terrible fears and should be reassured about pain, mutilation and death. The phrase 'put to sleep' may be misunderstood (Korsch 1975). The general principles are:

1. never lie
2. restrain the urge to give too much information
3. use simple language (Francis & Cutler 1957).

Offering the child the opportunity to participate and thus develop some mastery helps, for example by giving the child a choice of induction method.

Simple verbal preparation may be supplemented by hospital-related play and the use of books. A more sophisticated method is the use of a film. Melamed & Siegal (1975) in a controlled trial used a film of a coping model: 'Ethan has an operation'. The children who saw the film initially became more anxious, but then showed a marked reduction in pre- and postoperative anxiety.

The alternative approach is the use of premedication to modify the child's mental state in the anaesthetic room. It has been suggested that an unsatisfactory induction is associated with a high incidence of postoperative behavioural disturbance (Eckenhoff 1953). Meyers & Muravchick (1977) reported that premedication assisted in this respect only if it was heavy enough to permit an asleep induction. Other studies (Beeby & Morgan Hughes 1980, Brzustowicz et al 1984) have failed to show any major reduction in the child's distress in the anaesthetic room after light premedication. There would therefore seem to be two satisfactory alternatives from the psychological point of view: in the ideal paediatric unit, with careful preoperative preparation and gentle handling, no premedication is necessary; alternatively in more trying situations heavy oral premedication is best.

The elderly

The elderly are particularly at risk from postoperative delirium. There are several reasons for this. The elderly often have difficulty in coping emotionally with a change in their environment. They already have a degree of arterial hypoxaemia which is accentuated by the physical stress of surgery and anaesthesia (Berggren et al 1987). Their physical state may be poor due to inadequate nutrition, coexisting disease or side effects of drugs they are taking. Additionally they are prone to develop unwanted effects from drugs given to them during anaesthesia, such as hyoscine and morphine. The role of medication in causing and increasing confusion must be remembered, and one must resist the temptation to add to this by treating the symptoms with even heavier sedation.

More seriously, Bedford (1955) suggested that irreversible brain damage may follow an operation under general anaesthesia in this age group. It is a widely held belief that anaesthesia, surgery and the elderly do not mix. Simpson et al (1961) investigated this in a prospective study of 741 patients aged 65 years and over awaiting elective surgery. The patients were carefully assessed prior to admission, in hospital and on their return home. Their degree of social integration was measured, with a subsample of 250 also undergoing psychological testing. The results demonstrate that anaesthesia had no effect on the patients' physical activity, mental ability or personality. The majority showed improved social integration. Where deterioration did occur the authors believe this was for reasons unrelated to anaesthesia or organic brain damage. The authors suggested that the contrast between their findings and those of Bedford may have been due to improved care of surgical patients following advances made during the intervening period, such as altered prescribing habits, early ambulation of patients and so forth. Additionally, they noted that their sample underwent elective surgery, whereas in Bedford's sample some had emergency surgery, which is more commonly associated with complications. A further study, using formal psychometric testing, confirmed these findings (Blundell 1967), but did demonstrate some transient impairment in psychomotor performance. Flatt et al (1984) and Smith et al (1987) found no relationship between age and postoperative mental performance, although the latter group demonstrated that those with a marked preoperative mental deficit were at particular risk of at least short-term deterioration in their mental functioning. In conclusion, general anaesthesia for surgery which may improve the elderly patient's quality of life should not be denied, although techniques likely to further embarrass the patient's cerebral circulation, such as induced hypotension, should be avoided.

In the light of these considerations the use of regional anaesthesia is an attractive alternative. It should be noted that the use of sedative premedication prior to regional anaesthesia may induce restlessness and confusion in elderly patients. In terms of recovery of neuropsychological skills, regional anaesthesia plus sedation is indistinguishable from general anaesthesia (Chung et al 1989).

THE POSTOPERATIVE PATIENT

Many patients recovering from anaesthesia will experience psychological disturbance. This may be relatively transient, for example the mild confusional state associated with the hangover effects of anaesthetic agents, or it may be more severe and prolonged, as, for instance, has been reported following ketamine (see p. 453). While drugs undoubtedly contribute to a patient's postoperative mental state, other features are important too. The role of the patient's preoperative mental state in this respect has already been addressed (see p 447). The nature of the surgery and the postoperative environment must also be considered. These areas have been studied mainly in relation to cardiac surgery.

Delirium

During the early 1960s in association with the rapid increase in open-heart surgery came several reports of a high incidence of postoperative mental disturbance. In one series (Egerton & Kay 1964), 41% of patients became delirious in the first postoperative week, over half of these being delirious for 2 or more days and some for up to 3 weeks. In addition, 10% of patients were severely depressed. A number of workers (Blachly 1964, Kornfield et al 1965, Rubenstein & Thomas 1969) have examined postcardiac surgery delirium further and have found it to be associated with preoperative organic brain disease, preoperative physical state (as assessed by degree of surgical risk) and with the nature of the procedure, that is a higher incidence occurred in patients with mitral valve replacements. There was no association between postoperative delirium and the type of oxygenator used or the duration of bypass (although closed-heart surgery is not particularly associated with delirium). A more recent study by Sotaniemi et al (1981) contradicts this last finding: 49 patients undergoing heart valve replacement were given pre- and postoperative psychological testing (including tests of learning, psychomotor speed, visual memory, attention and mental flexibility), neurological examination and EEGs. Clinical examination 10 days after surgery revealed new neurological abnormalities in 47% of patients. This correlated well with the results of psychological testing. Such changes were associated with length of perfusion time (unlike previous studies which used less sensitive measures of psychological disturbance), mitral valve replacement, and unexpected intraoperative events such as massive bleeding, hypoxia or air embolism. Surprisingly, prolonged periods of hypotension in nine patients of less than 40 mmHg mean arterial pressure for longer than 25 min was associated with neuropsychological deterioration in only one patient. A modified Stroop colour test, primarily a test of mental agility, was found to be prognostically significant, a poor preoperative performance being related to postoperative neuropsychological deficit. Intraoperative monitoring revealed positive correlations between the mean frequency and percentage delta activity of the processed EEG with neuropsychological outcome.

Delirium following bypass surgery usually occurs after 2 days of lucidity. This timescale has led to an investigation of the postoperative environment and physical state of the patient. Egerton & Kay (1964) and Kornfield et al (1965) stress the role of sleep deprivation in the intensive care unit, recovery from delirium frequently occurring after a good night's sleep on the general ward. An alternative explanation for the timing of this delirium is that it follows a period of opioid induced rapid eye movement (REM) sleep deprivation. Features in the environment may affect the nature of the perceptual abnormalities. Egerton & Kay (1964) suggested that the rhythmic bleeping of monitors may account for some of the auditory phenomena experienced, and that, similarly, therapeutic dehydration is associated with paranoid features relating to fluid deprivation. They also reported that patients complaining of thirst postoperatively were more likely to suffer delirium than those who did not complain, thereby suggesting a causal link. Other organic features identified by them in this context were hyponatraemia, digitalis toxicity and a history of alcoholism. More recently a prospective study of neuropsychiatric complications following heart surgery (Smith et al 1986) found that at 24 h postoperatively 64% of patients had new neurological signs most of which had disappeared by 8 days, although 65% of patients still had deficits on neuropsychological testing. Such deficits were correlated with long bypass times and hypotension. They had largely resolved by 8 weeks. Nussmeier et al (1986), in a study of patients undergoing open-heart surgery, were able to demonstrate a significant reduction in postoperative neuropsychological complications by prophylactically treating patients with high-dose barbiturates during the bypass period. In view of the small numbers involved these results do have to be treated with caution. However, if confirmed, they offer hope for the future.

Morse & Litin (1969) reported similar findings for delirium following other types of surgery. They compared 60 patients who experienced postoperative delirium with a control group, matched on the basis of type of surgery, age and sex, who did not experience delirium. Organic factors were again relevant, such as metabolic disturbance, infection and so forth, as well as surgical factors in that those undergoing emergency surgery were more likely to have a history of alcoholism, depression, functional gastrointestinal disturbance, paranoid personality, retirement-adjustment problems and to have undergone previous psychiatric treatment. This was a retrospective study. Ideally these findings should be confirmed by a prospective study.

Influence of drugs

Many of the drugs used by the anaesthetist may provoke psychological disturbance, such as preoperative dreams and postoperative alterations in mood, impaired psychomotor performance and hallucinations. The sight of the restless, confused patient in the recovery room is common. However, it is less often realized that psychological disturbance may persist for several days or, in certain circumstances, even up to a year. Ketamine anaesthesia has been particularly implicated in this respect.

Ketamine is a unique anaesthetic agent derived from phencyclidine, a drug that produces anaesthesia but at the cost of a pronounced psychomimetic effect in the recovery period, making it unsuitable for clinical use. Ketamine retains some of these psychological effects. It produces 'dissociative anaesthesia' by excitation of the thalamus and limbic system combined with an effect on the relay nuclei associated with pain transmission. This provides profound analgesia even at subanaesthetic doses. Ketamine also has a depressive action on the visual and auditory relay nuclei as well as reducing skin and musculoskeletal sensation. These effects may be responsible for the emergence reactions described with ketamine, in which patients misinterpret stimuli, have the sensation of bodily detachment or floating, and experience psychedelic dreams and hallucinations (White et al 1982). These phenomena are graphically described by Collier (1972). The perceptual abnormalities tend to be visual or proprioceptive in nature, auditory phenomena being less common. There are several reports (Johnson 1971, Fine & Finestone 1973, Perel & Davidson 1976) of recurrent flashbacks to the original hallucinations experienced following ketamine anaesthesia. These may persist for up to 1 year, although they more commonly last only a few days. They are often very distressing. Meyers & Charles (1978) describe two such cases in children. The incidences reported for these various psychic disturbances cover a wide range, from less than 5% to greater than 30% (White et al 1982). This disparity is partly due to confused terminology, as to what constitutes a hallucination (Jago & Restall 1983) and also due to widely differing populations being studied. In a review of the literature, White et al (1982) report that women are more prone than men to develop these problems, as are those over 16 years of age. Dosage may also be an important parameter, although complaints of a floating sensation still occur when ketamine is used as an adjunct to local anaesthesia. Patients find the psychic disturbances associated with ketamine unpleasant. Lilburn et al (1978) report that 64% of patients would not want the same anaesthetic again. Consequently, various efforts have been made to reduce the incidence of these phenomena. One approach has been to control the postoperative environment. Hejja & Galloon (1975) reduced sensory input by placing the patient in a quiet, darkened room. Other researchers, however, point to the usefulness of actively orientating the patient. Garfield et al (1972) found that the patients in their study reported how much they appreciated being orientated by the recovery staff, and concluded that deliberate isolation may increase anxiety. An alternative approach to reducing the emergence phenomena following ketamine is to combine its use with other drugs. Llang & Llang (1975) reported a low incidence of emergence reactions and a high patient acceptability when low-dose ketamine was used as part of a balanced anaesthetic technique. The addition of droperidol has been investigated (Sandove et al 1971, Erbguth et al 1972, Coppel et al 1973), but it is associated with the occurrence of dizziness and unpleasant dreams so its use cannot be recommended. The most successful agents studied are the benzodiazepines, in particular lorazepam. Dundee & Lilburn (1978) found that the administration of 4 mg of lorazepam prior to ketamine anaesthesia reduces the incidence of psychic sequelae to acceptable levels but prolongs the recovery time.

Psychological disturbances are not exclusive to ketamine. Dreams occur in about 8% of patients undergoing surgery with a wide variety of anaesthetic techniques, including inhalational anaesthesia (Wilson et al 1975). Garfield et al (1972) reported a high incidence of illusions following thiopentone, nitrous oxide and halothane anaesthesia.

Many studies have been conducted to delineate the severity and duration of the hangover effects of anaesthetic drugs, including those done on volunteers without surgery who have then undergone careful psychological assessment. In one such study (Davison et al 1975) looking at halothane and isoflurane, intellectual performance was impaired for several days and subjects reported a depressed mood for up to a month. These effects were particularly marked after halothane. Similar findings have been reported following cyclopropane anaesthesia using subjective and objective measures (James 1969). Kortilla et al (1975, 1977) studied simulated driving skills after anaesthesia. Marked differences were found between the various agents. The earliest recovery occurred after inhalational anaesthesia, with prolonged effects occurring after the barbiturate intravenous agents methohexitone and thiopentone. These latter agents produced a marked reduction in performance at 8 h, although the majority of the subjects were unaware of this and felt their driving ability was normal. In view of these findings Kortilla and his colleagues recommended that patients should not drive for 24 h following administration of these drugs.

Awareness

One of the major anxieties of patients prior to anaesthesia is that of awareness during surgery. This is unfortunately not a totally unrealistic fear. In two large series a 1% incidence of awareness was reported (Hutchinson 1960, Wilson et al 1975). During anaesthesia for caesarean section, using thiopentone and unsupplemented nitrous oxide, figures as high as 9% have been quoted (Wilson & Turner 1969). For details of the causes, incidences and prevention of awareness, see Chapter 26.

Awareness may cause not only acute distress, but also a prolonged and disabling psychological state. Bergstrom & Bernstein (1968) described six patients given nitrous oxide and oxygen only for caesarean section, all of whom reported psychological disturbances. Three were still having problems a year later. For example one woman was 'almost daily tormented by the fear associated with a dream' she had had during surgery. Meyer & Blacher (1961) outlined a syndrome of 'traumatic neurosis' in patients that have awoken paralysed during surgery. Blacher (1975) elaborated this, reporting on several patients who complained of anxiety, irritability, preoccupation with death and repetitive nightmares. A striking feature of this syndrome is the reluctance of patients spontaneously to discuss their problem. They are not sure whether they were awake or not and are afraid of being thought insane. He suggested that these problems are caused by the state of helplessness experienced, and that the repetitive dreams are an attempt to master the experiences. Cundy (1978) describes the patients as feeling degraded and humiliated. Evidence from women undergoing caesarean section (Guerra 1980), and children having scoliosis surgery (Abbot & Bentley 1980), suggests that this syndrome does not occur in patients forewarned that they may be aware during surgery and the reasons for it. The difficulty in management of the 'traumatic neurosis' is primarily one of identification, in view of the patients' reluctance to discuss their experience. Blacher (1975) reports that a direct explanation of the cause may cure the patient, vividly describing the relief patients obtain on confirmation of their suspicions. Occasionally patients will require referral to a psychiatrist. It is clear that serious psychological disturbances can be caused by unexpected awareness and that these problems are usually easy to treat. It is important that the anaesthetist has a high index of suspicion and visits any patient in whom awareness is thought to have occurred, to provide reassurance and an explanation. Patients who complain of awareness should not be brushed off with the suggestion that they must have imagined it, and other defensive remarks, by the anaesthetist.

Another aspect of awareness is unconscious perception whereby it is hypothesized that even properly anaesthetized patients are able to absorb information subconsciously. This has been used to produce improved postoperative recovery by providing positive auditory messages perioperatively (Evans and Richardson, 1988). The other side of this is the possibility that negative comments made by theatre staff may be harmful.

REFERENCES

Abbot T R, Bentley G 1980 Intraoperative awakening during scoliosis surgery. Anaesthesia 35: 298–302

Bedford P D 1955 Adverse cerebral effects of anaesthesia on old people. Lancet 2: 259–263

Beeby D G, Morgan Hughes J O 1980 Behaviours of unsedated children in the anaesthetic room. Br J Anaesth 52: 279–281

Berggren D, Gustafson Y, Eriksson B, Bucht G, Hansson L I, Reiz S, Winblad B 1987 Postoperative confusion after anaesthesia in elderly patients with femoral neck fractures. Anesth Analg 66: 497–504

Bergstrom H, Bernstein K 1968 Psychic reactions after analgesia with nitrous oxide for Caesarean section. Lancet 2: 541–542

Blacher R S 1975 On awakening paralysed during surgery: a syndrome of traumatic neurosis. J Am Med Assoc 234: 67–68

Blachly P H 1964 Post-cardiotomy delirium. Am J Psychiatry 121: 371–375

Blundell E 1967 A psychological study of the effects of surgery on eighty six elderly patients. Br J Soc Clin Psychol 6: 297–303

Boyle P, Parbrook G D 1977 The inter-relation of personality and postoperative factors. Br J Anaesth 49: 259–263

Brice D D, Heatherington R, Utting J E 1970 A simple study of awareness and dreaming during anaesthesia. Br J Anaesth 42: 535–542

Brzustowicz R M, Nelson D A, Betts E K, Rosenberry K R, Swedlow D B 1984 The efficacy of oral premedication for pedeatric outpatient surgery. Anesthesiology 60: 475–477

Chapmn C R, Cox G B 1977 Anxiety, pain and depression surrounding elective surgery: a multi-variate comparison of abdominal surgery patients with kidney donors and recipients. J Psychosom Res 21: 7–15

Chung F F, Meier R H, Lautenschlaeger E, Seyone C 1989 Comparison of perioperative mental function after general anesthesia and spinal anesthesia with intravenous sedation. Can J Anaesth 36: 382–387

Clark G, Erwin D, Yate P, Burt D, Major E 1982 Temazepam as premedication in elderly patients. Anaesthesia 37: 421–425

Cohen F, Lazarus R S 1973 Active coping dispositions and recovery from surgery. Psychosom Med 35: 375–387

Collier B B 1972 Ketamine and the conscious mind. Anaesthesia 27: 120–134

Coppel D L, Bovill J G, Dundee J W 1973 The taming of ketamine. Anaesthesia 28: 293–296

Cundy J M 1978 Awareness during anaesthesia. Br J Anaesth 50: 1266

Davenport H T, Werry J S 1970 Effect of general anaesthesia, surgery and hosptialisation upon the behaviour of children. Am J Orthopsychiatry 40: 806–824

Davison L A, Stenhelber J C, Eger E I II, Stevens W C 1975 Psychological effects of halothane and isoflurane anaesthesia. Anesthesiology 43: 313–324

Dundee J W, Lilburn J K 1978 Ketamine-lorazepam attenuation of psychic sequelae of ketamine by lorazepam. Anaesthesia 33: 312–314

Eckenhoff J E 1953 Relationship of anaesthesia to postoperative personality changes in children. Am J Dis Child 86: 587–591

Eckenhoff J E, Helrich M 1958 Study of narcotics and sedatives for use in pre-anaesthetic medication. J Am Med Assoc 167: 415–421

Egbert L D, Battit G E, Turndorf H, Beecher H K 1963 The value of the preoperative visit by an anesthetist. J Am Med Assoc 185: 553–555

Egbert L D, Battit G E, Welch G E, Bartlett M K 1964 Reduction of postoperative pain by encouragement and instruction of patients. N Engl J Med 270: 825–827

Egerton N, Kay J H 1964 Psychological disturbances associated with open heart surgery. Br J Psychiatry 110: 433–439

Erbguth P H, Reiman B, Klein R L 1972 The influence of chlorpromazine, diazepam and droperidol on emergence from ketamine. Anesth Analg 51: 693–698

Evans C, Richardson P M 1988 Improved recovery and reduced post-operative stay after therapeutic suggestions during general anaesthesia. Lancet 2: 491–493

Feldman S A 1963 A comparative study of four premedications. Anaesthesia 18: 169–184

Fine J, Finestone S C 1973 Sensory disturbances following ketamine anesthesia: recurrent hallucinations. Anesth Analg 52: 428–430

Flatt J R, Binnel P C, Hobbes A 1984 Effects of anesthesia on some aspects of mental functioning of surgical patients. Anaesth Intensive Care 12: 315–324

Forrest W H, Brown C R, Brown B W 1977 Subjective responses to six common preoperative medications. Anesthesiology 47: 241–247

Francis L, Cutler R P 1957 Psychological preparation for pediatric anaesthesia. Anesthesiology 18: 106–109

Garfield J M, Garfield F B, Stone J G, Hopkins D 1972 A comparison of psychologic responses to ketamine and thiopental-nitrous oxide-halothane anesthesia. Anesthesiology 36: 329–338

Guerra F 1980 Awareness during anaesthesia. Can Anaesth Soc J 27: 178

Hanallah R S, Abramowitz M D, Oh T H, Ruttiman U E 1984 Residents' attitudes towards parents' presence during anesthesia induction in children: does experience make a difference? Anesthesiology 60: 598–601

Hejja P, Galloon S 1975 A consideration of ketamine dreams. Can Anaesth Soc J 22: 100–105

Hutchinson R 1960 Awareness during surgery: a study of its incidence. Br J Anaesth 33: 463–469

Jago R H, Restall J 1983 Postoperative dreaming. Anaesthesia 38: 438–441

James F M III 1969 Effects of cyclopropane anesthesia without surgical operation on mental functions of normal man. Anesthesiology 30: 264–272

Janis I L 1958 Psychological stress. Wiley, New York

Johnson B D 1971 Psychosis and ketamine. Br Med J 4: 428–429

Johnstone M 1971 Effects of oral sedatives on the vasoconstrictive reaction to fear. Br J Anaesth 43: 380–384

Kimball C P 1969 Psychological responses to the experience of open heart surgery. Am J Psychiatry 126: 348–359

Kornfield D S, Zimberg S, Malm J R 1965 Psychiatric complications of open heart surgery. N Engl J Med 273: 287–292

Korsch B M 1975 The child in the operating room. Anesthesiology 43: 251–257

Kortilla K, Linnoila M, Ertama P, Hakkinen S 1975 Recovery and simulated driving after intravenous anesthesia with thiopental, methohexital, propanidid or alphadione. Anesthesiology 43: 291–299

Kortilla K, Tammisto T, Ertama P, Pfaffli P, Blomgren E, Hakkinen S 1977 Recovery of psychomotor skills and simulated driving after brief inhalational anesthesia with halothane or enflurane combined with nitrous oxide and oxygen. Anesthesiology 46: 20–27

Krantz D S, Arabian J M, Davis J E, Parker J S 1982 Type A behaviour and coronary artery bypass surgery: intraoperative blood pressure and perioperative complications. Psychosom Med 44: 273–283

Langer E J, Janis I L, Wolfer J A 1975 Reduction of psychological stress in surgical patients. J Exp Soc Psychol 11: 155–165

Leigh J N, Walker J, Janganathan P 1977 Effect of preoperative anaesthetic visit on anxiety. Br Med J 2: 987–989

Levy D M 1945 Psychic trauma of operations in children. Am J Dis Child 69: 7–25

Lilburn J K, Dundee J W, Nair S G, Fee J P H, Johnson H M L 1978 Ketamine sequelae evaluation of the ability of various premedicants to attenuate its psychic actions. Anaesthesia 33: 307–311

Llang H S, Llang H G 1975 Minimising emergence phenomena: subdissociative dosage of ketamine in balanced surgical anesthesia. Anesth Analg 54: 312–316

Lucente F E, Fleck S 1972 A study of hospitalisation anxiety in 408 medical and surgical patients. Psychosom Med 34: 304–312

MacNaughton-Jones H 1908 Scopolamine-morphine and chloroform anaesthesia. Br Med J 2: 809–810

Melamed B G, Siegal L J 1975 Reduction of anxiety in children facing hospitalisation and surgery by use of filmed modelling. J Consult Clin Psychol 43: 511–521

Meyer B C, Blacher R S 1961 A traumatic neurotic reaction induced by succinylcholine. N Y State J Med 61: 1255–1261

Meyers E F, Charles P 1978 Prolonged adverse reactions to ketamine in children. Anesthesiology 49: 39–40

Meyers E F, Muravchick S 1977 Anesthesia induction techniques in pediatric patients: a controlled study of behavioural consequences. Anesth Analg 56: 538–542

Morse R M, Litin E M 1969 Postoperative delirium: a study of etiologic factors. Am J Psychiatry 126: 388–395

Murray W J, Bechtoldt A A, Berman L 1968 Efficacy of oral psychosedative drugs for pre-anesthetic medication. J Am Med Assoc 203: 89–94

Norris W, Baird W L M 1967 Preoperative anxiety: a study of the incidence and aetiology. Br J Anaesth 39: 503–509

Nussmeier N A, Arlund C, Scoguff S 1986 Neuropsychiatric complications after cardiopulmonary bypass: cerebral protection by a barbiturate. Anesthesiology 64: 165–175

Perel A, Davidson J T 1976 Recurrent hallucinations following ketamine. Anaesthesia 31: 1081–1083

Perry E K 1986 The cholinergic hypothesis: ten years on. Br Med Bull 42: 63–69

Prugh D G, Staub E M, Sands H H, Kirchbaum R M, Lenihan E A 1953 A study of the emotional reactions of children and families to illness and hospitalisation. Am J Orthopsychiatry 23: 70–106

Ramsay M A E 1972 A Survey of preoperative fear. Anaesthesia 27: 396–402

Reading A E 1981 Psychological preparation for surgery: patient recall of information. J Psychosom Res 25: 57–62

Reynolds A C, Raether D J, Fetterman C E, Davidson A J 1983 Assessment of severity of preoperative anxiety and dose response effectiveness of diazepam in preoperative anxiety reduction. Anesthesiology 59: A377

Rubenstein D, Thomas J K 1969 Psychiatric findings in cardiotomy patients. Am J Psychiatry 126: 108–117

Sandove M S, Hatano S, Zahed B, Redlin T, Arastounejad P, Roman V 1971 Clinical study of droperidol in the prevention of the side effects of ketamine anesthesia. Anesth Analg 50: 388–393

Simpson B R, Williams M, Scott J F, Crampton-Smith A 1961 The effects of anaesthesia and surgery on old people. Lancet 2: 887–893

Simpson K H, Smith R J, Davies L F 1987 Comparison of the effect of atropine and glycopyrrolate on cognitive function following general anaesthesia. Br J Anaesth 59: 966–969

Sington H 1926 Discussion on anaesthetics in children. Proc R Soc Med 19: Parts I and II.

Smith C M, Carter M, Loughnan B, Marks R, Sebel P S, Yate P M 1987 Effects of general anaesthesia on reaction time in elderly patients undergoing endoscopic urological surgery. Br J Anaesth 59: 1330P

Smith P L C, Newman S P, Ell P J, Treasure T, Joseph P, Schneidau A, Harrison M J G 1986 Cerebral consequences of cardiopulmonary bypass. Lancet: 823–825

Sotaniemi K A, Juolasmaa A, Kokkanen E T 1981 Neuropsychologic outcome after open heart surgery. Arch Neurol 38: 2–8

Vernon D T A, Schulman J L, Foley J M 1966 Changes in children's behaviour after hospitalisation. Am J Dis Child 111: 581–593

White P F, Way W L, Trevor A J 1982 Ketamine: its pharmacology and therapeutic uses. Anesthesiology 56: 119–136

Wilson J, Turner D J 1969 Awareness during Caesarean section under general anaesthesia. Br Med J 1: 280

Wilson S L, Vaughan R W, Stephen C R 1975 Awareness, dreams and hallucinations associated with general anesthesia. Anesth Analg 54: 609–617

30

Waste anaesthetic gases and antipollution equipment

T. H. Taylor

INTRODUCTION

This book describes the potential hazards to the patient during the practice of anaesthesia, but this chapter introduces a concept that is ethically unusual in medicine. The use of volatile agents and nitrous oxide in anaesthesia may not only present a hazard to the patient, but the presence of traces of anaesthetic vapours within the atmosphere of anaesthetic rooms, operating theatres and recovery rooms has been thought for many years to have an adverse effect on the staff working in these areas. Much has been written about the dangers of this environmental pollution, but there is no general agreement on the overall seriousness of the problem, nor on its long-term effects. Most authorities are, however, agreed that the presence of waste gases in the atmosphere in any quantity cannot be beneficial to the staff working in those places. As a result, and because of greater awareness of the need to promote Health and Safety at Work, reinforced by law, apparatus has been designed to minimize the escape of unwanted anaesthetic gas into the atmosphere of the workplace, and thus eliminate the problem from operating suites. Unfortunately, in so doing, fresh hazards have been created for the patient undergoing an anaesthetic. Antipollution devices must be the only example in anaesthetic practice of equipment connected to the patient not intended entirely for his benefit. Therefore three matters have to be considered:-

1. The hazard of workplace pollution to staff. This is not strictly within the compass of this book, but the subject must be briefly reviewed to place the whole matter in context. For the sake of completeness some references are appended for interested readers.
2. The effect of waste anaesthetic gases on the environment as a whole: atmospheric pollution.
3. The additional hazard to the patient due entirely to the introduction of apparatus designed to scavenge waste anaesthetic gases. It is clearly necessary to ensure that such apparatus is totally safe. If any doubt of this exists, then surely the patient's interest must be paramount.

THE HAZARD OF WORKPLACE POLLUTION

The nature of the work carried out in the operating theatre, and the fact that procedures are often performed on infected individuals, can lead to contamination of the atmosphere with bacterial organisms or viruses. In this context perhaps the most important contaminants are the viruses of hepatitis and HIV. Operations carried out with power tools and involving bone cutting are particularly dangerous. It is now routine procedure to minimize the effects of this pollution by the correct extraction and recirculation of air in the theatre, and the wearing of suitable protective clothing including gloves and goggles.

However it is the release into the atmosphere of waste anaesthetic gases that has in the past given rise to most concern. Despite a lack of firm evidence that traces of anaesthetic agents cause definite harm to people working in an operating theatre environment, the Department of Health (DOH; 1976) issued instructions that all possible measures should be taken to keep contamination to a minimum, including the provision of scavenging systems. Pregnant staff should, if possible, be employed elsewhere. In the USA the National Institute of Occupational Safety and Health (NIOSH) has issued firm guidelines in a Criteria Document (1977). The full implementation of both these sets of instructions adds considerably to the cost of anaesthetic apparatus, and to some extent increases the complexity of the apparatus. In other situations, for example in areas where anaesthetics are given in the dental chair, or in the anaesthetic recovery room, the removal of patients' exhalations is virtually impossible in a way that is tolerable to all concerned. The apparatus currently available to scavenge in these places could add considerably to the hazards facing the patient, as the watching staff have only limited access to the airway. Thus they are not in general use.

EVIDENCE OF HAZARDS TO STAFF

Spontaneous abortion

Spontaneous abortion is historically the oldest suggested complication and is the best documented, although the correlation between the effect and the cause has not always been shown to be close. It could be the nature of the work, which is stressful, that causes any increased abortions, and not necessarily the theatre pollution. Such a relationship could not be established by Knill-Jones et al (1972), and other studies reach the same conclusion. Later studies, however, both here and in the USA, seemed to suggest that there is indeed a higher spontaneous abortion rate in women exposed to traces of anaesthetic waste (by a factor of between 50–200%). This was not supported by Pharoah et al (1977), but a link must be presumed until convincingly disproved. This can only be done by extended prospective studies, which have been instituted in both the UK and the USA. In 1977, Spence & Knill-Jones commenced a prospective study of these effects by a postal survey on all women doctors below the age of 40 working in the UK. The response rate was over 80% and listed 13 000 pregnancies in 11 000 women. Although the collection of data ended in 1986, it has not so far been published in full. The interim analysis indicates that there was no connection between medical specialty and hours in the operating theatre, and the miscarriage rate (Spence et al 1989).

Congenital malformation

Again there is a considerable problem in obtaining reliable data on the topic of congenital malformation, for all studies have been retrospective, and the natural desire to blame outside influences for these sad events makes the mother's (or father's) work a convenient scapegoat. Thus analysis of these data presents considerable difficulty. No firm pattern of defect has been determined and many of the defects reported are minor. Pharoah (1977) found an increase in abnormalities, but this was not statistically significant in his sample. Again the results of the definitive prospective study is awaited, but it seems that congenital abnormalities are not influenced by the occupational factors surveyed (Spence et al 1989).

Infertility

A previous suggestion by Knill-Jones et al (1972) that there was an increase in infertility, both in women working in a theatre environment and in the wives of men who work in theatres, has not been substantiated by the recent survey (Spence et al 1989).

Carcinogenicity

In a retrospective survey, Bruce et al (1968) found an increase in deaths from lymphatic tumours. This led to speculation that the halogenated hydrocarbon volatile agents may have been implicated.

No firm evidence has been adduced to confirm this in man, and a further prospective study among anaesthesiologists (Bruce et al 1974b) failed to demonstrate an increased incidence of malignancy, although some animal work is available to support the link.

Deterioration in standard of work during exposure

Over the last 50 years, studies of the amount of anaesthetic vapour to be found in the atmosphere of an operating theatre have shown that significant quantities are present. Linde & Bruce (1969) found that the end-expired gas of anaesthetists contained significant amounts of halothane, and that the wash-out time could be as long as 64 h. This means that during a normal working week the blood levels of volatile agents are cumulative, and this accumulation will only recede if a work-free weekend intervenes. This should have some significance in the arrangements for the off-duty hours of personnel working in unscavenged environments, especially those working in recovery areas, as mentioned on page 460.

Although this accumulation has some bearing on the alleged adverse effects discussed on page 460, it will be of much greater significance if it can be shown that a person's work performance falls off as the blood levels rise. Bruce et al (1974a) in Chicago have consistently found such a deficit in work performance of people exposed to traces of an anaesthetic vapour. This finding is consistent with the known effects of other drugs, such as alcohol. Other workers have failed to demonstrate this effect in the range of concentrations likely to be found in scavenged operating theatres, unless the anaesthetist is subjected to very high concentrations emanating from the apparatus while in close proximity. This effect should be minimal in apparatus with properly fitting joints and efficient seals. Davenport et al (1980) thought that no anaesthetist's perform ance would be adversely affected even in an unscavenged theatre.

However it is clear that any such a deterioration in performance cannot be in the patient's best interest, increasing as it does the likelihood of error. If the effects are to render less rapid the recognition of and response to alterations in an established anaesthetic, this deterioration in response, together with fatigue, may be responsible for some of the many anaesthetic tragedies that are known to be a result of human error. If there is any possibility that this deterioration does occur, there is good reason to take every measure to reduce theatre pollution provided the added hazard to the patient is acceptable.

ACCEPTABLE LEVELS OF TRACE GASES

The monitoring of traces of anaesthetic vapours in the operating theatre suite is difficult because levels will clearly vary according to the position from which the sample is taken, as well as with the time of day. The only accurate method would be to measure the actual level in the staff concerned. This would also allow for the varying exposure time of the different members of staff. Such a study is likely to reveal that, in a well-scavenged theatre, the recovery room staff are most at risk. However, such estimations are tedious and expensive to perform, and routine monitoring is therefore simply not available in this country.

In an unscavenged theatre, atmospheric nitrous oxide levels are likely to reach 500 parts per million, and halothane 15 parts per million, near the anaesthetic effluent. The aim should be to reduce this to 25 parts per million for nitrous oxide and between 0.5 and 2 parts per million for halothane. These figures are taken from the NIOSH Criteria Document (1977). The criticism of this document is that it sets an exceedingly high standard that is very difficult to achieve. There is considerable danger in setting by law, standards that are virtually unobtainable in normal practice. This error has not been made in the UK. The threshold of perception of the smell of halothane lies between 3 and 100 parts per million. 50% of individuals can recognize 33 parts per million, but only 25% the lower level of 15 parts per million. The significance of this is in the suggestion of Bruce et al (1974a) that perceptual cognitive and motor skills may be lost at this level, and therefore 75% of anaesthetists would not be able to detect significant pollution without aid. It also implies that if the odour is detectable, the recommended NIOSH levels have been exceeded (Fleming & Johnstone 1977).

METHODS OF REDUCING THEATRE POLLUTION

Considerable attention should be paid to the atmospheric environment in operating theatres, where it is necessary to maintain full staff efficiency at all times during long procedures. Many operating suites in the UK are without the means to provide these conditions. This must have an adverse effect on the staff performance and ultimately on patient welfare. However, close attention to the following points will effectively reduce the loss of waste gases into the theatre atmosphere, and hence ensure the lowest possible levels of pollution:

1. Frequent air changes with ventilation so arranged that all areas of the operating theatre are equally well-served with the appropriate number of air changes per hour. This should include all corridors, patient waiting areas and recovery rooms. This airflow system should not be turned off when the suite is in use, and should be continued out of working hours for a sufficient time to ensure clearance of all traces of the contaminants from the atmosphere.
2. Complete removal of waste gases from the patient circuit to a point outside the theatre. This can be achieved by ensuring that there are no leaks from the patient connections, either at the mask or the endotracheal tube, and by the use of a suitable scavenging system attached to the spill valve. It is more difficult to remove the patient's direct exhalations from the atmosphere, especially in the recovery area, for here the apparatus required is more cumbersome and quite frightening to the recovering patient, and certainly does nothing to enhance his safety. The preferred solution in these areas is frequent air changes, and to see that the staff are not exposed for long periods during the working week. Similar problems are encountered in the dental surgery when 'dental gases' are being administered.
3. Prevention of all anaesthetic spillage and leaks, including care in the filling of vaporizers, which should be done at the end of a session and not at the beginning. Flowmeters should be turned off as soon as the patient is disconnected from the machine. Nitrous oxide cylinders and volatile agent vaporizers should not be turned on indiscriminantly for testing. Regular maintainance should ensure that there are no leakages from components within the apparatus itself.
4. Methods of anaesthesia should be employed that reduce the possibility of atmospheric pollution. Greater use should be made of reduced gas flows with carbon dioxide absorbers, total intravenous anaesthesia and regional anaesthesia.
5. The ultimate safeguard would be regular determination of pollution levels in the operating theatres, and the institution of corrective measures should they prove to be higher than approved safety levels. These measures have not been universally adopted in the UK.
6. Ideally, all staff working in the theatre environment should have regular monitoring of their individual blood levels. If levels are found to be consistently high, the scavenging system used, and other procedures and practices employed in the theatres should be examined for faults. If these are not implicated there may be a need to adjust the duty rotas of the staff concerned. Again, this policy has not been adopted in the UK.

ATMOSPHERIC POLLUTION

The contribution of waste anaesthetic gases to the 'greenhouse effect' and to destruction of the ozone layer was the subject of a review by Logan & Farmer (1989). We are all now aware that chlorofluorocarbons (CFCs) have a damaging effect on the ozone layer of the Earth's atmosphere, and considerable effort is being directed at reducing these emissions. Halothane, enflurane and isoflurane are, of course, hydrofluorocarbons (HCFCs). These agents are thought to have less potential for ozone destruction than CFCs, partly because their molecules are inherently less stable. In addition, the anaesthetic contribution to overall CFC and HCFC release is thought to be less than one ten thousandth of the total. Chlorine atoms released from CFCs are potent catalysts of ozone destruction, while fluoride atoms from HCFCs are less reactive and thus less damaging. Exposure of halothane to daylight causes bromine release which is potentially very damaging to the ozone layer. Fortunately the halothane molecule probably survives no more than 2 years in the atmosphere, and released bromine atoms are thought to form inorganic molecules which quickly return to the Earth's surface. The net effect, therefore, is of a very modest contribution to ozone depletion by waste anaesthetic gases.

Nitrous oxide poses a different problem, however. This is a 'greenhouse gas' which lasts a very long time in the atmosphere. Although the anaesthetic source represents only a small proportion of the nitrous oxide reaching the atmosphere, this gas is an increasingly important contributor to global warming. In addition, production of nitric oxide by photodissociation in the stratosphere acts as a powerful catalyst to ozone destruction. Since the concentration of nitrous oxide used in anaesthetic practice is so high, anaesthetists should consider carefully the implication of its continued use.

HAZARDS OF SCAVENGING SYSTEMS

To be effective the method of disposing of the effluent gas from the patient circuit must be to take it from the spill valve of the anaesthetic apparatus to a point outside the building by means of a closed duct. Special care has to be taken to achieve this when inflammable agents are employed. The danger of removing flammable agents by such a system is another factor making their use unsatisfactory in a modern operating theatre, and which will lead to their complete withdrawal from the armamentarium of the anaesthetist in the future. To facilitate the removal of gases the standard Heidbrink expiratory valve has been modified to provide a hood and a take-off point for the effluent so that this can be ducted away. Such a valve can be placed either in a Magill circuit or in most circle systems, but has the serious disadvantage that the increased size and weight of the valve and the extra piping increases the difficulty of holding a mask on the face or of fixing an endotracheal tube firmly. This has led to the increased use of coaxial, double tube systems, such as the Bain or Lack circuits, which enable the rather clumsy valve to be mounted directly on the anaesthetic machine.

The Association of Anaesthetists produced a document giving advice on methods of pollution control in operating theatres (Association of Anaesthetists 1975). The original should be consulted for the full details, but among its recommendations were:

1. Attempts to reduce pollution in operating theatres need not wait for the development of adequate monitoring programmes, nor for agreed standards of maximum levels that should be permitted.
2. Antipollution systems should be fitted with non-standard fittings or a 30 mm male cone to minimize the risk of misconnection.
3. Outlet vents should be clearly labelled 'Danger: Anaesthetic gases'.
4. The use of existing hospital piped medical vacuum systems is not recommended.

The DOH endorsed this report a year later (DHSS 1976). Subsequently the apparatus required for gas scavenging has been the subject of a British Standard (British Standards Institution 1987). The American National Standards Institute (ANSI) published similar guidelines for the use of the manufacturers of anaesthetic apparatus in 1982.

In conducting the waste gas away from the operating theatre atmosphere to the outside, two systems are currently in use. These are either active or passive according to the method used to propel the gases along the duct. The former requires the aid of an outside source of power; the latter relies on the patient's own expiratory efforts.

Gray (1985) described four components of a scavenging system: the collecting system, transfer system, receiving system and disposal system. The disposal system is outside the operating theatre, but the other parts are usually within and in close proximity to the anaesthetic apparatus.

The collecting system removes the gases from the expiratory valve or port of the anaesthetic apparatus and delivers them to the transfer system. This then permits the gases to flow to a receiving system. The tubing used for the transfer system should be non-kinkable, have a low resistance to flow and be kept as short as possible. A compromise has to be reached between the safety of corrugated tubing and its higher resistance to flow. The system should have a means of releasing positive pressure above 1–2 kPa to prevent the patient circuit from being over-pressurized. The receiving system should incorporate a reservoir and be capable of limiting both the positive and negative pressures within it. The American anaesthetist refers to this function of the receiving system as the 'scavenging interface' because of its importance in protecting the breathing circuit or ventilator from the effects of excessive positive or negative pressure. These 'interfaces' can assume many forms and may be open (without valves) or closed (when the pressure is regulated by means of valves). The former are probably safer for the patient. Finally the gases are delivered to a disposal system which passes them to the outside atmosphere. This may be done passively, that is by the patient's own power, or actively, when assisted by an air-pumping system of some sort.

Passive scavenging

Passive scavenging depends on the patient being able to propel the gas along the duct by his own expiratory efforts. The resistance of the duct must be low and must be incapable of occlusion by outside forces. It is usual to provide a 'break' in the system, usually in the form of an aperture or valve that will prevent a pressure build up but which discharges into a reservoir bag to prevent loss to the theatre atmosphere. The outside terminal or 'ventile' of the system must be away from any air intake into the theatre, or elsewhere, and be well protected from occlusion. Occlusion of such an outlet can occur by such simple means as a change in wind force or direction if the outlet is in an exposed position. The outlet must always be guarded. Such a system must not be branched to provide many inlet ports and should contain few bends. A well-constructed passive system probably presents less hazard to the patient than an active system, but two serious problems remain:

1. Resistance to expiration is increased. This will increase the work of breathing and may cause a rise in $P\text{aCO}_2$. Such expiratory resistance, even if only moderate, may adversely affect the pattern of gas flow within the breathing circuit by altering the pressure required to open the expiratory valve. If a partial rebreathing circuit is in use the proportion of rebreathed gases will be increased. It is recommended that resistance to gas flow along the pipe should not exceed 0.5 cm of water at a flow of 30 l/min. Such a resistance is found with 50 m of unbent smooth bore pipe of 1" diameter. Corrugated tubing increases resistance by a factor of 8, and bends will impose further increases.
2. Complete obstruction of the exhaust pipe close to the patient (if undetected in a circuit without leaks) will inevitably lead to overpressure on the lung and consequential cardiac arrest. The tubing should be able to resist compression by any force that may be applied to it in the operating theatre, such as impact by trolley wheels. However, such reinforced tubing is very heavy and therefore unsuitable for attachment to the patient's end of the circuit. The use of corrugated tubing is a compromise that reduces the risk of obstruction but increases the total resistance of a given length of pipe.

Thus there is no completely safe method of passive scavenging.

Active scavenging

The active scavenging system utilizes a source of power to draw the effluent from the patient's spill valve along a pipe to the outside atmosphere. Such a system should be constructed so as to prevent excess negative pressure being applied to the patient's airway. It is recommended that the negative pressure does not exceed 1 cm of water. A safety device to do this is built into the 'scavenging interface' referred to on page 463. It usually incorporates a system of valves on a closed reservoir which open if certain pressure limits are exceeded, or relies on the provision of an aperture so that the negative pressure is not applied directly to the patient circuit. This aperture is contained within a sleeve large enough to prevent the escape of gases into the theatre, which thus effectively acts as a reservoir for the waste gas. Active scavenging overcomes the problem of resistance to expiration seen with the passive system, but with some types valve failure exposes the patient to excess negative pressure. To achieve efficient scavenging, very high gas flows of the order of 250 l/min may be required.

The problem of complete obstruction of the exhaust-pipe near to the patient still remains, even with an active system that incorporates an aperture to allow spillover in the event of pump failure. The only method of overcoming this potentially serious and very common hazard is to position the spill-valve or aperture immediately adjacent to the expiratory valve, but this is very rarely seen in practice. The outside terminal of an active system must also be away from any other air intake, but is not so subject to wind problems as a passive system outlet.

Active scavenging systems tend to be noisy in operation, and for this reason are not liked by some theatre users, and of course are subject to power failure.

The chief criticism of scavenging apparatus is that it adds considerably to the complexity of the standard Boyle's anaesthetic machine and thus must increase the hazard to the patient. Many practising anaesthetists feel that it is time the whole concept of this machine is reviewed to reduce the many possibilities of incorrect connections, although the female and male connections of a scavenging system should be of a different size to the breathing systems. The transfer tubing can be fitted with either 30 mm or 19 mm tapered connections, but the disposal apparatus, where not permanently fitted, should employ tapers of dimensions other than 30 mm, 19 mm or 22 mm to prevent incorrect assembly.

CONCLUSION

Thus we return to the problem outlined at the start of this chapter, namely the addition of many hazards to the patient in order, perhaps, to protect the staff from an as yet unquantified risk to themselves. This increased risk to the patient would be justified if the reduction of theatre pollution could be proved to protect the staff from adverse effects and the patient from mistakes made by staff whose blood levels of trace anaesthetic vapours were too high.

REFERENCES

American National Standard for Anesthetic Equipment: Scavenging systems for excess anesthetic gases (ANSI Z79 11 1982). American National Standards Institute. New York.

Association of Anaesthetists of Great Britain and Ireland 1975 Advice to members from council: pollution of the atmosphere of operating theatres. Anaesthesia 30: 697–699

British Standards Institution 1987 British Standard 6834: Active anaesthetic gas scavenging systems. British Standards Institution, London

Bruce D L, Eide K A, Linde H W, Eckenhoff J E 1968 Causes of death among anesthesiologists: a 20 year survey. Anesthesiology 29: 565–569

Bruce D L, Bach M J, Arbit J 1974a Trace anesthetic effects on perceptual cognitive and motor skills. Anesthesiology 40: 453–458

Bruce D L, Eide K A, Smith N J, Seltzer F, Dykes M H M 1974b A prospective survey of anesthesiologist mortality 1967–1971. Anesthesiology 41: 71–74

Davenport H T, Halsey M J, Wardley-Smith B, Bateman P E 1980 Occupational exposure to anaesthetics in 20 hospitals. Anaesthesia 35: 354–359

Department of Health 1976 Pollution of operating theatres, etc. by anaesthetic gases. HC(76)38 or SHHD/DS(76)65. DHSS, London

Fleming D C, Johnstone R E 1977 Recognition thresholds for diethyl ether and halothane. Anesthesiology 46: 68–69

Gray W M 1985 Scavenging equipment. Br J Anaesth 57: 685–695

Knill-Jones R P, Rodrigues L V, Moir D D, Spence A A 1972 Anaesthetic practice and pregnancy: controlled survey of women anaesthetists in the United Kingdom. Lancet 1: 1326–1328

Linde H W, Bruce D L 1969 Occupational exposure of anesthetists to halothane, nitrous oxide and radiation. Anesthesiology 30: 363–368

Logan M, Farmer J G 1989 Anaesthesia and the ozone layer. Br J Anaesth 63: 645–647

NIOSH 1977 Criteria for a recommended standard: occupational exposure to waste anaesthetic gases and vapors. DHEW Publication No. 77–140. US Government Printing Office, Washington D.C.

Pharoah P O D, Alberman E, Doyle P, Chamberlain G 1977 Outcome of pregnancy among women in anaesthetic practice. Lancet 1: 34–36

Spence A A, Wall R A, Nunn J F 1989 In: Nunn J F, Utting J E, Brown B R (eds) General anaesthesia, 5th edn. Butterworths, London, ch 47, p 598

FURTHER READING

Davey A, Moyle J T B, Ward C S 1992 Ward's anaesthetic equipment, 3rd edn. W B Saunders, London, pp 279–292

Vessey M P 1978 Epidemiological studies of the occupational hazards of anaesthesia: a review. Anaesthesia 33: 430–439

SECTION 5

Hazards of anaesthesia procedures

31

Airway manipulations

M. R. Patrick

INTRODUCTION

General anaesthesia is always attended by risk. Nowhere in the practice of anaesthesia is this more true than in the context of the airway. The conscious animal is protected by a battery of reflex mechanisms that prevent obstruction of the airway and prevent foreign matter entering the lungs. General anaesthesia always depresses these reflexes, exposing the animal to risk. This chapter deals with the hazards that relate to difficulty with the airway during anaesthesia, and the complications that arise from efforts and techniques used to maintain the airway.

MASK ANAESTHESIA

The clear airway

Unobstructed spontaneous respiration is quiet. It is never noisy nor silent. The chest and abdomen of a supine patient move up and down synchronously and without apparent effort. The larynx, seen externally most easily as the apex of the thyroid cartilage, stays in the same position during inspiration and expiration, there being no inspiratory laryngotracheal descent. There is no indrawing of supraclavicular or suprasternal structures, no intercostal or subcostal recession and no use of the accessory muscles of respiration.

The opposites to the above become apparent when the airway is obstructed. Total respiratory obstruction is always silent since there is no movement of air to generate noise. Conversely, partial obstruction is accompanied by noises such as snoring, grunting, stridor or wheezing. There is inspiratory laryngotracheal descent, indrawing, recession and use of accessory muscles. Cyanosis may accompany the picture and this can be especially difficult to detect in dark-skinned patients who require special vigilance, and in whom pulse oximetry is particularly useful. Some of the signs of airways obstruction may be produced in other situations. For example residual neuromuscular blockade or bronchospasm can both superficially mimic upper airway obstruction and an accurate diagnosis must be made quickly.

Failure to maintain a clear airway at all times constitutes a serious danger to the patient. Quite apart from the impairment of gas exchange that occurs in airway obstruction there are other risks. Regurgitation and aspiration of gastric contents, pulmonary oedema and cardiovascular disturbances can all be precipitated by airway obstruction.

Causes of airway obstruction during anaesthesia

Upper airway obstruction, which can occur at several sites, and laryngospasm are the two common and treatable causes of an obstructed airway during anaesthesia. There is also evidence that anaesthetic agents cause an alteration in the pattern of activation of the muscles which maintain the upper airway. This too can contribute to upper airway obstruction (Drummond 1989).

Upper airway obstruction: maintaining the airway

When the head is in a neutral position the principal axes of the mouth and pharynx lie approximately at right angles to each other. The two axes can be aligned by flexing the neck while at the same time extending the head at the occipitoatlantoaxial complex. In practice this is achieved by placing the head on one generous pillow while holding up the chin. The above manoeuvre has two consequences. First, it pulls the tongue anteriorly away from the soft palate and away from the posterior wall of the pharynx. Second, it causes the hyoid bone to move anteriorly in relation to the thyroid cartilage, and this lifts the epiglottis up away from the glottis and the posterior pharyngeal wall (Boidin 1985). Both these effects improve upper airway patency, and this position is accepted as being the best for maintenance of the airway. However, obstruction sometimes persists despite the above positioning. In these patients the above manoeuvre can be augmented by applying forward pressure behind the mandibular rami, a move that often causes the temporomandibular joints to dislocate. This is not usually a problem, but isolated cases of facial nerve palsy have occurred. Occasionally, rotating the head to one side or the other may improve the airway. Great care must be taken while moving the head and neck in patients with cervical spine pathology in whom spinal cord compression can occur (Edelist 1964).

Laryngospasm

Laryngospasm – forced closure of the glottis by the action of the intrinsic laryngeal muscles – occurs very commonly during general anaesthesia. There are many causes. These include attempts at performing laryngoscopy under light anaesthesia, performance of surgery (particularly of the perineum and anus) under light anaesthesia, the presence of foreign matter such as blood, saliva, sputum or vomitus on or near the vocal cords and the inhalation of irritant vapours. Laryngospasm occurs commonly in children in whom it is particularly dangerous because their high oxygen consumption leads rapidly to hypoxaemia.

Premedication with anticholinergic drugs to reduce secretions, and topical analgesia of the airway, reduce the incidence of laryngospasm. Administration of muscle relaxants prevents and abolishes laryngospasm because the intrinsic laryngeal muscles are of the striated type.

Clinically, laryngospasm may be partial or complete. In partial spasm the patient makes a typical ‘crowing’ sound during inspiration. The tighter the spasm, the higher the frequency of the sound generated. When the spasm is complete the patient makes no sound at all. Both forms are accompanied by the hallmarks of respiratory obstruction.

Treatment must be instituted immediately. Initially this consists of administering 100% oxygen with the expiratory valve of the anaesthetic circuit almost closed to produce positive pressure: the so-called ‘tight bag’. If this is ineffective, as evidenced by continuing respiratory obstruction or a fall in arterial oxygen saturation, the safest course of action is to administer a muscle relaxant and controlled ventilation. Suxamethonium is the relaxant of choice because of the rapidity of onset of its action.

Prolonged, tight laryngospasm never occurs in an awake patient who will always reflexly attempt to remove the cause of the spasm, either by coughing if the cause is foreign material on the larynx or by attempting to get away from the source of an irritant vapour. Similarly, laryngospasm never occurs during deep surgical anaesthesia because the laryngeal reflexes are obtunded by such anaesthesia. This has important consequences in relation to the timing of extubation (see extubation, p. 496).

Pharyngeal airways

Frequently, despite correct positioning of the head, a clear airway cannot be produced, even with anterior dislocation of the temporomandibular joint, and it is necessary to use an artificial airway. A variety of such devices exist for both oral and nasal use, including the laryngeal mask airway which will be discussed separately (see p. 473). Of the remaining types, the Guedel pattern has become the standard for oral use. It is an excellent device although there are two hazards that may be encountered during its use. First, during insertion it is possible for the advancing tip of the airway to push the tongue back into the pharynx so that it lies behind the airway rather than below its concave lower surface. This invariably results in respiratory obstruction. It is best avoided by inserting the airway upside down until the tip reaches the hard palate and then rotating the airway through 180° before advancing it into the final position. Second, a check should always be made that neither the lips nor the tongue are interposed between the teeth and the airway to prevent trauma due to biting.

A nasal airway can be made by cutting an appropriately sized endotracheal tube to the required length. Alternatively there are proprietary devices both reusable and disposable. It is vital that nasal airways are the correct length. If they are too short they simply do not work; if too long they may irritate the larynx causing laryngospasm. For most adults the correct length is 12–15 cm. For males the diameter should be 7.0–7.5 mm and for females 6.5–7.0 mm. Diameters for children are the same as for endotracheal tubes (see Table 31.1, p. 490). The use of larger diameter nasal airways than these is unnecessary, causing trauma to the nasal passages and possibly fracturing the turbinates.

Other measures are also necessary to minimize trauma. Airways, and indeed any hardware introduced into the respiratory tract, should be lubricated with a sterile water soluble jelly (such as K-Y). Insertion should be as gentle as possible and force should not be used. If the airway will not easily pass the other nostril should be tried. If this fails a smaller size should be used. The airway should be rotated back and forth as it is advanced as this reduces the likelihood of stripping the nasal mucosa. Mucosal trauma causes bleeding and the blood may track back into the pharynx. If the blood then reaches the larynx, laryngospasm may occur. With either nasal airways or nasotracheal tubes there is an incidence of pharyngeal perforation and retropharyngeal abscess formation (Tintinalli & Claffey 1981). This is a serious complication as it can lead to upper airway obstruction several days later. Conversely, nasal airways should not be used in the presence of such an abscess since abscess rupture may occur leading to soiling of the lungs.

Actual disappearance of the airway is potentially a problem. This can be overcome either by transfixing the proximal end of the airway with a safety pin or by using a flanged airway. The Portex nasal airway, although flanged, should be used with a transfixing pin as the flange is not very large. The device is supplied with a safety pin for this purpose.

Facemasks

The most important goal with a facemask is to achieve a good seal on the face as easily as possible. Failure to produce a seal causes dilution of the gases being delivered through the anaesthetic circuit with ambient air, leading to a reduction in the inspired oxygen concentration and inadequate delivery of anaesthetic. Artificial ventilation by facemask is impossible in the presence of a large leak with constitutes a line of least resistance through which the gases escape. This is potentially hazardous, especially in a paralysed patient and in the presence of an obstructed airway where sustained positive pressure is sometimes necessary to help overcome the obstruction.

Correct use of a facemask therefore starts with selection of the appropriate size and shape. The former is often a case of trial and error. The latter rests with the preference of the anaesthetist. I prefer the McKesson pattern which has a very soft inflatable rim and provides a good seal in most patients. Sometimes, however, a seal is genuinely difficult to achieve. Bearded men are notoriously difficult in this respect. The edentulous are another difficult group, particularly if much bony resorption has occurred in the mandible. Often the best approach to the use of a facemask in the edentulous patient is to close the mouth (inserting an airway if necessary) and to hook the facemask around the underneath of the mandible rather than the usual position in front of the chin. This manoeuvre requires a large mask to be successful.

Infants, but not those below about 6 months of age who should virtually always be intubated, may be satisfactorily anaesthetized by facemask for short procedures. The often cited danger of excessive mask deadspace with some designs is less of a hazard than failure to produce a seal, therefore facemasks with inflatable rims are sometimes better than the theoretically superior Rendell–Baker types for this reason. Neonates should never be anaesthetized, nor ventilated by facemask. The latter merely succeeds in inflating the stomach due to the relatively high compliance of the abdomen compared with the thorax in this age-group (Hatch & Sumner 1981). The only use for a facemask in neonatal anaesthesia is for preoxygenation.

Patients with epidermolysis bullosa dystrophica (a rare inherited skin condition in which bulla formation occurs with subsequent scarring in response to mechanical trauma), especially of a shearing nature, require special care. Facemask rims must be coated with paraffin gauze. Endotracheal anaesthesia is often preferable to facemask anaesthesia for, no matter how gentle the handling of the patient's skin, traction is always required to hold on a facemask. All items (facemasks, tubes, laryngoscopes, etc.) should be liberally lubricated all over to minimize trauma to the mouth and airway, which may also be involved in the disease process. Many anaesthetists utilize the special properties of ketamine, with its tendency to preserve muscle tone, to enable the airway to be maintained under anaesthesia without the need for hazardous manual interference in these patients (Reddy & Wong 1972).

Harnesses

A harness is a useful adjunct to facemask anaesthesia as it frees the anaesthetist's hands. However, particular care needs to be paid to maintaining the airway when using a harness as obstruction is much more likely to pass unrecognized than when the facemask is being held on by hand. When using the Clausen type, which is the most common variety, it is important to ensure that the harness is truly centrally placed behind the head, otherwise it tends to slip off. Straps should be just tight enough to produce a seal. Excessively tight straps cause unsightly marks and may obstruct the venous drainage of the face and scalp. Much more serious, facial nerve palsy has been attributed to tight straps, as have sporadic cases of blindness due to retinal artery thrombosis. Tight lower straps frequently cause airway obstruction by pulling the mandible, and therefore the tongue, in a posterior direction. Finally, a check should always be made, before attaching the straps, that the eyes are fully closed and that neither the lips nor the tongue are caught between the teeth and an airway.

Dental damage

Damage to teeth during anaesthesia is one of the most common causes for litigation in anaesthetic practice. Dental crown and bridge work is time consuming and very expensive, and the distress produced by damage to these items is therefore hardly surprising. Certain features, notably loose teeth, and crowns and bridges, especially if involving the incisors, should alert the anaesthetist, for these are at greatest risk from mishap. However, even a normal healthy tooth can be chipped or broken by a carelessly wielded laryngoscope both during insertion and removal. Poor laryngoscopy technique, using the upper incisors as a fulcrum, is also a potent cause of damage.

If a patient has dentition that is likely to be fragile, it is correct practice to warn the patient before the anaesthetic that there is the possibility of damage. This fact and the warning should be recorded in the notes. If this is done and the patient is reassured that all possible care will be taken, the likelihood of resentment later is less.

In addition to cosmetic damage there is the hazard of inhalation or swallowing of broken teeth, an inhaled tooth requiring bronchoscopic removal. The use of a tooth shield and of a foam strip on the laryngoscope blade have been advocated to help avoid damage to the upper teeth (Lisman et al 1981). If there is any difficulty in intubating a patient with fragile dentition, my practice is to intubate with a long gum-elastic or neoprene oesophageal bougie, which is far easier to pass under difficult conditions than a tube, and then to railroad the tube down the bougie.

Fragile front teeth can be regarded as an indication to avoid an oral airway for, though it may be inserted atraumatically, damage may occur at the end of the anaesthetic when muscle tone returns and the airway is bitten on to. This is especially likely after inhalational anaesthesia with spontaneous respiration.

Ocular damage

Damage to eyes is always serious. The most common problem is the production of corneal abrasions as a result of physical trauma. Surgical drapes, instruments, hands and anaesthetic hardware have all been implicated as causes. Cleaning solutions may inadvertently enter the eyes causing irritation. Facemasks and the use of the prone position may produce orbital and periorbital compression. This can lead to retinal detachments and retinal artery thrombosis causing blindness, though this is very rare.

If the eyes are hidden from the anaesthetist's view, or if they do not remain closed, they should be taped to prevent them opening inadvertently, especially if a surgical drape is to lie directly on the face. The placing of drops or ointment in the eyes for lubrication does not alter the necessity to ensure that the eyes are at all times closed.

If a patient awakes with a painful eye, early diagnosis is essential to rule out serious conditions, especially acute glaucoma. Simple abrasions usually heal rapidly and spontaneously, and patient comfort can be improved by covering the eye with a patch until healing has occurred.

THE LARYNGEAL MASK AIRWAY

The laryngeal mask airway (LMA) is a major landmark in the progress of evolution of equipment in anaesthesia. First described by Brain (1983), it has rapidly become established in anaesthetic practice and is now a major part of the technical armamentarium of many anaesthetists. Both structurally and functionally it occupies a position intermediate between the facemask and the endotracheal tube, and it may be used in circumstances in which either of the latter might previously have been used, during both spontaneous and controlled ventilation (Brain et al 1985). The LMA comes in four sizes, of which sizes 1 and 2 are for paediatric use, and sizes 3 and 4 are for adults. Neonates and infants below 6 months of age should not in my opinion be anaesthetized using an LMA. The relative difficulty of maintaining the airway and the speed of onset of hypoxaemia in this age-group mean that these children should always be intubated with a standard endotracheal tube. The LMA has been advocated for use in patients that for various reasons have proved difficult to intubate (Brain 1985, Calder et al 1990), and for use in emergency situations (Brain 1984).

Insertion of the LMA is not always easy and practice with the device is required to achieve a high level of success. One difficulty frequently encountered is folding back of the tip of the inflatable cuff as the device is advanced into the pharynx. Thorough lubrication of the posterior surface can help avoid this difficulty, as can injection of a small amount of air into the cuff before insertion. Alternatively the device can be inserted facing posteriorly until it reaches the pharynx and then rotated through 180°.

Malpositioning of the LMA once inserted can also occur. Rotation through 180° so that the orifice faces posteriorly was reported in 2 out of 100 patients in one series using prototype LMAs (Brodrick et al 1989). Down-folding of the epiglottis appears to be a common problem but is only infrequently associated with airway obstruction. Failure to secure a clear airway following insertion of an LMA happens in only a minority of cases, but the presence of unobstructed respiration must always be verified. If there is any doubt whatsoever about airway patency the device should be removed and, if appropriate, reinserted.

Laryngospasm in the presence of an LMA is always a potential problem as the device does not cross the vocal cords. During spontaneous respiration this will be manifested in a similar manner to laryngospasm during facemask anaesthesia (see p. 470). During controlled ventilation, laryngospasm is a potential hazard as the effect of the muscle relaxant wanes towards the end of a procedure. This hazard can be minimized by the use of appropriate monitoring, consisting of a capnograph and an airway pressure monitor to detect obstruction.

The LMA should never be regarded as a substitute for an endotracheal tube in a patient with a full stomach or in any circumstance in which regurgitation is a possibility. However, if intubation has proved impossible in such a patient, an LMA can be used to maintain the airway. In this situation a small endotracheal tube can be inserted through the LMA to secure the airway against regurgitated material. A 6.0 mm Mallinckrodt tube will pass through a size 4 LMA, and a 5.0 mm will pass through a size 3 LMA (see Fig. 31.1).

The endotracheal tube should be rotated 90° anticlockwise to prevent snagging on the grille of the LMA during insertion, and securely fastened once in position.

The pressor response to laryngoscopy and intubation appears also to occur in response to LMA insertion, but the response is attenuated (Braude et al 1989). The LMA therefore has a possible advantage in this respect over an endotracheal tube in patients with coronary artery disease or hypertension, in whom increases in heart rate and arterial pressure are best avoided.

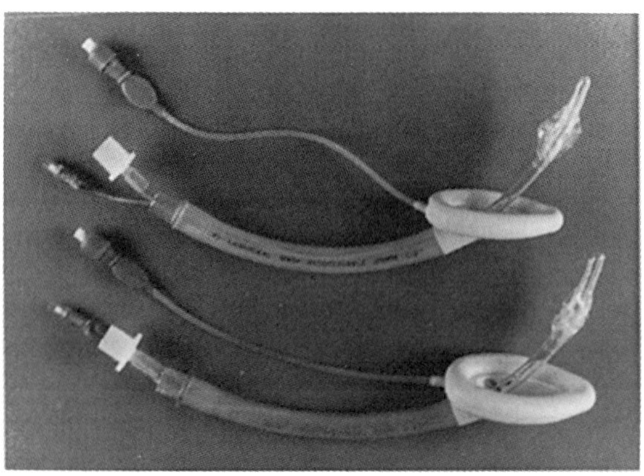

Fig. 31.1 Size 5.0 and 6.0 Mallinckrodt endotracheal tubes railroaded down size 3 and 4 laryngeal mask airways, respectively.

LARYNGOSCOPY AND TRACHEAL INTUBATION

Positioning the patient for laryngoscopy

Correct positioning for laryngoscopy is the same as positioning to achieve a clear airway. The neck should be flexed and the head extended at the occipitoatlantoaxial complex by placing the head on one generous pillow and pulling the mandible upwards (Magill 1930). It has been shown that extension at the occipitoatlantoaxial complex is near maximal during laryngoscopy (Horton et al 1989). While this is safe for the majority of patients, great care has to be exercised when there is cervical spine pathology, for these patients may suffer spinal cord compression when the cervical spine is moved (Norton & Ghanma 1982). The following list indicates the conditions in which cervical spine instability occurs:

- rheumatoid arthritis
- cervical spine fractures
- osteoporosis
- tumour deposits
- congenital malformations: Morquio's syndrome.

By far the most important group numerically comprises those patients with rheumatoid arthritis. Approximately 25% of such patients have instability of the atlantoaxial joint, and in some of these there are no symptoms or clinical signs of cervical spine disease (Norton & Ghanma 1982). The pathological picture of bony destruction of the odontoid process and weakening of the transverse ligament of the atlas allows the odontoid process to move posteriorly, compressing the cord against the posterior arch of the atlas. Fortunately the instability is usually worsened by flexion of the head, not extension. Nevertheless, great care is required during positioning not only for laryngoscopy, but also for surgery, especially where this involves turning the patient. One approach to safe positioning for laryngoscopy is to ask the patient to extend his own neck as far as possible. The position can then be maintained by an assistant holding the head firmly during laryngoscopy.

In view of the lack of correlation between clinical manifestations of cervical spine disease and actual pathology in rheumatoid arthritis, it is advisable to obtain preoperative lateral radiographs of the neck in both flexion and extension in all such patients. It is important to look for forward movement of the anterior arch of the atlas away from the odontoid process, or separation of the process from the body of the axis.

Patients with cervical spine fractures constitute another group requiring great care during laryngoscopy. Many of these patients wear a supportive collar that may itself make the procedure more difficult. All such patients should be laryngoscoped with an assistant firmly holding the neck in a neutral position. Exposure of the larynx may therefore be difficult and a selection of tubes and bougies should be available should problems arise. Muscle relaxants should be used to aid intubation in these patients, but suxamethonium is best avoided because displacement of the fracture can theoretically occur with the fasciculations produced by this drug (Norton & Ghanma 1982). Alternatively, an awake fibreoptic intubation can be performed.

The other causes of cervical spine instability are all rare but should be remembered as possible sources of hazard during laryngoscopy.

Trauma during laryngoscopy

Correct laryngoscopy technique cannot be learned from a book; it has to be achieved through practice in the clinical setting. There are, however, one or two points worth mentioning. A check should always be made prior to use that the laryngoscope bulb is properly attached and working, and that a second laryngoscope is available. The laryngoscope needs to be used with care. A carelessly wielded or dropped laryngoscope may traumatize any part of the face, eyes, lips, teeth, palate, pharynx or larynx. Always ensure that neither the lips nor the tongue is caught between the teeth and the laryngoscope blade. Gingival damage commonly occurs in edentulous patients as a result of the laryngoscope blade pivoting on and cutting the upper gum. This can be avoided by placing a folded gauze swab over the gum. Correctly placed, the swab does not impair the view of the larynx. Lingual nerve damage has been reported following laryngoscopy (Loughman 1983) but this seems to be a rare complication. It is thought to occur by compression of the nerve by the laryngoscope blade and is therefore presumably less likely if the tongue is displaced to the left by the blade rather than trapped by it.

Laryngeal reflexes

Various reflex disturbances are known to occur in response to laryngoscopy and endotracheal intubation. These disturbances are a source of morbidity and mortality. They are worsened by inappropriate or inadequate anaesthesia, and by hypoxia and hypercarbia (Blanc & Tremblay 1974). Coughing, gagging, vomiting and laryngospasm commonly occur when anaesthesia is too light in patients who have not received muscle relaxants. Tachycardia and hypertension almost invariably accompany laryngoscopy, but occasionally bradycardia and asystole occur. Although reports are scarce, bradycardia and asystole following laryngoscopy are almost certainly more common when a combination of a potent opioid and a muscle relaxant devoid of vagolytic activity is used without vagolytic drugs prior to intubation. Bradycardia and laryngospasm are less likely in an atropinized patient, though the use of this drug is not always appropriate, especially in the presence of ischaemic heart disease.

Plasma noradrenaline levels have been shown to rise in association with laryngoscopy, and this increase is at least in part responsible for the hypertension, tachycardia and sometimes pathological tachyarrhythmias that occur during the procedure. This type of cardiovascular disturbance is potentially life-threatening in patients with coronary artery disease, cerebral vascular disease and pre-existing arterial hypertension, especially if untreated. Hypertensive patients are additionally at risk because they produce an exaggerated response (Prys-Roberts et al 1971). This subject is dealt with in Chapter 3. Suffice it to say here that proper assessment and treatment of cardiovascular disease, coupled with a technique of anaesthesia based on intravenous opioid analgesics prior to laryngoscopy to reduce the cardiovascular response, is the key to safer intubation in these patients. Beta-adrenergic antagonists are particularly valuable in obtunding the reflex haemodynamic responses to laryngoscopy, and these drugs should not be discontinued prior to anaesthesia.

Intraocular pressure increases in response to laryngoscopy. In part this is due to the increase in arterial pressure mentioned above, but it is also related to an increase in venous pressure caused by gagging and straining during laryngoscopy. The increase in pressure is therefore exaggerated in the presence of inadequate anaesthesia and muscle relaxation. This is important in the presence of a penetrating eye injury when permanent blindness may result from extrusion of the contents of the eye. Patients with such an injury should be laryngoscoped following adequate anaesthesia and full muscle relaxation. However, it is well established that suxamethonium, which itself causes a rise in intraocular pressure, should not be used in these patients.

Bacteraemia associated with laryngoscopy

Manipulations inside the mouth, notably dental extractions, are known to produce transient bacteraemia. The act of laryngoscopy has also been implicated as a cause of bacteraemia, but the incidence is low (about 2%) in the presence of healthy teeth (Gerber et al 1980). When dental sepsis is present the incidence of bacteraemia is likely to be higher. Transient bacteraemia from any source is important in patients with structural heart disease who are susceptible to the development of infective endocarditis. Even in the era of antibiotics and heart-valve replacement, the mortality from this disease is still high. It is my practice to administer appropriate antibiotic prophylaxis to all patients with structural heart disease regardless of the operative procedure, on the basis that endotracheal intubation may be required even though it was not thought necessary preoperatively. Advice as to what constitutes appropriate prophylaxis, which will vary from one patient to another, can be obtained from a microbiologist.

Difficult laryngoscopy

Ease of laryngoscopy hinges on two vital points of head and neck anatomy. First, it must be possible to extend the head on the neck at the occipitoatlantoaxial complex (Nichol & Zuck 1983). Normally, approximately 35° of extension is possible from the neutral position at these upper two cervical joints with the majority occurring at the atlantooccipital joint. Extension at these joints aligns the axes of the mouth and the pharynx, and is essential if the larynx is to be visualized. Although extension also takes place at the remainder of the joints of the cervical spine, this is not helpful to the laryngoscopist since extension at these joints causes a forward bowing of the cervical spine leading to a condition known erroneously as 'anterior larynx'. The second essential ingredient is adequate space inside the mouth to be able to angulate a laryngoscope blade, and pull the tongue forward and to the left. How to obtain this information at the bedside is discussed below.

Given appropriate anaesthetic conditions, laryngoscopy is an easy procedure in the great majority of patients. Occasionally, despite good conditions, it is impossible to visualize the vocal cords and insertion of an endotracheal tube becomes very difficult. Cormack & Lehane (1984) have classified the view obtained at laryngoscopy into four grades of difficulty. In grade 1 all or most of the glottis is visible. In grade 2 only the posterior extremity of the glottis is visible. In grade 3 only the epiglottis can be seen. In grade 4 not even the epiglottis is visible. The approximate percentages of patients falling into the above grades are: 1: 99%; 2: 1%; 3: 1

per 2000; 4: 1 per 10 000. The above classification suggests that the incidence of difficult intubation in skilled hands should be around 1%. This figure, however, depends entirely on the skill of the anaesthetist and the criteria used to define difficulty, and some workers quote a much higher figure (Mallampati et al 1985).

Both failed and successful but difficult intubations are often accompanied by periods of hypoxia which may cause cerebral damage with or without cardiac arrest. Aspiration of gastric contents is a further hazard, especially in obstetric anaesthesia and in other patients with full stomachs, and the incidence of aspiration is higher when intubation is difficult. Indeed, the combination of a difficult intubation and a patient with a full stomach is a particularly dangerous and demanding one to handle. Anticipation of difficult laryngoscopy and intubation, and the adoption of an appropriate technique, are essential if this frequent cause of anaesthetic mortality and morbidity is to be avoided.

Anticipation of difficult laryngoscopy

Certain anatomical features and pathological conditions are known to be causes of difficult laryngoscopy. These can be subdivided as follows:

- conditions in which there is difficulty opening the mouth
- conditions in which there is difficulty extending the head at the occipitoatlantoaxial complex
- conditions causing airway obstruction
- miscellaneous conditions causing difficult laryngoscopy.

Conditions causing difficulty opening the mouth

Difficulty opening the mouth (trismus) is encountered in the conditions listed below:

1. conditions causing temporomandibular joint fixity:
   - rheumatoid arthritis
   - ankylosing spondylitis
   - postsurgical
   - post-traumatic
2. fibrosis due to burns or irradiation
3. local acute infections
4. local bulky tumours
5. scleroderma
6. tongue flaps.

Many of those listed are associated with difficulty extending the head. Local infective conditions and bulky neoplasms may also cause airway obstruction. Some neoplasms are friable, bleeding occurring when the tumour is traumatized by any foreign body such as a laryngoscope. Trismus that is due to pain disappears once the patient is asleep, therefore the distinction between this and trismus due to physical restriction is an important one since the latter persists in the anaesthetized patient.

Conditions causing difficulty extending the head

Conditions causing difficulty extending the head are listed below:

- variants of normal: small atlantooccipital gap
- rheumatoid arthritis
- ankylosing spondylitis
- cervical spondylosis
- cervical fusion
- fibrosis due to burns or irradiation
- scleroderma
- tube pedicle grafts
- cystic hygroma
- encephalocele
- hydrocephalus.

Again there is overlap between these conditions and those in the other groups. Patients who have undergone cervical fusion may cause difficulty, but are often relatively easy to laryngoscope provided good mobility has been preserved at the occipitoatlantoaxial complex. Patients with an unstable cervical spine, although not strictly difficult to position, need to be considered in this group because extension of the head, while not impossible, may be extremely hazardous. The patient with an unstable cervical spine may be asked to extend his own head as far as possible, the position then being maintained by an assistant, or a neutral position may be adopted. In either case, less than ideal conditions are likely to be achieved. In a patient with a pedicle graft connecting the mandible to the anterior chest wall it may be necessary to cut the pedicle in order to intubate the patient.

Conditions causing airway obstruction

Conditions causing airway obstruction are listed below:

1. conditions causing upper airway obstruction:
   - foreign bodies
   - infections
     - diphtheria
     - quinzy (peritonsillar abscess)
     - retropharyngeal abscess
     - Ludwig's angina
   - oedema due to
     - burns
     - trauma
     - insect stings
   - tumours of
     - tongue
     - tonsil
     - nasopharynx
     - floor of mouth
     - upper or lower jaw
   - micrognathia
   - macroglossia.
2. conditions causing laryngeal obstruction:
   - foreign bodies
   - infections
     - acute epiglottitis (supraglottitis)
     - laryngotracheobronchitis (croup)
     - laryngeal diphtheria
   - oedema due to
     - burns
     - trauma
     - allergy
   - tumours
     - carcinoma, papilloma and haemangioma of larynx
   - inflammatory diseases
     - rheumatoid arthritis
     - polychondritis
   - postextubation subglottic oedema and stenosis
   - recurrent laryngeal nerve palsy
   - laryngomalacia
   - laryngeal cysts
   - laryngeal polyps
   - laryngeal webs.
3. conditions causing tracheal obstruction:
   - foreign bodies
   - tumours
     - carcinoma and papilloma of trachea
   - external compression due to
     - thyroid enlargement of tumours
     - thymic tumours
     - mediastinal lymph nodes
     - haematomata (notably after thyroid and carotid surgery)
   - tracheomalacia
   - vascular rings
   - post-traumatic strictures.

The management of the patient with airway obstruction is difficult and hazardous whatever the cause of the obstruction. Management is considered later in this chapter.

Miscellaneous conditions causing difficult laryngoscopy

The remaining conditions causing difficult laryngoscopy are listed below:

1. variants of normal
   - small mouth (large tongue, receding jaw)
2. acromegaly
3. thyroid enlargement
4. thyroglossal cysts
5. bulky tonsils
6. facial injuries
7. cleft palate
8. inherited and congenital facial abnormalities
   - Hurler's syndrome, Pierre–Robin anomalad.

Attempts have been made by many workers to correlate variations in clinical and radiological anatomy of the head and neck with difficult laryngoscopy. In this context it is important to have simple bedside questions and tests that can be applied to all patients at the preoperative visit, with a more thorough examination, and investigations, should these appear necessary. Unfortunately, no single bedside test to assess ease of intubation is accurately predictive all of the time. As was stated above, the two important pieces of information to be obtained are the extent of occipitoatlantoaxial extension and the amount of space inside the mouth. Extension of the head can be assessed by asking the patient to sit up with the head facing straight forward and the mouth wide open. The occlusal surfaces of the upper teeth should be in a horizontal plane in this position. The patient is then asked to extend his head as far as possible without moving the neck, and the angle of the upper teeth relative to the horizontal plane is again noted. On this basis, Bellhouse & Doré (1988) have developed a grading system. Patients in grade 1 have full (35°) extension. In grade 2 there is a one-third reduction. In grade 3 there is a two-thirds reduction. In grade 4 there is a total absence of extension. Further information about extension of the head can be obtained by performing a lateral radiograph of the neck with the head in a neutral position. White & Kander (1975) have implied that, if the distance between the occiput and the posterior tubercle of the atlas is 5 mm or greater, laryngoscopy is likely to be easy. Conversely, if the distance is 4 mm or less than laryngoscopy will be difficult. Samsoon & Young (1987) have described a simple test to assess the size of the mouth. The patient is asked to sit up straight, open his mouth wide and protrude the tongue as far as possible. Patients can be divided into four grades by this means. In patients in grade 1 the entire uvula can be seen. In grade 2 part of the uvula can still be seen. In grade 3 none of the uvula can be seen and only the soft palate is visible. In grade 4 only the hard palate is visible.

The above two bedside tests allow patients to be allocated a degree of likely difficulty; the higher the aggregate score of grades the greater the difficulty. Edentulous patients are always easier than the score would predict, although those with partial upper dentition are notorious for being difficult because the laryngoscope often rests in the gap between the teeth, thus reducing the effective mouth opening afforded by the laryngoscope.

Management of difficult laryngoscopy and intubation

Assessment

The management of patients likely to be difficult to intubate is made safer by adequate preoperative assessment and all patients should always be assessed prior to anaesthesia. Assessment must include the variables mentioned above, namely head extension, mouth size and dentition. In addition the presence of stridor, cyanosis and the use of the accessory muscles of respiration must be noted, these being signs of upper airway obstruction. If there are clinical signs of upper airway obstruction, radiographs of the chest, thoracic inlet and neck, both anteroposterior and lateral, can be obtained to help localize the site of obstruction. In emergencies, such as acute epiglottitis, where complete airway obstruction can occur at any time, radiography may well be both dangerous and unhelpful. If, however, radiography is felt necessary, the patient should be accompanied by an anaesthetist during the process.

The use of antisialogogues

In any case of anticipated difficult laryngoscopy it is good practice to use antisialogogue premedication. There are two reasons for this. First, the presence of excessive saliva may make the larynx even more difficult to visualize than it already is. Second, if induction of anaesthesia without muscle relaxants is being employed, the likelihood of laryngospasm occurring is greatly reduced by antisialogogue premedication. The antisialogogue should be administered intramuscularly 45 min preoperatively, not intravenously in the anaesthetic room.

Sedative premedication

Sedative premedication should never be used in patients with airway obstruction, in whom frank respiratory failure may be precipitated. It is also safer to avoid opiates in any patient who is likely to be a serious intubation problem, in whom spontaneous ventilation is being maintained after induction prior to intubation. Patients with trismus or a mass lesion in the upper airway would fall into this category. The combination of opiates and other anaesthetic agents may produce unwanted apnoea. Patients to be intubated under local analgesia may be safely sedated, except, again, in the presence of airway obstruction. Sedation must also be used with caution in the patient with a full stomach being intubated under local analgesia, because depression of upper airway reflexes may allow the patient to aspirate gastric contents.

The use of muscle relaxants

The use of muscle relaxants in some cases of difficult intubation may be hazardous. A clear distinction must therefore be made between when and when not to use relaxants. The decision is based on whether the anaesthetist believes the patient will be able to maintain a patent upper airway once anaesthetized, with or without a pharyngeal airway, and whether intermittent positive pressure ventilation (IPPV) by mask can then be achieved. Only if the answer to both questions is yes can a muscle relaxant safely be administered. From the practical standpoint, patients that are likely to be difficult to intubate because of difficult anatomy may be safely given a relaxant. The incidence of failure to both intubate and ventilate by mask in these patients is of the order of one in 15 000. Conversely, in the presence of airway obstruction, muscle relaxants are absolutely contraindicated until ventilation by mask has been shown to be feasible. In between these two extremes lies a grey area. If there is any doubt, muscle relaxants should be avoided.

The choice of technique in difficult situations

Assuming that intubation is necessary, the choice lies between performing it under local analgesia with or without sedation, or under general anaesthesia, or, rarely, whether preoperative tracheostomy under local analgesia should be performed. With the increasing excellence and availability of fibre-optic intubating laryngoscopes and increasing familiarity with their use, more patients with difficult airways will be intubated by this method and tracheostomy should become unnecessary.

Adults with severe upper airway obstruction, as evidenced by stridor at rest, cyanosis and the use of the accessory muscles of respiration should be intubated awake with the fibre-optic laryngoscope. Awake intubation for children with severe upper airway obstruction is difficult both for the child and the anaesthetist, excepting those anaesthetists that frequently use the technique. General anaesthesia is usually required in these patients. Almost all other patients can safely be intubated under general anaesthesia provided the correct technique is used.

Patients with mild degrees of difficulty in opening the mouth or extending the head, and those with facial and neck anatomy likely to result in a difficult laryngoscopy, may be safely anaesthetized by any method, the object being to provide the best possible conditions for intubation. Muscle relaxants should be used in these patients. Provided the patient does not have a full stomach, I believe it is safer and easier to intubate using a large dose of a non-depolarizing relaxant rather than suxamethonium. This provides excellent intubating conditions, and the requirement to keep giving additional suxamethonium with its attendant side effects is eliminated.

A selection of different endotracheal tubes, laryngoscopes and bougies should be available. Smaller sizes of the long flexible gum elastic or neoprene bougies used for dilating the oesophagus (e.g. the Negus bougie) and steerable bougies are particularly helpful. The patient is intubated with the bougie and the tube is 'railroaded' down, taking care to rotate the tube 90° anticlockwise as it passes through the larynx. Intubation under local analgesia is neither necessary nor appropriate in these patients.

Patients with severe difficulty opening the mouth or extending the head, those with mass lesions distorting the airway and those with lesser degrees of airway obstruction should be intubated under local analgesia with the fibre-optic laryngoscope, or should receive an inhalational induction with spontaneous ventilation until IPPV by mask is shown to be feasible. If this is the case, a relaxant may be administered. Partial closure of the expiratory valve of the anaesthetic circuit to produce positive end expiratory pressure (PEEP), the so called 'tight bag', may help to maintain airway patency in obstructed cases.

Halothane in oxygen is suitable for inhalational induction and is at least as good as, if not better than, the newer fluorinated ethers, the theoretical advantages of which are negated by their pungent odour. Very small doses of an intravenous induction agent may sometimes help an inhalational induction, but doses large enough to produce apnoea should not be used. A full range of intubating equipment should be available, and in cases of airway obstruction a surgeon should be ready to perform a tracheostomy as an emergency, if necessary.

Intubation under local analgesia

For intubation under local analgesia the entire upper airway must be anaesthetized. Prior to administration of the antisialogogue, the patient can be asked to suck a benzocaine lozenge. This will help to anaesthetize the mouth and pharynx. The mouth or nasal passages can then be sprayed with 4% lignocaine or prilocaine. The maximum safe dose of either of these drugs is 3 mg/kg body weight. This can be followed by either a superior laryngeal nerve block (using pledgets soaked in local analgesic solution introduced into the pyriform fossa with Krause's forceps), or a cricothyroid puncture with injection of local analgesic direct into the airway during a deep inspiration.

Fibre-optic laryngoscopy

Prior to performing fibre-optic laryngoscopy, a check should be made that the laryngoscope is clean and working correctly, and that the suction channel is patent. The endotracheal tube, which must be well lubricated, is mounted on the laryngoscope. Awake fibre-optic laryngoscopy requires topical analgesia of the airway as has been described above, and appropriate sedation should be given. Additional local analgesic can be injected through the laryngoscope if required.

Fibre-optic intubation is much easier to perform nasally. There are two approaches that can be used. Either the patient can lie flat with the anaesthetist standing at the head of the bed, or he can recline at 45° with the anaesthetist standing at the side of the bed facing him. The procedure is much easier to perform with the head extended, and the patient should also be asked to protrude the tongue, or it should be held forward with a gauze swab by an assistant. It may be helpful to dilate gently the nasal passages with nasal airways coated in lignocaine jelly, and then to advance the nasotracheal tube as far as the pharynx before inserting the laryngoscope. Nasal fibre-optic laryngoscopy under general anaesthesia is made easier by the use of an oral airway with a 'tower', to which a breathing circuit can be attached. The airway can be sealed to the face with adhesive tape, and the patient can be kept asleep while laryngoscopy is performed. Visualization of the tracheal rings confirms entry into the trachea, and the tube is then railroaded down the laryngoscope.

Aspiration of gastric contents during the procedure is a theoretical risk in patients who have received topical analgesia of the airway prior to intubation, and this must be borne in mind. Laryngospasm during fibre-optic laryngoscopy under general anaesthesia is a risk and pulse oximetry should be always be used. Bleeding from the nose, while not necessarily hazardous in an awake patient, is disastrous since it makes fibre-optic laryngoscopy almost impossible. Great care should be taken to try to avoid this difficulty.

Fibre-optic laryngoscopy is a technique that requires much practice to achieve consistent results. There is evidence that a graduated programme of teaching, initially using a teaching model, achieves a higher success rate more rapidly than unrehearsed attempts on patients (Ovassapian et al 1988).

Tracheostomy under local analgesia

In the absence of a fibre-optic laryngoscope, pre-operative tracheostomy under local analgesia may be required in cases of severe facial injuries, in which general anaesthesia is made hazardous by the presence of blood and debris in the airway and in the most severe cases of upper airway obstruction. However, tracheostomy may be unusually difficult under such circumstances because of patient distress. Breathing a helium/oxygen mixture may help a severely obstructed patient during performance of the tracheostomy.

Other special techniques

There are three other techniques that can help in difficult circumstances: intubation through the LMA, the retrograde method and transtracheal ventilation. Intubation through the LMA has already been discussed (see p. 474). Both of the other methods are likely to become rarities with increasing use of fibre-optic techniques.

The retrograde method involves puncture of the cricothyroid membrane with a suitable needle through which is threaded a Seldinger wire (or epidural catheter) in a rostral direction. The wire is retrieved from the mouth. A soft rubber or plastic suction catheter is inserted through the nose and retrieved from the mouth, and is tied to the upper end of the wire. The suction catheter is then pulled back through the nose together with the attached wire. The endotracheal tube is now inserted nasally over the wire and 'railroaded' down using the wire as a guide.

Transtracheal ventilation involves inserting a suitable plastic cannula either through the cricothyroid membrane, or through the gap between the second and third tracheal rings, in a downward direction. In practice a standard venipuncture trocar and cannula are used. The correct sizes are 16 gauge for adults, 18 gauge for adolescents and 19–20 gauge for children. The method is inappropriate for infants. A suitable jetting source of oxygen or entonox at pipeline pressure (405 kpa) with a manual or automatic on–off valve is attached to the cannula. Alternatively a high frequency ventilator may be used. Pulmonary barotrauma can easily be produced during transtracheal ventilation, especially if an oversized cannula is used or if there is upper airway obstruction from any cause, and a close watch must be kept on chest movements to ensure that hyperinflation does not occur.

Total intubation failure

Provided the anaesthetist has access to the equipment and techniques mentioned, total intubation failure is unlikely. Unfortunately, fibre-optic laryngoscopes are expensive and not universally available, nor are facilities for jet ventilation, and very few anaesthetists are practised in techniques only occasionally required. The overall incidence of failed intubation therefore never reaches the minimum possible.

The action to take in failed intubation depends on the circumstances. With a clear airway, and in the absence of a full stomach, there are several possibilities. If only an induction agent and suxamethonium have been administered, the patient can be woken up after a few minutes and a local analgesic technique used to perform the surgery if this is possible. Alternatively, anaesthesia may be continued with spontaneous ventilation after recovery of neuromuscular conduction. If a non-depolarizing relaxant has been administered, ventilation by mask or laryngeal mask airway may well be feasible. Occasionally, particularly if a major and urgent procedure is contemplated, tracheostomy under general anaesthesia may be required.

In the presence of airway obstruction, there is little time to waste. The patient must be oxygenated. If a tube cannot be passed, the only way to oxygenate is directly into the trachea with a cannula, either by insufflation or with a jetting source.

Failed intubation drill

Obstetric patients and other patients with a full stomach require the use of a failed intubation drill, similar to that described by Tunstall (1976).

In these patients, prolonged attempts at intubation should not be made because of the risk of aspiration of gastric contents. Should intubation not succeed with one dose of suxamethonium, a second dose should not be given. If necessary, expert help should immediately be summoned. Cricoid pressure must be maintained and the patient turned onto the left side, head down, and the pharynx should be aspirated. Oxygen should be given with IPPV and an oral airway inserted if necessary. If the airway is obstructed, cricoid pressure should be removed at this stage. If the airway remains obstructed, either a laryngeal mask can be inserted (remembering that it does not protect against aspiration), or a cricothyroid puncture can be performed and oxygen insufflated into the trachea, using a cannula, three-way tap, male-to-male connector and oxygen tubing. If a jetting source is used to oxygenate via the cannula, it has to be used very gently in the presence of an obstructed upper airway to prevent barotrauma occurring. Having successfully restored oxygenation, the decision has to be taken whether to wake the patient up and proceed with a local analgesic technique or to continue with general anaesthesia using a facemask or LMA. If the latter is chosen, inhalational anaesthesia should be commenced and continued as spontaneous ventilation returns, which it will when the effect of suxamethonium wears off. Halothane is the agent of choice. With general anaesthesia well established, a wide bore (16 French gauge) orogastric tube can be passed to empty the stomach and instil 30 ml of 0.3 molar sodium citrate. However, this manoeuvre is not universally accepted as it has the potential to induce laryngeal spasm if anaesthesia is insufficiently deep. Surgery can be performed under inhalational anaesthesia by facemask, or, if an LMA has been used, a non-depolarizing muscle relaxant could be administered and IPPV instituted. Whenever general anaesthesia is chosen following a failed intubation, regurgitation and aspiration remain a risk until the patient has woken up at the end of the operation.

A suggested plan of action following failed intubation is shown in Figure. 31.2.

Complications of endotracheal intubation

Complications of intubation overlap with those of laryngoscopy. The latter have been described earlier in this chapter. There are some hazards, however, that relate specifically to the act of tube insertion. The use of excessive force may perforate the pyriform fossa (Blanc & Tremblay 1974), or the posterior pharyngeal mucosa which can lead to retropharyngeal abscess formation (Majumdar et al 1982), or the cervical oesophagus (see Fig. 31.3).

Dislocation of the left arytenoid cartilage may occur, but this is a rarity. It is associated with severe sore throat lasting several days (Quick & Merwin 1978). Overinflation of the cuff may result in rupture of the trachea.

Nasal intubation is associated with additional complications, the most common being trauma to the nasal passages. This includes mucosal stripping causing epistaxis and fractures of the turbinates. Before nasal intubation the patient should, if possible, be asked which nostril is easier to breathe through, and this nostril should be used for intubation. Gentle insertion, coupled with a little rotation from side to side, a well-lubricated tube and the use of the correct size all help to minimize trauma. In children the sizes are the same as for oral intubation (see Table 31.1, p. 490). Adults require smaller tubes nasally, 7.5 mm and 7.0 mm tubes being adequate for men and women, respectively. Hard PVC endotracheal tubes cause more nasal trauma than soft varieties and there are soft tubes manufactured specially for this purpose. Soft tubes are, however, more prone to compression between the conchae and the nasal septum, and this may cause significant obstruction of the lumen. Cuffed varieties, especially high-volume cuffs, are relatively traumatic because the folds of the cuff produce a rough surface. Laceration of the posterior pharyngeal mucosa has been reported to occur in 3% of nasal intubations (Tintinalli & Claffey 1981).

Following long-term intubation, erosion of the alae nasi and ulceration of mucosa over the turbinates which can cause massive haemorrhage

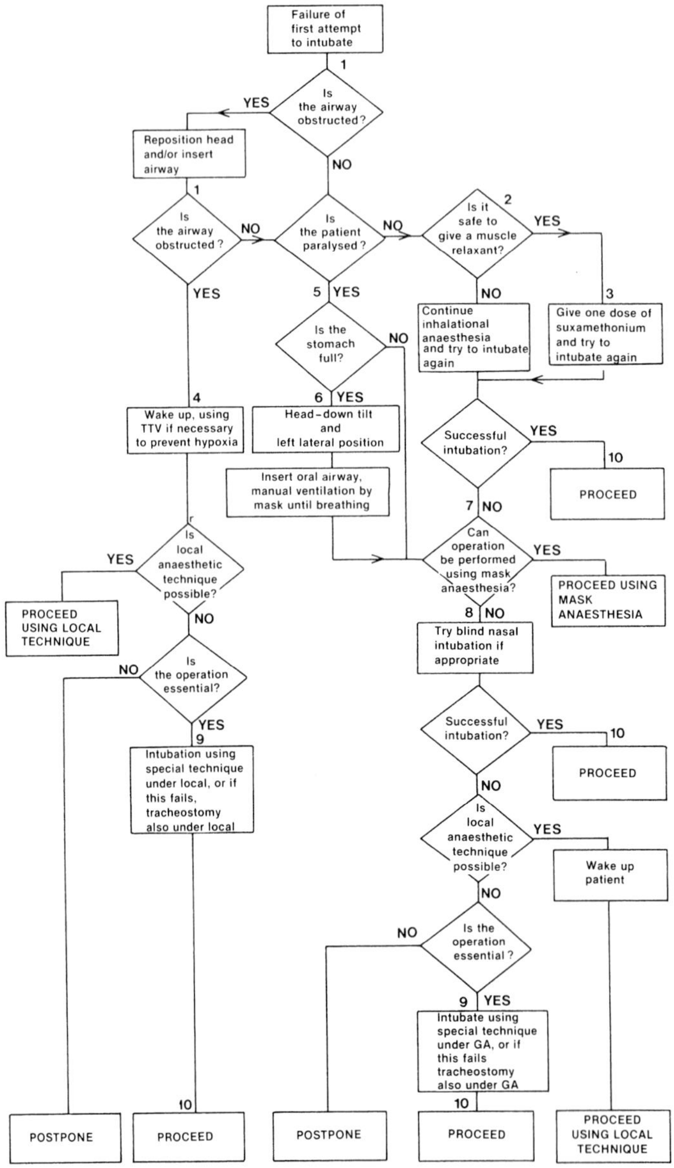

Fig. 31.2 A suggested course of action to take after failing to intubate at the first attempt:

1. If the obstruction is due to persistent laryngeal spasm a muscle relaxant should be administered.
2. This decision depends on the feasibility of ventilation by facemask. If mask ventilation can be achieved, a muscle relaxant may be administered.
3. The patient should receive atropine prior to the repeat dose of suxamethonium to prevent bradycardia.
4. TTV: transtracheal ventilation.
5. It is assumed that suxamethonium has been administered.
6. Cricoid pressure should be maintained until the patient has been turned.
7. This may not be appropriate if the stomach is full or if the surgery is complex.
8. This is inappropriate if the stomach is full or if the difficulty is due to distortion of the airway.
9. Special techniques are – fibre-optic laryngoscopy, the retrograde method and transtracheal ventilation.
10. Always extubate awake or transfer the patient to the intensive care unit to be extubated awake.

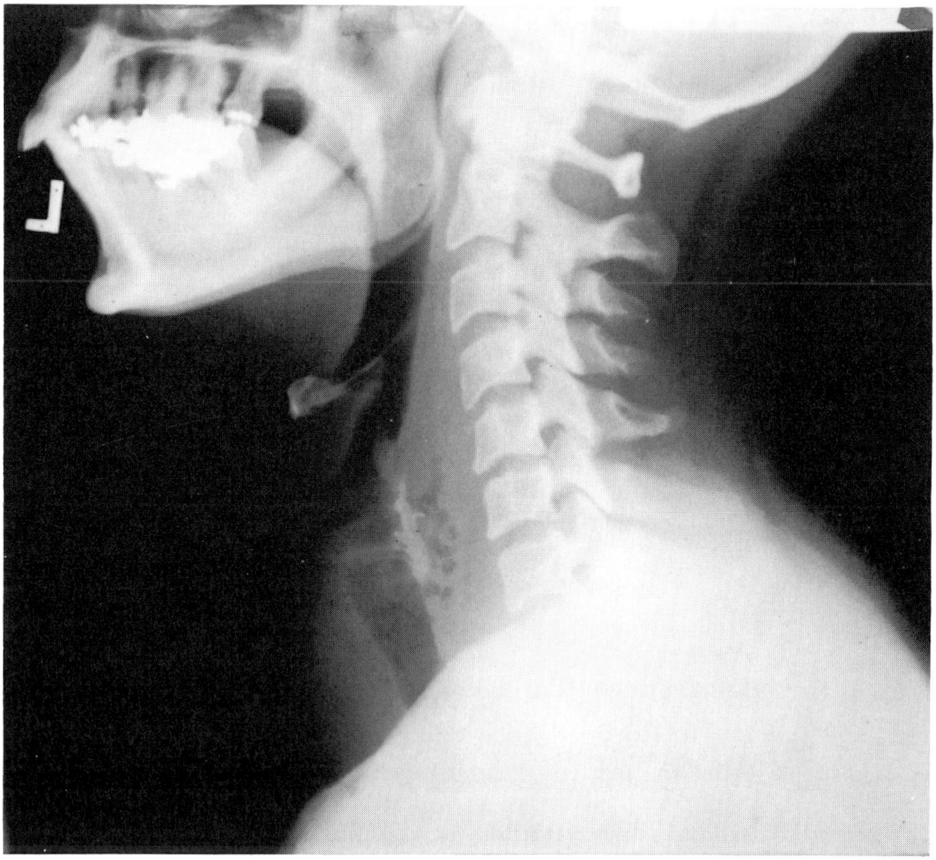

Fig. 31.3 Perforation of the cervical oesophagus by an endotracheal tube. Lateral radiograph of the neck showing air bubbles in the soft tissues around the larynx (with kind permission from Dr M Charlesworth).

have been reported (Sherry 1983a). Maxillary sinusitis, which is thought to occur from obstruction of the maxillary ostium due to oedema, is reported to occur in about 2% of nasally intubated patients in intensive care units (Pope et al 1981).

Trauma to the larynx is much more frequent following blind nasal intubation than after intubation under direct vision. Blind nasal intubation in children is potentially hazardous because the endotracheal tube may remove adenoidal tissue which may then block the lumen causing obstruction or enter the bronchial tree (Keane et al 1982). Nasal intubation should not be performed in the presence of fractures of the floor of the anterior cranial fossa. Not only is the risk of intracranial infection likely to be increased by the tube, but also the anterior fossa has actually been intubated on occasions (see Fig. 31.4).

Oesophageal intubation

One of the greatest dangers to the anaesthetized patient is unrecognized intubation of the oesophagus. The anaesthetist must always satisfy himself that this has not occurred. The best method of ensuring tracheal intubation is to visualize the tube entering the larynx. This is not always easy, for the tube often obscures the view. One method of obtaining a view of the larynx following intubation is to depress the tube posteriorly while lifting the laryngoscope. This usually allows the tube to be seen passing through the glottis (Ford 1983).

In the spontaneously breathing intubated patient, clear movements of the reservoir bag

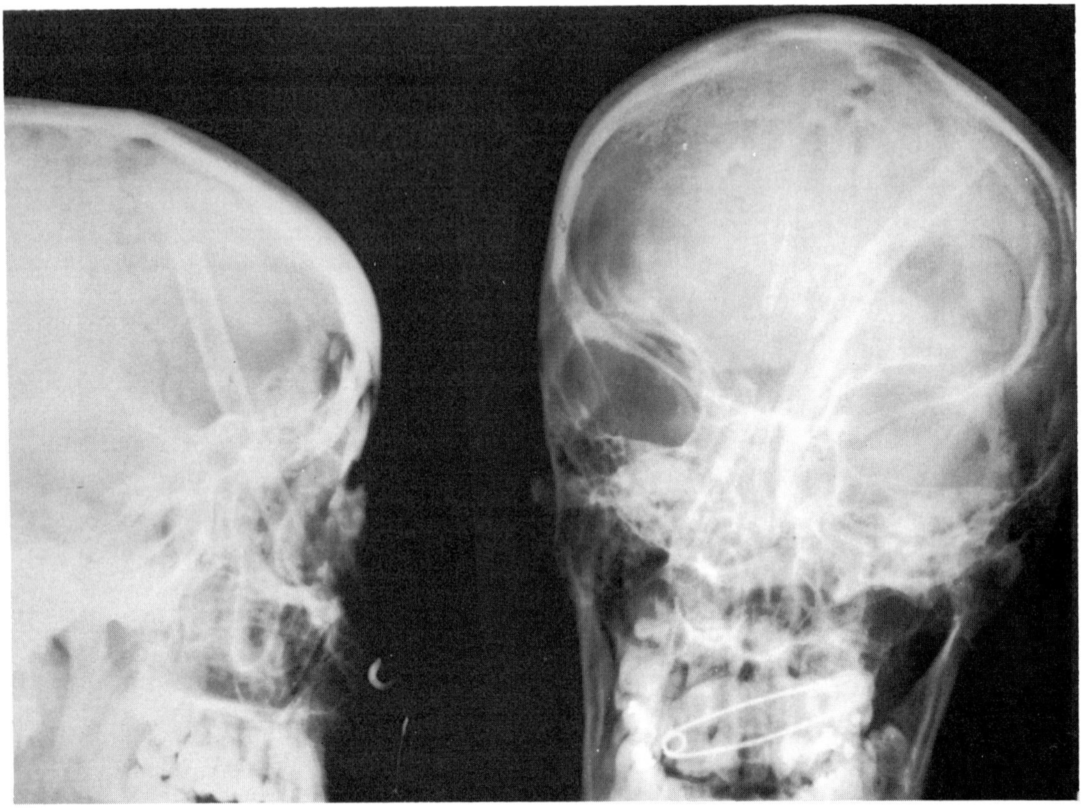

Fig. 31.4 Endotracheal tube in the anterior cranial fossa following nasal intubation in a patient with facial injuries. The patient made a good recovery (with kind permission from Dr M Charlesworth).

should be seen with respiration. In the apnoeic patient, tracheal intubation can be confirmed by manually compressing the sternum while listening or feeling for air exiting from the endotracheal tube. When the reservoir bag is squeezed, the chest should be seen to rise and fall synchronously, and auscultation should reveal bilateral clear breath sounds.

When the trachea has been intubated, the reservoir bag almost always has a compliant feel when squeezed, and rapid refilling of the bag from the patient in early expiration is typical. When the tube is in the oesophagus the bag is non-compliant, does not refill rapidly in early expiration and there is often audible belching heard when the bag is squeezed. Auscultation over the upper abdomen usually reveals air entering the stomach.

Unfortunately, oesophageal intubation can sometimes so mimic tracheal intubation that real confusion arises (Howells & Riethmuller 1980). If, despite signs of tracheal intubation, oxygen saturation falls or, in the absence of an oximeter, increasing cyanosis occurs, and provided the cyanosis is not due to circulatory collapse or the delivery of a hypoxic gas mixture, the proper action is to remove the endotracheal tube and administer 100% oxygen by facemask. If there is any doubt about the inspired oxygen concentration, whether or not an oxygen analyser is being used, disconnection of the pipelines and opening of the oxygen cylinder only will provide 100% oxygen.

An alternative method for confirming tracheal intubation is the oesophageal detector device (Wee 1988). This consists of a 60 ml bladder syringe connected in an airtight manner to a catheter mount and tube connector. The plunger of the syringe is depressed fully and the device is attached to the tube. The syringe is then aspirated. If the tube is in the trachea, 60 ml of air can easily be aspirated from the patient's lungs. However, if the tube is in the oesophagus, no air can be withdrawn because the oesophagus collapses around the tip of the tube. This device is almost always reliable.

Capnography is a highly reliable way of confirming tracheal intubation. If the trachea has been intubated, a typical capnogram is obtained when the patient is ventilated, and this capnogram continues to be present every breath. Conversely, following oesophageal intubation, no carbon dioxide is present in the expired gas except when mask ventilation has filled the stomach with air, and this disappears after a few breaths (Linko et al 1983).

Direct visualization of the tracheal rings through a fibre-optic laryngoscope inserted into the endotracheal tube can provide confirmatory evidence of tracheal intubation, though the usefulness of this method depends on the immediate availability of the laryngoscope.

Finally, it can never be repeated too often that if there is doubt about the placement of any endotracheal tube, the tube must be removed. Patients only come to harm if an incorrect intubation passes unrecognized.

Intubation of neonates

Neonates present additional difficulties to those already discussed. For a number of reasons, I believe that neonates under about 3 weeks of age should almost always be intubated awake, though this may not be possible with very vigorous babies. The neonate has an oxygen consumption in relation to body weight twice that of the adult. This means that hypoxia develops rapidly in the absence of an oxygen supply. Intubation of the neonate is not easy, and the risk of hypoxia is great in failed intubation since maintaining the airway may also be difficult. Attempts at intubation under light anaesthesia without muscle relaxants are particularly likely to induce laryngospasm which is potentially dangerous. Mask ventilation in neonates is useless; it merely succeeds in filling the stomach with gas because the abdominal compliance is greater than that of the respiratory system (Hatch & Sumner 1981).

All these factors make awake intubation safer, especially for the anaesthetist who only occasionally encounters this age-group. The neonate should be preoxygenated to prevent hypoxia which can result from breath-holding during intubation. When intubating the awake neonate, correct positioning is essential. An assistant should place the palms of both hands on the shoulders and press down firmly while the fingers immobilize the head. The tube should be passed through the larynx during inspiration when the laryngeal aperture is at its widest. Although the neonate, unlike the older infant, is not particularly prone to develop bradycardia during laryngoscopy, the use of preoperative atropine is recommended and this has the additional benefit of reducing secretions.

Monitoring during induction and intubation

The Association of Anaesthetists (1988) has recently made recommendations regarding monitoring. Induction and intubation can be achieved with greater safety if monitoring is employed during the procedure. Monitoring is useful in two areas, these being the assessment of cardiovascular function, and the confirmation of correct tube placement and adequate oxygenation. The former is achieved by the use of electrocardiographic and blood pressure monitoring, and these should be established prior to inducation of anaesthesia. Confirmation of adequate oxygenation requires the measurement of the inspired oxygen concentration and the use of pulse oximetry. The latter should also be in place prior to induction. Correct tube placement is accurately confirmed by a capnograph, and ideally this instrument should be available in any area where general anaesthesia takes place.

ENDOTRACHEAL TUBES

The principal hazards of endotracheal tubes are obstruction, displacement and disconnection of the tube. Additionally there are problems associated with specific designs and materials of tubes and cuffs. Selection of correct size and length is also very important. The greatest hazard of endotracheal tube malfunction is hypoxia. Because cyanosis is so difficult to detect in dark-skinned patients, hypoxia can easily pass undetected. Such patients should always be monitored with pulse oximetry and this is especially true in the presence of an endotracheal tube.

Endotracheal tube obstruction

Obstruction occurs as a result of external compression, kinking, blockage with foreign matter, faults with the cuff and incorrect alignment in the trachea. Airway obstruction occurring in an intubated patient is far more likely to be due to one of the faults with endotracheal tubes described above than to bronchospasm. Insertion of an appropriately sized suction catheter will confirm the presence of an obstruction in tube. If there is ever any doubt about the cause of airway obstruction in an intubated patient, the safest course of action is to replace the endotracheal tube rather than give bronchodilators in the first instance.

External compression

External compression by Dott or Boyle–Davis gags sometimes occurs when the gag is inserted and opened. If adjustment does not correct the problem, the gag should be removed and replaced. Sometimes it may be necessary to replace the tube with one of a different type. Compression of nasal tubes by the bony structures of the nose has already been mentioned (see p. 483).

Kinking of endotracheal tubes

Kinking of oral tubes usually occurs at the back of the mouth. This can often be felt by an examining finger. Nasal tubes rarely kink unless the tube protrudes from the nose. Under these circumstances kinking is common. Nasal tubes, excepting special designs such as the RAE tube, should therefore not protrude from the nose.

Blockage of endotracheal tubes

Blockage is usually due to blood, sputum, pus (in suppurative pulmonary diseases) and lubricating jelly, though many other causes have been described. The connector may also become blocked. Small tubes and connectors block more easily than large ones, paediatric and endobronchial tubes are therefore at greatest risk.

Faulty endotracheal tube cuffs

Faulty cuffs can cause obstruction in three ways. Cuffs, particularly on older latex armoured tubes, occasionally inflate asymmetrically. This can alter the alignment of the tube in the trachea so that the bevelled orifice is against the tracheal wall resulting in obstruction, particularly during expiration. Pressures in overinflated cuffs can reach very high levels (up to several hundred cmH_2O) and can cause compression of the lumen of the tube. Cuff overinflation can easily occur when nitrous oxide is being used because this gas diffuses into the cuff, causing an increase in intracuff volume and pressure during the course of the anaesthetic (Mehta 1981). The inward diffusion can be prevented by filling the cuff with the anaesthetic gas mixture being used, or filling it with physiological saline (Patel et al 1983). Uncommonly, overinflated cuffs herniate over the tube orifice causing obstruction. Again, this problem is worst with ageing latex armoured tubes.

Incorrect tube alignment in the trachea

Incorrect alignment of the tube in the trachea, causing orifice obstruction, occasionally occurs in children (Brasch et al 1981), and probably in adults when the position of the head is changed. It occurs particularly when the head is flexed and turned to the side away from the bevel. One method of preventing this and the similar problem that occurs with asymmetric cuffs is to cut away the bevel, leaving the end of the tube squared off. This manoeuvre makes insertion of the tube more difficult and potentially traumatic, and care is required during intubation. The 'Murphy eye', a hole cut in the wall of the distal end of the tube opposite the bevel, is an alternative solution.

Endotracheal tube displacement

Displacement generally occurs following adjustment of the tube, movement of the head or surgical manipulation inside the mouth and pharynx. Tubes may displace upwards out of the larynx or downwards into a bronchus, usually the right main bronchus. Incorrect tube length increases the likelihood of displacement. Inadequate or inappropriate fixation of tubes also predisposes to displacement, and this is particularly important when the patient is face down or the head is inaccessible, for example in posterior fossa surgery. Under such circumstances, saliva may dribble onto the adhesive tapes securing the tube causing adhesion failure. Great care with tube fixation is needed for such procedures. Displacement out of the larynx is also more likely when the Trendelenburg (head-down) position is being used, due to the weight of the anaesthetic circuit dragging on the endotracheal tube. The practice of not securing the tube at all and relying on gravity and cuff adhesion in the trachea for fixation is hazardous and should be avoided.

Disconnection of endotracheal tubes

Disconnection of endotracheal tubes is a very common occurrence. It is always potentially lethal during controlled ventilation, but during spontaneous ventilation the effect of a disconnection depends upon where it occurs. If the disconnection is close to the patient he will breathe room air and wake up, which is more undesirable than dangerous. However, if it occurs at the anaesthetic machine there will be an enormous increase in apparatus dead space, to the point at which it approaches or exceeds the tidal volume. The patient will therefore rebreathe expired gas and become hypoxic and hypercarbic. Disconnection can easily pass unnoticed if it occurs beneath surgical drapes. Cessation of movement and deflation of the reservoir bag in spontaneously ventilating patients and cessation of chest movement in mechanically ventilated patients should alert the anaesthetist to a disconnection.

All three major types of tube malfunction – obstruction, displacement and disconnection – are common and potentially fatal. The single expedient of using a correctly calibrated capnograph with appropriate alarm settings will detect all types of tube malfunction at an early stage, and this should be routine.

Diameter of endotracheal tubes

The use of the correct diameter tube is important. In the absence of abnormal anatomy or airway pathology which may necessitate reducing the size of the tube, a size 7.5–8.0 mm is suitable for adult females, and 8.5–9.0 mm for adult males for intubation by the oral route. Excessively small tubes cause several hazards, the most important being the high resistance to gas flow that they impose. During spontaneous ventilation through too small a tube the patient has to generate large swings in intrathoracic pressure to overcome tube resistance. This leads to impairment of gas exchange, cardiovascular disturbance and pulmonary oedema.

A small tube occupies a smaller volume in the trachea above the cuff than a large one. This space constitutes a collecting point for blood, saliva, gastric contents and other debris, and the smaller the tube the more that can collect. This space is generally inaccessible to suction, therefore the contents may enter the lungs when the tube is removed. Extubation with application of positive pressure to the reservoir bag helps blow this debris up and out of the trachea. Small tubes are also more likely to kink and become blocked.

Excessively large tubes may compress and traumatize the arytenoids, vocal cords, subglottis and trachea, causing mucosal ulceration and oedema. Oversize tubes are particularly dangerous in children, in whom the resulting oedema can lead to airway obstruction (see below).

Length of endotracheal tubes

Generally, adult females require a tube 21–22 cm long and adult males one of 23–24 cm. Occasionally, tubes outside this range are required. During intubation the cuff must be seen to pass through the vocal cords in its entirety. Apart from the danger of displacement out of the larynx with a short tube, inflation of a cuff lying within the larynx compresses the recurrent laryngeal nerves between the laryngeal cartilages and can cause a nerve palsy, which is usually unilateral and has an incidence of around 0.5% (Peppard & Dickens 1983). This can lead to dysphonia, laryngeal incompetence and, when both nerves are damaged, even airway obstruction (Gibbin & Egginton 1981).

Excessively long tubes pass beyond the carina usually into the right main bronchus with failure to ventilate the left lung. This is particularly important because the origin of the right upper lobe bronchus is only 2.5 cm below the carina and the orifice could be obstructed by the tube, leaving only the right middle and lower lobes ventilated. This is not adequate to maintain blood gas homeostasis. A check should always be made visually and by auscultation that both lungs ventilate equally.

Particular care is needed when using preformed tubes such as the Oxford and RAE types, which cannot be cut to length. Oxford tubes are occasionally too short and may displace into the pharynx. RAE tubes are relatively long and intubation of the right main bronchus may be a problem. This is especially so if one of these tubes is used in connection with a Boyle–Davis gag, for the gag may displace the tube downwards. Under these circumstances the tube must be repositioned or one of a different type substituted.

Endotracheal tube sizes in children

The use of the correct diameter and length tubes in children is especially important. A guide to tube diameters in children is given in Table 31.1. Diameters for nasal and oral tubes are the same. A guide to oral tube length is given by the following formula (Levin 1958) (see also p. 192):

$$\frac{\text{Age in years}}{2} + 12 = \text{tube length in cm}$$

Occasionally, different diameters and lengths will be required.

The greatest hazard is the use of tubes of excessive diameter. The narrowest part of the prepubertal child's lower airway is at cricoid (subglottic) level. In adults, by contrast, the glottis is the narrowest part. The cricoid cartilage is the only cartilage of the lower airway that is a closed ring. The mucosa at cricoid level is loosely attached to the underlying cartilage and is therefore prone to oedema formation. Passage of an oversize tube will cause pressure-induced ischaemia and oedema of the subglottic mucosa. Since no outward expansion can occur, the oedema forms at the expense of the tracheal lumen and may cause airway obstruction on removal of the tube. Subglottic oedema of 1 mm thickness in a neonate has been calculated to reduce the area of the lumen of the airway by two-thirds (Hatch & Sumner 1981). Oedematous mucosa heals by formation of granulation tissue and this can eventually lead to a fibrous subglottic stenosis. Tracheostomy and reconstructive surgery to the larynx and trachea may be needed to cure the problem.

Table 31.1 Endotracheal tube sizes in infants and children

Age	Metric sizes
0–2 months	2.5 & 3.0
3–5 months	3.0 & 3.5
6–9 months	3.5 & 4.0
10–12 months	4.0 & 4.5
1–4 years	4.5 & 5.0
5 years	5.0 & 5.5
6–7 years	5.5 & 6.0
8–9 years	6.0 & 6.5
10 years	6.5 & 7.0
11–12 years	7.0 & 7.5
13–14 years	7.5 & 8.0
15–16 years (boys)	8.0 & 8.5
17+ years (boys)	8.5 & 9.0

There are generally accepted rules for avoiding this disastrous situation. Cuffed tubes should never be used in the prepubertal child and there should always be an audible leak around the tube when the reservoir bag is squeezed. The 'Cole' pattern shouldered tube, often used during neonatal resuscitation, is particularly likely to produce laryngeal damage and should be used with great care. If a child develops post-extubation stridor, intravenous dexamethasone (0.25 mg/kg) may produce relief. There is a suggestion that postextubation stridor after long-term intubation may be more common in Down's syndrome (Sherry 1983b).

Because of the relatively high incidence of tube blockage and kinking, and because of the speed with which lung mechanics can change in neonates, a very strong case can be made for hand ventilating all neonates and as many infants as possible. The 'educated' hand can detect changes in lung and tube function very rapidly, whereas such changes easily pass unnoticed during mechanical ventilation. Ventilators with expired minute volume displays are no solution, for compression of gases in the ventilator circuit during inspiration can lead to the generation of the same expired minute volume by re-expansion in expiration whether the tube is clear or totally obstructed. Capnography, however, will always detect an obstructed tube.

Construction materials of tubes

Construction material is an important consideration in tubes intended for long-term use. Red rubber and latex are not biologically inert substances and will initiate an inflammatory reaction if in contact with living tissue. Polyvinylchloride, the material of most plastic tubes, is relatively inert. The situation, however, is complicated because many substances (stabilizers, antioxidants, plasticizers, hardeners, catalysts, pigments, etc.) are added to plastic tubes to improve their physical properties and many of these substances are toxic. Any tube for long-term use should bear the mark 'IT', meaning implant tested, which indicates that the construction material has been subjected to in vivo testing of biological inertness.

Shape of endotracheal tubes

Most tubes are in the form of a simple arc. This shape does not correspond to the overall shape of the upper airway, and the tube exerts excess force onto the upper teeth, the posterior part of the larynx and the anterior tracheal wall, leading to ulceration at the latter two sites in long-term use (see Fig. 31.5). Red rubber tubes which are stiff at body temperature are worse in this respect than PVC tubes which soften as they warm, a property termed thermolability. The Lindholm

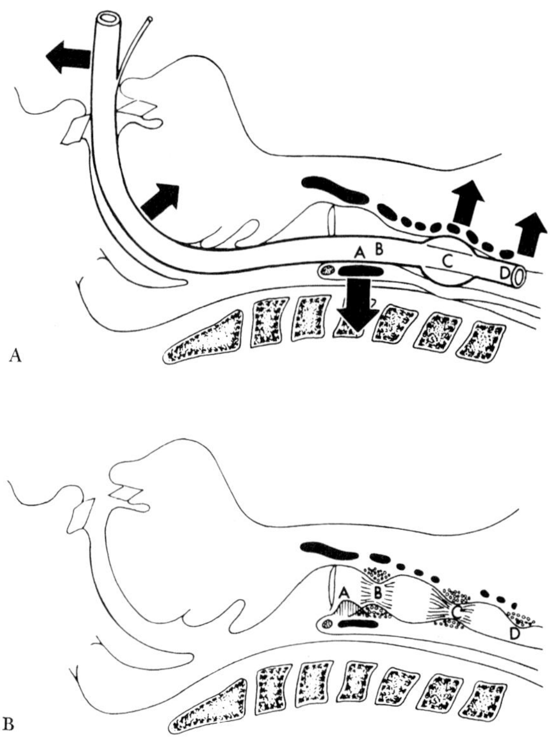

Fig. 31.5 (A) Arrows show direction of forces exerted by a standard shaped endotracheal tube on the teeth, tongue, posterior laryngeal wall and anterior wall of the trachea. A: posterior laryngeal wall, B: level of cricoid ring, C: cuff, D: tube tip. (B) Corresponding sites of lesions caused by standard-shaped endotracheal tubes. Scar tissue at A is on the posterior wall between the arytenoid cartilages. B and C are circumferential stenoses. Scar tissue at D is on the anterior wall of the trachea (from Lindholm & Grenvik 1982).

tube, which has a sigmoid shape, offers a theoretical advantage (Lindholm & Grenvik 1982).

Endotracheal tube cuffs

In the early days of intensive care, many patients (up to 20%) suffered serious tracheal damage following prolonged intubation (Grillo 1970). That this was due to the cuff is now well established. The cuffs in use were low volume, high pressure types, and it is now known that such cuffs exert a pressure greatly in excess of intravascular pressure on the tracheal mucosa. This results in cessation of mucosal perfusion and leads to ischaemic necrosis of the tracheal wall. Rarely this can lead to a tracheo-oesophageal fistula. The healing process can cause formation of fibrous strictures, and where there has been cartilaginous erosion acquired tracheomalacia occurs.

The use of thin-walled, non-elastic, low-pressure cuffs, such as are found on many disposable types, has largely eradicated the problem. It is, however, important that these tubes are used properly. Use of the correct size of tube and careful attention to cuff pressure are essential. Cuff pressure, which can be measured using a water manometer attached via a three-way stopcock, should be 20–30 cmH_2O (approximately 2–3 kPa) during expiration. Such a pressure offers the best compromise between preservation of mucosal perfusion and protection against aspiration.

Whether the use of such cuffs is desirable for short periods of intubation (up to a few hours) is debatable for there are some disadvantages. High-volume cuffs do not lie flat against the tube when fully deflated and the resulting ridges can traumatize the larynx during intubation. Such cuffs also impair the ease of visualization of the larynx, and there is evidence that postoperative sore throat is more common after intubation with a high-volume cuffed tube. It is likely, however, that the low pressure cuff, which produces less tissue damage in long-term use, is also less harmful in the short term.

Hazards associated with specific endotracheal tubes

The principal features of commonly used types of endotracheal tubes are shown in Table 31.2. Possible hazards are indicated.

Bronchospasm

Wheezes (rhonchi) heard on auscultation of the lungs are a common event during anaesthesia and are usually of little consequence. Occasionally, wheezes signify the presence of serious bronchospasm with clinically important airway obstruction. This requires urgent treatment.

With airway obstruction, accurate and rapid diagnosis of the cause is essential. Bronchospasm is a rarity compared with other forms of airway obstruction mentioned earlier. In the unintubated patient, obstruction by the tongue and laryngospasm are both far more common and must be excluded (by intubation if necessary) before a diagnosis of bronchospasm is made. In the intubated patient tube-related obstruction is more common than bronchospasm and this too must be excluded. This may necessitate a change of tube. Furthermore, bronchospasm is extremely uncommon in patients who do not have asthma.

Prevention and treatment

Vitalography provides a simple and useful indication of the degree of airway obstruction and its reversibility with bronchodilators. This should be performed if there is doubt about the diagnosis or the severity of the airway obstruction. Correct preoperative preparation of asthmatic patients is essential. This includes avoiding general anaesthesia in any asthmatic patient who has had a chest infection within the previous 3 weeks, since bronchospasm is more common at this time (Morgan & Gillbe 1985). Optimization of bronchodilator treatment and its continuation right up to the point of anaesthesia is important. Steroids undoubtedly have a place in the prevention of bronchospasm and a single preoperative dose is unlikely to do harm. It should be given at least 1.5 h preoperatively. Avoidance

Table 31.2 Principal features of major types of endotracheal tubes

Tube	Material	Cuff type	Bevel direction	Kink resistance	Comments
Magill	Red rubber	None, or low volume high pressure	Left	No	Not suitable if kinking likely to occur
Magill, flexometallic	Red rubber, stainless steel coil	None	Depends on orientation	Yes	Coil integrity must be checked. Insufflation port must be occluded
Latex, Armoured	Latex around stainless steel coil, or nylon coil, or nylon coil, or nylon mesh	None, or low volume high pressure	Depends on orientation	Yes	Cuff prone to asymmetric inflation and herniation on older tubes. Laminated structure with potential spaces between laminae, especially if vacuum autoclaved. N_2O can diffuse into spaces causing bulges in wall and obstruction of the lumen
Oxford	Red rubber	None, or low volume high pressure	Posterior	Yes	Right angle pharyngeal bend. Fixed length, sometimes too short. Cuff situated rather high. Orifice can obstruct if head flexed. Distal taper makes it easy to insert oversized tubes in children
Disposable types, standard pattern and Lindholm	PVC	None, or variable mostly low pressure	Left, some have Murphy eye	Partial	Only types suitable for long-term use. Cole pattern tube (designed for neonates) with distal shouldered taper causes serious laryngeal trauma
RAE oral and nasal	PVC	None, or low volume low pressure	Left with Murphy eye	Partial	Excellent in many maxillofacial and ENT procedures. Preformed bends. Fixed length. Sometimes too short

of drugs such as morphine, which can produce bronchospasm in susceptible individuals, is sensible since there are alternative agents.

Bronchospasm is more common during endotracheal anaesthesia than when other methods are used. The tube is presumed to act as an irritant foreign body, though there is little evidence that one type of tube is better than any other. In many cases the use of the tube is unavoidable.

Treatment of established bronchospasm depends upon its severity. Simple measures such as deepening the level of anaesthesia may suffice in mild cases. Halothane, enflurane and isoflurane have all been shown to have bronchodilator activity, and this is clinically useful. When bronchospasm is severe this type of treatment is less effective because it may be difficult to get adequate levels of inhaled anaesthetic into the patient. In such cases a systemic bronchodilator is required. Aminophylline (250 mg given over 5–10 min) is usually effective. The main side effects of aminophylline are sinus tachycardia and occasionally other tachyarrhythmias. The latter are more common in the presence of halothane, hypoxia and hypercarbia. The electrocardiogram should always be monitored. If signs of myocardial irritability occur, halothane should be replaced with another inhalational agent and the aminophylline given more slowly. Oxygen saturation should be monitored. If there are signs of hypoxia (including arrhythmias), 100% oxygen must be given and ventilation should be assisted in the spontaneously breathing patient to reduce the arterial $P\text{CO}_2$.

If aminophylline is ineffective, salbutamol may be used. It is usually given by infusion, starting at 5 μg/min and increasing in steps to 20 μg/min if necessary. This drug does not produce arrhythmias as commonly as aminophylline, but it has a marked tendency to produce sinus tachycardia due to stimulation of atrial beta2-adrenergic receptors.

In really severe cases unresponsive to the above drugs, adrenaline still has a place in treatment. Although it has an alpha adrenergic agonist (bronchoconstrictor) action, this is weak compared to the potent beta2-adrenergic agonism it produces. It may be given subcutaneously in a dose of 0.25–0.5 mg, but the dose should be reduced to 0.1–0.2 mg in the presence of halothane because the combination produces myocardial irritability. Adrenaline may also be given by intravenous bolus injection of 10–20 μg (1–2 ml of a 1:100 000 solution) or by infusion. 1 mg adrenaline in a burette containing 100 ml 5% dextrose at 5 drops/min is a suitable starting dose for infusion. Although adrenaline results in fewer arrhythmias than aminophylline it can produce a marked rise in arterial pressure. It is therefore essential to monitor accurately the arterial pressure during adrenaline administration.

Steroids should be given in the form of hydrocortisone (200–500 mg) in severe bronchospasm, but the bronchodilator effect is not immediate.

If bronchospasm has occurred as part of an allergic response and there is associated cardiovascular collapse, treatment needs to be modified. Adrenaline becomes the treatment of choice because its vasoconstrictor action is useful to restore arterial pressure. Hydrocortisone is particularly useful to counteract the associated bronchial oedema. Antihistamines (H_1-receptor antagonists) have no place in the treatment of cardiovascular collapse in an allergic reaction, but are useful to control the cutaneous symptoms and signs of histamine release. Intravenous chlorpheniramine (10 mg) is effective.

The airway obstruction in bronchospasm is mainly expiratory. It may be necessary in a ventilated patient to reduce the respiratory rate, increase the tidal volume and increase the duration of the expiratory phase to prevent overdistension of the thorax due to gas trapping. This will necessitate higher inflation pressure, but a peak inflation pressure of 50 cmH_2O should not be exceeded. Because of the high airway resistance the high pressure is only partially transmitted to the small airways. By contrast, overdistension caused by too short an expiratory phase can cause pulmonary barotrauma and can lead to acute right ventricular failure secondary to the increase in pulmonary vascular resistance which occurs. In severe cases, frequent arterial blood gas analysis is required.

It may be considered prudent to continue ventilation postoperatively in severe cases of bronchospasm where respiratory failure is likely to occur during recovery. A difficulty arises here out of the fact that part of the trouble may be caused by the presence of the tube, removal of which might be expected to help the bronchospasm. In practice, if a decision is made to extubate and the patient continues to have respiratory difficulty, there should be no hesitation in replacing the tube and ventilating the patient until the problem resolves.

Throat packs

Throat packs inserted into the pharynx to prevent blood and debris entering the larynx and oesophagus should always be used when there is any possibility of bleeding into the upper airway during surgery. The only exception to this rule is if a mouth gag is in place and any bleeding that occurs can be seen and dealt with by the surgeon. The use of a cuffed tube does not remove the necessity for a pack. Packs are also sometimes used to reduce leaks around uncuffed tubes in ventilated patients.

Packs may be used dry or moistened with water. They should not be moistened with liquid paraffin which may enter the lungs causing damage, particularly when an uncuffed tube is being used. Packs are associated with a high incidence of postoperative sore throat and insertion of the pack should be as gentle as possible. Whatever material (most commonly ribbon gauze or sponge) is used for the pack, it should not be subject to shredding or breakage in use. It is advisable to leave the tail of a ribbon gauze pack outside the mouth if this does not interfere with surgery. Alternatively, the patient should be labelled clearly to indicate that a pack is in place and to remind the anaesthetist to remove it.

The greatest danger attending the use of a throat pack is failure to remove it prior to extubation, for this results in complete airway obstruction and is potentially fatal. Packs should be removed under direct vision, if possible and any remaining debris should be suctioned clear.

ENDOBRONCHIAL TUBES

The requirements of a tube for thoracic surgery are that it should permit control of pulmonary secretions and occasionally pulmonary haemorrhage, and that it should allow independent ventilation of the two lungs. Double-lumen tubes alone satisfy these conditions, and have now largely replaced earlier types.

The bronchial anatomy of the two lungs is different. The left main bronchus is 5 cm long and is long enough to accommodate the bronchial lumen of a tube with ease. The right main bronchus is only 2.5 cm long and is too short to accommodate a cuff between the carina and the right upper lobe bronchus. Right-sided tubes therefore have a slotted bronchial cuff to allow ventilation of the right upper lobe. The position of this cuff in relation to the right upper lobe orifice is critical, for when the left lung is collapsed for surgery only the right middle and lower lobes will be ventilated if the tube is incorrectly sited, and this is inadequate for blood gas homeostasis. Left-sided tubes are therefore more satisfactory than right-sided ones and should be used whenever possible.

It is preferable to bronchoscope all patients prior to inserting a right-sided tube to ascertain the site of origin of the right upper lobe bronchus. This arises from the trachea in 0.5% of the population and in these patients a right-sided tube should not be used.

The same complications relating to intubation apply to these tubes as to endotracheal tubes, but there are some additional hazards. Tubes with carinal hooks require a special intubating technique. When the tip of the tube has entered the larynx the tube must be rotated through 180° to bring the hook anteriorly. The tube can then be advanced through the larynx and rotated to its final position. Failure to do this causes the hook to traumatize the transverse arytenoid muscle. Overinflation of the bronchial cuff leading to bronchial rupture has been reported with both disposable and reusable types of tube (Burton et al 1983, Foster et al 1983). 2–4 ml is usually enough to produce a seal.

Correct tube position is sometimes very difficult to achieve. Reasons for this include the use of the incorrect size, faulty cuffs that inflate asymmetrically and tracheal distortion due to external compression. Occasionally the tube passes into the opposite bronchus to that intended. Usually these difficulties can be overcome by trying a different size or type of tube. Whatever the problem it is essential to verify that the tube is correctly sited, allowing clear independent ventilation of the lungs once the patient is positioned for surgery. Changing the tube in mid-operation is difficult and dangerous. If there is doubt about the position of a tube, and especially of the bronchial cuff of a right-sided tube, the position can be assessed by passing a fibre-optic laryngoscope down the tube. Viewing down the bronchial lumen of a right-sided tube allows visualization of the right upper lobe bronchus. The tube position can then be adjusted as necessary.

So great is the danger of a malfunctioning endobronchial tube that, if there is any doubt about the tube, it should be replaced, if necessary with an ordinary endotracheal tube.

Endobronchial suction

During pulmonary surgery, blood, secretions and sometimes pus spill into the bronchial tree. This is particularly a problem when there is a bronchopleural fistula. To prevent soiling of the lower lung a suction catheter should be inserted into the lumen to the upper lung during one-lung anaesthesia and left on gentle suction until the tube is removed or the remaining part of the upper lung is re-expanded.

EXTUBATION AND POSTOPERATIVE AIRWAY MANAGEMENT

The moment of extubation is a hazardous one. Correct timing and good technique are the key to success. The fundamental requirement for extubation is that the patient is able to produce an appropriate tidal volume and respiratory rate without effort, with no signs of residual neuromuscular blockade or hypoxia.

No apnoeic patient should ever be extubated unless there is a clear reason, such as replacement of the tube with another. Extubation should be timed in such a way that the patient is either awake or in a state of established surgical anaesthesia at the moment of removal of the tube. In this way postextubation laryngospasm can be avoided. Conversely, removal of the tube during a light plane of anaesthesia frequently precipitates laryngospasm.

Oropharyngeal or nasopharyngeal suction should be employed to prevent debris entering the lungs after extubation. Sometimes this will have been performed by the surgeon, in which case it may be inappropriate to undertake further suctioning. Gentleness and the avoidance of suckers with sharp edges help to minimize trauma. Movement of the head during suction is best avoided, for it may make the patient cough, breath-hold or bite on the tube. This is particularly undesirable following intracranial or intraocular procedures, where the rise in intracranial or intraocular pressure so produced may have disastrous results. Rapid extubation to prevent coughing may be needed in these patients.

The routine use of endotracheal suction prior to extubation is most unwise. Quite apart from the risk of introducing infection and traumatizing the trachea, suctioning produces a dramatic fall in the functional residual capacity (FRC) with consequent hypoxaemia. This is the very last thing to be desired prior to extubation, which should be undertaken with the lungs filled with oxygen, not collapsed by suction (see Fig. 31.6). The risk of hypoxia can also be lessened by administering 100% oxygen for 2–3 min prior to extubation.

The application of positive pressure by squeezing the bag during the removal of the tube has two beneficial effects. It not only fills the lungs with oxygen, but also tends to blow any debris that may have collected in the larynx and upper trachea upwards into the pharynx, from whence it can be removed by gentle suction post-extubation. It should always be ensured that the cuff is fully deflated. This means that high-volume, non-compliant cuffs, which do not spontaneously empty, should be actively evacuated. After extubation, oxygen should be administered by facemask from the anaesthetic circuit to ensure that the patient continues to breathe well through a clear airway.

Special precautions need to be taken in some patients at extubation. Neonates and younger infants, who are particularly likely to develop laryngospasm and who become hypoxic extremely rapidly, should always be extubated wide awake. This means that the child should be moving all its limbs and opening its eyes before the tube is removed.

Patients with potentially full stomachs should be extubated awake because of the risk of aspiration of gastric contents while still anaesthetized. This is particularly true after obstetric anaesthesia. Patients in whom difficulty was experienced with laryngoscopy and intubation are another group in which awake extubation is safer, for if laryngospasm develops, rapid reintubation may be needed and this may be very difficult.

Patients who have undergone surgery following which there is likely to be bleeding into the upper airway need not be extubated awake. They should, however, be nursed in a lateral position, and the mouth should be below the level of the larynx. In this way, any blood will collect in the mouth, which can be kept clear by gentle suctioning with a catheter, thus preventing blood from reaching the vicinity of the larynx.

Major oral surgery produces a particular set of problems. The most important sources of trouble are postoperative oedema of the floor of the mouth causing airway obstruction and wiring of the jaws for immobilization of mandibular fractures. Patients should be extubated when fully awake after such procedures and nursed in an

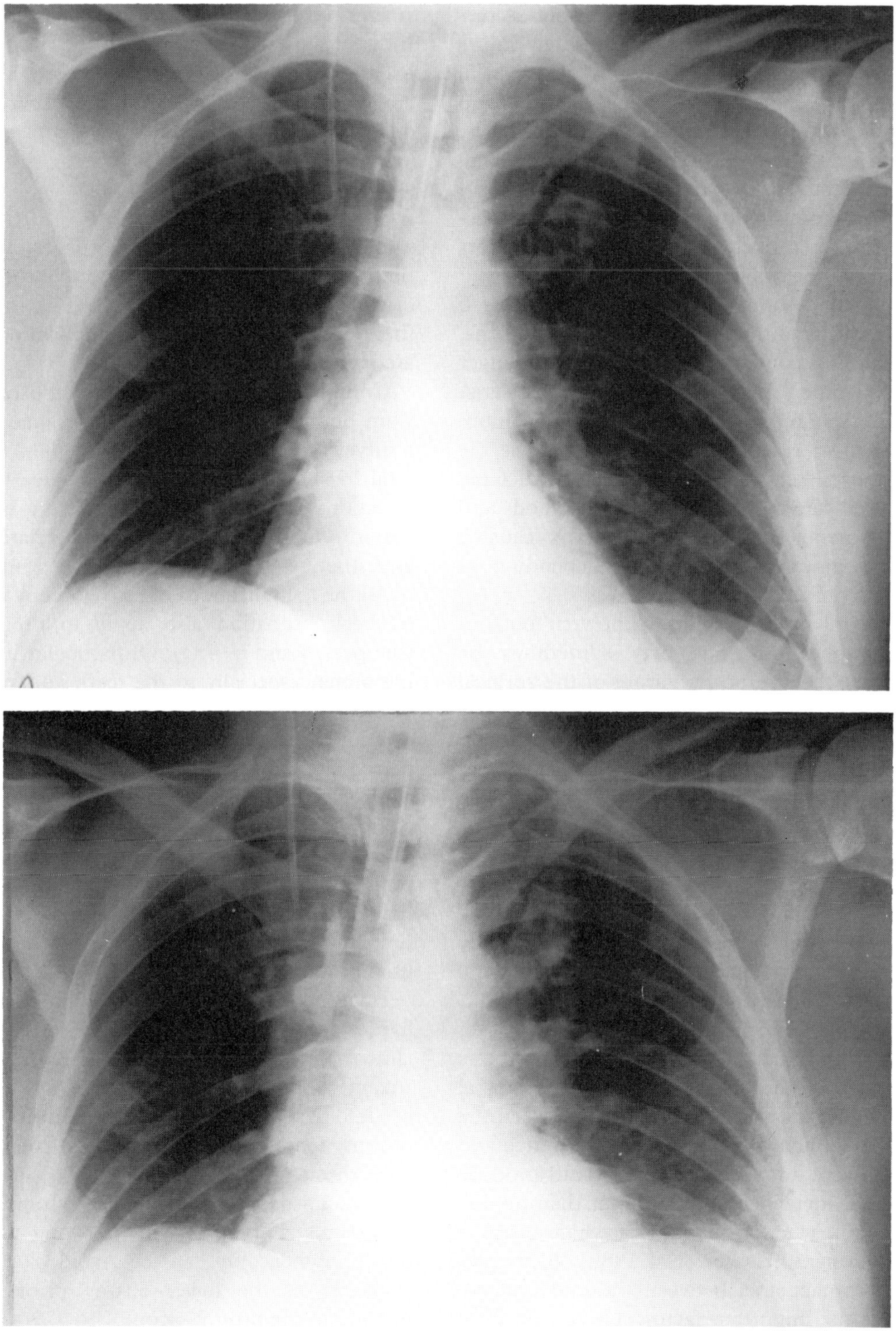

A

B

Fig. 31.6 Chest radiographs showing effects of endotracheal suction. Note the reduction in lung volume. (A) before suction, (B) after suction.

intensive care unit for 24 h if possible. Alternatively they may be ventilated for a few hours until fully recovered. The possibility of laryngeal spasm makes extubation while still anaesthetized hazardous in the presence of wired jaws. Vomiting is also a major hazard in these patients and a potent antiemetic such as droperidol should be administered before the end of anaesthesia. Postoperatively a set of wire cutters should always be available near the patient.

All patients should be individually nursed postoperatively until full consciousness returns, because airway obstruction is always a danger during this time. The supine position is less satisfactory for safe recovery than the lateral position. There are two reasons for this. Not only is the tongue more likely to fall back and obstruct the airway, but debris such as saliva, blood and gastric contents may reach the larynx causing either laryngospasm or aspiration, depending on the integrity of the laryngeal reflexes.

The lateral position helps to prevent both of these complications but may sometimes be undesirable because of the nature of the surgical procedure. Snoring, a sign of partial airway obstruction, is dangerous in the recovering patient. If it occurs, the patient should be aroused or repositioned to prevent the situation progressing to complete obstruction.

Postoperative sore throat

Sore throat, a minor though often distressing side effect, is a common accompaniment to general anaesthesia. The incidence ranges from 10–90% depending on the technique used. It is lower after mask anaesthesia than endotracheal anaesthesia and is more common in women (Jensen et al 1982). There is a strong correlation between the type of endotracheal tube and the incidence and severity of sore throat. High-volume cuffs produce a far higher incidence of sore throat than do low volume cuffs, whether the latter are high- or low-pressure designs (Loeser et al 1980). It appears that the contact area between the cuff and the trachea is the important factor. The use of local analgesic lubricants has a variable effect. Prolonged severe sore throat with dysphonia is suggestive of dislocation of an arytenoid cartilage. Indirect laryngoscopy should be performed to exclude this and direct laryngoscopy under general anaesthesia may be required to reduce the dislocation (Quick & Merwin 1978).

BRONCHOSCOPY

Other than for intubation purposes, the anaesthetist rarely uses the fibre-optic bronchoscope outside the intensive care unit. The following is therefore confined to the complications associated with rigid bronchoscopy.

Complications of rigid bronchoscopy arise from both the procedure and the anaesthetic. In a survey of nearly 3500 bronchoscopies (Lukomsky et al 1981), 173 (5%) were associated with complications, of which 48 (1.4%) were considered major. One-third of these were related to the anaesthetic and two-thirds to the procedure.

All the complications of laryngoscopy and endotracheal intubation also apply to bronchoscopy (see p. 474 and p. 483). Of particular importance is trauma, especially to the teeth and gums. The bronchoscope should not pivot on the upper teeth or gum but should rest on the anaesthetist's finger placed along the upper lip. Trauma to the pharynx can be avoided by advancing the instrument slowly along the tongue while viewing through it until the epiglottis is reached. The bronchoscope should be rotated through 90° before insertion into the larynx to minimize laryngeal trauma. Tracheal and bronchial rupture can occur if excessive force is used or if the patient coughs.

Haemodynamic changes – notably arterial hypertension, tachycardia and arrhythmias – almost invariably occur during barbiturate and suxamethonium anaesthesia which is commonly used. These changes can be reduced by intravenous fentanyl or alfentanil at induction of anaesthesia (Wark et al 1986).

Bronchospasm during the procedure is a risk in asthmatics. Laryngospasm following removal of the bronchoscope can be avoided by topical analgesia of the lower airway prior to introduction of the bronchoscope.

Virtually all bronchoscopy in adults is now performed using the Sanders technique (Sanders

1967). This utilizes an injector attached to the instrument, or the sidearm, to which is connected an oxygen or entonox supply at pipeline pressure. The method utilizes the Venturi (entrainment) principle and gas flow is controlled with a manual or automatic on–off valve. Maintenance of adequate gas exchange is not usually a problem. Pulmonary barotrauma is, however, a risk. It is more likely to occur in patients predisposed to pneumothorax, such as those with apical bullae. It is also more likely to occur if chest movements are not monitored closely for signs of overinflation, and if an excessively large injector is used. The correct sizes are 16 gauge in an adult, 18 gauge in an adolescent and 19–20 gauge in a child. Injector methods are unsuitable in infants in whom the Storz telescopic bronchoscope is used. This instrument is a ventilating bronchoscope and can be attached to a T-piece circuit via an adaptor.

The injector technique presents additional hazards to the bronchoscopist. Bacteria may be ejected into the face of the bronchoscopist in infected cases, and during such cases a hat, mask, glasses and gloves should be worn. This is especially important in patients with active tuberculosis.

The Luer lock between the oxygen delivery tube and the bronchoscope may disconnect during inflation, causing the delivery tube to fly through the air at great speed. This is potentially hazardous to the eyes and faces of nearby personnel. The Luer lock should be held on by hand during ventilation.

Bronchoscopic biopsy can occasionally result in serious haemorrhage into the airway. This usually occurs if a vascular tumour, such as a bronchial adenoma, is biopsied, or if a branch of the pulmonary circulation is entered. Massive haemorrhage can seriously interfere with ventilation and it may be necessary to insert a bronchus blocker to rescue the situation. A large Fogarty vascular catheter will double as a bronchus blocker.

LASER SURGERY

The carbon dioxide laser is increasing being used in the treatment of some respiratory tract disorders, notably for resection of laryngotracheal papillomata, localized vocal cord carcinomata and subglottic stenoses. The laser beam acts as a surgical scalpel, is easily controllable and inherently haemostatic. The device is used in conjunction with a suspension microlaryngoscope to visualize the operative field with magnification.

In addition to general hazards to personnel working in the vicinity of a laser, the anaesthetist is confronted with the problem of fires within the airway caused by endotracheal tube ignition. Most rubber and plastic materials used in the manufacture of tubes are easily ignitable by the carbon dioxide laser beam, especially in the presence of high local concentrations of oxygen or nitrous oxide. Such fires can cause both thermal and smoke injury to the airway with mucosal oedema and sloughing as well as pulmonary oedema. Irritant carbonaceous material may also be deposited in the tracheobronchial tree. Fires must be prevented from occurring, either by avoiding the use of an endotracheal tube altogether (a method attended by its own hazards) or by using a non-combustible tube. In addition, high concentrations of oxygen and nitrous oxide should be avoided, and oxygen in nitrogen, or better still helium, should be used.

Non-flammability of the endotracheal tube can be achieved either by wrapping an ordinary endotracheal tube with reflective tape or by using a tube made of metal. Adhesive copper or aluminium tape can be wound around the tube in a spiral starting at the tip with a plain tube, or above the cuff and working proximally. Tape of width 0.5–1.0 cm should be used. Although the carbon dioxide laser cannot penetrate metal tape, burning tissue fragments can ignite the exposed inner surface of the tube (Hermens et al 1983; see Fig. 31.7). PVC tubes should therefore never be used for this purpose if high concentrations of oxygen or nitrous oxide are being administered, because the products of PVC combustion are more toxic than those of red rubber. However, PVC is probably safe if oxygen in helium is used and the oxygen concentration is below 40% (Pashayan et al 1988).

Cuffs cannot be wrapped with tape and contact between the beam and the cuff should

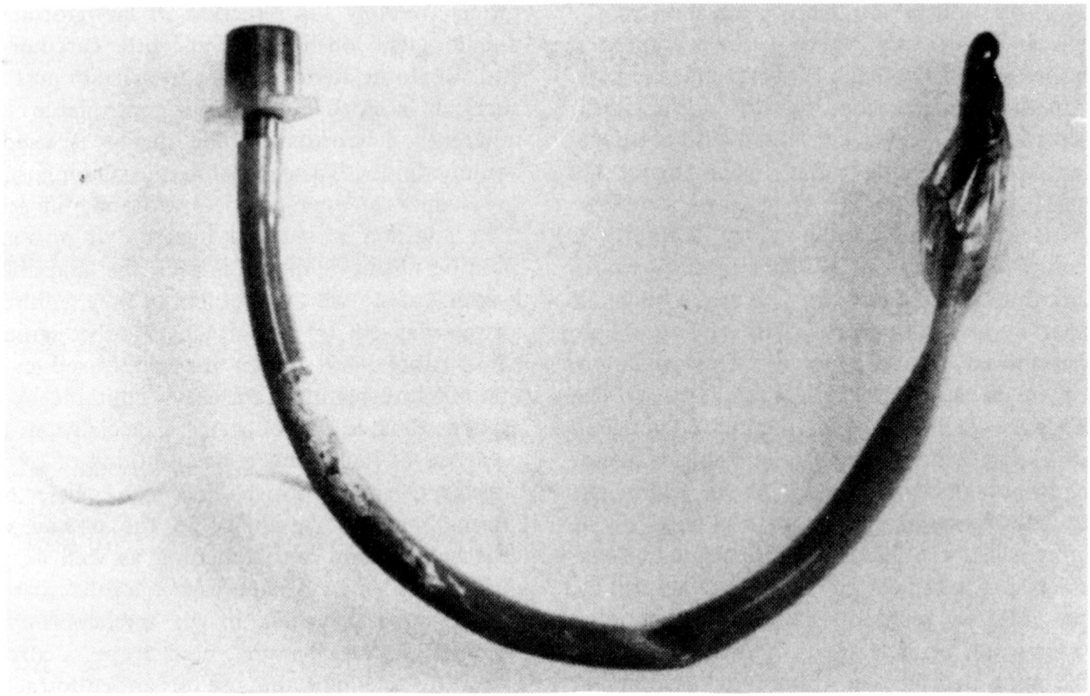

Fig. 31.7 PVC endotracheal tube which has been ignited by burning tissue on the inside of the tube (from Hirshman & Smith 1980).

therefore be prevented by placing moist ribbon gauze around the tube above the cuff. Alternatively, the cuff can be filled with physiological saline to act as a heat sink should the cuff be lasered (LeJeune et al 1982).

Tape-covered tubes are potentially traumatic to the larynx and trachea if the edges of the spiral become rough, and pieces of tape may break off and cause airway obstruction, necessitating bronchoscopic removal (Kaeder & Hirshman 1979).

Metal tubes are entirely non-flammable, but are thick walled and only semi-flexible (see Fig. 31.8). Because of the small size of the lumen in relation to the external diameter, some tubes are only suitable for use in conjunction with jet ventilation. None of these tubes is cuffed and none can be used in children.

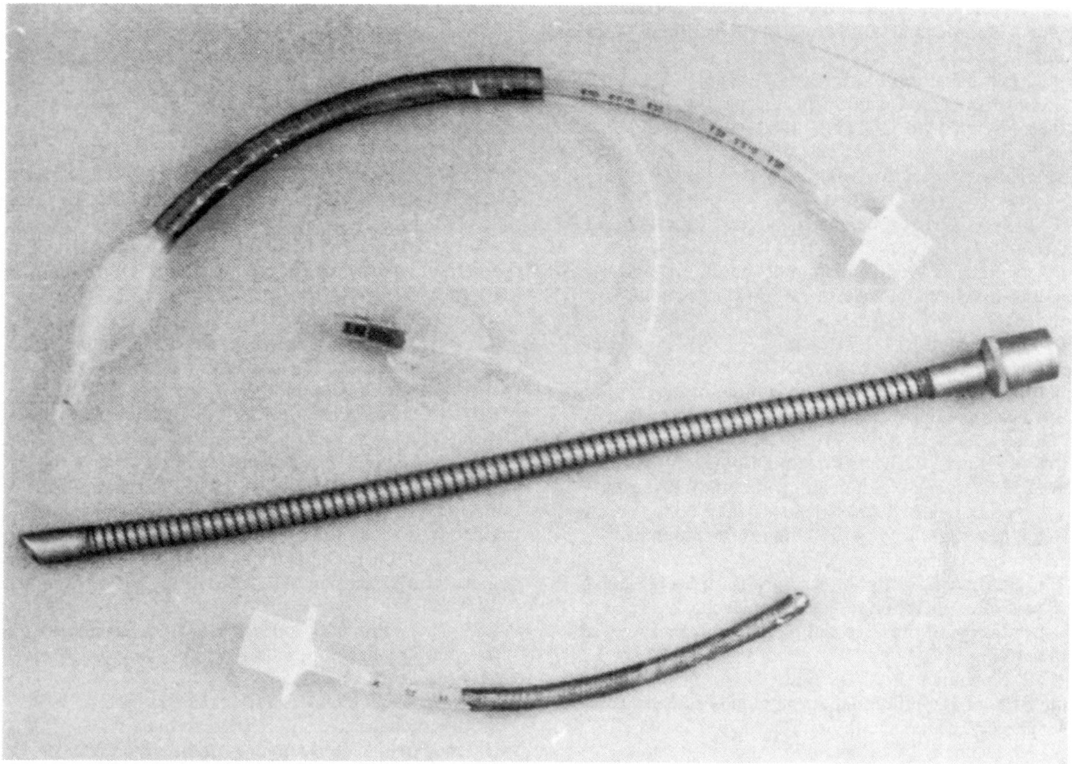

Fig. 31.8 Two PVC endotracheal tubes, the upper wrapped with copper and the lower with aluminium tape, and a metal tube (the Norton tube) in the centre (from Hermens et al 1983).

REFERENCES

Association of Anaesthetists of Great Britain and Ireland 1988 Recommendations for standards of monitoring during anaesthesia and recovery. Association of Anaesthetists, London

Barton N A, Fall S M, Lyons J, Graeber G M 1983 Rupture of the left main-stem bronchus with a polyvinylchloride double-lumen tube. Chest 83(6): 928–929

Bellhouse C P, Doré C 1988 Criteria for estimating likelihood of difficulty of endotracheal intubation with the Macintosh laryngoscope. Anaesth Intensive Care 16(3): 329–337

Blanc V F, Tremblay N A G 1974 The complications of endotracheal intubation: a new classification with review of the literature. Anesth Analg 53(2): 202–213

Boidin M P 1985 Airway patency in the unconscious patient. Br J Anaesth 57(3): 306–310

Brain A I J 1983 The laryngeal mask: a new concept in airway management. Br J Anaesth 55(8): 801–805

Brain A I J 1984 The laryngeal mask airway: a possible new solution to airway problems in the emergency situation. Arch Emerg Med 1: 229–232

Brain A I J 1985 Three cases of difficult intubation overcome by the laryngeal mask airway. Anaesthesia 40(4): 353–355

Brain A I J, McGhee T D, McAteer E J, Thomas A, Abu-Saad M A W, Bushman J A 1985 The laryngeal mask airway. Anaesthesia 40(4): 356–361

Brasch R C, Heldt G P, Hecht S T 1981 Endotracheal tube orifice abutting the tracheal wall: a cause of infant airway obstruction. Pediatr Radiol 141: 387–391

Braude N I, Clements E A F, Hodges U M, Andrews B P 1989 The pressor response and laryngeal mask insertion. Anaesthesia 44(7): 551–554

Brodrick P M, Webster N R, Nunn J F 1989 The laryngeal mask airway. Anaesthesia 44(3): 238–241

Calder I, Ordman A J, Jackowski A Crockard H A 1990 The Brain laryngeal mask airway: an alternative to emergency tracheal intubation. Anaesthesia 45(2): 137–139

Cormack R S, Lehane J 1984 Difficult tracheal intubation in obstetrics. Anaesthesia 39(11): 1105–1111

Drummond G B 1989 Influence of thiopentone on upper airway muscles. Br Anaesth 63(1): 12–21

Edelist G 1964 Principles of anaesthetic management in rheumatoid arthritic patients. Anesth Analg 43(3): 227–231

Ford R W J 1983 Confirming tracheal intubation: a simple manoeuvre. Can Anaesth Soc J 30(2): 191–193

Foster J M G, Lau O J, Alimo E B 1983 Ruptured bronchus following endobronchial intubation. Br J Anaesth 55(7): 687–688
Gerber M A, Gastanaduy A S, Buckley J J, Kaplan E L 1980 Risk of bacteremia after endotracheal intubation for general anesthesia. South Med J 73(11): 1478–1480
Gibbin K P, Egginton M J 1981 Bilateral vocal cord paralysis following endotracheal intubation. Br J Anaesth 53: 1091–1092
Grillo H C 1970 Current problems in surgery. Chicago Year Book, p 3–59
Hatch D J, Sumner E 1981 Induction of anaesthesia and intubation. In: Neonatal anaesthesia. Edward Arnold, London, ch 3
Hermens J M, Bennett M J, Hirshman C A 1983 Anesthesia for laser surgery. Anesth Analg 62: 218–229
Hirshman C A, Smith J 1980 Indirect ignition of the endotracheal tube during carbon dioxide laser surgery. Arch Otolaryngol 106: 639–641
Horton W A, Fahy L, Charters P 1989 Disposition of cervical vertebrae, atlanto-axial joint, hyoid and mandible during X-ray laryngoscopy. Br J Anaesth 63(4): 435–438
Howells T H, Riethmuller R J 1980 Signs of endotracheal intubation. Anaesthesia 35(10): 984–986
Jensen P J, Hommelgaard P, Sondergaard P, Eriksen S 1982 Sore throat after operation: influence of tracheal intubation, intracuff pressure and type of cuff. Br J Anaesth 54: 453–457
Kaeder C S, Hirshman C A 1979 Acute airway obstruction: a complication of aluminium tape wrapping of tracheal tubes in laser surgery. Can Anaesth Soc J 26: 138–139
Keane W M, Dennehy J C, Rowe L D, Atkins J P 1982 Complications of intubation. Ann Otol Rhinol & Laryngol 91: 584–587
LeJeune F E, Guice C, LeTard F, Marice H 1982 Heat sink protection against lasering endotracheal cuffs. Ann Otol Rhinol & Laryngol 91: 606–607
Levin J 1958 Endotracheal tubes in children. Anaesthesia 13: 40
Lindholm C-E, Grenvik A 1982 Tracheal tube and cuff problems. Int Anesthesiol Clin 20(3): 103–151
Linko K, Paloheimo M, Tammisto T 1983 Capnography for detection of accidental oesophageal intubation. Acta Anaesthesiol Scand 27: 199–202
Lisman S R, Shepherd N J, Rosenberg M 1981 A modified laryngoscope blade for dental protection. Anesthesiology 55(2): 190
Loeser E A, Bennett G M, Orr D L, Stanley T H 1980 Reduction of sore throat with new endotracheal tube cuffs. Anesthesiology 52(3): 257–259
Loughman E 1983 Lingual nerve injury following tracheal intubation. Anaesth Intensive Care 11: 171
Lukomsky G I, Ovchinnikov A A, Bilal A 1981 Complications of bronchoscopy. Chest 79(3): 316–321
Magill I W 1930 Technique in endotracheal anaesthesia. Br Med J 2: 817–820
Majumdar B, Stevens R W, Obara L G 1982 Retropharyngeal abscess following tracheal intubation. Anaesthesia 37(1): 67–70
Mallampati R S, Gatt S P, Gugino L D, Desai S P, Waraksa B, Freiburger D, Liu P L 1985 A clinical sign to predict difficult tracheal intubation: a prospective study. Can Anaesth Soc J 32(4): 429–434
Mehta S 1981 Effects of nitrous oxide and oxygen on tracheal tube cuff gas volumes. Br J Anaesth 53: 1227–1231
Morgan C, Gillbe C 1985 Anaesthetising the asthmatic. Br J Hosp Med 34(6): 326–330
Nichol H C, Zuck D 1983 Difficult Laryngoscopy: the 'anterior' larynx and the atlanto-occipital gap. Br J Anaesth 55: 141–143
Norton M L, Ghanma M A 1982 Atlanto-axial instability revisited: an alert for endoscopists. Ann Otol Rhinol & Laryngol 91: 567–570
Ovassapian A, Yelich S J, Dykes M H M, Golman M E 1988 Learning fibreoptic intubation: use of simulators v. traditional teaching. Br J Anaesth 61(2): 217–220
Pashayan A G, Gravenstein J S, Cassisi N J, McLaughlin G 1988 The helium protocol for laryngotracheal operations with CO_2 laser: a retrospective review of 523 cases. Anesthesiology 68(5): 801–804
Patel R I, Oh T H, Epstein B S 1983 Effects of nitrous oxide on pressure changes of tracheal tube cuffs following inflation with air and saline. Anaesthesia 38(1): 44–46
Peppard S B, Dickens J H 1983 Laryngeal injury following short term intubation. Ann Otol Rhinol & Laryngol 92: 327–330
Pope T L, Stelling C B, Leitner Y B 1981 Maxillary sinusitis after nasotracheal intubation. South Med J 74(5): 610–612
Prys-Roberts C, Greene L T, Meloche R, Foëx P 1971 Studies of anaesthesia in relation to hypertension. II. Haemodynamic consequences of induction and endotracheal intubation. Br J Anaesth 43: 531–547
Quick C A, Merwin G E 1978 Arytenoid dislocation. Arch Otolaryngol 104: 267–270
Reddy A R R, Wong D H W 1972 Epidermolysis bullosa: a review of anaesthetic problems and case reports. Can Anaesth Soc J 19(5): 536–548
Samsoon G L T, Young J R B 1987 Difficult tracheal intubation: a retrospective study. Anaesthesia 42(5): 487–490
Sanders R D 1967 Two ventilating attachments for bronchoscopes. Delaware Medical Journal 39: 170
Sherry K M 1983a Ulceration of the inferior turbinate: a complication of prolonged nasotracheal intubation. Anesthesiology 59(2): 148–149
Sherry K M 1983b Post-extubation stridor in Down's syndrome. Br J Anaesth 55(1): 53–55
Tintinalli J E, Claffey J 1981 Complications of nasotracheal intubation. Ann Emerg Med 10(3): 142–144
Tunstall M E 1976 Failed intubation drill. Anaesthesia 31: 850
Wark K J, Lyons J, Feneck R O 1986 The haemodynamic effects of bronchoscopy. Effect of pretreatment with fentanyl and alfentanil. Anaesthesia 41(2): 162–167
Wee M Y K 1988 The oesophageal detector device. Assessment of a new method to distinguish oesophageal from tracheal intubation. Anaesthesia 43(1): 27–29
White A, Kander P L 1975 Anatomical factors in difficult direct laryngoscopy. Br J Anaesth 47: 468–473

32

Vascular catheterization

T. M. Savege

(Reprinted from the 1st edition)

INTRODUCTION

Catheterization of either arteries or veins has become a universal practice so that most patients admitted to hospital will have an intravascular needle or catheter inserted at some time during their admission. Unfortunately this practice has been associated with a large number of complications, some of them lethal.

The range of complications is discussed in this chapter, divided into those related to venous and those related to arterial catheterization.

COMPLICATIONS OF VENOUS CATHETERIZATION

Complications of venous catheterization can be divided into seven main headings:

- phlebitis
- thrombus formation
- infection
- trauma
- catheter embolus
- air embolus
- failures.

Phlebitis

Phlebitis is usually defined as an area of erythema, tenderness and induration over the vein associated with a palpable 'cord' along the vein and sometimes with perivenous oedema (Tully et al 1981). It is a common complication of intravenous infusion with a reported incidence of between 15 and 70%. The usual incidence is around 20%. The wide variation in incidence is probably due to the number of factors that influence its development. It usually occurs between 24 and 72 h after cannulation and lasts some 24–72 h (Hershey et al 1984). It is very unusual for it to occur within 12 h of cannulation, and if it has not developed by 10 days it will almost certainly not occur later. Most catheters are placed in a vein for a relatively short time, consequently more than half the cases of phlebitis develop over 12 h after catheter removal. Phlebitis tends to develop rapidly so that 24 h before the diagnosis is made there will be few, if any, warning signs, although about 30% of patients will complain of pain at the infusion site (Hershey et al 1984).

Aetiology

In animal studies the first change is one of intimal damage with initial vacuolization of the endothelial cells proceeding to destruction of intimal lining. It is probable therefore that the main cause is one of physical or chemical trauma, or both, caused either by (1) the catheter or (2) the infusion fluid.

1. It is likely that phlebitis is in part a response to a foreign body. The reaction is seen despite the use of a wide variety of materials used in the manufacture of cannulae, including stainless steel, and might be

initiated by movement of the cannula in or out of the vein resulting in mechanical trauma. The material associated with most phlebitis was rubber infusion tubing (Handfield et al 1952), and the lowest incidence is seen with stainless-steel needles (8.8%), at about half that of Teflon (Tully et al 1981). Toxic plasticizer (di-2-ethylhexylphthalate) may account for some of the phlebitis caused by plastic catheters (Collin et al 1975). Curelaru et al (1984) could not demonstrate any significant difference in the incidence of thrombophlebitis with the use of seven different types of plastic catheter.

2. Solutions that are hypertonic, for example 50% glucose and amino acid solutions or those that have a low pH, are associated with an increased incidence of phlebitis. Dextrose that is heat-sterilized has to be prepared at a pH of between 3 and 5 to prevent carmelization. If it is then buffered to a more physiological pH the incidence of phlebitis is reduced by 60% or more. Similarly, if dextrose solutions are sterilized by filtration the pH is higher and the incidence of phlebitis is reduced. Drugs such as vancomycin, pethidine, barbiturates and benzodiazepines are associated with a high incidence of phlebitis.

Phlebitis and infection

As phlebitis often occurs after a catheter is removed, and sometimes 10 days later, it has been suggested that it must be an infective process. There is no doubt that an infected infusion site, contaminated catheter tip or even septicaemia can be associated with phlebitis. Furthermore, phlebitis is more severe and lasts longer in patients who are immunosuppressed, or who have some other concurrent infection. On the other hand, there is much evidence to suggest that phlebitis can occur in the absence of local and systemic infection, and one is led to assume that infection exacerbates and prolongs phlebitis rather than initiates it.

Other factors associated with the incidence and severity of phlebitis. It has been said that phlebitis is less likely if a catheter is inserted into a peripheral vein so that its tip lies in a central vein (Wilmore et al 1965). This may be explained on the basis that any effect induced by infusion fluids and drugs would not be visible. However, long lines do cause phlebitis of the superficial veins and the incidence at 21% is similar to that of short catheters (Curelaru et al 1984).

Prevention of phlebitis

If catheter insertion, maintenance and removal is supervised by a specialized intravenous team the incidence of phlebitis can be halved (Tomford et al 1984). It seems likely that the single most important factor is the removal of all catheters at between 48 and 72 h. The use of heparin as ointment or in the infusion does not prevent phlebitis. The avoidance of irritant drugs and fluids is obviously a useful preventative factor whenever this is possible.

Thrombus formation

Thrombus is formed as part of the natural response to the presence of a foreign body in a vessel. Platelets adhere to plastic catheters and a thrombus rapidly forms. Catheters placed in the internal jugular veins of dogs have significant amounts of clot attached to their surface within 30 min. Similarly, a number of reports have shown that catheters placed in the central venous system of man, or in an artery, are 85% (or more) covered by a thin layer of thrombus after being in the vessel for only 2 h (Hoar et al 1978, Kido et al 1982).

Curelaru et al (1984) have tried to assess whether various types of plastic material encourage different degrees of platelet adhesiveness in vitro. Their findings suggest that, of the catheters tested, platelet adhesion was greatest in plain silicone elastomer and least in satiny surface polyurethane (Table 32.1). The type of plastic probably does not make a great deal of difference to the amount of thrombus formed. However, it may be that stiffer material induces greater intimal damage and therefore initiates more thrombus formation.

Table 32.1 Plastic materials listed in order of platelet adhesiveness

Platelets	Catheter material
Most adhesive	Plain silicone elastomer
↓	Polyethylene
	Plain soft urethane
	Plain soft polyvinyl chloride
	Heparinized polyethylene
	Heparinized soft polyurethane
Least adhesive	Stiff, satiny surface polyurethane

Modified from Curelaru et al 1984

Heparin can be bonded to the surface of plastic catheters, and has been shown to reduce the incidence and volume of thrombus formation. In one study, thrombus formation was detected in 44% of heparin-treated catheters 2 h after insertion into the carotid artery, compared with a higher incidence of 85% in non-heparin-treated catheters (Kido et al 1982). Heparin leaches out of the catheter, probably over a period of 12 h. Even so, heparin-bonded pulmonary artery catheters left in place for 24 h show a lower incidence of thrombus formation: 10% compared with 100% incidence in non-heparin-treated catheters (Mangano 1982).

Thrombus also forms over areas of intimal damage and inflammation, whether caused by trauma of the needle insertion, mechanical movement of the catheter or the irritant effect of transfusion fluids and drugs. Some sort of thrombotic process was demonstrated in 95% of patients by venography in whom a 16-gauge polyvinyl chloride catheter was placed in the central venous system. Most commonly a sheath of thrombus adherent to the catheter was noted, but in 13% of patients a mural thrombus was demonstrated (Ahmed & Payne 1976).

Chastre et al (1978) reported an incidence of asymptomatic internal jugular vein thrombosis in 66% of a series of consecutive patients, all critically ill and catheterized with Swan–Ganz catheters for just over 3 days. The diagnosis was established by contrast venography or at postmortem. The one feature that distinguished the patients was that those with thrombosis had had a cardiac output some 30% lower, measured at 12 h after insertion, and it remained lower for a longer period of time.

Thrombus, once formed, can be expected to propagate at a rate that will depend on such factors as the rate of blood flow in the vein, the size of the catheter (which becomes wider as thrombus forms over its length), whether it is doubled over, and the general condition of the patient. The latter broad term includes such conditions as hypercoagulability of the blood and low cardiac output. Patients with severe burns are particularly susceptible to catheter-related thrombus formation.

Thrombus formation is so frequently associated with phlebitis that in the presence of signs of the latter one can assume there is thrombus formation. Commonly, however, venous thrombus is only diagnosed at postmortem or when one of its complications occurs.

In one series of postmortem examinations of patients with hydrocephalus who had had long-term ventriculovenous plastic shunts in situ, extensive thrombus formation was seen extending along the length of the catheter in each case. In one patient a large fibrin clot was seen wedging open the tricuspid valve, rendering it incompetent. Six of these patients had mural thrombus in the atrium, and another had clot propagated throughout the superior caval system. Few of these findings had been suspected before death (Emery & Hilton 1960).

On removing a catheter it can look remarkably free of clot. Clot on the outside is wiped off as the catheter is pulled out, and is released into the vascular system as an embolus. Clot on the inside of the catheter is more often visible, but this too can be dislodged when the catheter is flushed with fluids or when a guidewire reinserted.

The principal complications of venous thrombus formation are venous occlusion, thromboembolism, suppurative thromobophlebitis and catheter occlusion.

Venous occlusion

Thrombus formation leading to a superficial vein occlusion has a reported incidence of between 0 and 19%. It is a very frequent complication of phlebitis, and is said to be more common in superficial veins because blood flow is slower and the narrow vein is more obstructed by the catheter. Furthermore, a catheter in a peripheral vein is more likely to be in contact with the vessel wall so that the effects of mechanical and chemical trauma are greater. However, it seems more likely that deep-vein thrombosis is just not observed by clinicians, because the vein cannot be palpated and because venous obstruction leading to clinical signs of oedema seldom result owing to the presence of an adequate collateral circulation. The incidence of deep-vein occlusion by thrombosis is said to be about 7%, but this will depend on the clinical condition of the patient (Ahmed & Payne 1976), the technique of insertion, the type of catheter used, the duration of catheterization and the method used to establish the diagnosis (Smith & Hallett 1983).

Deep-vein thrombosis can sometimes lead to tissue swelling and oedema. In the upper part of the body this is known as the superior vena cava syndrome, and is characterized by suffusion and swelling of the face, neck and upper extremities; cough; dyspnoea and dysphagia with or without the presence of visible dilated collateral veins over the upper part of the thorax. Pyrexia and shoulder pain are also commonly found.

The mechanism for the development of this syndrome is presumably the same as for thrombus formation. Reports refer to patients who have had catheters in for a long time, or alternatively have had Swan–Ganz catheters inserted to investigate poor cardiovascular function. This suggests that clot builds up with the passage of time and its formation may be accelerated in conditions of low flow (Gore et al 1984).

Infection of the catheter tip may facilitate occlusion of the vein. In one series, 30% of tips were shown to be infected (Smith & Hallett 1983). It seems more likely, however, that infection complicates thrombus formation rather than the other way around.

The diagnosis is confirmed by contrast venography. Treatment includes removal of the catheter and the elevation of the swollen limb. Antibiotics should be given only if there is evidence of sepsis. The patient should be fully anticoagulated with heparin for 7–10 days, followed by warfarin for 3–6 months. Unfortunately, heparin may not prevent progression of the thrombus. Streptokinase given as a loading dose of 250 000 units, and followed by infusion of 100 000 units/h, can lead to lysis of the clot and subsidence of symptoms (Rubenstein & Creger 1980) and may be more effective than heparin (Marder 1979). Dramatic clearing of thrombus has been reported after the use of a much smaller dose of streptokinase (500 units/h for 24 h) (Jacobs & Yaeger 1984). Fibrinolytic and anticoagulant agents can increase the risk of haemorrhage. They should not be used where bleeding could result and be inaccessible to control, for example in a head injury.

Thrombosis affecting the inferior vena cava used to be thought more common than thrombosis of the superior caval system. Possibly as a result of this impression, catheters have been passed almost exclusively into the superior caval system. It seems likely that the frequency of thrombosis in the great veins is proportional to the frequency of selection of any particular vein.

Thromboembolism

Bits of clot may break free from the vein or catheter and form emboli in the pulmonary circulation. The incidence of clinically demonstrable pulmonary embolism is low, but it is probable that symptomless emboli occur much more frequently. The incidence during parenteral nutrition is about 5% (Jeejeebhoy et al 1976). Ryan et al (1974) examined 200 patients with central lines inserted for parenteral nutrition. Although none showed signs of venous obstruction, eight of the 34 deaths had superior vena caval thrombosis and three had demonstrable pulmonary emboli. It is important to realize that thrombus formation can continue after removal of a catheter, and that pulmonary emboli may result at a much later date. One report described a patient who was catheterized in May following a myocardial infarction. Subsequently, pulmonary embolism occurred in September, but was diagnosed as pneumonia and the correct diagnosis was made only at postmortem. Thrombi of the right internal jugular, innominate, subclavian vein and part of the superior vena cava were noted, and the lungs contained signs of old and new pulmonary emboli with multiple infarction (Snow 1980).

Emboli can originate from superficial veins, although they are very rare from arm veins unless the thrombus has suppurated. Small emboli can be released from a catheter as it is removed. This is unlikely to be significant with venous lines, but can be a potentially serious complication of arterial lines.

Catheter occlusion

Thrombus building up on the inside of a catheter can ultimately cause blockage. Prior to occlusion, sampling becomes difficult and venous pressure measurements become unreliable, often necessitating removal of the catheter. Tully et al (1981) reported an incidence of 15% for steel needles and 16.8% for Teflon catheters. It is probably a less frequent complication today when a constant flow of infusion fluid is so frequently ensured by the use of infusion pumps. A small dose of heparin (5–10 mg/l) added to the infusion fluid may also help prevent this complication.

Sometimes it is impractical to replace a very valuable catheter, for example during the treatment of acute renal failure by haemodialysis. The incidence of complete block of such catheters has been variously reported between 7% and 24%. The use of guidewires to dislodge thrombus is often not successful and probably undesirable. Streptokinase (250 000 units diluted in 6 ml of saline and placed in the catheter for 20 min) has been reported as an effective method of unblocking such catheters (Chillar et al 1980).

Prevention of thrombus formation

It is probably impossible to prevent the formation of a thrombus on a catheter or over damaged intima. Heparin, administered either intravenously or subcutaneously, is not effective, although full heparinization will reduce the rate of thrombus formation. The use of Dextran 70 to reduce the rate of platelet adhesion is also not reliably effective.

Thrombus formation can be kept to a minimum if a strict aseptic technique is used for inserting the catheter, if the insertion technique is performed expertly with minimum trauma and if soft catheters are used, possibly bonded with heparin. Small catheters placed in veins of high blood flow for the shortest possible time are likely to minimize the extent of thrombus formation, as is the use of intravenous fluids that do not initiate phlebitis.

The practice of changing an inadequately functioning catheter by passing a guidewire and threading up a new catheter is probably unwise. It prolongs the duration of catheterization of a vein that already has thrombus forming along it.

Infection

Bacterial and fungal penetration of the skin during intravenous therapy

Organisms probably gain access to the circulation in two ways. The first is via the catheter, either at the time of insertion or later by migrating from the skin up the outer surface of the catheter into the bloodstream. Movement of the catheter in and out of the catheter–skin entry site, such as when the limb is flexed, could well encourage bacterial entry, although anchoring the catheter firmly has not been shown to reduce infection.

The second way in which organisms enter the patient is from the infusion fluids, the giving set and associated ports. It has been estimated that some 10% of infusion fluids contain small amounts of bacteria (<1/ml), but such low concentrations are not likely to cause septicaemia, which is probably ten times less common from the infusion fluid than from the catheter (Maki et al 1977).

Bacteria can contaminate the sterile infusion system by gaining entry through unprotected air ports, for example the CVP measuring lines, when infusion sets or bottles are replaced, or when drugs are administered through open injection ports (three-way taps). Very occasionally the infusion fluid itself has not been correctly sterilized and catastrophic septicaemia can result. Dextrose and dextrose saline solutions will not support bacterial growth, probably because of the low pH of the solutions. However, organisms can grow in Hartman's solution and in normal saline. Amino acid solutions support the growth of both bacteria and fungi within a temperature range of 25–37°C, although bacteria and fungi do not grow as readily in synthetic amino acid dextrose solutions as they do in casein hydrolysate dextrose solutions. Lipid solutions also support bacterial and fungal growth. Bacterial filters placed in line are effective at filtering out bacteria but frequently become blocked and have to be replaced. This necessitates breaking open the system and risks further contamination.

Once an infusion system is contaminated it may become a self-perpetuating source of infection, so it is important that bottles and plastic tubing are all changed once every 24 h. It has been suggested that bacteria from the infusion system lodge and multiply in the hub of the catheter, then infect the patient from there. If this is so, eradication of contamination will prove more difficult than has been hoped.

Contamination of skin and wound infection

Normally, skin harbours only harmless flora. However, in ill and debilitated patients, colonies of pathogens may be cultured from the skin, and some of the so-called harmless commensals can be responsible for serious infection. The catheter–skin entry site rarely becomes colonized within 48 h of inserting the catheter, but thereafter the incidence of colonization rises rapidly. Contamination may occur as a result of medical and nursing personnel handling the site. Furthermore, bacteria may be transferred from other infected superficial sites, such as a tracheostomy wound. If a dressing is applied over the catheter–skin entry site it must not be allowed to become wet or contaminated with blood because this will encourage the growth of organisms.

Even the cleaning fluid can be a source of catheter–skin entry site contamination: both benzalkonium chloride and cetrimide kept in corked bottles can support bacterial growth.

Catheter colonization and infection

Organisms can be cultivated from about 10–30% of catheters, although the incidence varies greatly from one source to another and has even been reported to be as much as 88%. The incidence of positive cultures can be correlated with the duration of catheterization, and is very unusual if the catheter has been in place for less than 2 days. In one study where needles or catheters were removed by 72 h, only 1.5% grew organisms (Tully et al 1981). In another study 13% of patients with central venous catheters in position for less than 8 days developed infected catheters compared to 43% of patients where the catheter was in place for 8 days or more (Prager & Silva 1984).

Organisms can get to the catheter in a number of ways. Contamination may occur at the time of insertion or on removal of the catheter through an infected skin entry site. Organisms may be carried to the catheter in the blood from other infected tissues. Although catheter-tip cultures are more often positive in patients with pre-existing infection, attempts to correlate the organisms at the catheter site with those causing infection elsewhere are often unsuccessful.

As mentioned earlier, the most common source of catheter organisms is thought to be from the catheter–skin entry site. Inflammation of this site is more frequent in patients with catheter-tip infection (60%) than in those with catheter-tip contamination (30%), although, unfortunately, the absence of inflammation does not rule out the possibility of catheter infection (Maki et al 1977).

Even with the use of longer venous lines inserted in the subclavian or internal jugular vein, 35% of patients with organisms grown on their catheters also had inflammation of the catheter–skin entry site (Prager & Silva 1984).

The organisms grown on the catheter can be found at the skin entry site or at sites of other superficial skin wounds in 75% of instances, and they are frequently of a type that is considered a normal skin commensal (Keohane et al 1983). Furthermore, catheter infection is a frequent complication of burns patients, where huge colonies of organisms can be found cultured on the damaged skin surface.

The terms 'catheter infection' and 'catheter contamination' lead to considerable confusion in the literature. Clearly a few bacteria that become attached to a catheter at the time of its removal would amount to contamination, and have little significance for the patient, whereas a catheter tip covered in thrombus and containing a huge number of organisms, multiplying rapidly and possibly breaking off into the bloodstream to be carried elsewhere, would present a grave risk to the patient. It is also clear that a mild contamination might lead to a life-threatening infection if the catheter were to remain in position for long enough. Attempts have been made to differentiate between contamination and infection by applying semiquantitative culture techniques. A length of catheter is rolled across a blood agar plate and if 15 or more colonies are subsequently cultured, infection is said to be present (Maki et al 1977). Clearly this is no real help to the clinician, for whom the diagnosis of catheter infection is very difficult. The diagnosis should always be in one's mind when a catheter has been in position for several days, and if the patient shows signs of generalized infection or even septicaemia but where no other source of infection can be found. In addition the presence of inflammation of the catheter–skin entry site increases the likelihood of catheter infection.

A number of other factors may influence the incidence of catheter infection:

- thrombus formation
- catheter material
- catheter length
- site of insertion.

Thrombus formation. It has been suggested that thrombus formation on the catheter encourages bacterial growth and subsequent catheter-tip infection. Stillman et al (1977) reported a correlation between the presence of visible thrombus at a catheter tip on removal and the culture of organisms at the tip. It was concluded that catheter tip infection was most unlikely if the catheter appeared completely free of thrombus after removal from the patient. The use of a catheter made of ethylene acrylic acid delayed the development of visible thrombus by 2 days in each instance, and in only 31% of catheters could thrombus be seen on removal at 12 days compared with 100% of catheters made of other materials. The ethylene acrylic acid catheters were associated with a lower frequency of catheter-tip infection (2.6% compared with 17.9%). Therefore the active prevention of thrombus formation along the length of a catheter may significantly reduce the incidence of catheter infection.

Catheter material. It is commonly stated that stainless steel needles are less likely to become infected than plastic catheters. This finding is probably associated with the fact that metal needles are left in veins for a shorter period of time than plastic catheters. Recent studies suggest that needles are just as susceptible to infection if they are left in place for a similar time (Tully et al 1981).

There is no evidence that infection is more commonly associated with any specific plastic material except where it is associated with more or less thrombus formation.

Catheter length. Longer catheters may be associated with more phlebitis and a greater incidence of infection than with the use of shorter ones (Collin et al 1975).

Site of insertion. It has been suggested that central catheters inserted via the internal jugular vein are less likely to develop infection than those passed via the subclavian vein (Prager & Silva 1984).

Suppurative thrombophlebitis

Infection along a vein or a catheter that becomes established in a thrombus can lead to suppuration, with pieces of infected clot breaking off and being disseminated to other organs. The incidence of suppurative thrombophlebitis is about 5% in cannulated patients with burns, and has been reported as the most common cause of death from sepsis in these patients (Pruitt et al 1970). In Pruitt et al's study, 76 cases of suppurative thrombophlebitis were diagnosed out of 1929 patients with burns, of whom 25 died as a result. Suppurative thrombophlebitis is a much less frequent complication in patients without burns, and it is not clear why this should be. It may be that patients with burns are particularly prone to bacteraemia as a result of damaged and infected skin, and as a consequence of the suppression of immune mechanisms.

Suppurative thrombophlebitis is difficult to diagnose because it frequently occurs after the catheter has been removed; furthermore there may be no clinical signs related to the affected vein. It should always be suspected in patients with persistent septicaemia who have an indwelling venous catheter, or who have recently had one removed. Sometimes, if the overlying skin is massaged, pus can be 'milked' down the vein to appear at the catheter-skin entry site and to confirm the diagnosis. Apart from septicaemia the most serious complication is that of septic embolus leading to multiple abscesses in the lungs, liver or spleen, and acute bacterial or fungal endocarditis.

Once again the incidence of infection is reduced if a scrupulous aseptic technique is used for the insertion and maintenance of the catheter, and if it is removed within 72 h of insertion. Catheters should not be inserted through broken skin. The condition is said to be more frequent if catheters are placed in lower limbs. Once the diagnosis is established the catheter must be removed. Local or systemic antibiotics are seldom of value in this condition. Ligation of the infected vein, or its complete removal, may be the only effective treatment (O'Neill et al 1968).

Bacteraemia and septicaemia

The terms 'bacteraemia', 'septicaemia' and 'sepsis' are often used confusingly in the literature, so accurate assessment of incidence is impossible. Bacteraemia is a term that should be reserved for the positive culture of organisms in the blood without overt clinical signs, whereas septicaemia is a bacteraemia or fungaemia accompanied by a variable number of clinical signs such as rigours, pyrexia, leucocytosis or leucopenia, hypotension, oliguria, disseminated intravascular coagulation and possibly changes in the patient's state of consciousness. The diagnosis of septicaemia can be notoriously difficult. It is often missed and at other times presumed without confirmation from blood cultures.

It is difficult to know whether a septicaemia originates from the infusion system or from some other primary site, but it is generally accepted that the infusion system is responsible if the same organisms are isolated from the blood and the catheter or infusion equipment. The incidence of septicaemia due to the placement of an intravenous catheter for between 4 and 72 h is in a range between 2% and 5%, and is said to account for 20–30% of all septicaemias detected in hospital practice (Maki 1981). The incidence rises with the duration of catheterization. In one study it was 1.6% in patients where the catheter was in situ for up to 7 days and 25% in patients where the catheter was in position for 8 days or more (Prager & Silva 1984). These figures may underestimate the true incidence. The mortality from such septicaemia has been reported at 40% (Maki 1981). In one study, 40% of the patients with infected catheters developed septicaemia, but in only about half of these was the organism in the blood correlated with the catheter organism. There are two possible explanations. It is possible that the infusion system is responsible and one has merely failed to culture the causative organism in the system. In addition, or alternatively, patients who require long-term vascular catheterization are usually very ill, and are more susceptible to the potentially lethal effects of any bacteraemia from whatever source. Many of the risk factors associated with septicaemia are present in patients who require prolonged vascular catheterization (Table 32.2).

The organisms that are most frequently found in catheter-related septicaemias are staphylococci (*S. aureus*, *albus* and *epidermidis*), *streptococci*, *E. coli* and *proteus*, *diphtheroides*, *Klebsiella*, *Bacteroides* and *Candida albicans*).

Table 32.2 Risk factors for nosocomial septicaemia

Host factors	Therapeutic factors
Newborn	Corticosteroid and immunosuppressive therapy
Elderly	Systemic antimicrobial therapy
Multiple trauma	Confinement to an intensive therapy unit
Burns	Invasive intravascular device
Fatal underlying disease	Administration of large volumes of parenteral fluids or blood products
Granulocytopenia	Haemodialysis

Septicaemia complicated total parenteral nutrition in about 20% patients in the early 1970s, but with strict attention to sterile technique by keeping to a meticulous nursing protocol the incidence has fallen to about 5% or even less. *Candida albicans* accounts for about half of the cases that occur. The large incidence of septicaemia during parenteral nutrition is in part due to the long duration of venous catheterization in these debilitated patients (Ladefoged & Jarnum 1978). Attempts at tunnelling the catheter so as to separate the catheter–skin entry site from the entrance of the catheter into the vein was initially thought to reduce the incidence of catheter infection and septicaemia. However more recent controlled studies have shown that tunnelling is only really advantageous if the nursing procedures for the management of the infusion are lax. Where a detailed protocol for the management of the system is meticulously followed the septicaemia rates can be cut to 4% or less, and in such circumstances tunnelling is of little benefit (Keohane et al 1983).

It needs to be stressed that intravenous nutrition should be avoided whenever possible because of the high risk of infection. If it seems likely that a patient will be absorbing nutrition form the enteral route in a few days' time it is probably preferable to omit intravenous nutrition altogether.

The complications of septicaemia can include cardiovascular collapse, acute respiratory distress syndrome, disseminated intravascular coagulation, renal failure and intrahepatic cholestasis. Infection can be spread to other organs via the blood, and a wide range of sites have been reported for metastatic infection including, for example: osteomylitis; septic arthritis; perisplenic, myocardial and mediastinal abscesses; and septic pulmonary emboli. Fungal and bacteraemic endocarditis have been reported as a complication of catheter-based septicaemia and are especially likely if one of the heart valves is already diseased.

Prevention and treatment of infection

Site of infusion. Inflamed, infected and burned areas should be avoided, as should zones normally colonized by a large number of organisms, such as the groin. There is some evidence to suggest that catheters in the internal jugular vein are less likely to become infected than those in the subclavian vein. There is no obvious explanation for this finding at present and it has not yet been confirmed.

Method of insertion of catheter and maintenance of infusion. It is constantly emphasized that the insertion of intravenous catheters should be carried out under full aseptic conditions and that such standards should apply to percutaneous as well as cut-down procedures. This may be impractical where infusions are being set up in healthy patients for periods of less than 48 h. When the patient is seriously ill and/or debilitated and/or it is expected that infusion will be required for more than 48 h, full sterile precautions are mandatory. The skin should be washed with soap and water to remove dirt and organic debris, defatted with ether or alcohol and then scrubbed with an effective antiseptic, such as 1% iodine in 70% alcohol. The operator should scrub up, wear a mask, gown and gloves, and isolate the skin site with sterile towels. A single needle puncture will be associated with less infection than a case where the vein is difficult to locate and repeated needling is required. The catheter should be effectively anchored once it is in position to prevent movement in and out of the wound. Secure anchorage does not necessarily require a skin suture, and silk sutures should be avoided because they have been associated with stitch abscesses at a later date. The catheter–skin entry site should be sprayed with an antiseptic containing iodine and covered with a sterile occlusive dressing. The purpose of the dressing is to isolate the catheter–skin entry site from the rest of the skin; it should therefore provide an effective seal. It should not be made up of bulky absorbent material which can become wet with infusion or body fluids, thus providing a culture medium for organisms, and it should allow the skin beneath the dressing to dry out so that it does not become macerated. A transparent dressing is useful because the catheter–skin entry site can be observed for signs of inflammation and swelling without disturbing the dressing.

Inspection of the site should be carried out regularly and the infusion site changed once inflammation is apparent. It is probably best not to change the dressings regularly, only once the material shows signs of not being occlusive, for example rolling up at the edges. A 'no touch' sterile technique should be used when the dressing is changed. A swab of the wound should be taken, the site resprayed with antiseptic solution and resealed.

The entire infusion system, including taps and bungs, should be replaced once every 24 h, and care should be taken not to contaminate the hub of the catheter during this procedure.

As infection is thought to get to the catheter–skin entry site from other infected superficial areas or from contaminated hands of medical or nursing attendants, great care should be taken to keep the body surface of the patient clean. Secretions from superficial wounds, sputum from the tracheostomy, pus from drainage wounds, faeces, etc., must be effectively removed and not allowed to contaminate the catheter–skin entry site. Attendant staff should avoid handling the infusion system, and when handling is necessary must wash their hands in antiseptic beforehand or wear sterile gloves.

Duration of catheterization. Catheters should be left in place for the minimum time. The incidence of infection, phlebitis and thrombosis is correlated with duration of cannulation. As infection is uncommon if the catheter has been in situ for less than 2 days it is often recommended that the entry site should be changed every 48 h. In many instances this is impractical and the infusion has to be left at one site until signs of a complication develop.

Sterility of infusion fluids and equipment. Infusion fluids must be correctly sterilized and should not be used if they contain foreign particles. Fluids that are normally clear should not be used if they become cloudy.

The infusion set should be arranged taking care to avoid contamination of sterile surfaces (and keeping disconnections to a minimum). The use of taps or cannulae with injection side-ports should be avoided if possible. Covered injection ports that can be scrubbed with antiseptic before injection of drugs are preferable (Saloheimo et al 1984).

Antibiotic agents. Antibiotic cream placed at the catheter–skin entry site has been shown to reduce infection. However it may encourage resistant strains of bacteria to develop, may not be effective against fungi and can cause local allergic reactions. Consequently, antibiotic cream is not used today. Antiseptic sprays, such as povidone iodine, are effective against a wide range of fungi and bacteria in vitro and are frequently applied to the catheter–skin entry site. It is still too early to assess the advantage of such measures. There are reports that they make no difference to the incidence of catheter contamination and infection. Systemic antibiotics administered via the infusion system often fail to prevent colonization of the catheter tip and may encourage the growth of resistant organisms or fungal infection.

Wound and blood cultures. Regular culture of the skin close to the catheter–skin entry site is a useful method of monitoring infection. In one study, 67% of catheter–skin entry sites that were culture-positive also grew organisms at the proximal intravascular segment of the catheter, and 10% of patients developed septicaemia, whereas no catheter-related infection could be identified in patients with sterile catheter-skin entry sites (Snydman et al 1982).

Blood cultures should be routinely taken from patients who have intravascular lines in place for more than 2 days, and segments of the catheter should be sent for culture once it has been removed.

Trauma

Damage to vessels

Close to the site of catheterization. Trauma at the insertion site of peripherally placed catheters is a common complication, although it usually only involves damage to veins with resultant haematoma and is seldom reported. Bleeding is easily noticed and stopped by the application of pressure.

Stainless steel needles and plastic catheters can 'cut out' of a vein, although needles are far more likely to do this. In one study the incidence was 40%: more than twice as frequent for needles as for catheters (Tully et al 1971). As a consequence of the catheter or needle cutting out of the vein, large volumes of infusion fluid may be transfused subcutaneously if the leak is not noticed, as, for example, when an area is covered with sterile towels during surgery. Ischaemic necrosis of skin can occur after subcutaneous infusion of either large quantities of fluid or solutions containing certain drugs, such as adrenaline, sodium bicarbonate and calcium chloride.

Local pain at the infusion site in the absence of inflammation has been described. Transient limb ischaemia has been reported after puncture of the femoral vein, and during rapid infusion into the long saphenous vein the skin blanches, pulses disappear and limb temperature falls. The aetiology of this condition is unknown, although reflex arterial spasm has been suggested.

Far more serious and more varied complications may result from attempts to cannulate large veins in the neck, thorax and groin. If vessels at these sites are damaged there may be considerable haemorrhage, which is either revealed as a haematoma or concealed with the development of haemomediastinum, a haemothorax or a retroperitoneal haematoma. Large arteries run close to the veins at these sites and they can be accidentally punctured or torn by guidewires or needles. Haemorrhage into the thorax or abdomen may not be recognized until the patient has lost a large quantity of blood and the signs of hypovolaemia become apparent. If haemothorax or haemomediastinum develops, breathlessness, deviation of the trachea to one side and reduced breath sounds over the lung fields may be detected. The diagnosis can be confirmed by chest radiography. Alternatively if a retroperitoneal haematoma develops, the lower abdomen may be tender and distended, a mass may be felt on palpation and bowel sounds are likely to be absent. Radiography of the abdomen may show displacement of the bladder or colon (Sharp et al 1983). Pelvic and rectal examination may confirm the diagnosis.

The incidence of serious complications from haemorrhage is probably less than 1%. Haemorrhage is more likely if the patient is taking anticoagulant therapy or has a coagulation defect. As a later consequence of vessel trauma, arteriovenous fistulae and arterial aneurysms may develop in the subclavian and femoral vessels.

Far from the site of catheterization. The tips of long catheters may perforate the vessel walls just as can short catheters and needles. If this occurs it is usually some 24–48 h after the initial cannulation. Several litres of blood may be lost from the circulation, and surgery is sometimes necessary to evacuate clot and repair the damaged vessel. One probable mechanism of this damage is that the catheter gets bound to the vessel wall by thrombus. Hyperosmolar infusion fluid, brought into close contact with a section of vessel wall, then initiates phlebitis and necrosis of the vascular tissue (McDonnell et al 1984). Once a catheter tip has perforated the vessel, large quantities of intravenous solution can be transfused outside the vein. A case of fatal hydrothorax that compressed both lungs has been reported (Adar & Mozes 1970). As much as 2700 ml of glucose solution has been successfully aspirated from the thorax (Pruitt et al 1970). Hydrothorax can occur bilaterally as a consequence of one catheterization procedure and should be suspected if a patient becomes breathless some 24–48 h after the catheter is inserted. Clinical evidence of pleural effusion should be sought and a radiograph of the chest will reveal the diagnosis (McDonnell et al 1984).

A catheter tip sited in the right atrium can perforate into the pericardial cavity and lead to hydro- or haemopericardium. Thomas et al (1969) described a patient that had been catheterized via the basilic vein and the catheter tip located in the right atrium. The patient collapsed some 36 h later, hypotensive and pulseless. It was decided to inject intracardiac adrenaline. A needle was inserted into the heart and aspirated to check its position. To their surprise and consternation, clear fluid was aspirated. Finally, 250 ml of clear fluid was removed from the pericardial sac with immediate improvement in the patient's condition (Thomas et al 1969).

There have been several reports of atrial perforation and pericardial tamponade, often with fatal results. Catheter tips should be sited in the vena cavae and not in the heart. The end of the catheter should not be cut for any reason as this may leave a sharp point.

There are some 50 documented cases of pulmonary artery trauma caused by Swann–Ganz catheters and an incidence of 1–2 per 1000 has been suggested (McDaniel et al 1981). The haemorrhage that results can be uncontrollable, with a mortality estimated at 50%. In those that do not exsanguinate immediately about half require pulmonary resection or vascular repair (Stone et al 1983). The cause of this damage is often due to the fact that the balloon on the catheter has been inadvertently left inflated, or the catheter has migrated distally until it wedges in the vessel. Perforation is most likely during cardiac surgery, when the low body temperature makes the catheter more rigid and repeated manipulation of the heart and vessels by the surgeon increases catheter trauma. Prolonged wedging of a catheter in a pulmonary vessel can also lead to a pulmonary infarction. This problem is prevented if the pulmonary artery pressure is continuously displayed on a monitor so that accidental wedging can be seen immediately. The diagnosis of pulmonary artery trauma may be aided by the presence of haemoptysis and radiological evidence of either pulmonary haemorrhage or infarction (Stone et al 1983, Colvin et al 1975). If a Swann–Ganz catheter is left in place during cardiac surgery it should be withdrawn by some 15 cm using the sterile sleeve that is provided. Inflation of the balloon once the catheter is withdrawn ensures the tip of the catheter is blunt and atraumatic.

Trauma to other tissues

Any structure lying within about 8 cm of the cannulation site can be, and probably has been, damaged by intravenous needles. One of the most serious complications of subclavian and internal jugular vein puncture is pneumothorax. It is relatively rare if the internal jugular vein is used and a 'high approach' is adopted. Pneumothorax as a consequence of subclavian vein catheterization has an incidence of 3–4% and is much more frequent if the operator is inexperienced. Several attempts may be needed to cannulate the vein, and this increases the hazard. On occasion the operator has failed to puncture the vein on one side and so has attempted to use the vein on the other side, leading to bilateral pneumothoraces that proved fatal on at least two recorded occasions (Matz 1965, Schapira & Stern 1967, Bernard & Stahl 1971).

Shapira & Stern (1967) reported a case where they failed to enter the subclavian vein in a patient that had pneumonectomy on the same side. An attempt was made to cannulate the vein on the other side, a pneumothorax was induced and the patient died.

Reports of damage to other tissues include permanent and transient paralysis to the diaphragm, brachial plexus injury, vagal nerve injury including damage to the recurrent laryngeal nerve leading to hoarseness, Horner's syndrome, perforation of the trachea and injury to the thoracic duct. Subcutanous emphysema may occur and be so extensive as to encroach on the upper airway, causing severe airway obstruction and necessitating tracheostomy (Smith et al 1965).

Catheters that pass through the heart, or whose tip lies in one of its chambers, can cause arrhythmias (Colvin et al 1972). This is a further reason for ensuring catheter tips are sited in the vena cavae. When a Swann–Ganz catheter is being passed through the heart, cardiac rhythm should be continuously monitored by electrocardiogram.

Prevention

The best way to avoid the effects of trauma is to avoid central veins. If this is not possible the high approach to the internal jugular vein or cannulation of the femoral vein are probably the safest techniques. Subclavian vein cannulation may be safe in experienced hands, but unfortunately there is a constant stream of people who need to be trained and to gain experience in catheterization techniques. Consequently it is probably best to avoid using the subclavian vein whenever possible.

Catheter embolism

In the 1960s and 1970s there were over 60 case reports published of catheter embolism, that is loss of part or all of the catheter into the circulation. By far the most common cause was shearing of the catheter by the needle in systems where the catheter was inserted through the intravenous needle. Shearing could occur at any time of insertion, especially if the catheter was pulled back through the needle, or later if the needle remained around the catheter. Movement of the patient's arm, for example, could result in the catheter shearing on the needle.

Decline in the use of such a catheter system has greatly reduced this complication. However, any catheter can be accidentally cut with scissors when the dressing is applied, or by tension at some time after it has been inserted. Alternatively the catheter can separate from the hub and then embolize into the circulation.

The catheter may remain in the peripheral vein, but more commonly it is carried to the heart where it is usually located trailing from the vena cavae through the right atrium, right ventricle and occasionally the pulmonary artery.

Further complications include:

1. catheter trauma leading to perforation of the heart
2. thrombus formation on the catheter
3. infection of the thrombus
4. septic emboli from the infected thrombus causing abscesses elsewhere, such as in the lung
5. fungal and bacterial endocarditis.

These complications may be fatal.

Prevention of catheter embolism

The following should help to avoid catheter embolism:

1. Catheters should never be passed through needles.
2. Potential catheterization sites near joints should be avoided whenever possible and if used the limb should be immobilized.
3. Catheters should be effectively fixed to the skin close to the catheter–skin entry site.
4. All catheters should be radio-opaque.

Removal of catheter embolus

Every catheter that is withdrawn at the end of infusion therapy should be checked to ensure that it is complete. In view of the mortality as a result of catheter embolism, embolised catheter fragments must be removed (Blair et al 1970). If possible, a tourniquet should be placed around the limb proximal to the catheter insertion site to trap the catheter at the periphery of the circulation. Some authors have thought they could palpate the catheter in the superficial vein, and local explorations were often carried out, but this is usually fruitless. The exact position of the catheter must be established by radiography. For this to be successful the catheter must be radio-opaque. If a catheter is still in the limb, surgical cut-down on the vein is possible. Once it has passed into the thorax it must be removed by open surgery if thrombus can be demonstrated on the catheter or in the heart. Otherwise the catheter can be removed by an intravascular snare technique (Massumi & Ross 1967). A length of 0.021 inch diameter, Teflon-coated guidewire can be fashioned into a loop by threading both ends through a size 6.5 French gauge catheter from the patient end before inserting the device via a long saphenous venotomy. The loop of guidewire can be closed on the embolus under radiographic control by pulling the ends through the 6.5 French gauge catheter. The difficult task of catching the embolus in the loop guidewire can be made easier by using a catheter with a right-angled bend at its tip (Davies et al 1984).

Knotting of catheters

Knotting of the intravascular part of the catheter is an unusual complication seen if the catheter is thin and very flexible (Moncrief 1958). A knotted catheter can usually be removed by gently pulling the knot tight, although there is a risk that the catheter will break.

I once inserted a fine pulmonary artery catheter via the internal jugular vein in a patient with a pre-existing central catheter placed via a 'cut-down' in the antecubital fossa. The pulmonary catheter became knotted around the larger central venous pressure line, and could not be removed until it was divided at its skin entry site and pulled out via the anticubital fossa attached to the end of the central venous catheter.

Air embolus

Air can be sucked into any vein through an open-ended needle or catheter if the pressure in the vein is below atmospheric. It is particularly likely to complicate cannulation of veins in the neck and thorax if the patient has not been positioned head-down (Duffy 1949). About 100 ml air/s can flow through a needle of internal diameter 2 mm when a pressure difference of 5 cmH_2O exists between the two ends of the needle. Hypovolaemic patients with hypoxaemia may generate considerably higher pressure gradients between their central veins and the atmosphere, and are therefore more at risk. Flanagan et al (1969) described a fatal case of air embolism during subclavian vein puncture. Air could be heard passing through the needle, the patient developed tachypnoea and the characteristic millwheel rumour over the praecordium was heard. If a patient has a septal defect in the heart, air can cross to the left side and lead to cerebral air embolism (Calverley et al 1971).

Air embolism has been reported to develop up to 1 h after removal of the catheter, the air entering through the subcutaneous track left by the catheter (Hanley et al 1984).

Prevention of air embolus

To avoid air embolus the following should be ensured:

1. The vein chosen for cannulation should always be positioned below the level of the heart.
2. Veins should not be catheterized with needles that are open to the atmosphere, and care should be taken to ensure that air cannot be sucked into the vein through loose-fitting or badly maintained infusion sets. A combination of an infusion clamp placed high up on the giving set and a hole in the plastic infusion tubing below it can lead to entrainment of air, as can a blocked filter in the drip chamber.

Therapy

The patient should be placed in the left lateral decubitus position and closed cardiac massage started if necessary (Gottleib et al 1965). If a central venous catheter is in position attempts should be made to aspirate the air out of the heart.

Failures

Failure to puncture the vein

Failure to puncture the vein may be due to obesity, abnormal anatomy, the shocked condition of the patient or the inexperience of the operator. Percutaneous puncture of central veins has a failure rate of less than 10%. In one study the easiest vein to cannulate was the subclavian (5.1% failure rate), and the most difficult was the external jugular (16.7% failure rate) (Malatinsky et al 1983).

Mechanical failure of the catheter

The end of the catheter may become kinked, pinched or stuck against the wall of the vessel. Catheters easily become blocked with a thrombus.

Failure to position the catheter in a central vein

There may be difficulty in advancing a catheter from a peripheral vein to a central vein. Sometimes the catheter may be easily fed up the vein and fail to reach a central position within the thorax. The failure to position correctly catheters passed from peripheral veins is of the order of 15–20%. If one looks at the failure to position correctly central lines inserted from all sites, the failure rate is between 6% and 9% (Nordlund & Thoren 1964, Malatinsky et al 1983). Quite frequently the catheter loops back and moves peripherally (2% incidence). The sites that allow the lowest incidence of incorrect position of the catheter tip are the supraclavicular subclavian approach, the internal jugular and the brachiocephalic. The worst site in this respect is the external jugular with a failure rate of 30% (Malatinsky et al 1983).

The correct measurement of central venous pressure does depend on the exact position of the catheter tip (Johnson & Clarke 1972); however absolute pressure is irrelevant because the external reference point normally used is arbitrary and the pressure difference between the right atrium and the internal jugular vein is very small (Bell et al 1973). Catheters in the abdominal part of the inferior vena cavae can give inaccurate readings of central venous pressures in abdominal distension (Wilson et al 1962). Furthermore, in the newborn child a central venous catheter placed through the umbilical vein can be accidentally positioned in the liver. If an alkaline infusion is given, massive liver necrosis may result. The position of central venous catheter tips should always be checked by radiography.

Conclusion

The complications of venous catheterization contribute substantially to patient morbidity and mortality. Catheters should be inserted under aseptic conditions into superficial veins for a minimum period. Central venous and pulmonary artery catheterization should be used only when absolutely necessary.

COMPLICATIONS OF ARTERIAL CATHETERIZATION

The complications of arterial catheterization are less frequent than those of venous catheterization. Serious long-term effects are rare, having an estimated incidence of 0.3% (Zorab 1969). Principal complications are thrombus formation, in some cases leading to arterial occlusion or the release of emboli; ischaemia; haemorrhage; infection; haematoma; aneurysm; and arteriovenous fistula formation. By far the most common complication is thrombus formation, sometimes associated with arterial occlusion and occasionally associated with embolism and ischaemia.

Thrombus formation

Thrombus forms at the puncture site or downstream at the site of maximum blood turbulence (Kim et al 1975). The factors that allow thrombus formation are similar to those discussed under venous catheterization. Angiography can be used to demonstrate that clot forms rapidly along most arterial catheters, and in nearly 50% of cannulated arteries the amount of clot present can be described as moderate or more, up to a stage of complete thrombosis (Bedford 1977).

Conditions that slow blood flow past the catheter are likely to increase the risk of thrombus formation and eventual arterial occlusion. These are:

- vasoconstriction
- partial obstruction of the vessel
- factors that alter characteristics of blood.

Vasoconstriction

As many as 50% of cannulated radial arteries go into spasm shortly after catheterization, possibly as a response to the presence of a foreign body and/or to the trauma of puncturing the vessel. Some have demonstrated that multiple puncture of an artery at the time of cannulation can nearly double the risk of arterial thrombosis (Davis & Stewart 1980); others failed to show any significant hazard (Slogoff et al 1983). The flushing of the artery with room-temperature fluid may exacerbate spasm. Temporary pallor of the hand and forearm is more commonly seen when a radial artery catheter is flushed manually, probably because a larger volume of fluid is administered under pressure.

Changes in blood flow to the hand can be monitored by the use of a pulse volume plethysmograph or an ultrasonic flow probe sited close to digital or palmar arteries. Flow changes resulting from radial artery spasm can be studied if the collateral circulation from the ulnar artery is temporarily stopped by manual pressure over the vessel.

Initial radial artery spasm usually lasts some 30 min after cannulation and does not in itself result in long-term radial artery occlusion. However, in some patients spasm persists far longer and increases the risk of arterial thrombosis (Kim et al 1975). For example, arterial thrombosis has been shown to be far more frequent in patients who are systemically vasoconstricted as a result of a low cardiac output, hypothermia or the use of vasoconstrictor drugs (Davis & Stewart 1980, Slogoff et al 1983).

The inadvertent administration of a drug or an inappropriate intravenous fluid into an arterial line may be responsible for intense arterial spasm and thrombosis. The cannulation of peripheral arteries of patients with Raynaud's disease has long been presumed to increase the risk of arterial occlusion.

Partial obstruction of the vessel

The catheter partially obstructs the artery and flow is slowed according to the degree of obstruction. Some studies have reported that the use of 15 or 18 gauge catheters increases the incidence of arterial thrombosis compared with the use of small-diameter catheters (Little et al 1973, Davis & Stewart 1980, Downs et al 1973). Catheters that are tapered along their length have been reported by Downs et al (1973) to have a higher risk of arterial occlusion than those that are not tapered; however others have been unable to distinguish any difference in the incidence of arterial thrombosis when comparing the use of 18 and 20 gauge catheters, tapered or otherwise (Bedford & Wollman 1973, Evans & Kerr 1975, Slogoff et al 1983). Conversely it has been suggested that occlusion of the femoral artery rarely complicates catheterization because the catheter takes up such a small proportion of the cross-sectional area of the vessel. Russell et al (1983) reported a comparable incidence of digital ischaemia following radial artery (4%) and femoral artery (3.4%) cannulation. This marginally reinforces the argument, because in their study a size larger and longer catheter was used, and was placed in the femoral artery for a longer period of time than that placed in the radial artery.

It has been consistently reported that radial artery thrombosis is more frequent in women than men, although the differences in incidence vary from being just significant to a frequency twice as great in females (Davis & Stewart 1980, Slogoff et al 1983). Bedford (1978) correlated the incidence of radial artery thrombosis with lumen diameter as measured using arteriography. He also correlated the incidence of arterial thrombosis with wrist circumference, showing that this complication was more than twice as frequent in patients with wrist circumference below 18 cm. Women who have smaller wrists fell into this latter group.

Haematoma formation at the puncture site is also associated with a greater incidence of subsequent arterial occlusion and has been shown to double the risk of reducing or occluding blood flow in the artery (Davis & Stewart 1980, Slogoff et al 1983). Presumably haematomata contribute to vessel narrowing. Haematoma formation is more likely if a patient is anticoagulated or has a bleeding disorder, if multiple punctures of the artery precede successful cannulation or if a surgical cut-down is necessary to gain access to the artery. Haematomata occur more frequently following femoral artery catheterization because it is more difficult to apply effective pressure once the catheter has been removed (Colvin et al 1977). Enthusiastic pressure applied in order to prevent haematoma formation may also play a part in encouraging thrombus extension, the pressure narrowing the vessel and slowing flow.

Peripheral vascular disease, in the form of either atheromatous plaques (Colvin et al 1977) or Raynaud's disease, may contribute to arterial thrombus formation, although again once can find reports where such conditions seem to cause no significant effect (Russell et al 1983).

Factors that alter characteristics of blood

A number of factors can alter the physical properties of blood. For example an increase in viscosity due to hyperglycaemia (Cannon & Meshier 1982) will slow peripheral blood flow and increase the risk of thrombosis. In conditions of slow flow, red cells may clump together, predisposing to thrombus formation (Vaughan 1980). Increases in fatty acid levels of blood have been shown to increase thrombus formation and platelet aggregation (Luscher 1975). Arterial occlusion is also more frequent in hypocoagulable states such as disseminated intravascular coagulation (Baker & Nyhus 1976).

Other factors may increase the risk of thrombus formation and eventual arterial occlusion. These are:

- the duration of catheterization
- the chemical composition of the catheter
- the amount of intimal trauma.

Duration of catheterization

The duration of catheterization is associated with the incidence of thrombosis. Thrombosis is less likely to occur if the catheter has only been in position 4–6 h (Evans & Kerr 1975, Davis & Stewart 1980) and more likely to occur if the catheter has been in position for more than 30 h (Bedford & Wollman 1973, Baker & Nyhus 1976). It has not been possible to correlate the incidence of arterial occlusion against duration of catheterization for those catheters that have been in place for between 6 and 30 h (Singh et al 1982, Russell et al 1983).

Catheter material

There is little agreement about the effect of catheter material on the incidence of arterial occlusion. Some studies suggest that Teflon catheters result in a significantly lower incidence of arterial occlusion than polypropylene (Bedford 1975, Kim et al 1975, Davis & Stewart 1980). Others have been unable to distinguish any difference (Evans & Kerr 1975, Slogoff et al 1983).

Intimal trauma

Repeated punctures of the artery may lead to an increased incidence of thrombus formation; on the other hand there is no evidence that transfixion of the artery at the time of cannulation results in any subsequent reduction in hand blood flow compared with single arterial wall puncture (Jones et al 1981).

The clinician can easily become bemused by the diversity of findings and the variety of factors that may or may not lead to arterial thrombosis. In many reports the number of patients studied and the duration of cannulation are insufficient to establish significant differences between various techniques, catheters and events. It is probably wise to assume that all the factors mentioned above may increase the risk of thrombus formation and that this risk increases in proportion to the number of causative factors present in any particular patient.

Incidence, detection and clinical signs of arterial thrombosis

The incidence of arterial thrombosis leading to complete occlusion of the radial artery is about 20–30% (Evans & Kerr 1975, Kim et al 1975, Davis & Stewart 1980, Slogoff et al 1983). Normal blood flow is restored within 10–20 days, although in a few instances the artery remains permanently occluded. In some cases the radial artery is apparently patent immediately following decannulation, but occlusion subsequently occurs some 4–5 days later. In the vast majority of instances of arterial thrombosis there are no clinical consequences of occlusion and an adequate distal blood flow is achieved by collateral vessels such as the ulnar artery. Consequently, arterial occlusion is not diagnosed because there are no symptoms or signs. Furthermore in 60% of instances of arterial thrombosis the pulse remains palpable, albeit slightly reduced, when compared with that of the other limb (Evans & Kerr 1975, Slogoff et al 1983).

Arterial narrowing or occlusion is therefore assumed if there is evidence of reduced or absent blood flow to the downstream tissues once all collateral vessels have been temporarily occluded by external manual pressure. The quality of flow can be assessed by the use of either plethysmography or an ultrasonic probe placed near digital or palmar arch vessels. Alternatively the quality of flow can be assessed using a modified Allen's test.

The development of thrombus formation when the catheter is still in place may be manifest by a repeat damping of the arterial blood pressure trace after flushing, or difficulty in obtaining blood samples through the catheter (Downs et al 1973).

Kim et al (1975) suggested that symptomless radial artery occlusion that developed while a catheter is still in place can be detected by applying manual pressure over the artery distal to the catheter. If the artery is thrombosed there will be no change in the pressure trace being recorded through the catheter; whereas if the artery is patent the pressure trace will change in configuration and with an increase in amplitude as blood flow is stopped downstream.

Occasionally, arterial thrombosis may contribute to the development of peripheral ischaemia, and this is likely if there is an inadequate collateral circulation.

Ischaemia and necrosis

Clinical symptoms and signs of ischaemia complicating arterial catheterization include pallor or cyanosis, discolouration of the skin, fall in skin temperature, paraesthesia, weakness, poor capillary refill and oedema. Occasionally there is pain which may be severe. The incidence of peripheral ischaemia complicates some 2.0–3.5% of radial and femoral artery catheterization. Catheterization of the femoral artery has been claimed to result in a lower incidence of downstream ischaemia (Colvin et al 1977). This is probably true under comparable conditions, but the femoral artery is usually cannulated in more seriously ill patients. Relatively larger lines are inserted and left in for a longer period of time. Consequently the incidence of ischaemia due to thrombosis of the femoral artery is not much different from that of radial artery cannulation (Russell et al 1983).

Quite often, signs develop hours or even days after the catheter has been removed (Mangano & Hickey 1979). Ischaemia usually resolves after some time if suitable measures are taken (see later). Rarely, the skin affected will become gangrenous and tissue is permanently lost. The extent of necrosis will vary from a small patch of skin to a complete hand. The incidence of such severe complications is of the order of 0.07% (Dalton & Laver 1971).

The ischaemia is due either to the development of thrombosis in the presence of an inadequate collateral circulation or to peripheral embolism. Downs et al (1973) were able to identify thrombotic emboli in 23% of patients with indwelling radial artery catheters using arteriograms. Emboli were observed in the forearm, hand and fingers, but in only two instances were there signs of ischaemia. In both cases there were resolved within 2 h of the removal of the catheter.

Emboli may also result from other causes, such as atheroma dislodged at the time of catheterization or the flushing of air and clot from the pressure measurement system into the artery.

Emboli originating from other sites of the circulation, such as the heart, might occlude an artery already narrowed by a catheter and attendant thrombus, possibly leading to ischaemia.

Although ischaemia usually occurs downstream from the catheterization site it can also occur upstream. Areas of skin discolouration and necrosis 1–5 cm across have been reported in the forearm proximal to the radial artery catheter (Wyatt et al 1974). It is likely that one of the few vessels that supply the skin of the forearm becomes obstructed by the catheter, by thrombus or by an embolus (Wyatt et al 1974).

Forceful flushing of an arterial catheter may allow emboli to be carried a considerable distance upstream as flow is temporarily reversed. Cerebral damage has been reported following the freeing of a clot in a Scribner shunt and unexplained neurological deficits have been noted in patients with indwelling arterial catheters (Lowenstein et al 1971). Temporal artery catheterization became fashionable, especially in infants, until reports suggested that cerebral emboli had been a consequence of such catheterization. In two cases rhythmic twitching or flexion contraction of the limbs occurred down one side while a temporal artery catheter was in position. In one instance a clot had just been flushed through the catheter and in the other small clots had been removed on a number of previous occasions. In both patients, small areas of low-density penetration suggesting infarction were demonstrated on the CAT scan in the parietal region of the cortex (Priam et al 1978). In a prospective study of 39 infants who had had temporal artery catheterization followed up over a period of 9 months, 11 patients had neurological abnormalities. In eight of these there was evidence of hemiparesis on the side contralateral to the catheterization. In four of these the catheter had been removed because it had clotted. Not all patients received a CAT scan but in four there was evidence of a cerebral infarction on the same side of the catheterization site (Bull et al 1980). The temporal artery is very close to the origin of the carotid artery. Flushing of the former may allow emboli to be pushed into the latter (Simmons et al 1978, Bull et al 1980).

Lowenstein et al (1971) flushed various volumes of radioisotope-tagged saline into radial arteries at a rate of 12–15 ml/s and measured gamma-emitting activity over the area of the subclavian/vertebral artery junction. As little as 3 ml of flush produced a positive response in some patients, and the average volume that produced a response was 6.6 ml.

Precautions to minimize thrombotic and embolic complications of arterial catheterization

Selection of the artery. If catheterization is primarily for the purpose of obtaining blood samples the dorsalis pedis artery is probably the safest vessel to use, provided there is flow in the posterior tibial artery. Radial artery cannulation will usually give a more reliable blood pressure trace and is a satisfactory site, provided there is a good blood flow to the hand and an effective collateral circulation through the ulnar artery. It is sensible to select the artery of the non-dominant hand.

In cases of extreme collapse and vasoconstriction the femoral artery is easier to catheterize, will give more reliable measurement of blood pressure and will avoid the potential hazards of cannulation of a radial artery in the presence of severe vasoconstriction and low cardiac output. Brachial artery catheterization is probably best avoided because of the lack of an effective collateral circulation. The temporal artery should not be used.

Assessment of collateral blood flow. Arteries of the foot and hand should not be catheterized unless adequate collateral blood flow can be demonstrated. For the hand a modified Allen's test is used (Bedford & Wollman 1973). The patient clenches his fist, and radial and ulnar arteries are occluded by manual pressure of the examiner's fingers. The patient then opens his hand and the examiner releases the ulnar artery compression. Adequate collateral flow is shown by a hyperaemic flush within 7 s over the palmar surface of the hand. Collateral flow is considered slow if it takes 8–15 s for the skin to flush. Cannulation should not normally be performed if a flush onset time exceeds 15 s. Use of the Doppler ultrasonic flow probe to detect arterial flow in the palmar arch is probably more reliable than observing the rate of onset of the flush. Little et al (1973) demonstrated reduced palmar arch flow in 6% of hands tested by this method, although only 3% of hands had negative Allen's tests.

Cannulation should be avoided in limbs subjected to previous injury that may have threatened blood supply. Careful assessment is necessary in patients with Raynaud's phenomenon and peripheral vascular disease.

Techniques. Cannulation should be carried out as a sterile technique. A single puncture without transfixion and with the minimum number of attempts is ideal. Small Teflon catheters (20 gauge) should be inserted for the shortest time necessary. Lines and transducers should be kept free of air and clots. A continuous flush (3–4 ml/h) of Hartmann's solution containing 4 units heparin/ml should be used to keep the end of the catheter clear of blood. Bolus flushes with a syringe should be avoided if possible, and those made from a pressure bag via a continuous-flow device should be kept to a minimum volume, ideally less than 3 ml (Lowestein et al 1971).

Catheters should be removed as soon as their use is no longer necessary.

Malfunction. If a catheter repeatedly blocks, or if the pressure trace rapidly becomes damped after flushing, the catheter should be removed.

Ischaemia. A catheter should be removed if clinical signs of local ischaemia develop, for example cooling of the limb, oedema, pallor, cyanosis or blotchy discoloration of the skin, poor capillary refill, paraesthesia or pain.

Withdrawal of clot. An attempt should be made to withdraw clot at the time of decannulation by applying pressure over the artery proximally and distally to the catheter and then aspirating the catheter as it is removed (Bedford 1977).

Manual pressure should be applied over the puncture site once the catheter has been removed, for 5 min or until haemorrhage ceases.

A followed-up examination should be made on the seventh postcannulation day.

Management of distal ischaemia

If the blood flow to an extremity becomes markedly reduced, 500 units of heparin may be injected into the catheter followed by 20 mg of papaverine diluted in 10 ml of normal saline. The catheter should then be removed. If the affected tissue does not rapidly improve, arterial angiography should be undertaken early, and the site and extent of the block established. If thrombectomy or small vessel repair is indicated, this should be undertaken early. At the same time ancillary treatment should be instituted. This includes anticoagulation with heparin if not otherwise contraindicated, continuous sympathetic blockade (for example, axillary plexus block using a catheter; Selander 1977) and the administration of low molecular weight dextran in a dose of 50 g of 10% dextran over 3 h every 12 h for 3 days (Baker & Nyhus 1976).

Axillary plexus block not only promotes vascular dilatation but also relieves the pain of ischaemia (Cannon & Meshier 1982). Injections of reserpine (1.5 mg diluted with 10 ml of saline) into the affected artery to cause maximum dilatation of the vessel has been suggested, as has intra-arterial infusion of fibrinolysin (Samaan 1971).

Infection

Factors that lead to contamination and infection associated with arterial lines are probably very similar to those associated with intravenous catheters. Organisms have been cultured from some 16% of skin swabs in one study (Singh et al 1982). Catheter tips grew organisms in 2–8% of cases (Gardner et al 1974, Colvin et al 1977, Singh et al 1982, Thomas et al 1983) and positive blood cultures associated with a positive catheter-tip culture have been found in 2–5% of patients (Band & Maki 1979, Singh et al 1982, Thomas et al 1983). Local inflammation at the skin–catheter entry site is more frequent in patients that have catheter-tip infection.

It is widely assumed that femoral artery catheters are more prone to contamination than radial artery catheters because they are sited in the groin, 'a dirty area'. Some workers have been unable to confirm this, finding that infection rates between femoral and radial catheters are comparable (Colvin et al 1977, Thomas et al 1983). Infection rates increase with the duration of catheterization, and cut-down techniques are associated with a greater incidence of infection (Band et al 1977). The general impression is that infection is less of a problem with arterial lines than with intravenous lines, and this may reflect the shorter duration of cannulation of arteries and the limited type of solutions administered. However, the dangers of infection are equally present. Samples of blood are regularly removed from arterial lines, and cultures taken from tap ports grow organisms in up to 16% of instances (Shinozaki et al 1983). Furthermore, the fluid in transducer domes has been shown to grow organisms in 11% of samples (Maki & Hassemer 1981). Infection may be encouraged if the continuous-flush device is placed close to the arterial catheter and the transducer is separated distally by a length of tubing. The fluid in this tubing is static and may never be flushed through. One recommendation that all transducer domes, manometer tubes and continuous-flush devices should be replaced every 48 h may reduce contamination and the risk of infection, but would be an extremely expensive precaution. Strict aseptic precautions and minimum handling of the lines, as described for intravenous catheters, can keep infection at an acceptably low incidence (Russell et al 1983, Shinozaki et al 1983, Thomas et al 1983).

Other complications

Haemorrhage, disconnection and haematoma formation

Accidental disconnection of an arterial line with consequent severe haemorrhage is an entirely avoidable complication that occurs from time to time in most units. It is least likely to occur if all the in-line connections are secured by luer locks.

Occasionally, following routine decannulation, there is frank haemorrhage through the puncture hole despite a period of firm pressure.

Haematomata commonly occur, either at the time of attempting cannulation or after decannulation. Much depends on the experience of the operator and the effectiveness of the pressure applied after decannulation. Haematomata may occur in up to 10% of radial artery punctures (Russell et al 1983) but are most common after femoral artery decannulation (45%) (Colvin et al 1977).

Accidental decannulation

Catheters are sometimes accidentally removed by the activity of the patient. This can result in blood loss if it is not noticed. All patients with arterial cannulae in position require close nursing attention.

Malfunction

Some 10–18% of catheters malfunction, that is the pressure trace becomes repeatedly damped and/or blood sampling becomes impossible. The cause of these problems is either kinking of the catheter or thrombus forming along its length. Such catheters are best removed.

Aneurysm and arteriovenous fistula formation

Pseudoaneurysm of the radial artery has been described on a number of occasions (Mathieu et al 1973, Woolf & Mangano 1980): a pulsatile mass is observed over the course of the radial artery some time following decannulation. It can be months before the swelling is noticed. There is a tendency for the aneurysm to enlarge progressively, therefore surgical treatment is necessary. It is not recommended that the artery be tied off because of the risk of precipitating downstream ischaemia. Rather, the aneurysm should be resected and the artery rejoined end-to-end. If necessary a small venous patch can be incorporated (McLeskey 1980).

Trauma affecting the artery and a vein, where these run closely together, can occasionally cause an arteriovenous fistula.

CONCLUSIONS

Arterial catheterization for the purpose of blood pressure measurement and blood sampling has become an essential part of the treatment of severely ill patients. If the cannulation technique is expertly performed and the indwelling lines carefully managed, serious complications are comparatively rare and are often preceded by warning signs. As with venous catheters, arterial lines must be removed as soon as they cease to form an essential part of treatment.

REFERENCES

Adar R, Mozes M 1970 Hydromediastinum. J Am Med Assoc 214: 372

Ahmed N, Payne R F 1976 Thrombosis after central venous cannulation. Med J Aust 1: 217

Baker R J, Nyhus L M 1976 Severe ischemia of the hand following radial artery catheterization. Surgery 80: 449

Band J D, Maki D G 1979 Infection caused by arterial catheters used for hemodynamic monitoring. Am Med J 67: 735

Bedford R F 1975 Percutaneous radial artery cannulation. Anesthesiology 42: 219

Bedford R F 1977 Removal of radial artery thrombi following percutaneous cannulation. Anesthesiology 46: 430

Bedford R F 1978 Wrist circumference predicts the risk of radial artery occlusion. Anesthesiology 48: 377

Bedford R F, Wollman H 1973 Complications of percutaneous radial artery cannulation. Anesthesiology 38: 228

Bell J A, Bradley R D, Jenkins B S 1973 Malpositioning of central venous catheters. Lancet 1: 105

Bernard R W, Stahl W M 1971 Subclavian vein catheterization. Ann Surg 173: 184

Blair E, Hunziker R, Flanagan M E 1970 Catheter embolism. Surgery 67: 457

Bull M J, Schreiner R L, Garg B P, Hutton N M, Lemons J A, Gresham E L 1980 Neurologic complications following temporal artery catheterization. J Paed 96: 1071

Calverley R K, Dodds W A, Trapp W G, Jenkins L C 1971 Hyperbaric treatment of cerebral air embolism. Can Anaesth Soc J 18: 665

Cannon B W, Meshier W T 1982 Extremity amputation following radial artery cannulation. Anesthesiology 56: 222

Chastre J, Courvand F, Bouchama A, Viau F, Benacerraf R, Gilbert C 1982 Thrombosis as a complication of pulmonary artery catheterization via the internal jugular vein. N Engl J Med 306: 278

Chillar R K, Farbstein M, Ellington O B et al 180 Use of right atrial catheter for prolonged i.v. support in cancer patients. Cancer Treat Rep 64: 243

Collin J, Collin C, Constable K L et al 1975 Infusion thrombophlebitis and infection with various catheters. Lancet 2: 150

Colvin M P, Blogg C E, Savege T M, Jarvis J D, Strunin L 1972 A safe long-term infusion technique? Lancet 2: 317

Colvin M P, Savege T M, Lewis C T 1975 Pulmonary damage from a Swan Ganz catheter. Br J Anaesth 47: 1107

Colvin M P, Curran J P, Jarvis D, O'Shea P J 1977 Femoral artery pressure monitoring. Use of the Seldinger technique. Anaesthesia 32: 451

Curelaru I, Bylock T, Gustavsson B, Hultman E, Linder L E, Stefansson T, Stenquist O 1984 Dynamics of thrombophlebitis in central venous catheterization via basilic and cephalic veins. Acta Chir Scand 150: 285

Dalton B, Laver M B 1971 Vasospasm with an indwelling radial artery cannula. Anesthesiology 34: 194

Davies P, Graham T R, Walker E 1984 A simple snare for the retrieval of an embolised central venous cannula. Br J Radiol 57: 87

Davis F M, Stewart J M 1980 Radial artery cannulation. Br J Anaesth 52: 41

Downs J B, Rackstein A D, Klein E F, Hawkins I F 1973 Hazards of radial artery catheterization. Anesthesiology 38: 283

Duffy B J 1949 The clinical use of polyethylene tubing for intravenous therapy. Ann Surg 130: 929

Emery J L, Hilton H R 1960 Lung and heart complications of the treatment of hydrocephalus by ventriculo-auriculostomy. Surgery 50: 309

Evans P J D, Kerr J H 1975 Arterial occlusion after cannulation. Br Med J 3: 197

Finholt D A 1984 Superficial temporal artery cannulation is not benign. Anesthesiology 62: 93

Flanagan J P, Gradisar I A, Gross R J, Kelly T R 1969 Air embolus: a lethal complication of subclavian venepuncture. N Engl J Med 281: 488

Gardener R M, Schwartz R, Wong H C et al 1974 Percutaneous indwelling radial artery catheters for monitoring cardiovascular function. N Engl J Med 290: 1227

Gore J M, Matsumoto A H, Layden J J, Haffajee C I, Love J C, Alpert J S, Dalen J E 1984 Superior vena cava syndrome. Arch Intern Med 144: 506

Gottleib J D, Ericsson J A, Sweet R B 1965 Venous air embolism: a review. Anesth Analg 44: 773

Handfield Jones R P C, Lewis H B M 1952 Superficial thrombophlebitis caused by rubber drip sets. Lancet 1: 585

Hanley P C, Click R L, Tancred R G 1984 Delayed air embolism after removal of venous catheters. Ann Intern Med 101: 401

Hershey C O,Tomford J W, McLaren C E, Porter D K, Cohen D I 1984 The natural history of intravenous catheter associated phlebitis. Arch Intern Med 144: 1373

Hoar P F, Stone J G, Wicks A G et al 1978 Thrombogenesis associated with Swan Ganz catheters. Anesthesiology 48: 445

Hoar P F, Wilson R M, Mangano D T, Avery G J, Starnick R J 1981 Heparin bonding reduces thrombogenicity of pulmonary artery catheters. N Engl J Med 305: 993

Jacobs M B, Yeager M 1984 Thrombotic and infection complications of Hickman-Broviac catheters. Arch Intern Med 144: 1597

Jeejeebhoy K N, Langer B, Tsallas G T et al 1976 Total parenteral nutrition at home. Gastroenterology 71: 943

Johnston A O B, Clarke R G 1972 Malpositioning of central venous catheters. Lancet 2: 1395

Jones R M, Hill A B, Nathrwold M L, Bolles R E 1981 The effect of method of radial artery cannulation on post-cannulation blood flow and thrombus formation. Anesthesiology 55: 76

Keohane P P, Attrill H, Northover J, Jones B J M, Cribb A, Frost P, Silk D B A 1983 Effect of catheter tunnelling and a nutrition nurse on catheter sepsis. Lancet 1388

Kido D K, Paulin S, Alenghat J A, Waternaux C, Riley W D 1982 Thrombogenicity of heparin and non-heparin coated catheters. Am J Roentgenology 139: 957

Kim J M, Arakawa K, Bliss J 1975 Arterial cannulation factors in the development of occlusion. Anesth Analg Curr Res 54: 836

Ladefoged K, Jarnum S 1978 Long term parenteral nutrition. Br Med J 2: 262

Little J M, Zylstra P L,West J et al 1973 Circulatory patterns in the normal hand. Br J Surg 60: 652
Lowder J N, Lazarus H M, Herzog R H 1982 Bacteremias and fungemias in oncologic patients with central venous catheters. Arch Intern Med 142: 1456
Lowenstein E, Little J W, Lo H H 1971 Prevention of cerebral embolization form flushing radial artery cannulas. N Engl J Med 285: 1414
Luscher E F 1975 The effect of lipids and fatty acids on blood coagulation and platelets in relation to thrombosis. Adv Exp Med Biol 60: 107
McDaniel D D, Stone J G, Faltas A N, Khambatta H J, Thys D M, Antunes A M, Bregman D 1981 Catheter induced pulmonary artery haemorrhage. J Thor Cardiovasc Surg 82: 1
McDonnell P J, Qualman S J, Hutchins G M 1984 Bilateral hydrothorax as a life threatening complication of central venous hyperalimentation. Surg Gynecol Obstet 158: 577
McLesky C H 1980 Radial artery pseudoaneurysm. Anesthesiology 53: 226
Maki D D 1981 Nosocomial bacteremia. Am J Med 70: 719
Maki D G, Weise C E, Sarafin H W 1977 A semi quantitative culture method for identifying intravenous catheter related infection. N Engl J Med 296: 1305
Maki D G, Hassemer C A 1981 Endemic rate of fluid contamination and related septicaemia in arterial pressure monitoring. Am J Med 70: 733
Malatinsky J, Faybik M, Griffith M, Majek M, Samuel M 1983 Venepuncture catheterization and failure to position correctly during central venous cannulation. Resuscitation 10: 259
Mangano D T 1982 Heparin bonding and long term protection against thrombogenesis. N Engl J Med 207: 894
Mangano D T, Hickey R F 1979 Ischaemic injury following uncomplicated radial artery catheterization. Anesth Analg 58: 55
Marder V J 1979 The use of thrombolytic agents. Arch Intern Med 90: 802
Massumi R A, Ross A M 1967 Atraumatic non-surgical technique for removal of broken catheter from cardiac cavities. N Engl J Med 277: 195
Mathieu A, Dalton B, Fischer J E, Kumar A 1973 Expanding aneurysm of the radial artery. Anesthesiology 38: 401
Matz R 1965 Complications of determining central venous pressure. N Engl J Med 273: 703
Moncrief J A 1958 Femoral catheters. Ann Surg 147: 166
Nordlund S, Thoren L 1964 Catheter in the superior vena cava for parenteral feeding. Acta Chir Scand 127: 39–45
Oh T E, Davis N J 1975 Radial artery cannulation. Anesth Intensive Care 3: 12
O'Neill J A, Pruitt B A, Foley R D, Moncrief J A 1968 Suppurative thrombophlebitis: a lethal complication of intravenous therapy. J Trauma 8: 256
Prager R L, Silva J 1984 Colonization of central venous catheters. South Med J 77: 458
Priam G W, Wright G B, Rumack C M, O'Meara O P 1978 Apparent cerebral embolization after temporal artery catheterization. J Pediatr 93: 115
Pruitt B A, Stein J M, Foley F D, Moncrief J A, O'Neill J A 1970 Intravenous therapy in burn patients. Arch Surg 100: 399
Rubenstein M, Creger W P 1980 Successful streptokinase therapy for catheter induced subclavian vein thrombosis. Arch Intern Med 140: 1370
Russell J A, Joel M, Hudson R J, Mangano D T, Schlobohm R M 1983 Prospective evaluation of radial and femoral artery catheterization. Crit Care Med 11: 936
Ryan J P, Abel R M, Abbott W M et al 1974 Catheter complications in total parenteral nutrition. N Engl J Med 290: 757
Saloheimo S, Henning C, Hillborgh U 1984 Infection risk from cannulae used to maintain intravenous access. Acta Anaesthesiol Scand 28: 199
Samaan H 1971 The hazards of radial artery pressure monitoring. J Cardiovasc Surg 12: 342
Savege T M 1973 The complications associated with the use of plastic intravenous catheters. Resuscitation 2: 83
Schapira M, Stern W Z 1967 Hazards of subclavian vein cannulation for central venous pressure monitoring. J Am Med Assoc 201: 327
Selander D 1977 Catheter technique in axillary plexus block. Acta Anaesthesiol Scand 21: 324
Sharp K W, Spees E K, Selby L R, Zachary J B, Ernst C B 1983 Diagnosis and management of retroperitoneal haematomas after femoral vein cannulation. Surgery 95: 90
Shinozaki T, Deane R S, Mazuzan J E, Hamel A J, Hazelton D 1983 Bacterial contamination of arterial lines. J Am Med Assoc 249: 223
Simmons M A, Levine R L, Lubchenco L O, Guggenheim M A 1983 Serious sequelae of temporal artery catheterization. J Paed 92: 284
Singh S, Nelson N, Acosta I, Check F E, Puri V K 1982 Catheter colonization and bacteremia with pulmonary and arterial catheters. Crit Care Med 10: 735
Slogoff S, Keats A S, Arlund C 1983 On the safety of radial artery cannulation. Anesthesiology 59: 42
Smith B E, Modell J H, Gamb M, Moya F 1965 Complications of subclavian vein catheterization. Arch Surg 90: 228
Smith V C, Hallett J W 1983 Subclavian vein thrombosis during prolonged catheterization for parenteral nutrition. South Med J 76: 603
Snow P 1980 Swan Ganz catheter and the superior vena cava syndrome. J Am Med Assoc 243: 1525
Snydman D R, Pober B R, Murray S A, Gorbea H F, Majka J A, Perry L K 1982 Predictive value of surveillance skin cultures in total parenteral nutrition-related infection. Lancet 1: 385
Stamm W E, Colella J J, Anderson R L, Dixon R E 1975 Indwelling arterial catheters as a source of nosocomial bacteremia. N Engl J Med 1099
Stillman R M, Soliman F, Garcia L, Sawyer P N 1977 Etiology of catheter-associated sepsis. Arch Surg 112: 1497
Stone J G, Khambatta H J, McDaniel D D 1983 Catheter-induced pulmonary artery trauma. J Thor Cardiovasc Surg 86: 146
Thomas F, Burke J P, Parker J, Orme J F, Gardner R M, Clemmer T P, Hill G A, MacFarlane P 1983 The risk of infection related to radial vs femoral sites for arterial catheterization. Crit Care Med 11: 807
Thomas C S, Carter J, Lowder S C 1969 Pericardial tamponade from central venous catheters. Arch Surg 98: 217
Tomford J W, Hershey C O, McLaren C E, Porter D R, Cohen D I 1984 Intravenous therapy team and peripheral venous catheter associated complications. Arch Intern Med 144: 1191

Tully J L, Friedland G H, Baldini L M, Goldmann D A 1981 Complications of intravenous therapy with steel needles and Teflon catheters. Am Med J 70: 702
Vaughan P B 1980 Local cold injury: menace to military operations. Mil Med 145: 305
Wilmore D W, Dudrick S J 1969 Safe long term catheterization. Arch Surg 98: 256
Wilson J N, Grow J B, Demong C V, Preuedel A E, Cuthbert-Owens J 1962 Central venous pressure in optimal blood volume maintenance. Arch Surg 85: 563
Woolf S, Mangano T D 1980 Pseudoaneurysm, a late complication of radial artery catheterization. Anesthesiology 52: 8
Wyatt R, Glaves I, Cooper D J 1974 Proximal skin lesions after radial artery catheterization. Lancet 1: 1135
Zorab J S M 1969 Continuous display of the arterial pressure. Anaesthesia 24: 431

33

Induced hypotension

P. J. O'Shea

INTRODUCTION

Hypotension must only be induced in the honest belief that some good to the patient will accrue.

Larson 1964

The aim of induced hypotension is to reduce significantly blood loss, and to improve the surgical field. Benefits from this technique in anaesthesia can be obtained for operations in head and neck surgery (including cosmetic), middle ear surgery and some neurosurgical operations (Yashon et al 1975).

Properly conducted prospective studies show the incidence of complications to be similar for normotensive and hypotensive techniques (Warner et al 1970, Hygosson & Högströtm 1973). The incidence of complications is relatively low, being of the order of 0–0.34% as discussed by Pasch & Huk (1986). However, these complications can be devastating. Pasch & Huk (1986) also point out that a request by the surgeon for induced hypotension should not be the 'sole reason for employing this technique'.

Lindop (1975), and more recently Pasch & Huk (1986), have reviewed the literature on the morbidity of controlled hypotension. McDowall (1985) has written about induced hypotension and brain ischaemia. These authors are recommended reading for anaesthetists using this technique and when considering the precautions.

PREOPERATIVE ASSESSMENT

The conditions listed below may be regarded as absolute contraindications to hypotensive anaesthesia:

- cerebrovascular disease
- coronary artery disease
- systemic hypertension
- congestive cardiac failure
- anaemia
- hypovolaemia
- renal disease
- liver disease
- pregnancy
- old age
- lack of proper monitoring facilities.

It has not been definitely established that there is an increased risk with hypotensive anaesthesia in ischaemic heart disease, renal and liver disease. However, careful consideration and extreme caution must be exercised before using the technique in such a patient. During the preoperative clinical examination it is also important to check that carotid bruits are not present.

Whatever the technique or combination of drugs used, anaesthesia with controlled hypotension must be carried out with full monitoring. Since the publication of the recommendations by the Association of Anaesthetists of Great Britain and

Ireland (1988) on standards of monitoring, lack of proper monitoring must be regarded as a contraindication. Utting et al (1979) found that in the period 1970–1977, 348 cases of death or cerebral damage were reported to the Medical Defence Union and 47% of these were associated with faulty technique.

It is important to note that morbidity and mortality are unpredictable (Lindop 1975, Pasch & Huk 1986, Leigh & Tytler 1990) and only become apparent in the postoperative period. The factors arising during anaesthesia and recovery that increase the risk of complications are:

- hypocapnia
- mean arterial pressure below 70 mmHg
- rapid reduction of blood pressure
- cardiac output reduced by hypovolaemia
- cardiac output reduced by depressant drugs.

CEREBRAL CIRCULATION AND INDUCED HYPOTENSION

The cerebral circulation autoregulates to maintain a constant cerebral blood flow between mean arterial pressures of 50 and 150 mmHg (Lassen 1959). However, there are individual variations due to age, condition of cerebral vasculature and whether or not systemic hypertension or hypovolaemia are present. As the blood pressure is lowered the cerebral vasculature vasodilates until maximal vasodilatation has occurred. If the blood pressure is lowered further the cerebral blood flow decreases proportionally. Finnerty et al (1954) have suggested that, in normotensive, normocapnic and awake volunteers, cerebral hypoxic symptoms appear at a mean arterial pressure of 35 mmHg. Moyer & Morris (1954) found hypoxic symptoms appearing at a mean arterial pressure of 55 mmHg, and Finnerty et al (1954) found that hypoxic symptoms also appeared at higher mean arterial pressures in hypertensive subjects. The latter suggest that cerebral autoregulation fails when the mean arterial pressure has fallen by a third, corresponding to a systolic value of 60 mmHg in normotensive subjects. Fitch et al (1976) demonstrated in baboons that the cerebral autoregulatory curve shifted to the right when the baboons were made hypertensive. This and the previous work (Moyer & Morris 1954) suggest that cerebral circulation will fail at a higher mean arterial pressure in hypertensive patients, who are therefore more vulnerable to hypotension.

Cerebral blood flow autoregulation relates to the cerebral blood flow as a whole and does not take into account regional variations that occur, irrespective of the presence of cerebral vascular disease. 'Boundary zones' (Graham 1985) are areas between the vascular distribution of the major cerebral arteries. The local arterial pressure in these zones is lower than normal and they are therefore at greater risk of ischaemic damage due to hypoperfusion.

Anatomical variations of vascular supply

The vascular supply to the brain can be affected by congenital variations in the Circle of Willis, degenerative arterial disease or vasospasm following subarachnoid haemorrhage.

Congenital variations in the Circle of Willis may cause shifts in the 'boundary zones' so that the areas most susceptible to ischaemia during induced hypotension may be changed. If there is atheromatous narrowing in one carotid artery and induced hypotension causes low intravascular pressure and flow, the cerebral hemisphere becomes reliant on the collateral circulation through the Circle of Willis and the cortical surface arteries. Pasch & Huk (1985) reported a case in which the patient never regained consciousness after hypotensive anaesthesia and autopsy confirmed a hypoplastic right vertebral artery. Another patient in their series suffered left hemiparesis 1 h postoperatively with almost complete recovery. Cerebral angiography revealed unexpected stenosis of the internal carotid artery.

The anaesthetist will not be aware of any cerebral insult during the operation for the only way of detecting the lowest arterial pressure tolerated by the patient is by monitoring the surface electrical activity of the brain.

Induced hypotension and neurosurgical anaesthesia

Vasospasm following subarachnoid haemorrhage will increase the ischaemic area in the presence of hypotension and the use of vasodilator drugs may cause local areas of 'steal' when there is spasm.

In the presence of raised intracranial pressure (ICP), even a small decrease in blood pressure may result in serious ischaemic damage (mean cerebral perfusion pressure = mean arterial pressure – mean intracranial pressure). There is no place for deliberate hypotension in patients with raised ICP unless the dura is open or the intracranial pressure is directly monitored. Even then it must be remembered that there may be regional variations in ICP (e.g. cerebral tumour). Retraction of the brain during intracranial surgery causes local pressure on cerebral tissue and this may reduce blood flow to that region, causing ischaemic damage and localized oedema (equivalent to cytotoxic oedema). This effect will be enhanced by hypotension.

Some anaesthetists, when inducing hypotension for non-neurosurgical operations, maintain spontaneous respiration to promote normocarbia or slight hypercarbia, aiming at cerebrovascular dilatation to provide good perfusion and to assess medullary function. Evidence shows, however, that during both haemorrhagic and induced hypotension there is reduced carbon dioxide responsiveness (McDowall 1985) and the desired result may not be achieved.

If the blood pressure is reduced to a level below the autoregulatory limit, autoregulation remains impaired for a time after the return to normotension (Keaney et al 1972, 1973). This may have deleterious effects if rebound hypertension occurs, especially in neurosurgical anaesthesia as the vascular distension may lead to vasogenic cerebral oedema. This can occur particularly after halothane or sodium-nitroprusside-induced hypotension with rapid return to normal blood pressure, therefore return to normal pressure should be carried out slowly. In neurosurgical anaesthesia, where cerebral tissue is vulnerable, some protection may be afforded by hypocapnia as there is still some responsiveness to changes in the arterial carbon dioxide tension where autoregulation has not been lost (McDowall 1976).

Choice of hypotensive drug in neurosurgical anaesthesia

Some agents cause cerebral vasodilatation and, if used in patients with raised ICP prior to the skull flap and dura being raised, lead to an increase in ICP. Turner et al (1977), in their study of the relationship between ICP and mean blood pressure, showed that with either normocapnia or hypocapnia, sodium nitroprusside caused a significant increase in ICP when mean arterial pressure was reduced to 90% or 80% of the pretreatment value. However, further reduction of blood pressure to 70% of control was accompanied by a reduction in ICP, but this was not the case when trimetaphan was used. The explanation is that sodium nitroprusside affects all vessels, including the cerebral vessels, whereas the ganglion blocker, trimetaphan, only affects those vessels under autonomic control. Autonomic control extends to only a small proportion of the intracranial vasculature. Nitroglycerine has an even greater effect on the ICP (Rogers & Traystman 1979). Thus if hypotension has to be induced for neurosurgery before the skull flap and dura have been raised, trimetaphan should be used (e.g. removal of meningioma).

CORONARY CIRCULATION

Blood flow through the coronary circulation varies according to the metabolic demands of the myocardium and this is determined by the myocardial workload. There is some autoregulation but not to the same degree as in the cerebral circulation, and flow through the coronary circulation depends mainly on the diastolic arterial pressure. Consequently, if diastolic arterial pressure and systemic vascular resistance are simultaneously lowered, the workload and hence metabolic demands are lower.

The situation changes if there is high metabolic demand or insufficient coronary flow to meet the myocardial demands for oxygen. For example if there is coronary artery disease and the arterial pressure falls, there will be insufficient coronary flow with consequent myocardial ischaemia and failure. It is well known in anaesthesia for coronary artery surgery that, if the main stem of the left coronary artery is stenosed, a significant fall in the aortic pressure will reduce the coronary flow. This will lead to hypoperfusion of the left side of the heart which will not receive the oxygen required for its metabolic needs, leading to a further fall in the blood pressure which then causes further myocardial failure.

In the literature review by Lindop (1975) the incidence of complications due to coronary thrombosis is very low but, as he points out, electrocardiogram (ECG) monitoring was not routine. Rollason & Hough (1960) found ischaemic changes on the ECG when the arterial pressure fell below 60 mmHg systolic. They also found that the changes were more likely in hypertensive patients. Rollason & Hough (1969) found an association between rapid lowering of the arterial pressure with earlier ECG changes.

CIRCULATION TO OTHER ORGANS

As yet there have been no definite reports of morbidity or mortality due to liver or renal failure resulting from induced hypotension. Apart from an increase in the physiological dead space, no pulmonary complications have been reported due to hypotensive anaesthesia.

POSTURE

Patients may be placed in the head-up position as an adjunct to induce hypotension, since pooling of blood below the heart will reduce venous return and hence cardiac output. This position also aids venous drainage from the surgical field. The height of the head above the heart can be critical: for every 11 cm above the heart the arterial pressure will be lowered by approximately 10 mmHg. This must be taken into account to ensure adequate cerebral perfusion pressure.

In the head-up position, venous pressure will be lowered in the deep venous channels which remain patent and become the main venous drainage as the internal jugular veins tend to collapse (Epstein et al 1970). If these are exposed at operation venous air embolism may well occur.

HYPOTENSIVE AGENTS

Volatile agents

Halothane has been used as a sole hypotensive agent or as an adjunct to hypotensive agents. The actions of halothane and hypotensive agents summate and make the patient more sensitive to both. A severe fall in blood pressure may occur if the full effects of the hypotensive agents have been allowed to take place when the halothane concentration is too high. Similarly, if a hypotensive agent is added as an adjunct to halothane hypotensive anaesthesia, the same severe fall in blood pressure may occur. Therefore it is prudent to use a small concentration of halothane at the start, if other agents are to be used as the principle hypotensive drug, and then to vary the concentration of halothane when the full effect is known. Alternatively, the concentration of the halothane can be set around 1 × MAC and the hypotensive agent titrated in reduced doses to achieve the desired effect. If ganglion-blocking agents are to be used it is probably better to keep the halothane concentration around 0.5% until the effects of the ganglion blockers are established. The same principles apply to other volatile agents if used instead of halothane.

Sodium nitroprusside

Sodium nitroprusside (SNP), which is usually administered in a 0.01% solution in dextrose or normal saline, is used because of its rapid action and evanescence. It has been extensively studied but has disadvantages in that it is unstable in solution and sensitive to light. If there is green or blue discolouration, as opposed to its normal light-brown colour, it must be discarded. It is also highly toxic. The hypotensive action of SNP is due to its nitroso radical interfering with the excitation–contraction mechanism of the smooth muscle fibres in vessel walls. It is also believed to interfere with the calcium influx and intracellular activation of calcium. Sodium nitroprusside is broken down in vitro to release cyanide with sulphydryl radicals supplied by endogenous sodium thiosulphate. The cyanide is converted by the enzyme rhodanase (found mainly in the brain, liver and kidneys) into the harmless form of thiocyanate. The alternative pathway for rendering the cyanide harmless is by in vivo combination with hydroxycobalamin to form cyanocobalamin which is then excreted. Sodium nitroprusside also interferes with vitamin B_{12} metabolism and iodine uptake by the thyroid.

The toxic effects of SNP are due to liberated cyanide reacting with the haemoglobin forming cyanomethaemoglobin and toxic effects on the cellular cytochrome oxidases. Since the reported fatalities have been due to large doses of SNP (Jack 1974, Merrifield & Blundell 1974) the rate of infusion and the patient response to SNP are important. The conversion of liberated cyanide into thiocyanate is limited by the availability of endogenous thiosulphate and the slow rate of the rhodanase reaction. These two factors are probably the reasons for toxic effects being manifest 1–3 h post-SNP infusion. It has also been suggested (Davies et al 1975) that the red blood cell enzyme, thiocyanate oxidase (which converts thiocyanate to cyanide), may be partly responsible. If the patient has cooled due to vasodilatation this reaction is slowed, but when the patient rewarms in recovery the rate of the reaction is increased, thus 'overwhelming' the patient with cyanide.

Signs of SNP toxicity

The signs of SNP toxicity are tachyphylaxis, respiratory and central nervous system depression, metabolic acidosis and bradycardia. If untreated, death may follow.

Rate of infusion of SNP

McDowall et al (1974) suggested an infusion rate of 1.6 mg/kg/h and Merrifield & Blundell (1974) suggested a maximum total dose of 3 mg/kg, but these doses are now regarded as too high. Vesey et al (1974), Greiss et al (1976) and Bennett & Abbott (1977) recommend that SNP be infused at less than 10 μg/kg/min as rates above this are associated with metabolic disturbance 'or, more often, disaster'. If higher rates of infusion are needed because of tachyphylaxis, the infusion should be stopped immediately, the acid-base status of the patient checked and an alternative method of induced hypotension used.

To reduce the chance of SNP toxicity some anaesthetists administer hydroxycobalamin (0.1 mg/kg) intravenously, prior to SNP administration, to increase the amount of substrate for the cyanide-cyanocobalamin pathway. Since this drug has no ill-effects it is probably advisable to give it.

There are several absolute contraindications to nitroprusside itself, in addition to those for induced hypotension generally. These are Leber's optic atrophy, tobacco amblyopia, malnutrition, vitamin B_{12} deficiency and hypothyroidism.

Cyanide antidote therapy

Cyanide antidote therapy comprises four components:

1. Sodium nitrite for intravenous administration (5 mg/kg in 20 ml sterile water) over 3–4 min. Alternatively, amyl nitrate inhalations every 2 min. (This is to form methaemoglobin which has greater affinity for cyanide than the cellular cytochrome oxidases.)
2. Sodium thiosulphate infusion (150 mg/kg in 50 ml of sterile water) given over 15 min.
3. Hydroxycobalamin (0.1 mg/kg) intravenously.
4. Calcium (either as gluconate or chloride) to raise the blood pressure (Bennett & Abbott 1977).

If the patient has been, or is being, given a prolonged SNP infusion, daily blood thiocyanate levels should be monitored and if greater than 10 mg/100 ml the infusion must be stopped.

Nitroglycerine

Nitroglycerine has been used successfully for induced hypotension in neuroanaesthesia as 0.01% at 2–4 mg/kg/min. Chestnut et al (1978) feel that there are advantages in using nitroglycerine over SNP. Nitroglycerine is not toxic and affects the capacitance vessels rather than the resistance vessels so reducing venous resistance, but at the same time allowing arterial tone to remain. Thus it should not affect intracranial pressure or increase the rate of cerebral oedema formation that would follow arteriolar distension. However, Rogers & Troystman (1979) have shown that, in the experimental animal, nitroglycerine can cause a rise in ICP while the dura is still intact.

Ganglion blockers

Ganglion blockers cause sympathetic blockage at the postsynaptic membrane of the ganglia and are used with positioning (e.g. head up, etc.) to lower the blood pressure. Pentolinium and hexamethonium have prolonged action times of 20–40 min and up to 4 h, respectively, whereas trimetaphan is rapidly metabolised and can therefore be more conveniently administered in a dilution of 1 mg/ml.

If peripheral vasoconstrictors are to be used to raise the blood pressure, the dosage should be reduced or titrated as they are more effective following the loss of autonomic tone. The tachycardia that occurs is due to the action of baroreceptors and parasympathetic blockade of the heart may be troublesome. Parasympathetic block also causes dilatation of the pupils which is not popular with neurosurgeons postoperatively.

Trimetaphan is the most practical of these agents as on ceasing the infusion the blood pressure usually returns to normal within a few minutes. The principal disadvantages are tachycardia (which may persist) and sometimes delay in the return of blood pressure (which may be due partly to histamine release). The response of the blood pressure to the administration or withdrawal of trimetaphan is not as rapid as sodium nitroprusside or nitroglycerine. The activity recorded on a cerebral function monitor is depressed at higher mean arterial pressure with trimetaphan than with sodium nitroprusside (McDowall 1985, Prior 1985) and brain surface oxygen tension is better with sodium nitroprusside than with trimetaphan. Neither drug, however, affects brain surface oxygen tension as adversely as hypotension due to haemorrhage (Mackawa et al 1979).

Beta blockers

Beta blockers may be used to reduce the tachycardia in response to hypotension, especially in the younger patient. Care should be taken during administration as an excess may induce prolonged bradycardia with possible difficulty in raising the blood pressure and cardiac output. The new beta-receptor blocking drug, esmolol, with a short half-life would be the most appropriate drug in this case. It should be remembered that these agents may cause severe bronchospasm in susceptible patients, even leading to death.

CONCLUSION

The incidence of complication is low and the general consensus on induced hypotension is that deaths and complications cannot be attributed solely to the technique. To predict which patient is going to suffer complications is almost impossible. However, there are certain conditions where there are greater risks of complications and these patients should be excluded. Lastly, patients undergoing hypotensive anaesthesia must be monitored very closely. Direct arterial pressure, ECG oximetry and capnography must be the minimum level of monitoring.

REFERENCES

Association of Anaesthetists of Great Britain and Ireland 1988 Recommendations for standards of monitoring during anaesthesia and recovery. Association of Anaesthetists, London

Bennett N R, Abbott J R 1977 The use of sodium nitroprusside in children. Anaesthesia 32: 456–459

Chestnut J S, Albin N S, Gonzalez-Aboda E, Newfield P, Maroon J C 1978 Clinical evaluation of intravenous nitroglycerine for neurosurgery. J Neurosurg 48: 704–711

Davies D W, Greiss L, Kadar 1975 Metabolic observations during normal and abnormal responses to sodium

nitroprusside during anaesthesia in children. Can J Anaesth 22: 547–553
Enderby G E H 1980 Hypotensive anaesthesia. In: editors General anaesthesia, 4th edn. Butterworths, London vol 2, p 1149–1169
Epstein H M, Linde H W, Crampton A R, Civic I D, Eckenhoff J I 1970 The vertebral plexus as a major outflow tract. Anesthesiology 32: 332–337
Finnerty F A, Wilkin L, Fazekas F J 1954 Cerebral haemodynamics during cerebral ischaemia induced by acute hypotension. J Clin Invest 33: 1227–1231
Fitch W, Mackenzie E T, Jones J V, Harper A M 1976 Effect of halothane on the autoregulation of cerebral blood flow in normotensive and chronically hypertensive baboons. Br J Anaesth 48: 1123
Graham D I 1985 The pathology of brain ischaemia and the possibilities for therapeutic intervention. Br J Anaesth 57: 3–17
Greiss L, Trembley N A G, Davies D W 1976 The toxicity of sodium nitroprusside. Can Anaesth Soc J 23: 480–485
Hygosson R, Högström S 1973 Factors disposing to morbidity in surgery on intracranial aneurysms with special regard to deep controlled hypotension. J Neurosurg 38: 561–567
Jack R D 1974 Toxicity of sodium nitroprusside. Br J Anaesth 46: 952
Keaney N, Pickerodt V W A, McDowall D G, Coroneos N J, Turner J M, Shah Z P 1972 Cerebral effects of hypotension produced by deep halothane anaesthesia. Br J Anaesth 44: 623–624
Keaney N, McDowall D G, Turner J M, Lane J R, Okuda Y 1973 The effects of profound hypotension induced with sodium nitroprusside on cerebral blood flow and metabolism in the baboon. Br J Anaesth 45: 639
Larson A G 1964 Deliberate hypotension. Anesthesiology 25: 682–706
Lassen N A 1959 Cerebral blood flow and oxygen uptake. Physiol Rev 39: 197
Leigh J M, Tytler J A 1990 Admissions to the intensive care unit after complications of anaesthetic techniques over 10 years. II. The second 5 years. Anaesthesia 45: 814–820
Lindop M J 1975 Complications and morbidity of controlled hypotension. Br J Anaesth 47: 799–803
McDowall D G 1976 Neurosurgical anaesthesia and intensive care: Mewer L, Atkinson R (eds) In: Recent advances in anaesthesia and analgesia. Churchill Livingstone, Edinburgh
McDowall D G 1985 Induced hypotension and brain ischaemia. Br J Anaesth 57: 110–119
McDowall D G, Keaney N P, Turner J M, Lane J R, Okunda Y 1974 Toxicity of sodium nitroprusside. Br J Anaesth 46: 327
Mackawa T, McDowall D G, Okunda Y 1979 Brain surface oxygen tension and cerebral cortical blood flow during haemorrhage and induced hypotension in the cat. Anesthesiology 51: 313–321
Merrifield A J, Blundell M D 1974 Toxicity of sodium nitroprusside. Br J Anaesth 46: 324–326
Moyer J H, Morris G 1954 Cerebral haemodynamics during controlled hypotension induced by continuous infusion of ganglion blocking agents. J Clin Invest 33: 1081
Pasch T, Huk W 1986 Cerebral complications following induced hypotension. Europ J Anaesthesiol 3: 299–312
Prior P F 1985 EEG monitoring and evoked potential in brain ischaemia. Br J Anaesth 57: 63–81
Rogers M C, Traystman R J 1979 Cerebral haemodynamic effects of nitroglycerine and nitroprusside. Anesthesiology 51: 5199
Rollason W N, Hough J M 1960 A study of hypotensive anaesthesia in the elderly. Br J Anaesth 32: 276–291
Rollason W N, Hough J M 1969 An examination of some electrocardiographic studies during hypotensive anaesthesia. Br J Anaesth 41: 985–986
Turner J M, Powell D, Gibson R M, McDowall D G 1977 Intracranial pressure changes in neurosurgical patients during hypotension induced with sodium nitroprusside and trimetaphan. Br J Anaesth 49: 419–425
Utting J E, Gray T C, Shelley F C 1979 Human misadventure in anaesthesia. Can Anaesth Soc J 26: 472–478
Vesey C J, Cole P V, Linnell J C, Wilson J 1974 Some metabolic effects of sodium nitroprusside in man. Br Med J 2: 140–142
Warner W A, Shumrick D A, Caffrey J A 1970 Clinical investigation of prolonged induced hypotension in head and neck surgery. Br J Anaesth 42: 39–44
Yashou D, Magness A P, Vise W M 1975 Systemic hypotension in neurosurgery. J Neurosurg 43: 579–589

34

Patient position

M. P. Colvin and K. Wilkinson

INTRODUCTION

This chapter describes some of the effects on patients that are a consequence of their position on the operating table and how they can be avoided. These effects are important because of the significant impact they make on intra-operative and postoperative morbidity and mortality. There is a brief account of injuries from other apparatus, including blood warmers, heating blankets and tourniquets, but the particular problems caused by position in obstetric and dental anaesthesia, and injuries to peripheral nerves, are not included as they are dealt with in detail in other chapters.

THE PRINCIPLES OF POSITIONING

The position of the patient is usually chosen by the surgeon to make the operative procedure as technically easy as possible. The actual positioning and the treatment of the immediate physiological effects of the chosen position are almost invariably delegated to the anaesthetist and the theatre staff. It is therefore the duty of the anaesthetist to protect the patient by anticipating the anatomical and physiological consequences of the proposed position and, if necessary, to modify it by tactful negotiation.

Safe positioning requires meticulous attention to detail. This is achieved by patience and concentration, and no anaesthetist, however junior, should allow himself to be rushed during this procedure by an impatient surgeon anxious to start the operation. Any uneasiness that remains about aspects of the position or physiology of the patient when the operation starts is greatly magnified after the incision and access becomes difficult or impossible. At best the anaesthetist will suffer a great deal of unnecessary anxiety; at worst, poor preparation may lead to the death of the patient. Before the surgeon is allowed to approach the patient the anaesthetist must be satisfied that all aspects of the patient's position, anaesthetic and surrounding apparatus are in a perfect condition. These aspects will be considered in turn. The only circumstance under which this rule can be broken is when immediate surgical intervention is necessary to prevent the death of the patient.

THE OPERATING TABLE SURFACE

The surface of the operating table is made of smooth, soft, antistatic rubber which serves both for comfort and electrical safety. If the patient is to be subjected to a steep head-down tilt, during abdominoperineal resection for instance, a corrugated surface may be used that prevents slipping (Hewer 1953).

During long operations, when heat loss is anticipated or the temperature is to be lowered deliberately, it is usual to have a heating blanket under the patient. Heating blankets in common use in adult anaesthetic practice comprise two types. The first is an electric element covered with washable plastic. The second is a plastic sheet approximately the size of the operating table made up of tubes through which warm or cold water can be circulated from a separate, thermostatically controlled, pump or heat exchanger. All such devices must have a double thermostat, nonetheless one must always be alert to the possibility of malfunction, overheating and burns. Of the two, the warm water type is probably the safer. Electric blankets have the added disadvantage that an electrical fault can itself cause electrocution or burns of both the patient and his attendants. It is necessary to monitor the temperature of the patient if there is a need for a warming blanket, and it is good practice to use a second temperature probe between the patient and the blanket so that the blanket temperature can be checked regularly from an independent source.

The table top is then covered with a clean, smooth, wrinkle-free linen sheet. In addition a drawsheet about 20 cm wide may be laid across the table to be folded over to pinion the arms.

The heels, which are particularly vulnerable to pressure necrosis, are supported on foam rubber pads. These serve a double purpose in that they raise the calf muscles off the table, preventing pressure on the deep veins which may initiate deep venous thrombosis.

The patient may be an unusual shape, for example with kyphoscoliosis, or may have to assume a potentially unstable position during thoracotomy or renal exploration. Under these circumstances a mouldable mattress may be used. This device is an operating-table-shaped bag filled with polystyrene granules rather like a domestic 'bean bag'. When the patient is placed on the bag, the granules shift and the bag assumes the exact shape of the patient. Suction is then applied to the valve in the bag which is then fixed in that shape. The patient therefore has a rigid mattress, tailor-made to his own shape. Because he is surrounded by it rather than on top of it, he remains in a stable position provided the bag is not punctured and the valve does not leak. The disadvantage of this device is that following evacuation it is rather hard, and slight movement of the patient could allow undetected and unsuspected pressure points to develop. While these could to some extent be anticipated and padded, this device is probably not suitable for very long operations in excess of 3–4 h.

PATIENT COMFORT AND POSSIBLE INJURIES

Within the limits imposed by the operative procedure, the patient should lie in a position that he would find reasonably tolerable if he were awake. To achieve this the anaesthetist should try to visualize how long he would be able to tolerate the position himself. This principle is illustrated in a case report by Swerdlow et al (1988) in which they describe a technique for positioning a morbidly obese (177 kg) patient in the prone position. Following awake intubation under local anaesthesia in the supine position, the patient positioned himself prone on an orthopaedic frame with his pannus freely suspended. Only when the patient was comfortable and breathing satisfactory, as measured by pulse oximetry and capnography, was general anaesthesia and controlled mechanical ventilation initiated. This technique could easily be applied to any patient of unusual shape, or in whom a potentially uncomfortable position is necessary.

Pressure on soft tissues overlying bony points must be avoided, especially in the elderly or emaciated. These points include elbows, knees, the greater trochanter of the femur, the head of the fibula and the heels. All of these can be padded with foam rubber. Around the head, the nose, malar prominences, ears and teeth are all vulnerable and particular attention must be paid to the eyes. Scratching of the cornea is not uncommon. Lincoln & Sawyer (1961) cite a number of examples of pressure damage to the eyeball including blurred vision, severe pain, and retinal artery thrombosis and blindness. If the patient is to be face down or the eyes otherwise inaccessible, the eyes must be taped closed, then padded and covered, if necessary, with plastic eye shields. The use of the padded horseshoe rest in the face-down position in neurosurgery can very easily cause eye pressure if the face is not accurately positioned within it. A safe way to achieve such accuracy is for the anaesthetist to lie flat on his back on the floor directly below the patient's face so that a close personal assessment can be made.

Stretching of soft tissues and joints can also cause postoperative pain and morbidity. Lincoln & Sawyer (1961) suggest that a D-shaped wedge may help maintain the normal lumbar lordosis and may reduce the incidence of postoperative backache associated with the supine, and more commonly the lithotomy, position which accentuates rotation of the pelvis. The lumbar spine can also be supported in the same way with a full 3 l bag of irrigation fluid such as glycine that readily conforms to the right shape. The adoption of the lithotomy position with extreme flexion of the hips and knees may cause sacroiliac strain and both legs must be moved in unison. Personal experience has shown that patients with kyphoscoliosis must be carefully evaluated before medial sternotomy or open-heart surgery. The necessary wide retraction of the sternal edges may distort the spine sufficiently to cause paraplegia. This possibility must be explained and fully understood by the patient before such surgery is undertaken.

It is possible to dislocate joints and fracture bones during positioning if limbs are allowed to move unsupported. Fractures are most likely if patients with osteoporosis, secondary tumours of the bone or osteogenesis imperfecta are handled carelessly.

Vascular injury giving rise to thrombophlebitis or phlebothrombosis may follow direct pressure on veins or arteries, or distortion of the vessel, for long periods of time, especially in the presence of peripheral vascular disease. Vulnerable atheromatous vessels include the femoral, popliteal and carotid arteries. Extreme abduction of the arm may compromise the circulation by stretching the axillary vessels, even in healthy individuals. Hovagim et al (1989) describe eight cases in which pulse oximetry of the arm warned the anaesthetist that the patient was positioned incorrectly. In seven of these the circulation of the limb was temporarily compromised. The mechanisms of potential injury were all common situations in everyday anaesthesia and included hyperabduction of the arm, insertion of an axillary roll, suspension of the arm from an anaesthetic screen, securing of the arms in forward flexion in the prone position, hyperextension of the wrist to facilitate radial artery cannulation and the use of a Favaloro retractor for internal mammary artery dissection. These descriptions suggest that the pulse oximeter should be used to check the position of any limb that is to be strapped in an abnormal position. In the same way an arterial monitoring line may become damped or otherwise fail to detect blood pressure. While there are several possible explanations for this, the possibility of external distortion, occlusion or disconnection must always be borne in mind.

Hypothermia by surface cooling is no longer commonly employed. Severe cold injury to the skin and subcutaneous tissue can occur if ice is allowed to come into direct contact with the skin. This can be avoided by wrapping the ice in wet cloths, frequent movement of the ice packs and constant vigilance.

PATIENT STABILITY AND FIXATION

The head, trunk and limbs must all be in a stable position, particularly if changes in position are anticipated during the operation. The possible consequences of sudden, violent, uncontrolled movements of the head and neck are so serious that, in any movement of the patient, the anaesthetist must himself take charge of the head and neck in order to maintain the correct relationship to the trunk. The lifting of the patient should be done by personnel employed for that purpose.

The arms, being underneath the drapes in most instances, are the most likely to fall off the table unnoticed. This accident could give rise to damage to the brachial plexus or shoulder joint and to diathermy burns if the limb becomes earthed. The arms can be held down either by a drawsheet lying behind the patient folded over the arms and tucked behind his back, or by inserting padded, shaped, plastic supports under the edge of the rubber mattress.

If the trunk or position of the legs is likely to be unstable, in the lateral decubitus position for example, it is necessary to pass straps over two points of the body or to use a mouldable mattress in order to achieve total security.

If a steep head-up position is to be used, a foot rest may be placed at the bottom end of the table and a corrugated mattress used. The steep head-down position is now rarely used, but if it is necessary it must be remembered that shoulder supports can cause brachial plexus damage.

DIATHERMY AND METAL CONTACT

The diathermy plate must be fixed firmly to a clean, hairless area, if possible on the thigh. Although the buttock is often used, this has the disadvantage that, if a burn does occur, it is very difficult to position and maintain a skin graft in that area. During preparation of the skin, spirit must not be allowed to trickle underneath the diathermy plate. Care must also be taken to avoid the skin of the patient touching metal that could be grounded to earth. Vulnerable areas include the fingers slipping below the mattress to touch the operating table and the shoulders touching an un-insulated anaesthetic screen. Adequate protection can be afforded by liberal padding with foam rubber. The problem of electrical safety is considered in greater depth in Chapter 43.

ANAESTHETIC APPARATUS

Movement of the patient during positioning may cause a displacement of the endotracheal or double-lumen tube. This may lead to obstruction of the airway, total extubation, inadvertent intubation of the right main bronchus and, in the case of a right double-lumen tube, occlusion of the right upper lobe bronchus. If the patient is turned into the lateral or prone position, the anaesthetist, while attending to the position of the head and neck, must at the same time look after the tube. When the manoeuvre is completed he must also recheck its position. If the patient's head is to be held in a position that may kink the endotracheal tube within the pharynx, an armoured tube must be used.

The tubing connecting the patient to the anaesthetic machine is often heavy and, if unsupported, may not only displace the endotracheal tube, but also cause undue pressure on the face or forehead. Before draping the patient the anaesthetic tubing connections must be checked obsessively and, if necessary, taped together to prevent disconnection. A 'loss of pressure alarm' must always be in the circuit and a final check made that it is switched on before the patient is draped for surgery.

MONITORING, INTRAVENOUS INFUSIONS AND BLOOD WARMING

Once the patient has been satisfactorily positioned, the final check must be of the monitoring and infusion apparatus.

The integrity and continuity of the airway, whether the connections are in view or not, must always be monitored by ventilator alarm, pulse oximeter and capnograph. The measurement of blood pressure using a cuff on the arm, whether by oscillotonometer or by automatic apparatus, is readily subject to interference. It is sensible to place the cuff where it is least likely to suffer interference from the unpredictable movements of the surgeon, which may make blood pressure recording impossible for long periods at a time. If blood pressure is recorded from a line in the radial artery, it may be necessary to hyperextend the wrist slightly with a splint in order to achieve a satisfactory trace.

Radial artery lines must be flushed under direct vision before surgery begins, as prolonged blanching of the thumb and thenar eminence is an indication for immediate removal. Femoral artery lines can be kinked if the patient is sat up.

ECG electrodes must be checked to confirm that they are properly adhesive, and that the signal is good and without interference. Finally the arm containing the intravenous infusion should be positioned in such a way that it runs freely. It goes without saying that the correct time to detect a poorly functioning intravenous cannula is the beginning and not the middle of an operation, especially if heavy blood loss is anticipated.

If a blood warmer is available it should always be used for blood transfusion. Modern blood warmers, whether of the dry heat or hot water type, have two thermostats and a prominently displayed thermometer in order to eliminate, as far as possible, damage to the blood and haemolysis caused by overheating. It is better to run cold blood into the patient than to risk overheating it, and the practice that still exists in some places of prewarming bags of blood in a bowl of warm water can only be condemned.

POSITIONING IN SPECIAL CIRCUMSTANCES

Paediatric surgery

Although positioning is usually easier in children, several points should be made concerning the operating theatre environment and facilities available. Theatre suites that have regular, designated paediatric lists may elect to have a single theatre committed for paediatric use and properly equipped for this purpose. This is a luxury rarely afforded outside major centres, therefore the anaesthetist and surgical team will need to spend some time and thought anticipating the needs of the small patient with reference to the planned procedure.

Simple adjuncts to anaesthetic equipment such as a variety of small sand bags, head rings and wedges of foam rubber are invaluable when stabilizing the position of the infant in whom the head is relatively large. If nothing else is available, a 0.5 l infusion bag is an excellent means of extending the neck in the infant weighing less than 10 kg in preparation for internal jugular vein cannulation.

Many centres have developed special bars and frames to minimize the problem (particularly in neonatal work) of the surgeon impinging on the small space allowed to the anaesthetist for direct observation and monitoring of the child (Yamashita 1988). Anaesthetic tubing should be stabilized in such a way as to avoid traction on the endotracheal tube and pressure on the delicate skin.

Temperature

Avoidance of cold stress is basic to good paediatric surgical and anaesthetic management (Dilworth 1973, Friesen & McIlvaine 1989). However, the provision of a warm, draught-free theatre may be difficult to achieve. Vale (1973) has stated that 'the modern operating room environment . . . is designed for the comfort of the surgical team'. Unfortunately this is still too often the case with minimal facility for altering the temperature quickly and efficiently for the paediatric patient.

In the unclothed term neonate, an ambient temperature of 33–35°C needs to be achieved to provide a neutral thermal environment (Hey & Katz 1970, Hey & O'Connell, 1970). Some authors continue to recommend these temperatures for the preterm infant (Gregory 1989). However, provided the infant is additionally clothed and the environment draught-free, an environmental temperature of 25–27°C is felt by others to be sufficient (Friesen & McIlvaine 1989) and is usually the maximum at which theatre personnel are able to work. Therefore the provision of additional equipment, such as safe and efficient warming mattresses (Hatch 1985) and warming devices for infusions, become all the more important in the paediatric age-group. Goudsouzian et al (1973) demonstrated that children weighing less than 10 kg are particularly likely to lose heat under surgical conditions and derived most benefit from the use of external warming devices, such as a water circulating warming blanket. More recently the circulating air mattress has been recommended (Hatch 1985).

Humidification of inspired gases will also minimize heat and fluid loss in these patients, and can be provided optimally by the use of a heated water-bath humidifier. Heat and moisture exchange devices suitable for paediatric use are also readily available. Their efficiency has been improved by the incorporation of a hygroscopic element, and they have the advantages of portability and simplicity. Heat loss during paediatric surgical procedures may also be avoided by:

1. making sure the child is adequately clothed and covered on what may be a draughty journey to theatre. Infants up to about 5 kg in weight can be efficiently transported in incubators and this should be routine

practice with all neonates. Incubator temperature should be between 32°C and 34°C. This same incubator should be kept warm and made available for the return journey.

2. minimizing heat loss when the infant is exposed, for example for neck-line insertion by the use of servo-controlled overhead heaters. These may also be employed during surgery, but increased fluid loss is incurred and must be replaced. Others have advocated a policy of the surgeon operating on the smallest and sickest neonates in the incubator in the neonatal ICU (Besag et al 1984). In the author's experience this works extremely well on the open cot with overhead servo heater, as long as the surgeon can be provided with adequate light and the anaesthetist allowed sufficient access to the patient.
3. wrapping the infant's limbs and head in domestic foil which cuts down on radiant loss (Friesen & McIlvaine 1989). Insulation of the head is particularly important and may be most efficiently provided by the use of gamgee-lined woollen bonnets (Stothers 1981), or those made from a composite of olefin and polyester which also prove to be extremely efficient if correctly applied (Rowe et al 1983). The use of insulating wrap such as gamgee and the warming of surgical cleaning fluids and drapes are all simple measures that even a hospital unused to paediatric surgery can easily employ.

The lateral position

Davies et al (1985) looked at regional ventilation in infants and very young children (ranging in age from eleven days to 27 months) with lung disease. They found ventilation to be preferentially distributed to the uppermost lung, the reverse of the adult situation. This finding may have important implications for the infant with unilateral lung disease. However another more recent paper has shown that, in anaesthetized infants and children with previously normal lungs, the distribution of ventilation in the lateral position is that reported previously in anaesthetized adults (Larsson et al 1989).

Paediatric orthopaedic surgery

In the paediatric age-group several orthopaedic procedures are carried out in positions taxing to the unprepared anaesthetist. The Harrington and Luque posterior spinal fusion procedures for kyphoscoliosis are carried out with the patient in the prone position which can be facilitated by the use of special frames (Relton & Hall 1967). As with all procedures in the prone position, it is important to avoid inferior vena caval compression which may, if significant, impede venous return and thus reduce cardiac output, as well as lead to engorgement of vertebral venous plexuses making surgery on the spine impossible.

The use of additional monitoring equipment to assess intact long-tract function (somatosensory cortical evoked potentials) is replacing the traditional wake-up test still employed in some centres, but requires skilled interpretation. It is imperative that sufficient personnel are available to allow safe turning from supine to prone position. An anaesthetic technique that allows for the quick recovery of laryngeal reflexes is important and the use of an antiemetic at this stage may also be helpful.

Hip surgery in children is usually performed with the patient in the supine position using a conventional operating table. Change of hip spica, though a minor surgical procedure, requires careful preparation. It involves the use of a special frame onto which the child's legs and buttocks are placed. Adequate support for the head, neck and trunk must therefore also be ensured. The provision of a 'belly pad' is essential if the plaster is to extend to waist level. This consists of a piece of foam or cotton-wool placed on the lower abdomen before the plaster is applied which will prevent it being strapped too tightly and thus impeding diaphragmatic respiratory function.

Adult orthopaedic surgery

Positioning the patient for orthopaedic procedures demands, as always, provision for safe access by both surgeon and anaesthetist. Positioning may prove to be a particularly time-consuming process and should be carried out with considerable care to avoid potential morbidity.

Surgery on the hip joint and femur

Positioning the adult patient for hip surgery involves the use of the lateral decubitus or, when dealing with fractured neck or shaft of femur, the use of a modified supine posture on a fracture table.

Surgery for replacement of the femoral head may be carried out in a full lateral decubitus position. In this posture a cylindrical padded support may be provided anteriorly and placed cephalad to the iliac crests. Additional padding in the form of foam or cotton-wool should be interposed between patient and support. This is particularly important in the elderly patient susceptible to pressure-sore injury. The patient's arms can be conveniently placed on lateral arm boards.

Venous access, if possible, should be achieved in the upper arm. Placement of the blood pressure cuff is more of a problem since, if on the lower arm it may be compressed and artificially high readings obtained; if on the upper arm the intravenous infusion may be repeatedly obstructed. In practice one's decision is influenced by the patient's general body build and in the obese, in whom venous access and indirect blood pressure measurement are usually problematic, one usually has to compromise. Some surgeons will elect to use a half lateral position with a sand bag supporting the ipsilateral buttock which makes positioning a far simpler task.

In the case of fracture to the femoral neck or shaft, the patient is transported to theatre in traction. The anaesthetist must ensure, before anaesthesia is induced, that the bed can be tipped easily and traction taken down if turning the patient becomes essential. Following induction of anaesthesia, temporary disconnection of infusions and monitoring equipment will be necessary. It is wise to ensure secure placement of lines and adequate cardiovascular stabilization prior to this manoeuvre as well as sufficiently deep anaesthesia.

The patient should then be lifted directly onto the fracture table, plenty of skilled help being required to minimize the duration of the manoeuvre and ensure patient safety. The anaesthetist controls head and neck movement while the surgeon maintains traction on the hip. At least two other trained personnel will be needed. The patient's trunk is placed on a modified operating table and his legs are supported in free-moving supports which allow the use of the image intensifier.

Padding of the knees, particularly over the head of the fibula, and in the popliteal fossa and the ankles is essential. The ipsilateral arm is strapped across the chest, flexed and adducted so as to be removed from the screening field and thus obscuring the hip joint. This may make some slight difference to the inflation pressures required to ventilate the chest and may also mean that the blood pressure cuff is best placed on the contralateral arm.

The fact that the patient is approximately 1.5 m from the ground during surgery makes observation and the use of regional techniques alone difficult, not least because the position would prove worrying for the conscious patient. At the end of surgery the patient will need to be lifted carefully back onto the bed. It is inadvisable to turn off anaesthetic gases and reverse muscle relaxation too early.

As with many orthopaedic procedures, turning the patient into the customary lateral 'coma' position on recovery may be considered undesirable from the surgical standpoint. This being the case it may be useful to retain a surgical presence at the time of recovery so that, if turning is felt to be necessary, this is achieved rapidly and with optimal attention to the surgical site.

Spinal surgery

Surgical indications for the prone position include all types of spinal surgery, craniotomy for lesions involving the posterior fossa and, less commonly, rectal and varicose vein surgery. The problems of the classic prone position are shown on page 550. They principally relate to cardiovascular decompensation due to inferior vena cava compression, and respiratory embarrassment from abdominal compression. Nerve or plexus injury due to inadvertent pressure over bony prominences or excessive traction is also a risk. In addition, serious upper airway obstruction may occur due to kinking of the endotracheal tube and many anaesthetists now routinely employ one of an excellent range of disposable armoured tubes.

If inferior vena caval compression is allowed to occur in the prone position, obstruction of the normal routes of venous drainage can make surgery on the spine virtually impossible because of attendant bleeding. This is particularly difficult to avoid in the obese patient, in whom the lateral position may be an acceptable alternative. Certainly the obese patient should not be subjected to the risks of the prone position without very careful planning. Various modifications of the classic prone position have also been described to help minimize the adverse effects, the best being the use of various supporting frames.

Common to all these techniques, however, is the transfer of the patient into the prone position. This needs to be undertaken by a minimum of four skilled personnel to ensure the patient's safety. It is recommended that the patient be relatively lightly anaesthetized at this point, and paralysed to avoid coughing and straining. In addition it may be advisable for the table initially to be placed in a slight head-down tilt to reduce the effects of any hypotension incurred.

Attention to detail at each stage is probably more important to the safety of the manoeuvre than whether the patient is turned on the operating table, or transferred into the prone position between trolley and table. During this period, monitoring is necessarily minimal but should be readily available for reconnection, as should the intravenous infusions. Simple continuous monitoring in the form of an oesophageal stethoscope, for example, is helpful in the relatively young and fit patient. One should consider the need for continuous intra-arterial monitoring of blood pressure when turning the patient with a potentially unstable cardiovascular system in spinal shock, for example.

Cervical instability

Particular mention should also be made of the special circumstances involved when dealing with the unstable cervical spine. Patients with an unstable cervical fracture should be in some form of secure traction, which may lead to problems with intubation. Others, in whom protection of the cervical cord is no less of a problem (for example subluxation of the atlantooccipital joint in the patient with rheumatoid arthritis or Down's syndrome), may arrive in theatres with little more than a soft collar which gives minimal protection. Intubation of such patients may be difficult and should be carried out with extreme care. In particular, extension of the neck is to be avoided (Doolan & O'Brien 1985) since this can most easily lead to additional cervical cord trauma.

Fibre-optic intubation is a possibility in most centres if difficulties are anticipated (Hemmer et al 1982). In the emergency situation, when cervical trauma has occurred or severe atlantooccipital instability exists, necessary neck traction should be provided by no less than two skilled assistants, one of whom should be the neurosurgeon familiar with the case. Turning such a patient prone is a particular worry and again requires the direct attention of the neurosurgeon. In some situations it will be felt advisable to insert special head and neck traction screws into the skull before the manoeuvre can be safely attempted.

Particular mention should be made of patients with ankylosing spondylitis who seem to be at particular risk of fracture of the cervical spine, sometimes after minor trauma (Salathé & Jöhr 1989). Careless manipulation of the neck, and even skilled intubation, may result in quadriplegia which carries a poor prognosis. Awake fibre-optic intubation is suggested as a safe technique.

Shoulder surgery

Positioning the patient to afford adequate exposure of the shoulder joint may be particularly taxing and should only be performed after full discussion with the surgeon. Access to as much of the joint circumference as possible is usually required. Two alternatives exist. The first is the so-called 'barbers chair' position in which the head, neck and upper trunk are about 35–45° to the horizontal and the knees gently flexed to provide the 'chair'. The second is a modified supine position in which the surgeon will operate seated. In both situations, to facilitate access to the shoulder, the patient is shifted to the ipsilateral edge of the operating table so that the limb is free. Care is required so that enough of the patient remains on the table to prevent him falling. The ipsilateral arm is then strapped across the body until it can be supported by a surgical assistant. The head is turned away from the side of surgery and should be supported by a small ring, but in so doing should not produce stretch on the brachial plexus. Intravenous cannulae, blood pressure cuff, etc., will need to be secured in the contralateral arm. The advantage of the modified position for shoulder surgery is that it avoids the theoretical risk of entrainment of air into open veins above heart level while operating on the joint.

The arterial tourniquet

The arterial tourniquet is used extensively in orthopaedic surgery to provide a bloodless field during peripheral operations on upper and lower limbs. The history, use and complications of the tourniquet have been reviewed by Fletcher & Healey (1983). The application of the tourniquet is very often supervised by the anaesthetist and some responsibility for its safe use may devolve on him.

The equipment

The tourniquet, whether of the bicycle pump or automatic type, of which there are a number on the market, must have an accurate pressure gauge so that the pressure applied to the limb is measured continuously and accurately. Although it has been recommended that the gauge of the tourniquet should be calibrated daily against a mercury manometer, it is doubtful whether this practice is ever carried out (Bruner 1970).

At one time it was common practice to occlude the circulation of the limb by wrapping an Esmarch exsanguinating rubber bandage tightly around the limb and tucking it in at the top. However this method gives no indication of the pressure applied to the tissues and, with the ready availability of accurate tourniquets, this practice must now be regarded as being unacceptably dangerous and legally indefensible if damage to soft tissues occurs.

For short operations on the digits, arterial occlusion can be achieved by winding a short piece of rubber tubing around the base of the digit and holding the ends in a clamp. This is acceptable only for short operations provided both the surgeon and the anaesthetist check that it has been removed at the end of the procedure.

Before inflating the tourniquet, it is usual to exsanguinate the limb by wrapping it from the distal end upwards with a rubber bandage, such as the Esmarch (red rubber) or Martin (latex). An alternative is the pneumatic exsanguinator which is an inflatable sleeve and may be less traumatic than a bandage (Burchell & Stack 1973).

Application of the tourniquet

Before starting to apply the tourniquet, the identity of the patient and the site and side of the operation should have been checked verbally with the patient and with the hospital notes and operating list. After padding the upper arm or thigh with orthopaedic wool or towelling, the tourniquet is applied firmly and evenly to avoid pinching the skin or subcutaneous tissues. The area chosen must be well covered with muscle and fat, and any bony prominence that would compress tissue between bone and the tourniquet must be avoided.

After elevating the limb, it is exsanguinated by rubber bandage or inflatable tube, the tourniquet is inflated, the time noted and the bandage or tube removed. The tourniquet is inflated rapidly to avoid any venous congestion. Automatic tourniquets usually indicate that the pressures adopted should be 250–350 mmHg for the upper limb and 500–550 mmHg for the lower limb.

These figures appear to have been more or less arbitrarily selected.

A number of authors suggest that a range between 30 and 150 mmHg above the systolic blood pressure should be used in order that the padding effect of fat and muscle can be overcome, particularly in the thigh (Fletcher & Healey 1983). In children and the elderly it would seem sensible to limit the pressure to that required to achieve haemostasis, and a pressure of 75 mmHg above systolic for the arm and 100 mmHg above the systolic pressure for the leg would be appropriate.

Tourniquet time

There is a long tradition that tourniquet time is limited to 1 h for the upper limbs and 2 h for the lower limbs. Although these figures appear at first sight to be arbitrary, they nonetheless represent a distillation of experience over the many years since the first description of the technique (Cushing 1904). There is also an extensive literature of animal and human research into functional, histological and metabolic changes associated with tourniquet application which is reviewed in detail by Fletcher & Healey (1983).

What does emerge however, is that the time should be as short as possible, particularly in the elderly. In a long operation, up to 10–15 min can be saved by exsanguination and tourniquet inflation after draping the patient. In the event of the operation taking longer than the agreed time, a choice must be made between prolonging the inflation time, with an increasing risk of permanent nerve or muscle damage, and temporary deflation, which is understandably unpopular with the surgeon. If deflation is necessary a further decision must be made as to the time necessary for recovering before reinflation. Shaw Wilgis (1971) suggests a recovery time of 15–20 min based on venous blood gas measurements in 50 patients. A study of eight awake volunteers, in whom arm tourniquets were inflated for a mean time of 36 min, showed that lactate and venous blood gas levels all took 30 min to return to near baseline levels.

In the same study somatosensory evoked potentials measured at the elbow, neck and cortex all recovered by between 15 and 30 min in the subjects who tolerated 25 to 45 min of inflation, but in one subject who tolerated 55 min inflation, recovery at elbow and neck took more than 1 h (Benzon et al 1988). These studies support the view of Fletcher and Healey that at least 15–20 min should elapse before a tourniquet is reinflated after an initial 2 h inflation, and may suggest that 30 min would be more prudent in the elderly.

Complications and side effects

Despite the thousands of tourniquets applied each year, the complications of such a crude procedure are surprisingly uncommon, probably because they are, in general, carefully applied and supervised and for the most part used in operations of comparatively short duration. There are several possible complications and side effects, described below.

Bruising, haematoma or degloving of skin or subcutaneous tissues can be caused by the tourniquet itself or by careless application of the exsanguinating bandage. In particular, the Esmarch bandage can cause severe damage to delicate skin and should not be used in those with primary or secondary disorders associated with skin fragility. These include rheumatoid arthritis, epidermolysis bullosa and prolonged steroid therapy.

Damage to muscle. Muscle damage may be caused by the pressure of the tourniquet, both directly and indirectly, by damaging the blood vessels supplying the muscle. This may lead to post ischaemic contracture.

Vascular injury. Damage to an artery, followed by arterial occlusion can cause variable ischaemic damage to all tissues up to and including loss of the limb. Venous damage may induce venous thrombosis, which may in turn lead to peripheral oedema or pulmonary embolus.

Nerve injury may be caused by direct pressure or ischaemic injury. Nerve injury may lead to temporary or permanent sensory or motor loss (Larsen & Hommelgaard 1987).

Tourniquet pain. In the absence of a general anaesthetic or sedation, pain may be felt at the site of the tourniquet even when a regional anaesthetic has been properly established. Abolition of this pain has been described after the use of intrathecal clonidine (Bonnet et al 1989), epidural fentanyl (Solanki 1987) and application of local anaesthetic cream to the skin before tourniquet application (Lowrie et al 1989). The pain associated with the release of the tourniquet lasts only a few minutes and is not usually important.

Intracranial pressure changes. A tourniquet is often used for limb surgery in a patient with multiple injuries, including head injuries. A significant rise in end-tidal $P\text{CO}_2$ has been shown to occur following the release of a peripheral tourniquet (Dickson et al 1989). This is presumed to be the likely cause of increased intracranial pressure associated with release of the tourniquet in head-injured patients. A decrease in cerebral perfusion pressure may be exacerbated by any associated fall in blood pressure (Conaty & Klemm 1989, Eldridge & Williams 1989). Such a potentially damaging rise in intracranial pressure might be prevented by hyperventilation, adequate circulating blood volume and prophylactic mannitol before tourniquet release.

Acute heart failure may be caused by increased circulating blood volume, particularly if more than one limb is occluded at the same time. This complication is rare and only likely in the elderly or infirm.

Contraindications to the use of a tourniquet are:

- peripheral vascular disease
- extensive muscle injury caused by laceration or crushing that might be associated with ischaemic tissue
- proven or suspected venous thrombosis
- sickle-cell disease
- anticoagulant therapy
- haemophilia and other disorders of coagulation
- infection of the limb. This is only a relative contraindication and relates mainly to avoiding the use of an Esmarch bandage over the infected area. Exsanguination should be by elevation only
- severe peripheral vascular disease
- conditions associated with bone or soft-tissue fragility.

Tourniquets in paediatric patients

Use of the tourniquet for orthopaedic and plastic surgery in infants is theoretically likely to be less desirable. As a result of the increased basal metabolic rate and hence oxygen requirements of this age-group, it is possible that the products of anaerobic metabolism produced in tissues distal to the tourniquet will be inadequately dealt with and lead to prolonged acidosis. This concern has been addressed by Lynn et al (1986) and led the authors to provide the following recommendations:

1. Attempt to limit inflation time to less than 75 min.
2. Use controlled ventilation prior to and after tourniquet deflation to remove the respiratory component of acidosis.
3. Check arterial blood gases within 5 min of tourniquet deflation in infants in whom the tourniquet has been inflated for more than 75 min, or when bilateral tourniquets are deflated simultaneously or within 30 min of each other.

It is important to note that in all but two patients studied, the lower limb was under tourniquet. Tourniquet release was associated with less haemodynamic change than in adults; however there was a small but statistically significant fall in blood pressure at 1 and 3 min.

Positioning for urological surgery

The lithotomy position, the most common position for both urological and gynaecological procedures, is discussed on page 550. Special mention should be made, however, of the so-called 'kidney position' in which the flank is exposed by providing lateral spinal flexion over a 'broken' table (in which the break should be just above the level of the iliac crest), or with the aid of an inflatable pillow positioned under the dependent flank. Stability in this position is maintained by flexing the lower leg (providing padding and separation of the legs with pillow) and using a padded central support (the kidney brace), adhesive strapping or both. Care should be exercised to avoid pressure over bony prominences such as the iliac spines, and also the external genitalia. The arms should be placed in a neutral posture, to avoid traction on the brachial plexus, and a bar may be helpful to prevent the surgeon and assistants inadvertently leaning on the infusion lines or blood pressure cuff.

Respiratory problems in this position include those related to ventilation of the dependent lung which is largely solved by intubation and intermittent positive pressure ventilation (IPPV), but the potential also exists for producing a pneumothorax if exposure of the left kidney is undertaken. Inadequate venous return can occur in this position, either as a result of pooling of blood in the lower limbs if they are placed at a level below the heart, which can be corrected by raising the foot of the table, or as a result of direct compression on the inferior vena cava by the surgeon or by incorrect positioning of the table break. This may not be apparent unless hypovolaemia coexists.

Positioning in ear, nose and throat surgery

During ear, nose and throat (ENT) procedures the anaesthetist and surgeon will need particularly good communication, since there exists the constant problem of the shared airway and both teams need to be at pains to ensure it is clear at all times. More often than not the anaesthetist will need to occupy a relatively distal position in relation to the head and neck. Kinking or misplacement of the endotracheal tube is a real possibility during such procedures and one that the team needs to bear in mind at all times.

Adenotonsillectomy

Positioning the patient for adenotonsillectomy involves moderate extension of the head by placement of a sandbag or roll underneath the shoulders. If this is excessive or the oral endotracheal tube is rather short, accidental extubation may result. A more common occurrence, however, is partial obstruction of the endotracheal tube by the divided tongue plate used by the surgeon.

Ear surgery

Grommet insertion and myringotomy can usually be carried out with the patient breathing spontaneously via a mask. The head should be positioned on a small ring to aid stability. Major ear surgery, including tympanoplasty and surgery involving the middle ear, requires carefully controlled conditions. As an adjunct to close control of blood pressure in this situation, venous drainage is improved by a slight 15° head-up tilt. The anaesthetist is best positioned on the contralateral side to the surgery as are the venous and arterial cannulae, if used.

Thyroidectomy

The surgeon will usually desire a degree of neck extension for thyroidectomy, but care should be exercised particularly in the elderly, and the patient asked to demonstrate his usual range of comfortable neck movement on the preoperative visit. This should be noted by the anaesthetist and should not be exceeded in positioning. A sandbag under the shoulders and a suitable head ring is required. Towards the end of the surgical procedure, prior to skin closure, the surgeon may request that extension is reduced to allow easy skin apposition. This will necessitate either raising the head of the table independently, or removal of the shoulder sand bag which is awkward and risks desterilizing the operative fields. A novel solution is provided by placing an inflated 1 l infusion bag under the shoulders for surgery. This can be deflated when skin sutures or clips are about to be inserted.

Tracheostomy

For tracheostomy the patient is again carefully positioned with a sandbag under the shoulders and the head fully extended to produce prominence of the trachea. A ring is required to stabilize the head. The anaesthetist must ensure that easy access to the endotracheal tube is maintained by positioning himself at the head of the table, being careful not to contaminate the site. Once the trachea is open, the endotracheal tube should be carefully pulled back but not removed. Ventilation is continued via the tracheostomy tube once it is in place. Before tapes to secure this tube are tightened, the sandbag should be removed from under the shoulders, and the head placed in a normal degree of slight flexion.

Unusual bone and soft tissue fragility

Osteogenesis imperfecta

Osteogenesis imperfecta may present in two broad forms: the severe recessive forms often lead to fractures present at birth, and those forms presenting later in life usually exhibit dominant inheritance, and with less severe and less frequent injuries. Associated features which should be noted when positioning these patients and preparing them for anaesthesia and surgery are dental fragility, joint hypermobility and thin skin. They have also been noted on several occasions to demonstrate temperature instability and case reports of malignant hyperpyrexia have appeared (Rampton et al 1984). During positioning of the patient, all movements must be carried out with the utmost care. It is probably safest to anaesthetize the patient on a well-padded operating table and to avoid transfers if possible, particularly while the patient is unconscious.

Anaesthetic management has been reviewed by Libman (1981). Of particular note is the fact that application of blood pressure cuffs and tourniquets for venous cannulation has been associated with fractures, and the latter at least should be avoided. If blood pressure monitoring is felt to be important, an arterial cannula should be inserted with care because of an increased tendency to soft tissue and vascular trauma due to a generalized collagen defect. In the severe forms the head is relatively large in comparison with the contracted body and padding around it is important, not just for protection but also to improve stability. Airway control and intubation may be difficult. They must be executed with due attention to jaw and cervical spine which can be fractured during the manoeuvres. Recovery is no less an important period than initial positioning. The patient should ideally be recovered on his own bed which is suitably padded, or on the operating table to minimize transfers.

Ehlers–Danlos and Marfans syndromes

Soft tissue fragility exists in other inherited diseases of collagen synthesis such as the several forms of Ehlers–Danlos and Marfans syndromes. In both these conditions, hypermobility and increased bruising tendency are associated problems. Careful positioning to avoid trauma and abnormal joint posture is thus imperative. In the case of Marfans syndrome, positioning may be more difficult because the subjects are so tall and the operating table needs to be modified accordingly. Once more this is a case for proper positioning and limb support prior to induction of anaesthesia, and any subsequent handling of the patient should be very gentle.

Epidermolysis bullosa

Several forms of epidermolysis bullosa exist with different degrees of severity and patterns of inheritance. However the form most important to the anaesthetist is epidermolysis bullosa dystrophica (EBD), for which the prevention of friction and soft tissue trauma is essential. The use of adhesive tape, sticky electrocardiogram (ECG) pads and diathermy plates should be avoided at all costs and replaced with crepe or cotton-wool wrapped around intravenous cannulae, non-adhesive ECG plates and bland ointment to protect the eyes. Blood pressure cuffs should be carefully padded, and for long procedures properly secured arterial lines may cause less trauma (Smith & Shribman 1984).

As with the other conditions of increased soft tissue fragility already discussed, the number of transfers in theatres should be kept to a minimum and if possible the patient should position himself on the table prior to anaesthesia and be allowed to recover on the same table. The operating surface should be carefully padded with foam or cotton-wool under all pressure points. Several excellent reviews on the subject of anaesthesia in EBD exist and it behoves the anaesthetist to familiarize himself with these prior to even the most minor surgical procedure (Young & Hardwick 1968, James & Wark 1982, Smith & Shribman 1984).

POSITIONING IN THE RECOVERY ROOM

The positioning of patients with unstable cervical spines and after some types of orthopaedic procedures has been discussed on page 542. Some general points, however, should be made about the transfer and care of all patients in the recovery room.

Both the anaesthetist and the surgeon take responsibility for the safe conduct of the unconscious patient in theatre and should insist on the provision of equipment to facilitate patient transfer. The practice of leaving the anaesthetist and theatre technician to transfer the patient is to be deplored.

Patients are usually transferred from operating table to bed or trolley using any one of a number of systems:

1. Canvas is placed underneath the patient and poles are threaded laterally. Although widely employed, this method has obvious risks inherent to both the patient and the theatre personnel. Split canvases and fractured poles are relatively common occurrences.
2. The patient is lifted bodily from the operating table to the recovery bed. This may be necessary after several orthopaedic procedures (see above). It may also be undertaken if the canvas on which the patient is lying is severely soiled or wet. This method obviously requires more personnel, is more time consuming and is of considerably greater risk to the patient.
3. A commercially available 'roller' is placed half way under the patient in the semilateral position and stretched across onto the trolley or bed which should be placed at the same level. The patient is manoeuvred onto the roller which is then gently moved onto the bed or transfer trolley and removed from underneath the patient. The roller mattress is made of a soft material and covered with a non-static, antislip surface.
4. A commercially available 'board' may be used. This is made of a smooth, extremely strong plastic and has strips of a gripping material on one side which improve stability. The patient is preferably 'swaddled' in a sheet to protect the limbs and enable smooth transfer. The board is placed half way under the patient with the bed or trolley adjacent and at the same level. The patient is then 'slipped' across. In practice this proves to be very efficient, needing only two personnel even for adult patients, and awake subjects have commented on its comfort.

The proper use of such transfer systems avoids back strain in theatre personnel and improves patient safety.

The recovery bed

The requirements for patient positioning should be just as rigid in the recovery area as in theatre. They should involve specific instructions and care on the part of the anaesthetist in the form of verbal and written advice to the recovery and ward staff. Ideally the patient should be recovered on his own bed which should be easily tipped (preferably by one operator at the head end). The head of the bed should be detachable so that access to the patient's airway is not inhibited. The advantages are that patient transfers are minimized and the patient awakes on a comfortable surface from which he is less likely to sustain injury while unconscious. Unfortunately only very few recovery areas have the space to accommodate beds for all their patients; even fewer hospitals have been planned with sufficient space for their routine use in corridors, lifts and anaesthetic rooms. The usual compromise involves the provision of the bed if the recovery period is likely to be prolonged.

The anaesthetist should anticipate such a need and make sure that the patient's bed is used. The relatively rigid surface of the standard operating trolley with metal supporting sides is not only extremely uncomfortable, but is an additional cause of nerve and soft tissue injury. One could also postulate that postoperative analgesia requirements are likely to be greater if the patient recovered on such a trolley.

THE EFFECTS OF POSTURE ON CARDIORESPIRATORY FUNCTION DURING ANAESTHESIA

In the anaesthetized patient the effects of posture on cardiorespiratory function may be difficult to predict in that they depend on a host of interacting variables. These include drugs, the use of spontaneous or positive pressure ventilation, the presence of obesity or an intra-abdominal mass, and a variety of pre-existing cardiovascular and respiratory pathology that may influence the response of the body to a change in circulating blood volumes.

The extraordinary adaptability of the physiological reflexes in the body usually ensures that any changes in cardiovascular and respiratory function are transient and of little practical importance. Nonetheless the anaesthetist must monitor the patient attentively and be ready to give assistance to these reflexes if it becomes necessary. Possible exceptions to this general statement occur in neurosurgery and thoracic surgery. These will be considered in more detail after a summary of the problems associated with each of the common positions in surgery. The cardiorespiratory effects of changes of body position have been reviewed by Coonan & Hope (1983).

Supine position

This basic position is well tolerated and causes no important effect on cardiovascular or respiratory function in normal patients.

The presence of a large abdominal tumour may mimic the effect of the pregnant uterus. As anaesthesia is induced and muscle tone is lost the tumour may partially compress the inferior vena cava, and reduce venous return, cardiac output and blood pressure. This can usually be corrected by the slight left lateral tilt that has been described for Caesarean section. (Crawford et al 1972). The particular problem of the supine hypotension syndrome in pregnancy is discussed in detail in Chapters 11 and 40.

Supine head-down (Trendelenburg)

The steep head-down position for long periods is now rarely necessary but slight degrees of head-down are commonly used for all kinds of pelvic surgery.

If spontaneous breathing is allowed, the compression of the diaphragm by the abdominal contents will cause a fall in functional residual capacity (FRC) and respiratory difficulty, particularly in the obese, in patients with ascites or abdominal tumours, and pregnancy. Studies carried out in spontaneously breathing, lightly anaesthetized young patients in the head-down position have shown no significant effect on blood gases, pH or minute volume (Scott et al 1966, Scott and Slawson 1968). It is usual to use positive pressure ventilation in the head-down position except for very short procedures.

The moderate head-down position increases venous return and may improve cardiac output. If the head-down position is very steep this effect is lost, venous blood tends to accumulate in the head and neck, and cardiac output falls (Coonan & Hope 1983). The resultant high venous pressure and fall in blood pressure will lead to a decrease in cerebral perfusion pressure, a fall in cerebral blood flow and even cerebral oedema, particularly in a patient with a pre-existing brain injury.

The careless use of the head-down position, even for short periods to facilitate insertion of a central venous cannula, must therefore be avoided in patients with brain injury, congestive cardiac failure or other instability of the circulation.

Head-up position (reverse Trendelenburg)

A slight head-up position, as distinct from the full sitting up position, is commonly used in operations on the head and neck or trunk as it improves venous drainage and may reduce bleeding.

There is often a slight fall in blood pressure. This is easily corrected and may actually be an advantage, provided it does not fall so far as to impair cerebral perfusion. For this reason the position should be used with caution and full monitoring in the elderly hypertensive patient.

Respiration is either unaffected or may even be improved as the abdominal contents fall towards the pelvis and allow the diaphragm more freedom of movement. All these effects apply whether the patient is head-up lying in the supine or prone position.

Lithotomy position

The lithotomy position usually causes no significant effect in normal patients. In the obese patient the flexed thighs will push the abdominal contents up, which in turn compress the diaphragm and reduce FRC. This process is often exacerbated by the use of a slight head-down tilt in this position. The problem can be overcome by positive pressure ventilation which is the method of choice except in short operations.

The increase in venous return associated with elevation of the legs may help to maintain the blood pressure in this position. Great care must therefore be observed when the legs are lowered at the end of the operation, particularly if there has been heavy blood loss. If a degree of hypovolaemia persists a fall in blood pressure may occur.

Prone position

Provided the abdomen is lifted clear of the table by a frame, or by pillows under the shoulders and pelvis, the abdominal contents including the vena cava are not compressed and cardiovascular effects are for the most part trivial in the prone position. FRC increases, although this does not appear to cause any changes in ventilation parameters (Stone & Khambatta 1978). Ventilation should always be controlled in this position.

Perhaps the greatest danger to the patient in the prone position lies in the handling and positioning of the head and neck as the patient is turned and transferred onto one of the frames used for lumbar laminectomy. Twisting and hyperextension of the head and neck could cause damage to the cervical vertebrae, particularly in patients with ankylosing spondylitis (Salathé & Jöhr 1989). Danger can also occur from the subsequent kinking of the airway, or from undetected accidental disconnection of the ventilator. The use of a non-kinking, armoured endotracheal tube and a ventilator alarm are mandatory.

Lateral position

The lateral, or lateral decubitus, position is used in thoracic surgery and in the lateral approach to the kidney. The only problem directly associated with surgery on the kidney that is not covered later in this section is that of hypotension. To expose the flank fully the patient is placed in the lateral position stretched over an inflatable pillow. The table is then 'broken' under the pillow. Although this causes no difficulties with the patient lying on the left side, in the right lateral position for surgery to the left kidney this manoeuvre may be associated with a sudden, significant fall in blood pressure. This is caused by partial obstruction of the inferior vena cava and a reduction of venous return to the heart.

To understand the cardiovascular complications associated with the lateral position, it is first necessary to understand the complex varying interrelationship between blood flow and ventilation in the lungs. The physiology, theory and practice of anaesthesia in the lateral position in general, and in thoracic anaesthesia in particular, have been described in detail by Benumof (1983).

Pulmonary blood flow

Blood flow in the lungs is essentially dependent on the force of gravity. In the upright position the greater part of the blood flow is distributed to the dependent, lower part of the lungs with less flow at the apex (West 1970). In the lateral position, by the same mechanism, the upper lung is relatively poorly perfused and the lower lung is well perfused (Denlinger et al 1972). This distribution is common to all lateral positions except the special case of one-lung anaesthesia which is discussed on pages 553–554.

Pulmonary ventilation

The changes associated with ventilation in the lateral position are more complex than those of the pulmonary blood flow. The problems will be familiar to thoracic anaesthetists, but apply equally to anaesthesia for other operations in the lateral position.

Benumof (1983) based his description of lung ventilation in the lateral position on the regional transpulmonary pressure–alveolar volume curve (Figs 34.1 & 34.2). In these diagrams the flat parts of the curve, at the top and bottom, represent low compliance or a relatively large change in pressure for a small change in volume. The middle, steep part of the curve represents high compliance or a small change in pressure for a large change in volume.

In the upright position, alveoli in the apex of the lung are relatively large in volume and low in

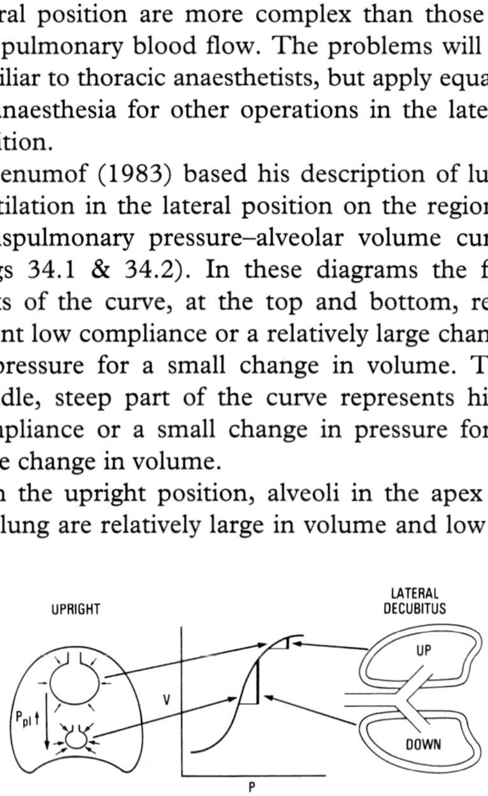

Fig. 34.1 Curve of the regional transpulmonary pressure (P) and alveolar volume (V) in the awake patient in the upright and lateral decubitus positions. Pleural pressure (Pp1) in the awake patient (closed chest) is least negative at the base of the lung. Alveoli in this region are therefore the most compressed, have the least volume and are most compliant. Pleural pressure is most negative at the apex of the lung. Alveoli in this region are least compressed, have the largest volume and are less compliant. In the diagram the steeper the curve the greater the compliance. For a given change in pressure the alveoli at the base of the lung will receive a greater proportion of the tidal volume. In the lateral decubitus position the upper lung behaves in the same way as the apex of the upright lung and the lower lung like the base. The lower lung will therefore receive the greater share of the tidal volume (from Benumof 1983 with permission).

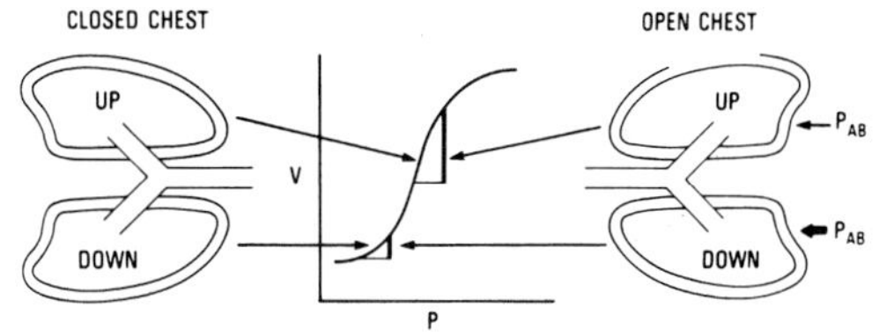

Fig. 34.2 Curve of the regional transpulmonary pressure (P) and alveolar volume (V) in the anaesthetized patient in the lateral decubitus position. Following the induction of anaesthesia, both lungs suffer loss of volume. If the left-hand side of the diagram is compared with the right-hand side of Figure 34.1 it can be seen that the upper lung has moved from the flat, non-compliant part of the curve, to the steep, compliant part of the curve. The lower lung has moved from the steep, compliant part of the curve to the lower, flat, non-compliant part. Thus in the anaesthetized patient with a closed chest the greater proportion of the ventilation will go to the upper lung where the perfusion is less and the rest of the ventilation will go to the lower lung that is better perfused. When the upper pleura is opened (right of diagram) the upper lung, free of the constraint of the chest wall, becomes even more compliant. This increases further the proportion of tidal volume going to the upper lung. Paralysis exacerbates this tendency since the pressure of abdominal contents (Pab) against the upper lung diaphragm is less than that against the lower lung and it is easier to displace the diaphragm by positive pressure ventilation (from Benumof 1983 with permission).

compliance since pleural pressure is more negative. At the base of the lung, pleural pressure is less negative and the alveoli are smaller and more compliant. For a given change in pressure, therefore, the base of the lung will expand more than the apex and will be better ventilated (Fig. 34.1).

In someone lying awake in the lateral position, the upper lung assumes the characteristics of the apex of an upright lung and lies in the same, less-compliant part of the pressure–volume curve. The lower lung, like the base of the upright lung, lies on the more compliant part of the curve and is therefore better ventilated than the upper lung (Fig. 34.1), a characteristic that is reinforced by the fact that the lower lung diaphragm is pushed up higher than the upper lung diaphragm and is able to contract more forcibly.

In summary, the awake person in the lateral position will experience relatively poor ventilation and blood flow in the upper lung and relatively good ventilation and blood flow in the lower lung.

Effects of anaesthesia in the lateral position

In the anaesthetized patient, distribution of blood flow remains unchanged and dependent on gravity. There are, however, major alterations in the distribution of ventilation. Anaesthesia induces a fall in the FRC of both lungs. This effect is greater on the lower lung as it is compressed by the mediastinum sagging down from above and the abdominal contents pushing up the lower diaphragm. Further pressure is provided from outside the chest wall by the practice of breaking or angulating the table under the patient, which is commonly used in thoracic procedures or operations through the flank. If the patient is paralysed and ventilated, all diaphragmatic tone will be lost and the compression of the diaphragm increased.

These various factors conspire to induce a greater fall in FRC in the lower lung than in the upper lung. This has the effect of moving the upper lung down to the more compliant part of the pressure–volume curve and the lower lung further down to a less compliant part of the curve (Fig. 34.2). Most ventilation is therefore directed to the upper lung where there is less blood flow. The lower lung, though still well-perfused with blood, is less well-ventilated. The result is an increase in the ventilation/perfusion mismatch.

For short, closed chest procedures in the lateral position in healthy people, it is acceptable to allow them to breath spontaneously under these circumstances. For longer procedures this situation cannot be tolerated.

It has been shown (Rheder et al 1973) that artificial ventilation with the use of positive end-expiratory pressure (PEEP) improves ventilation to the lower lung, thus restoring a more even matching of ventilation and blood flow throughout both lungs. This would seem to be the technique of choice if the chest is to remain closed, in the lateral approach to the kidney, for example.

The open chest

Once the chest and parietal pleura have been opened, spontaneous ventilation is no longer acceptable and paralysis and positive pressure ventilation must be used. The reason for this is simple. When the chest is still closed the negative pressure in the upper pleura not only helps the lung to remain expanded, but also serves to counteract the tendency of the mediastinum to sag downwards.

When the chest is open this suspensory effect is lost. The mediastinum drops downwards, causing a reflex fall in blood pressure that may be exacerbated by distortion of the superior and inferior vena cava, and a reduction of venous return to the heart. Furthermore, as the mediastinum descends, not only does the upper lung collapse by elastic recoil but the lower lung collapses as it is crushed downwards. This effect occurs whether for a large, deliberate thoracotomy or from the accidental breach of the pleura that frequently occurs during the lateral approach to the kidney.

The open chest with positive pressure ventilation of both lungs

The solution to the problem of the open chest wall is positive pressure ventilation through an endotracheal tube. This maintains the volume of the dependent lung, holds the mediastinum in the horizontal position, preserves the cardiac output and overcomes the tendency of the exposed upper lung to collapse. It is possible to apply PEEP to the lower lung through a special valve (Brown et al 1977). This technique is experimentally successful in maintaining dependent lung volumes and improving oxygenation, but is rarely used in routine thoracic surgery.

Following a wide thoracotomy, the upper lung, already more compliant than the lower lung (Fig. 34.2), becomes even more compliant as it is freed from the constraints of the chest wall. In theory, therefore, the upper lung will receive an even greater share of the available ventilation in the face of a continuing predominance of perfusion in the lower lung. In practice this phenomenon is modified by the partial collapse of the upper lung caused by the surgical retraction necessary to perform the operation. This restores the balance of ventilation and perfusion to some extent.

One-lung anaesthesia

The use of the double-lumen tube allows the upper lung to be collapsed with all ventilation directed to the lower lung. In thoracic surgery one-lung anaesthesia has a number of advantages, indeed many intrathoracic procedures are impossible without it.

At first sight it would appear that collapse and non-ventilation of the upper lung would result in severe hypoxia as a large proportion of the cardiac output is shunted through that lung. However, a number of studies have shown (Khanam & Branthwaite 1973a, Kerr et al 1974) that the amount of shunt and fall in Pa_{O_2} varies considerably from patient to patient. When the upper lung is first collapsed the Pa_{O_2} may fall to low levels, but as the upper lung becomes hypoxic the proportion of the cardiac output shunting through that lung decreases in response to the hypoxic pulmonary vasoconstriction that occurs (Torda et al 1974, Benumof 1979). For this reason the Pa_{O_2} often improves quite rapidly as the shunt decreases. There is usually no difficulty in eliminating carbon dioxide during one-lung anaesthesia (Kerr et al 1973).

One-lung anaesthesia with a double lumen tube is usually safe if the following principles are observed:

1. Bronchoscope the patient before inserting the tube. This confirms that the bronchial anatomy is normal and that no plugs of sputum are present that could cause difficulties in ventilating the lower lung.
2. The double-lumen tube must be carefully positioned if it is to perform safely and efficiently. This is relatively easy for a left endobronchial tube as the left upper lobe bronchus branches off 4–6 cm from the carina and allows some room for error. On the right side, however, the upper lobe bronchus branches off only 1.2 cm from the carina and is easily occluded. Although a side hole is cut in right endobronchial tubes to allow ventilation of the right upper lobe, this may be difficult to position correctly by clinical observation and the routine use of a fibre-optic bronchoscope is recommended (Watson 1987).
3. After the patient has been placed in the lateral position, or there is any other change in the relative position of the head, neck or trunk, the position of the tube must be rechecked. Repositioning of the tube after the chest is open is extremely difficult.
4. The patient must be monitored continuously with pulse oximeter and capnograph as well as ECG and an intra-arterial line through which blood pressure and blood gases can be measured.
5. Tidal volume is usually set at 10–12 ml/kg. When the upper lung is collapsed, Pa_{CO_2} is maintained by ventilating the lower lung at the same minute volume. Initially the tidal volume is maintained, but if the airway pressure rises significantly it may be necessary to decrease tidal volume and increase respiratory rate.
6. Ventilation of both lungs should be continued for as long as possible.
7. When the upper lung is collapsed the lower lung should be ventilated initially with 100% oxygen. Anaesthesia and analgesia can be easily maintained if a total intravenous technique is used. A combination of propofol and alfentanil is particularly suitable.
8. Continued use of 100% oxygen will cause absorption atelectasis in the lower lung. Some attempt to avoid this can be made by ventilation with an air/oxygen mixture. The concentration of oxygen can be varied from minute to minute by observation of oxygen saturation. A total intravenous technique will allow the anaesthetist to avoid nitrous oxide and make a small contribution to the reduction of global warming and the 'greenhouse effect'.
9. If the lung is to be removed, the surgeon should try to occlude the blood supply to that lung as soon as possible.
10. The position of the mediastinum must be observed. Any tendency for it to sag downwards may be counteracted by inflating the lower lung with 5 cm H_2O of PEEP.

11. Hypoxia. If the patient becomes cyanosed or bradycardic, it must be assumed that acute hypoxia has occurred and the upper lung must be reinflated immediately with 100% oxygen. If, on the other hand, hypoxia occurs as measured by oxygen saturation or blood gas measurement, but the patient remains otherwise stable, several measures can be taken to improve oxygenation without inflating the upper lung:
    - The inspired oxygen can be increased to 100%.
    - The lower lung can be ventilated with 5–10 cm of H_2O of PEEP. The effect of this has been shown to be variable (Khanam & Branthwaite 1973b, Katz et al 1982) and may improve, worsen or make no difference to $Pa\text{O}_2$. The complex reasons for this variability have been discussed by Benumof (1982).
    - The upper, non-ventilated lung can be insufflated, but not ventilated with oxygen under a pressure of 5 cm H_2O. This technique has been shown to improve overall oxygenation (Capan et al 1980) by causing oxygen exchange with what blood continues to run through the collapsed lung. Surprisingly, this does not cause a significant change in the amount of blood running through the lower ventilated lung by reversing hypoxic pulmonary constriction. The disadvantage of this technique is that the upper lung remains slightly distended which could make surgery difficult. However, Benumof (1988) points out that using 5 cm H_2O pressure on a lung with a compliance at near residual volume of only 10 ml/cmH_2O causes a lung volume change of only 50 ml which is unlikely to be of any significance.

Sitting position

Patients are anaesthetized in the sitting position for neurosurgery and in dental anaesthesia. The problems peculiar to dentistry are discussed in Chapter 37.

The sitting position is used as an approach to the surgery of the posterior fossa. Ingram (1987) discusses in detail the advantages and disadvantages of this position in neurosurgery. He also compares it with the two alternatives: prone position and the park-bench position, a lateral, slightly head-up position that resembles the posture of somebody sleeping on a park bench.

Although the hazards of air embolism have caused the sitting position to be abandoned in favour of the prone position by some neurosurgeons and anaesthetists, a survey of 37 neurosurgical centres in the UK (Campkin 1981) showed that 19 (52.7%) used the sitting technique and a further four (11%) used the technique at least some of the time. Only 30.5% used the approach routinely for cervical surgery, but this may simply reflect the fact that the sitting position has less of an advantage over the prone in operations on the cervical vertebrae.

With the patient upright and the head flexed forward, the surgeon can get a good view of the posterior fossa. Arterial blood pressure is easy to control and venous drainage is good, both of which should minimize blood loss. This position should, if anything, improve CSF drainage and keep brain swelling to a minimum.

In a retrospective study of 579 patients having posterior fossa craniectomies between 1981 and 1984 (Black et al 1988), 333 (57.5%) were sitting (60–90° head-up) and 246 (42.5%) were in a horizontal position (0–20° head-up). Venous air embolus occurred in 45% of sitting patients and 12% of horizontal, but no mortality or morbidity could be attributed to any air embolism. Hypotension during positioning occurred in 19% of the sitting patients and 24% of the horizontal patients.

Blood loss was lower, therefore the need for transfusion was lower in the sitting patients. Postoperative cranial nerve function was significantly better in the sitting group and there was no significant difference in cardiopulmonary complications between the two groups.

Despite these figures, which would, on the whole, tend to favour the sitting-up group, neurosurgeons (who ultimately choose the position) have changed dramatically between 1981 when 82% of patients were sat up and 18% placed horizontally, and 1984 when 35% were sat up and 65% placed horizontally. The reason for this change is not clear, nor is it discussed, but it is tempting to suggest that the increasingly threatening medico–legal climate may have influenced their choice.

Ventilation

There has long been controversy about the use of spontaneous or controlled ventilation in the sitting position. The principle argument for preserving spontaneous respiration is that changes in the pattern of breathing may indicate surgical interference with vital structures in the medulla or brainstem. In a study of 110 patients in the sitting position, Millar (1972) ventilated half his patients and allowed the other half to breathe spontaneously. In his series, only two showed respiratory changes in the absence of other signs during surgical dissection.

Blood pressure was better maintained in the spontaneous ventilation group. The ventilated group needed more frequent intervention for hypotension with fluids or vasopressors. Despite this, he felt that the disadvantages of spontaneous ventilation (which included hypercapnia, swelling of the brain, coughing and straining, increased bleeding and an increased likelihood of air embolus with a lower mean intrathoracic pressure) suggested that mechanical ventilation was the method of choice in the sitting position. It would also seem likely that the incidence of atelectasis of the lung which might persist into the postoperative period would increase in patients breathing spontaneously. The argument for controlled ventilation is also supported by Campkin (1981).

Hypotension

Millar (1972) reported that, of the 110 patients in his series, only four developed hypotension on assuming the sitting position to a degree that required the position to be abandoned. All four showed moderate or marked systolic hypertension preoperatively. In most of his patients a fall in systolic pressure of 10–20 mmHg occurred and this would accord with my experience. These falls are usually transient and respond to a reduction in the level of anaesthesia, an increase in blood volume or, as a last resort, injection of a vasopressor. Millar (1972) also noted that persistent instability of systolic blood pressure, which was presumably of manageable proportions, occurred in nine of his patients in the sitting position.

Air embolus

Air embolus can occur not only in the sitting position, but also when the patient is only slightly head-up. The reported incidence varies from 2% (Millar 1972) to 45% (Black et al 1988), but these figures are probably of doubtful value as they depend on the sensitivity of the monitoring equipment. The operation of suboccipital craniotomy may carry a higher risk of embolism (Matjasko et al 1985, Standefer et al 1984). Katz & Mayhew (1985) describe a group of 18 patients with achondroplasia undergoing suboccipital craniotomy. Seven (60%) of 12 in the sitting position and one (17%) of six in the prone position suffered air embolus though none was fatal. They suggest that achondroplasia may constitute a particular risk factor.

It is perhaps significant that both the patients in the work by Leivers et al (1971) were undergoing removal of a meningioma near the foramen magnum. The authors suggest that such operations are more likely to produce air embolus than operations on the cerebellum. The prevention, detection and treatment of air embolus has been reviewed by Leivers et al (1971) and Brodrick (1987).

Prevention of air embolus

Preventative measures must be taken whenever there is a negative pressure gradient between the head and the right atrium. The first line of prevention must be communication between surgeon and anaesthetist when dangerous territory is entered.

Brodrick (1987) suggests that the best form of prevention lies in a consistent rise in central venous pressure (CVP). Maintenance of a high CVP by transfusion alone is extremely difficult and, even if successful, carries a risk of inducing right heart failure, particularly in the elderly. It is therefore of limited practical value. The use of transfusion can be reinforced by the antigravity or G-suit used in aviation medicine (Hewer & Logue 1962).

Brodrick & Ingram (1988) have shown that inflation of a G-suit to 60 mmHg can sustain a statistically significant rise in CVP of about 6 mmHg. The concomitant rise in systolic blood pressure of 10 mmHg will at the same time help prevent hypotension. They also showed that the addition of PEEP of 5.0–7.5 mmHg caused a small but significant further rise in CVP. The use of 10 cmH_2O PEEP is also discussed by Lee et al (1981). The incidence of air embolus in their series was reduced when compared with a group of controls. An alternative to the G-suit is the medical antishock trouser (MAST) designed for lower body compression in trauma which produces a similar effect (Toung et al 1980).

Additional, rapid changes in venous pressure if air embolus is suspected can be achieved in a number of ways. Manual compression of the jugular veins in this position is possible, but if it is to be maintained for any length of time it requires more agility and strength than is possessed by most anaesthetists. The use of a piece of Paul's tubing threaded through rubber tube and pulled tight around the neck is slightly more practical (Buckland & Manners 1976), but its use may be limited if the incision extends down the neck. An inflatable venous neck tourniquet has been described that has the advantage of simplicity and precise control, but may, like Paul's tubing, interfere with the incision (Sale 1984). Personal experience has shown that a rapid rise in venous pressure can be achieved and maintained by pushing a fist firmly into the epigastrium, which is a great deal more accessible than the neck in a sitting position.

Detection of air embolus

Careful, continuous monitoring is necessary for the early detection of air embolus. Apart from the methods used by the anaesthetist, a careful and communicative surgeon will usually be aware that a large vein has been opened and that air may have entered the venous circulation before any other signs are apparent. Devices for diagnosis of air embolus rely on detection of the presence of air in the circulation and observing its effects on the cardiopulmonary system.

Monitoring must include an intra-arterial pressure line, ECG, pulse oximeter and capnograph for measurement of end-tidal carbon dioxide. In the venous circulation, a central line is an absolute minimum, but a multifunction pulmonary artery catheter is to be preferred (Munson et al 1975). A pulmonary artery catheter is capable of measuring CVP, cardiac output by thermodilution, pulmonary artery pressure and left atrial pressure through the pulmonary artery wedge pressure. A rise in pulmonary artery pressure is an early sign of air embolus (English et al 1978) as pulmonary vascular resistance rises.

Special large bore, pulmonary artery catheters have been designed so that air can be aspirated rapidly from the venous circulation (Noel 1989). Bowdle & Artru (1988) have demonstrated how a long introducer sheath and the proximal port of the catheter can be accurately positioned at the junction of the superior vena cava and atrium by using an ECG trace. The saline-filled catheter is used as an exploring electrode which demonstrates inversion of the P-wave as the tip passes the junction of cava and right atrium.

The precordial ultrasonic Doppler detector is capable of monitoring small quantities of air (Edmonds-Seal & Maroon 1969, Martin & Colley 1983). It is, if anything, too sensitive but has been widely used clinically (Standefer et al 1984, Matjasko et al 1985). Continuous end-tidal carbon dioxide measurement shows a fall in CO_2 after air embolus but will detect it later than the other methods (Bethune & Brechner 1968).

The oesophagus can be used for monitoring through a transeosophageal Doppler (Martin & Colley 1983), and an oesophageal stethoscope, if properly positioned, may detect a 'mill wheel' murmur, but it is a tedious task to listen continuously for the many hours that a posterior fossa operation lasts. This technique may anyway not detect small amounts of air.

In both cases described by Leivers et al (1971), the first sign of air embolus was sudden ventricular fibrillation. Both in this report and that of McComish & Thompson (1968) it is suggested that, in patients breathing spontaneously, the change in respiratory pattern in air embolus may be a series of large gasps which may themselves encourage aspiration of air. These reports reinforce the view that controlled ventilation should be used in the sitting position.

Treatment of air embolus

Once air embolus is thought to have occurred, the surgeon must be informed, and the venous pressure must be induced to rise further by intravenous infusion and by one of the methods already described. Further air embolus is prevented by diathermy, bone wax, flooding the wound with normal saline, or a saline-soaked pack.

A significant fall in blood pressure is treated with intravenous fluids or even a vasopressor. If the fall is extreme or cardiac arrest occurs, external cardiac massage must be started in the sitting position and the patient lowered horizontal as soon as possible while every effort is made to avoid contamination of the open wound.

The pressure of nitrous oxide will increase the size of air embolus as it replaces nitrogen in the air bubbles (Munson1971) and should be discontinued immediately in favour of 100% oxygen. This may be a strong argument for abandoning nitrous oxide altogether in the sitting position and for the routine use of air/oxygen mixtures for ventilation.

It has been traditional to advocate that a patient should be placed in the left lateral position following an air embolus to prevent air entering the pulmonary artery (Hamby & Terry 1952). However, Leivers et al (1971) point out that this advice is based on a false assumption. The anatomy of the heart in man is such that the right lateral position is more appropriate in positioning the foam that forms in the right ventricle away from the pulmonary artery outflow tract. Although attractive in theory, in practice the adoption of the lateral position from sitting in a patient with cardiac arrest is difficult, time-consuming, of little practical value, and must greatly increase the chance of contaminating the wound.

Paradoxical air embolus

Paradoxical air embolus is a potential further complication of venous air embolus in the presence of a patent foramen ovale where the right atrial pressure is higher than the left atrial pressure. Matjasko et al (1985) report an incidence of 2.3% of patients that experienced venous air embolus or 0.5% of all patients in his series.

Once the air has entered the left side of the heart it can cause serious damage to the heart through the coronary circulation or to the brain through the cerebral circulation.

Although, in theory, the efforts to prevent venous air embolus through increased venous pressure may make paradoxical air embolus more likely, Zasslow et al (1988) have shown that PEEP does not increase the gradient between right and left atrium in a series of 20 patients. Prevention is best achieved: by an attempt at preoperative diagnosis of a right–to–left shunt by contrast echocardiography in the patient in which the sitting-up position is to be used; and the frequent monitoring of pulmonary artery wedge pressure in all patients, to be sure of early detection of a rise in right atrial pressure above that of the left.

Summary

The mortality and morbidity of the sitting position is remarkably low in the work quoted in this text. This is probably due to the high measure of vigilance brought to such a case by the anaesthetist, a good understanding of the physiology of air embolus and the battery of sophisticated monitoring devices used. Ingram (1987) is of the opinion that the risk of the sitting position is acceptable in otherwise fit patients, if the surgeon feels it is necessary to facilitate the operation and all the evidence would support this view.

Changes in position during anaesthesia

Ramsay et al (1976) described measurements of blood pressure, CVP, heart rate and blood gases that occurred following rapid changes in posture in patients anaesthetized and strapped into an isocentric chair for pneumoencephalography. Despite movements from supine, to sitting, to prone and back to supine, no cardiovascular or respiratory changes attributable to alteration of position could be detected. In this series all the patients were normovolaemic and it is likely that changes in position that occur at the end of an operation might cause hypotension in hypovolaemic patients.

REFERENCES

Benumof J L 1979 Mechanism of decreased blood flow to the atelectatic lung. J Appl Physiol 46: 1047–1048

Benumof J L 1982 One-lung ventilation: which lung should be PEEPed? Anesthesiology 56: 161–163

Benumof J L 1983 Physiology of the open chest and one-lung ventilation. In: Kaplan J A (ed) Thoracic anaesthesia, 1st edn. Churchill Livingstone, New York, ch 8, p 287–316

Benumof J 1988 Anaesthesia for one-lung ventilation Anesthesiology 69: 631

Benzon H T, Toleikis J R, Meagher L L, Shapiro B A, Ts'ao C, Avram M J 1988 Changes in venous blood lactate, venous blood gases and somatosensory evoked potentials after tourniquet application. Anesthesiology 69: 677–682

Besag F M C, Singh M P, Whitelaw A G L 1984 Surgery of the ill, extremely low birth weight infant: should transfer to the operating theatre be avoided? Acta Paediatr Scand 73: 594–595

Bethune R W M, Brechner V L 1968 Detection of venous air embolism by carbon dioxide monitoring. Anesthesiology 29: 178

Black S, Ockert D B, Oliver W C, Cucchiara R F 1988 Outcome following posterior fossa craniectomy in patients in the sitting or horizontal positions. Anesthesiology 69: 49–56

Bonnet F, Diallo A, Saada M, Belon M, Guilbaud M, Boico O 1989 Prevention of tourniquet pain by spinal isobaric bupivacaine with clonidine. Br J Anaesth 63: 93–96

Bowdle T A, Artru A A 1988 Positioning the air aspiration pulmonary artery catheter introducer sheath by intravascular electrocardiography. Anesthesiology 69: 276–279

Brodrick P M 1987 The sitting position: monitoring diagnosis and treatment of air embolism. In: Jewkes D A (ed) Baillière's clinical anaesthesiology. Anaesthesia for neurosurgery 1(2): Baillière Tindall, London, Ch 10, p 419–440

Brodrick P M, Ingram G S 1988 The antigravity suit in neurosurgery: cardiovascular response in seated neurosurgical patients. Anaesthesia 43: 762–765

Brown D R, Kafer E R, Roberson V O, Wilcox B R, Murray G F 1977 Improved oxygenation during thoractomy with selective PEEP to the lower lung. Anesth Analg 56: 26–31

Bruner J M 1970 Time pressure and temperature factors in the safe use of the tourniquet. Hand 2: 39–42

Buckland R W, Manners J M 1976 Venous air embolism during neurosurgery: a comparison of various methods of detection in man. Anaesthesia 31: 633–643

Burchell G Stack G 1973 Exsanguination of the arm and hand. Hand 5: 124–126

Campkin T V 1981 Posture and ventilation during posterior fossa and cervical operations: current practice in the United Kingdom. Br J Anaesth 53: 881–884

Capan L M, Turndof H, Chandrakant P, Ramanathan S, Acinapura A, Chalon J 1980 Optimization of arterial oxygenation during one-lung anaesthesia. Anesth Analg 59: 847–851

Conaty K R, Klemm M S 1989 Severe increase of intracranial pressure after deflation of a pneumatic tourniquet. Anesthesiology 71: 294–295

Coonan J C, Hope C E 1983 Cardio-respiratory effects of change of body position. Can Anaesth Soc J 30: 424–437

Crawford J S, Burton M, Davies P 1972 Time and lateral tilt at Caesarean section. Br J Anaesth 44: 477–484

Cushing H 1904 Pneumatic tourniquets with special reference to their use in craniotomies. The Medical News 84: 577–580

Davies H, Kitchman R, Gordon I, Helms P 1985 Regional ventilation in infancy: reversal of adult pattern. N Engl J Med 313: 1626–1628

Denlinger J K, Kallos T, Marshall B E 1972 Pulmonary blood flow in man anaesthetized in the lateral position. Anesth Analg 51: 260–263

Dickson M, White H, Kinney W, Kambam J R 1989 Effect of tourniquet extremity deflation on end tidal $P\text{CO}_2$ values. Anesth Analg 68: S71

Dilworth N M 1973 The importance of changes in body temperature in paediatric surgery and anaesthesia. Anaesth Intensive Care 1: 480–485

Doolan L A, O'Brien J F 1985 Safe intubation in cervical spine injury. Anaesth Intensive Care 13: 319–324

Edmonds-Seal J, Maroon J C 1969 Air embolism diagnosed with ultrasound. Anaesthesia 24: 438–440

Eldridge P R, Williams S 1989 Effect of limb tourniquet on cerebral perfusion pressure in a head injured patient. Anaesthesia 44: 973–974

English J B, Westenskow D, Hodges M R, Stanley T H 1978 Comparison of venous air embolism monitoring methods in supine dogs. Anesthesiology 48: 425–429

Fletcher I R, Healey T E J 1983 The arterial tourniquet. Ann R Coll Surg Engl 65: 409–417

Friesen R H, McIlvaine W B 1989 Basic techniques of paediatric anaesthesia. In: Sumner E, Hatch D J (eds) Textbook of paediatric anaesthesia, 1st edn. Baillière Tindall, London, ch 6, p 113–149

Goudsouzian N G, Morris R H, Ryan J F 1973 The effects of a warming blanket on the maintenance of body temperature in anaesthetized infants and children. Anesthesiology 39: 351–353
Gregory G A 1989 Induction of anaesthesia. In: Gregory G A (ed) Paediatric anaesthesia, vol 1, 2nd edn. Churchill Livingstone, New York, ch 16, p 539–560
Hamby W B, Terry R N 1952 Air embolism in operations done in the sitting position: a report of 5 cases and one of rescue by a simple maneuver. Surgery 31: 212–215
Hatch D J 1985 Paediatric anaesthetic equipment. Br J Anaesth 57: 672–684
Hemmer D, Tai-Shoin Lee, Wright B D 1982 Intubation of a child with cervical spine injury with the aid of a fibreoptic bronchoscope. Anaesth Intensive Care 10: 163–165
Hewer A J H, Logue V 1962 Methods of increasing the safety of neuroanaesthesia in the sitting position. Anaesthesia 17: 476–481
Hewer C L 1953 Maintenance of the Trendelenburg position by skin friction. Lancet 1: 522–524
Hey E N, O'Connell B 1970 Oxygen consumption and heat balance in the cot nursed baby. Arch Dis Child 45: 335–343
Hey E N, Katz G 1970 The optimum thermal environment for naked babies. Arch Dis Child 45: 328–334
Hovagim A R, Backus W W, Manecke G, Lagasse R, Sidhu U, Poppers P J 1989 Pulse oximetry and patient positioning: a report of eight cases. Anesthesiology 71: 454–456
Ingram S 1987 Posterior fossa surgery: patient position and mode of ventilation. In: Jewkes D A (ed) Baillère's clinical anaesthesiology. Anaesthesia for Neurosurgery 1(2): Baillière Tindall, London, Ch 9, p 405–417
James I, Wark H 1982 Airway management during anaesthesia in patients with epidermolysis bullosa dystrophica. Anesthesiology 56: 323–326
Katz J A, Laverne R G, Fairley H B, Thomas A N 1982 Pulmonary oxygen exchange during endobronchial anaesthesia: effect of tidal volume and PEEP. Anesthesiology 56: 164–171
Katz J, Mayhew J F 1985 Air embolism in the achondroplastic dwarf. Anesthesiology 63: 205–207
Kerr J H, Smith A C, Prys Roberts C, Meloche R 1973 Observations during endobronchial anaesthesia. I. Ventilation and carbon dioxide clearance. Br J Anaesth 45: 159–167
Kerr J H, Smith A C, Prys Roberts C, Meloche R, Foëx P 1974 Observations during endobronchial anaesthesia. II. Oxygenation. Br J Anaesth 46: 84–92
Khanam T, Branthwaite M A 1973a Arterial oxygenation during one-lung anaesthesia. 1. A study in man. Anaesthesia 28: 132–138
Khanam T, Branthwaite M A 1973b Arterial oxygenation during one-lung anaesthesia. 2. Anaesthesia 28: 280–290
Larsen V T, Hommelgaard P 1987 Pneumatic tourniquet paralysis following intravenous regional analgesia. Anaesthesia 42: 526–528
Larsson A, Jonmarker C, Lindahl S G E, Werner O 1989 Lung function in the supine and lateral decubitus positions in anaesthetized infants and children. Br J Anaesth 62: 378–384
Lee D S, Litchmann M W, Weintraub H D 1981 Effect of PEEP on air embolism during sitting neurosurgical procedures. Anesth Analg 60: 262
Leivers D, Spilsbury R A, Young J V I 1971 Air embolism during neurosurgery in the sitting position. Br J Anaesth 43: 84–90
Libman R H 1981 Anaesthetic considerations for the patient with osteogenesis imperfecta. Clin Orthop Relat Res 159: 123–125
Lincoln R J, Sawyer H P 1961 Complications related to body position during surgical procedures. Anesthesiology 22: 800–809
Lowrie A, Jones M J, Eastley R J 1989 Effect of a eutectic mixture of local anaesthetic agents (EMLA) on tourniquet pain in volunteers. Br J Anaesth 63: 751–753
Lynn A M, Fischer T, Brandford H G, Pendergrass T W 1986 Systemic responses to tourniquet release in children. Anesth Analg 65: 865–872
Martin R W, Colley P S 1983 Evaluation of transoesophageal Doppler detection of air embolism in dogs. Anesthesiology 58: 117–123
Matjasko J, Petrozza P, Cohen M, Steinberg P 1985 Anesthesia and surgery in the seated position: analysis of 554 cases. Neurosurgery 17: 695–702
McComish P B, Thompson D E A 1968 Respiratory disturbances in air embolism. Anaesthesia 23: 259–263
Millar R A 1972 Neurological anaesthesia in the sitting position. Br J Anaesth 44: 495–505
Munson E S 1971 Effect of nitrous oxide on the pulmonary circulation during venous air embolism. Anesth Analg Cur Res 50: 785–793
Munson E S, Paul W L, Perry J C, De Padua C B, Rhoton A L 1975 Early detection of venous air embolism using a Swan Ganz catheter. Anesthesiology 42: 223–226
Noel T A 1989 Air embolism removal from both pulmonary artery and right atrium during sitting craniotomy using a new catheter: report of case. Anesthesiology 70: 709–710
Rampton A J, Kelly D A, Shanahan E C, Ingram G S 1984 Occurrence of malignant hyperpyrexia in a patient with osteogenesis imperfecta. Br J Anaesth 56: 1443–1446
Ramsay M A E, Colvin M P, Taylor T H, Gil-Rodriguez J A, Morris J L, Wylie I G 1976 Cardiorespiratory changes during pneumoencephalography. Anaesthesia 31: 1179–1185
Relton J E S, Hall J E 1967 An operation frame for spinal fusion. J Bone Joint Surg 49: 327–332
Rheder K, Wenthe F M, Sessler A D 1973 Function of each lung during mechanical ventilation with ZEEP and with PEEP in man anaesthetised with thiopentameperidine. Anesthesiology 39: 597–606
Rowe M I, Weinberg G, Andrews W 1983 Reduction of neonatal heat loss by an insulated head cover. J Pediatr Surg 18: 909–913
Salathé M, Jöhr M 1989 Unsuspected cervical fractures: a common problem in ankylosing spondylitis. Anesthesiology 70: 869–870
Sale J P 1984 Prevention of air embolism during sitting neurosurgery. Anaesthesia 39: 795–799
Scott D B, Lees M M, Taylor S H 1966 Some respiratory effects of the Trendelenburg position during anaesthesia. Br J Anaesth 38: 174–178
Scott D B, Slawson K B 1968 Respiratory effects of prolonged Trendelenburg position. Br J Anaesth 40: 103–107
Shaw Wilgis E F 1971 Observations on the effects of tourniquet ischaemia. J Bone Joint Surg 53: 1343–1346
Smith G B, Shribman A J 1984 Anaesthesia and severe skin disease. Anaesthesia 39: 443–455

Solanki D R 1987 Epidural fentanyl for relief of lower extremity tourniquet pain in orthopaedic surgery. Anesth Analg 66: S161
Standefer M, Bay J W, Trusso R 1984 The sitting position in neurosurgery: a retrospective analysis of 488 cases. Neurosurgery 14: 649–658
Stone J G, Khambatta H J 1978 Pulmonary shunts in the prone position. Anaesthesia 33: 512–517
Stothers J K 1981 Heat insulation and heat loss in the new born. Arch Dis Child 56: 530–534
Swerdlow B N, Brodsky J B, Butcher M D 1988 Placement of a morbidly obese patient in the prone position. Anesthesiology 68: 657–658
Torda T A, McCulloch C H, O'Brien H D, Wright J S, Horton D A 1974 Pulmonary venous admixture during one-lung anaesthesia. Anaesthesia 29: 272–279
Toung T J K, Alano J, Nagel E L 1980 Effects of MAST suit on central venous pressure in the siting position. Anesthesiology 53: S188
Vale R J 1973 Normothermia: its place in operative and post-operative care. Anaesthesia 28: 241–245
Watson C B 1987 Fibreoptic bronchoscopy in thoracic anaesthesia. In: Gothard J W W (ed) Baillière's clinical anaesthesiology 1: No 1 Thoracic Anaesthesia Baillière Tindall, London, ch 3, 33–60
West J B 1970 Inequality of blood flow and ventilation in the normal lung. In: Ventilation/blood flow and gas exchange, 2nd edn. Blackwell Scientific, Oxford, ch 2
Yamashita M 1988 Modified anesthetic screen for pediatric surgery. Anesthesiology 69: 636–637
Young D A, Hardwick P B 1968 Anaesthesia for epidermolysis bullosa dystrophia. Anaesthesia 23: 264–267
Zasslow M A, Pearl R G, Larson P, Silverberg G, Shuer L F 1988 PEEP does not affect left atrial-right atrial pressure difference in neurosurgical patients. Anesthesiology 68: 760–763

35

Nerve injury

J. Payan

INTRODUCTION

The subject of this chapter is the injury to peripheral nerve which occurs as a consequence of anaesthesia but is not a direct result of anaesthetic or surgical technique. Such injury occurs when those upon whom the unconscious patient must rely for protection of his nerves are not aware of the danger or alert enough to prevent it.

In attempting a rational approach to prevention, this chapter takes into account the pathological changes to which nerves are subject, the factors that predispose to injury and the mechanisms that bring it about. Attention has also been paid to the role of electromyography, which is indispensable in prognosis.

INCIDENCE

There are two major retrospective studies in the literature. Parks (1973) recorded that 72 out of 50 000 patients operated on at the Colorado General Hospital between 1957 and 1969 developed postoperative peripheral nerve complications, of which 23 were lesions of the brachial plexus after open-heart surgery. Since we now know that splitting the sternum is itself liable to stretch the brachial plexus (p. 566), this leaves only one adverse consequence of anaesthesia per 1000 operations. I believe this figure to be an underestimate, although it agrees exactly with Dhunér's (1950) finding of 31 peripheral nerve palsies following 30 000 operations at the Karolinska Institute between 1940 and 1945.

Kroll et al (1990) analysed the American Society of Anaesthesiologists Closed Claims Study database and found that 227 out of 1541 claims (15%) were for anaesthesia-related nerve injury. Injury to the ulnar nerve was the most common and represented one third of all injuries. Brachial plexus injury had an incidence of 23% and lumbosacral roots 16%.

A continuing prospective study is needed wherever surgery is practised. This would not only give a truer incidence, but would also result in greater preventive efforts and provide early warning of which personnel and procedures were mainly at fault.

PATHOLOGY

Nearly all peripheral nerve lesions occurring as a consequence of anaesthesia are due to compression or stretching brought about in ways to be discussed. In a very few cases, intravenous or intramuscular injection results in needle trauma or chemical irritation. Excellent line drawings of some of the ways in which nerves can be damaged are provided by Britt & Gordon (1964) and Dornette (1986).

It has long been known that paresis lasting days or weeks may follow nerve compression, as in 'Saturday night palsy' but the nature of the pathological change causing block of conduction did not begin to be appreciated until Seddon (1943) proposed that this type of lesion be called 'neurapraxia', implying that there was no axonal degeneration. Denny-Brown & Brenner (1944) showed that the explanation lay in loss of myelin at the site of compression. This change, now referred to as segmental demyelination, was also shown to be responsible for the effects of stretching.

Segmental demyelination was, until quite recently, thought to be due to ischaemia, by mistaken analogy with the rapidly reversible form of conduction block that occurs when a limb 'goes to sleep'. There is now good evidence that Saturday night palsy, tourniquet paralysis and, by inference, many of the lesions suffered by anaesthetized patients are due to distortion and subsequent degeneration of myelin where a localized compressive force applied to the nerve has set up a steep pressure gradient. Thus, in the case of experimental tourniquet paralysis, there is demyelination at the edges of the cuff but not between (Ochoa et al 1972).

In most patients with acute nerve lesions sustained during sleep, intoxication or anaesthesia, remyelination leads to complete clinical recovery in 6–8 weeks, but there are a few in whom improvement only begins after 2 or 3 months, taking several more months to become complete. Such a patient was that described by Trojaborg (1977a) who took 13 months to recover fully from tourniquet paralysis caused by an Esmarch bandage. Such delays may occur when an unusually long segment of nerve has been demyelinated, or perhaps because intramyelin oedema has interfered with the normal processes of repair (Ochoa et al 1972). Severe compression may also result in an element of Wallerian degeneration (Trojaborg 1977a), which can never be excluded with certainty in even the mildest case, but is generally found to be important only where secondary ischaemia has resulted from obliteration of vasa nervorum by a rise in tissue pressure. This may be seen when a low pressure has acted for a long time, as when patients are found drugged or comatose, and it is therefore not strictly relevant to a discussion of the effects of anaesthesia. The best reviews of the subject of acute nerve compression are by Gilliatt (for example 1981), who with his colleagues was responsible for most of our knowledge in this field.

PROGNOSIS AND THE ROLE OF ELECTROMYOGRAPHY

The question of prognosis is of great interest to all concerned. It depends above all on the pathology of the lesion, and this can be determined only by neurophysiological study. In brief, the electromyographer must discover whether nerve fibres supplying weak or paralysed muscles are simply not conducting, or whether they have degenerated. In the first case he must determine the degree of block, in the second the approximate proportion of surviving fibres. In the first few days it is not possible to make the distinction, but thereafter the finding of normal muscle and nerve responses when stimulating and recording distal to the lesion must mean that most, if not all, fibres have survived, and that the clinical picture is due to a localized failure of the nerve to conduct. The importance of arriving at this conclusion is difficult to exaggerate, since spontaneous recovery from even severe conduction block can be confidently expected to occur in due course.

Further reference to the help to be expected from electromyography will be made in connection with lesions of specific nerves.

PREDISPOSING CAUSES

When a patient who has just had a general anaesthetic is found to have a peripheral nerve lesion, the first questions to be asked should be whether the affected nerve was normal before the anaesthetic was given, and whether there was a general condition that rendered individual nerves more vulnerable.

Local predisposing causes

Such superficial nerves as the ulnar and the common peroneal are relatively unprotected in those who are naturally thin, or whose illness has caused them to lose weight. Many apparently normal subjects, moreover, can be shown by neurophysiological means to have subclinical lesions due to an habitual or occupational posture such as sitting with the legs crossed, compressing the common peroneal nerve, or holding the telephone receiver for long periods with the elbow in full flexion, stretching the ulnar. When a subclinical lesion is found in the absence of an obvious postural factor it is usually assumed that the anatomical course of the nerve is in some way marginally unfavourable to it, and that in either case a stable balance is being preserved between the effects of daily wear-and-tear and the normal processes of repair. A brief episode of otherwise innocuous stress may then exceed the lowered tolerance of the nerve and result in a clinical lesion.

Specific local anatomical peculiarities that predispose to peripheral nerve injury under anaesthesia will be referred to when the relevant nerve at risk is being considered.

General predisposing causes

A very important factor predisposing to focal peripheral nerve damage is the presence of a generalized polyneuropathy (Gilliatt & Harrison 1984). Thus, not only are conditions such as carpal tunnel compression of the median nerve and ulnar nerve entrapment at the elbow more common in diabetic patients than in the general population, but the occurrence of such a lesion may be the first sign of a polyneuropathy, indeed of the disease responsible for the polyneuropathy. There is also a rare inherited condition of nerves that renders them unduly susceptible to external pressure (Behse et al 1972).

Hypothermia for cardiac operations has been held responsible for peripheral nerve palsies (Swan et al 1955) and it is reasonable to assume that in any condition of general physiological disturbance, such as dehydration or hypoxia the peripheral nerves, in common with other tissues, will be less resistant to some forms of stress.

The lessons for the anaesthetist are clear: he should satisfy himself that there is no clinical evidence of a mononeuropathy or polyneuropathy before operation, take even greater care than usual to protect the nerves if either is present, and suspect an underlying disorder if his patient develops a peripheral nerve lesion.

RECOGNITION OF THE LESION

In the immediate postoperative period it may not be obvious that peripheral nerve injury has occurred. Even when inability or reluctance to move has been overcome, the patient may be unsure of, or unable to communicate precisely, what disturbs him. There may be pain from various sources, paraesthesiae, numbness or weakness, and if an affected limb is being, or has been, used for intravenous infusion, he may believe this to be the cause. At this early stage reluctance to complain of something seemingly trivial can delay recognition that a complication has arisen. After a few days, however, competent clinical examination (if necessary with the aid of a manual such as that published by HMSO), should leave no doubt as to which nerve is involved and how severe is the deficit. The precise level and extent of a brachial plexus traction injury may be more difficult to ascertain. The findings must be recorded most carefully, quantitating weakness according to the MRC scale and mapping sensory loss.

LESIONS OF SPECIFIC NERVES

Brachial plexus

The first report of a brachial plexus injury associated with general anaesthesia appeared in 1894 (Büdinger). In a valuable paper, Trojaborg (1977b) has reviewed the subsequent literature and analysed 50 lesions drawn from it with regard to distribution, degree of severity and rate of recovery. He found that the whole plexus had been involved in 36, of whom 24 had suffered a complete palsy. Lesions were confined to the upper trunk in nine, to the lower in three, and in a rare instances to a single cord. Bilateral damage was sometimes present. Complete recovery had taken less than 5 months in 29, more than 5 months in 14, and had remained incomplete in three.

Dhunér (1950) reported that the shortest period in the operating theatre after which brachial plexus palsy had occurred was 40 min. Sunderland (1968) has reminded us that, although such palsies are usually referred to as 'postoperative', the damage is done on the operating table. The relaxation of muscles under general anaesthesia allows joints to be put in extreme positions for periods beyond the tolerance of nerve, and it is reasonable to suppose (Wylie & Churchill-Davidson 1972) that the advent of relaxant drugs has increased the risk. Anatomical variation at the thoracic outlet, in particular the presence of an extra rib on the seventh cervical vertebra, or a band running from its transverse process to the first rib (Gilliatt & Harrison 1984), may provide a local predisposing cause.

Mechanisms of injury

In most instances of brachial plexus injury occurring under anaesthesia a combination of stretching and compression is brought about in one of the following ways:

1. When the arm is in any extreme position, but particularly when it is abducted and externally rotated, with elbow extended and forearm supinated. This gives access to the axilla, makes arm veins available and accommodates surgeon, assistant or bystander, who may unintentionally increase the displacement of the limb. Sunderland paints a detailed picture of the anatomical consequences of this position. The head of the humerus comes forward from the glenoid fossa so that the cords of the plexus are bowed or stretched across it and the trunks are compressed in the reduced space between clavicle and first rib. Displacement of the humeral head will be even greater if:
   - the arm is abducted beyond a right angle and forced posteriorly
   - the weight of the patient lying on his back fixes the scapula and prevents its rotation from contributing to abduction of the arm
   - the arm drops away from the side of the body
   - the body is raised still higher by means of a gall-bladder rest. The latter is said (Kiloh 1950) to stretch the cords of the plexus under the tendinous attachment of pectoralis minor to the coracoid process.

   Other positions unfavourable to the plexus are suspension of the arm from a bar when the patient is in the lateral position, and extreme abduction of the arms above the head with the patient supine.
2. When the patient is in the Trendelenberg position and is being prevented from slipping by:
   - wristlets which pull on the arms and stretch the upper plexus
   - shoulder braces which are inadequately or badly positioned. If too medial they compress the plexus between clavicle and first rib; if too lateral they force the shoulders down, dragging on the plexus. In either case the ill-effect will be compounded by abduction of the arm.
3. When the neck is extended and flexed to the opposite side.

Diagnosis and prognosis

Clinical examination will indicate whether the palsy is complete and, if not, which part of the plexus has been affected. The lesion of the lower plexus caused by splitting the sternum will be considered later with ulnar lesions, with which it is more often confused. The electromyographer may enable the extent and level of damage to be more precisely known, but his usefulness lies mainly in the assessment of prognosis. The best example of this is to be found in the description by Trojaborg (1977b) of a 50-year-old housewife who awoke from a 3½ hour operation for lumbar disc with a completely paralysed and analgesic left arm and a weak right arm. The latter had virtually recovered within a week, but after a month there was still paralysis of the whole left upper limb, except for a flicker of movement in small hand muscles. Electromyography at this time showed that, while hardly any motor units could be voluntarily activated, stimulation of motor fibres in the axilla gave normal muscle responses. Sensory function was also severely disturbed, and yet normal sensory responses were picked up in the axilla on stimulating the radial and musculocutaneous nerves. The importance of these findings was that, even in the presence of such severe disability, it would have been justifiable to reassure the patient that full recovery was almost certain to occur in due course. In the event, clinical and neurophysiological recovery was complete 4 months after injury. Trojaborg points out that, in general, sensory function recovers faster than motor, and that muscles innervated by lower cervical roots tend to recover before those supplied through the upper roots, particularly C5 and 6.

Prevention

This flows from a consideration of the mechanisms of injury. A survey of texts, in particular those of Wylie & Churchill-Davidson (1972), Atkinson et al (1977) and Martin (1978), suggests that the following measures would meet the requirements of most experienced anaesthetists:

1. Support in the Trendelenberg position should be achieved where possible by means of the Hewer or other non-slip mattress (Hewer 1953). Otherwise, well-padded shoulder braces should be placed at the acromion processes. Wristlets should not be used.
2. Abduction of the arm on a board should be avoided where possible. When the use of a board is unavoidable it should be built up to prevent backward displacement of the arm, fitted with a locking device to prevent abduction beyond a right angle, and maintained at a higher horizontal plane than the body.
3. Intravenous injections should be given with the arm at the patient's side or folded across the chest.
4. When the patient is prone his arms should be by his side.
5. When the patient is in the lateral decubitus position the head should be properly supported so that the cervical and thoracic portions of the vertebral column are kept in the same horizontal plane.

Ulnar nerve

Injury to the ulnar nerve after anaesthesia is more common, in my experience, than brachial plexus palsy, yet it has received comparatively little attention in the literature. De Léon (1901) reported a lesion that followed laparotomy under chloroform, and Gurdjian (1931) another after herniotomy, early suggestions of an association with abdominal surgery which has been confirmed by experience (Payan 1970, Miller & Camp 1979). Of the 31 patients reported by Dhunér (1950), eight had ulnar nerve lesions, one of which was caused by a mere ½ hour on the operating table. An alternative view of causation was held by Mumenthaler (1960) who, observing that the lesion in bedridden patients was nearly always on the side on which the bed-table stood, concluded that recumbency and the bearing of weight on the elbow were responsible, not narcosis or fixation of the limb during operation. The timing and severity of many postoperative ulnar lesions make this an implausible explanation. The importance of general predisposing conditions is illustrated by Jones' (1967) case of a 50-year-old man who complained of cramp in the hand 5 min after coming round from anaesthesia. A severe ulnar lesion developed in the course of a few days and diabetes was then diagnosed. The vulnerability of the nerve may be increased by its tendency to leave the cubital sulcus and ride up to, or even over, the tip of the medial epicondyle when the elbow is flexed, an anatomical peculiarity said to occur in 16% of the normal population (Childress 1956).

Mechanisms of injury

If the patient is supine and the elbow allowed to sag, the ulnar nerve is liable to be compressed between the medial epicondyle of the humerus and the edge of the operating table. To the weight of the arm may be added that of the surgeon or his assistant standing up against the table. Miller & Camp (1979) point out that pressure may be focused on a very small area of the nerve by the fibrous bridge which bounds the cubital tunnel (Feindel & Stratford 1958). Wadsworth & Williams's statement (1973) that pronation is much more dangerous than supination is supported by Aita's (1981) account of three patients who suffered ulnar palsies after lying supine for 13–48 h with the prone or semiprone arm taped to the side or to an armboard. Atkinson et al (1977) refer to reports of injury to the nerve occurring as a result of prolonged acute flexion of the elbow when the arm is placed in front of the chest. Finally, it seems possible that the nerve could receive a blow from the end of a pole thrust too vigorously up the lateral sleeve of the carrying sheet, or from a support for the opposite arm pushed under the patient's body.

Diagnosis

A lesion of the ulnar nerve is likely to be present if the patient complains of paraesthesiae, numbness or pain in the little finger, and on examination there is impairment of sensation over the volar surface of the last two phalanges. It is important to remember that sensory symptoms along the medial border of the forearm from the elbow downwards implicate the medial cutaneous nerve of the forearm and hence the lower fibres of the brachial plexus. The distinction from specifically ulnar involvement can be made if weakness of hand muscles includes those supplied by the median nerve. I have seen several patients referred after cardiac surgery with sensory and motor symptoms in the hand thought to be due to ulnar nerve damage. Electromyography has then revealed partial denervation of abductor pollicis brevis, suggesting that the medial cord of the plexus has been stretched in the act of splitting the sternum (Vander Salm et al 1980). Such a discovery does not, of course, exclude coincident ulnar damage at the elbow, but this can be identified only by nerve conduction studies.

Prognosis

Mild, exclusively sensory symptoms will usually disappear after a few days or weeks provided that unnecessary, prolonged or repetitive elbow flexion be avoided. The prognosis for motor function depends on the pathological nature of the lesion at the elbow. If stimulation of the nerve below the elbow gives a normal or nearly normal muscle response, even the weakest hand will recover fully, as in the well-documented patient (Harrison 1976) whose paralysed muscles took 20 weeks to recover completely.

Unfortunately, in contrast to the brachial plexus lesions discussed above, ulnar nerve compression during an operation can result in lesions of quite remarkable severity in which axonal degeneration is predominant and from which recovery is very slow and incomplete (Miller & Camp 1979). When it has been established that such a lesion is present, and that neither clinical nor neurophysiological improvement is taking place at the hoped-for rate, or indeed at all, the question arises as to whether surgical exploration should be performed at the presumed level of damage. In principle there is no reason for this unless it is believed that the nerve was compromised even before the episode of compression, and in practice the results of surgery for this type of lesion are not demonstrably better than those of careful conservative management (Payan 1970, Miller & Camp 1979).

Prevention

The severity and permanence of many postoperative lesions of the ulnar nerve make it imperative that every precaution be taken to prevent their occurrence. The arm should be kept on the operating table, preferably supine, and applied to the side of the body by means of a draw sheet extending to well above the elbow. If it is necessary to have the arm on a board there should be sufficient padding. A padded shield similar to that used to prevent bedsores on the heel has been recommended in certain circumstances (Murphy & Deevers 1974).

Radial nerve

The lesion that occurs as a consequence of anaesthesia is very similar to that of 'Saturday night palsy', being in most cases due to compression of the nerve between the hard edge of the operating table or armboard and the shaft of the humerus. It is also said to occur when the uppermost arm of a patient in the lateral position is abducted to beyond 90° and suspended from a vertical screen support. Tourniquet palsy usually involves radial, median and ulnar nerves, but the radial may be affected alone (Eckhoff 1931).

The classical manifestation is wrist-drop, but in most cases brachioradialis is weak as well as wrist and long finger extensors. Triceps weakness implies high axillary damage and is rare in these circumstances. Sensory impairment may be present in the distribution of the radial nerve, of the posterior cutaneous nerve of the forearm, or of both. Such variations in the extent of motor and sensory involvement reflect mainly differences in the level of branching from the main trunk. The prognosis is almost invariably good, the only question being how long recovery will take. If normal motor and sensory responses are obtained when the electromyographer stimulates distal to the level of compression, recovery is likely within 6–8 weeks. To the extent that evidence of axonal degeneration can be demonstrated, the course will be longer, occasionally many months, rarely over a year. A useful indication is sometimes provided by comparison of radial nerve sensory action potentials at the two wrists. For the duration of severe weakness the wearing of a simple cock-up splint is recommended.

Sciatic nerve

The sciatic nerve is at risk if the patient is thin, the table hard and the operation long. The compressive force will be increased if the opposite buttock is raised, as in hip-pinning. In the lithotomy position, maximal external rotation of the flexed thigh may damage the nerve not only by stretching it (Burkhart & Daly 1966) but also, as in one remarkable case, by subjecting it to compression by a mass of heterotopic calcification (Reinstein & Eckholdt 1983).

In the most severe lesions there will be no voluntary movement below the knee, and hamstrings may also be affected. When the lesion is less severe, dorsiflexion of the foot is nearly always weaker than plantar flexion.If stimulation of the common peroneal and tibial nerves results in full movement at the ankle it may be taken that the lesion is one of demyelination, with a correspondingly good prognosis. Evidence of severe denervation is more than usually disturbing, because the time taken by axons to grow so far may be such that replacement of muscle by fibrous tissue has already taken place.

Common peroneal nerve

The common peroneal nerve is the most frequently damaged nerve in the lower limb. In a very early report, Pershing (1897) described a patient that took several months to recover from palsy due to compression of the nerve between the fibula and the operating table, a particular risk attached to the lateral position. The more usual cause is compression between fibula and lithotomy pole or stirrup, resulting in foot-drop and a variable patch of sensory impairment. Voluntary dorsiflexion is usually weaker than eversion but, even when both are absent, stimulation of the nerve just distal to the fibular head almost always results in full movement. It is necessary to wear a right-angled splint until remyelination reverses the conduction block and adequate voluntary movement returns.

Stretching of the last part of the deep branch of the nerve at the ankle, where it is called the anterior tibial, can occur because of forced plantar flexion in the prone position. It is prevented by supporting the ankles on a roll.

Less commonly injured nerves

Tibial nerve

The other main division of the sciatic nerve, the tibial nerve, can suffer compression in the popliteal fossa if the legs of a patient in the lithotomy position are supported by stirrups behind the knees. This will lead to temporary weakness of plantar flexion.

Femoral and obturator nerves

Klempner (1906) quoted by Sunderland (1968) described palsies of the femoral and obturator nerves, apparently due to acute angulation when the thighs were fully flexed upon the abdomen. When a patient is lying in bed after an abdominal operation the precise nature of weakness of thigh movements may be uncertain and the spinal anaesthetic blamed. I have delivered an anaesthetist from suspicion by showing that symmetrical weakness without denervation was present only in quadriceps. Inadvertent surgical retraction of the femoral nerves was responsible and recovery ensued.

Saphenous nerve

The saphenous nerve may be compressed between the medial condyle of the tibia and the lithotomy post or stirrup, causing sensory impairment over the medial calf (Slocum et al 1948).

Pudendal nerve

Loss of perineal sensation and faecal incontinence may result from pressure of the pudendal nerve against an inadequately padded perineal post (Lembcke 1947).

Lateral cutaneous nerve of the thigh

When the patient is lying prone with the pelvis supported on a hard pillow transient meralgia paraesthetica may follow as a result of pressure on the lateral cutaneous nerve of the thigh.

Supraorbital nerve

The supraorbital nerve may be compressed by a metal endotracheal connector or tight head harness, causing photophobia, numbness of the forehead and pain in the eye (Barron 1955).

Facial nerve

The anaesthetist's fingers may compress the facial nerve against the ascending ramus of the mandible when holding the jaw forward to maintain an airway (Fuller & Thomas 1956). The buccal branch is sometimes compressed by a head strap that is too tight (Conway 1978).

Long thoracic nerve of Bell

Sunderland (1968) states that paralysis of the long thoracic nerve of Bell has followed compression by an unpadded shoulder rest badly applied to a patient in the Trendelenberg position. Presumably transient winging of the scapula resulted.

INVESTIGATION OF NERVE DAMAGE: TECHNICAL CONSIDERATIONS

When a patient's symptoms include weakness, wasting, sensory impairment or paresthesiae it is usually desirable to supplement clinical examination by the study of electrical activity in nerve and muscle. This form of investigation is known as clinical electromyography and has its origin in eighteenth-century speculation and experiment concerning the nature of 'animal electricity'. It aims to detect, and distinguish between, disorders of anterior horn cell, root, plexus, peripheral nerve, neuromuscular junction and muscle, to determine their extent and severity and to relate neurophysiological abnormality to the clinical context in which it is found. It is rarely of value when clinical examination gives normal results, especially when the only complaint is of pain.

The electromyographer does two things. He puts needle electrodes into muscles to detect spontaneous activity and to observe the nature of voluntary motor unit potentials. By this means it is possible to demonstrate denervation, fall-out of motor units and changes in the structure and function of surviving motor units. Secondly he stimulates nerves with brief electric shocks, recording the responses evoked in sensory fibres, mixed nerve trunks and muscles. When nerve damage occurs during general anaesthesia the cause is almost always conduction block over a small segment of nerve, and the role of the electromyographer is to discover the location and severity of the lesion. Since such lesions are more likely to occur when there is an underlying and perhaps unsuspected polyneuropathy, no investigation is complete until the electromyographer has satisfied himself as to the state of other, apparently healthy nerves. Finally, serial investigation can become necessary when the expected clinical improvement fails to occur or is unduly protracted.

Spontaneous activity

When motor nerve fibres degenerate, the membrane properties of the muscle fibres they supply undergo changes that result after a few days or weeks in spontaneous activity called fibrillation. This cannot be seen through the skin. There is some evidence that severe focal demyelination, by cutting off the flow of normal impulses to muscle, can result in fibrillation even when axonal degeneration has not taken place. The prognosis is therefore not invariably rendered worse by the finding of fibrillation. A common mistake is to confuse fibrillation, which is pathological, with endplate activity, which occurs in all normal muscles.

Voluntary activity

A voluntary motor unit potential is the sum of action potentials from those muscle fibres belonging to the unit that happen to lie near the electrode tip. The reliable analysis of such properties as amplitude, duration, form and stability requires training and much experience. It is not for the occasional or self-taught performer.

Nerve conduction velocity

The principle of measurement can be illustrated by reference to the median nerve. A supramaximal stimulus (capable of exciting all underlying fibres) applied to the nerve at the wrist crease will be followed by a thenar muscle action potential after, say, 3 ms, an interval called the distal motor latency. If the nerve is now stimulated at the level of the elbow and the response follows after 7 ms, conduction from elbow to wrist has taken 4 ms and the conduction velocity, given a distance between the two points of 240 mm, will be 60 mm/ms, or 60 m/s. Slowing of conduction may be focal, as in the conduction block which is our principal concern in the present context, or general, as in polyneuropathy. The velocity in fast-conducting fibres is normally 50–70 m/s in the upper limb and 40–60 m/s in the lower limb. Maximum conduction velocity slows by about 2 m/s per degree celsius, so that conduction studies performed on a cold limb are valueless. Apparent slowing of maximum conduction velocity will occur when the disease process selectively affects the largest diameter, fast-conducting fibres.

Conduction block

As already discussed (p. 563), peripheral nerve lesions that occur under general anaesthesia are almost always due to compression or stretching causing focal demyelination. When this affects all the motor fibres supplying a given muscle or muscle group, complete paralysis will be the result. Lesser degrees of conduction block will result in proportionately less severe degrees of weakness. The detection of conduction block depends on comparison of the size and shape of evoked compound muscle action potentials when stimulating proximal and distal to the lesion. When there is complete block of conduction, stimulation distal to the site of the lesion will result in a normal evoked potential and in normal contraction of the muscle, which is usually evident. Stimulation proximal to the site of the lesion will result in neither an evoked potential nor a muscle contraction. When there is partial conduction block it will be possible to evoke a potential and a muscle contraction by stimulating proximal to the lesion, but it will be smaller than the potential evoked when stimulating distal to the lesion by a certain percentage. With recovery this percentage gradually declines. The point is illustrated by Figure 35.1 which shows that immediately after a period of compression of the ulnar nerve there was no certain response from hypothenar muscles when stimulating above the elbow. A year later it was possible to obtain such a response, though it was still significantly reduced by comparison with the potential obtained on stimulating at the wrist.

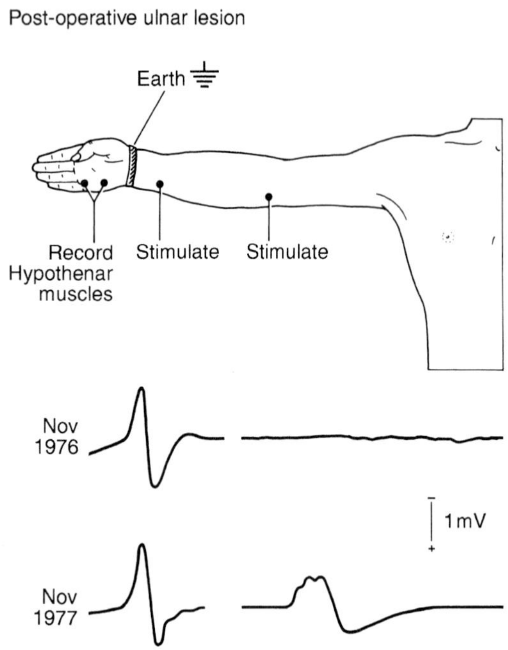

Fig. 35.1 Recovery of nerve transmission over a 12-month period following intraoperative ulnar nerve damage, using stimulating electrodes distal and proximal to the lesion.

Had there been an opportunity to re-examine the patient after a further year, there is little doubt that the proximally evoked potential would have returned to normal.

Several points have to be borne in mind. In the first place, even when the nerve is healthy a proximally evoked muscle action potential will be a little smaller than the distally evoked potential because of gradual dispersion of the volley of impulses as it passes down the nerve. Such a decrement should not normally exceed 10% in the case of the thenar muscles, for example. With surface electrodes over the extensor digitorum brevis, however, it can reach 20% when stimulating in the popliteal fossa. Second, the more severe a nerve lesion the more readily error arises. For example a very strong stimulus can fail to excite the nerve under consideration but spread to a neighbouring nerve and thus activate a muscle near the recording site. Strong stimulation of the median nerve in midarm can activate the ulnar nerve, causing adductor pollicis to contract, so that recording electrodes on the thenar eminence will appear to have picked up a response from a median-innervated muscle. Third, it is a general principle in studying nerve injuries that the more severe degrees of injury, in this context axonotmesis, cannot be identified with accuracy until at least 10 days after injury, that is when all fibres that are going to degenerate have done so. Unless such a period has elapsed, paralysis may incorrectly be attributed to neurapraxia alone. If significant axonotmesis has occurred the muscle action potential will be of reduced amplitude, or even absent, when stimulating distal to the lesion.

The foregoing discussion should leave no doubt in the reader's mind that, invaluable as clinical electromyography can be, the opportunities for acquiring erroneous and misleading data are manifold. The belief that a few lessons are sufficient to equip any normally intelligent person is oddly prevalent, occurring even in professors of neurology. It is mistaken.

CONCLUSION

For nearly a century the literature has contained reports of damage to the peripheral nerves of patients undergoing general anaesthesia. The anaesthetist has not always been entirely to blame: in some cases there has been a pre-existing lesion or a general increase in susceptibility to pressure and stretch; in others the damage has been done after the patient has left the theatre, especially in bed. It is nevertheless true, and regrettable, that such lesions can nearly always be prevented: witness their rarity after neurosurgery, when anaesthetist and surgeon pay meticulous attention to positioning the patient in expectation of many hours in the theatre.

It is clear that some positions, such as abduction of the arm, are particularly hazardous, and that the function of some nerves, notably the ulnar, can be permanently impaired. The likelihood of recovery can be assessed by the electromyographer, who is usually in the happy position of being able to reassure patient and doctor. That this is so must never allow complacency to take the place of vigilance.

REFERENCES

Aita J F 1981 Postoperative ulnar neuropathy. J Am Med Assoc 245: 2295

Atkinson R S, Rushman G B, Lee J A 1972 A synopsis of anaesthesia, 8th edn. John Wright, Bristol, p 829

Barron D W 1955 Supraorbital neurapraxia. Anaesthesia 10: 374

Behse F, Buchthal F, Carlsen F, Knappeis G G 1972 Hereditary neuropathy with liability to pressure palsies: electrophysiological and histopathological aspects. Brain 95: 777–794

Britt B A, Gordon R A 1964 Peripheral nerve injuries associated with anaesthesia. Can Anaesth Soc J 11: 514

Büdinger K 1894 Ueber Lähmungen nach Chloroformnarkosen. Arch Klin Chir 47: 121–145

Burkhart F L, Daly J W 1966 Sciatic and peroneal nerve injury: a complication of vaginal operations. Obstet Gynecol 28: 99

Childress H M 1956 Recurrent ulnar nerve dislocation at the elbow. J Bone Joint Surg 38A: 978–984

Conway C 1978 Neurological and ophthalmic complications of anaesthesia. In: Churchill-Davidson H C (ed) A practice of anaesthesia, 3rd edn. Lloyd-Luke, London, p 1021

De Léon 1901 Paralysie du nerf cubital et contracture consecutive. Main en pince. (quoted by Sunderland 1968)

Denny-Brown D, Brenner C 1944 Paralysis of nerve induced by direct pressure and by tourniquet. Arch Neurol Psychiatry 51: 1–26

Dhunér K-G 1950 Nerve injuries following operations: a survey of cases during a six-year period. Anesthesiology 11: 289–293

Dornette W H L 1986 Compression neuropathies: medical aspects and legal implications. Int Anesthesiol Clin 24: 201–209

Eckhoff N L 1931 Tourniquet paralysis. Lancet 3: 343–345

Feindel W, Stratford J 1958 The role of the cubital tunnel in tardy ulnar palsy. Can J Surg 1: 287–300

Fuller J E, Thomas D V 1956 Facial nerve paralysis after general anaesthesia. J Am Med Assoc 162: 645

Gilliatt R W 1981 Physical injury to peripheral nerves: physiologic and electrodiagnostic aspects. Mayo Clin Proc 56: 361–370

Gilliatt R W, Harrison M J G 1984 Nerve compression and entrapment. In: Asbury A K and Gilliatt R W (eds) Peripheral nerve disorders: a practical approach. Butterworth, London, ch 10, p 245, 255

Gurdjian E S 1931 Traumatic ulnar neuritis due to strapping of the elbow and the forearm to the operating table. J Am Med Assoc 96: 944 (quoted by Sunderland 1968)

Harrison M J G 1976 Pressure palsy of the ulnar nerve with prolonged conduction block. Neurol Neurosurg Psychiatry 39: 96–99

Hewer C L 1953 Latest pattern of non-slip mattress. Anaesthesia 8: 198

HMSO 1976 Aids to the examination of the peripheral nervous system. HMSO, London

Jones H D 1967 Ulnar nerve damage following general anaesthetic: a case possibly related to diabetes mellitus. Anaesthesia 22: 471–475

Kiloh L G 1950 Brachial plexus lesions after cholecystectomy. Lancet 258(1): 103–105

Klempner S 1906 Ueber Narkoselähmung des N Cruralis und obturatorius. 25: 107 (quoted by Sunderland 1968)

Kroll D A, Caplan R A, Posner K, Ward R J, Cheney F W 1990 Nerve injury associated with anaesthesia. Anesthesiology 73: 202–207

Lembcke W 1947 Rare nerve paralysis due to pressure while lying on an extension table: two cases. Chirurgie 17–18: 264–265

Martin J T 1978 Positioning in anaesthesia and surgery. Saunders, Philadelphia

Miller R G, Camp P E 1979 Postoperative ulnar neuropathy: J Am Med Assoc 242(15): 1636–1639

Mumenthaler M 1960 Die Ulnarislähmungen. Ueber 314 "nicht traumatische" eigene Beobachtungen. Schweiz Med Wochenschr 90: 815–820

Murphy J P, Deevers J C 1974 Prevention of post-surgical ulnar neuropathy. J Am Med Assoc 227: 1123–1124

Ochoa J, Fowler T J, Gilliatt R W 1972 Anatomical changes in peripheral nerves compressed by a pneumatic tourniquet. J Anat 113: 433–455

Parks B J 1973 Postoperative peripheral neuropathies. Surgery 74: 348

Payan J 1970 Anterior transposition of the ulnar nerve: an electrophysiological study. J Neurol Neurosurg Psychiatry 33: 157–165

Pershing 1897 (quoted by Sunderland 1968)

Reinstein L, Eckholdt J W 1983 Sciatic nerve compression by pre-existing heterotopic calcification. Arch Phys Med Rehabil 64(2): 65–68

Seddon H J 1943 Three types of nerve injury. Brain 66: 237–288

Slocum H C, O'Neal K C, Allen C R 1948 Neurovascular complications from malposition on the operating table. Surg Gynecol Obstet 86: 729

Sunderland S 1968 Nerves and nerve injuries. Churchill Livingstone, Edinburgh

Swan H, Virtue R W, Blount S G Jr, Kirchner L T 1955 Hypothermia in surgery. Ann Surg 142: 382

Trojaborg W 1977a Prolonged conduction block with axonal degeneration: an electrophysiological study. J Neurol Neurosurg Psychiatry 40: 50–57

Trojaborg W 1977b Electrophysiological findings in pressure palsy of the brachial plexus. J Neurol Neurosurg Psychiatry 40: 1160–1167

Vander Salm T J, Cereda J-M, Cutler B S 1980 Brachial plexus injury following median sternotomy. J Thor Cardiovasc Surg 80: 447–452

Wadsworth T G, Williams J R 1973 Cubital tunnel external compression syndrome. Br Med J 1: 662–666

Wylie W D, Churchill-Davidson H C 1972 A practice of anaesthesia, 3rd edn. Lloyd-Luke, London, p 1262

36

Day-case anaesthesia

G. Cooper

INTRODUCTION

Although day-case surgery has been performed efficiently and enthusiastically by a small number of surgeons since the beginning of this century, the recent drive for economic savings has led to greatly increased popularity. The actual savings are hard to quantify but appear to be in the region of 50–75% (Flanagan & Bascom 1981, Rockwell 1982, Burn 1983), and accrue because of the need for fewer staff, especially the saving of night staff. The benefits are not purely economic: the patient has less disruption to his life, a shorter wait for his operation, a greater likelihood of a convenient date for surgery and a lower risk of infection if the operating theatre is one used solely for elective minor procedures. Morale is increased when an efficient service is provided. The daytime working hours make it a popular job and hence nursing recruitment is of a high standard.

Where day-case work is performed in an autonomous unit the nursing staff devote all their attention to the day-stay patients without the distraction of sick patients that may require urgent care. As a result, day-unit nurses tend to be adept at discovering and sorting out the many minor problems that can occur with benefits in patient safety. Another advantage of the autonomous unit is that the medical staff are able to see the patients briefly immediately before surgery, which is not possible during a major operating list.

In order to be viable, a separate day-stay unit needs an adequate volume of suitable work (Davis 1973). Long waiting lists for hospital beds, a high demand for minor surgical procedures and the variable enthusiasm of individual surgeons make out-patient surgery more common in some areas. An autonomous unit does have the disadvantage that it is more difficult to admit the patient overnight if complications arise.

THE OUT-PATIENT APPOINTMENT

The key to safe and successful day-care surgery lies in the out-patient department. To maximize the use of theatre space and avoid wasting the patient's time it is vital that there is minimal chance of the operation being delayed or cancelled. This means taking extra care at the out-patient appointment to ensure that the patient and the procedure are appropriate for treatment as a day-case. The three main factors that determine this are:

- the type of operation
- the medical condition of the patient
- the social circumstance of the patient.

Type of operation

There is usually little doubt which operations are suitable. In general they should be of short duration, have little likelihood of postoperative complications and be unlikely to result in severe pain which would make postoperative analgesia difficult to achieve.

It is important that common sense is used when deciding which operations are suitable rather than adhering to a preordained list. Therapeutic abortion may be suitable in the early stages of pregnancy, but postoperative bleeding is a real risk at advanced gestation. The estimated gestation by dates needs to be confirmed by scan or vaginal examination, and only those in the first trimester booked as day-cases.

There is no doubt that the longer the duration of an operation the greater is the likelihood of postoperative complications. A reasonable upper limit from the point of view of the anaesthetic is 1 h.

Improved surgical technique has reduced the likelihood of immediate complications after cataract surgery, thus many surgeons discharge patients the same day provided the patient can be examined the following day (Editorial 1983).

Medical condition

Essentially patients need to be either completely healthy or only have mild disease that does not interfere with normal life (i.e. ASA I or II). It is wise to adhere to this principle because of the increased likelihood of complications from anaesthesia in patients that have serious systemic disease. There has been a recent move in the USA to include ASA III patients for day-care: we await evidence of the safety of this practice.

In the case of the well-controlled diabetic patient, if the operation is unlikely to produce a severe stress response or postoperative anorexia or vomiting, the intelligent patient is likely to benefit from managing his insulin requirements himself at home on the day of surgery. Conversely, there are potential hazards of hypoglycaemia or hyperglycaemia which would prejudice against day-case surgery in the patient unable to predict and respond to these problems. Bad management on the part of the patient or anaesthetist, even in those on oral therapy, can result in severe hypoglycaemia (Ainsworth & Wittman 1987).

Age itself is not a bar to day-case surgery, but concurrent illness is more frequent in elderly patients and the social circumstances are less often satisfactory. Children are frequently ideal candidates for day-case surgery because parents usually give their offspring even more care and attention than they would receive in hospital, and there is less psychological trauma for both parents and children.

Any coexisting disease must be detected before the patient is booked as a day case. As it is frequently impractical to perform a full clerking in out-patients, a questionnaire filled in by the patient before he sees the surgeon helps to suggest which patients might be suitable for consideration. An example is given in Figure 36.1. This form has the advantage of emphasizing the positive replies to individual questions, thus saving time in finding the relatively rare condition that might preclude treatment as a day-case (e.g. malignant hyperpyrexia, suxamethonium apnoea: see Question 4). Question 6 is a reminder to do a sickle test in those of black African extraction. Other useful screens at this stage are urinalysis, examination of the pulse and blood pressure measurement, the results of which could be added to the form. It is also valuable to take blood for a full blood count so that the results will be available on the day of surgery. Two surveys (Ogg 1976, Moxon & Jago 1987) have confirmed the usefulness of such questionnaires and show that about 40% of those accepted for day care have significant medical conditions.

Social circumstances

The safety of day-case surgery lies in the low likelihood of serious complications after going home, but also in ensuring that, in this unlikely event, help can be summoned. Thus it is essential that the patient will be in the company of a responsible adult, for both returning home and the first postoperative night. Provided this is explained in out-patients, many patients are prepared to make special arrangements to avoid unnecessary hospitalization. The need to be accompanied home and *not* to drive is highlighted by the report (Fahy 1987) of a non-epileptic that had a grand mal seizure in the car on the way home, 5 h after day-case surgery. Fortunately his

Name: Today's date is....................
Address: What is your age?.............. yrs
What is your approximate weight?....

1. Have you ever suffered from any of the following?
   - Heart trouble (e.g. angina, heart failure, murmurs etc)............... Yes ☐ No ☐
   - High blood pressure .... Yes ☐ No ☐
   - Breathing problems (e.g. asthma, bronchitis, pneumonia)............ Yes ☐ No ☐
   - Jaundice or liver disease .... Yes ☐ No ☐
   - Kidney disease .... Yes ☐ No ☐
   - Diabetes.. Yes ☐ No ☐
   - Thyroid disorder.. Yes ☐ No ☐
   - Bleeding tendency (apart from heavy periods)........................ Yes ☐ No ☐
   - Thrombosis (blood clots)... Yes ☐ No ☐
   - Severe arthritis (including neck and jaws).......................... Yes ☐ No ☐
   - Severe anxiety or depression....................................... Yes ☐ No ☐
   - Epilepsy, convulsions or blackouts .... Yes ☐ No ☐
   - Any other serious illness.. Yes ☐ No ☐

   Please give details.
2. Have you taken any medicine or tablets, used an inhaler or received any injections in the past 3 months?............................. Yes ☐ No ☐
   If YES, please give details.
3. Have you had an anaesthetic previously?.......................... Yes ☐ No ☐
   If YES, please give details of operations and approximate dates below:
4. To your knowledge, have you or your family had any problems connected with anaesthesia or operations?................................. Yes ☐ No ☐
   If YES, please give details.
5. Are you allergic to anything that you know of?..................... Yes ☐ No ☐
   If YES, please give details.
6. Are your parents of black African or eastern Mediterranean origin? ... Yes ☐ No ☐
   If YES, have you or any of your family had sickle cell disease?....... Yes ☐ No ☐
7. Do you smoke? If YES, how much?.................................... Yes ☐ No ☐
8. Do you drink alcohol? If YES, how much?........................... Yes ☐ No ☐

Questions 9–15 to be answered on arrival in day unit.

Fig. 36.1 Preoperative assessment questionnaire. Questions 1–8 can be answered in the outpatient clinic.

wife was driving. The presence of a telephone at home may also be relevant. The distance of home from hospital may also be important as a long journey may be impractical and uncomfortable. The patient's wishes should be borne in mind when booking for day care as a well-motivated patient is more likely to recover well.

INSTRUCTIONS TO THE PATIENT

Having decided that both the procedure and the patient are suitable, it is vital to stress to the patient that the process must be taken as seriously as an in-patient operation. It is preferable that the patient is given a definite date for operation in the near future, so that personal arrangements can be made. In addition, the medical condition is unlikely to have altered significantly, and the instructions given are less likely to be forgotten or mislaid.

An instruction sheet is invaluable to reinforce verbal explanations. An example is given in Figure 36.2. Note the use of bold face to emphasize the necessity for starving. The form

FIX IT QUICK HOSPITAL

It has been arranged for you to come into hospital to have your operation as a day case on .... 19... Follow these instructions for a safe and pleasant stay.

1. **Do not eat or drink** anything after 12 midnight the night before your operation.
2. Have a bath.
3. Bring a specimen of urine with your name on the bottle.
4. Arrive at the hospital between 8 and 8.30 a.m. Bring nightdress/pyjamas, washing things and a book to read, and your dressing gown.
5. For the 24 hours after your anaesthetic you will be advised not to drive, operate machinery, sign important papers or drink alcohol. Make arrangements to be collected by a responsible adult and to have a responsible adult at home for the night following surgery.
6. If, for any reason, you need to change the date of your operation, or if there is a change in your general health (e.g. a cold or sore throat) please telephone between 8 a.m. and 4 p.m. to take advice about rescheduling your operation.

Fig. 36.2 Instruction sheet to be given to the patient in the out-patient clinic.

can be suitably adjusted for an afternoon operation by allowing a light breakfast before 8 a.m. and a later time for arrival at hospital. The need for starving before operations expected to be performed under local anaesthesia is controversial. I am of the opinion that, in the interests of safety, *all* patients should be starved. There is always the possibility of toxicity of injected local anaesthetics causing convulsions, with an unguarded airway leading to inhalation of gastric contents. This implies that the need to starve is especially important when large doses of local anaesthetic are required (e.g. Bier's block, field blocks) and less important when only small doses are needed (e.g. ring block of a finger). However, if the block proves to be inadequate, local anaesthesia can be safely converted to general anaesthesia in the starved patient.

LETTER TO GENERAL PRACTITIONER

A letter sent to the general practitioner (GP), informing him of the nature of operation on his patient and the proposed date, forewarns him in case of possible complications. Any requests for wound dressing or removal of sutures can be communicated through the GP to the district nurse. It is also helpful for the GP to have all the instruction sheets available so that he knows what the patient has been warned about and can give further explanation if requested.

THE DAY OF OPERATION

Preoperative assessment

The major part of the preoperative assessment should be done at the out-patient booking appointment. On arrival in the day unit the nurses should analyse the urine brought by the patient, and measure the patient's temperature, pulse and blood pressure. The preoperative assessment sheet should be checked and the patient asked if there have been any changes since the out-patient appointment. The second part of the preoperative questionnaire (Fig. 36.3) should be completed. The patient should be undressed, prepared for theatre and, if appropriate, the operative site shaved.

The surgeon and the anaesthetist then make their assessments. The surgeon should check the operative site and side with the notes and the patient, and confirm the suitability for treatment as a day case. The surgeon then explains the nature of the operation and obtains signed consent.

9. What time did you last eat?.......................................
   What time did you last drink?....................................
   Have you arranged to be collected?.............................. Yes ☐ No ☐
10. Since you were seen in the outpatient clinic has your complaint changed?... Yes ☐ No ☐
11. Apart from minor coughs and colds, have you had any illnesses since you were seen in the outpatient department?................ Yes ☐ No ☐
    If YES, please give details:
12. Do you have a cold or sore throat at the moment?................. Yes ☐ No ☐
13. Are you bringing up phlegm from your chest at the moment?....... Yes ☐ No ☐
14. Do you suffer from shortness of breath or wheezing?.............. Yes ☐ No ☐
15. Do you have any false, crowned or loose teeth?................... Yes ☐ No ☐

For gynaecological patients only:

16. What was the date of your last period?..........................
17. What method of contraception are you currently using?

Fig. 36.3 Preoperative assessment questionnaire. Questions 9–17 (which would be found on the reverse of the single sheet) can be answered on arrival in the day unit. Questions 16 and 17 are for gynaecological patients only.

Any positive replies on the questionnaire filled in by the patient should be followed up by the anaesthetist. The results of any tests done in outpatients must be checked for abnormal values. The anaesthetist may also wish to discuss the pros and cons of local and general anaesthesia and enquire about previous experience with anaesthesia. This is also a suitable time to mention possible minor postoperative side effects (e.g. scoline pains, sore throat) which may trouble the patient after he has gone home. The anaesthetist should not be afraid to turn a patient away from day-care surgery if this is felt to be the safest course. Postponement may result from inadequate preparation, intercurrent illness (e.g. colds, fever, general malaise) or unsuitable selection. Safety is paramount.

ANAESTHETIC TECHNIQUE

Above all, day-case patients must receive the same quality of care as in-patients. The aim of a day-case anaesthetic is to provide adequate operating conditions with minimal complications and a swift recovery.

Premedication

Premedication is usually omitted for day-case surgery to avoid prolonged postoperative sedation and drowsiness. It may be helpful to administer an anticholinergic to minimize vagal responses to surgery and excessive salivation, but this can usually be administered intravenously on induction of anaesthesia.

The problem patient is the one that is so nervous that he will not consider treatment as an in-patient but nonetheless is terrified on arrival in the day unit. Temazepam (20 mg orally, 1 h preoperatively) can be very useful in this situation. Its short duration of action means that it does not appreciably impair recovery (Beechey et al 1981), especially as it may reduce intraoperative anaesthetic requirements. The longer-acting benzodiazepine, lorazepam, is not recommended because of prolonged postoperative dizziness (Loach & Fisher 1975). Just as for in-patients, the need for premedication must be judged for each case and sympathetic explanation of what is to happen is better than blind drug premedication. Premedicated patients should never be left alone, allowed to walk to theatre or climb onto trolleys and tables unaided.

Local anaesthesia

The advantage of local anaesthesia is a low incidence of postoperative complications such as nausea and vomiting. It may not always be appropriate, either because of the operative site or because of the patient's personality. Infiltration with local anaesthetic, in doses well below the toxic level, provides good operating conditions with minimal risk and excellent postoperative recovery. Nevertheless, local anaesthetics are not completely devoid of after effects and produce some central nervous impairment, certainly for a few hours (Korttila 1974).

There is continued debate about the suitability of epidural and spinal techniques for day-case surgery. The disadvantages of epidurals are the slow onset of surgical anaesthesia and the uncertainty that full recovery of motor, sensory and autonomic function will occur before the anticipated time of discharge home. Nevertheless, clinical practice (Sarma & Lundstrom 1989) has found that 90% of patients can be discharged within 5 h.

The speed of onset and shorter recovery time of spinal analgesia makes it more favourable, but the frequent occurrence of spinal headache has been a serious disadvantage. Using 26 gauge needles the incidence of headache in young patients having day-case surgery is 39% (Clarke & Power 1988). The recent introduction of 29 gauge needles and ogival (Sprotte) and pencil (Whittaker) pointed needles may make spinal anaesthesia in the day-case unit a more attractive proposition (Mudie & Cooper 1991). A written explanation of the nature and treatment of spinal headache (and provision of facilities for blood patching) given to patients has been of value in our obstetric service and has similar principles to day-case work.

General anaesthesia

All anaesthetic agents have psychomotor effects that last many hours after initial awakening. The choice of suitable drugs has been reviewed by Korttila (1988).

Induction agents

Propofol has rapidly become the agent of choice for day-stay surgery because of the rapid, clear-headed nature of recovery. This clinical observation was difficult to demonstrate but there is some objective evidence (Heath et al 1988, Millar & Jewkes 1988, Puttick & Rosen 1988). The antiemetic effect of propofol (McCollum & Milligan 1988) is an important factor in the well-being following surgery. One reservation is the rare observation of opisthotonus and other neurological sequelae where propofol has been implicated as the causative agent (Saunders & Harris 1990).

The pharmacokinetic profile of propofol, with a high clearance and short elimination half-life, predicts rapid recovery and indeed makes it a suitable agent for total intravenous anaesthesia, thus it is often used for maintenance as well as induction (Cooper 1991).

Methohexitone is a suitable alternative to propofol although the pharmacokinetic profile does not predict as rapid recovery, especially when used as a total intravenous technique. Although thiopentone is still the most popular induction agent in general use, there have been misgivings about its use (and that of methohexitone) for day-case work because full psychomotor recovery after a single induction dose of these barbiturates takes at least 24 h (Korttila et al 1975). This and the known synergistic effect of the barbiturates with alcohol are the basis for advising patients not to drive, operate machinery or drink alcohol for 24 h following anaesthesia. There may be specific indications for using other induction agents which may outweigh the differences in recovery.

The possibility of reversing benzodiazepines with the antagonist flumazenil might have been expected to increase their use for induction of anaesthesia, but there has not been a great change in clinical practice. Although flumazenil effectively reverses the sedative effects of diazepam and midazolam (Jensen et al 1989), its duration of action is short and resedation can be a problem.

Maintenance agents

For such short anaesthetics the differences in recovery between halothane, enflurane and isoflurane are too small to be of clinical importance, and the incidence of nausea and vomiting is similar with all three agents. Therefore the choice rests on other considerations.

Analgesics

Intraoperative use of analgesics can be important where postoperative pain is anticipated, but needs to be balanced against the increased likelihood of nausea and vomiting. Local anaesthetic blocks, non-steroidal anti-inflammatory agents and non-opioid analgesics play an important role in postoperative analgesia.

Muscle relaxants

There has been debate (Goold 1983) about whether it is safe to send patients home after endotracheal intubation because of the potential development of laryngeal oedema. The risk of this happening several hours later is small and must be weighed against the risks of not intubating for procedures such as those involving intraoral surgery. The laryngeal mask (Brain 1983) has enabled control of the airway, without endotracheal intubation, for spontaneous or controlled ventilation and reduces the incidence of postoperative sore throat to a level comparable to that seen after the use of a face mask (Alexander & Leach 1989). It has had a significant impact on the practice of out-patient anaesthesia. The choice of muscle relaxant is influenced by the anticipated duration of the operation. The incidence of 'muscle pains' is very much greater in patients that are ambulant. If suxamethonium is used, the severity of the pains can be reduced by pretreatment with a small dose of non-depolarizing muscle relaxant. If suxamethonium is used regularly a sixth point can be added to the instructions given on leaving the unit (Fig. 36.4) warning the patient about possible pains.

Provided they are used in a dose that will reverse without difficulty at the end of the procedure, none of the non-depolarizing agents shows great advantages over the others. Atracurium and vecuronium have better return of muscle power than other non-depolarizing agents. This may be important in minimizing postoperative diplopia, a distressing complication which might prejudice safety while going home.

ASSESSMENT OF FITNESS TO GO HOME

With suitable patient selection the need for admitting patients should be of the order of 1% (Levy & Coakley 1976, Ogg 1987, Cloud 1987). Admission related to anaesthesia is of the order

After your operation:

1. Go straight home with a responsible adult. Do not drive, operate machinery or sign important papers for the next 24 hours.
2. Do not remain alone in your home the night following your operation.
3. You may eat and drink as you wish, but avoid alcohol for 24 hours.
4. If you develop complications (such as severe bleeding) phone and ask for the doctor on call. For minor problems call your GP the following morning and if possible go to his surgery.
5. If needed, for pain relief take aspirin, paracetamol or codeine.

Fig. 36.4 Instructions given to patients as they leave the day unit. Additional information for the particular operation (e.g. for cystoscopy; recommend drinking 3 pints of non-alcoholic fluid daily for the next 3 days) can be added.

of 0.25% and is mainly due to nausea and vomiting or excessive drowsiness.

The stages of recovery can be divided into:

1. Immediate clinical recovery, such that the patient has regained protective reflexes and can be left unattended.
2. Fit to go home if supervised by a responsible adult. This recognizes that recovery is incomplete but, in the absence of complications, should proceed uneventfully over a period of time. The important criteria are that the patient can stand without falling (with the eyes open and with them shut) and that he can walk satisfactorily (in a straight line without staggering or swaying). It is helpful if the patient can eat and drink before going home as it prevents hypoglycaemia and demonstrates well-being. Complications such as haemorrhage should be checked for. Although there have been many tests used to assess recovery, none is simple and reliable enough to predict safety to leave the premises and are only applicable as research tools.
3. Street fitness, where psychomotor recovery is well advanced and the patient is unlikely to step out inadvertently in front of traffic.
4. Complete psychomotor recovery, where the patient is fit to undertake all aspects of daily life, including major decision-making and driving.

It is self-evident that the divisions between these stages are very arbitrary and ill-defined. Complex psychomotor tests which elicit a variety of performance-related tasks show that full recovery takes many hours, and the current recommendation is that driving should be avoided for 24 h. This takes no account of the severity of the surgery and it seems most appropriate to request patients to be sensible and abstain from driving for longer if they do not feel totally well. It is also worth pointing out the great disparity in the time it takes to regain normality when it is assessed by the patients themselves, being anything up to 21 days (Brindle & Soliman 1975, Routh 1979).

The usual duration of stay in the day-unit is a few hours, and need be less after local anaesthesia. Indeed, provided there is no limb paralysis making walking difficult, it can be beneficial to allow the patient to go home while still deriving benefit from the analgesia. Patients should be warned to expect some tingling and pain after the block wears off.

On discharge the patient should be given a sheet explaining the recommendations following surgery (Fig. 36.4). Patients are more likely to comply with written than verbal instruction (Malins 1978) and perhaps by emphasizing the importance by repetition, more patients will adhere to them. This type of sheet can be modified to include specific instructions to be followed after certain types of operation. It may also be useful to explain any minor complications that may occur, and what can be done to alleviate them. It is most important that the patient is aware of whom to contact in case of problems, and this should be included on the discharge sheet.

ORGANIZATION OF THE DAY-STAY UNIT

Equipment

Despite the fact the surgery may be minor, *there is no minor anaesthesia*. Indeed, a mishap is all the more catastrophic when the surgery is relatively trivial. This emphasizes the fact that the equipping of the unit must *not* be second rate, applying to both anaesthetic equipment and surgical instruments.

The equipment available for the anaesthetist should include an adequate modern anaesthetic machine with vaporizers, a full range of oral and nasal endotracheal tubes, a range of introducers and other aids for difficult intubation. All drugs needed for resuscitation, and a defibrillator, must be instantly available. Facilities must be there for indirect measurement of blood pressure and electrocardiogram (ECG) recording. Capnography and oximetry are also desirable aids to safe practice of anaesthesia. A good case can be made for having a bronchoscope available because the patient's starve has not been supervised. Occasionally, surgical disasters occur and the anaesthetist must be able to transfuse a patient rapidly.

This implies that large cannulae, blood warmers, blood filters, a supply of plasma expanders and facilities for central venous pressure measurement must be readily available. It is preferable for emergency apparatus to be kept in a separate, clearly labelled box whose location is known by all the theatre staff. The surgical instruments needed for an urgent laparotomy should be available. Finally in dire emergency a method must be available to summon more appropriate assistance.

Staffing

Good use can only be made of such equipment if the calibre of staff is also good. The daytime hours make nursing posts attractive but the regrading of nurses' pay has had a detrimental effect on nurse recruitment in some units. The number of nursing staff must be sufficient for safe working. An assistant is needed for the scrub nurse and the anaesthetist needs a trained operating department assistant or nurse. In the recovery area at least two trained staff are needed. In addition there should be portering and secretarial staff available.

A consultant should be in overall charge of the unit and have a special interest in it. This could be either a surgeon or an anaesthetist. The operations should be performed only by fully trained surgeons or by trainees under supervision. In particular, operations need to be performed speedily. The anaesthetic staff should be of sufficient experience to foresee the problems and forestall them. Thus unsupervised junior anaesthetists should not be deployed there and, above all, there must be some continuity of medical staff to ensure rapport with the nursing staff.

REFERENCES

Ainsworth Q, Wittman F W 1987 Day case surgery in a diabetic. Today's Anaesthetist 2: 184

Alexander C A, Leach A B 1989 Incidence of sore throats with the laryngeal mask. Anaesthesia 44: 791

Beechey A P G, Eltringham R J, Studd C 1981 Temazepam as premedication in day surgery. Anaesthesia 36: 10–15

Brain A I J 1983 The laryngeal mask: a new concept in airway management. Br J Anaesth 55: 801–805

Brindle G F, Soliman M G 1975 Anaesthetic complications in surgical out-patients. Can Anaesth Soc J 22: 613–619

Burn J M B 1983 Responsible use of resources: day surgery. Br Med J 286: 492–493

Clarke G A, Power K J 1988 Spinal anaesthesia for day case surgery. Ann R Coll Surg Engl 70: 144–146

Cloud D T 1987 Major ambulatory surgery of the pediatric patient. Surg Clin North Am 67: 805–817

Cooper G M (1991) Recovery from total intravenous anaesthesia. In: Kay B (ed) Total intravenous anaesthesia. Elsevier Science Publishers, Amsterdam, pp 175–186

Davis J E 1973 Ambulatory surgical care. Surgery 73: 483–488

Editorial 1983 Day-case cataract surgery. Lancet 2: 383–384

Fahy L T 1987 Delayed convulsions after day-case anaesthesia with enflurane. Anaesthesia 42: 1327–1328

Flanagan L, Bascom J U 1981 Herniorrhaphies performed upon out-patients under local anaesthesia. Surg Gynecol Obstet 153: 557–560

Goold J E 1983 Anaesthesia for day-case surgery: a review. J R Soc Med 76: 415–420

Heath P J, Kennedy D J, Ogg T W, Dunling C, Gilks W R 1988 Which intravenous induction agent for day surgery?: a comparison of propofol, thiopentone, methohexitone and etomidate. Anaesthesia 43: 365–368

Jensen S, Knudsen L, Kirkegaard L, Kruse A, Knudsen E B 1989 Flumazenil used for antagonizing the central effects of midazolam and diazepam in outpatients. Acta Anaesthesiol Scand 33: 26–28

Korttila K 1974 Psychomotor skills related to driving after IM lidocaine. Acta Anaesthesiol Scand 18: 290–296

Korttila K 1988 Choice of drugs. Curr Opin Anaesthes 1: 54–59

Korttila K, Linnoila M, Ertama P, Hakkinen S 1975 Recovery and simulated driving after IV anaesthesia with thiopental, methohexital, propanidid or alphadione. Anesthesiology 43: 291–299

Levy M L, Coakley C S 1976 Organisation and experience with outpatient anaesthesia in a large university hospital. Int Anaesthesiol Clin 14: 131–142

Loach A, Fisher A 1975 Lorazepam as a premedicant for day-case surgery: an assessment. Anaesthesia 33: 832–835

McCollum J S C, Milligan K R 1988 The antiemetic action of propofol. Anaesthesia 43: 239–240

Malins A F 1978 Do they do as they are instructed?: a review of outpatient anaesthesia. Anaesthesia 33: 832–835

Millar J M, Jewkes C F 1988 Recovery and morbidity after daycase anaesthesia: a comparison of propofol with thiopentone-enflurane with and without alfentanil. Anaesthesia 43: 738

Moxon M A, Jago R H 1987 Day stay surgery: Evaluation of a preoperative anaesthetic questionnaire. Today's Anaesthetist 2: 170–172

Mudie L L, Cooper G M 1991 Spinal anaesthesia for day case surgery. Curr Anaesth Crit Care 2: 130–134

Ogg T W 1976 Assessment of preoperative cases. Br Med J 1: 82–83

Ogg T W 1987 An anaesthetist's view of day case surgery. In: Hindmarsh I, Jones J G, Moss E (eds) Aspects of recovery from anaesthesia. John Wiley, London, p 9–15

Puttick N, Rosen M 1988 Propofol induction and maintenance with nitrous oxide in pediatric outpatient dental anaesthesia: a comparison with thiopentone-nitrous oxide-halothane. Anaesthesia 43: 646–649

Rockwell E 1982 Out-patient repair of inguinal hernia. Am J Surg 143: 559–560

Routh G S 1979 Day care surgery under general anaesthesia in a purpose built unit. Anaesthesia 34: 809–811

Saunders P R I, Harris M N E 1990 Opisthotonus and other unusual neurological sequelae after outpatient anaesthesia. Anaesthesia 45: 552–557

Sarma V J, Lundstrom J 1989 Epidural anaesthesia for day care surgery: a retrospective study. Anaesthesia 44: 683–685

37

Dental chair anaesthesia

J. H. Sheldrake

INTRODUCTION

The first general anaesthetic given in the UK on 19 December 1846 at a house in Gower Street, London was for a dental extraction. Indeed, the pioneers of general anaesthesia, Horace Wells and William Morton, were both dentists in the USA. Ever since that time there has been a close and unique association between general anaesthesia and the dental profession.

The administration of anaesthetics was considered to be within the capabilities of any qualified doctor in the early days. The advent of the National Health Service in 1948 led to the recognition of anaesthesia as a speciality and rapid development of skills and techniques. Increasingly, anaesthesia became a postgraduate skill in the medical profession and anaesthetics were administered by full-time specialists.

There was still a great need to provide painless surgery in the dental chair and a shortage of specialist anaesthetists, so dentists continued to practise general anaesthesia following undergraduate training. The practice of one person as operator and anaesthetist was stopped as recently as 1983 by the General Dental Council. Many reports have examined aspects of dental anaesthesia and another working party is presently reviewing the position in the light of many changes during the 1980s. These reports are listed below:

- 1967: Report of the Joint Subcommittee on Dental Anaesthesia of the Standing Medical and Dental Advisory Committees of the Central Health Services Council.
- 1969: Report of the Committee of the Association of Anaesthetists, Faculty of Dental Surgery and Faculty of Anaesthetists of the Royal College of Surgeons of England and the British Dental Association (Windeyer Report).
- 1978: Report of the Working Party on Training in Dental Anaesthesia (Wylie Report).
- 1981: Report of the Working Party formed to consider the Implementation of the Wylie Report (Seward Report).
- 1990: Report of an Expert Working Party on General Anaesthesia, Sedation and Resuscitation in Dentistry (Poswillo Report).

Recent changes

There have been a number of important changes that impinge on the practice of dental chair anaesthesia:

1. Dental caries has declined by 35–50% in most industrialized countries in the past 10–15 years. The evidence suggests that the use of fluoride toothpastes has been the factor largely responsible for the reduction of caries in the UK (Jenkins 1985). This has led to a sharp decline in the number of anaesthetics given in the community (Table 37.1) and in dental hospitals. One consequence of this is a dilution of

Table 37.1 Deaths associated with dental treatment in England and Wales

Years	Total deaths	Number known to include general anaesthesia	Place of operation		No. of general anaesthetics administered outside hospital
			Dentist	Hospital	
1986–1988	12	8	5	5	1 319 255
1983–1985	12	12	7	5	1 566 386
1980–1982	18	15	8	6	2 272 679
1977–1979	32	26	15	11	2 980 961

Figures courtesy of Mr C Howard, Senior Dental Officer, DHSS.

experience both for dental students and anaesthetic trainees. In addition, dental surgeons now qualify with very little experience of tooth extraction under general anaesthesia (Padfield 1989).

2. The range and availability of monitoring has increased greatly in the last decade. Despite any conclusive evidence that modern monitoring has reduced mortality, it is widely felt that some tragedies may be averted by the addition of equipment monitoring to clinical monitoring. The Association of Anaesthetists has published Recommendations for Standards of Monitoring during Anaesthesia and Recovery (1990) and strongly supports the use of continuous monitoring devices. Adhering to these standards may prove costly for surgeries and clinics giving small numbers of anaesthetics.
3. Attention has been focused on resuscitation with the awareness that health staff are often incapable of providing basic life-support procedures (Skinner et al 1985). This has led to improved organization and resuscitation training in some hospitals and the increased use of simulated cardiac arrest procedures. All personnel involved with dental chair anaesthesia will now be expected to be familiar with and have practised cardiac arrest procedures. The General Dental Council, in May 1989, amended its guidance on general anaesthesia and sedation, and stated that dentists 'must ensure that all those assisting them know precisely what is required of them, should an emergency arise, and that they regularly practise their routine in a simulated emergency'. These guidelines have been further updated in the light of the Poswillo Report (General Dental Council 1992).

MORTALITY

The mortality from general anaesthesia in community and general dental practices is small at about 1 in 260 000 anaesthetics. This compares with a rate of 1 in 185 000 in 1986 as a result of anaesthesia in all hospital procedures (Buck et al 1987). The comparison is misleading because most dental chair patients are young and fit. Death during or following a dental chair anaesthetic is always a tragedy, but the greatest concern arises from the many reports that suggest the death was avoidable. One coroner has called for patients to be sent to hospital if they need a dental operation, following the death of a 9-year-old boy apparently given too much methohexitone (Brahams 1989). In this and other cases, criticism has been made of the resuscitation, in particular the failure to intubate and to use a defibrillator even when it is available.

Avoiding morbidity or mortality from the complications of dental chair anaesthesia depends on the application of three principles:

- preventing the complication by the application of a correct and safe technique
- detecting complications swiftly and efficiently
- acting promptly and correctly.

PREOPERATIVE ASSESSMENT

General anaesthesia for dentistry is not a minor procedure and should be given the same consideration as in other settings. As for day-case anaesthesia, the patients must be fit and the use of questionnaires (as in Chapter 36) will be very useful in providing an initial screening of fitness. It would seem sensible to apply stricter criteria to anaesthesia in the community only taking on ASA I patients. Stable asthmatics and diabetics, for example, are better treated as day-cases in hospital. Examination of the heart and chest should be done prior to obtaining consent and, in the case of children, the anaesthetist should discuss the anaesthetic with the parents.

Cancelling patients

It is often difficult for parents and patients to understand why inadequate starvation or a common cold should lead to refusal to give a general anaesthetic for a dental procedure. The need for safety should be stressed; they will find it even harder to understand a complication resulting from less than ideal preoperative conditions. Uncooperative patients can sometimes be delayed and improved by a benzodiazepine premedication. Postponing the procedure may be necessary but can lead to reinforcement of the difficult behaviour. The use of EMLA (Eutectic Mixture of Local Anaesthetics) cream may be beneficial in children who are excessively frightened of needles and masks, provided an hour is allowed for it to be effective.

EQUIPMENT

Anaesthetic machine

It is important to check thoroughly any piece of anaesthetic equipment before use, but this becomes vital in community dental practice where assistants might not be familiar with anaesthetic apparatus. A large number of different anaesthetic machines are used in dental practices: one survey found 14 different types in 75 practices. In addition, the standard of maintenance was poor with more than 50% serviced irregularly or not at all (Hutchinson 1975). The delivery of an hypoxic mixture to a patient from a Quantiflex RA apparatus in a dental surgery may have been due to the failure to service the apparatus according to the manufacturer's advice (Simpson & Lacey 1987).

Resuscitation

The May 1989 guidelines from the General Dental Council on general anaesthesia and sedation stated that equipment necessary for basic life-support, including suction apparatus, oral airways and positive pressure equipment with appropriate attachments to inflate the lungs with oxygen, must be to hand. In addition to these guidelines, laryngoscopes, endotracheal tubes, an electrocardiogram (ECG), defibrillator and cardiac arrest drugs should be mandatory.

Dental chair

One piece of equipment the anaesthetist must always check and be familiar with is the dental chair. Moving the chair from the sitting, to the supine, to the head-down position must be practised so that it can be achieved quickly and without harm to the patient, should the need arise.

Scavenging

There is an awareness that long-term exposure to nitrous oxide and volatile agents may be harmful, and very high levels have been measured close to the dental chair. Effective scavenging can be difficult with mask anaesthesia because of leaks and the need to operate on the mouth. However, successful devices have been described for efficient scavenging (Andersson-Wenkert et al 1989, Jastak 1989).

GENERAL ANAESTHESIA

Drugs and methods

Anaphylaxis and malignant hyperpyrexia are life-threatening hazards common to all anaesthetic settings and are discussed elsewhere. Although rare, all personnel involved with the procedure should be aware of their significance, be able to run through intravenous infusions and know how to locate the nearest source of dantrolene and ice.

Until recently, nitrous oxide and halothane have been the main inhalational agents used and methohexitone the main intravenous agent. A dental hospital survey over a 25-year period revealed that a nitrous oxide, oxygen, halothane induction and maintenance was used in 75% of anaesthetics and a methohexitone induction followed by nitrous oxide, oxygen, halothane maintenance in about 20% (McLaughlin et al 1987). The addition of enflurane and isoflurane together with the introduction of propofol has broadened the range of agents suitable for dental chair anaesthesia.

Propofol has impressed many anaesthetists with the quality of recovery it produces. During a dental-chair session it may be important to have a rapid recovery in order to be able to complete the list without overloading or compromising safety in recovery. As a sole agent for dental extractions it produces a lower incidence of excitatory phenomena than methohexitone, and very similar recovery characteristics (Logan et al 1987). The pharmacokinetic profile of propofol suggests it would be a useful maintenance agent, and this has been successfully demonstrated in out-patient dental anaesthesia (Puttick & Rosen 1988).

Inhalational inductions are commonly used in out-patient dental anaesthesia and until recently halothane has been the volatile agent of choice. There is an incidence of cardiac dysrhythmias between 18–60% with halothane when used during dental anaesthesia (Rodrigo et al 1987), and also a very rare but often fatal incidence of hepatitis. The properties of isoflurane and enflurane suggest these complications would be reduced and, in addition, the lower blood/gas partition coefficients indicate a quicker induction and recovery.

Isoflurane has been used frequently for dental-chair anaesthesia, but there is disagreement about its suitability (Cattermole et al 1986, McAteer et al 1986). Isoflurane produces a far lower incidence of dysrhythmias than halothane (Cripps 1987), and a change to isoflurane from halothane during dental anaesthesia results in a very rapid decrease in the frequency of ectopic beats (Hutchison et al 1989). The irritant effect of isoflurane on the airways leads to more difficult inductions, and this is associated with longer induction times and more frequent episodes of oxygen desaturation (Sampaio et al 1989, Simmons et al 1989).

Enflurane is associated with as low an incidence of dysrhythmias as isoflurane, but produces less respiratory problems, fewer episodes of desaturation and has the most rapid recovery time. This makes it a very suitable agent for inhalational induction in the dental chair (Simmons et al 1989).

Airway maintenance

A survey of dental anaesthetic mortality indicated that hypoxia was the most common single cause of death (Tomlin 1974). Maintenance of a satisfactory airway at all times is essential to avoid hypoxia. The anaesthetist needs to keep a seal on the nasal mask at the same time as allowing the dentist good access to the mouth and maintaining the airway. To maintain a good airway:

1. The patient must be sufficiently deep to allow the mouth to be relaxed and open easily.
2. The pack and dental prop should be inserted carefully and the airway checked for 2–3 breaths before allowing the procedure to start.
3. The airway must be watched continuously and the dentist must be informed and asked to stop whenever obstruction or apnoea occurs.
4. The airway must be checked again whenever the prop is moved.

The anaesthetist may be more used to maintaining an airway in the supine position although it might maintain itself better in the sitting position. Dental extraction often involves a lot of force and it is important for the anaesthetist to provide counter pressure to provide a base for efficient extraction. It can be difficult to maintain an airway under these circumstances. There should be no hesitation in stopping the procedure and either intubating the patient, or waking him up and rescheduling the procedure if the airway is unsatisfactory.

Intubation

Intubation secures and protects the airway but has the potential for causing laryngeal oedema, the effects of which will be more significant and dangerous in the small airways of children. Oral intubation reduces the operating field and nasal intubation may not be advisable in children because of their adenoidal tissue. Intubation is advisable in cases that are taking longer and proving more difficult than predicted. Cases that are expected to take longer than 20 min are not suitable for dental-chair anaesthesia. Intubation should be used readily and at an early stage in resuscitation, and all dental anaesthetists should be skilled at intubation and be practising it regularly.

The laryngeal mask airway

The laryngeal mask airway (LMA), which is now available in a range of paediatric and adult sizes, has revolutionized dental-chair anaesthesia. Although the LMA is bulky and difficult to fix to the patient during dental extractions, the markedly improved airway allows unhurried surgery which is to everyone's benefit. In my experience, episodes of desaturation are almost eliminated by the use of an LMA and placement of an oropharyngeal pack is relatively easy. The use of the nasal mask, held with difficulty by a struggling anaesthetist, should be a thing of the past.

Dysrhythmias

Dysrhythmias can be provoked by dental surgery. The particularly significant ventricular dysrhythmias occur commonly during general anaesthesia with halothane. The more benign supraventricular dysrhythmias occur occasionally with enflurane and isoflurane. Many techniques are described for preventing dysrhythmias, including beta blockers, flecanide and local infiltration of the operating site (Clyburn ct al 1989).

Should dysrhythmias occur during halothane anaesthesia, enflurane or isoflurane can be substituted. Failing this, lowering the $P\text{aCO}_2$ by assisted ventilation is often successful. Then 1 mg/kg of lignocaine should be used and, if ventricular dysrhythmias are still present, it would be wise to terminate the procedure.

Monitoring

The widespread use of continuous ECG monitoring, and the increasing availability of pulse oximeters in other fields of general anaesthesia, led to the examination of their role in dental-chair anaesthesia. Pulse oximeters are non-invasive and easy to use during quick procedures in the dental chair. They are sensitive indicators of decreases in oxygen saturation before the development of cyanosis and so give a warning of hypoxia before it is clinically apparent (Clapham & Mackie 1986). It is self-evident that the relationship between oxygen saturation and $P\text{aO}_2$ should be understood and remembered when using oximetry data. Hypoxic episodes are frequently associated with the placement of the prop and pack in patients anaesthetized via nasal mask, as well as with extractions. Not surprisingly, they occur more frequently in patients anaesthetized and operated on by supervised students (Bone et al 1987). To prevent these hypoxic episodes, a minimum inspired oxygen concentration of 50% has been advocated (Parbrook 1988), but no significant difference in the incidence of hypoxaemia between 33% and 50% inspired oxygen has been found (Allen et al 1989). A pulse oximeter can be a sensitive detector of dysrhythmias and may be the only monitor required, provided an ECG is readily available. It seems likely that pulse oximetry will soon be regarded as minimal monitoring for general anaesthesia.

Capnography, via a nasal catheter, has proved valuable in out-patient dental anaesthesia as an instant monitor of apnoea or airway obstruction and a trend indicator of progressive hypoventilation (Anderson et al 1987).

Posture

The position of the patient in the dental chair is a controversial subject. An emotional faint during general anaesthesia in the sitting position has been postulated as a common cause of morbidity and mortality in the dental chair. This has led to a call for any degree of head-up tilt to be outlawed to prevent cardiac arrest (Bourne 1988). The supine position does not prevent fainting but lessens the likelihood of serious sequelae.

Advocates of the sitting position argue that there is less risk of regurgitation, and blood and debris from the operation fall out of the mouth and are less likely to be aspirated. An analysis of dental mortality revealed roughly equal numbers of anaesthetics given in the sitting and supine positions with no evidence of a difference in safety (Coplans & Curson 1982). An emotional faint during a general anaesthetic is only likely to be harmful if it is not immediately recognized.

Interestingly there appear to be no significant differences in the oxygen saturation changes during dental-chair anaesthesia in the sitting and supine positions (Evans & Dawson 1990).

Recovery

Almost 30% of deaths associated with dental surgery appear to occur in the recovery period (Tomlin 1974). An adequately staffed recovery area should be available, and the patient should be recovered in the lateral position on a tipping trolley with suction and oxygen available. Just over 20% of children significantly desaturate (SaO_2 <90%) on arrival in recovery following dental anaesthesia, so initial oxygen supplementation is indicated (Young & Bosco 1989). The stages of recovery are as for any day-case surgery and the criteria for discharge are the same. The patients should be given the same instructions as for any other day-case procedure. These are given in detail in Chapter 36.

SEDATION

Sedative techniques combined with local anaesthesia are becoming more popular and can be administered by the operator. Conscious sedation maintains protective reflexes and verbal contact with the patient. States of deep sedation are described in which protective reflexes are partially lost and verbal contact with the patient is lost, but in my view this should be regarded as general anaesthesia.

Sedation is not without risk (Jastak & Pallasch 1988). Coplans & Curson (1982) described a case of a motorcyclist killed in a road traffic accident 6 h after receiving 16 mg of intravenous diazepam (Coplans & Curson 1982). This emphasizes the need for giving the same postoperative advice to the sedated patient as to the general anaesthetic patient.

Many sedative techniques have been used and nitrous oxide has retained its popularity as a safe and effective sedative. Recently the newer anaesthetic agents have been tried:

1. Propofol produces reliable sedation with good operating conditions. It has the advantages of easy alteration of the degree of sedation and quick recovery, but the disadvantages of pain during injection and increased talkativeness (Rodrigo & Jonsson 1989).
2. Isoflurane also produces good operating conditions. It is preferred by patients to nitrous oxide (Rodrigo & Rosenquist 1988) and produces a quicker recovery than midazolam (Parbrook et al 1989).
3. Enflurane appears to be equally favourable and is currently cheaper than isoflurane (Ryder & Wright 1988).
4. Midazolam is an effective sedative for dental patients and is readily reversed by flumazenil, the benzodiazepine antagonist (Rosenbaum & Hooper 1988, Ochs et al 1990). This might improve immediate recovery, but resedation is always possible because of the shorter half-life of flumazenil. Flumazenil should be available wherever benzodiazepine sedation is the administered, but sedation should still be titrated against the response. Reliance should not be placed on the ability of flumazenil to reverse an overdose.

It is very easy to oversedate patients, especially with intravenous boluses and also in response to agitation in the middle of a procedure. For this reason all the resuscitation apparatus appropriate for a general anaesthetic is required whenever a sedative technique is used.

THE FUTURE

The end of general anaesthesia in the general and community dental service has been predicted within the next few years (Parbrook 1986). This might occur through a continuing fall in demand, due to economic difficulties of increased standards or by imposition. The Poswillo Report (1990) made many recommendations principally with regard to general anaesthesia, sedation and resuscitation. A reduction in the number of general anaesthetics is urged with sedation, under a strict protocol, being used as an alternative. Standards were laid down for monitoring and resuscitation. Whatever the future it is unacceptable to read case reports of deaths in the dental chair that imply lack of vigilance in both technique and monitoring together with poor resuscitation standards.

REFERENCES

Allen N A, Rowbotham D J, Nimmo W S 1989 Hypoxaemia during outpatient dental anaesthesia. Anaesthesia 44: 509–511

Anderson J A, Clark P J, Kafer E R 1987 Use of capnography and transcutaneous oxygen monitoring during outpatient general anaesthesia for oral surgery. J Oral Maxillofac Surg 45: 3–10

Andersson-Wenkert I, Haggmark S, Johansson G, Lindkvist R, Reiz S 1989 Anevac-D, a new system for close scavenging of anesthetic gases in dental practice. Scand J Dent Res 97: 456–464

Association of Anaesthetists of Great Britain and Ireland 1988 Recommendations for standards of monitoring during anaesthesia and recovery. Association of Anaesthetists, London

Bone M E, Galler D, Flynn P J 1987 Arterial oxygen saturation during general anaesthesia for paediatric dental extractions. Anaesthesia 42: 879–882

Bourne J G 1988 A cardiac arrest in the dental chair. Br Dent J 164: 34

Brahams D 1989 Death in the dentist's chair. Lancet 2(8669): 991–992

Buck N, Devlin H B, Lunn J N 1987 The report of a confidential enquiry into perioperative deaths. The Nuffield Provincial Hospital Trust and King's Fund, London

Cattermole R W, Verghese C, Blair I, Jones C J H, Flynn P J, Sebel P S 1986 Isoflurane and halothane for outpatient dental anaesthesia in children. Br J Anaesth 58: 385–389

Clapham M C C, Mackie A M 1986 Pulse oximetry. Anaesthesia 41: 1036–1038

Clyburn P A, Fassoulaki A, Rosen M, Webster J 1989 Flecainide and cardiac dysrhythmias during dental extraction under anaesthesia. Eur J Anaesthesiol 6: 39–48

Coplans M P, Curson I 1982 Deaths associated with dentistry. Br Dent J 153: 357–362

Cripps T P 1987 Isoflurane for anaesthesia in the dental chair: a comparison of the incidence of cardiac dysrhythmias during anaesthesia with halothane and isoflurane. Anaesthesia 42: 189–191

Evan C S, Dawson A D G 1990 Oxygen saturation during general anaesthesia in the dental chair: a comparison of the effect of position on saturation. Br Dent J 168: 157–160

General Dental Council 1989 Amendment to the notice for guidance of dentists.

General Dental Council 1992 Professional conduct and fitness to practise.

Hutchinson R I 1975 The accuracy and efficiency of general anaesthetic machines in dental practice. Br Dent J 139: 187–189

Hutchison G L, Davies C A, Main G, Gray I G 1989 Incidence of arrhythmias in dental anaesthesia: a cross-over comparison of halothane and isoflurane. Br J Anaesth 62: 518–521

Jastak J T 1989 Nitrous oxide in dental practice. Int Anesthesiol Clin 27: 92–97

Jastak J T, Pallasch T 1988 Death after chloral hydrate sedation: report of a case. J Am Dent Assoc 116: 345–348

Jenkins G N 1985 Recent changes in dental caries. Br Med J 291: 1297–1298

Logan M R, Duggan J E, Levack I D, Spence A A 1987 Single-shot i.v. anaesthesia for outpatient dental surgery. Br J Anaesth 59: 179–183

McAteer P M, Carter J A, Cooper G M, Prys-Roberts C 1986 Comparison of isoflurane and halothane in outpatient paediatric dental anaesthesia. Br J Anaesth 58: 390–393

McLaughlin W, Broomhead L, Hill C M 1987 A 25-year review of general anaesthesia at the Leeds Dental Hospital. Br Dent J 163: 317–320

Ochs M W, Tucker M R, Owsley T G, Anderson J A 1990 The effectiveness of flumazenil in reversing the sedation and amnesia produced by intravenous midazolam. J Oral Maxillofac Surg 48: 240–245

Padfield A 1989 The future of general anaesthesia in the dental surgery. J R Soc Med 82: 30–32

Parbrook G D 1986 Death for anaesthesia in the general and community dental service? Br J Anaesth 58: 369–370

Parbrook G D 1988 Arterial oxygen saturation during general anaesthesia for dental extraction in children. Anaesthesia 43: 67

Parbrook G D, Still D M, Parbrook O 1989 Comparison of i.v. sedation with midazolam and inhalational sedation with isoflurane in dental outpatients. Br J Anaesth 63: 81–86

Puttick N, Rosen M 1988 Propofol induction and maintenance with nitrous oxide in paediatric outpatient dental anaesthesia. Anaesthesia 43: 646–649

Rodrigo M R C, Moles T M, Lee P K 1987 A comparison of the incidence and nature of cardiac dysrhythmias occurring

during enflurane and isoflurane anaesthesia for dental surgery. Anaesth Intensive Care 15: 179–184
Rodrigo M R C, Rosenquist J B 1988 Isoflurane for conscious sedation. Anaesthesia 43: 369–375
Rodrigo M R C, Jonsson E 1989 Conscious sedation with propofol. Br Dent J 166: 75–80
Rosenbaum N L, Hooper P A 1988 The effects of flumazenil, a new benzodiazepine antagonist, on the reversal of midazolam sedation and amnesia in dental patients. Br Dent J 165: 400–402
Ryder W, Wright P A 1988 Dental sedation: a review. Br Dent J 165: 207–216
Sampaio M M, Crean P M, Keilty S R, Black G W 1989 Changes in oxygen saturation during inhalational induction of anaesthesia in children. Br J Anaesth 62: 199–201
Simmons M, Miller C D, Cummings G C, Todd J G 1989 Outpatient paediatric dental anaesthesia. Anaesthesia 44: 735–738
Simpson K H, Lacey V 1987 Hypoxia during general anaesthesia for dental extractions involving a Quantiflex RA apparatus. Br Dent J 162: 378
Skinner D V, Camm A J, Miles S 1985 Cardiopulmonary resuscitation skills of pre-registration house officers. Br Med J 290: 1549–1550
Tomlin P J 1974 Death in outpatient dental anaesthetic practice. Anaesthesia 29: 551–570
Young E R, Bosco D 1989 The use of pulse oximetry in the immediate recovery phase following dental extractions under general anaesthesia in children. J Can Dent Assoc 6: 39–48

38

Hazards of local and regional anaesthesia

A. P. Rubin

INTRODUCTION

Local and regional anaesthesia may cause less interference with patient's vital functions than general anaesthesia, and reduce the risk of intraoperative and postoperative complications (Modig 1982, Kehlet 1984). Blood loss and thromboembolic complications are reduced, especially with spinal and epidural anaesthesia. However, the use of local anaesthetics is not without complications, although these arise mostly from inappropriate patient selection or incorrect management. There is always a danger of systemic toxic reactions, hence they must not be given without intravenous access and adequate monitoring. A doctor trained to use resuscitative drugs and equipment must be available immediately. If large doses of local anaesthetic are being administered, a doctor other than the operator should be available to monitor the patient closely. Local anaesthetics can only be used safely after careful patient evaluation, considering age, weight, systemic disease, psychological state, any contraindications to local anaesthetic drugs or vasoconstrictors and the particular block technique. The characteristics of the local anaesthetic, its concentration, volume (and therefore dose) and the dose of any additional vasoconstrictor must all be checked carefully.

LITIGATION

Permanent complications may result in litigation. In a review of medical negligence cases brought against anaesthetists in the State of Washington, USA, during the period 1971–1982, there were 57 cases involving regional anaesthesia compared with 135 general anaesthesia (Solazzi & Ward 1984). Twenty-five (44%) regional anaesthesia cases had suffered cardiac arrest, brain damage or death, 22 (39%) permanent nerve damage and six (11%) convulsions. Many different blocks were implicated: spinal in 33%, caudal in 25% and femoral sciatic blocks in 2%. Even when good standards had been maintained, only 18% of regional anaesthesia cases were defended successfully compared with 50% when general anaesthesia alone had been used. These cases cause great distress to the patient and considerable anguish to the doctor. (In the USA as many as one in 45 anaesthetists sued committed suicide.) The potential for complications is great, although most are preventable and many are incidental. Good patient communication and informed consent must be emphasized. A careful explanation should include: the reasons for the choice of method; what the patient will experience during the induction, maintenance and recovery from the block; and the estimated duration of sensory and motor dysfunction. An impeccable technique should be used, and an understanding of conditions that may mimic the sequelae of regional anaesthesia helps to ensure correct clinical management and should avoid inappropriate litigation.

In a recent study of 900 closed claims for anaesthetic mishaps in the USA, 14 (1.6%) were associated with spinal anaesthesia (Caplan et al

1988). This may be compared with 193 (31%) where difficulty in the management of the respiratory system was the single most common cause of injury under general anaesthesia. While these results are obviously biased by the relative number of the different anaesthetic techniques used, there is considerable data to support the relative safety of regional compared with general anaesthesia.

HAZARDS OF INFILTRATION AND NERVE BLOCKS

Local anaesthetics differ from most other drugs in that they are injected into particular anatomical sites to produce a local effect. The maximum amount should remain locally to improve the quality of the block. Absorption and resultant blood level is unwanted and potentially toxic. Many peripheral nerve blocks involve the use of large doses of local anaesthetic and the choice of an appropriate drug with low toxicity is vital.

Choice of local anaesthetic

Lignocaine, an amide introduced in 1948, is used often when short or medium duration is required. However, lignocaine plain has rather poor blocking characteristics and a short duration of action. Not more than 4 mg/kg should be used. If adrenaline is added to the solution, up to 7 mg/kg should be safe, and the quality and duration of the block are increased.

Prilocaine is an alternative amide, has less vasodilator action and is more rapidly metabolized. The result is lower blood levels with equivalent doses and less toxicity than lignocaine (Englesson et al 1965a,b). Twice the blood level is needed to produce convulsions. It is the agent of choice for intravenous regional anaesthesia, and may be preferred for infiltration and peripheral nerve blocks when relatively large doses are required. More than 7 mg/kg may produce methaemoglobinaemia due to a metabolite, orthotoluidine. Methaemoglobinaemia is unlikely to cause clinical problems and can be reversed rapidly with 1 mg/kg methylene blue.

Bupivacaine is a long-acting amide with a relatively poor safety record. Its particular danger lies in its capacity to produce cardiac arrhythmias, and there is less safety margin between the cardiac toxicity and central nervous system toxicity doses than with lignocaine or prilocaine (Morishima et al 1983). The total dose of bupivacaine should not exceed 2 mg/kg. Etidocaine is another long-acting amide useful when motor block is essential. The dose should be limited to 5 mg/kg.

Ropivacaine is an interesting new local anaesthetic undergoing clinical trials. It seems to be similar to bupivacaine in blocking characteristics but has lower cardiotoxicity (Reiz et al 1989).

Mixtures of local anaesthetics are often advocated to shorten latency, prolong duration and prevent toxicity. Their action may not be as satisfactory as expected because the components of the mixture may fall below a suitable blocking concentration. The pH of the mixture may be suboptimal and the toxicity will be additive. Any mixing of solutions runs the risk of contamination and increases the risk of wrong solutions being administered.

The prolongation of action can be achieved by using long-acting highly protein-bound agents, such as bupivacaine, or continuous methods which can be applied to most nerve blocks.

Site of injection

The blood level depends on the vascularity of the site of injection, being higher after intercostal, caudal and lumbar epidural injections than after brachial plexus, sciatic, femoral or subcutaneous infiltration (Tucker & Mather 1979). The same doses may be potentially toxic in one area and not in another, making it impossible to state exact safe dose for all types of administration (Scott 1989). High blood levels may be associated with a relative overdose injected into the correct site or an inadvertent intravascular injection. It is essential to aspirate carefully, but small veins may collapse when negative pressure is applied. It can never be assumed that the injection will not be intravenous because of negative aspiration. High blood levels rapidly follow intravenous injection, but after correct injection the peak blood concentration may occur 20–30 min later, so vigilance is essential for a long period.

Total dosage

The total dose administered is the product of the volume and concentration. An awareness of the mass of drug (in mg) is essential to prevent overdose. The lowest concentration likely to achieve the intended blockade should always be used. Nerve fibres vary in size in relation to their function. Only when large fibres, for example motor nerves, need to be blocked are higher concentrations such as 2% lignocaine or 0.5% bupivacaine essential.

Speed of injection

The blood level is not only proportional to the dose, but also to the speed of injection. The slow injection of about 5–10% of the total dose initially should be followed by a pause to assess its effect. If there are no signs of toxicity the full dose may be administered slowly or in fractionated volumes. Constant verbal contact should be maintained with the patient and the cardiovascular and central nervous system (CNS) signs should be monitored carefully throughout the operation and recovery period.

Vasoconstrictors

Adrenaline added to lignocaine shortens onset time and increases the intensity, extent and duration of sensory and motor block. Adrenaline will reduce absorption of local anaesthetic and hence the peak plasma level, and increase safety. The adrenaline concentration should be 5 μg/ml (1 in 200 000) which is the lowest that produces local vasoconstriction. The adrenaline dose should not exceed 3–4 μg/kg. Prilocaine, bupivacaine and etidocaine are influenced less by adrenaline. Adrenaline must not be used when there is impaired local circulation, or where there are end-arteries. It is contraindicated therefore in ischaemic tissues and in digital nerve blocks. Its use must be avoided in patients with cardiac disease and those on tricyclic antidepressants (Boakes et al 1973).

It has not proved possible to make a mixture of prilocaine and adrenaline. Felypressin (Octapressin) is often used with prilocaine, particularly for dental work. Felypressin is a less effective vasoconstrictor but reduces the likelihood of cardiovascular effects and can be used even in patients with cardiac problems (Aelig et al 1970).

General condition of the patient

Absorption will be decreased in hypovolaemia, decreased tissue perfusion and heart failure. A hyperkinetic circulation, for example in anaemia, will increase absorption and hence blood level, and decrease the duration of the block.

There is now evidence that the individual susceptible to malignant hyperthermia may be given amide local anaesthetics safely (Adragna 1985).

PREVENTION AND TREATMENT OF LOCAL ANAESTHETIC REACTIONS

There are several different types of reaction to local anaesthetics. These are described below.

Vasovagal and psychogenic reactions

Vasovagal and psychogenic reactions tend to occur rapidly, occasionally even before the injection, and produce anxiety, sweating, pallor, faintness, nausea and vomiting, bradycardia or hypotension. They should be prevented by gentle technique, good rapport and careful observation of the patient. The treatment is to stop the injection, place the patient supine and elevate the legs. The reactions will resolve rapidly.

Allergic reactions

Allergy to amide local anaesthetics is extremely rare, cross-sensitivity is unlikely and reactions occur only occasionally to the preservative methylparaben in the solution (Larson 1977). Allergic reactions arise more commonly with the ester group, which includes procaine, 2-chloroprocaine and amethocaine, and are due usually to the paraaminobenzoic acid group (Aldrete & Johnson 1970). Reaction may be immediate, causing severe anaphylaxis with bronchospasm, oedema and hypotension. Treatment includes volume replacement, steroids, adrenaline and other vasoactive drugs. There may also be milder delayed allergic reactions, such as urticaria, which may be treated with antihistamines. Suspected allergic reactions should be investigated fully, so that a conclusive diagnosis is reached and future management is clear.

Reactions associated with high blood level of drug

To achieve a high success rate, many nerve blocks require local anaesthetic doses close to the safe maximum. There is always a risk, therefore, of high blood levels. Features include sedation, dizziness and tinnitus, followed by anxiety, restlessness, tremor and tonic-clonic (grand mal) convulsions. The treatment is to clear the airway, give oxygen and ensure adequate ventilation to prevent hypoxia and hypercarbia. Hypercarbia and metabolic acidosis increase the uptake of local anaesthetic into the central nervous and cardiovascular systems, and lower the convulsant and arrhythmia thresholds.

The convulsions should be stopped with either a benzodiazepine or thiopentone. Suxamethonium must only be used by those skilled in intubation. Lignocaine has myocardial depressant and anti-arrhythmic properties, while bupivacaine and etidocaine may depress cardiac contractility, conduction velocity and produce malignant ventricular arrhythmias and fibrillation (Albright 1979). In the event of cardiovascular collapse the legs should be elevated and intravenous fluids administered. Bradycardia may require treatment with an isoprenaline drip or 0.3–0.6 mg atropine, and hypotension with 10–25 mg ephedrine. Cardiac arrhythmias require specific anti-arrhythmic drugs or cardioversion. With long-acting local anaesthetic drugs, resuscitation may need to be continued for a long time until the myocardial concentration falls to a safe level.

Reactions to vasoconstrictor drugs

High blood levels of adrenaline may cause apprehension, tachycardia, palpitations, pain in the chest and hypertension, and may require treatment with alpha- or beta-blocking agents.

Retrograde arterial spread

Retrograde arterial spread can follow high-pressure injections, especially with dental syringes in the head and neck region, and may lead to convulsions (Aldrete et al 1978).

OTHER COMPLICATIONS

A detailed knowledge of anatomy and techniques, as well as pharmacology and toxicity, is essential to ensure a high success rate and to avoid complications. Reported incidence of neuropathies following regional anaesthesia varies from zero to more than 5% (Usubiaga 1975, Selander et al 1979). These may be mechanical, toxic or ischaemic in origin (Selander 1988). Complications may follow the technique itself, or the need for additional medication due to inadequate anaesthesia (Nolte 1989). Unexpectedly extensive anaesthesia may follow nerve blocks in the region of the vertebral column if the drug is injected inadvertently into the epidural or subarachnoid space as might occur with the interscalene brachial plexus or paravertebral blocks, or if it finds access to the subarachnoid space along dural cuffs as may occur with a retrobulbar block.

Direct trauma

Direct needle trauma to a nerve or intraneural injection may occur. Fine needles with short bevels, inserted with the bevel parallel to the nerve fibres, are advised, as they will produce the least trauma (Selander et al 1977). Paraesthesiae should not be used deliberately as a means of locating nerves (Selander et al 1979b). If paraesthesiae occur, their exact distribution should be recorded, both as a guide to the likely extent of the block and also so that their relevance to any subsequent deficits can be evaluated. Utilizing surface and bony landmarks and the feel of tissue planes rather than seeking paraesthesiae reduces the likelihood of nerve trauma.

A nerve stimulator may be helpful, particularly with deep nerves, for example the sciatic. The nerve stimulator should have a very low current amplitude that will elicit responses when the needle is in close proximity to the nerve without the risk of damage to it. However, false-positive results may occur when the nerve is on the other side of a fascial plane, which allows stimulation but not local anaesthetic to pass. Intraneural injection must be avoided as it causes up to 12% postblock neuropathies (Loftstrom et al 1966, Mogensen & Mattson 1980).

The nerve may be damaged by the solution injected, and this may be due to the local anaesthetic itself, excess added adrenaline, antioxidant such as sodiun bisulphite, or some contaminant or incorrect solution (Selander 1988). Obsessively careful checking of all solutions injected in the region of nervous tissue must be stressed. Neurological deficits are blamed very commonly on nerve blocks, but often other factors are involved, such as stretching or compression of a nerve during surgery. This may be due to faulty position, inadequate support of arms and legs, surgical trauma including the use of retractors, tourniquets or haematoma formation producing pressure effects, or tight bandages or plasters. Certain patients, such as those with pre-existing neurological disease, diabetes mellitus or systemic lupus erythematosus, are more likely to develop neurological sequelae. Nerve blocks should be used in these subjects only when the preoperative neurological status has been evaluated and documented carefully, and the benefit to the patient outweighs the risks.

Infection

Infection following regional anaesthetic procedures is extremely unusual. It may rarely be due to contamination, but most local anaesthetic solutions are made up with preservatives that have potent antimicrobial activity. It is safer to use single-dose ampoules rather than multidose vials, which once opened can no longer be guaranteed to be sterile. Aseptic precautions should be taken and there should be no touch or contamination of the needle or solution.

More often, infection is due to local spread. For this reason, nerve blocks should not be done in the presence of local sepsis, and if the patient has a systemic infection there remains a risk of haematogenous spread. The spontaneously occurring extradural abscess is the classic example.

Broken needles

Modern needles break very rarely, and then usually at the junction of needle and hub. Needles should be long enough so that they are not inserted as far as the hub, but not so long as to risk damage to distant structures. Leverage should not be applied to change direction; instead the needle should be withdrawn to the subcutaneous tissue and reinserted. Needles may have a security bead placed a short distance form the hub attachment. If the needle should break there will be a portion outside the body and it can be removed easily. Once they disappear into the tissues they can migrate large distances, especially if the area is palpated repeatedly.

COMPLICATIONS OF SPECIFIC BLOCKS

Brachial plexus blocks

The concept that the brachial plexus is surrounded in a fascial sheath, from its origin at the C5–T1 roots right down to the axilla, has resulted in the development of several routes of brachial plexus block, including the interscalene, the supraclavicular, the infraclavicular and the axillary approaches (Winnie 1984). Choosing an appropriate approach will result in the need for less drug and a higher success rate. The interscalene approach blocks the upper part of the plexus preferentially, and is indicated for the shoulder region and upper arm. By contrast the axillary approach is more likely to block the lower part of the plexus and is thus preferred for the distal part of the limb, including the hand. All approaches may result in nerve injury with persistent postoperative paraesthesiae or neuritis. The incidence should be reduced by the use of short-bevel needles and by not seeking paraesthesiae. The close proximity to major vessels means that intravascular injection is possible and that haematomas may occur.

Interscalene

In the interscalene approach the roots of the plexus are close to the vertebral artery. The local anaesthetic might be injected inadvertently into it, producing a rapid rise in brainstem concentration with convulsions. The interscalene is a lateral approach, and the needle might miss the cervical transverse process and pass through the intervertebral foramen into the epidural or subarachnoid space. Extensive anaesthesia, including total spinal, may result and there is even a small possibility of damage to the spinal cord. The needle should be inserted in a caudal direction so that it will strike the transverse process and cannot enter the foramen. The recurrent laryngeal nerve may be blocked, leading to hoarseness.

Supraclavicular

The dome of the pleura rises above the level of the thoracic inlet, and if the needle passes inside the first rib it may enter the pleural cavity. There is about a 2% incidence of pneumothorax following supraclavicular block, and at least 25% of these will require treatment by underwater seal drains. It follows that the supraclavicular route should not be used for patients who are soon to leave hospital. Damage to the subclavian vein or artery and intravascular injection of local anaesthetic are also hazards. The subclavian perivascular, which is a low interscalene technique, appears much safer than the classical supraclavicular. Bilateral interscalene or supraclavicular blocks are not advisable in view of the possible complications, including extensive blockade, recurrent laryngeal nerve paralysis, pneumothorax and paralysed hemidiaphragm.

Axillary

The most likely complication is direct nerve trauma. The classical description suggests a needle insertion at right angles to the axillary sheath, but it is preferable to insert it tangentially so that it enters the sheath and passes a short distance within it. This makes the axillary sheath easier to detect and ensures that the needle lies securely in it. The injection will also tend to spread cephalad, ensuring better blockade of the plexus, including the musculocutaneous nerve. It also enables a cannula or catheter to be passed for prolonged blockade, although this can be achieved often with one dose of a long-acting agent such as bupivacaine. The duration of action of bupivacaine in peripheral nerve blocks averages 12–14 h, but in up to 1% may last 24–36 h (Brockway et al 1989). Patients should be warned about this possibility, and bupivacaine should not be used if there is any possibility of nerve damage associated with injury or surgery.

Ulnar, median, radial and ankle nerve blocks

As these nerves tend to lie superficially, paraesthesiae are likely to be induced and persistent neuritis is a potential sequela. The nerves lie mostly close to blood vessels and there is a small risk of vascular damage or intravascular injection. Aponeuroses, such as the palmar (carpal tunnel), may compress the nerve and if the pressure rises following the injection neuritis may follow.

Sciatic nerve block

Several approaches to the sciatic nerve have been described, including posterior, lateral and anterior. The nerve is very deep and the success rate of sciatic nerve block can be increased markedly by seeing dorsiflexion of the foot following nerve stimulation. Less anaesthetic will achieve adequate blockade, while the risk of neuritis will be reduced. The innervation of the lower limb being complicated, it may be necessary to block the sciatic, femoral, lateral cutaneous and obturator nerves to achieve complete anaesthesia of the knee area. This will inevitably lead to a tendency to use large volumes of local anaesthetic and constant awareness of the risks of high volumes in relation to toxicity has been stressed repeatedly.

Digital nerve blocks

The digital nerves are related closely to the arteries which are end-arteries, and vasoconstrictors are contraindicated as any vascular spasm may result in ischaemia of the digit. Small volumes of local anaesthetic and proximal injections should be used to prevent pressure effects on the nerves.

The eye

Complications of ophthalmic regional anaesthesia are usually local but may occasionally be distant and life-threatening. Careful patient selection allows sedative drugs to be avoided altogether or used in very low doses so that complications related to their use need not be discussed. Contraindications to local anaesthesia include the young, psychological or psychiatric problems, uncontrolled cough, inability to lie still and flat, head tremor and long operations.

Long-acting local anaesthetics, such as bupivacaine, are needed, but in view of its slow onset time this drug is often combined with lignocaine. High concentrations, for example 0.75% bupivacaine or 2% lignocaine, are required to produce adequate akinesia of the external ocular muscles and an immobile globe. The total dose should be below that liable to produce systemic toxicity but intravascular injections might occur.

Hyaluronidase is often added to the local anaesthetic solution to promote spread and reduce orbital pressure. There is a potential for allergic reaction (Kind & Roffler 1961, Taylor & Pollowitz 1984) and it should be used in low concentration not exceeding 7.5 i.u. per ml.

Adrenaline is advocated to diminish bleeding, promote orbital tissue pressure reduction, and to augment the duration of anaesthesia and the intensity of akinesia of the external ocular and orbicularis oculi muscles. It will also delay absorption and hence reduce systemic local anaesthetic blood level. It is usually added on the day of operation to produce a higher pH than commercially available solutions.

Short needles reduce the risk of complications associated with injections at the apex of the orbit, such as retrobulbar haemorrhage or optic nerve trauma, and the peribulbar technique is gaining popularity as it is safer and does not require a separate facial nerve block. Fine needles cause less pain and are less traumatic. Injections tangential to the globe and with the bevel facing the globe make globe perforation less likely. Central spread of local anaesthetic along the optic-nerve dural sheath is a recognized complication of the retrobulbar block with an incidence of up to 0.79% (Hamilton et al 1990). Symptoms usually occur within 10 min and include mild confusion, shivering, convulsions, brainstem palsies, loss of consciousness, apnoea and marked cardiovascular depression.

The involvement of an anaesthetist allows a rational choice of technique, preoperative assessment, preparation and counselling, careful monitoring, and attention to the patient's psychological and physical well-being during the operation (Rubin 1990).

Stellate ganglion block

There are many approaches to the stellate ganglion and an extensive list of possible complications includes haematoma formation, intravenous or intra-arterial injection, vasovagal reactions and pneumothorax. Horner's syndrome, the main features of which are ptosis, meiosis and enophthalmos, is an inevitable side effect. The meiosis can be reversed with 10% phenylephrine eyedrops. Blockade of the recurrent laryngeal and phrenic nerves may also occur if the solution is not injected in the correct fascial plane, thus bilateral blocks should not be performed at the same time.

The anterior approach passing between the trachea and carotid sheath should be used whenever possible as this has the lowest incidence of complications. Anterolateral and posterior approaches might lead to epidural or subarachnoid injections.

Coeliac plexus block

The most common side effect is hypotension, due to splanchnic vasodilatation. Neurolytic solutions should only be injected if X-ray control is available so that the solution can be seen to spread in the correct tissue plane, and not backwards towards the intravertebral foramen, or even into the epidural or subarachnoid space.

The close relation of the plexus to the aorta and origin of the coeliac artery makes intravascular injection a possibility. A risk of impotence in the male must also be considered if a neurolytic block is contemplated for a benign condition, such as chronic pancreatitis. Large volumes of neurolytic solutions are required, therefore 50% alcohol is usually preferred to phenol.

Lumbar sympathetic block

Hypotension may occur, particularly if bilateral blocks are performed in elderly patients. These blocks should not be performed in anticoagulated patients, as retroperitoneal haematomata may arise. As in coeliac plexus blocks, X-ray control must be used with neurolytic solutions to prevent serious neurological complications.

The genitofemoral nerve (lying on the psoas fascia) is closely related to the chain, and may get damaged by neurolytic solution, leading to neuritis in the groin and genitalia. Some patients also get a cramp-like denervation pain in the quadriceps area. These may resolve spontaneously, or respond to a course of carbamazepine or transcutaneous nerve stimulation.

TOPICAL ANAESTHESIA

Intact skin

The eutectic mixture of the local anaesthetics lignocaine and prilocaine (EMLA) can penetrate the skin slowly (Lundh 1984). This has the disadvantages of taking an hour to work effectively and causing local vasoconstriction which may make venepuncture more difficult. Occasional erythematous reactions may occur, but these usually resolve rapidly.

Mucous membranes

Topical anaesthesia usually refers to mucous membranes, including the conjunctiva, nasal and buccal cavities, the pharynx, larynx, trachea, bronchial tree and the urethra. Many preparations are available, but as absorption from mucous membranes is rapid a safe dose must not be exceeded. The local anaesthetic blood level achieved will depend on the anatomical site, the volume and concentration, and whether it is applied by ointments or gels, or by sprays, aerosols or nebulizers which may disperse the solution over a very wide area. A vasoconstrictor does not retard the absorption of topical local anaesthesia.

Conjunctiva

Local anaesthetic eyedrops usually contain amethocaine or oxybuprocaine, both of which are esters and carry a small risk of hypersensitivity reaction. Alternatives contain lignocaine or cocaine. Cocaine may produce occasional clouding or even ulceration of the cornea. The total amount used is small so there is little danger of toxicity. The main risk is damage to the anaesthetic eye, which should be closed and protected with a pad and shield.

The respiratory mucosa

Local anaesthetics are often used in the nose for their vasoconstrictor as well as their anaesthetic action. They are useful prior to nasal intubation and for minor procedures such as nasal polypectomy or antral washouts. Cocaine, which has a very rapid onset and produces intense vasoconstriction, is still very popular. It may be applied as a 4%, 10% or 20% solution, a paste or an ointment. The dose of cocaine must not exceed 2 mg/kg. Signs of toxicity include excitation with euphoria and tremor, and an increased heart rate, blood pressure and respiratory rate. Very high blood levels may lead to convulsions, then medullary depression and coma.

Local anaesthetic techniques are useful for endoscopies including oesophagogastroduodenoscopies, fibre-optic and rigid bronchoscopies, and for the insertion of endotracheal tubes. Not more than 3 mg/kg or about 5 ml of 4% lignocaine (200 mg) in an adult should be used during any one procedure (Curran et al 1975, Scott et al 1976). If larger volumes are required the concentration of lignocaine must be reduced to 2% or even 1%. With these doses the blood level should not exceed 2–3 μg/ml and systemic toxicity is unlikely. While anaesthesia is present, care must be taken to prevent trauma, and there remains a risk of aspiration into the bronchial tree.

Urethra

Local anaesthetic gels or ointments may be used for catheterization or the passage of urethral bougies, and enable a cystoscope to be passed. However, not much bladder filling will be possible nor the performance of painful procedures within the bladder. Lignocaine (2%) is the most useful anaesthetic as it is effective rapidly and rarely causes hypersensitivity. It may be made up with chlorhexidine antiseptic. A tube contains 20 ml (400 mg of lignocaine), but it is not usually necessary to use the whole quantity.

Local anaesthetic ointments are not advised for the treatment of pruritus vulvae or ani. These are usually esters and may produce an allergic dermatitis and even more pruritus.

INTRAVENOUS REGIONAL ANAESTHESIA

Intravenous regional anaesthesia was introduced by August Bier in 1908 (Bier 1908) and repopularized by Holmes (1963). It is very simple but has caused morbidity and even mortality. Local anaesthetic is injected intravenously into an exsanguinated limb that has been isolated by a tourniquet from the general circulation. The local anaesthetic spreads through the venous system producing effective sensory and motor blockade. High systemic blood levels of local anaesthetic may follow overdosage, failure of the tourniquet cuff to prevent the drug entering the general circulation, or the tourniquet being released inadvertently or too early. Failure to monitor the patient continuously during and after the technique might allow local anaesthetic toxicity to go undetected and untreated.

Technique

It is essential that venous access is secured in the opposite limb so that anticonvulsant or resuscitative drugs may be administered without delay. A winged needle or a cannula is also inserted into a distal vein in the limb to be blocked.

Choice of cuff

The cuff site should be well padded with Orthoband, and a cuff of correct width and length placed snugly and secured so that it cannot undo suddenly. It should be on the upper arm or thigh as there is a small risk of drug passing through the interosseous circulation if the cuff is applied to a limb with a double bony anatomy. Single cuffs should be used. Double cuffs are narrow individually and it is more difficult to apply sufficient pressure to ensure continuous arterial occlusion.

Exsanguination

The limb should be exsanguinated completely, preferably using an Esmarch bandage or Rhys–Williams exsanguinator. In some painful states exsanguination may not be tolerated, and then the limb must be elevated for at least 5 min. It should appear pale and the venous system empty before any local anaesthetic is injected. If the limb is congested there is a greater rise in pressure during injection and the drug may pass under the tourniquet (Duggan et al 1984). If the arterial tourniquet is seen to fail at any time, as judged by increasing engorgement of the limb, then no more local anaesthetic should be injected.

Cuff pressure

Blood pressure fluctuates dramatically and cuff inflation must be sufficient to prevent arterial ingress at all times. The pressure to prevent arterial flow should be measured with the apparatus being used and the cuff pressure inflated to at least 100 mmHg above the measured occlusion pressure. Obviously it must remain at that level and must be monitored continuously. The patient must be able to tolerate the inflated tourniquet, as it will not be possible to let it down safely for at least 15 min (Thorn-Alquist 1969).

Choice of local anaesthetic

There has been great controversy about the best drug for intravenous regional anaesthesia. Over the past 30 years 0.5% or 1% lignocaine has been the most widely used. The advent of bupivacaine and its popularity for many nerve blocks led to its use in this technique. This drug was believed to produce excellent analgesia and even some residual analgesia after tourniquet release (Ware 1979). However, the residual anaesthesia is unreliable and patchy, and sufficient information has accumulated about the relative cardiotoxicity of bupivacaine to contraindicate it for this technique.

Prilocaine has been shown to be as effective a local anaesthetic as lignocaine, to be very much less toxic at equivalent blood levels and is thus the most suitable (Wildsmith et al 1979). Preservative-free prilocaine should be used to avoid painful injection or the risk of allergic reactions. For the upper limb, 20 ml of 1% or 40 ml of 0.5% is used. This amounts to 200 mg of prilocaine, which is well below the level that might produce methaemoglobinaemia.

Site and speed of injection

The drug should be injected slowly through a distal vein to reduce the rise in venous pressure and make it unlikely that the drug will pass under the cuff.

Intravenous regional anaesthesia is dangerous as its simplicity leads to complacency and tempts doctors to become operator-anaesthetists. It demands considerable attention to detail and very careful monitoring of the apparatus and patient. Continuous rapport should be maintained with the patient so that early signs of local anaesthetic toxicity will be appreciated, the injection can be stopped and appropriate treatment started. It is essential that the cuff remains inflated for at least 15 min to allow time for the drug to become fixed sufficiently in the tissues, so that excessive blood levels do not follow cuff release.

Continuous observation must continue following cuff release. The arm should be kept still as this reduces the local anaesthetic blood level (Hargrove et al 1966). There will usually be a rapid return of sensory and motor function following reperfusion of the limb, thus there is less risk of injury than when brachial plexus or lower limb peripheral nerve blocks render the limb anaesthetic for a longer time.

The technique is unsuitable when the surgeon releases the tourniquet to ensure haemostasis before closing the wound, as the anaesthesia will regress while it is still needed.

Intravenous regional guanethidine block

This is a development of Bier's block, using 10–20 mg guanethidine in 20–40 ml saline in place of local anaesthetic to produce prolonged sympathetic block (Hannington-Kiff 1974). The same precautions are essential for its safe use, as complications may follow high blood levels of guanethidine or of released noradrenaline.

SPINAL AND EPIDURAL

Complications associated with spinal or epidural anaesthesia are mostly preventable or even incidental. In a review of 542 complications following spinal anaesthesia, 538 were found to be due to other causes (Marinacci 1960).

The subject of neurological complications following epidural anaesthesia was the subject of an excellent monograph (Usubiaga 1975). A survey of obstetric epidurals analysed 505 000 epidural blocks. Five patients suffered permanent disability, three following cardiac arrest and two after nerve damage (Scott & Hibbard 1990).

Selection of patients

Spinal and epidural anaesthesia may be considered as an alternative technique for fit, healthy patients having appropriate surgery, as well as indicated particularly for some patients in poor physical condition. However the concept that a patient unfit for general anaesthesia is fit automatically for a spinal or epidural must be challenged. A careful assessment of the psychological as well as the physical status of the patient is essential, and contraindications must be respected.

Contraindications

Haemorrhagic diseases or anticoagulant therapy

Spinal and epidural needles or catheters may damage epidural veins. The bleeding normally stops rapidly, but in the presence of abnormal coagulation, epidural haematoma and neurological complications might result. Even without anaesthesia, spontaneous epidural haematoma has occurred in patients on anticoagulant therapy.

The response to low-dose heparin varies, but, once the first dose has been given, neither epidural nor spinal anaesthesia should be used unless coagulation is normal. Epidurals may be advocated for major vascular surgery, as it has been shown that sympathetic blockade increases blood flow through the graft (Cousins & Wright 1971). The risks of subsequent anticoagulation must be weighed against the benefit of increased flow. It should also be remembered that major aortic surgery under general anaesthesia has been followed by paraplegia, as a result of either prolonged clamping of the aorta or damage to lumbar arteries that supply the spinal cord.

Patient refusal

Unwilling patients should not be persuaded against their will, as other techniques are usually acceptable. If regional anaesthesia is particularly indicated then a full explanation of the advantages and disadvantages should be given, what they will experience and why they are being advised to have it. The patient will then usually agree.

Infection

Introducing needles through local areas of skin sepsis may lead to deeper infection. Severe systemic infections might result in extradural abscess via haematogenous spread.

Neurological disease

Neurological disease, particularly of an active or unstable type, may progress after surgery and lead to diagnostic and medico–legal difficulties. However, some peripheral nerve diseases such as diabetic neuropathy or burnt-out neurological diseases such as poliomyelitis need not be absolute contraindications and the advantages to the individual patient should be considered.

Lumbosacral spine abnormalities

Lumbosacral spine abnormalities may lead to considerable technical difficulties and neurological problems, and other forms of anaesthesia may be preferred.

Cardiovascular problems

Fixed cardiac output states, such as aortic stenosis, may make it impossible for the patient to compensate for any resulting hypotension. However, myocardial ischaemia is not an absolute contraindication, provided the diastolic blood pressure can be maintained. In fact, the reduction in afterload and the bradycardia may decrease the work of the heart and help improve myocardial oxygenation. Uncorrected hypovolaemia in the presence of sympathetic block may lead to severe hypotension, which may resist rapid correction. Blood volume must be restored before spinal or epidural anaesthesia is induced.

Choice of sedation or general anaesthesia

The required level of sedation or anaesthesia should be assessed so that an appropriate technique can be planned. Many procedures, such as hernia repairs, cystoscopies and minor anorectal or orthopaedic operations involving soft tissues, may be performed easily in conscious or mildly sedated patients. Propofol is useful as it allows good sleep control and rapid recovery. Additional use of intravenous analgesics, such as opiates, should be unnecessary if the block is successful. However, intraperitoneal operations, major orthopaedics or operations performed with the patient in abnormal positions (such as head-down, lateral or prone) are likely to require deep sedation or additional general anaesthesia. These additional techniques may cause problems including airway obstruction, and respiratory and cardiovascular depression. Light general anaesthesia with a controlled airway may be safer than deep sedation. Adequate monitoring is essential. Cardiovascular effects are likely to be increased by positive pressure ventilation.

Preparation

An intravenous infusion must be set up so that fluid may be given to maintain blood volume, prevent hypotension and for the possible urgent administration of vasoactive drugs. The blood pressure and pulse rate must be measured very frequently so that changes, which occur very suddenly, can be detected rapidly and appropriate treatment instituted.

Technique

There is little doubt that these techniques are safer if performed in the awake or lightly sedated patient, as any pain resulting from trauma to nervous structures or the injection of inappropriate solutions is likely to be reported immediately and before any serious damage ensues. Strict asepsis is essential, and the skin should be cleaned carefully with antiseptic solution which should be coloured to prevent any possible confusion with the local anaesthetic.

Locating the epidural space

An exact method, based on a detailed understanding of the anatomy and technique, should enable the needle to be placed accurately in the epidural space. Partial or complete failure to produce epidural anaesthesia often results in the need for additional anaesthesia, often under more difficult circumstances than if it had been planned from the beginning.

The strict midline approach is easiest to understand and perform. In the lateral position the back of the patient should be vertical and along the edge of the table so that the assessment of the correct angle of needle insertion will be easier. Liberal infiltration is carried out with up to 5 ml of 1% lignocaine so that no pain is felt during the Tuohy needle insertion. In the midline the needle will be gripped by the ligaments and this is a good guide that it is following its intended direction. A continuous method, in which the needle is advanced constantly while pressure is applied to the plunger of the syringe, is safer than an intermittent technique, where the needle is advanced step by step and repeated tests made for loss of resistance. The ligamentum flavum is very tough, and once the needle has stopped it requires a big push to overcome the inertia. This may lead to inadvertent dural puncture. In the continuous method with saline, the fluid is injected automatically as the bevel of the needle pierces the ligamentum flavum and enters the epidural space. This may help to push away veins, nerve roots or even the dura mater. The use of saline rather than air for the loss of resistance test gives a much better feel and reduces the incidence of dural puncture (McDonald 1983).

The only disadvantage of saline is that a small amount may return, particularly in elderly patients who tend to have higher epidural pressures, and it could be confused with cerebrospinal fluid (CSF). In practice this should not be a problem, as a dural puncture with a large needle is usually followed by a continuous flow of CSF, whereas if the fluid is injected saline it will rapidly slow and stop. If there is any doubt, the temperature or glucose content of the fluid may be assessed. Methods based on the existence of a subatmospheric pressure in the space, such as the hanging drop or Macintosh balloon, are much less reliable.

Injection of solution

The therapeutic dose may be injected through the epidural needle as there is a greater incidence of successful blocks (98%) than if it is injected through a catheter (90%) (Cousins & Bromage 1988). A test dose of 3–4 ml of local anaesthetic, such as 0.5% bupivacaine or 2% lignocaine, may be used to detect subarachnoid injection, provided sufficient time is allowed to elapse.

It may take up to 10 min after intrathecal injection for motor blockade of the legs to be seen, and the level of sensory blockade may not rise above L1 with glucose-free solutions. The injection should be made as slowly as possible to minimize the rise in blood level if an intravenous injection is occurring. Animal studies elucidated the greater cardiotoxicity of bupivacaine (Kotelko et al 1984) and its intravenous injection is very dangerous.

Intravascular injection may be identified if the test dose contains adrenaline (5 μg/ml) which will cause a tachycardia. However, false-positives are common (Dain et al 1987). Constant verbal contact should be maintained with the patient so that early signs of toxicity can be recognized.

Epidural catheters

Epidural catheters have become popular as they increase flexibility, allowing reinforcing and incremental doses to extend, intensify and maintain the area of blockade, and to provide effective postoperative analgesia. However, their use increases the risk of complications. The increased possibility of damage to an epidural vein or the dura mater makes intravascular or intrathecal injection more likely, and the catheter may cause trauma to nerve roots, a transient paraesthesia often occurring as the catheter is passed. The exact site of the paraesthesia should be recorded. Sometimes the patient complains of pain in the distribution of a nerve root and the catheter will not pass. It is unwise to persist as permanent damage might ensue. Sufficient catheter should be left in the space to ensure that it cannot become dislodged, but not so much that it may pass round to the anterior aspect or even exit through an intervertebral foramen. About 5 cm seems to be optimal and is associated with the highest incidence of successful blocks.

Catheter migration

Very rarely an epidural catheter may migrate from a correct position to become intravascular or subarachnoid, and an unexpected dramatic response follows a top-up injection. This rare event means that epidural top-ups should only be given by those capable of dealing rapidly with all side effects and complications, and the patient should be carefully supervised whenever epidural top-ups or infusions are used.

Catheter fracture

The catheter must never be withdrawn through the needle, as the bevel may cut through the catheter and a portion may be retained. The catheter may also get pinched between two closing laminae as the spine extends, and, during removal, it does not come out easily. If excessive force is used the catheter breaks. If the back is flexed the catheter will come out easily. It is essential to check that the catheter is complete. A retained portion is unlikely to do any harm as it is inert and sterile. Although the occurrence should be recorded, and the patient advised and reassured, there is no indication for surgical removal unless it is causing a neurological problem.

Local anaesthetic for epidural anaesthesia

There is a wide variation in the effect of a given volume of local anaesthetic, therefore to ensure a high success rate it is usual to use volumes greater than probably necessary to achieve effective blockade. The surgical patient requires about 2 ml per segment to be blocked, although this may decrease with age, atherosclerosis, diabetes and other causes of debility (Bromage 1962, 1969). There is therefore a risk of high blood levels, even in the absence of inadvertent intravenous injection. Lignocaine (1.5% or 2%) and bupivacaine (0.5%) each produce excellent sensory and reasonable motor block. The use of lignocaine (2%) with adrenaline, or bupivacaine (0.75%) or etidocaine (1.5%) with adrenaline, is necessary if intense motor block is required. An accurate assessment of the extent of blockade should be made before deep sedation or general anaesthesia is given. The anticipated course of anaesthesia and surgery should be appreciated so that incremental doses of local anaesthetic can be given in good time to maintain anaesthesia. In this way unnecessary supplementary medication may be avoided.

Use of adrenaline in epidural solutions

Adrenaline should be used only when the local anaesthetic action is improved or the systemic toxicity reduced. The addition of adrenaline to lignocaine results in more intense sensory and motor blocks, a longer duration of action and a reduction in blood levels of local anaesthetic by 25%. However, bupivacaine in normal concentrations is affected less, and, with the possible exception of its use for the test dose, adrenaline is unnecessary. It is never necessary to use a concentration in excess of 5 μg/ml. There has been a fear that, by producing vasoconstriction, adrenaline may jeopardize the blood supply to the spinal cord, but there is no conclusive evidence to support this contention.

Reinforcing or repeated doses

Lignocaine has a high liver extraction, 60–70% being removed in the first passage. Its half-life is approximately 90 min, so if a further dose is given within 90 min is should be reduced by at least 50%. It has low fat-solubility so that the blood level increases with repeated doses.

Bupivacaine and etidocaine have greater fat-solubility, thus there is less cumulation in the blood. For this reason these drugs are safer for repeat injections or continuous techniques. The use of long-acting amides increases the interval between doses and therefore decreases the number of reinjections.

There is less chance of a time lag between the return of sensation and the re-establishment of the block, and this likely to reduce the incidence of tachyphylaxis. The advent of tachyphylaxis means a larger dose of local anaesthetic will be required and the chance of systemic toxicity is increased. Prolonged epidural analgesia may be maintained by intermittent injection or by continuous infusion devices. Intermittent injections allow each dose to be adjusted according to need, but usually mean periods of pain between top-ups and frequent cardiovascular side effects. Constant infusion allows analgesia to be achieved with concentrations of local anaesthetic as low as 0.1% bupivacaine, and a more constant level of analgesia with a more stable blood pressure should result. However, the patient may still require additional bolus injections, and there remains the remote possibility of catheter migration into the subarachnoid space. To prevent toxic manifestations, not more than 30 mg bupivacaine/h should be administered. Epidural analgesia should only be used in the postoperative period when the level of nursing supervision is high and an anaesthetist is easily available.

Technique of spinal puncture

Fine needles, such as a 22 swg needle for older patients and a 25, 26 or 29 swg or a 24 swg pencil are used in young adults to minimize the size of the dural hole and reduce the incidence of headache. These fine needles are very flexible and an introducer needle (20 swg) is helpful. It is usual to insert the spinal needle with the bevel laterally so that the fibres of the dura mater are separated rather than cut across (Mihic 1985). This should reduce CSF leakage, allow the dural rent to heal more quickly, and thereby reduce the incidence and severity of headache. The technique follows the principles outlined for epidural puncture, and the anaesthetist should be aware of the likely position of the needle tip throughout the procedure. An awareness of the moment the needle tip pierces the dura will prevent the needle from being inserted too far into or through the subarachnoid space. Although the spinal cord ends usually at the lower border of the first lumbar vertebra, the space below this level contains the nerve roots of the cauda equina which can be easily damaged.

Spinal needles with good flow characteristics and transparent hubs aid in the rapid identification of the fluid (Messahel et al 1983). Local anaesthetic should not be injected until there is a free flow of clear fluid, and a small aspiration and reinjection should be made at the beginning and end of the injection to indicate that all the solution has gone into the subarachnoid space.

Choice of local anaesthetic

Hyperbaric solutions

Bupivacaine (0.5% in 8% glucose) produces excellent sensory and motor blockade of at least 2 h duration. If a shorter-acting agent is required, hyperbaric lignocaine (5%) may be chosen. Volumes of 3 ml heavy bupivacaine can be expected to produce blocks to about T6 height, although there is considerable variation. Increasing the volume results in a small increase in height, but a considerable prolongation of action.

Glucose-free solutions

Bupivacaine (0.5%) without glucose is mildly hypobaric and is a useful solution if low blocks are required, as for lower limb orthopaedic and perineal surgery, although the spread is very variable (Cummings et al 1984). Bupivacaine (3 ml of 0.5%) will produce blockade up to at least L1, and glucose-free solution is helpful if the patient cannot be placed on the painful side, for example fractured neck of femur. Because of the lower blocks achieved it is likely that the magnitude of the fall in blood pressure will be less, but this cannot be guaranteed and constant vigilance is essential.

Prevention and treatment of complications

Cardiovascular system

Very rapid changes may occur in cardiovascular function. These may be a cause of morbidity, mortality and litigation. A review of closed claims in the USA described 14 patients with sudden cardiac arrest during spinal anaesthesia (Caplan et al 1988). Bradycardia or hypotension were the intitial clinical clues in nine of the 14. The sympathetic outflow arises from T1 to L2. The more rapid the onset and the greater the number of preganglionic fibres blocked, the more vasodilatation will occur and the greater will be the fall in blood pressure.

If the block passes the sixth thoracic segment it will affect the cardiac accelerator sympathetic nerves, resulting in bradycardia and a further fall in cardiac output. Considerable venous pooling, particularly in association with inappropriate posture or aortocaval occlusion, may result in a sudden decrease in venous return with reflex bradycardia and a fall in cardiac output. In the conscious or lightly sedated patient a vasovagal reaction may follow, leading to nausea, pallor, sweating, fainting, bradycardia and a dramatic drop in cardiac output (Wetstone & Wong 1974, Scott 1975). A sudden change in position, for example lowering the legs from lithotomy, may produce severe hypotension if the block is high or there is hypovolaemia. With epidural anaesthesia, further factors are the effects of inadvertent intravenous injection of local anaesthetic or vasoconstrictor, or high blood levels following absorption.

Blood pressure and pulse rate must be monitored continuously, and the significance assessed in relation to the patient's general condition and the needs of anaesthesia and surgery. It cannot be assumed that as the blood pressure falls the flow to vital organs will be maintained. There is evidence that both hepatic and renal blood flows fall in direct proportion to the hypotension (Kennedy et al 1969, 1971), and ischaemia of the spinal cord and vital neural structures is possible, particularly in elderly patients.

A fall in blood pressure of less than 30% is unlikely to be harmful, while excessive treatment that increases cardiac work may reduce myocardial oxygenation. Fluid preloading with at least 1 l of crystalloid or colloid may help to minimize the fall in blood pressure. Excessive intravenous fluid could lead to overload when the sympathetic block wears off, and to urinary complications. The response to fluid is slow and, if an immediate pressor effect is required, vasopressors are preferred. Ephedrine, a combined alpha and beta agonist, is usually recommended. It may be titrated in 5 mg increments, or 15 mg intravenously and 15 mg intramuscularly given as bolus doses. An acute rise in blood pressure may lead to increased absorption and a sudden rise in plasma concentration of local anaesthetic (Mather et al 1976). Dihydroergotamine (0.5 mg) injected slowly intravenously is an alternative vasoconstrictor as it acts primarily on the venous capacitance vessels. Its disadvantage is an incidence of nausea and vomiting. Atropine can restore blood pressure to normal levels, but only by increasing heart rate and cardiac work. Thus the net result may be a decrease in myocardial oxygenation. It may have a place in the treatment of a severe vasovagal attack, and reduces the incidence of nausea and vomiting arising from intraperitoneal stimuli.

A particular problem is the cardiovascular effects of high blood levels of local anaesthetic, especially bupivacaine. This drug becomes fixed to the myocardium and its effects may be substantial and prolonged. Hypoxia and acidosis must be avoided, and the circulation supported with vasopressor drugs, antiarrhythmics and inotropes, as indicated. Bretylium (5–10 mg/kg injected over 20 min) may be indicated as it raises the ventricular tachycardia and fibrillation thresholds (Kasten & Martin 1985).

The respiratory system

Very high blockade is needed before the respiratory function of a normal individual is affected. However, debilitated or very obese patients, those with respiratory or intra-abdominal pathology, and those receiving other respiratory depressant drugs, may get into respiratory difficulties. Patients under spinal or epidural anaesthesia should be monitored with oximetry and, if intravenous sedation is employed, capnography may be valuable. High blockade abolishes proprioceptive input from the intercostal and abdominal muscles and may lead to a sensation of dyspnoea. However as study of 68 000 patients has demonstrated the safety of spinal anaesthesia in patients with chronic lung disease (Tarhan et al 1975).

High levels of blockade are associated with reductions in maximal expiratory pressure and flow rates, although blood gas levels are unlikely to change (Pitkanen 1987). The patient finds it difficult to take a deep breath or to cough effectively. Very high blocks may have an effect on the muscles of respiration, but apnoea is more often secondary to brainstem ischaemia.

The treatment of respiratory inadequacy follows well-established principles of intubation and positive pressure ventilation with appropriate oxygen concentrations. Intraperitoneal upper abdominal operations performed with spinal or epidural anaesthesia should be accompanied by endotracheal intubation and positive pressure ventilation.

Total spinal

A total spinal is recognized by unconsciousness, respiratory difficulty or apnoea, cardiovascular depression and fixed dilated pupils. Oxygenation, urgent intubation and positive pressure ventilation are required, as well as rapid support of the circulation as previously described. If it is recognized and treated instantly it should not cause complications, but there is very little time to spare and successful treatment depends on the presence of someone able to identify the condition and skilled in immediate resuscitation.

Massive epidural

Occasionally the block ascends very high but rather more slowly than after a subarachnoid injection. Respiration may not be affected and hypotension is less severe than would be expected. The pupils do not become fixed and dilated. It has been suggested that this is due to a subdural extra-arachnoid injection (Boys & Norman 1975).

Nausea and vomiting

Nausea and vomiting are very commonly warning signs of hypotension. They may also result from inadequate anaesthesia, particularly of structures with visceral innervation.

Shivering

Shivering is relatively common under spinal and epidural anaesthesia. Warming the intravenous fluids and local anaesthetic drugs reduces its incidence.

Urinary system

Retention of urine is common as the bladder may become overdistended, the sacral autonomic fibres unblock, and the detrusor muscle contraction returns, very late (Axelsson et al 1984). Urinary catheters must be used when necessary to prevent overdistension of the bladder.

Backache

Backache may follow spinal or epidural anaesthesia and is usually due to positioning during surgery, for example the lithotomy position. It seems a particular, although mild, problem in day-case surgery where the incidence may be as high as 55% (Flaaten & Raeder 1985). Severe or persistent backache should demand a detailed neurological examination to exclude rare causes.

Dural puncture headache

Dural puncture allows a cerebrospinal fluid (CSF) leak, low CSF pressure and traction on the dura and blood vessels of the brain. The headache tends to be more severe in younger and obstetric patients, and in those who are dehydrated. It is occipital, becomes worse when the head is raised and is relieved by the supine position. Temporary cranial nerve palsies occur occasionally, but using fine needles the incidence is only about one in 5000. They are due to the low CSF pressure causing dragging, particularly on the abducens (sixth) cranial nerve which has a long intracranial course.

Treatment of dural puncture headache should include hydration and measures to raise the epidural pressure, such as the prone position or tight abdominal binders: 500 mg caffeine sodium benzoate in 1 l of Hartmann's solution infused intravenously has been advocated (Jarvis et al 1986).

There is no evidence that bed rest in the supine position reduces the incidence, although it provides symptomatic relief (Caarbaat & Van Crevel 1981). Incapacity or prolonged headache is an indication for an epidural blood patch in which 10–15 ml autologous blood is injected into the epidural space under aseptic conditions. The headache is usually relieved within 1 h, although there may be a small incidence of minor temporary neurological sequelae. Blood patches should not be performed if the patient has a temperature, is on anticoagulants or declines the technique.

Other headaches

It is dangerous to assume that all headaches following spinal and epidural anaesthesia are in fact due to dural puncture. Headache should warrant a detailed neurological examination to exclude rare causes, such as subdural haematoma or aseptic meningitis.

Neurological complications

Not all neurological complications that follow spinal and epidural anaesthesia are in fact due to these procedures. Other causes must always be sought, such as: incorrect position during surgery; surgical trauma; vascular problems resulting from surgery, particularly in the region of the aorta; use of retractors, for example femoral palsy following the circular lower abdominal retractor; pre-existing neurological disease becoming apparent at this time; and in obstetrics complications from the use of instruments or pressure from the fetal head. Very early assessment by a competent neurologist, accompanied by relevant investigations, should help to elucidate the true aetiology of the complication.

Neurological sequelae may be due to:

- injury to the spinal cord, nerve roots, or blood vessels in the area by the needle or catheter
- ischaemia due to hypotension, venous pressure raised in relation to arterial pressure, thrombosis or embolization of the spinal arteries and vasoconstrictor drugs
- damage due to the toxic effects of the agents injected, especially when excessive concentrations are used, preservatives such as sodium bisulphite are included, the pH is very low, chemical contamination occurs, or wrong solutions are injected
- bacterial contamination

- haemorrhage
- an exacerbation of a pre-existing neurological disease.

It is apparent that most of these neurological complications can be prevented by careful patient selection and good technique. Contraindications, such as active neurological disease, must be respected and a baseline neurological status should be recorded in any patient who has a neurological deficit. Strict asepsis and avoidance of carrying material from the skin into deeper structures are important. Injections into the subarachnoid or epidural space should not be painful, and very traumatic or difficult punctures should be abandoned early in favour of a different anaesthetic technique.

Strict attention must be paid to methods of sterilization, the use of preservatives and the pH of the solution. Sequelae of spinals and epidurals will usually result in neurological complications that can be related to the lower part of the body. In addition there may be general complications resulting from excessive hypotension and possible cardiac arrest, leading to brain ischaemia and hypoxic brain damage.

Types of neurological complication

Cauda equina syndrome usually manifests as sphincter disturbances, altered perineal and lumbosacral sensation and variable loss of motor power in the legs. It may be due to an adhesive arachnoiditis in which the subarachnoid space becomes obliterated. There is an occlusive inflammatory reaction in the vessels which leads to ischaemic damage to the cord. The condition may deteriorate over a prolonged period.

Anterior spinal artery syndrome is a primary ischaemic lesion of the cord. It is manifested by a flaccid paralysis the lower extremities, with or without sensory loss and loss of bladder and rectal function. this might arise when there is severe hypotension. Constant vigilance about the level of blood pressure is essential, particularly in the elderly, and in this age-group it is probably unwise to allow prolonged hypotension and to use local vasoconstrictor drugs.

Aseptic chemical meningitis produces headache and neck stiffness, nausea and vomiting, and slight pyrexia. Unlike the dural puncture headache it is not affected by posture. The diagnosis is usually confirmed by lumbar puncture which will show a leucocytosis with a normal sugar and raised protein concentration. Culture of the CSF will be sterile. It may be due to:

- pyrogens
- local toxicity of the injected solution
- the introduction of minute amounts of antiseptic solution, skin, metal or glass particles.

Septic meningitis is extremely rare, but produces headache, fever, tachycardia, tachypnoea, nausea and vomiting, neck stiffness, head retraction, and positive Kernig's and Brudzinski's signs. Meningitis requires a lumbar puncture and antibiotic therapy should be started urgently.

Extradural haematoma may occur spontaneously, after lumbar puncture or epidural anaesthesia. It is more likely to occur in anticoagulated subjects, and presents usually with backache and increasing paraplegia.

Extradural abscess is usually due to haematogenous spread in septicaemia, and only rarely due to infection introduced percutaneously. It usually presents with backache, fever and an increasing neurological deficit. Vertebral tenderness is often present. Extradural haematoma or abscess may necessitate urgent surgical decompression.

Spinal opiates

Ever since the first description of a direct spinal action of morphine (Yaksh & Rudy 1976) and the first successful relief of pain by intrathecal morphine (Wang 1977), there has been great enthusiasm for the use of spinal opiates for the relief of acute and chronic pain. However, this has been expressed mostly by authors of uncontrolled studies. Well-controlled prospective studies (Chambers et al 1981, Rutter et al 1981) have tempered the enthusiasm and brought to light several problems.

There are opiate receptors in the substantia gelatinosa of the posterior horn of the spinal cord and in the dorsal root ganglion cells. Opiates affect particularly C-fibre input which is responsible for 'dull pain'. They have less effect on A delta fibres (mediating sharp pain) and practically no effect on A alpha and A beta fibres (motor and autonomic function) (Yaksh & Rudy 1977). This means they should be indicated particularly for postoperative pain where autonomic or motor interference is undesirable. They are likely to be ineffective in producing anaesthesia for surgery, in blocking severe postoperative pain, especially that associated with movement, and are disappointing in the management of labour pain unless combined with local anaesthetic. As well as relieving postoperative pain, function should be maintained or restored. Studies looking at restoration of function have often shown spinal opiates to be less effective than local anaesthetics (Kehlet 1982). A clear advantage is that spinal opiates can produce a longer duration of analgesia at smaller doses than by other methods of administration.

Choice of drug

Most studies of spinal opiates have been with morphine. However, this drug is poorly lipid-soluble and is highly ionized at physiological pH. This means that it is relatively poorly transferred from the epidural to the subarachnoid space, and into the spinal cord, causing a slow onset of action. High CSF levels persist for a long time and the drug may migrate rostrally to the brain, causing late, severe respiratory depression. However, morphine has a long duration of action, with a mean of about 16 h. If spinal opiates are to be used for postoperative pain relief they should achieve excellent analgesia of considerably longer duration and with fewer side effects than systemic opiates.

The highly lipid-soluble opiates that are mostly ionized at physiological pH, for example pethidine and fentanyl, are rapidly conveyed to the CSF, probably via arachnoid granulations in dural root sleeves (Cousins et al 1979). From the CSF there is rapid uptake into the substantia gelatinosa causing a rapid onset of pain relief (Cousins & Mather 1984). The residual cerebrospinal fluid levels remain low so that the duration is correspondingly brief (mean 5–7 h). Blood level studies comparing systemic and epidural administration of opiates have confirmed the spinal action of the drug (Cousins et al 1979), but a systemic contribution to this action cannot be ruled out (Justins et al 1983).

The selection of the correct opiate in the correct dose is still empirical and for the most part experimental.

Side effects

Side effects of spinal opiates are dose-related, and usually due to the migration of the drug to the brainstem. They include respiratory depression, pruritus, nausea and vomiting, and urinary retention. These side effects can be reversed mostly by naloxone, while analgesia remains.

Respiratory depression. The exact frequency of this complication is unknown, and it may be overlooked if the numbers in a series are small. It may occur if there is summation with other CNS depressant drugs given before, during or after the anaesthetic, and care must be taken in the use of other opiates if the spinal opiate fails to produce adequate analgesia.

With epidural administration there remains the risk of unrecognized dural puncture and an intrathecal injection of an epidural dose. Respiratory depression may be early, and is probably due to absorption and a rising opiate concentration in the plasma which will depress the CO_2 response curve. It may also be late, occurring up to 24 h after the administration, and is almost certainly due to rostral spread of opiate to the fourth ventricle. The highly lipid-soluble drugs, such as pethidine or fentanyl, are less likely to produce late respiratory depression. Respiratory depression is an unpredictable complication that to be treated successfully, must be recognized quickly. Thus it is recommended that spinal opiates should only be given to patients in high-dependency nursing areas. While constant supervision by the nursing staff is desirable, some form of respiratory or apnoea monitor should be considered. Continuous naloxone infusions may reduce the severity of some complications but may also antagonize the analgesia, making the technique more complicated and therefore less widely applicable (Gowan et al 1988).

Pruritus. The itching can be generalized or segmental, dose-dependent, is often very distressing and may last for several days. It may respond to naloxone, but antihistamines are unhelpful.

Urinary retention The incidence of urinary retention is increased following spinal opiates, and is more likely to occur in males than females. There is a marked relaxation of the detrusor muscle with an increase in bladder capacity leading to retention (Rawal et al 1983). This is probably a spinal action, possibly due to interference with the sacral parasympathetic outflow. It is antagonized by 0.8 mg of intravenous naloxone.

Neurological sequelae. There is a small possibility of neurological sequelae, such as arachnoiditis, as the local effect of opiates on the spinal cord, nerve roots and meninges are largely unknown. It has been recommended that preservative-free drugs should be used as some of the preservatives, such as chlorocresol, are known to have neurolytic properties.

Nausea and vomiting. There is a baseline incidence of 30% nausea and vomiting after parenteral opiates, but this is likely to be increased after spinal opiates.

Combination of local anaesthetic and opiate

It has been suggested that the combination of local anaesthetetic and opiate produces a better effect with a lower risk of side effects. The combination may be useful to intensify spinal and epidural block during surgery (Müller et al 1984), as well as providing longer postoperative analgesia. That there is a synergistic action between the two has been confirmed in animals and humans (Abouleish et al 1988, Akerman et al 1988, Preston et al 1988).

It is likely that spinal opiates will find a definite place in the management of postoperative pain, but epidural local anaesthetics will probably remain more suitable for obtunding the stress response and for maintaining graft blood flow after vascular surgery. The advent of acute pain services, including a joint nurse education programme, would extend the range of techniques that could safely be applied in general wards, as well as in high-dependency areas (Ready et al 1988).

At present, individual anaesthetists in conjunction with the resident medical and nursing staff must decide how and where to manage postoperative pain. It must be emphasized that close supervision is required for up to 24 h after morphine, and resident staff must understand the indications for urgent administration of naloxone.

REFERENCES

Abouleish E, Narinder R, Fallon K, Hernandez D 1988 Combined intrathecal morphine and bupivacaine for cesarean section. Anesth Analg 67: 370–374

Adragna M G 1985 Medical protocol by habit: the avoidance of amide local anesthetics in malignant hyperthermic patients. Anesthesiology 6: 99–100

Aelig W H, Laurence D R, O'Neil R, Verrill P J 1970 Cardiac effects of adrenaline and felypressin as vasoconstrictors in local anaesthesia for oral surgery under diazepam sedation. Br J Anaesth 42: 174–176

Akerman B, Arweström E, Post C 1988 Local anesthetics potentiate spinal morphine antinociception. Anesth Analg 67: 943–948

Albright G A 1979 Cardiac arrest following regional anesthesia with etidocaine or bupivacaine. Anesthesiology 51: 285–287

Aldrete J A, Johnson D A 1970 Evaluation of intracutaneous testing for investigation of allergy to local anaesthetic agents. Anesth Analg 49: 173–181

Aldrete J A, Romo-Salas F, Arora S, Wilson R, Rutherford R 1978 Reverse arterial blood flow as a pathway for central nervous system toxic responses following injection of local anesthetic agents. Anesth Analg 57: 428–443

Axelsson K, Möllefors K, Olssen J O, Lingardh 1984 Bladder function in spinal anaesthesia. Linkoping University Medical Dissertations No 184: vols 3–21

Bier A 1908 Über einen neuer weg Lokalanästhesie an den Gliedmassen zu erzeugen. Arch Klin Chir 86: 1007–1112

Boakes A J, Laurence D R, Teoh P C, Barar F S K, Benedikter L T, Prichard B N C 1973 Interactions between sympathomimetic amines and antidepressant agents in man. Br Med J 1: 311–315

Boys J E, Norman P F 1975 Accidental subdural analgesia: a case report, possible clinical implications and relevance to 'massive extradurals'. Br J Anaesth 47: 1111–1113

Brockway M S, Winter A W, Wildsmith J A W 1989 Prolonged brachial plexus block with 0.42% bupivacaine. Br J Anaesth 63: 604–605

Bromage P R 1962 Spread of analgesic solutions in the epidural space and their site of action: a statistical study. Br J Anaesth 34: 161–178

Bromage P R 1969 Ageing and epidural dose requirements: segmental spread and predictability of epidural analgesia in youth and extreme age. Br J Anaesth 41: 1016–1022

Caarbaat P A T, Van Crevel H 1981 Lumbar puncture headache: controlled study on the preventive effects of twenty-four hours bed rest. Lancet 2: 1133–1134

Caplan R A, Ward R J, Posner K, Cheney F W 1988 Unexpected cardiac arrest during spinal anesthesia: a closed claim analysis of predisposing factors. Anesthesiology 68: 5–11

Chambers W A, Sinclair C J, Scott D B 1981 Extradural morphine for pain after surgery. Br J Anaesth 53: 921–925

Cousins M J, Bromage P R 1988 Epidural neural blockade. In: Cousins M J, Bridenbaugh P O (eds) Neural blockade. Lippincott, Philadelphia, p 319

Cousins M J, Mather L E 1984 Intrathecal and epidural administration of opioids. Anesthesiology 61: 42–71

Cousins M J, Wright C J 1971 Graft, muscle and skin blood flow after epidural block in vascular surgical procedures. Surg Gynecol Obstet 133: 59–65

Cousins M J, Mather L E, Glynn C J, Wilson P R, Graham J R 1979 Selective spinal analgesia. Lancet 1: 1141–1142

Cummings G C, Bamber D B, Edstrom H H, Rubin A P 1984 Subarachnoid block with bupivacaine: a comparison with cinchocaine. Br J Anaesth 56: 573–579

Curran J, Hamilton C, Taylor T 1975 Topical analgesia before tracheal intubation. Anaesthesia 30: 765–768

Dain S L, Rolbin S H, Hew E M 1987 The epidural test dose in obstetrics: is it necessary? Can J Anaesth 34: 601–605

Duggan J, McKeown D W, Scott D B 1984 Venous pressures in intravenous regional anesthesia. Reg Anesth 9: 70–72

Englesson S, Eriksson E, Ortengren B, Wahlqvist S 1965a Differences in tolerance to intravenous xylocaine and citanest. Acta Anaesthesiol Scand Suppl 16: 141–145

Englesson S, Paymaster N J, Hill T R 1965b Electrical seizure activity produced by xylocaine and citanest. Acta Anaesthesiol Scand Suppl 16: 29–35

Flaaten H, Raeder J 1985 Spinal anaesthesia for outpatient surgery. Anaesthesia 40: 1108–1111

Gowan J D, Hurtig J B, Fraser R A, Torbicki E, Kilts J 1988 Naloxone infusion after prophylactic epidural morphine: effects on incidence of post-operative side effects and quality of analgesia. Can J Anaesth 35: 143–148

Hamilton R C, Gimbel H V, Javitt J C 1990 The prevention of complications of regional anesthesia for ophthalmology. In: Zahl K, Mettzer M A (eds) Regional anesthesia for ophthalmology. Ophthalmol Clin North Am 3: 111–125

Hannington-Kiff J G 1974 Intravenous regional sympathetic block with guanethidine. Lancet 1: 1019–1020

Hargrove R L, Hoyle J R, Parker J B R, Beckett A H, Boyes R N 1966 Blood lignocaine levels following intravenous regional analgesia. Anaesthesia 21: 37–41

Holmes C McK 1963 Intravenous regional analgesia: a useful method of producing analgesia of the limbs. Lancet 1: 245–247

Jarvis A P, Greenawalt J W, Fagraeus L 1986 Intravenous caffeine for postdural puncture headache. Anesth Analg 65: 316–317

Justins D M, Knott C, Luthman J, Reynolds F 1983 Epidural versus intramuscular fentanyl: analgesia and pharmacokinetics in labour. Anaesthesia 38: 937–942

Kasten G W, Martin S T 1985 Bupivacaine cardiovascular toxicity: comparison of treatment with bretylium and lidocaine. Anesth Analg 64: 911–916

Kehlet H 1982 The modifying effect of general and regional anesthesia on the endocrine metabolic response to surgery. Regional Anesthesia Suppl 7: 538–548

Kehlet H 1984 Influence of regional anaesthesia on post-operative morbidity. Ann Chir Gynaecol 73: 171–176

Kennedy W F, Sawyer T K, Gerbeshagen H U, Cutler R E, Allen G D, Bonica J J 1969 Systemic cardiovascular and renal hemodynamic alterations during peridural anesthesia in normal man. Anesthesiology 31: 414–421

Kennedy W F, Everett G B, Cobb L A, Allen G D 1971 Simultaneous systemic and hepatic hemodynamic measurements during high peridural anesthesia in normal man. Anesth Analg 50: 1069–1078

Kind L S, Roffler S 1961 Allergic reactions to hyaluronidase. Proc Soc Exp Biol Med 106: 734–735

Kotelko D M, Schnider S M, Dailey P A et al 1984 Bupivacaine induced cardiac arrhythmias in sheep. Anesthesiology 60: 10–18

Larson C E 1977 Methylparaben: an overlooked cause of local anesthetic hypersensitivity. Anesth Prog 24: 72–74

Loftstrom B, Wennberg A, Widen L 1966 Late disturbances in nerve function after block with local anaesthetic agents. Acta Anaesthesiol Scand 10: 111–122

Lundh R 1984 Topical anaesthesia from Koller to the present. In: Scott D B, McClure J, Wildsmith J A W (eds) Regional anaesthesia 1884–1984. ICM AB, Sweden, p 72–73

Macdonald R 1983 Dr Doughty's technique for the location of the epidural space. Anaesthesia 38: 71–72

Marinacci A A 1960 Neurological aspects of complications of spinal anesthesia: with medicolegal implications. Bull Los Angel Neurol Soc 24: 170–192

Mather L E, Tucker G T, Murphy T M, Stanton-Hicks M d'A, Bonica J J 1976 Hemodynamic drug interaction: peridural lidocaine and intravenous ephedrine. Acta Anaesthesiol Scand 20: 207–210

Messahel F M, Robinson J J, Mathews E T 1983 Factors affecting cerebrospinal fluid flow in two spinal needles. Br J Anaesth 55: 169–175

Mihic D N 1985 Postspinal headache and relationship of needle bevel to longitudinal dural fibers. Reg Anesth 10: 76–81

Modig J 1982 Thromboembolism and blood loss: continuous epidural block versus general anesthesia with controlled ventilation. Reg Anesth 7: 584–585

Mogensen B A, Mattson H S 1980 Post-traumatic instability of the metacarpophalangeal joint of the thumb. Hand 12: 85–90

Morishima H O, Pedersen H, Finster M, Tsuji A, Hiraoka H, Feldman H S, Arthur G, Covino B G 1983 Is bupivacaine more cardiotoxic than lidocaine. Anesthesiology Suppl 59(3): A409

Müller H, Borner V, Gips H, Stoyanov M, Hempelmann G 1984 Intraoperative peridurale opiatanalgesie: neue Aspekte in der Regional-anaesthesia. In: Wust H, Stanton-Hicks M D'a, Zindler M (eds) Anaesthesiology and intensive care medicine, p 152–158

Nolte H 1989 Sedation and regional anaesthesia. Curr Opin Anaesthesiol 2: 612–613

Pitkanen M T 1987 Body mass and spread of spinal anesthesia with bupivacaine. Anesth Analg 66: 127–131

Preston P G, Rosen M A, Hughes S C, Glosten B, Ross B K, Daniels D, Shinder S M, Dailey P A 1988 Epidural anesthesia with fentanyl and lidocaine for cesarean section: maternal effects and neonatal outcome. Anesthesiology 68: 938–943

Rawal N, Millefors K, Axellson K, Lindgardh G, Widman B 1983 An experimental study of urodynamic effects of epidural morphine and naloxone reversal. Anesth Analg 62: 641–647

Ready L B, Olden R, Chadwick H S, Benedetti C, Rook G A, Caplan R, Wild L M 1988 Development of an anesthesiology-based post-operative pain management service. Anesthesiology 68: 100–106

Reiz S, Haggmark S, Johansson G, Nath S 1989 Cardiotoxicity of ropivacaine: a new amide local anaesthetic agent. Acta Anaesthesiol Scand 33: 93–98

Rubin A P 1990 Anaesthesia for cataract surgery: time for change? Anaesthesia 45: 805–806

Rutter D V, Skewes D G, Morgan M 1981 Extradural opioids for postoperative analgesia. Br J Anaesth 53: 915–920

Scott D B 1975 Management of extradural anaesthesia during surgery. Br J Anaesth Suppl 47: 271–272

Scott D B 1989 'Maximum recommended doses' of local anaesthetic drugs. Br J Anaesth 63: 373–374

Scott D B, Hibbard B M 1990 Serious non-fatal complications associated with extradural block in obstetric practice. Br J Anaesth 64: 537–541

Scott D B, Littlewood D G, Covino B G, Drummond G B 1976 Plasma lignocaine concentrations following endotracheal spraying with an aerosol. Br J Anaesth 48: 899–902

Selander D, 1988 Nerve toxicity of local anaesthetics. In: Loftstrom J B, Sjostrand U (eds) Local anaesthesia and regional blockade. Elsevier Science Publishers, Amsterdam

Selander D, Dhuner K G, Lundbord G 1977 Peripheral nerve injury due to injection needles used for regional anaesthesia. Acta Anaesthesiol Scand 21: 182–188

Selander D, Brattsand R, Lundborg G, Nordborg C, Olsson Y 1979a Local anaesthetics: importance of mode of application, concentration and adrenaline for the appearance of nerve lesions. Acta Anaesthesiol Scand 23: 127–136

Selander D, Edshage S, Wolff T 1979b Paraesthesiae or no paraesthesiae: nerve lesions after axillary blocks. Acta Anaesthesiol Scand 23: 27–33

Solazzi R W, Ward R J 1984 The spectrum of medical liability cases. In: Pierce E C Jr, Cooper R B (eds) Analysis of anesthetic mishaps. Int Anesthesiol Clin 22: 43–59

Tarhan S, Moffitt E A, Sessler A D et al 1975 Risk of anaesthesia and surgery in patients with chronic bronchitis and chronic obstructive pulmonary disease. Surgery 74: 720–726

Taylor I S, Pollowitz J S 1984 Allergy to hyaluronidase. Ophthalmology 91: 1003

Thorn-Alquist A M 1969 Blood concentration of local anaesthetics after intravenous regional anaesthesia. Acta Anaesthesiol Scand 13: 229–240

Tucker G T, Mather L E 1979 Clinical pharmacokinetics of local anaesthetics. Clin Pharmacokinet 4: 241–278

Usubiaga J E 1975 Neurological complications following epidural anesthesia. Int Anesthesiol Clin 13: 19–50

Wang J K 1977 Soulagement de la douleur par injection intrathécale de serotonine ou de morphine. Ann d' Anesthesie Francaise 5: 371–372

Ware R J 1979 Intravenous regional anaesthesia using bupivacaine: a double blind comparison with lignocaine. Anaesthesia 34: 231–235

Wetstone D L, Wong K C 1974 Sinus bradycardia and asystole during spinal anesthesia. Anesthesiology 41: 87–89

Wildsmith J A W, Scott D H T, Brown D T 1979 Intravenous regional analgesia using bupivacaine. Anaesthesia 34: 919–920

Winnie A P 1984 Perivascular techniques of brachial plexus block. In: Lennart Hakansson (eds) Plexus anesthesia, Churchill Livingstone, Edinburgh, vol 1

Yaksh T L, Rudy T A 1976 Analgesia mediated by a direct spinal action of narcotics. Science 192: 1357–1358

Yaksh T L, Rudy T A 1977 Studies on the direct spinal action of narcotics in the production of analgesia in the rat. J Pharmacol Exp Ther 202: 411–428

39

Emergency anaesthesia

A. J. Sutcliffe

THE DEFINITION OF EMERGENCY ANAESTHESIA

There is no doubt that there is a higher incidence of mortality and morbidity after emergency anaesthesia than after elective anaesthesia. The reasons for this are complex and are often interrelated. Comparisons between different mortality and morbidity studies are difficult because usually only one or two of the many possible factors influencing outcome have been studied. The discussion is confused still further by the absence in the older literature of a clear definition of emergency anaesthesia and surgery. Buck et al (1988) have recently produced a set of definitions which, if universally adopted, would clarify the situation considerably. A true emergency requires instant action. There are only three emergencies requiring anaesthesia which fall into this category. These are severe haemorrhage from the heart or an inaccessible major blood vessel, life-threatening intracranial haemorrhage and life-threatening upper airway obstruction. Most other emergency anaesthetics are better described as urgent. Urgent operations are performed as soon as possible after resuscitation and usually within 24 h. Where possible, this chapter makes a clear distinction between emergency and urgent anaesthesia. Most published statistical data, however, combine emergency and urgent anaesthesia and are referred to as 'emergency'.

The mortality rate after 'emergency' anaesthesia varies between series (Table 39.1). The risk of death after 'emergency' anaesthesia ranges from three times greater than for elective anaesthesia to 36 times greater. The difference is probably because the mortality rate is assessed at different times after anaesthesia. Mortality rates assessed later after the anaesthetic and operation are probably more realistic. Anaesthesia can contribute to deaths occurring days or weeks after an operation. A hypoxic insult during anaesthesia, for example, may cause prolonged coma. The ultimate cause of death is usually pneumonia, but the importance of the anaesthetic insult cannot be denied.

Table 39.1 The mortality rate after 'emergency' and elective anaesthesia

Date	Authors	Mortality rate/1000 anaesthetics		Time of postoperative assessment
		Emergency	Elective	
1970	Vacanti et al	12.0	2.4	48 h
1973	Marx et al	39.0	11.0	7 days
1988	Bradley et al	10.9	0.3	24 h
1988	Bradley et al	26.8	1.8	7 days

FACTORS INFLUENCING MORTALITY AFTER GENERAL ANAESTHESIA

ASA status

Many studies have shown that mortality after anaesthesia increases as physical fitness decreases (Table 39.2). There is a marked increase in mortality in patients with ASA status IV or V. This is to be expected because these patients either have a disease which is a constant threat to life or are moribund. Vacanti et al (1970) have analysed mortality in relation to ASA status and the urgency of anaesthesia. For patients with ASA status I, II or III, the mortality rate for elective anaesthesia is 0.17% and for 'emergency' anaesthesia is 0.47%. The mortality rate is increased almost three-fold for 'emergency' cases. For patients with ASA status IV or V, the mortality rates are 7.5% and 9.0% for elective and 'emergency' anaesthesia, respectively. The cause of death is not identified, but it is notable that the excess mortality occurs mainly among the fitter patients. This implies that the severity of their disease was not recognized or that they were inadequately treated.

Type of anaesthetic

Local anaesthesia is sometimes administered as a safe alternative to general anaesthesia, particularly if the stomach is full or there is pre-existing respiratory disease. This may be true but, even after local anaesthesia, deaths occur. Marx et al (1973) have estimated a mortality rate of 0.8% following spinal anaesthesia, 1.4% following extradural anaesthesia, 12.6% following local infiltration and 1.8% following general anaesthesia. When the patients are assessed by anaesthetic technique and ASA status, an increase in mortality with decreasing physical fitness is demonstrated similar to that associated with general anaesthesia. It is possible that a significant proportion of the deaths occurring after local anaesthesia are related more to the severity of the patients' illnesses than to the type of anaesthesia. Indeed, the choice of anaesthesia was probably made because of the severity of the patients' illnesses.

Dripps et al (1961) have studied postoperative deaths where anaesthesia was thought to have caused or contributed to the death. They calculated that spinal anaesthesia caused or contributed to 1 in 780 postoperative deaths and general anaesthesia to 1 in 259 postoperative deaths. In a similar study, Memery (1965) estimated that spinal anaesthesia caused or contributed to 1 in 2037 postoperative deaths, therapeutic blockade to 1 in 36 deaths, regional anaesthesia to 1 in 687 deaths and general anaesthesia to 1 in 833 deaths. There are no data available comparing emergency and elective anaesthesia. It should be stressed that the groups are not strictly comparable because not all techniques are suitable for every operation.

Vasodilatation, secondary to spinal or extradural anaesthesia, may cause profound hypotension, particularly if hypovolaemia has not been corrected preoperatively. Vasodilatation is a common cause of death after this type of anaesthesia (Marx et al 1973, Dripps et al 1961). In addition to rendering the myocardium ischaemic, hypotension also causes vomiting and unconsciousness with the loss of protective airway reflexes. In this situation there is a grave risk that inhalation of gastric contents will occur.

Peripheral nerve blocks can be performed safely on patients who are inadequately starved, provided the maximum safe dose of local anaesthetic is not exceeded. If, however, the block

Table 39.2 ASA status related to mortality per 1000 anaesthetics (elective and emergency cases combined)

Date	Authors	ASA I	ASA II	ASA III	ASA IV	ASA V
1970	Vacanti et al	0.8	2.7	18.0	78.0	94.0
1973	Marx et al	0.1	4.7	45.5	249.0	510.0
1988	Bradley et al	0.0	2.5	7.3	56.0	287.0

fails, there is a strong temptation to proceed immediately to general anaesthesia with potentially fatal consequences if gastric contents are inhaled. Postponing the operation is far easier if this possibility has been explained to the patient and surgeon beforehand.

Intravenous regional anaesthesia is also used for 'emergency' operations and has caused deaths. The most important contributory factors are the operator-anaesthetist, the use of automatic tourniquets with multiple switches and confusing gauges, bupivacaine, and failure to recognize early signs of local anaesthetic toxicity. It has therefore been suggested that prilocaine and a simple tourniquet inflated by a bicycle pump should be used (Heath 1982). One person must administer, and be solely responsible for, the anaesthetic. This point should be stressed to surgeons who sometimes wish to administer intravenous regional anaesthesia themselves when the emergency anaesthetist is occupied elsewhere.

Light sedation, using a combination of an opiate and benzodiazepine, is often requested for the reduction of dislocations in patients who are not starved. In young fit patients, sedation is relatively safe but often inadequate. For frail elderly patients, sedation is likely to be effective but the risk of overdose is ill-appreciated. Loss of protective airway reflexes may result in sputum retention or inhalation of vomit. The risks are increased because sedation usually persists after the procedure is complete and the opiate may cause vomiting. Little nursing attention is given to the patient because he has not had an 'anaesthetic'. The use of sedation probably requires more, not less, care than a formal anaesthetic, and has little or no place as an adjunct to emergency surgery.

Operation site

Mortality varies according to the operation site. Intrathoracic, intra-abdominal and intracranial operations are each associated with a mortality rate of approximately 10%, whereas operations at all other sites have a mortality rate of less than 5% (Marx et al 1973). Although the operation site influences mortality indirectly by limiting the choice of anaesthetic techniques available, the site of the incision and adequacy of postoperative analgesia are far more important in determining outcome (Otto 1980).

FACTORS INFLUENCING MORBIDITY AFTER ANAESTHESIA

Death is a clear endpoint which is useful for comparative studies of anaesthetic risk. It is, however, only a crude indicator of outcome. The use of morbidity to assess outcome is more useful because the incidence of complications following anaesthesia is far higher, but it is far more difficult to make comparisons between studies because different authors use different indicators of morbidity. They also vary considerably in their definitions of major and minor complications. In most, but not all, studies, death is excluded as a major complication of anaesthesia! It is also very difficult to relate complications such as chest infection to anaesthesia when there is a gap between the anaesthetic and the onset of the complication which may have several possible causes. Zelcer & Wells (1987) studied all patients admitted to a recovery room and found that 30% had complications for which the anaesthetist, if not the anaesthetic, was responsible. Complications for which the anaesthetist was considered responsible included pain and hypovolaemia. Of the patients with complications, 58% had had a general anaesthetic with long-acting muscle relaxant, 25% had had a general anaesthetic without long-acting relaxant and 17% had had a regional local anaesthetic, although in some cases this was combined with general anaesthesia. No attempt was made to relate recovery room complications to urgency of anaesthesia. Cooper et al (1989) have studied patients admitted to an intensive care unit as a result of anaesthetic complications. The complication rate was 1 per 1543 anaesthetics, and approximately half of the patients had undergone 'emergency' anaesthesia. Following 'emergency' anaesthesia there was a seven-fold increase in risk of complications requiring admission to the intensive therapy unit (ITU). Pedersen & Johansen (1989) have studied the incidence of all serious complications of anaesthesia with a substantial negative outcome, that is death or severe disability. They showed that severe complications occur in 0.69% of elective patients and 0.41% of 'emergency' patients.

PREVENTABLE MORTALITY AND MORBIDITY AFTER ANAESTHESIA

Several studies conclude that death was entirely due to, or associated with, anaesthesia. Until recently, the incidence of anaesthesia-associated deaths was around 6% (Dripps et al 1961, Memery 1965, Marx et al 1973). More recent studies have found a much higher incidence. Holland (1984) found that 27.2% of deaths were associated with anaesthesia and that 19.4% of the deaths were preventable. Buck et al (1988) found that 14% of deaths were related to anaesthesia and 0.1% of deaths were solely due to anaesthesia. The reasons for this increase are not clear but could be due to the fact that more seriously ill patients are being operated on or that standards in general are rising. When studying the complications of anaesthesia causing admission to an intensive care unit, Cooper et al (1989) concluded that 26% were preventable and Pedersen & Johansen (1989) considered that one third of all serious complications were preventable. It is notable that deaths often occur as a result of more than one error (Memery 1965, Lunn et al 1983, Holland 1987). Errors occur during local as well as general anaesthesia (Dripps et al 1961, Memery 1965, Utting 1987). In general terms, errors occur in four broad categories. These are inadequate preoperative preparation, faulty anaesthetic technique, inadequate monitoring and inadequate postoperative care. These may be grouped together as lack of care, which was considered a contributory factor in 30% of the deaths in the Confidential Enquiry into Perioperative Deaths (Buck et al 1988). Other contributory factors included lack of knowledge in 15.1%, lack of experience in 23.7% and failure to apply knowledge in a staggering 75.1% (Buck et al 1988). In many studies the most common causes of death are airway problems associated with hypoxia, unrecognized or untreated hypovolaemia and inhalation of gastric contents (Utting et al 1979, Lunn et al 1983, Holland 1984, Utting 1987). Hypovolaemia and inhalation of gastic contents are commonly regarded as problems associated with 'emergency' anaesthesia. They can and do, however, cause death after elective anaesthesia. In fact, all complications of anaesthesia can occur at any time, which is perhaps why there is a dearth of information relating specifically to 'emergency' anaesthesia. Over the years the same risks have been identified over and over again without an apparent effect. Holland (1987) has shown, however, that it is possible to identify specific causes of morbidity and mortality, and that a concerted effort will reduce the incidence of these causes.

PREOPERATIVE PREPARATION OF THE EMERGENCY PATIENT

An operation is the treatment of choice for a wide variety of conditions and is performed in the expectation that the patient will be cured of his disease or relieved of distressing symptoms. Anaesthesia allows surgery to be performed painlessly with optimal operating conditions. It does not cure the patient, but subjects him to numerous hazards that are not necessarily associated with his presenting complaint or its surgical treatment. When choosing the optimum time for anaesthesia and surgery, the anaesthetist must first establish how long the operation can be delayed without risk of death or the development of irreversible damage. Consultation with surgical colleagues may be necessary. Having decided when the operation will be performed it is the anaesthetist's duty to reduce, as far as possible, the risks of anaesthesia. Ideally the operation should be performed when the risks of delaying surgery outweigh the risks of administering an anaesthetic. Every patient requires individual assessment and opinion. Anaesthetists and surgeons are also individuals. In some cases the anaesthetic risks can be greatly reduced if an anaesthetist with greater experience is asked to administer the anaesthetic. Similarly, greater surgical expertise may shorten the operation, minimize tissue trauma and reduce blood loss, thus lessening the problems faced by the anaesthetist.

The preoperative visit

With the exception of the three genuine emergencies mentioned previously, all patients should be visited preoperatively. A few patients, notably those with major haemorrhage, may require immediate resuscitation (see p. 620). Once resuscitative measures have been effective, all patients should have a full history taken and should undergo a complete physical examination. This rarely takes longer than 20 min and the information obtained is invaluable in identifying problems likely to complicate anaesthesia (Sutcliffe 1983). Numerous drugs, for example, have potentially hazardous interactions with anaesthetic agents. Potential interactions, if recognized, can be avoided by choosing a suitable anaesthetic technique. Similarly, a family history of malignant hyperpyrexia or suxamethonium apnoea may influence the choice of anaesthetic. There are also several important non-surgical problems that should be treated, if time permits, before induction of general anaesthesia. These are listed below:

- hypovolaemia
- full stomach
- dysrhythmias, particularly rapid atrial fibrillation and complete heart block
- uncontrolled heart failure
- hypertension
- pneumothorax
- acute chest infection
- endocrine imbalances (e.g. diabetic ketoacidosis, myxoedema, thyrotoxicosis, adrenal insufficiency)
- electrolyte imbalance.

It is rarely possible to change a patient's ASA category. Within a category, however, it may be possible to improve the patient's condition. The advice of a physician concerning treatment of medical conditions can be invaluable. Failing this, Hutton & Cooper (1985) provide excellent advice on the preoperative management of medical problems.

Preoperative investigations

Emergency investigations should only be performed if an abnormal result is expected and precise knowledge of the abnormality will influence the management of the patient. Blery et al (1986) have identified and evaluated a protocol for ordering preoperative tests. The parameters used include type of surgery, age, associated disease and medication. Using this protocol, only 0.2% of tests not actually ordered would have been useful to anaesthetists.

It is traditional to insist on a haemoglobin of 10 g/dl prior to routine surgery. There is little scientific evidence to support this view. Jenkins (1986) and Bevan (1978) have suggested that oxygen demand can be met with a haemoglobin of 8 g/dl if the patient is normovolaemic. Higher values are probably required for patients who have suffered severe injuries or are septic. These patients are hypercatabolic and have increased oxygen demands. Furthermore, they may have been given stored blood which has altered oxygen-carrying characteristics. Preoperative haemoglobin values in emergency patients should be interpreted with caution. Normal values occur prior to resuscitation following acute haemorrhage, and may also be found in dehydrated patients with chronic anaemia. Even if chronic anaemia is correctly diagnosed, a blood transfusion will not, in the short term, fully restore the oxygen-carrying capacity of the blood, and may precipitate cardiac failure in the normovolaemic patient. The diagnosis of hypovolaemia is far better made using physical signs, although measurement of haemoglobin, packed cell volume and urea may be used as an adjunct to management, particularly if dehydration is present. Biochemical tests should only be requested if an abnormal result is expected. Routine requests rarely produce unexpected, abnormal and anaesthetically important results (Whitehead & Wootton 1974).

The preoperative chest radiograph is imperative if a pneumothorax is suspected. For other patients it may confirm the clinical diagnosis but is unlikely to alter decisions already made regarding the most suitable anaesthetic technique. Seymour et al (1982) studied routine preoperative chest radiographs in patients aged more than 65 years. 40.3% had significant preoperative cardiac or respiratory abnormalities and there was an increased incidence of pulmonary but not cardiac abnormalities in 'emergency' patients. The radiographic findings altered management in 2.3% of cases. Postoperative complications were not predicted by the preoperative radiograph, although it was useful in some cases as a baseline investigation.

Irregularities of the pulse can only be accurately diagnosed if an electrocadiogram (ECG) is taken. An ECG is useful, but not mandatory, as a baseline in patients over the age of 65 because 30% develop new ECG abnormalities postoperatively (Seymour et al 1983). Rabkin & Horne (1983) have shown that an ECG abnormality alone is unlikely to result in the delay or cancellation of surgery, although it may in 2% of cases influence the choice of anaesthesia.

Table 39.3 shows a modified version of the protocol devised by Blery et al (1986) which may be helpful for emergency anaesthesia.

MINIMIZING THE RISKS OF EMERGENCY AND URGENT ANAESTHESIA

Prior to emergency and urgent anaesthesia the anaesthetist may have a limited amount of time to prepare the patient. It is therefore important that this time is used profitably. Pedersen et al (1986) have shown that ASA status III or worse, cardiac failure, a Goldman score of greater than 13, pulmonary disease, pulmonary abnormalities confirmed on X-ray, ECG abnormalities and emergency operation are important indicators of a poor outcome. These are listed in order of importance. Goldman et al (1977) published a multifactorial index of cardiac risk. Treatable risk factors include cardiac failure, dysrhythmias, and abnormal electrolytes and blood gases. It is notable that, although 'emergency' surgery is identified as a risk factor, it is the least important

Table 39.3 Guidelines for investigations prior to emergency and urgent anaesthesia

Considerations	XMatch	Hb	PT/PTT	Plts	Na/K	BUN	BS	CXR	ECG	Sickle
Surgery										
Major	+	+								
Minor										
Age (years)										
<40										
40–60									+	
>60					+	+			+	
Associated disease										
Cardiovascular									+	
Respiratory								+	+	
Malignancy		+								
Hepatobiliary			+							
Renal		+			+	+				
Bleeding disorder			+	+						
Diabetes					+	+	+			
Drugs										
Diuretics					+	+				
Digitalis					+					
Steroids					+		+			
Anticoagulants			+							
Ethnic origin										
Black African										+

with regard to outcome. It is clear from these studies that, if time is available, cardiac and respiratory disease should be treated preoperatively. Myocardial infarction in the 6 months prior to surgery places patients at increased risk of perioperative or postoperative reinfarction. With aggressive management, which includes invasive monitoring, the mortality rate for these patients can be reduced from 7.7% to 1.93% (Rao et al 1983). The effects of other treatments for cardiac and respiratory problems have not been quantified.

Chronic respiratory infection is associated with 26.4% incidence of postoperative respiratory complications, whereas active infection has a 44% risk. Active infection with a productive cough is associated with a 57.5% incidence of postoperative complications (Otto 1980). Stein & Cassara (1970) have suggested that physiotherapy, bronchodilators, antibiotics and education about breathing exercises will reduce the incidence of postoperative complications by two thirds if surgery can be delayed long enough for these to be effective.

Bearing in mind the factors that are associated with postoperative complications, the anaesthetist must decide for each individual patient the best plan for preoperative management. It may, for example, be better for the patient to spend the preoperative period receiving bronchodilators and physiotherapy rather than wasting time in the X-ray department having the diagnosis of chronic bronchitis confirmed. In most cases it is best for the anaesthetist to institute therapy rather than relying on the surgeons. This may take time, but should ensure that necessary treatments are commenced as soon as possible.

SPECIFIC PREOPERATIVE PROBLEMS RELATING TO EMERGENCY AND URGENT ANAESTHESIA

Hypovolaemia

Inadequately treated hypovolaemia appears as a preventable cause of death in most surveys of anaesthetic mortality and is probably responsible for 2–3% of preventable deaths (Marx et al 1973, Lunn et al 1983). Following fluid loss, vasoconstriction and an increase in heart rate may maintain the blood pressure. However, hypotension will occur in the presence of anaesthetic agents which cause vasodilatation or myocardial depression. Intraoperative hypotension has been implicated in as many as 30% of preventable anaesthetic deaths (Dripps et al 1961), although it is not clear whether this was associated with hypovolaemia in all cases. Blood loss associated with hypotension was reported as a specific cause of death in 1.8% of cases referred to the Medical Defence Union by anaesthetists (Utting et al 1979).

Failure to treat hypovolaemia not only puts the patient at risk intraoperatively, but may also lead to life-threatening multiple organ failure postoperatively. The immediate effect of sudden blood loss is the activation of a variety of homeostatic mechanisms. These include activation of the sympathetic nervous system and the release of a number of humoral mediators. Initially these mechanisms are protective and help to preserve life. In excess they cause severe tissue hypoxia, cellular damage and release of toxic substances which increase microvascular permeability and ultimately multiple organ failure. Furthermore, vasoconstriction of the splanchnic bed causes ischaemia of the gut mucosa which becomes permeable to microorganisms and endotoxins. These enter the portal circulation and damage Kuppfer cells in the liver, thus rendering the patient at increased risk of infection (Redl & Schlag 1990). At present, rapid and accurate restoration of circulating blood volume is the only effective means of reducing the incidence of multiple organ failure secondary to hypovolaemia.

Direct measurement of fluid loss is rarely possible. Estimations of the average losses after trauma (London 1968) and burns (Cason 1981) have been made, but should only be used as a guide. Losses due to intestinal obstruction, peritonitis or gastrointestinal haemorrhage are variable. The diagnosis of hypovolaemia is best made on clinical grounds, bearing in mind that the speed of fluid loss as well as the volume of loss influence the clinical picture. The effects of acute blood loss are summarized in Table 39.4. Misinterpretation of these parameters is an ever-present danger, especially if only one or two are measured. A tachycardia and peripheral venous constriction are classical signs of hypovolaemia, but may also be found in normovolaemic patients who are in pain or are frightened. The vasoconstriction caused by pain often contributes to the maintenance of blood pressure in hypovolaemic patients. In this situation, analgesia should not be withheld but should be administered in conjunction with resuscitation fluid. Primary water loss causes intracellular dehydration and circulatory failure does not occur until the patient is grossly dehydrated. The presence of thirst indicates a water deficit of at least 1.5 l. Water loss in association with sodium depletion causes an extracellular deficit and leads to the traditional clinical picture of hypovolaemia.

There has been a lengthy debate concerning the best type of fluid for resuscitation. It revolves around clinical aspects such as the efficacy of volume replacement, or the possibility of long-term side effects such as the adult respiratory distress syndrome, and, sadly, the financial aspects and relative costs of the various fluids available. The duration of the debate indicates that there is merit in both arguments (Fisher 1990).

Speed of resuscitation is far more important than the type of fluid chosen. One limitation to the rapid resuscitation of patients with major haemorrhage is the availability of blood. In life-threatening situations, O-Rhesus negative blood is given, but otherwise doctors tend to wait for full compatibility testing. ABO compatibility can, however, be assessed in less than 10 min using a saline cross-match technique which gives a 99.4% probability of the blood being compatible with the recipient. Testing for Rhesus compatibility as well as ABO compatibility increases the chance of compatability with recipient to 99.8%. The further addition of negative Rhesus antibody screening increases the chances of recipient compatibility to 99.84% and complete pretransfusion screening to 99.95%. Even randomly selected blood has a 64.4% probability of recipient compatibility (Isbister 1984). The key step in the cross-match procedure is, therefore, ABO compatibility testing. If this is done the risks to the patient are minimal compared to the risks in delaying the administration of blood if the haemorrhage is severe.

Another technique that is gaining popularity is small-volume resuscitation using hypertonic-hyperoncotic solutions. The most commonly used solutions are Dextran 60/70 in hypertonic saline or glucose. These solutions have the advantages that they restore circulating blood volume rapidly and that they are cheap. Furthermore they are relatively free from the risk of volume overload (Kreimeier & Messmer 1988). It is probable that hypertonic-hyperosmotic solutions will find a routine place in resuscitation regimes, particularly for prehospital resuscitation.

It is important that resuscitation commences as rapidly as possible. Initially the administration of fluid is more important than the accuracy of monitoring. A diagnosis compatible with major fluid loss in combination with tachycardia, hypotension and peripheral vasoconstiction is sufficient cause to commence fluid resuscitation. When resuscitation has begun, attention can be given to monitoring the accuracy of volume replacement. Basic parameters such as urine output, skin temperature and the filling of peri-

Table 39.4 Signs of acute blood loss

Sign	Blood loss		
	<1500 ml	1500–2000 ml	> 2000 ml
Heart rate	N–120 bpm	120–140 bpm	>140 bpm
Systolic BP	120 mmHg	70–90 mmHg	<70 mmHg
Peripheral vasoconstriction	+–++	+++	+++
Urine output	>50 ml/h	<50 ml/h	0–20 ml/h
Mental status	Mildly anxious	Anxious or confused	Confused or semiconscious

pheral veins can be immensely useful. Palpation of the skin rather than formal measurement of great toe temperature is particularly helpful. A cold foot indicates a deficit of approximately 500 ml, whereas a leg that is cold below the knee indicates a deficit of 2 l or more. Central venous pressure measurement is also helpful if the response to repeated fluid challenges is noted. Isolated readings are of little value because the central venous pressure can be normal in the presence of intense vasoconstriction. Total restoration of circulating blood volume requires reversal of the vasoconstriction which, if allowed to happen naturally, may take several hours, during which time replacement of fluid should continue. If time is limited, controlled vasodilatation using small doses of chlorpromazine or sodium nitroprusside and simultaneous administration of fluid may be preferable to precipitous vasodilatation at induction of anaesthesia.

If there is major blood loss or hypovolaemia occurs in a patient with myocardial disease, a pulmonary artery flotation catheter can be extremely helpful. It is also useful when surgery is likely to be lenghthy and bloody. Use of the catheter allows measurements of cardiac output and vascular filling to be made, and thus improves the accuracy of resuscitation. The prime purpose of resuscitation is to restore tissue oxygenation. For this reason all patients should be given oxygen during resuscitation and, if necessary, controlled mechanical ventilation should be used. It is not yet possible to measure at the bedside the adequacy of oxygenation of individual tissues. A global assessment of tissue oxygenation can be obtained by estimating oxygen delivery and consumption using arterial and mixed venous blood samples. Above a critical lower value, oxygen consumption is independent of oxygen delivery in well-oxygenated tissues (Bihari 1988). Pulmonary artery flotation catheters are associated with an appreciable incidence of complications. They should only be used in situations where the additional information obtained is likely to influence the patient's clinical management. For these patients, Shoemaker (1988) has produced an algorithm for emergency resuscitation which he has demonstrated increases the speed and effectiveness of resuscitation.

The full stomach

The inhalation of gastric contents is a problem that nearly always indicates faulty anaesthetic technique. It is responsible for between 15 and 40% of deaths associated with anaesthesia (Marx et al 1973, Holland 1984, Utting 1987).

The stomach may contain either solids, such as food and blood clot, or liqid. Pulmonary aspiration of solid may obstruct the trachea, bronchi or bronchioles, causing distal pulmonary collapse. If the operation is urgent a small area of collapse may be left untreated until the operation is complete. More serious obstructions should be removed immediately at bronchoscopy, or death from hypoxia may rapidly ensue. Aspiration of liquid blood causes severe hypoxia. The patient may require mechanical ventilation with high concentrations of oxygen for up to 72 h. Blood is usually cleared efficiently by the lungs and long-term problems are rare. Aspiration of acidic stomach contents causes severe lung damage, particularly if the pH is less than 2.5. Bronchospasm and pulmonary oedema develop within a few hours. Reflex cardiac arrest may be precipitated as acid enters the lungs. More commonly, death occurs later as a result of severe prolonged hypoxia.

Prevention is better than cure. The first step is recognition of patients at risk. The risk factors are listed below:

1. inadequate protective airway reflexes:
    - severe illness
    - debilitation
    - old age
    - opiate analgesics and sedative drugs
    - loss of consciousness:
        - head injury
        - alcoholic intoxication
        - general anaesthesia
        - shock
        - hypothermia
2. delayed gastric emptying:
    - trauma

- alcohol/nicotine
- hypothermia
- pain
- anxiety
- drugs, including opiate analgesics, benzodiazepines, anticholinergics and beta agonists
- gastrointestinal obstruction
- paralytic ileus

3. insufficient gastro-oesophageal sphincter tone:
   - hiatus hernia
   - nasogastric tube in situ
   - increased intra-abdominal pressure:
     - gastrointestinal obstruction
     - paralytic ileus
     - large abdominal masses, including the pregnant uterus
     - ascites
     - obesity.

On the ward and during transportation to theatre these patients should be nursed in the head-down lateral position. If a patient is deeply unconscious, or head injury contraindicates the head-down position, endotracheal intubation may be necessary.

There are many causes of delayed gastric emptying and huge variations between patients (Rose 1979, Horowitz & Pounder 1985). Ideally the induction of general anaesthesia should be delayed until it is certain that the stomach has emptied, but this may take 24 h. If the operation cannot be delayed for this length of time, measures to empty the stomach should be taken. Liquids may be aspirated through a nasogastric tube. If solids are present a large-bore stomach tube should be used. Stomach emptying can be hastened pharmacologically using metoclopramide (Olsson & Hallen 1982).

Complete stomach emptying is almost impossible to achieve. Further measures are necessary to neutralize acid stomach contents. Magnesium trisilicate is marginally more effective than colloidal aluminium hydroxide (Taylor & Pryse Davies 1966) or 0.3 molar sodium citrate (Hester & Heath 1977), although sodium citrate mixes more easily with the stomach contents, particularly if the patient is rolled through 360° (Holdsworth et al 1980). If inhalation of gastric contents occurs, sodium citrate is less toxic to the lungs than particulate antacids (Gibbs et al 1982). Cimetidine (Brock-Utne et al 1983) and ranitidine (Andrews et al 1982) are effective in reducing gastric acidity, but neither neutralizes acid already present in the stomach.

None of the aforementioned guarantees that the stomach is empty or that its contents are neutral; still more precautions are necessary. An awake intubation is sometimes possible if the patient's reflexes are diminished. It must be done skillfully because pharyngeal stimulation may cause vomiting. Intubation under local anaesthesia is an alternative, but postoperative inhalation may occur if the patient is extubated before the local anaesthetic has worn off. Usually, anaesthesia is induced intravenously and suxamethonium given to allow rapid intubation. Cricoid pressure is regarded by many as one of the most important measures available to prevent regurgitation of stomach contents. It is alarming to note that, in a study by Howells et al (1983), only half of the participants applied sufficient force to prevent regurgitation and 50% of the anaesthetists questioned had noted inadvertent release of cricoid pressure before the airway was protected. If an unfamiliar assistant is about to apply cricoid pressure, tactful instructions should be given prior to induction of general anaesthesia. The presence of a nasogastric tube probably prevents occlusion of the oesophagus by cricoid pressure, but may still be helpful because the stomach is decompressed so the likelihood of regurgitation is less. Some anaesthetists give a small dose of non-depolarizing muscle relaxant in an attempt to reduce suxamethonium-induced muscle fasciculations and hence a rise in intra-abdominal pressure. If this is done, failure to administer suxamethonium in a dose of 1.5 mg/kg may make intubation extremely difficult, thus increasing rather than decreasing the risk of vomiting and inhalation (Freund & Rubin 1972). Suxamethonium is contraindicated if there is an open eye injury as the rise in intraocular pressure may cause loss of eye contents and permanent blindness. Atracurium and vecuronium both act reasonably rapidly. With preoxygenation, secure intravenous access and careful timing it is possible to administer the relaxant before the induction agent and to secure the airway safely and smoothly without significant risk of inhalation.

Extubation is best delayed until protective airway reflexes are adequate. Coughing may provoke vomiting but, if the patient is extubated in the head-down lateral position, inhalation of gastric contents is unlikely. Patients with raised intracranial pressure or who have had open-eye operations are exceptions to this rule as the dangers of coughing or vomiting are greater than the risk of inhalation.

Aspiration of liquid stomach contents sometimes occurs in spite of precautionary measures. If acid aspiration does occur, colloids, not crystalloids, should be used for resuscitation. The use of steroids is sometimes advocated, but they are probably ineffective and certainly increase the risk of pulmonary infection and death from gram negative septicaemia (Wolfe et al 1977). Other aspects of management are supportive and are discussed in Chapter 16.

Alcohol abuse

More than 50% of patients who have suffered severe trauma are acutely intoxicated with alcohol. This in true both in the USA (Edwards & Mosher 1980) and in the UK. Alcohol-induced vasodilatation reduces the ability of these patients to compensate for blood loss and increases their susceptibility to hypothermia. Urine output is a poor guide to the adequacy of resuscitation because alcohol causes a diuresis by inhibiting antidiuretic hormone secretion. Alcohol delays stomach emptying by as much as 24 h (Rose 1979). Local anaesthesia may therefore seem an attractive alternative to general anaesthesia, but there will be practical difficulties if the patient is confused and uncooperative. This is not a problem if the patient is unconscious, but alcohol can cause vomiting and, if the airway is unprotected, the vomit may be inhaled. Alcohol is an excellent analgesic and it is sometimes possible to manipulate fractures or dislocations in acutely intoxicated patients without anaesthetic.

Prior to general anaesthesia the acutely intoxicated patient requires careful evaluation. Alcohol inhibits gluconeogenesis (Edwards & Mosher 1980) and these patients are susceptible to hypoglycaemic episodes which may occur up to 30 h after the last intake of alcohol. The risk of hypoglycaemia is increased if food is withheld in preparation for general anaesthesia. Smaller doses of barbiturates, sedatives and opiates are required. If recovery from anaesthesia is delayed this may be due to the effect of the alcohol or the anaesthetic drugs. It should never be assumed that this is so until other potentially fatal causes, such as hypoglycaemia or an extradural haematoma, have been excluded.

Chronic alcoholics are usually, but not always, acutely intoxicated on admission to hospital. The problems of chronic alcoholism should be sought in all patients who are acutely intoxicated and all those giving a history of heavy alcohol intake. In particular, they may suffer from megaloblastic anaemia, thrombocytopenia, clotting factor deficiencies, chronic respiratory infections, hypertension, beri-beri, alcoholic cardiomyopathy and autonomic neuropathy (Caldwell 1981). Alcoholics require increased doses of induction agents, opiates, sedatives and inhalational agents. These drugs should, however, be used with caution in the presence of alcoholic heart disease, autonomic neuropathy or hypovolaemia. The risk of awareness must be balanced against the risk of severe hypotension. Alcoholics also require increased doses of non-depolarizing muscle relaxants. Atracurium is probably the most suitable relaxant because it does not depend on hepatic metabolism for excretion (Stoetling et al 1988). Spinal and epidural anaesthesia should also be used with caution because the risk of hypotension is as much a problem as it is with general anaesthesia. In addition, unless blood clotting is known to be normal, excessive bleeding may cause a haematoma and spinal cord compression.

PREMEDICATION FOR EMERGENCY ANAESTHESIA

The preoperative assessment should include an evaluation of the need for premedication. Most patients are frightened or in pain and benefit from anxiolytic or analgesic drugs. Some will require other drugs such as steroids or prophylactic antibiotics.

ANAESTHESIA FOR EMERGENCY SURGERY

Choice of technique

There are three surgical emergencies that require emergency anaesthesia. The first is severe haemorrhage from the heart or an inaccessible major blood vessel. Patients with uncontrollable severe haemorrhage are usually shocked and unconscious, and can frequently be intubated without anaesthesia. Muscle relaxation may be required to aid surgical access. The patient should be ventilated with 100% oxygen until the source of haemorrhage has been controlled. A small dose of fentanyl or ketamine may also be given to provide analgesia. The second emergency is life-threatening upper airway obstruction unrelieved by manipulation of the jaw, or endotracheal intubation with or without local anaesthesia. Minitracheotomy (Matthews & Hopkinson 1983) through the cricothyroid membrane will provide immediate relief of the obstruction if it is above this level. The procedure is painless provided the skin is infiltrated with local anaesthetic, and is easy to perform. The alternative is a traditional tracheostomy. This can also be made under infiltration anaesthesia but is technically more difficult and therefore more time-consuming. Total obstruction of the trachea by a foreign body is rare and will not be relieved by a tracheostomy. Foreign bodies can sometimes be removed through a rigid bronchoscope, but moribund patients may require emergency thoracotomy and intubation of the bronchi. A similar procedure is necessary for patients with ruptured trachea. In either situation there is rarely time for anaesthesia until the obstruction has been bypassed. The third emergency is drainage of an intracranial haematoma. These patients should be fully anaesthetized and intubated using a rapid sequence technique and cricoid pressure. There will be no time to empty stomach contents or to reduce acidity. Although trauma victims usually have full stomachs, it is surprisingly common to find that the pH is neutral.

With these exceptions, there is always a certain length of time available to prepare the patient for theatre. The preoperative preparation of the patient has already been discussed. The anaesthetist should also use this time to consider which is the most suitable anaesthetic technique and to anticipate potential anaesthetic problems. There is very little evidence to suggest that one technique is better than any other. It has been suggested that ketamine is a useful induction agent for hypovolaemic patients because the sympathetic nervous system is stimulated and the blood pressure is raised at induction. Although the blood pressure rises, cardiac output does not alter (Brown 1987). This suggests that blood flow is redistributed and vasoconstriction occurs in some parts of the circulation. It is not known whether this redistribution is beneficial, or whether it causes a mismatch of oxygen supply and demand in important tissues such as the gut and liver. Ketamine has, however, been shown to be extremely safe when used on the battlefield (Perel 1987).

Each patient should be assessed individually and, having considered the relative importance of all the risk factors, the anaesthetist should choose the most suitable technique. This may involve an easy choice between local and general anaesthesia, or a more complicated decision such as alternative methods of induction avoiding suxamethonium for a patient with a perforating eye injury and a full stomach. Adequate time should be allowed for the preparation and checking of anaesthetic equipment. Anticipation and prevention of potential disasters by a well thought out anaesthetic technique and careful preparation of equipment will go a long way towards reducing anaesthetic mortality and morbidity.

MONITORING FOR EMERGENCY AND URGENT ANAESTHESIA

The Association of Anaesthetists of Great Britain and Ireland (1988) has produced standards for monitoring. These include various electromechanical devices for monitoring the adequacy of the circulation and oxygenation of the tissues. The most important monitoring device is the anaesthetist himself. Not only must he be present at the patient's side, but he must also be able to interpret the information being offered by the monitoring equipment. Often, when unexpected information appears, it is the monitor and not the patient that receives the first attention. In numerous studies of anaesthetic mortality, deaths have occurred because anesthetists have failed to recognize and treat the signs of impending disaster (Memery 1965). The prime purpose of monitoring is to provide early warning of abnormal parameters. An explanation should be sought for all abnormalities by examining the patient. If the patient appears to be well, the monitors should be checked. Treatment should never be started on the basis of an abnormal monitoring parameter without seeking confirmatory evidence that something is truly amiss. This evidence may come from examining the patient or from other monitors. The effects of treating a monitoring abnormality when the monitor is malfunctioning can be as dangerous as ignoring the monitor altogether (see Ch. 44).

HAZARDS AND COMPLICATIONS OF ANAESTHESIA OCCURING IN THE POSTOPERATIVE PERIOD

Approximately 30% of deaths related to anaesthesia occur as a result of complications occuring in the postoperative period (Dripps et al 1961, Lunn et al 1983). Many of these deaths are due to inadequately treated respiratory failure which is usually due to laryngeal stridor or the depressant effects of anaesthetic drugs. Depressant anaesthetic drugs are also responsible for loss of protective airway reflexes and an appreciable incidence of inhalation of gastric contents postoperatively. Most other deaths are due to circulatory collapse as a result of myocardial failure or untreated hypovolaemia.

Hypothermia, defined as a core temperature of less than 35°C, can cause several problems in the postoperative period. It may delay recovery from anaesthesia due to reduced metabolism and excretion of drugs, or cause intense shivering which increases oxygen demand by as much as 500% (Bay et al 1968), and may increase pain and anxiety. It also causes vasoconstriction which may mask hypovolaemia. In trauma patients, hypothermia has been shown to be associated with an increase in mortality rate and this effect is independent of other factors such as major blood loss or shock (Jurkovich et al 1987).

Some patients, such as the elderly and those involved in road traffic accidents, may already be hypothermic when admitted to hospital. Body temperature may drop still further in the Accident and Emergency department. It is essential to remove the patient's clothes to make a complete physical examination, but this should be completed as quickly as possible and the patient covered with warm blankets immediately after the examination. Numerous factors contribute to heat loss during anaesthesia:

- ambient temperature <24°C
- low basal metabolic rate (e.g. the elderly, myxoedema)
- large area relative to body weight for heat loss (e.g. children, abdominal and thoracic operations)
- vasodilatation produced by anaesthetic drugs
- abolition of shivering reflex by anaesthetic drugs
- ventilation with cold, dry gases
- intravenous infusion of cold fluids
- cold irrigation fluids
- prolonged operating time.

Of these factors, transfusion of cold blood is probably the most important. When blood at 4°C is transfused at rates of 50 ml/h or more, the postoperative mortality rate is nearly 60%. It can be reduced to 7% simply by warming the blood to 32°C before transfusion (Boyan 1964). All anaesthetics, with the exception of ketamine, cause heat loss, but the type of anaesthetic does not seem to influence the degree of hypothermia (Vaughan et al 1981).

Core temperatures of less than 33°C are associated with major physiological disturbances. These include a reduction in cardiac output, conduction defects and dysrhythmias, abnormalities in serum potassium and glucose levels, increased viscosity of the blood and an increase in haemoglobin oxygen affinity, a decrease in glomerular filtration rate, a decrease in the level of consciousness, and an increase in sensitivity to sedative drugs, inhalational agents and long-acting muscle relaxants (Morley-Forster 1986). Furthermore, cold tissues, especially fat, skin and peripheral nerves, are particularly susceptible to trauma. Acute renal failure and pancreatitis may complicate hypothermia and are thought to be caused by prolonged vasoconstriction and tissue hypoxia during rewarming (McNicol & Smith 1964).

The body has numerous thermoregulatory mechanisms, most of which are abolished by anaesthesia. It is therefore the anaesthetist's responsibility to reduce heat loss during anaesthesia and surgery. Patients at particular risk should be identified and their temperature monitored carefully. Extremes of age, major haemorrhage, preoperative hypothermia, lengthy surgery, and abdominal and thoracic operations are all associated with hypothermia (Holloway 1988). Hypothermia can occur in adults if the ambient temperature in the operating theatre is less than 24°C (Hall 1978). Surgeons, however, are uncomfortable at this temperature and are likely to work more slowly. It is usual to maintain the theatre temperature at 21°C, which is a reasonable compromise between the surgeon's and the patient's needs. The use of warmed, humidified gases in conjunction with a warming blanket has been shown to be an effective means of maintaining body temperature (Tølløfsrud et al 1984), as has the warming of all infusion fluids (Roizen et al 1980). The speed with which these measures are commenced is probably more important than the methods used (Bernard et al 1987). Occasionally, measures to prevent hypothermia are so effective that hyperthermia occurs. It is therefore important to monitor body temperature closely. All heating equipment should be serviced regularly and have a temperature gauge. Haemolysis of blood, and skin and respiratory tract burns can occur if equipment overheats as a result of thermostat failure.

The duration of postoperative hypothermia correlates well with the mortality rate (Slotman et al 1985). Rewarming should, therefore, be as rapid as possible but should not exceed 1.2°C/h unless ventricular fibrillation has occurred. Fluctuations in serum potassium and glucose levels during rewarming require constant monitoring and treatment. Until rewarming is complete, relative hypovolaemia caused by fluid shifts should be treated with vasopressors if the patient is hypotensive. If fluids are given during rewarming, pulmonary and cerebral oedema may occur on recovery. Urine output and skin–core temperature difference do not reflect the adequacy of cardiac output which may require measurement with a flow-directed pulmonary artery catheter. This can also be used to measure the adequacy of tissue oxygenation. Tissue hypoxia can be reduced by increasing inspired oxygen concentration, reducing the work of breathing and preventing shivering. This is most easily achieved by paralysing and ventilating the patient with warmed, humidified gases until recovery is complete. Endotracheal intubation has the additional advantage of providing airway protection (Derek & Hockaday 1969).

Most complications in the recovery period are preventable. The anaesthetist should not leave until the patient is able to maintain his own airway, is breathing normally and cardiovascular parameters are stable. It is also essential to ensure that a plan of postoperative management, including the administration of intravenous fluids and analgesia, is agreed with the surgeons and that it is clearly understood who will be responsible for the patient's future management.

CONCLUSION

This chapter describes the hazards and complications of emergency anaesthesia. These problems are more common with emergency anaesthesia but can and do occur in association with elective anaesthesia. In almost all cases they can be prevented. The key factors that will lead to a reduction in mortality and morbidity after anaesthesia are listed as follows:

1. The anaesthetist in charge of the patient must be able to recognize, understand and deal with all possible problems associated with that patient.
2. A comprehensive preoperative assessment is necessary to establish the existence of potential problems.
3. Anticipation of potential problems allows preoperative treatment of the patient, choice of the most suitable anaesthetic technique, preparation of any special equipment and, most important of all, consultation with senior anaesthetic colleagues.
4. Monitoring should be comprehensive and vigilant. A cause should be identified for all abnormalities and prompt action taken to correct them.
5. The recovery period is associated with several problems directly related to anaesthesia. Continued vigilance is necessary until recovery from anaesthesia is complete and the patient has been transferred to the care of the surgeons.

REFERENCES

Andrews A D, Brock-Utne J G, Downing J W 1982 Protection against pulmonary acid aspiration with ranitidine. Anaesthesia 37: 22–25

Association of Anaesthetists of Great Britain and Ireland 1988 Recommendations for standards of monitoring during anaesthesia and recovery. Association of Anaesthetists, London

Bay J, Nunn J F, Prys-Roberts C 1968 Factors influencing arterial PO_2 during recovery from anaesthesia. Br J Anaesth 40: 398–407

Bernard J M, Pinaud M, Souron R 1987 Peroperative hypothermia prevention. Acta Anaesthesiol Scand 31: 521–523

Bevan D R 1978 Peri-operative care: intraoperative fluid balance. Br J Hosp Med 19: 445–453

Bihari D 1988 Oxygen delivery and consumption in the critically ill: their relation to the development of multiple organ failure. In: Kox W, Bihari D (eds) Shock and the adult respiratory distress syndrome. Springer-Verlag, London, p 95–122

Blery C, Szatan M, Fourgeaux B et al 1986 Evaluation of a protocol for selective ordering of preoperative tests. Lancet 1: 139–141

Boyan C P 1964 Cold or warmed blood for massive transfusions. Ann Surg 160: 282–286

Bradley J P, Beem M F, O'Donnell J E, Van de Meene A H 1988 Mortality audit in a large teaching hospital. Anaesth Intensive Care 16: 94–97

Brock-Utne J G, Downing J W, O'Keefe S J D, Gjessing J 1983 Protection against acid pulmonary aspiration with cimetidine. Anaesth Intensive Care 11: 138–140

Brown D L 1987 Anesthetic agents in trauma surgery: are there differences? Int Anesthesiol Clin 25(1): 75–90

Buck N, Devlin H B, Lunn J N 1988 Confidential enquiry into perioperative deaths. The Nuffield Provincial Hospitals Trust, London

Caldwell T 1981 Anaesthesia for patients with behavioural and environmental disorders. In: Katz J, Benumof J, Kadis L B (eds) Anesthesia and uncommon diseases, 2nd edn. Saunders, Philadelphia, p 672–777

Cason J S 1981 Shock. In: Treatment of burns. Chapman and Hall, London, p 24–27

Cooper A L, Leigh J M, Tring I C 1989 Admissions to the intensive care unit after complications of anaesthetic techniques over 10 years. Anaesthesia 44: 953–958

Derek T, Hockaday R 1969 Accidental hypothermia. Br J Hosp Med 2: 1083–1093

Dripps R D, Lamont A, Eckenhoff J E 1961 The role of anaesthesia in surgical mortality. J Am Med Assoc 178: 261–266

Edwards R, Mosher V B 1980 Alcohol abuse, anaesthesia and intensive care. Anaesthesia 35: 474–489

Fisher M M McD 1990 The crystalloid versus colloid controversy. Clinical Intensive Care 1: 52–57

Freund F G, Rubin A P 1972 The need for additional succinylcholine after d-tubocararine. Anesthesiology 36: 185–187

Gibbs C P, Spohr L, Schmidt D 1982 The effectiveness of sodium citrate as an antacid. Anesthesiology 57: 44–46

Goldman L, Caldera D L, Nussbaum S R et al 1977 Multifactorial index of cardiac risk in non-cardiac surgical procedures. New Engl J Med 297: 845–850

Hall G M 1978 Body temperature and anaesthesia. Br J Anaesth 50: 39–44

Heath M L 1982 Deaths after intravenous regional anaesthesia. Br Med J 285: 913–914

Hester J B, Heath M L 1977 Pulmonary acid aspiration syndrome: should prophylaxis be routine? Br J Anaesth 49: 595–599

Holdsworth J D, Johnson K, Mascall G, Roulston R G, Tomlinson P A 1980 Mixing of antacids with stomach contents. Anaesthesia 35: 641–650

Holland R 1984 Anesthesia-related mortality in Australia. Int Anesthesiol Clin 22(2): 31–42

Holland R 1987 Anaesthetic mortality in New South Wales. Br J Anaesth 59: 834–841

Holloway A M 1988 Monitoring and controlling temperature. Anaesth Intensive Care 16: 44–47

Horowitz M, Pounder D J 1985 Gastric emptying: forensic implications of current concepts. Medicine, Science and Law 25: 201–214

Howells T H, Chamney A R, Wraight W J, Simons R S 1983 The application of cricoid pressure. Anaesthesia 38: 457–460

Hutton P, Cooper G 1985 Guidelines in clinical anaesthesia. Blackwell Scientific, Oxford

Isbister J P 1984 Haemotherapy for acute haemorrhage. Anaesth Intensive Care 12: 217–228

Jenkins G C 1986 Haematological disorders. Clin Anesth 4(3): 651–666

Jurkovich G J, Greiser W B, Luterman A, Curreri W 1987 Hypothermia in trauma victims: an ominous predictor of survival. J Trauma 27: 1019–1024

Kreimeier U, Messmer K 1988 Small-volume resuscitation. In: Kox W J, Gamble J (eds) Fluid resuscitation. Clin Anesth 2(3): 545–578

London P S 1968 Traumatic Shock. Br J Hosp Med 1: 312–321

Lunn J N, Hunter A R, Scott D B 1983 Anaesthesia-related surgical mortality. Anaesthesia 38: 1090–1096

McNicol M W, Smith R 1964 Accidental hypothermia. Br Med J 1: 19–21

Marx G F, Mateo C V, Orkin L R 1973 Computer analysis of postanaesthetic deaths. Anesthesiology 39: 54–58

Matthews H R, Hopkinson R B 1983 Treatment of sputum retention by minitracheotomy. Br J Surg 70: 1–4

Memery H N 1965 Anesthesia mortality in private practice. J Am Med Assoc 194: 1185–1188

Morley-Forster P K 1986 Unintentional hypothermia in the operating room. Can Anaesth Soc J 33: 516–527

Olsson G L, Hallen B 1982 Pharmacological evacuation of the stomach with metoclopramide. Acta Anaesthesiol Scand 26: 417–420

Otto C W 1980 Respiratory morbidity and mortality. Int Anesthesiol Clin 18(3): 85–106

Pedersen T, Eliasen K, Ravnborg M et al 1986 Risk factors, complications and outcome in anaesthesia: a pilot study. Eur J Anaesth 3: 225–239

Pedersen T, Johansen S H 1989 Serious morbidity attributable to anaesthesia. Anaesthesia 44: 504–508

Perel A 1987 Battlefield anesthesia. Int Anesthesiol Clin 25(1): 175–189

Rabkin S W, Horne J M 1983 Preoperative electrocardiography: effect of new abnormalities on clinical decisions. Can Med Assoc J 128: 146–147

Rao T L K, Jacobs K H, El-Etr A A 1983 Reinfarction following anaesthesia in patients with myocardial infarction. Anesthesiology 59: 499–505

Redl H, Schlag G 1990 Pathophysiology of multi-organ failure: proposed mechanisms. Clinical Intensive Care 1: 66–71

Roizen M F, Sohn Y J, L'Hommedieu C S, Wylie E J, Ota M K 1980 Operating room temperature prior to surgical draping: effect on patient temperature in the recovery room. Anesth Analg 59: 852–855

Rose E F 1979 Factors influencing gastric emptying. J Forensic Sci 24: 200–206

Seymour D G, Pringle R, Shaw J W 1982 The role of routine preoperative chest X-ray in the elderly general surgical patient. Postgrad Med J 58: 741–745

Seymour D G, Pringle R, Maclennan 1983 The role of the routine preoperative cardiogram in the elderly surgical patient. Age Ageing 12: 97–104

Shoemaker W C, Kram H B 1988 Crystalloid and colloid fluid therapy in resuscitation and subsequent ICU management. In: Kox W J, Gamble J (eds) Fluid resuscitation. Clin Anesth 2(3): 509–544

Slotman G J, Jed E H, Burchard K W 1985 Adverse effects of hypothermia in postoperative patients. Am J Surg 149: 495–501

Stein M, Cassara E L 1970 Preoperative pulmonary evaluation and therapy for surgery patients. J Am Med Assoc 211: 787–790

Stoetling R K, Dierdorf S F, McCammon R L 1988 Diseases of the liver and biliary tract. In: Anaesthesia and co-existing disease, 2nd edn. Churchill Livingstone, New York, p 382–385

Sutcliffe A J 1983 Preoperative preparation. In: Handbook of emergency anaesthesia. Butterworths, London, p 3–13

Taylor G, Pryse Davies J 1966 The prophylactic use of antacids in the prevention of the acid pulmonary aspiration syndrome. Lancet 1: 288–291

Tølløfsrud S G, Gundersen Y, Andersen R 1984 Peroperative hypothermia. Acta Anaesthesiol Scand 28: 511–515

Utting J E 1987 Pitfalls in anaesthetic practice. Br J Anaesth 59: 877–890

Utting J E, Gray T C, Shelley F C 1979 Human misadventure in anaesthesia. Can Anaesth Soc J 26: 472–478

Vacanti C J, VanHouten R J, Hill R C 1970 A statistical analysis of the relationship of physical status to postoperative mortality of 68 388 cases. Anesth Analg 49: 564–566

Vaughan M S, Vaughan R W, Cork R C 1981 Postoperative hypothermia in adults: relationship of age, anaesthesia and shivering to rewarming. Anesth Analg 60: 746–751

Whitehead T P, Wootton I D P 1974 Biochemical profiles for hospital patients. Lancet 2: 1439–1443

Wolfe J E, Bone R C, Ruth W E 1977 Effect of corticosteroids in the treatment of patients with gastric aspiration. Am J Med 63: 719–722

Zelcer J, Wells D G 1987 Anaesthetic-related recovery room complications. Anaesth Intensive Care 15: 168–174

40

Anaesthesia for labour and operative delivery

R. A. Green

INTRODUCTION

Childbirth is inevitably associated with some degree of hazard for both mother and child, but during this century there has been a steady decline in both morbidity and mortality. In the 33 years from 1955–1987 the maternal death rate in the UK decreased from 67.1 to 7.6 per 100 000 total births. The percentage of deaths due to maternal causes also declined over the same period. In the 3 years between 1955 and 1957, pregnancy accounted for some 4.0% of all deaths in the age group 15 to 44 years. By the triennium 1985–1987, pregnancy was associated with only 0.7% of deaths in the same age-group (DOH 1991).

Although neonatal and maternal mortality is likely to continue declining with advancing medical techniques, there is always the danger that these techniques may bring with them their own inherent risks. It is these risks that have led to the belief by many groups of women that labour is dominated too much by medical interference and as a result there has been a resurgance of requests for natural childbirth which, by its very nature, has no iatrogenic hazards. However, experience shows that the majority of women, even those most dedicated to natural childbirth, seek some medical assistance before labour is completed.

It is the objective of this chapter to emphasize the risks to both mother and child of modern methods of pain relief during labour and operative delivery, and to discuss, first, how to avoid these hazards and second, how to treat any complications that may arise. This chapter should be read in conjunction with Chapter 11 which deals with the physiological changes of pregnancy that make provision of anaesthesia more hazardous. Quite apart from the hazards of pregnancy, however, there are specific problems related to operative delivery. It is these that will be dealt with here.

BASIC PHYSIOLOGICAL CONSIDERATIONS

The basic physiological changes during pregnancy with anaesthetic implications are discussed in detail in Chapter 11 and will only be dealt with superficially here.

Cardiovascular changes

In the last few months of pregnancy there is a 35–40% increase in blood volume and a 50% increase in cardiac output. In the healthy patient these changes are well compensated by a reduction in peripheral resistance and blood viscosity. Such changes therefore have very little influence on the hazards of general anaesthesia but, in the presence of heart disease and reduced myocardial reserve, full-term pregnancy may prove a considerable strain on the patient, particularly during labour when there is evidence of circulatory failure. Provided there is no evidence of circulatory failure when labour begins, these patients are best managed with well-monitored epidural analgesia and low forceps delivery to shorten the second stage. Caution should be exercised in the use of ergometrine after delivery (Johnstone 1973) as it may induce pulmonary oedema. Oxytocin is just as effective in the management of third-stage bleeding and is appreciably safer (Moir & Amoa 1979).

The delivery of women in circulatory failure when labour begins may present difficult problems, but on balance they are probably best delivered by caesarean section under general anaesthesia and moved to an intensive care unit postoperatively.

Effect on epidural analgesia

The cardiovascular changes during late pregnancy have a greater effect on the conduct of epidural analgesia than they do on general anaesthesia. The increase in blood volume and the compression of the lumbar venous plexus by the enlarged uterus may cause considerable engorgement of the venous plexus within the epidural space. This delays the absorption and increases the spread of fluid within the space, so smaller volumes of local anaesthetic are required to achieve the same height of block than would be necessary in the non-pregnant woman. As a corollary to this, if spinal (subarachnoid) anaesthesia is used during labour, particularly in the second stage, a unit dose of local anaesthetic may produce an abnormally high block owing to the fluctuation of CSF pressure during uterine contractions and bearing down efforts. Caution is therefore necessary.

Effect on blood pressure

The blood pressure may be profoundly affected by posture during late pregnancy. The supine posture combined with epidural block are well known to cause hypotension and reduced utero-placental blood flow. Less obviously, the aorta may also be compressed causing a reduction in placental blood flow and a threat to fetal oxygenation (Ekstein & Marx 1974, Joupilla et al 1978). Left lateral tilt is all that is necessary in most cases.

Respiratory changes

After the fifth month of pregnancy there is a significant progressive change in respiratory physiology which, if not recognized, may increase the hazards of general anaesthesia. At full term there is a 15–20% reduction in functional residual capacity (FRC) and expiratory reserve volume (ERV), and an appreciable increase in minute ventilation.

These factors will influence the speed of induction and recovery from general anaesthesia, causing them to be more rapid compared with anaesthesia in the non-pregnant woman. There is also a 20% increase in oxygen uptake in late pregnancy which leads to a rapid development of hypoxaemia during periods of apnoea or hypoventilation, hence the value of preoxygenation prior to the administration of general anaesthesia. This puts the patient at special risk during difficult intubation, a subject to be discussed later.

Artificial ventilation during caesarean section may also be influenced by these changes, as carbon dioxide washout is more rapidly achieved and the consequent respiratory alkalosis may produce a significant reduction in uterine blood flow with fetal hypoxaemia and subsequent failure of the neonate to breathe immediately after delivery.

TOXAEMIA OF PREGNANCY

The additional physiological changes that occur during toxaemia of pregnancy present special hazards to the anaesthetist and merit particular attention. When considering the safest method of management the following considerations are important:

- blood volume
- vascular reactivity
- generalized oedema
- drug interaction
- coagulopathy
- placental insufficiency.

Blood volume

In spite of the oedematous appearance, pre-eclampsia and eclampsia are accompanied by an overall decrease in blood volume with haemoconcentration producing an increased tendency to postural hypotension, and a catastrophic fall in blood pressure if epidural analgesia is used. However, provided there is no evidence of coagulation disorder, epidural analgesia may be helpful in the management of these patients (Moir et al 1972). Constant blood pressure monitoring and a fluid load is therefore particularly important. Fluid loading is best accomplished with a colloid rather than a crystalloid solution if further oedema is to be avoided. In severely ill patients a central venous line is important, but of course the presence of a coagulation disorder may make insertion more hazardous.

Vascular reactivity

There is a generalized increase in sympathetic activity and increased responsiveness to circulating catecholamines and other vasopressor substances (Grant et al 1973). Care must therefore be exercised to avoid a further increase in blood pressure due to the stimulation of intubation. It is important to have well-established general anaesthesia and good topical analgesia before attempting intubation (Hodgkinson & Hussain 1979).

Generalized oedema

The generalized oedema may cause intubation difficulties and the risk of laryngeal obstruction on extubation. Special attention must be paid to the airway during the postoperative period.

Drug interaction

Hypoproteinaemia

If general anaesthesia is used the low plasma protein concentration must be taken into consideration as drugs such as thiopentone and bupivacaine, which are highly protein-bound, will need to be given in reduced dosage.

Magnesium sulphate

As magnesium sulphate may be used in pre-eclampsia, its action in potentiating muscle relaxants must always be considered and its dosage must be carefully monitored (Gohoneim & Long 1970).

Coagulopathy

Eclampsia and pre-eclampsia often interfere with fibrinogen levels causing an increased tendency to bleeding. This is a contraindication to the use of spinal or epidural analgesia. Coagulation studies must always be carried out on pre-eclamptic and eclamptic women prior to conduction anaesthesia or the insertion of a central venous cannula in the neck.

Placental insufficiency

The fetus is at high risk in toxaemia due to prematurity and placental insufficiency, therefore the maintenance of maximum uterine blood flow and maternal oxygenation is particularly important during anaesthesia and analgesia in these patients. If conduction anaesthesia is used, blood pressure must be maintained with fluid preloading and ephedrine, if necessary.

Anaesthesia for patients with pre-eclampsia

Mild pre-eclampsia

Mothers with mild pre-eclampsia usually present no particular anaesthetic hazard, but every attempt must be made to use techniques that reduce the likelihood of increasing maternal blood pressure. Epidural analgesia not only avoids the sympathetic overactivity associated with pain, but also assists the use of low forceps delivery, thus reducing the period of straining in the second stage of labour (Crawford 1978). In addition, epidural analgesia reduces significantly the incidence and severity of neonatal depression in the fetus at risk as compared with systemic analgesia or general anaesthesia. As a means of controlling blood pressure, however, epidural analgesia has proved disappointing. Epidural analgesia must not be used if there is an abnormality of blood clotting.

Severe pre-eclampsia

The management of a patient with severe pre-eclampsia should involve discussion between obstetrician, paediatrician and anaesthetist, but the anaesthetist will play a major role in securing the safety of both the mother and baby during vaginal delivery or caesarean section as well as ensuring the mother's continuing well-being in the postoperative period. During vaginal delivery the anaesthetist has a number of responsibilities:

1. To maintain adequate pain relief at all times during labour as inadequate pain relief may provoke a further increase in blood pressure. This is best achieved with epidural analgesia provided the clotting mechanism is not seriously impaired.
2. To maintain adequate blood pressure during epidural analgesia by careful monitoring and fluid loading with colloid, plasma protein and crystalloid solution. Plasma protein fraction (250 ml) plus Ringer's lactate solution (250 ml) before inducing analgesia may be adequate , but the patient with hypertension, oedema and oliguria may need a large volume of fluid which should only be given under central venous pressure (CVP) monitoring. A CVP of 6–8 mmHg is reasonable for a spontaneously breathing patient.
3. Oxygen should be continuously administered to the mother in order to maintain optimal fetal oxygenation.

Many obstetricians favour delivery by caesarean section in these patients and, on balance, general anaesthesia is probably safest for this.

The main hazards of general anaesthesia occur during induction and intubation when a hypertensive crisis may develop (Hodgkinson and Hussain 1979). Although deep anaesthesia prior to intubation would help to avoid such a crisis, this is unsuitable for the obstetric patient. Stable anaesthesia and good topical analgesia of the larynx and trachea are essential prior to intubation, and continuous blood pressure monitoring is mandatory. Some workers advocate the use of a hypotensive agent prior to induction. Hydrallazine (20 mg intravenously) is recommended and beta blockers may also be used. A single bolus injection of 25–50 mg of labetalol (a combined alpha and beta blocking agent) may be preferred, but sodium nitroprusside or a similar infusion should be at hand to control any sudden or excessive rise in blood pressure during the induction of anaesthesia. Convulsions prior to induction are readily controlled by induction of anaesthesia with thiopentone.

THE ADMINISTRATION OF SEDATIVES AND NARCOTICS DURING LABOUR

It may occasionally be necessary to administer sedative drugs to the mother during labour. Such drugs are best avoided unless specifically indicated. However, if given at the right time and in minimal doses, they carry no appreciable risk to mother and baby, but it must always be remembered that all sedatives pass through the placental barrier and may accumulate in the baby.

Barbiturates

Barbiturates are best avoided immediately prior to or during labour as their prolonged action may lead to sluggish neonatal responses, particularly when attempting to establish feeding.

Tranquillizers

In the apprehensive and anxious mother, tranquillizers may afford a very positive benefit to the course of labour, but the possible effect on the neonate must never be forgotten.

Promethazine or Promazine in doses of up to 50 mg intramuscularly or 20 mg intravenously are probably the drugs of choice as they are good anxiolitics and carry the least hazard to the neonate. Benzodiazepines, such as diazepam and lorazepam, are popular sedatives during labour, particularly prior to epidural analgesia in the anxious mother. Diazepam, for example, presents little hazard to the neonate provided the dose is kept below 0.3 mg/kg over a 4–6 h period. These drugs pass the placental barrier rapidly and therefore accumulate in fetal tissues if large doses are used. This may produce hypotonia, lethargy and sluggish feeding for at least 48 h after delivery (Gamble et al 1977). Midazolam has a shorter half-life than diazepam and would seem to pass the placental barrier less readily than other benzodiazepines (Vree et al 1984), but it has not yet been investigated extensively in pregnancy.

Special care must be taken with the premature baby if benzodiazepines have been used because of the tendency to loss of temperature control.

Narcotics

Before the introduction of regional analgesia for relief of pain during labour, narcotic analgesics held the pride of place although many women have found 50% nitrous oxide in oxygen to be all that is required. In order to get optimal benefit from narcotic analgesia without undesirable side effects, the timing and dose of the drug must be carefully chosen. Pethidine is the drug most commonly used and, if adequate dosage is employed (1.5–1.8 mg/kg), satisfactory pain control can be achieved in about 70% of mothers without undue neonatal depression, provided the last dose is given at least 4 h before delivery.

For mothers that experience severe pain in the second stage of labour or with rapid progress of labour, pethidine is best given intravenously in a dose of about 0.5 mg/kg over a period of 10–15 min. A syringe pump is a satisfactory method of administration.

Meptazinol is claimed to have a less depressant effect on the neonate while providing analgesia equivalent to pethidine. Its true place in obstetric practice remains to be established. Nicholas & Robson (1982) claim better analgesia with less fetal depression than a similar dose of pethidine, whereas Morrison et al (1987) could detect no significant difference between the drugs. For some years, premixed solutions of a narcotic and a narcotic antagonist were employed with the false impression that these drugs gave good analgesia without the hazard of neonatal depression. Pethilorfan (Pethidine & Levallorphan 10:0.125) was the commonly used drug. These mixtures have no advantage and have mostly been abandoned (Campbell 1965).

If neonatal depression is thought to be due to narcotic depression, the narcotic antagonist naloxone (Narcan Neonatal^R) can be safely given to the infant in a dose of 5–10 mcg/kg intramuscularly. Dosage depends on the severity of the respiratory depression.

ANAESTHESIA AND ANALGESIA FOR OPERATIVE DELIVERY

General anaesthesia for operative delivery has always been treated with great respect by the trained anaesthetist, and often with trepidation by the trainee because of the specific hazards involved. These hazards may be compounded because the operation is frequently unplanned and therefore dealt with by relatively inexperienced junior staff. Efforts to increase the safety of obstetric anaesthesia must, therefore, involve not only good training in obstetric anaesthesia, but also special attention to the logistics of all obstetric anaesthesia services, so that junior staff are not left to manage emergencies unsupervised.

Progress has undoubtedly been prompted by many of the recommendations made in the regular Reports on Confidential Enquiries into Maternal Deaths in the United Kingdom, which have appeared every 3 years since 1954. It is pleasing to note that the contribution of anaesthesia to maternal mortality appears to be declining (from 10.8% of maternal deaths in 1970–1972 to 4.4% of maternal deaths in 1985–1987), in spite of an increasing number of anaesthetics being given during pregnancy. However the 1985–1987 triennial report points out that 'there is still a high incidence of tracheal tube problems', and it suggests that 'there is a need to concentrate resources in units where consultant cover can be provided continuously' (DOH 1991).

Choice of general anaesthesia or regional analgesia

Before discussing the hazards of obstetric anaesthesia for operative delivery, it may be helpful to give a general review of the relative merits of general anaesthesia compared with regional analgesia. It is appreciated that to some extent the choice will depend upon the competence of the anaesthetist in managing each technique but, given equal ability, there is probably little to choose between the two methods when the overall hazards to both mother and child are taken into consideration. There is, however, some evidence to suggest that the neonate that has become distressed by prolonged labour, maternal hypotension or an unforeseen intrauterine accident may be more adversely affected by the general anaesthetic agents that those born in similar stress under well-conducted regional analgesia, provided further maternal hypotension is avoided (Moir & Willcocks 1968).

The patient's preference

Provided the anaesthetist concerned is thoroughly competent in both methods, the preference of the patient must receive careful consideration. It should, however, be remembered that an anaesthetist trained in regional analgesia for general surgery is not necessarily familiar with the particular problems involved in the obstetric patient.

Unless there are very special circumstances, such as anticipated difficult intubation, it is generally unwise to use regional analgesia against the patient's wishes, as such an event will inevitably end in a stressful operation with an overall increase in the hazards involved.

For those parents that believe in the importance of immediate contact with their baby on delivery to improve the bonding between mother and child, every effort should be made to use regional analgesia for operative delivery. Provided the analgesia has been competently performed, the operation will almost certainly be a happy event. If the mother is feeling anxious, ill or sick and the father is feeling faint at the time of delivery, bonding will almost certainly not be enhanced by the experience. Although many anaesthetists might take pride in successful epidural anaesthesia for caesarean section and get a great deal of satisfaction from it, many patients will find it an almost intolerable ordeal and will not seek to repeat the experience. The secret of success apart from competent administration is good communication between patient and anaesthetist.

In conclusion, the choice between these two methods of anaesthesia for elective caesarean section, provided there is no absolute contra-indication to either method, must be influenced mainly by the mother's preference and the anaesthetist's skill in each procedure. For operative vaginal delivery, regional analgesia is always to be preferred unless there is an emergency that will not wait for the delay in inducing a satisfactory block. Regional analgesia in unquestionably less hazardous than general anaesthesia for this procedure.

Hazards of general anaesthesia for caesarean section

The hazards of general anaesthesia for caesarean section are greater than in any other group of healthy patients. The reasons for this are not difficult to find. First, the presence of a pregnant uterus, altered sphincter activity and emergency surgery means an increased risk of gastric regurgitation. Second, the ever present fear of gastric regurgitation often leads to hurried induction of anaesthesia, with consequent increased risk of oesophageal intubation and failure to maintain adequate fetal and maternal oxygenation. Third, the presence of the unborn child demands that premedication and anaesthesia must be kept to a minimum, thus there is always a risk of awareness during the operative procedure. Fourth, the anaesthetic drugs and hypocarbia from hyperventilation may cause fetal depression and/or hypoxia (Moya et al 1965, Levinson et al 1974).

Regurgitation of gastric contents

The problem of regurgitation and inhalation of stomach contents during the induction of anaesthesia was described by Mendelson (1946), but did not appear as a major hazard in obstetric anaesthesia until after the introduction of muscle relaxation for intubation. The true incidence of Mendelson's syndrome is unknown but the mortality rate due to it fortunately appears to be declining. In the 1985–1987 triennial report on

Maternal Mortality in the UK (DOH 1991), only one woman died from inhalation of gastric contents in association with anaesthesia. This is in marked contrast to the situation in the early 1970s when 14 mothers died of the same cause over a similar period of time. Whether this improvement is temporary or due to improvements in the delivery of anaesthesia in the UK is unclear. Disturbingly the woman died in spite of administration of ranitidine and sodium citrate and the presence of a skilled anaesthetic assistant. Cricoid pressure was administered, but still the patient regurgitated and inhaled at induction.

The main weakness of the standard induction technique is that it involves the use of suxamethonium, the only muscle relaxant known to increase the intragastric pressure, thus potentially increasing the risk of regurgitation in the obstetric patient (Anderson 1962). Since the pregnant woman starts with a considerably increased intragastric pressure before induction of anaesthesia (Lind et al 1968), it would seem logical to use a technique that avoids suxamethonium and therefore will not exacerbate the problem (Green 1978). The dependence on correct cricoid pressure is then not so great. In an attempt to avoid this problem I have used the technique described below for many years.

Prior to surgery the patient is given standard antacid prophylaxis (see Table 40.1) This is designed to increase the pH of gastric juice above the critical level of 2.5 (Taylor & Pryse-Davies 1966, Husmeyer & Davenport 1980). In addition, premedication with metoclopramide increases the tone of the aesophageal sphincter and aids gastric emptying. The maximum effect on gastric emptying is achieved by giving an intravenous dose (Murphy et al 1984). Atropine antagonizes the beneficial effect on the oesophageal tone (Cotton & Smith 1978) and is not used.

Table 40.1 Antacid prophylaxis

Drug	Quantity	Method	Time
Ranitidine	150 mg	Orally	6 hourly throughout labour
Ranitidine	50 mg	Intravenously	As soon as decision to operate is taken
Sodium citrate (0.3 M)	30 ml	Orally	Prior to induction

Before induction of anaesthesia the patient is placed on the operating table with 25° head-up tilt. Oxygen is administered and intravenous access is secured. A non-depolarizing muscle relaxant (0.1 mg/kg vecuronium, for example) (Martin et al 1990) is injected into a running infusion. This is followed a few seconds later by a sleep dose of the induction agent. During the next 60–90 s a nitrous oxide/oxygen mixture (60/40) is administered by face mask and cricoid pressure is applied. The patient is intubated, then placed horizontally with a lateral wedge inserted and surgery begins.

In the rare event of immediate intubation proving difficult, an airway is inserted. The patient's lungs are inflated with nitrous oxide, oxygen and a low concentration of a volatile agent to re-establish good oxygenation before a second attempt is made and the procedure for difficult intubation is adopted (see Ch. 31). The use of a laryngeal mask may get over a difficult situation should tracheal intubation prove impossible.

Additional methods of reducing the risk of gastric regurgitation may be necessary when gastric distension is suspected or the patient has had a recent meal. Under such circumstances the passage of a gastric tube, although unpleasant, may be advisable. Prior to induction the use of apomorphine to initiate vomiting has been advocated (Holdsworth 1978) but, as with gastric aspiration, this will not guarantee to empty the stomach and has lost popularity (Nimmo 1985). Whichever method is used the basic precautions should not be relaxed.

Inhalation of gastric contents

Inhalation of gastric contents is a potentially hazardous and frequently fatal event in which 'prevention is better than cure'.

There is some evidence to support the theory that a properly conducted regimen of antacid therapy, which maintains a gastric pH above 3, will reduce the mortality resulting from inhalation, but this is by no means proven. To obtain the required reduction of gastric acidity, at least two doses of an antacid are usually required but antacids do not reduce gastric volume and it is now generally thought best to combine an H_2 receptor antagonist with antacid treatment. The use of magnesium trisilicate is no longer considered satisfactory as it often fails to reduce gastric acidity and the particulate matter, if inhaled, can itself cause lung irritation (Holdsworth et al 1980).

If regurgitation does occur before intubation, even if inhalation has not obviously occurred, a regime of treatment for chemical pneumonitis must be adopted immediately. At the first sign of gastric regurgitation the pharynx and trachea should be thoroughly sucked out with the patient in the head-down or lateral position. The patient must be intubated immediately to prevent further contamination. Some anaesthetists recommend bronchoscopic suction and pulmonary lavage with an alkaline solution. There is no evidence, however, that this does anything but increase the period of hypoxia and is therefore not recommended. Hydrocortisone (300 mg/6 h for 48 h) should be commenced immediately as this may hasten recovery in those patients where the inhaled gastric juice has a pH above 1.5 (Downs et al 1974). When the pH is below 1.5, mortality may be as high as 100% (Moir & Thorburn 1986). The patient should be ventilated and the baby delivered as quickly as possible. Signs of respiratory distress and pulmonary oedema usually develop within 15–30 min following the inhalation and should be treated with artificial respiration, bronchodilators, antibiotics and other supportive measures demanded by the situation.

Difficult or impossible intubation

The hazards of difficult intubation in general are discussed fully in Chapter 31, but as this hazard has a special significance in obstetric anaesthesia it needs a separate mention here. In competent hands the inability to intubate the trachea is a rare event, but some difficulty or delay may be expected in about 5% of patients. Delay in intubation carries a particular risk in obstetric patients for the following reasons:

1. The reduced respiratory reserve associated with full-term pregnancy results in a more rapid development of hypoxaemia during periods of apnoea than in non-pregnant women.
2. Any delay in intubation will increase further the risks of regurgitation and inhalation.

The incidence of maternal and fetal damage caused by difficult intubation may be reduced by taking special precautions. Anaesthesia should not be induced under any circumstances unless a good assistant is available and all the necessary intubating equipment is at hand. This must include a working sucker, a range of laryngoscopes and tube sizes, a well-designed tube stillette or bougie and a guard for protecting the teeth against damage. The stillette or bougie is particularly important as it may make intubation possible without visualizing the larynx. The stillette should be malleable and blunt-ended, preferably with a light at the end. In short, safe obstetric anaesthesia requires a properly staffed and adequately equipped unit.

The Report on Confidential Enquiries into Maternal Deaths in the United Kingdom, 1985–87, clearly recommends that a failed intubation drill should be agreed and practised by all those involved in obstetric anaesthesia (see Table 40.2). It also makes specific recommendations that the following extra anaesthetic apparatus is available for the difficult intubation:

- a laryngoscope with a blade in line with the axis of the handle (polio blade)
- long introducers (gum elastic, rubber or plastic-coated malleable wire)
- laryngeal masks
- large-bore orogastric tubes
- a laryngotomy kit.

The anaesthetist should not attempt the impossible. The greatest hazard of difficult intubation in the obstetric patient is the anaesthetist that is determined to perform intubation no matter how long it takes, and consequently makes many attempts using repeated doses of suxamethonium. Between each attempt, hypoventilation and laryngeal spasm produces repeated and progressively

Table 40.2 Obstetric intubation drill

<table>
<tr><td colspan="2">Antacid prophylaxis
Preoxygenation
Induction and cricoid pressure
Wait for muscle relaxation
First attempt to intubate</td></tr>
<tr><td>Success
Release cricoid pressure
Continue anaesthesia</td><td>Failure
Maintain cricoid pressure
Gentle manual inflation with oxygen</td></tr>
<tr><td colspan="2">Second attempt to intubate</td></tr>
<tr><td>Success
Release cricoid pressure
Continue anaesthesia</td><td>Failure
Maintain cricoid pressure
Turn patient to left lateral
Oxygenate with manual inflation
Laryngeal mask airway (if needed)
Transtracheal ventilation (if needed)</td></tr>
<tr><td colspan="2">Decision</td></tr>
<tr><td>Surgery can be delayed
Release cricoid pressure
Wake patient
Seek help
Conduction anaesthesia</td><td>Surgery cannot be delayed
Maintain cricoid pressure
Seek help
Establish spontaneous respiration with inhalational anaesthesia
Return to supine
Position with 20° wedge</td></tr>
<tr><td colspan="2">SURGERY</td></tr>
</table>

See also Chapter 31, pp. 482 and 484.

more severe periods of hypoxia in the mother and fetus. No more than two separate attempts at intubation should be made. If the second attempt is unsuccessful, the procedure should be abandoned but cricoid pressure maintained until the patient is in a safe posture, that is head-down on the left side. Further management will depend on the degree of urgency of the procedure.

If time allows it might be appropriate to wake up the patient and establish a spinal or epidural block. However, should this be contraindicated or the operative procedure be urgent owing to fetal distress or severe haemorrhage, general anaesthesia must be continued. Usually this can be achieved by using manual ventilation with a mask and oral airway, or spontaneous respiration. Alternatively the use of a laryngeal mask airway (LMA) may be an easier and safer way of overcoming the problem. However, it must be emphasized that, although the LMA will provide unobstructed respiration and facility for positive pressure ventilation, it will not guarantee protection of the lungs against contamination (Brain et al 1985). Whichever method is used there is little doubt that the risks of hypoxia in the mother and baby from repeated attempts at a difficult intubation are far greater than the risks of caesarean section without intubation (McClune et al 1990). The passage of a large gastric tube may be desirable to empty the stomach and prevent inflation of the stomach with gas. The risks of having a hypoxic mother and neonate from repeated attempts at intubation are far greater than the risks of caesarean section without intubation. Finally, it must be remembered that oesophageal intubation is a common result of difficult intubation and in full-term pregnancy it can easily go unrecognized. It is recommended that, whenever possible, a capnograph is attached immediately after intubation.

Hazard of incorrect drug administration

The emergency obstetric anaesthetic is fruitful ground for the careless mistake.

The practice of preparing drugs in advance or using multidose bottles to save time is to be deprecated as such practices are potential sources of error. No operation can be so urgent that normal careful preparation has to be abandoned. It would be inappropriate to relate all the errors that could occur and have occurred, so it may suffice to remind the reader of two mistakes that are particularly relevant to obstetric anaesthesia. It is common and reasonable practice to draw up all drugs that are likely to be required before the induction of anesthesia. This includes the oxytocic as well as the anaesthetic drugs. However, this has led on a number of occasions to the injection of syntocinon or syntometrine instead of suxamethonium, with unfortunate consequences for both mother and baby. Not only should the syringes be labelled, but also the drugs in the same sized syringes should always be separated so that this mistake cannot occur. Undue haste can also lead to incorrect mixing of anaesthetic agents. For example failure to add methohexitone or thiopentone powder when preparing the induction agent has led to patients being paralysed while still awake. Urgency is no excuse for error.

Awareness

Awareness during surgery under general anaesthesia can in no circumstances be justified. The incidence of this hazard has considerably increased in recent years with the introduction of techniques involving intravenous analgesics and very light anaesthesia. The subject is fully reviewed in Chapter 26. There is a tendency to regard awareness as an acceptable risk in anaesthesia for operative obstetrics because of the desire to expose the fetus to minimal anaesthesia and maximum oxygenation. This attitude cannot be supported, as adequate anaesthesia can almost always be supplied for the mother without risking neonatal depression.

By adding up to 0.5% halothane, 1% enflurane or 0.6% isoflurane to the anaesthetic mixture, the problem can be prevented without harm to mother or fetus. Indeed, these drugs in low anaesthetic concentrations increase placental blood flow and thus improve fetal oxygenation (Palahnuik & Shnider 1974). To reduce the risk of awareness in the resistant patient, at least 60% nitrous oxide should be used during the induction period (Wilson 1982). This will increase the initial uptake of volatile agent by means of the second gas effect (Wylie & Churchill-Davidson 1978). In addition to these precautions the isolated forearm technique, designed to give warning of awareness, may be used (Tunstall 1979), or lower oesophageal contractility may be monitored (Bogod et al 1990). Neither is completely reliable.

Amniotic fluid embolism

Amniotic fluid embolism is now considered to be the most common cause of sudden death during the course of labour and operative delivery. It is a rare condition but it carries a mortality rate of about 86% (Morgan 1979). When sudden collapse occurs during general anaesthesia or analgesia for obstetrics, amniotic fluid embolism must always be considered. If the embolism arises during general anaesthesia it may be very difficult or impossible to make the diagnosis at the time. In consequence the anaesthetist may be accused of mismanagement of the anaesthetic. Oesophageal intubation, pulmonary aspiration or left ventricular failure due to drug misuse are often suggested as the cause of the problem. The only early sign pointing to the correct diagnosis is the development of a coagulopathy with excessive uterine bleeding. Definitive diagnosis requires the identification of amniotic fluid in the maternal circulation.

The main clinical feature presenting under anaesthesia is unexplained cardiovascular collapse with early cyanosis, despite the administration of adequate oxygen. In the conscious patient, respiratory distress is usually the first sign, followed by cardiovascular collapse and coma. If death occurs without a definite diagnosis it is important that the anaesthetist insists on a competent post mortem with thorough examination of lung sections and sputum for fetal squames.

HAZARDS ASSOCIATED WITH EPIDURAL INJECTION FOR THE RELIEF OF PAIN IN LABOUR

Although a regional block by epidural injection of local anaesthetic (Caudal or Lumbar) is the most efficient way of providing pain relief during labour, it is not without its hazards even in the most experienced hands. It is therefore the responsibility of the operator to ensure that these hazards are reduced to a minimum by using an impeccable technique. This can only be achieved by very thorough training and attention to careful detail at all times. The hazards will be outlined and the ways they can be reduced to a minimum discussed in detail below.

Before discussing the hazards themselves, it cannot be stressed too strongly that the training required to manage epidural analgesia for general surgery is not the same as that required to conduct an 'obstetric epidural' efficiently and safely. This is a fact often neglected.

Painful injection

The obstetric patient does not have the benefit of sedation prior to epidural injection, therefore every effort should be made to make it as comfortable as possible. Complaints during the induction of the epidural can be reduced to a minimum by attention to certain details:

1. Following skin preparation and towelling up, a generous quantity of local anaesthetic (2–5 ml of 1% lignocaine) should be injected down to the ligamentum flavum at the chosen space for epidural injection. At least 2–3 min should be allowed to establish good analgesia before the Tuohy needle is introduced. Bupivacaine is not a suitable drug for local infiltration.
2. If localization of the space proves difficult, no more than two or three attempts should be made before abandoning the procedure or seeking help. The anaesthetist must be constantly aware that this procedure is designed to relieve distress and not to produce it. He should also remember that the hazards of dural puncture and chronic postpartum backache more often than not follow repeated attempts to find a difficult epidural space.
3. Having entered the epidural space successfully, the passage of the catheter, particularly in the lumbar area, may cause acute discomfort. The incidence of this discomfort may be considerably reduced by injecting 2–3 ml of 1% lignocaine through the Tuohy needle before introducing the catheter. This injection has the additional advantage of acting as a test dose against unrecognized dural puncture.

Fainting

Fainting may occur during injections of any sort. It is for this reason, and for the general comfort of the patient, that the left lateral position is recommended in preference to the sitting position for lumbar epidural injection in obstetrics. It is appreciated that the sitting position makes the operation easier in some obese patients, but mastery of injection in the lateral position must lead to an overall increase in comfort and safety.

Intravascular injection

The epidural space, particularly during late pregnancy, is a very vascular area thus increasing the likelihood that the catheter will enter a venous sinus when being introduced. This complication occurs in about 3% of patients. If local anaesthetic is then injected into the catheter, some toxic effects will inevitably occur. Fortunately, because of the small dose of local anaesthetic used in obstetric epidurals, this seldom leads to serious consequences although convulsions have been reported. The incidence of this mishap can be considerably reduced by injecting saline through the catheter while advancing it into the epidural space and making sure that the catheter is free of blood before injecting local anaesthetic.

Epidural infection

Infection in the epidural space following epidural analgesia is a complication well-known to neurologists and neurosurgeons (Male & Martin 1973). Fortunately this complication following obstetric epidurals is almost unknown in the UK. This can possibly be attributed to the strict training given to obstetric anaesthetists in this country. There is absolutely no justification for performing an obstetric epidural without strict aseptic precautions. These should include:

- full surgical gowning technique
- the use of sterile ampoules whenever possible
- the employment of a bacterial filter for all top-up procedures.

Bacterial filters, although an important instrument for safety, are not 100% reliable and therefore must not be used as an excuse for relaxing other aseptic precautions. These filters may also prevent glass particles, dislodged when opening the ampoule, from entering the epidural space (Furgang 1974).

Skin infection in the area chosen for epidural injection must remain an absolute contraindication to the procedure. If an epidural abscess occurs the space must be drained as soon as the diagnosis is made and the appropriate antibiotic given. Any delay could lead to meningitis or permanent paraplegia.

Epidural haematoma

Bearing in mind the vascularity of the epidural space it is surprising that epidural haematoma does not occur more frequently. In 35 years of performing and teaching epidural analgesia, I have never experienced an epidural haematoma that has led to symptoms. All the cases reported in the literature have been associated with the concomitant use of anticoagulants. It is thus mandatory that the passage of an epidural catheter should be resisted in patients on anticoagulants or with any bleeding diathesis. To do so could not be defended in the event of a serious haematoma developing (Odoom & Sih 1983).

Catheter fracture

Catheter fracture within the epidural space is due to faulty technique and the incidence is not increased in obstetric epidurals. This complication is fully described in Chapter 38 and will not be discussed further here.

Dural tap

Dural tap has an overall incidence of about 4%. Even in the most experienced hands it is unusual to get an incidence below 0.5% (Dawkins 1969). This mishap cannot therefore be regarded as negligent, but failure to recognize it or treat it properly is inexcusable.

There are two notable hazards resulting directly from dural puncture during obstetric anaesthesia namely postpartum headache and total spinal anaesthesia.

Postpartum headache

Postpartum headache is not always due to dural puncture as about 14% of women who have not received an epidural complain of headache postpartum (Moir & Davidson 1972). However, if the headache is persistent and influenced by posture, a CSF leak must be suspected and treated appropriately. If the dura has been punctured with a Tuohy needle, it is inevitable that a low pressure headache will follow unless rigorous treatment is initiated after delivery. It is essential that a strict treatment regime is followed if this hazard is to be avoided. The following procedure is recommended:

1. The needle should be withdrawn and an epidural catheter inserted in the space above, if possible.
2. The incident must be clearly documented. If documentation is not clear and staff are unaware of the incident, it is possible that the patient will be discharged after a few days with only a mild analgesic prescribed for the headache. In such an event the patient is likely to suffer many days of acute distress and possibly neurological damage, such as paralysis of the sixth cranial nerve (Bryce-Smith & Macintosh 1951) or, rarely, intracranial subdural haematoma (Jack 1979). It is most important that proper communication between the doctor, nursing staff and patient is established, and that the cause and treatment of dural tap are carefully explained to the patient.
3. A strict supine posture should be maintained for at least 48 h, after which time the patient may be allowed to sit up but returned to the supine posture for a further 24 h if the headache recurs.
4. The epidural catheter should be kept in place, and a continuous drip of normal saline solution or lactated Ringer's solution given through the catheter for 24 h in an attempt to equalize the pressure between the CSF and epidural space. If this is unsuccessful and the patient is apyrexial a blood patch may be employed (Bromage 1978, Crawford 1980). There is some evidence, however, to suggest that a blood patch may limit the spread of epidural analgesia performed subsequently (Rainbird & Pfitzner 1983). To perform a blood patch, 15–20 ml of the patient's blood

is withdrawn from an arm vein under sterile conditions and injected into the epidural space. The patient is placed prone for 30 min and supine for the next 12 h.

5. High total fluid intake should be maintained either by mouth or intravenous infusion.
6. Analgesics should be prescribed regularly if required.

Total spinal anaesthesia

If the dura is damaged during the induction of epidural analgesia, there is the risk that the catheter will pass intrathecally and result in total or massive spinal anaesthesia when a standard dose of local anaesthetic is injected (Park 1984, Phillip & Brown 1976). This dose will lead to apnoea, loss of consciousness, dilated pupils and hypotension within 5–10 min of the injection. Treatment must be initiated immediately with intubation, positive pressure ventilation and intravenous fluids sufficient to maintain blood pressure. Should the systolic blood pressure fall 30% below normal and not be reversible with intravenous fluids within 2–3 min, ephedrine should be given in increments of 5–10 mg intravenously until the blood pressure has been restored to normal. Short periods of moderate hypotension are well tolerated by the neonate provided they do not exceed 2–3 min. It is unwise to employ other vasopressor drugs, such as metaraminol and methoxamine, as they are likely to reduce placental blood flow even when the normal blood pressure has been restored. If fetal distress is evident, immediate caesarean section may be indicated as the effect of total spinal anaesthesia is likely to last for at least 1 or 2 h. To avoid a tragedy from this rare but devastating hazard the following discipline is mandatory when performing obstetric epidurals:

1. An intravenous infusion must always be running before any local anaesthetic is injected into the epidural space.
2. The anaesthetist must never leave the patient within a period of 30 min after giving the first therapeutic dose of local anaesthetic.
3. Full resuscitation equipment must always be immediately available in the labour ward when epidural analgesia is being performed.
4. No doctor should establish epidural analgesia or top up an existing block unless he is experienced in intubation and capable of performing modern methods of resuscitation.
5. Because total spinal anaesthesia has been reported following the second and third top-up procedures, midwives that perform top-up injections must be competent in the management of simple resuscitation and an emergency team must always be available to give assistance.

Avoidance of dural puncture

The incidence of dural puncture during epidural analgesia can only be reduced by experience and a careful technique. Many methods and gadgets have been devised over the years in an attempt to reduce this hazard. These were fully described by Dawkins (1963) and need not be discussed here; however, it would not be out of place to discuss a simple loss of resistance technique described by Doughty (1982) which has proved to be 'almost' dural-puncture-proof.

After infiltrating with local anaesthetic, the Tuohy needle is inserted, with the stilette in place until it is firmly held by the ligamentum flavum, an endpoint readily recognized with experience. The stilette is then removed and a free-running glass syringe, loaded with saline, is attached to the end of the needle. The needle is then advanced through the ligamentum flavum by pressure of the right thumb, index and middle fingers gripping the rim of the syringe. At the same time, firm pressure is applied to the plunger of the syringe by a squeezing action with the ball of the index finger. The left hand controls and steadies the advance of the needle. As soon as the tip of the needle enters the epidural space, the finger pressure on the plunger of the syringe will discharge saline into the space and push the dura out of the way until all the needle tip enters the space and enables the catheter to be passed easily.

Maternal hypotension

By far the most common hazard of obstetric epidural analgesia is hypotension produced by a combination of the sympathetic blockade and venacaval compression by the gravid uterus. Fortunately the sympathetic blockade is usually slow in onset and its influence on the circulation can be easily controlled by attention to a few simple details:

1. The dose of local anaesthetic should be kept to the minimum required for a successful block. Such a dose will naturally vary with the individual patient, but I have found that 8 ml of 0.375% bupivacaine seldom has to be exceeded.
2. Fluid loading with at least 500 ml of Ringer's Lactate or similar is mandatory before the block becomes fully effective.
3. The patient should be placed in the left lateral position if any signs of hypotension develop, but in any case a lateral tilt should be maintained. Many anaesthetists prefer to have the mother in the lateral position at all times during labour under epidural analgesia. Half the local anaesthetic is injected while the patient is on one side, and half while on the other in order to get uniform spread within the epidural space.
4. Should hypotension persist despite the above measures, a vasopressor may be necessary. Ephedrine (5–10 mg) is the drug of choice under these circumstances as the effect on uterine blood flow is minimal (Ralston et al 1974). The prophylactic use of intramuscular ephedrine to prevent maternal hypotension during epidural analgesia would not appear to be very effective (Rolbin et al 1982).

Failure to achieve pain relief

Although failure of epidural analgesia during labour may not be a hazard in the true sense of the word, the patient may be justified in regarding it as such. She may be denied an alternative method of pain relief while the unbelieving anaesthetist attempts to sort out the problem. If the patient becomes distressed, a small dose of intravenous pethidine should be given while the problem is being sorted out. In experienced hands, 'failed' epidurals are uncommon during labour. When they do occur they usually do so for one of the following reasons:

1. Failure to identify the ligamentum flavum. In consequence the catheter is passed outside the epidural space.
2. Failure to limit the length of catheter inserted into the epidural space so that it either passes through an intervertebral foramen or, by its position within the space, produces a unilateral block. No more than 2 cm of catheter should lie in the space. This can be precisely calculated by observing the length of needle required to enter the space using a calibrated needle. This method was described in detail by Doughty (1974).
3. Anatomical obstruction within the epidural space. This is a rare event which cannot be avoided.

Instrumental delivery

Epidural analgesia during labour has been shown to increase the incidence of instrumental delivery. This is due to the relaxation of the pelvic floor muscles causing malrotation of the fetal head and must be regarded as a minor hazard of epidural analgesia. This minor hazard, however, is offset by avoidance of the greater hazard of general anaesthesia should operative delivery be required in the absence of a regional block.

The incidence of instrumental delivery can be considerably reduced by providing selective analgesia which reduces perineal pain but does not abolish it (Doughty 1969, Phillips & Thomas 1983). The simplest guideline is to adjust the concentration of local anaesthetic in such a way as to produce good analgesia without paralysis of the legs.

Urinary retention

Urinary retention following delivery is a recognized hazard of obstetrics and there is little evidence that regional analgesia increases this incidence. However, perineal anaesthesia may lead to over-filling of the bladder due to abolition of the micturation reflex with a consequent difficulty in reestablishing normal bladder function. Regular examination of the bladder is essential after all forms of regional analgesia. Catheterization should be performed if retention is prolonged.

Neurological damage

Serious neurological damage following epidural analgesia is the complication most feared by the patient who is often influenced by the publicity these tragedies receive. Such complications are very rare and occur for reasons that are usually obscure (Hargrove 1981). Because of their rarity, some have concluded they must be the result of error in technique. It is therefore essential that a meticulous technique is always used and is seen to be used.

Cranial nerve palsies

A reduction in CSF pressure due to fluid leak following dural puncture can lead to damage to the cranial nerves, particularly the sixth nerve, but trochlear, oculomotor and auditory nerves may also be involved. The paralysis of these nerves is usually transient, but prolonged failure to treat the CSF deficit following dural puncture may lead to permanent damage.

Isolated peripheral nerve injury

Most peripheral nerve injuries that occur during obstetric practice are due to traumatic instrumental delivery or the incorrect positioning of the legs in stirrups. However, injury to spinal nerves may be the direct result of trauma by a misplaced epidural needle or catheter. Such accidents often follow the induction of epidural analgesia on restless patients in strong labour when the correct positioning of the needle proves difficult. Fortunately the majority of injuries of this nature recover rapidly.

Postpartum intracranial subdural haematoma

Postpartum intracranial subdural haematoma is a very rare complication following dural puncture and prolonged CSF leak, but it must be considered as a possible cause of pesistent headache, despite every effort to restore normal CSF pressure.

Paraplegia

One or two cases of paraplegia have been reported following obstetric epidural analgesia. The cause of this serious complication is often obscure, which makes avoidance difficult. One can only repeat the advice given on page 638. and adhere to the basic principles of good technique, with particular attention to the identification and preparation of all drugs injected into the epidural space.

Caudal epidural analgesia

Caudal block was at one time the primary form of regional analgesia for labour and vaginal delivery, but in the last 10–15 years it has been almost totally replaced by the lumbar route because the latter has a much higher success rate, particularly in the control of labour pains. Its main advantage over the lumbar approach is a lower incidence of dural puncture, but to offset that there is a higher failure rate, greater risk of infection and a risk of accidentally injecting local anaesthetic into the fetal head if it is performed late in labour (Sinclair et al 1965).

When used in conjunction with a lumbar epidural during labour, caudal block can provide better control of the changing needs of pain relief in labour and reduce the total dose of local anaesthetic required. It will also limit the extent of the sympathetic block and minimize the hazard of hypotension. This technique is seldom used today as the disadvantages outweigh the advantages.

PARACERVICAL AND PUDENDAL BLOCKS

Paracervical block

Paracervical block for the relief of pain in labour, and pudendal block during the second stage of labour, were at one time commonly used by obstetricians and believed to be the safest way of providing pain relief during childbirth. However, in recent years, particularly since the introduction of the lumbar epidural, they have lost favour owing to a number of inherent hazards associated with the techniques.

These hazards include:

1. A failure rate of about 15%, even in skilled hands.
2. A significant incidence of toxic reactions due to rapid absorption of the local anaesthetic.
3. An alarmingly high incidence of fetal bradycardia due to direct myocardial depression from the high dose of local anaesthetic often required.

Pudendal block

Pudendal block is usually performed by the obstetrician and may be an effective way of providing perineal analgesia for episiotomy and low forceps delivery in the absence of an epidural or spinal block (Scudmore & Yates 1966). It has the advantage of producing no vasomotor blockade and therefore no risk of maternal hypotension. The block does entail, however, the use of large amounts of local anaesthetic and excessive doses have been reported on many occasion with consequent toxic effects. A total dose of 20 ml of 1% lignocaine should not be exceeded.

MASSIVE HAEMORRHAGE

Haemorrhage still remains a prominent cause of maternal mortality. In the triennium 1982–1984 a total of seven mothers died from antepartum or postpartum haemorrhage in England and Wales (3.5 per million pregnancies). This number increased to 10 (5.0 per million pregnancies) for the 3 years 1985 to 1987 (DOH 1991). Therefore the anaesthetist and obstetrician must, at all times, be prepared for this hazard, no matter how simple the case may seem. Blood loss in excess of 500 ml is officially classified as a postpartum haemorrhage (PPH), but as the pregnant woman increases her blood volume by a litre or more during pregnancy this loss seldom alters the haematocrit or has any clinical significance. The need for blood replacement must therefore be judged on clinical grounds rather than according to recorded blood loss.

If excessive blood loss does occur and signs of hypovolaemia develop, blood replacement should be prompt. Not only should fluid replacement maintain an adequate blood pressure and a haematocrit reading above 30%, but also a urinary output approaching 60 ml/h. If reasonably vigorous fluid replacement does not restore urinary output, it may be necessary and justified to set up a central venous line to avoid the risk of overloading as more fluids are given.

Coagulation defects

Disseminated intravascular coagulation (DIC) is one of the most alarming hazards of pregnancy leading to massive haemorrhage. The aetiology of the condition is still obscure, and a discussion of the factors that are believed to cause this condition are not within the scope of this chapter, except to say that it commonly follows placental abruption.

Treatment is often difficult, and when available the expert advice of a haematologist should be sought. As soon as excessive haemorrhage is noticed, blood should be taken for platelet count, and a coagulation screen including fibrinogen titre and fibrin degradation products.

Blood loss is best replaced by fresh whole blood, but this is rarely available. Fresh frozen plasma should be used to replace clotting factors and platelet transfusion may be necessary. Hypofibrinogenaemia may be corrected by direct fibrinogen replacement or cryoprecipitate.

The role of antifibrinolytic agents and heparin is doubtful, and they should only be used under the direction of an experienced haematologist.

DIABETES MELLITUS

Diabetes in late pregnancy presents many problems in care with which the anaesthetist must be fully familiar.

Hazards to the fetus

Placental insufficiency due to a decrease in placental blood flow and premature labour are common problems with the diabetic mother. Despite the onset of premature labour, the babies are often large and uterine contractions poor. In consequence long labours are common. All these factors contribute to the risks for the fetus.

It is the duty of the anaesthetist to take special precautions to ensure that maternal hypotension, hypoxaemia and excessive hyperventilation do not occur during anaesthesia.

Hazards to the mother

Anaesthetics that cause catecholamine release, hyperglycaemia and metabolic acidosis should be avoided. Halothane, enflurane and isoflurane are suitable agents, but fear, pain, hypoxia and hypercarbia should be avoided.

Most obstetricians will favour caesarean sections as the safest method of delivery for the diabetic mother. In skilled hands an epidural block is the best way of managing the anaesthesia, but special care has to be exercised to avoid maternal hypotension. General anaesthesia however, is not contraindicated. For vaginal delivery a lumbar epidural block or a combined lumbar and caudal block will give the safest conditions.

The price of safety is constant vigilance.

REFERENCES

Anderson N 1962 Changes in intragastric pressure following the administration of suxamethonium. Br J Anaesth 34: 363–367

Bogod D G, Orton J K, Yau H M, Oh Te 1990 Detecting awareness during general anaesthetic Caesarean section. Anaesthesia 45: 279–284

Brain R J, McGhee T B, McAteer E J, Thomas A, Abdu-Saad M A W, Bushman J 1985 The laryngeal mask airway. Anaesthesia 40: 356–361

Bromage P R 1978 Epidural analgesia. Saunders, Philadelphia, p 211–212

Bryce-Smith R, Macintosh R 1951 Sixth nerve palsy after lumbar puncture and spinal anaesthesia. Br Med J 1: 275–276

Campbell D, Masson A H B, Norris W 1965 A revaluation of pethidine and Pethilorfan. Br J Anaesth 37: 199–200

Cotton B, Smith G 1978 Lower oesophageal sphincter pressure. In: Kauffman L (ed) Anaesthesia review 1, ch 7

Crawford J S 1978 Principles and practice of obstetric anaesthesia, 3rd edn. Blackwell Scientific, Oxford, p 307

Crawford J S 1980 Experiences with epidural blood patch. Anaesthesia 35: 513–515

Dawkins C J M 1963 The identification of the epidural space. Anaesthesia 18: 67–69

Dawkins C J M An analysis of the complications of epidural block. Anaesthesia 24: 554–557

DOH 1991. Report on confidential enquiries into maternal deaths in The United Kingdom 1985–87. HMSO, London

Doughty A 1969 Selective epidural analgesia and the forceps rate. Br J Anaesth 41: 1058–1062

Doughty A 1974 A precise method of cannulating the epidural space. Anaesthesia 29: 63–64

Doughty A 1982 Finding the epidural space. Anaesthesia 37: 470

Downs J B, Chapman R L, Modell J H, Hood C I 1974 Evaluation of steroid therapy in aspiration pneumonitis. Anesthesiology 40: 129

Eckstein K L, Marx G F 1974 Aortocaval compression and uterine displacement. Anesthesiology 40: 92–96

Furgang F A 1974 Glass particles in ampules. Anesthesiology 41: 525–526

Gamble J A S, Moore J, Lamki H, Howard P J 1977 Study of diazepam levels in mother and infant. Br J Obstet Gynaecol 84: 588–591

Gohoneim M M, Long J P 1970 Interaction between magnesium sulphate and other neuromuscular blocking agents. Anesthesiology 32: 23–27

Grant N F, Daley G L, Chard S 1973 A study of angiotensin 11 response throughout primagravid pregnancy. J Clin Invest 52: 2682–2686

Green R A 1978 Anaesthesia for Caesarean section. Anaesthesia 33: 70

Hargrove R L 1981 The neurological complications of spinal and epidural analgesia. Anaesthesia 36: 454

Hodgkinson R, Hussain F J 1979 Systemic and pulmonary blood pressure in severe hypertensive parturients undergoing Caesarean section. Report of the Obstetric Anaesthetists Association Meeting. Birmingham, September 1979

Holdsworth J D 1978 The place of apomorphine prior to obstetric anaesthesia. J Intern Med Res Suppl 6(1): 26

Holdsworth J D, Johnson K, Marshall G, Roulston G, Tomlinson P A 1980 Mixing of antacids with stomach contents: another approach to the prevention of acid aspiration syndrome. Anaesthesia 35: 641–650

Husemyer R P, Davenport H T 1980 Prophylaxis for Mendelson's syndrome before elective Caesarean section: a comparison of cimetidine and magnesium trisilicate regimen. Br J Obstet Gynaecol 87: 565–570

Jack T M 1979 Postpartum intracranial subdural haematoma. Anaesthesia 34: 176–180
Johnstone M 1973 The cardiovascular effects of oxytocic drugs. Br J Anaesth 44: 826–838
Joupilla R, Joupilla P, Hollman A, Kuikka J 1978 Effect of segmental extradural analgesia on placental blood flow. Br J Anaesth 50: 563–567
Levinson G, Shnider S M, de Lorimer A A, Steffenson J L 1974 Effect of maternal hyperventilation on uterine blood flow, fetal oxygenation and acid base status. Anesthesiology 40: 340–347
Lind F J, Smith A M, McIver D K, Coopland A J, Crispin J S 1968 Heartburn in pregnancy. Can Anaesth Assoc J 98: 571–573
McClune S, Regan M, Moore J 1990 Laryngeal mask airway for Caesarean section. Anaesthesia 45: 227–228
Male C G, Martin R 1973 Puerperal spinal epidural abscess. Lancet 1: 608–609
Martin C, Guillen J C, Dupin J, Ragni J, Aknin P, Gouin F 1990 Lower oesophageal reflux during priming with vecuronium. Br J Anaesth 64: 33–35
Mendelson C L 1946 The aspiration of stomach contents into the lungs during obstetric anaesthesia. Am J Obstet Gynecol 52: 191–205
Moir D D, Amoa A B 1979 Ergometrine or oxytocin? Br J Anaesth 51: 113–117
Moir D D, Davidson S 1972 Postpartum complications of forceps delivery performed under epidural and pudendal nerve block. Br J Anaesth 44: 1197–1199
Moir D D, Thorburn J 1986 Obstetric anaesthesia and analgesia, 3rd edn. p 346
Moir D D, Willocks J 1968 Epidural analgesia in British obstetrics. Br J Anaesth 40: 129
Moir D D, Rodrigues V, Willocks J 1972 Epidural analgesia during labour in patients with pre-eclampsia. J Obstet Gynecol Br Commonw 79: 465–469
Morgan M 1979 Amniotic fluid embolism. Anaesthesia 34: 20–32
Morishima H, Pederson H, Finster M 1978 Influence of maternal psychological stress on the fetus. Am J Obstet Gynecol 131: 286
Morrison C E, Dutton D, Howie H, Gilmour H 1987 Pethidine compared with meptazinol during labour. Anaesthesia 42: 7–14
Moya F, Morishima H, Shnider S M, James L S 1965 Influence of maternal hyperventilation on the new born infant. Am J Obstet Gynecol 91: 76–84
Murphy D F, Nally B, Gardiner J, Unwin A 1984 Effect of metocloptamide on gastric emptying before elective and emergency Caesarean section. Br J Anaesth 56: 1113
Nicholas A D G, Robson J 1982 Comparison of meptazinol and pethidine in labour. Br J Obstet Gynaecol 89: 318–322
Nimmo W S 1985 Aspiration of gastric contents. Br J Hosp Med 34(3): 176
Odoom J A, Sih I L 1983 Epidural analgesia and anticoagulant therapy. Anaesthesia 39: 254–259
Palahnuik R J, Shnider S M 1974 Maternal and fetal cardiovascular and acid base changes during halothane and isoflurane anaesthesia in the pregnant ewe. Anesthesiology 41: 462–472
Park R 1984 A migrating epidural cannula. Anaesthesia 39: 289
Phillip J H, Brown H V 1976 Total spinal analgesia late in the course of obstetric bupivacaine epidural block. Anesthesiology 44: 340–341
Phillips S, Thomas T A 1983 Second stage labour with or without epidural analgesia. Anaesthesia 38: 972–976
Rainbird A, Pfitzner J 1983 Restricted spread of analgesia following epidural blood patch. Anaesthesia 38: 481–484
Ralston D H, Shnider S M, de Lorimer A A 1974 Effects of equipotent ephedrine, metaraminol, mephenteramine and methoxamine on uterine blood flow in the pregnant ewe. Anesthesiology 40: 354–370
Rolbin S H, Cole A F D, Hew E M, Pollard A, Virgint S 1982 Prophylactic intramuscular ephedrine before epidural analgesia for Caesarean section. Can Anaesth Soc J 29: 148–153
Scudmore J H, Yates M J 1966 Pudendal block: a misnomer. Lancet 1: 23
Sellick B A 1961 Cricoid pressure to control regurgitation of stomach contents during induction of anaesthesia. Lancet 2: 404–406
Sinclair J C, Fox H A, Lentz J F, Fuld C L, Murphy J 1965 Intoxication of the fetus by local anaesthetic. N Engl J Med 273: 1173–1177
Taylor G, Pryse-Davies J 1966 The prophylactic use of antacids in the prevention of acid pulmonary aspiration syndrome (Mendelson's Syndrome). Lancet 1: 288–291
Tunstall M E 1979 The reduction of amnesic wakefulness during Caesarean section. Anaesthesia 34: 316–319
Vree T B, Reekers-Ketting J J, Fragen R J, Arts T H M 1984 Placental transfer of midazolam and its metabolites in the pregnant ewe. Anesth Analg Curr Res 63: 31–34
Wilson M E 1982 Awareness. Anaesthesia 37: 263–265
Wylie W D, Churchill-Davidson H C 1978 A practice of anaesthesia, 4th edn. pp 308–310

41

Cardiovascular collapse under anaesthesia

J. Lumley and D. A. Zideman

INTRODUCTION

The publication of the results of the Confidential Enquiry into Perioperative Deaths (CEPOD) by the Association of Anaesthetists and Surgeons of Great Britain and Ireland (Buck et al 1987) was described by Spence (1988) 'as an important landmark in audit in the two disciplines'. Although anaesthesia was considered to have played some part in 14.1% of the 5081 deaths analysed from 485 850 operations, in only three individuals (0.1%) was it regarded as the sole cause of death. That the role of anaesthesia in surgical deaths was found to be small is in keeping with the findings of the previous UK study (Lunn & Mushin 1982), another national multicentre study from France (Tiret et al 1986) and the report from New South Wales (Holland 1987).

Cardiac arrest during anaesthesia could be a convenient marker of morbidity and mortality. It should be easily identifiable and its immediate cause can usually be determined. However, quantifying the problem of cardiopulmonary collapse during anaesthesia is extremely difficult. The studies alluded to above have all the problems encountered in performing such epidemiological studies as described by Derrington & Smith (1987). While there is difficulty in providing overall representative statistics, the major causes of the need for resuscitation following cardiopulmonary collapse can be identified from the above studies and from the report from Keenan & Boyan (1985) which looked prospectively at the incidence of cardiac arrest due solely to anaesthesia in one centre over a 15 year period. Out of 163 240 anaesthetics administered, there were 449 cardiac arrests. Only 27 events (1 per 6046 anaesthetics) were judged to be primarily due to anaesthetic practice: an incidence of 1.7 per 10 000 anaesthetics.

Major causes implicated in these reports are: age and physical status of the patient; inadequate preoperative preparation and inappropriate timing of the operation; and failure to apply knowledge or use of monitoring equipment.

Age

Keenan & Boyan (1985) found that the paediatric age-group had a three-fold higher risk than adults. This is in keeping with the findings of Tiret et al (1986). However, the greatest risk of arrest reported by Tiret et al occurred at an age greater than 75, and the CEPOD report also noted that 75% of deaths were over 70 years of age.

Physical status

For the purpose of comparison and assessment of risk, the American Society of Anesthesiologists' classification (1963) is of undoubted value. Keenan & Boyan (1985) excluded ASA grade V patients as they felt they were, by definition, moribund, and stated that the role of anaesthesia in the subsequent arrest was difficult to determine. Tiret et al's (1986) figures for the rate of complications were 0.41:1000 for ASA grade I patients, with a 37-fold increase in risk between ASA grade I and ASA grades IV and V. The CEPOD report showed that some very poor risk patients were subjected to elective surgery, and half of these elective procedures reported were ASA grade V.

Preoperative preparation

It is mandatory that all patients are visited by an anaesthetist preoperatively; only 82% of patients in the CEPOD report had been visited preoperatively. Surgical failure of preoperative management occurred in 13.9% of cases in the CEPOD report. The anaesthetic assessor noted that in 10.6% of cases, he would have refused to anaesthetize the patient. At the time of the anaesthetist's visit, careful preoperative assessment of the airway using the Mallampati et al classification (1985) is advocated.

Selection of premedicant drugs should be made in the light of the physical status of the patient, as the administration of the premedication may itself cause cardiac arrest.

Timing of the operation

All the studies agree that there is an increased risk of perioperative cardiac arrest with emergency procedures. One-fifth of the deaths in the CEPOD study were emergencies and 40% were urgent. A sobering comment on these figures by the authors was that more than 10% of these fatal operations were judged unnecessary.

Failure to apply knowledge

In Keenan & Boyan's (1985) study, failure to provide adequate ventilation and overdosage of anaesthetic agent accounted for 50% and 30% of anaesthetic cardiac arrests, respectively. The CEPOD study showed that 75% of anaesthesia-attributable deaths were due to failure to apply knowledge. Lack of knowledge, and lack of care and experience were also identified as additional major factors. Even detection of a principal factor leading to a cardiac arrest may not invoke an appropriate response. Tests of resuscitation skills of junior hospital doctors in the UK (Casey 1984, Skinner et al 1985) and the USA (Lowenstein et al 1981) showed that there was a uniform poor performance. Frequent training and testing of all personnel in the operating theatre suite and recovery room in resuscitation is therefore essential.

The use of monitoring equipment

All surveys stress the importance of monitoring. In 1986 the Harvard Medical School's Department of Anesthesia formulated a series of standards for minimal monitoring during anaesthesia to try to improve patient care, to enhance the detection of relatively low-frequency events and to provide a means of objective evaluation.

Conventionally, anaesthetists have observed the patient's colour, pulse rate and respiratory movements, and listened to the respiratory sounds, but it is generally accepted nowadays in the UK that the minimum monitoring requirements during anaesthesia conform with the Association of Anaesthetists' recommendations (1988).

Minimal, essential and desirable monitoring functions can provide the trained and experienced anaesthetist with a wealth of information and should commence prior to induction of anaesthesia (see Ch 44).

PERIOPERATIVE

At any time during the conduct of general anaesthesia (be it induction, maintenance or recovery) hypoxia, hypotension or arrhythmias may precipitate cardiopulmonary collapse. Drug usage, equipment hazards, respiratory problems and failure to secure circulatory homeostasis are four major areas of concern that need further consideration.

Drug usage

Anaesthetic agents

The inherent safety of anaesthetic agents was emphasized as long ago as 1970 by the report of the New South Wales Special Committee investigating deaths under anaesthesia. The committee stated that anaesthetic drugs were found to be lethal only when misused. However, intravenous induction agents can cause hypoxia and hypercarbia as a result of central respiratory depression or respiratory obstruction, even when used in correct dosage. Cardiopulmonary collapse can occur with errors in technique or overdosage of these agents in association with direct myocardial depression. The result is hypotension, especially if the drugs are administered to patients with an inability to increase cardiac output, for example heart block, severe valvular stenosis or hypovolaemia.

Allergic reactions to these agents commonly present on induction, but may be delayed in onset. They are sometimes difficult to differentiate from adverse reactions to other agents administered at the same time or late in the anaesthetic sequence, for example anaphylactic and anaphylactoid reactions may be reported with the neuromuscular blocking agents and plasma expanders. A sudden severe hypotensive episode at the time of induction is classed as the most common presenting feature of an anaphylactoid reaction (Fisher & Baldo 1984). Such reactions are an important cause of mortality and morbidity in anaesthesia. Thirty-one patients (1 in 4600) were reported by Tiret et al (1986) to have had an anaphylactic reaction.

During induction, failure of the masseter muscles to relax after the administration of suxamethonium should alert the anaesthetist to the possibility of malignant hyperthermia, although this is a rare occurrence. Overdosage of volatile anaesthetic agents should be avoided as this will lead eventually to respiratory and myocardial depression. This may also present in the immediate postoperative period, as may problems with the reversal of muscle relaxants.

Non-anaesthetic agents

Cullen & Miller (1979) stated that the average patient may receive eight different drugs during hospitalization and an additional 5–10 drugs during anaesthesia. They reviewed the mechanisms and specific drug interactions that may commonly present. The British National Formulary lists alphabetically, drugs and their interactions in its appendix (see also Appendix 2).

The use by surgeons of adrenaline infiltration in concentrations greater than 1:200 000 in an attempt to reduce bleeding should be discouraged. As the dose that provokes ventricular arrhythmias varies with the different halogenated agents, the question is posed as to whether they should be used at all or another anaesthetic technique employed if adrenaline is infiltrated.

Equipment hazards (see Ch. 42)

It is generally agreed that anaesthetists are entitled to assume that the correct gas will issue from the appropriate pipeline terminal and that a cylinder contains the gas that it is alleged to contain. The fact that this is not always true has to be noted. However, from the pipeline terminal or the cylinder contents onwards, the anaesthetist has to be responsible for trying to foresee problems.

Equipment failure appears to cause fewer mishaps than human error. However, adequate checks of the anaesthetic machine and any associated ventilators and respiratory equipment must be made prior to the commencement of anaesthesia (Association of Anaesthetists 1990), and vaporizers should not be resited once anaesthesia has started. Breathing systems may be incorrectly assembled and accidental disconnections or even failure to connect patients to the machine or breathing system have been reported.

Serious and occasionally fatal accidents can arise from the inadvertent application of excessive pressures direct from an anaesthetic machine to the patient's airways. Newton & Adams (1978) reported that there were sufficient examples of this problem in the literature to demonstrate that it is by no means uncommon. The effects produced are modified by the presence of the compliant reservoir bag which may act as a buffer to the system. Incorrect assembly of the breathing system, obstruction or kinking of the outlet tube (i.e. Bains or Ayres T-piece), sticking or closed antipollution systems, Heidbrink or non-return expiratory valves, oxygen flushing valves that stick open and the delivery of gas too rapidly, are all causes of outflow obstruction. The effects produced depend on the manner in which the pressure is applied, the characteristics of the lungs and the cardiovascular state of the patient. Raised intrathoracic pressure has a deleterious effect on the cardiac output within a matter of minutes and delayed effects may be caused by a pneumothorax.

Respiratory problems

While the induction of anaesthesia is regarded as a critical period, respiratory problems can occur at any time during the course of anaesthesia. Hypoxia at this time should alert the anaesthetist to respiratory depression, respiratory obstruction or hypotension. It is important to remember that cyanosis may not be manifest when haemoglobin is under 5 g, when lighting is indequate or in dark-skinned patients. A quick assessment should be made as to the level of the obstruction and its cause, while checking the patient's pulse and oxygen saturation and immediately changing the inspired gas mixture (to 100% oxygen if necessary). However, the patient must not be allowed to become aware as a result. If the obstruction is above the cords, the insertion of an oral nasopharyngeal airway may be all that is needed to allow administration of oxygen; if at the level of the cords, the possibility of laryngeal spasm due to secretions, regurgitation or even silent aspiration must be considered.

Dinnick (1973) and Harrison (1983) stressed that tracheal intubation is one of the more common accident and risk situations. Intubation may be difficult, indeed impossible, leading to the risk of hypoxia. Misplacement of the tube can occur, and there is an increased risk of aspiration particularly in the presence of a full stomach or hiatus hernia when hypoxia, bronchospasm and hypotension will present. Even if the tracheal tube is correctly placed it can become dislodged or kinked, the latter leading to severe respiratory obstruction. In Keenan & Boyan's (1985) study there was a direct failure of the intubation technique in eight patients, unrecognized oesophageal intubation occurring in four patients. These problems are fully discussed in Chapter 31.

If intubation has been attempted, increasing hypoxia and drop in oxygen saturation must alert the anaesthetist to a misplaced tube. This is where the use of capnography is to be advocated as an extra aid in detection, in addition to observation of respiratory movements and ausculating with a stethoscope. Difficulty in ventilating the patient manually at this time must suggest some form of obstruction. The possibility of kinking or obstruction of the tube by an overdistended cuff must be quickly assessed by feeling for kinks within the mouth and pharynx, deflating the cuff and passage of a suction catheter if the patient's condition permits. If necessary, the tube must be removed, especially if manual ventilation is difficult and it is known that the patient was easy to inflate by hand prior to insertion of the tube. Needless to say, the patient during any emergency situation must always be connected to a source of high oxygen concentration from the anaesthetic machine and awareness must be avoided by the use of other agents, for example a volatile agent or benzodiazepines. Tubes can be dislodged or kinked during the course of an anaesthetic, leading to hypoxia and hypotension.

Signs of pneumothorax should be looked for and a check made back from the patient to the machine in order to identify any obstruction within the breathing system. If the tube is found to be patent and signs of lower respiratory obstruction, that is bronchospasm, are present, then aspiration, asthma and pulmonary oedema must be considered.

Once patients are attached to mechanical ventilators, difficulty in inflation may be apparent from the increase on the pressure gauge if a constant volume ventilator is in use. Reverting to hand ventilation and 100% oxygen administration will help to identify where the level of obstruction is. Again the anaesthetist should remember to consider the possibility of a tension pneumothorax and institute drainage immediately.

Leaks within the breathing system should be constantly looked for. The patient's pulse rate, colour, respiratory movements and lack of movement of the reservoir bag if spontaneously breathing or, if paralysed, a fall in minute volume associated with absent respiratory movements and a fall in inflation pressure should alert the anaesthetist to impending problems.

Failure to secure homeostasis

Once again, preoperative assessment and preparation are of prime importance in the ability to achieve the aim of oxygen delivery to the tissues. A low haemoglobin is not a contraindication to anaesthesia if it is a result of chronic anaemia, such as occurs in renal failure, as long as an allowance is made for additional oxygen therapy and the cardiac output is maintained at all times. For all patients, dehydration and hypovolaemia should be corrected prior to anaesthesia, except perhaps in the most exceptional emergency situations. The hypotension occurring on induction is accentuated and may be severe enough to cause cardiopulmonary collapse if either of these two factors is present. The hypotension associated with anaesthesia in the dental chair and with inferior vena caval obstruction must be remembered, as must the possibility of myocardial infarction.

Air embolism is particularly associated with the introduction of lines for central venous pressure monitoring to assess the state of dehydration and hypovolaemia, especially in the shocked patient. Air embolus is manifested by severe hypoxia and hypotension. This must also be considered when surgical procedures are being undertaken which involve damage to veins in the neck, thorax, pelvis, or when neurosurgical operations are performed in the sitting position. Diagnostic and therapeutic injections of air into pleural and peritoneal cavities, large joints, the bladder and nasal antra are also responsible for causing air embolus. A hissing sound in the wound may precede severe hypotension and hypoxia. If an end-tidal carbon dioxide monitor is in use, the level falls rapidly as the blood fails to reach the lungs.

Other embolic phenomena occurring during general anaesthesia are more rare, but a massive pulmonary embolus will lead to severe hypotension, hypoxia and signs of electromechanical dissociation of the cardiac complex. This too may be detected by capnography.

The other main problem associated with the insertion of central venous lines is the production of a pneumothorax. This is more common when the subclavian route is used and may be insidious in onset. Nitrous oxide will cause an increase in volume of the space and eventually a tension pneumothorax may occur.

Arrhythmias

Arrhythmias associated with anaesthesia and surgery were first reported by Levine (1920). They may be associated with pre-existing cardiac pathology, for example heart block, electrolyte imbalance such as hyper- or hypokalaemia, hypercapnia, hypoxia, circulating catecholamines, vagal reflexes or drug therapy. Of importance in the aetiology of cardiopulmonary collapse are the following: bradycardia which may be associated with either vagal stimulation or overdose of anaesthetic agent, and which is also a feature of hypoxia; atrial or ventricular premature contractions which usually indicate the presence of some degree of hypercarbia; supraventricular and ventricular tachycardias which may lead to diminution of cardiac output.

Arrhythmias should be quickly detected by feeling the pulse and observation of the electrocardiogram (ECG) monitor. Any deviation from the patient's normal rhythm should be queried and assessment made of the cause. Is the patient too lightly or too deeply anaesthetized? In the case of a bradycardia, is vagal stimulation present, and is it related to drug therapy or hypoxia? Can it be prevented from progressing to asystole? Beware of adrenaline infiltration leading to ventricular fibrillation, either due to overdosage or direct injection into the vascular system.

Aystole, ventricular fibrillation and electromechanical dissociation are the three disastrous consequences to be avoided if at all possible. The latter occurs when the ECG complexes appear relatively normal but there is no cardiac output.

Electrical hazards

At present the proliferation of electrical apparatus around the patient has increased the risk of electrocution occurring, both to patients and staff. Not only does the danger arise from the use of mains electricity, but also the possibility exists of a current as small as 100 mamps causing ventricular fibrillation in the 'microshock' situation. This may arise particularly in patients who have external conductors for cardiac pacemakers or who have catheters containing electrolyte placed within or near the heart. Small differences in electrical potential between two pieces of apparatus may produce a flow of current that is concentrated near the heart, with disastrous effects (see Ch. 43).

Perioperative resuscitation

No matter what the cause or the timing of the event, there can be no excuse for delaying resuscitation of a pulseless patient in the operating theatre environment. As basic physiological monitoring is mandatory, even for the simplest of procedures, the signs of imminent cardiopulmonary collapse should be recognized early and measures taken to prevent a total cessation of cardiac function. A change in the electrocardiographic rhythm, a fall in oxygen saturation or a change in plethysmograph trace, an unexplained fall in blood pressure or the sudden absence of expired carbon dioxide tracings should warn the anaesthetist that trouble is afoot.

CARDIOPULMONARY RESUSCITATION

Resuscitation must begin immediately. It must not be delayed pending the arrival of equipment or personnel. Initially, resuscitation is performed without equipment: Basic Life Support. This progresses to Advanced Cardiac Life Support: the use of equipment and advanced protocols in resuscitation. The end result of resuscitation should never be forgotten, that is the temporary provision of an artificial circulation of oxygenated blood, especially to the brain. The ultimate aim is to convert from the artificial provision of this circulation to a patient self-maintained circulation.

Basic life support (BLS)

(BLS Working Party of the European Resuscitation Council)

Basic cardiac life support is a three-part sequence:

- airway
- breathing
- circulation.

Phase 1 – assessment

Airway. Assess and open the airway. The airway is opened by tilting the head back and supporting the jaw. The extension of the head on the neck opens the upper airway and is best performed by placing one hand on the forehead and the other on the chin. Supporting the jaw or lifting the mandible will displace the tongue from the back of the pharynx.

Breathing. With the airway held open, the absence of breathing is checked. Look at the chest wall for movement, listen over the airway and feel over the airway for effective air movement.

Circulation. The circulation is assessed by feeling for the carotid pulse in the neck.

Phase 2 – action

1. If the patient is unconscious, but breathing and with a pulse, maintain the airway and turn him into the recovery position. Then get help.
2. If the patient is unconscious, *not* breathing but with a pulse, give 10 (expired air respirations) mouth-to-mouth ventilations and then go to get help. On return repeat Phase 1 but this time continue ventilations until help arrives.
3. If the patient is unconscious, not breathing and with no pulse, go immediately to get help. On return repeat Phase 1 but now commence expired air resuscitation and chest compressions.

Expired air respiration is performed by mouth-to-mouth ventilation, blowing into the patient's mouth until the chest starts to expand. Two individual normal breaths are given at this time. Do not use excessive volumes or pressures as these will cause gastric distension and may cause vomiting.

Chest compressions are carried out on the lower third of the sternum, depressing the sternum 4–5 cm with each compression at a rate of 80 compressions/min. Fifteen compressions are followed by two ventilations.

This is basic life support in its most fundamental form as currently recommended by The European Resuscitation Council (1992a). In the operating theatre environment the above may be modified if the patient is already intubated and ventilated, or if there is a second person present that can perform compressions. In the latter case (two rescuer cardiopulmonary resuscitation [CPR], five compressions are followed by one ventilation, at a compression rate of 60 compressions/min. Basic Life Support can only be regarded as 'buying time'. The cardiac output achieved by chest compressions is only 10–15% of normal and it is therefore essential that Advanced Life Support is initiated as soon as possible.

Advanced life support (ALS)

(ALS Working Party of the European Resuscitation Council)

Airway

The Guedel airway is probably the simplest airway adjunct. Select the correct size: size 2 for an adult female or size 3 for an adult male. The airway is best inserted upside-down until the tip reaches the roof of the mouth, then it is gently rotated into position so that the teeth rest on the bite block. If too small a Guedel airway is selected then airway obstruction will result; if too large a size is used then this can result in trauma to the posterior pharyngeal wall. Nasopharyngeal airways are often forgotten. These are extremely useful, especially when the patient still has pharyngeal reflexes.

Tracheal intubation is the only guaranteed method of establishing a protected airway. Unfortunately, failure to intubate the trachea, either because of lack of experience or the failure to recognize an oesophageal intubation, is commonly reported. Keenan & Boyan's (1985) study reported eight cases of direct failure, four of which were unrecognized oesophageal placement. Failure to intubate should not mean loss of the airway. Redding & Pearson (1962) recognized the fact that any delay in establishing or maintaining an airway will adversely affect the eventual outcome of resuscitation. The use of simple manual methods of maintaining the airway are of primary importance and should never be forgotten.

Although preoperative airway assessment is widely recommended, a study by Samsoon & Young (1987) reported an inability to intubate 1 in 280 obstetric patients and 1 in 2230 surgical patients, but that none of these failed intubations were expected. Sia & Edens (1981) have recommended the use of fibre-optic laryngoscopy as useful in difficult intubation. They stress the point that this is not a technique to be learned at a time of crisis and recommend at least 30 practice attempts at the technique before attempting a difficult intubation. In a survey of anaesthetists, Ovassapian & Dykes (1982) found that only 16.5% had tried the technique more than 25 times.

Other techniques that may be considered when intubation fails are the use of a light wand to facilitate intubation (Rayburn 1979), transtracheal ventilation (Smith et al 1975, Attia et al 1975) and the use of the laryngeal mask (Brain 1983). Latto (1985) concluded that every clinician must have a clear plan of action when dealing with a difficult or failed intubation. This plan must be rehearsed at regular intervals and not tried for the first time on a difficult case. The position of the tracheal tube can be checked by simple observation, fibre-optic bronchoscopy down the tracheal tube or the detection or measurement of carbon dioxide in the expired gases. More recently Higgins et al (1990) described a simple chemical colour-change method of detecting expired carbon dioxide, but its success must be tempered by reports of similar colour changes occurring following the endotracheal administration of adrenaline.

Breathing

Expired air resuscitation by mouth-to-mouth respiration can provide an adequate concentration of oxygen in the emergency situation, but a self-inflating bag valve should be attached to the anaesthetic machine at all times. The self-inflating bag-valve-mask system is the advanced adjunct of choice. It can be used with a face mask provided the user is experienced at obtaining a tight seal of the mask on the face. Training is essential for the safe and efficient use of the resuscitation bag. There have been many studies showing how little ventilation is provided when it is placed in untrained hands (Elling & Politis 1983, Harrison et al 1982, Hess & Baron 1985). If the bag-valve-mask is not providing adequate ventilation the rescuer should return to a mouth-to-mouth technique. All self-inflating resuscitation bags now fit via a 22 mm connector directly onto the 15 mm connector of the tracheal tube.

When using the self-inflating resuscitation bag it is certainly worth providing additional inspired oxygen. This can be done by passing oxygen directly into the resuscitation bag or using an inspiratory reservoir system. The reservoir system is more satisfactory as its use results in an inspired oxygen concentration of up to 80% FIO_2.

There has been much discussion as to the use of mechanical ventilators (so-called artificial resuscitators) in cardiopulmonary resuscitation. In the operating theatre there can be no objection to the continued use of a mechanical ventilator during resuscitation, especially if the patient is already attached to such a device. It is, of course, of extreme importance to check that the ventilator is functioning properly and is adequately ventilating the patient's lungs. It is ideal to choose 100% inspired oxygen, but care must be taken that this does not result in patient awareness especially if the event occurs during a surgical procedure. Mechanical ventilators that are pressure cycled are not acceptable.

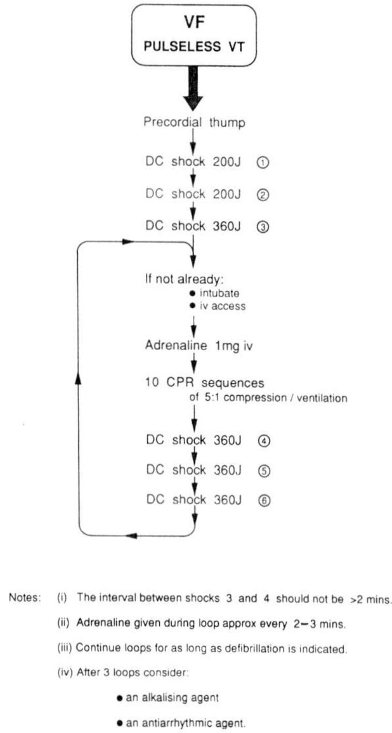

Fig. 41.1 Algorithm for ventricular fibrillation (VF) or pulseless ventricular tachycardia (VT). DC, direct current, CPR, cardiopulmonary resuscitation.

Circulation

The insertion of a wide-bore cannula into a large central vein is an essential part of the resuscitation procedure. The internal jugular, subclavian or femoral vein are all acceptable. The administration of resuscitation drugs by a subdiaphragmatic route have been shown to be less efficacious. Drugs and fluids can be administered by the intravenous route but, should this fail, drugs can be given down the tracheal tube for absorption by the pulmonary capilliary bed or by the intraosseous route via a cannula inserted into the tibia 1 cm below the tibial plateau.

Electrocardiographic diagnosis

There are three main rhythms associated with cardiac arrest. The European Resuscitation

Council (1992b) recommended treatment protocols are described below.

Ventricular fibrillation

The treatment of ventricular fibrillation is defibrillation. As most of the events in the perioperative period can be considered witnessed if not monitored, then cardioversion by a precordial chest thump is the most immediate therapy available. If this is not effective then two 200 J defibrillations followed by 360 J should be administered. Adrenaline (1 mg; 10 ml of 1 in 10 000 solution) is the first drug of choice. Adrenaline's alpha-adrenergic activity will raise the peripheral vascular resistance and thus improve coronary perfusion. Its beta-adrenergic effect on the heart increases automaticity. Basic Life Support is continued for 10 cycles of 5 compressions to 1 ventilation before attempting three more DC defibrillations at 360 J each. Adrenaline should be repeated every 2–3 minutes. After three loops an alkalising agent, sodium bicarbonate, or an antiarrhythmic agent should be considered. If ventricular fibrillation can be excluded or if it is treated by DC shock give adrenaline 1 mg intravenously followed by 10 cycles of 5 compressions to 1 ventilation. Atropine 3 mg given intravenously, during the first loop only, should then be given.

Asystole

A straight-line trace on the electrocardiogram should immediately alert the anaesthetist not only to check the pulse of the patient but also to check the switches, connections and gain of his electrocardiographic monitor.

It is not always possible to exclude the diagnosis of ventricular fibrillation from that of asystole. If any doubt exists, defibrillation must be attempted as the prognosis of asystole is extremely poor when compared with that of ventricular fibrillation.

Atropine, a parasympathetic blocking drug, will release the heart from the effect of the vagus nerve and from the parasympathetic chaos of cardiac arrest. If there is 'p' wave activity then

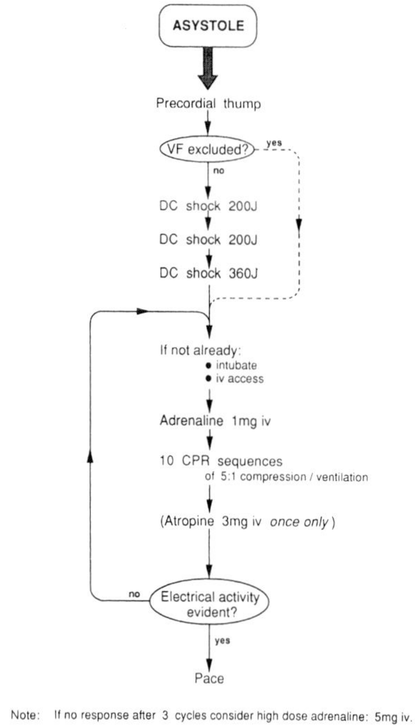

Fig. 41.2 Algorithm for astystole.

transthoracic pacing should be considered. The results of this carried out in the Emergency Department are reported as being disappointing, but this is believed to be because pacing was commenced too late. Early attempts at pacing are recommended.

Electromechanical dissociation

Adrenaline (1 mg) should be given immediately and basic life support commenced. The underlying cause of the electromechanical dissociation (EMD) should then be treated.

The primary causes of electromechanical dissociation are a failure of the excitation–contraction mechanism. These include hypovolaemia, tension pneumothorax, cardiac tamponade, pulmonary embolism, drug overdosage/ intoxication, hypothermia and electrolyte imbalance. Administration of calcium chloride is specifically indicated in hyper-kalaemia, hypocalcaemia or where calcium antagonist activity is suspected.

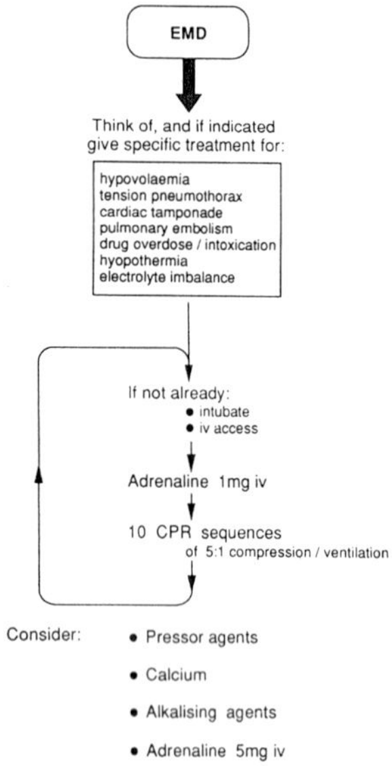

Fig. 41.3 Algorithm for electromechanical dissociation (EMD).

Prolonged resuscitation

Repeat administration of adrenaline (1 mg) is recommended every 2–3 min to maintain the high level of adrenergic activity needed for successful resuscitation. Sodium bicarbonate (50 ml of an 8.4% solution) can also be given according to arterial blood gas results. Sodium bicarbonate should only be given if effective ventilation has been established. Overenthusiastic bicarbonate administration may result in alkalosis, hypernatraemia and hyperosmolality and will lead to the eventual failure of resuscitation.

The operating theatre is, of course, the ideal environment to provide the optimum in resuscitation procedures. External chest compressions, although immediately effective, only produce a small fraction of normal cardiac output and cerebral perfusion. Internal cardiac compressions seem to have been forgotten, or if they are remembered they are often commenced too late to be effective. It only requires a simple incision in the fifth intercostal space to provide access to the heart. Internal cardiac compressions are much more effective and in the operating room should be a real alternative in providing an improved and realistic cardiac output.

POSTOPERATIVE PERIOD

Too often the postoperative period is forgotten. The essential minimal monitoring required during anaesthesia is either removed or handed on to recovery staff with insufficient training to make proper sense of it. The postoperative period is often one of the most vital periods and should provide the all-important link between the intensive observation and care in the operating theatre to the long-term postoperative care in the surgical ward. Monitoring must be maintained, and the patient airway checked and cleared at frequent intervals. The observation of effective breathing must be continued and a stable circulation established. If the condition of the patient warrants postoperative intensive care or high-dependency care, then these units must also be properly equipped and staffed to receive such patients.

Respiratory depression from opiate administration has been a well-known complication of postoperative analgesia. Specific antagonists have eased this situation but, although such drugs will reverse the respiratory depressions, they will also reverse the analgesia, thus leaving the patient in pain. Modern anaesthesia and analgesia techniques have proceeded down the epidural opiate line, but respiratory depression still remains a problem. This simple but important side effect, which is now recognized with a wide variety of agents, has limited the use of intrathecal or epidural administration of opiates. Gustaffson et al (1982) in Sweden reported a 1.0% incidence of associated respiratory depression. Such depression can occur up to 13 h following the initial treatment and is more commonly associated with prior or additional opiate administration by another route. The recommendation of Glynn (1987), that following intrathecal or epidural opiate administration the patient should be monitored and nursed in a high-dependency area for 24 h, is strongly endorsed.

PAEDIATRIC RESUSCITATION

Children are a special risk during anaesthesia. Although the majority have healthy hearts, children do not tolerate hypoxia at all well, the usual result being a profound bradycardia. Initially, perioperative paediatric resuscitation must therefore concentrate on establishing an airway and proper oxygenation. Chest compressions may be required during the bradycardic episode and before aystole ensues. Compressions are performed with the tips of two fingers on the lower third of the sternum at a rate of 100 compressions/min. Five compressions alternate with one breath.

Advanced Paediatric Life Support is complicated by the wide variety of equipment required to match the range of sizes of children encountered. Selection of equipment is usually made on a personal basis considering training and previous experience. Drugs and fluids are usually given in a dose per body weight. Although all children should be weighed before anaesthesia, in the emergency this may not be so. The chart in Figure 41.4 is recommended as a simple method of relating age or length/height of the child via a single graph to his weight. It also gives the recommended size and length of the tracheal tube and the recommended doses of drug (Oakley 1988).

Endotracheal tube

Length (cm)	Internal diameter (mm)
18–21	7.5–8.0
18	7.0
17	6.5
16	6.0
15	5.5
14	5.0
13	4.5
12	4.0
	3.5
10	3.0–3.5

Paediatric resuscitation chart

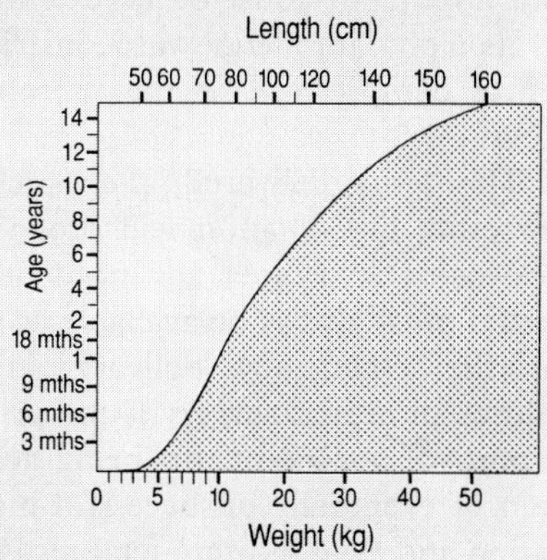

Adrenaline (ml of 1/10 000) intravenous or endotracheal	0.5	1	2	3	4	5
Atropine (mg) intravenous or endotracheal	0.1	0.2	0.4	0.6	0.6	0.6
Bicarbonate (ml of 8.4%) intravenous	5	10	20	30	40	50
Calcium chloride (mmol)* intravenous	1	2	4	6	8	10
Diazepam (mg) intravenous	1.25	2.5	5	7.5	10	10
per rectum	2.5	5	10	–	–	–
Glucose (ml of 50%) intravenous	10	20	40	60	80	100
Lignocaine (mg) intravenous or endotracheal	5	10	20	30	40	50
Salbutamol (µg) intravenous	25	50	100	150	200	250
Initial DC defibrillation (J)	10	20	40	60	80	100
Initial fluid infusion in hypovolaemic shock (ml)	50	100	200	300	400	500

* One millilitre calcium choride 1mmol/ml ≡ 1.5ml calcium chloride 10% ≡ 4.5ml calcium gluconate 10%

Fig. 41.4 Paediatric resuscitation chart (from Oakley 1988).

PREGNANCY

Cardiopulmonary collapse during pregnancy requires special care to be provided for the mother and the child. It is currently suggested that the management of such a collapse is determined by the gestational age of the pregnancy (Resuscitation Council (UK) 1990). The procedures for each gestational age are listed below:

1. Less than 25 weeks: Standard resuscitation is recommended.
2. Over 25 weeks: The first priority must be to position the mother on her side to diminish aorta caval compressions by the gravid uterus. Successful external chest compression has been reported using a 30° wedge to fit the mother. Further management then depends on whether the pregnancy has progressed further than 32 weeks.
3. Under 32 weeks: A thoracotomy should be performed, with internal cardiac compressions to maintain the maternal circulation until delivery of the fetus can be accomplished.
4. Over 32 weeks: An immediate caesarean section should be performed, possibly progressing to internal chest compressions following delivery.

Successful external defibrillation has been reported without adverse effect on the fetus. Intravenous lignocaine at maternal therapeutic levels has shown little effect on the fetal heart, but adrenaline must be used with some caution as its alpha-adrenergic vasoconstrictor effect may cause compromise of the uteroplacental blood flow.

The fetus delivered after such a period of maternal resuscitation will probably be hypoxic and acidotic. Proper advanced neonatal resuscitation must always be available as an integral part of the emergency delivery suite procedure. Although urgent surgery is the priority, there are reports of normal infants being delivered after 15 min of eventually unsuccessful maternal resuscitation and even in-utero fetal resuscitation.

AFTERCARE

Following a prolonged period of suboxygenation or cardiopulmonary collapse, attempts must be directed towards reducing cerebral oedema in order to obtain adequate cerebral function. Some authorities recommend steroid therapy which should be commenced early in the post resuscitation phase. Effective oxygenation, artificial ventilation and the use of dehydrating agents, such as mannitol, will have to be considered. Sedative agents have their place if restlessness and fits are a feature at this time, but the appropriateness of high-dose barbiturates is not proven, and these can lead to severe myocardial depression and a fall in cardiac output. At present, conflicting evidence exists as to the role of calcium blockers in extending cerebral survival time. It will be interesting to follow developments.

When all resuscitation attempts appear to have failed, the criteria laid down by the Conference of Royal Colleges and Faculties of the United Kingdom (1976) should be strictly adhered to when diagnosing brain death.

Meticulous attention to detail and almost obsessive care in relation to patients, drug therapy, machinery and monitoring will hopefully reduce the incidence of cardiopulmonary collapse during anaesthesia and its sometimes disastrous consequences.

REFERENCES

American Heart Association 1986 Standards and guidelines for cardiopulmonary resuscitation (CPR) and emergency cardiac care (ECC). J Am Med Assoc 255: 2905–2922

American Society of Anesthesiologists 1963 New classification of physical status. Anesthesiology 24: 111

Association of Anaesthetists of Great Britain and Ireland 1988 Recommendations for standards of monitoring during anaesthesia and recovery. Association of Anaesthetists, London

Association of Anaesthetists 1990 Checklist for anaesthetic machines. Association of Anaesthetists of Great Britain and Ireland, London

Attia R R, Battit G E, Murphy J D 1975 Transtracheal ventilation. J Am Med Assoc 234: 1152–1153

Brain A I J 1983 The laryngeal mask: a new concept in airway management. Br J Anaesth 55: 801–805

Buck N, Devlin H B, Lunn J N 1987 Report of a confidential enquiry into perioperative deaths. Nuffield Provincial Hospitals Trust, London

Casey W F 1984 Cardiopulmonary resuscitation: a survey of standards amongst junior staff doctors. Proc R Soc Med 77: 921–922

Conference of Royal Colleges and Faculties of the United Kingdom 1976 Diagnosis of brain death. Lancet 2: 1067–1070

Cullen B F, Miller M G 1979 Drug and interactios and anaesthesia: a review. Anesth Analg 58: 413–423

Derrington M C, Smith G 1987 A review of studies of anaesthetic risk, morbidity and mortality. Br J Anaesth 59: 815–833

Dinnick O P D 1973 Hazards of respiratory circuits. Ann R Coll Surg Engl 52: 349–354

Eichorn J H, Cooper J B, Cullen D J, Mair W R, Phillip J H, Seeman R G 1986 Standards for patient monitoring during anesthesia at Harvard Medical School. J Am Med Assoc 256: 1017–1020

Elling R, Politis J 1983 An evaluation of emergency medical technicians ability to use manual ventilation devices. Ann Emerg Med 12: 765–768

European Resuscitation Council (ERC) 1992a Basic Life Support Working Party of the ERC. Guidelines for basic life support. Resuscitation 24: 103–110

European Resuscitation Council (ERC) 1992b Advanced Life Support Working Party of the ERC. Guidelines for advanced life support. Resuscitation 24: 111–122

Fisher M M, Baldo B A, 1984 Anaphylactoid reactions during anaesthesia. Clin Anaesthesiology, 2 Adverse Reactions 677–692

Glynn C J 1987 Intrathecal and epidural opiate administration. In: Budd K (ed) Update in opioids, vol 1 no 4. Baillières clinical anaesthesiology. Saunders, London

Gustafsson L L, Schildt B F, Jacobson K J 1982 Adverse effects of epidural and intrathecal opiates: a nationwide survey in Sweden. Br J Anaesth 54: 479–486

Harrison G G 1983 Anaesthetic accidents. Clin Anaesth 1 (2): 415–429
Harrison R R, Maull, K I, Keenan R L, Boyan C P 1982 Mouth-to-mask ventilation: a superior method of rescue breathing. Ann Emerg Med 2: 74–76
Hess D, Baron C 1985 Ventilatory volumes using mouth-to-mouth, mouth-to-mask and bag-valve-mask techniques. Am J Emerg Med 3: 292–296
Higgins D, Hayes M, Denman P, Wilkinson D J 1990 Effectiveness of using end-tidal carbon dioxide concentration to monitor cardiopulmonary resuscitation. Br Med J 300: 581
Holland R 1987 Anaesthetic mortality in New South Wales. Br J Anaesth 59: 834–841
Keenan R L, Boyan C P 1985 Cardiac arrest due to anesthesia. J Am Med Assoc 253: 2373–2377
Latto J P 1985 Management of difficult intubation. In: Latto J P, Rosen M (eds) Difficulties in tracheal intubation. Baillière Tindall, London
Levine S A 1920 Acute Cardiac upsets, occurring during or following surgical operations. J Am Med Assoc 75: 749–799
Lowenstein S R, Libby L S, Mountain R D, Hansbrough J F, Hill D M, Scoggin C H 1981 Cardiopulmonary resuscitation by medical and surgical house officers. Lancet 2: 679–681
Lunn J N, Mushin W W 1982 Mortality associated with anaesthesia. Nuffield Provincial Hospitals Trust, London
Mallampati S R, Gatt S P, Gugino L D et al 1985 A clinical sign to predict difficult tracheal intubation: a prospective study. Can Anaesth Soc J 32: 429–434
Newton N I, Adams A P 1978 Excessive airway pressure during anaesthesia: hazards effects and prevention. Anaesthesia 33: 689–699
Oakley P A 1988 Inaccuracy and delay in decision making in paediatric resuscitation and a proposed reference chart to reduce error. Br Med J 297: 817–819
Ovassapian A, Dykes M H 1982 Difficult paediatric intubation: an indication for the fibreoptic bronchoscope. Anesthesiology 56: 412–413
Rayburn R L, 1979 Light wand intubation. Anaesthesia 34: 667–668
Redding J S, Pearson J W 1962 Resuscitation from asphyxia. J Am Med Assoc 182: 283–286
Resuscitation Council (UK) 1990 ABC of resuscitation, 2nd edn. Brit Med J
Samsoon G L T, Young J R B 1987 Difficult tracheal intubation: a retrospective study. Anaesthesia 42: 487–490
Sia R L, Edens E T 1981 How to avoid problems when using the fibreoptic bronchoscope for difficult intubations. Anaesthesia 36: 74–75
Skinner D V, Camm A J, Miles S 1985 Cardiopulmonary resuscitation skills of pre-registration house officers. Br Med J 290: 1549–1550
Smith R B, Schaer W B, Pfaeffle H 1975 Percutaneous transtreacheal ventilation for anaesthesia and resuscitation: a review of report of complications. Can Anaesth Soc J 22: 607–612
Special committee investigating deaths under anaesthesia 1970 Report on 745 classified cases 1960–68. Med J Aust 1: 473–595
Spence A A 1988 The lessons of CEPOD. Br J Anaesth 60: 753–754
Tiret L, Desmonts, J M, Hatton F, Vourch G 1986 Complications associated with anaesthesia: a prospective survey in France. Can Anaesth Soc J 33: 336–344

SECTION 6

Equipment hazards

42

Equipment to deliver inhaled agents

P. K. T. Nichols

Murphy's law

If anything can go wrong, it will, and at the most inconvenient opportunity.

Dickson 1978

INTRODUCTION

The scope for hazards and complications to occur as a result of the interaction of the anaesthetist, the equipment, the patient, the theatre and operating room environment is enormous.

Individual faults, omissions and errors of practice have been described on many occasions. It may, therefore, seem superfluous to repeat their categorization, but they continue to occur in the practice of experienced anaesthetists and junior anaesthetists alike. At best such incidents are merely annoying, but the potential for serious morbidity and even mortality is always present. This makes the reiteration and updating of these problems essential.

To avoid unnecessary duplication I will make no detailed reference to those hazards associated with the following:

- endotracheal tubes or airways
- fires and explosions
- monitoring.

MORBIDITY AND MORTALITY

It is unfortunate that there is little available data showing the incidence of either equipment failure, or associated morbidity or mortality. Indeed, some studies imply that equipment failure causes *no* mortality and therefore would seem not to be a problem worthy of any effort! This attitude can only lead to complacency. Vigilance on the part of the anaesthetist must be the patient's ultimate protection, therefore only in the most exceptional of circumstances should equipment failure lead to death.

Olsson & Hallén (1988), in a survey covering 17½ years and over a quarter of a million anaesthetics, looked at cardiac arrests during anaesthesia and their outcome. There were 170 cardiac arrests in all (with 115 anaesthesia-related) and nine patients died. Of the 115 anaesthesia-related arrests only one was equipment-related. This was due to disconnection of the ventilator tubing and the patient was successfully resuscitated.

In a study looking at the records of a professional liability insurance company (Taylor et al 1976), 41 cases of 'unexpected cardiac arrest' were reviewed. Of these, only one was definitely associated with equipment failure, where the patient had become disconnected for a prolonged period. The outcome of this incident is not stated, but only 11 (27%) of the patients left hospital and just three (7.3%) were capable of an independent existence.

In Holland's (1984) prospective survey of 20 years of postanaesthetic deaths in New South Wales, Australia, 2064 deaths were examined. Of these, 562 were anaesthetic-related, but in only 107 were anaesthetic-related incidents largely responsible for patient deaths. In this group equipment failure (19) constituted the third most common incident following inhalation of gastric contents (44) and airway complications (31). The breakdown of these incidents is given in Table 42.1 and includes those airway problems related to the endotracheal tube.

In a more recent prospective survey from France, Tiret et al (1986) reviewed 198 103 anaesthetics and their major complications. There were 268 major complications associated with anaesthesia, of which 163 were solely related to anaesthesia. There were 15 deaths and 10 prolonged comas in this group. The role of equipment failure is shown in Table 42.2.

Keenan & Boyan (1985) found 27 cardiac arrests solely due to anaesthesia in 163 240 anaesthetics. Two of these were due to equipment failure, both resulted from disconnections and both patients were successfully resuscitated.

It is also interesting to note that in the study of closed claims by Caplan et al (1990), claims resulting from respiratory equipment failure represented only 1% of the total database.

The Confidential Enquiries into Maternal Deaths in England and Wales (DHSS 1982, 1989) have pinpointed a small number of deaths related to anaesthetic equipment. In each case, death was related to misuse of, or a lack of understanding of, the equipment being used rather than equipment failure itself.

In the Report of a Confidential Enquiry into Perioperative Deaths (Buck et al 1988) 2928 deaths were reviewed, of which 400 were associated with anaesthesia. Seven deaths were related to equipment failure (Table 42.3). The relative frequencies of other factors are shown in Table 42.4

To provide a very crude estimate of equipment-related mortality I have combined data from a number of reviews and studies to produce an overall mortality rate (Table 42.5). The accuracy of this is severely limited by the small number of studies quoting the total number of anaesthetics administered. The overall mortality rate would appear to be almost 1:400 000 anaesthetics. I am a little surprised, but happy, that it should be as low as this given the number of events presented from many of the 'closed claim' analyses.

Table 42.1 Causes of equipment failure

Difficulty	Number of cases
Obstruction of endotracheal tube	8
Disconnection from ventilator	5
Misconnection of breathing system	4
Barotrauma from other cause	4
Exhausted oxygen cylinder	1
Crossed gas lines	1
Monitor malfunctions	1
Failure of transfusion lines	3

(from Holland 1984)

Table 42.2 Causes of major complications totally related to anaesthesia

Cause	Complications	Death	Coma
Respiratory failure or postanaesthetic respiratory depression	28	7	5
Inhalation of gastric contents	27	4	2
Complications of intubation	16	1	1
Bronchospasm	9	–	–
Equipment failure	5	1	1
Laryngospasm	3	–	–
Pneumothorax	2	–	–
Circulatory failure	73	2	1
Total	**163**	**15**	**10**

(from Tiret et al 1986)

CRITICAL INCIDENTS

Given the paucity of 'hard' data, many authors have used 'Critical Incidents' (CI) (Flannagan

Table 42.3 Causes of equipment-related deaths

Cause of failure	Number of deaths
Disconnections	2
Essential equipment not available	2
Misuse of equipment	2
Failure to test anaesthetic machine	1

(from Buck et al 1988)

Table 42.4 Anaesthetic assessors' opinions of which factors were involved in deaths associated with anaesthesia

Factor	% of total deaths (n = 2928)	% of cases where death associated with anaesthesia. (n = 410)
Failure to apply knowledge	10.5	75.1
Lack of care	4.2	30.0
Failure of organization	3.5	24.9
Lack of experience	3.3	23.7
Lack of knowledge	2.1	15.1
Drug effect	1.3	9.5
Failure of equipment	0.2	1.7
Fatigue	0.1	1.0
Impairment	0.0	0.0
Other	0.4	2.7

(from Buck et al 1988)

1954) as a means of highlighting problems. The general public are familiar with the 'near miss' in the field of aviation and of course the CI is similar.

In anaesthesia the technique has been adapted many times, but the most comprehensive definition is that supplied by Cooper et al (1978):

A Critical Incident is a mishap that was clearly an occurrence that could have led (if not discovered or corrected in time), or did lead to an undesirable outcome, that could range from an increased length of hospital (or recovery room) stay, to death or permanent disability, and which satisfies the following criteria:

1. It is an error by a member of the anaesthetic team, or a failure of their equipment to function properly.
2. It occurs whilst the patient is under the care of the anaesthetic team (including during the recovery period).
3. It is reported by someone who was either involved in, or witnessed, the episode.
4. It was clearly preventable.

The aim of the CI scheme, therefore, is to highlight problems with techniques, equipment or members of staff before they have an observable effect on patient morbidity or mortality. This is particularly important in the field of equipment where the overall mortality is very low and thus large changes in risk could easily be missed.

Cooper et al (1984) reported on three adaptations of the CI technique:

- voluntary reports from self-selected volunteers in four hospitals in the Boston Metropolitan area.
- volunteers in one of the Boston teaching hospitals.

Table 42.5 Resumé of the contribution of equipment failure to anaesthetic mortality

Source article	Number of anaesthetics	Cardiac arrests	Comas	Deaths
Olsson (1988)	250 543	1	0	0
Tiret (1986)	198 103	Unknown	1	1
Keenan & Boyan (1985)	163 240	2	0	0
Turnbull (1980)	195 232	0	0	0
Marx (1973)	34 145	0	0	0
Harrison (1978)	240 483	Unknown	Unknown	1
Chopra et al (1990)	113 074	1	0	1
Total	**1 194 820**	**3+?**	**1+?**	**3**

Therefore overall mortality rate = 1/398 270 anaesthetics.

- telephone reports, as soon as practicable after an occurrence had taken place.

In the first and second adaptations the reports were taken during interview by a trained interviewer who was not an anaesthetist. Following categorization of the incident, some strategies were suggested to 'close the loop' to minimize the risk of repetition. The data they presented also enables a comparison between the relative incidences of human error (in its many guises) and equipment failure. As can be seen from Table 42.6, human error as a source of CIs is more common than equipment failure (including disconnections).

Craig & Wilson (1981; see Table 42.7) confirm that human error is between two-and-a-half and three times more common than equipment failure, even when disconnections are included.

If the published data of Cooper et al (1978, 1984) (Tables 42.6, 42.8 & 42.9) are studied more closely it becomes apparent that the divisions are not as clear-cut as they appear. Examination of the equipment-related incidents shows that human error plays less of a role in certain areas than equipment failure, for example in respect of breathing circuits and ventilation. However, there are also areas where the converse is true. Human error is over eight times more likely than equipment failure to lead to a CI in anaesthetic-machine-related incidents. Awareness of such information should encourage us to redesign equipment to minimize actual problems. Table 42.10 shows the relative frequency of these incidents and the likelihood of what Cooper (1984) termed 'Substantive Negative Outcome', that is mortality, cardiac arrest, cancelled procedure or extended stay in theatre, recovery, ITU or hospital.

Table 42.6 Distribution of critical incidents according to type of failure

Type of failure	Number of incidents
Equipment failure	115
Human error	583
Disconnection	111
Other	46

(from Cooper et al 1984)

Before discussing specific equipment failures that have been reported, it is important to remember that everyone makes errors. This was well summarized by Allnutt (1987):

> For a pilot or a doctor to accept that he or she is as likely as anyone else to make a catastrophic error today is the first step towards prevention: to claim exemption on the grounds of being a test pilot, senior professor, commanding officer or consultant, or of having 30 years experience or 3000 accident free hours is the first step on the road to disaster.

Various studies from Australia (Williamson et al 1985, Currie et al 1988, Currie 1989) support the concept that human error is the most important cause of incidents (80–90%), but airway and circuitry events were numerous with 60% involving periods of non-ventilation of the patient. The most common causes of CIs are summarized in Table 42.11, in descending order of frequency.

Table 42.7 Breakdown of critical incidents by area of problem and source of error

Incident type	Miscellaneous	Human error	Equipment failure
Transmission of anaesthetic gases			
disconnections	0	0	7
leaks	0	3	3
gas supply	1	8	1
vaporizer	0	5	1
valve	0	5	1
Obstruction	0	0	1
Tracheal tube problems	0	16	5
Drug administration	2	10	0
Miscellaneous	0	11	1
Total	**3**	**58**	**20**

(from Craig & Wilson 1981)

Table 42.8 Distribution of human error and disconnection incidents by the nature of the activity or system involved

Activity or system	Human error	Disconnection
Drug administration	138	
Anaesthetic machine use	129	
Airway management	92	
Breathing system or ventilation	64	79
Fluid and electrolyte management	31	
Intravenous apparatus	33	22
Monitoring device use	26	10
Other	70	

With permission from Cooper et al (1984).

Another method of assessing frequency of equipment failure is a review of published articles in anaesthetic and technical journals. A search was undertaken in the journal, *Anaesthesia*, to find such reports over the last 5 years. It showed 53 instances of equipment failure (see Table 42.12). No doubt there is a bias towards unusual and exceptional events that make publication more attractive, but such articles can still act as timely reminders.

Because of the great variety of equipment failures described in the literature it is necessary to provide a framework on which to base a systematic categorization. This is most usefully done by looking at the problems the patient may suffer rather than the primary equipment failure, for this is the manner in which the fault will probably present itself to the anaesthetist. This categorization is shown in Table 42.13. The alternative classification based on the site of hazard is shown in Table 42.14.

Table 42.9 Distribution according to type of equipment involved

Equipment	Number of incidents
Breathing circuit	26
Monitoring device	22
Ventilator	17
Anaesthetic machine	16
Airway device	14
Laryngoscope	11
Other	9

(from Cooper et al 1984)

HYPOXIA

Failure of supply

Pipelines

In a survey by Feeley & Hedley-Whyte (1976), 31% of hospitals reported some difficulty with their pipeline systems, with the most common complaint being an unacceptably low or absent supply pressure. This may be caused by:

- damage during construction
- debris in the line following installation
- unannounced system shut-down
- unauthorized system shut-down (Wyant 1979)
- regulator malfunctions (Allberry 1989)
- damage to the bulk storage tank by bad weather (Johnson 1975)
- spontaneous closure of an isolation valve (Gibson 1979)
- low-pressure alarm failure or disregard from ignorance (Morrison 1981).

Moving further along the 'chain', the Schraeder valves may fail from obstruction (Morrison 1981) or may not connect (Anon. 1975). The hoses themselves may become completely or partially blocked, be unable to be inserted into the pipeline or become inadvertently disconnected. If there is a movable ceiling column or boom, then the flexible hoses in these may wear and leak or fail completely. Thus all machines using pipeline supplies should have a pressure gauge showing pipeline pressure (rather than the 'system' pressure of the anaesthetic machine), which obviously should be checked before use for these may also fail, showing full (or no) pressure.

Table 42.10 Distribution of frequent critical incidents and numbers of substantive negative outcome (SNOS)

Incident description	Number of incidents	Number of SNOS
Breathing system disconnection during mechanical ventilation	57	4
Gas flow control technical error	41	2
Loss of gas supply	32	
Vaporizer off unintentionally	22	
Drug overdose (vaporizer, technical)	20	2
Breathing system leak	19	
Unintentional extubation	18	
Misplaced endotracheal tube	18	3
Breathing system misconnection	18	5
Ventilator malfunction	15	
Breathing system control technical error	15	
Wrong choice of airway management technique	13	4
Hypoventilation (human error only)	11	
Drug overdose (vaporizer, judgemental)	9	
Drug overdose (syringe, technical)	8	4
Miscellaneous technical error	5	
Miscellaneous judgemental error	9	
Failure to detect	5	

(from Cooper et al 1984)

Cylinders

Failure of the cylinder supply may be due either to an empty cylinder or to the anaesthetist's inability to use the full cylinder supplied. In the first instance, failure may be due to natural emptying of the cylinder from use going unnoticed by the anaesthetist (in spite of the presence of an oxygen failure alarm, or due to its absence or failure). It may also follow failure of a pipeline supply when the oxygen cylinder valve has been left open and thus the cylinder has been allowed to empty. In the second case the failure may be due to the absence (or removal) of the cylinder valve key. Other causes of failure include the failure to remove the dust cover leading to the blockage of the yoke gas inlet or reducing valves with its material, or inserting the cylinder the wrong way round with concomitant escape of gas under high pressure.

Machines

In old anaesthetic machines that used rubber pipe to connect the internal components, kinking was possible causing obstruction to the flow of the gas concerned. With the return of non-metallic pipe materials it may be possible for this problem to recur.

Table 42.11 Critical incidents by area of failure in descending order of incidence

Airway	Circuit	Disconnection
		Misconnection
	Endotracheal tube	Misplaced
		Cuff
		Kinked
	Obstruction	Tongue
	Breathing	Inadequate
		Absent
Drugs	Syringe swap	
	Overdose	
	Adverse reaction	
	Wrong site	
Equipment	Misuse	Flow meters
		Vaporizer
	Malfunction	Vaporizer
		Ventilator
		Monitors
	Absence	
Circulation	Arrhythmia	
	Intravenous fluid errors	
Other	Malpositioning	

Table 42.12 Summary of equipment failure (Anaesthesia 1986–1990). Survey by area of failure and year of publication

Area of failure	1986	1987	Year 1988	1989	1990	Total
Pipelines	3	1	0	1	3	8
Anaesthetic machine	4	2	2	1	1	11
Vaporizer	4	3	0	1	3	10
Ventilator	0	0	5	0	1	6
Breathing system	2	4	3	6	2	17
Humidifier	1	0	0	0	0	1
Total	**14**	**10**	**10**	**9**	**10**	**53**

As stated above, the oxygen failure alarm itself may fail in the 'no fault' mode. The oxygen safety valve may also fail, leading to the continued delivery of the other gases and the rapid deoxygenation of the patient, whether he is breathing spontaneously or being ventilated.

Recently, 'advances' in anaesthetic machine design have led to the establishment of links between the oxygen and nitrous oxide flowmeters to establish a minimum supplied oxygen concentration of 25%. However, these may lead to a false sense of security for they may also fail, leading to the delivery of an hypoxic mixture (Richards 1989).

Pressure variation in the other gas supplies

Increases in the pressure of other gases will lead to an increase in flow through any associated flow meter that is open. If this gas contains no oxygen (e.g. nitrous oxide) this will lead (Finlay & Penlton 1971) to a decrease in inspired oxygen which may be sufficient to cause hypoxia.

Delivery of gas instead of oxygen

There have been many reports of morbidity and mortality resulting from the delivery of non-

Table 42.13 Classification of equipment failure by mode of presentation

Presentation	Equipment failure
Hypoxia	Oxygen supply problem
	Incorrect gas supplied
	Leaks
	Rebreathing
Hypercarbia	Absorber related
	Added carbon dioxide
	Rebreathing
Hypoventilation	Disconnections
	Leaks
	Ventilator failure
Hyperventilation	Ventilator leaks
Excessive airway pressure leading to:	Barotrauma
	Cardiovascular depression
	Gas embolism
Inhalation of foreign substances	Dusts
	Gas contaminants
	Bacterial
Excess inhalation agent	—
Insufficient inhalation agent	—

Table 42.14 Classification of equipment failure by site of failure

Equipment failure	Site of failure
Central storage facilities	Pipelines Cylinders
Anaesthetic machines	Internal gas
Connections	
	Flow meters Vaporizers Oxygen failure safety Devices
Breathing systems Ventilators Humidifiers Anaesthetic gas Scavenging systems	

oxygen-containing gas in place of oxygen, with the Westminster disaster (Kidner et al 1977) perhaps the most notable in British practice.

Pipeline crossovers

Crossovers may occur at any point within a pipeline network and at any time, but are most common following addition to, or alteration in, an existing system (Wyant 1979). The bulk storage vessel may be incorrectly filled with nitrogen (Sprague & Archer 1975), or the pipework may not have been flushed following testing after construction has been completed, and thus may remain full of air or, more usually, nitrogen.

Within the theatre suite the Schraeder valves may be wrongly inserted due to faulty design (Lane 1980, Russel & Snowdon 1986), wear and tear, and lack of maintenance (Forrester 1968), or due to errors in construction or maintenance leading to the presence of the wrong connection, hose (Kidner et al 1977) or pipeline inlet to the machine itself. In addition, connections in the machine (Klein & Lilburn 1980), or other ancillary equipment (Bageant et al 1980) such as air-oxygen mixer valves (Karmann & Roth 1982, Thorp & Railton 1982), may lead to contamination of the oxygen pipeline with the other gas.

Machine crossovers

In addition to the crossovers described above, many have occurred within the anaesthetic machine itself, the majority following servicing of the machine (Kalra & Doughty 1963).

Incorrect cylinder contents

Just as it is possible for central storage facilities to be wrongly filled, oxygen cylinders may also be mislabelled or incorrectly filled (Mazze 1972, Jawan & Lee 1990), or they may contain other substances, such as water (Schiller 1986, Coveler & Lester 1989). A number of episodes of incorrect labelling also occur on a regular basis (Jayasuriya 1986, Boon 1990). It is particularly important that anaesthetists should be aware of the colour coding of cylinders. The proposed international colour code is not yet implemented worldwide, so there may be inconsistencies in different countries. The anaesthetist moving between countries must therefore be particularly wary.

Incorrect attachment to machine yoke

For many years the Pin Index Safety System has existed to try to prevent the attachment of the incorrect cylinder to the anaesthetic machine yoke, but there is no limit to human endeavours to defeat such a system. One of the pins involved may be removed (Saposnick 1975), or they may be too short (Goebel 1980). Two Bodok seals have also been used to circumvent the system and the cylinders or, more often, the pipeline supply may be inserted upside-down. Fortunately, improvements in the design of yokes has led to a marked decrease in this type of fault. Alternatively, following service or otherwise, the incorrect control block may be inserted (Spurring & Small 1983), leading to potential disaster.

Flow meter hazards

The majority of hypoxic problems associated with the use of flow meters are operator errors where the anaesthetist has set the wrong flow rate, often (unfortunately) aided by poor and inconsistent design. Flow meters themselves have proved generally reliable. Some faults have, however, occurred and will, no doubt, continue to do so.

Leaks

The most common leak is now at the point of insertion of the vaporizer since there is potential for the interchangable types to be incorrectly seated.

With a normal design of flow meter blocks (i.e. with oxygen the first gas), leaks from any of the flow meters will lead to preferential loss of oxygen (unless the leak is beneath the bobbin in another gas's flow meter). This has been well summarized by Eger et al (1963). The leak may be caused by misassembly following service, or cracking or chipping of the flow meter tube (Liew & Ganedran 1973, Powell 1981). The risks of this may be minimized if oxygen is the last gas to enter the machine, when the other diluent or carrier gases will be lost rather than oxygen. This will obviously still lead to problems because the delivered fresh gas flow will be diminished, but the risks of hypoxia will be lessened.

Leaks may also be introduced by incorrect settings of the gas pathway where there are two or more outlets and fresh gas and the patient breathing system is connected to a different source. In some machines a dedicated oxygen supply to vaporizers may contribute a significant source of oxygen with agents of low volatility. If this is inadvertently turned off then hypoxia may well intervene. This type of problem, while not entirely due to the equipment itself, is related to the equipment-anaesthetist interface.

Inaccuracies

Inaccurate flow meters will obviously affect the delivered oxygen concentration. If the oxygen flow meter under-reads (or the other gases over-read), hypoxia may result. The inaccuracies may be caused by sticking of the flow meter bobbin due to the presence of static electricity (Clutton-Brock 1976), dirt, grease or oil (Bracken 1976). The effects are often greatest at the lowest flow rates (Saunders et al 1981). Inaccuracies may also be brought about by the transposition of flow meter, bobbin or scales (Chadwick 1974), calibration errors (Kelly & Gabel 1970) or loss of the bobbin from view at maximum flow, which may be a particular problem with flow meters for gases other than oxygen (Rendall-Baker 1976).

Air entrainment

In the presence of a leak in a breathing system and a machine that generates a negative pressure within the breathing system, for example a descending bellows ventilator, air may be entrained, thus leading potentially to hypoxia (Liston 1981).

Rebreathing

Rebreathing itself may lead to hypoxia, particularly in the presence of inadequate fresh gas flow (Waters 1968).

HYPERCARBIA

Hypercarbia most commonly occurs as a result of central respiratory depression from anaesthetic drugs. There are, however, a number of equipment problems that may also lead to it. With one exception they can, in essence, be described as originating with rebreathing, although this underlying mechanism hides many discrete failures that may occur. These are described below.

Inadequate fresh gas flow

Inadequate fresh gas flow is almost certainly the most common equipment-related cause and usually results from the anaesthetist setting the wrong flows on the anaesthetic machine. This is normally the result of 'human error', but sometimes, unfortunately, it is due to ignorance of the underlying physical mechanisms involved in the use of the chosen breathing system. This principally applies to Mapleson D systems used in the spontaneously breathing patient and the Mapleson A used when ventilating a patient.

Inadequate fresh gas flow may also result from a leak within the anaesthetic machine downstream of the flow meters. If the oxygen flow rate is sufficient, hypoxia may not appear until very late. The subject of anaesthetic machine leaks is discussed more fully on page 674.

Absorber related

In breathing systems that use intentionally low flows there must obviously be a mechanism for 'scrubbing' carbon dioxide from within the system. This is usually done by calcium hydroxide (soda-lime) or barium hydroxide (baralyme). If the absorbent becomes exhausted, partially or completely, then the patient will be at risk of hypercarbia. Partial exhaustion is the greater risk, as the indicator may not have started to change colour, 'rejuvenation' of the absorbent may have occurred (giving the appearance of fresh soda-lime) or the indicator may have been omitted from the mix (Barasch et al 1976). Exhaustion may also occur in isolated areas if the absorber has been improperly filled (Elam 1958), thus leading to preferential 'channelling' of gas down through a few areas of the canister. This is rather less of a problem now since circle systems have replaced Water's 'to-and-fro' systems.

Failure of the absorbent may also occur if no moisture is available to initiate the reaction, such as may occur if a heat and moisture exchange humidifier is used (Bellamy 1988).

In addition to failure of the absorbent, the absorber itself may be removed from the system. The ability to remove the absorber is very useful at the conclusion of anaesthesia to ensure that the carbon dioxide concentration is sufficient to provide a stimulus to respiration. This can be done by a simple on/off or bypass switch. This causes no problems until the anaesthetist omits to turn the bypass switch on prior to commencing low-flow anaesthesia in the next case. This risk of what is, in fact, human error rather than equipment failure has led anaesthetic machine manufacturers to withdraw this option, often without consultation, in spite of the almost universal presence of gas analysers within operating theatres.

Added carbon dioxide

The unintentioned and excessive addition of carbon dioxide to the fresh gas flow is another hazard more related to human error than equipment failure. It has altered the practice of anaesthesia and the design of anaesthetic machines. Bad design has resulted in high flow (up to, or greater than, 2 l/min) carbon dioxide flow meters being placed on our anaesthetic machines. This, coupled with a design fault that allows the bobbin to 'disappear' at the top of the flow meter's range (DHSS 1987), has led to some patients receiving an extremely high concentration of carbon dioxide and, potentially, a hypoxic anaesthetic gas mixture (Esplen 1956).

This is undesirable, to say the least, but instead of following the reasoned approach of limiting the maximum flow of carbon dioxide and ensuring that the bobbin is always prominently visible, there is pressure for complete removal of carbon dioxide from our machines.

Valve problems

Essential to the correct performance of any circle or one-way system is the presence and correct functioning of its unidirectional valves. Should these fail to act properly then rebreathing is certain to occur, as the respired gases will flow along the limb with the least resistance, that is the limb with the malfunctioning open valve. This is most marked when the faulty valve is in the inspiratory limb (i.e. closest to the site of bag, or ventilator hose connection in British practice), when as much as 90% of the tidal volume may be rebreathed (Nichols unpublished observations). Valve leaflets may be made ineffective by the surface tension of condensed moisture on the valve dome (Nunn & Rosewarne 1990) or guard, holding the leaflet away from its seating (Eger & Epstein 1964). Alternatively the seating or the valve leaflet itself may be damaged during cleaning or maintenance (Kerr & Evers 1958). The presence of a rough patch on the leaflet guard may cause the lightweight valve disc to catch. This may not become apparent for weeks following servicing and may then be only intermittent (Nichols unpublished observations).

In addition, care must be taken, if the valve leaflet needs replacement, that the correct new part is fitted, for there are a number of instances where either too large or too small a leaflet has been fitted, or the valve cage has been inadequately seated (Rosewarne & Wells 1988) and valve incompetence or other failure has resulted.

Finally, absence of the leaflet valve will obviously have similar but more marked effects (Smith & Volpitto 1959). This may occur if the system is used with a separate, external valve system (e.g. a Ruben's valve) and then taken for use by another anaesthetist for whom the external valve is removed. It is therefore, worth remembering that any absence of a valve leaflet must be fully explained before the system is repaired and used, for it may have become dislodged and go on to obstruct (Anon. 1982).

Non-rebreathing valves

If non-rebreathing valves fail to function correctly the inevitable result is significant rebreathing. The causes of such rebreathing are related to either of the following:

1. Gas leaks back through the inspiratory valve and down the inspiratory limb (Meyer 1972). The level of hypercarbia will depend on the size of the leak and the total fresh gas flow.
2. The rebreathing valve is assembled incorrectly following cleaning or repair. This leads to concurrent obstructed exhalation and incompetence of the inspiratory valve.

Coaxial systems

With all coaxial breathing systems the risk exists that the inner hose may become detached at the machine-end with a subsequent massive increase in dead space. While this problem is almost exclusively reported from the use of the Bain system there is no reason why the Lack should not also be at risk. Detachment of the inner tube of the Bain may be due to kinking, avulsion or puncture (Hewitt & Campbell 1986). In addition, the inner tube may be too short to reach the patient-end and a large dead space will effectively be added to the breathing system (Wildsmith & Grubb 1977, Fukunaga 1981).

Improper assembly of the breathing system

A number of examples of improper assembly leading to hypercarbia are known, related both to the Bain (Peterson 1978, Cundy & Baldock 1982) and the Magill system. No further comment should be necessary within the scope of this chapter.

HYPOVENTILATION

While equipment failure may lead to either hypoxia or hypocarbia as previously described, certain types of failure may lead to significant evidence of both and are therefore best described together in a discussion of hypoventilation.

Occlusion of inspiration and expiration

Occlusion of inspiration and expiration is most commonly due to blockage of the final common pathway, that is the catheter mount, endotracheal tube and connectors, particularly the endotracheal tube (problems of which are discussed elsewhere). It may, however, be due to failure of a non-rebreathing valve (Wisborg & Jacebson 1975), or incorrect assembly of a circle breathing system where both unidirectional and non-rebreathing valves are incorporated.

Low tidal volumes

Low tidal volumes are probably the most common cause of hypoventilation and may arise from a number of errors:

- disconnection
- leak
- failure of, or incorrectly adjusted, relief valve
- ventilator failures
- fresh gas flow problem
- occlusion of inspiratory pathway
- negative pressure generated within the system.

Disconnections

Disconnections are the most common source of equipment failure. One can define a disconnection as an unintentional break in the breathing system components that allows the gas intended for the ventilation of the patient to escape into the atmosphere. This is an example of a problem that we as anaesthetists have created for ourselves as a result of 'solving' another problem.

In the early years the patient self-ventilated or was ventilated by hand. In these circumstances any disconnection was apparent from changes in the bag of the breathing system, either in its compliance (if the patient was being 'bagged') or because it collapsed (if the patient was self-ventilating). Following the introduction and universal use of the anaesthetic ventilator, this warning disappeared.

Disconnection may occur at any junction in the breathing system, but is most common at the junction between the breathing system and the endotracheal tube (Dolan 1976), particularly when this connection is hidden under the drapes during ophthalmic, ear, nose and throat or neurosurgery. While the introduction of various monitoring apparatus, such as pressure-triggered devices and expired gas analysers, have done much to diminish the problems of disconnection, they have not and will probably never abolish them, particularly as the monitors themselves are not 100% reliable and may not respond in all situations (Levine et al 1989, Pryn & Crosse 1989).

Several systems have been developed to improve on the present friction fit, for instance that of Penlon by the addition of a locknut and thread. Unfortunately, none has achieved great acceptance.

Leaks

Leaks may occur from the anaesthetic machine, the breathing system or the ventilator. It is fair to say that the majority of leaks are small and clinically insignificant (assuming explosive or flammable agents are not being used), and outside certain low tolerance areas, for instance low-flow/closed breathing systems. The detection of leaks is best done by monitoring inspiratory and expiratory tidal volume, although the majority will be detected by exhaled carbon dioxide monitoring or expiratory spirometry.

Anaesthetic machine leaks. Leaks may occur at any point along the gas line but are commonly associated with vaporizers, flow meters or downstream piping.

Vaporizers. Vaporizer leaks may occur at the inlet, outlet or agent filling port due to loose connections, incorrect fitting (Eldrup-Jorgensen & Sprissler 1977, Anon 1973), a physical defect in the connection (Van-Besouw & Thurlow 1987) or missing seals on Selectatec blocks.

Flow meters. Faults leading to hypoventilation are similar to those described above with regard to hypoxia, and include leaks from within the flow meter (Bishop et al 1967) or backflow through an open flow meter with exit to the atmosphere (Edwards et al 1956, McQuillan & Jackson 1987).

Downstream leaks. Connections downstream of the flow meter are, in general terms, metal-to-metal and are thus susceptible to damage and leaks, particularly following service or abuse.

Breathing system leaks. Leaks from the breathing system are probably the most common source of leaks encountered in clinical practice. They may be particularly common with disposable breathing systems as up to 50% of these may leak (Kemen et al 1990), and they are less robust than the previous systems (Sosis & Payne 1989). Another common site in systems using an absorber is the absorber itself, where leaks can occur from around the rubber seals due to misalignment, distortion or interposition of the absorbent material itself. Humidifiers also provide a common source of leak (Raja & Geller 1986). In addition the attachment for various monitoring devices may crack due to mishandling (Lamarche 1985) or contamination with volatile agents (Ferdebar et al 1986). A forward leak may occur if a non-rebreathing valve is used when ventilating the patient.

Ventilator leaks. Leaks may occur within the ventilator itself (Higgs & Garrett 1979), at the attachment of the breathing system (Rolbin 1977) and at the selector-valve housing (Cooper 1978).

Pressure relief valve failure

Anaesthetic breathing systems (with a few notable exceptions, such as the enclosed Magill) preferentially lose gas during inspiration when they are being used for assisted or controlled ventilation. This leads to considerable difficulty is estimating the amount of gas reaching the patient and that proportion being vented through the pressure relief valve. This, therefore, can lead to the situation where, unbeknown to the anaesthetist, the vast majority (or all) of the ventilated volume escapes through the pressure relief valve. In this way complete airway obstruction may go unnoticed until the patient's cardiac arrest (Clinical Anaesthesia Conference 1963).

Ventilator failure

A ventilator fault leading to hypoventilation is most often due to 'operator error' from failure to connect correctly or accidentally turning the machine off (Ciobanu & Meyer 1980). However, true equipment failure may also be the cause, the ventilator failing to cycle (Sarnquist & Demas 1982) or delivering a smaller minute volume than preset (Jorgensen 1976).

Fresh gas flow failure

If the fresh gas flow provided by the anaesthetic machine should fail, hypoventilation may result. The site of this failure may be within the anaesthetic machine itself, at the connection of the machine to the breathing system or within the breathing system.

Failure of the oxygen supply will lead to shutting of the oxygen failure device and occlusion of the fresh gas supply. Normally the anaesthetist's attention would be drawn to this failure by the sound of the oxygen failure alarm, but this may fail, be absent or be missed in a noisy theatre environment.

Adventitious material within the piping of the machine may obstruct it and again result in hypoventilation (Chang et al 1980, Goddard & Abbott 1986).

In certain breathing systems a small-bore, high-pressure hose is used to connect to the anaesthetic machine. This in turn may become detached (Longmuir & Craig 1975), obstructed or kinked.

Faults within the breathing system are, in the main, related to the coaxial form of the Mapleson D (Bain), where the inner tube (fresh gas flow) may become obstructed by twisting (Mansell 1976) or kinking (Inglis 1980).

Occlusion of the inspiratory limb

If the gas pathway becomes occluded between the ventilator or reservoir bag and the patient, pressure generated therein will result in insufficient gas flow to the patient and hypoventilation will result. The fault may lie with misconnection of the ventilator hose or reservoir bag (Cobcroft 1978), collapse of the reservoir bag neck due to twisting, kinking of the hoses within the breathing system (Cottrell et al 1976, Goresky 1990), failure to remove the seals on a disposable carbon dioxide absorber package (Feingold 1976) or occlusion by tape (Frankel 1983).

The high temperature output of certain humidifiers may be sufficient to cause airway scalds or deformation and occlusion of disposable system components (Shroff & Skerman 1988).

Negative pressure within the breathing system

Active gas scavenging systems may result in hypoventilation due to the generation of negative pressure within the breathing system, especially when the pressure relief valve (expiratory valve) is fully open (Mostafa & Sutcliffe 1982).

HYPERVENTILATION

Hyperventilation may also be caused by equipment failure, although it is a far more unusual event. The only situations I have been able to identify relate either to misassembly (Love 1980), or to 'bag in the bottle' ventilators where a hole has developed in the bag (Waterman et al 1978).

Podraza et al (1991) found that the effect on ventilation was greatest with descending type bellows, large tidal volumes, holes greater than 2 cm long and low fresh gas flows.

EXCESSIVE AIRWAY PRESSURE

Before discussing equipment failures that lead to the generation of excessive airway pressure, it is necessary to describe the modes of presentation. Excessive airway pressure may present as pneumothorax, pneumomediastinum, pneumoperitoneum, surgical emphysema or possibly even gas embolus. Cardiovascular depression from the Valsalva effect and/or tamponade from raised mean intrathoracic pressure are, however, more common occurrences. Which system is affected will be determined by the duration and degree of raised airway pressure. Abnormally high airway pressure may result from excessive gas inflow or insufficient outflow.

Excessive gas inflow

Excessive gas inflow may be due to the inadvertent operation of the 'oxygen flush' or 'emergency oxygen' supply by damage (Puttick 1986), activation from other components of the breathing system, other items of theatre equipment or failure to close following its use during the anaesthetic (Anderson & Rendall-Baker, 1982). Similar accidents may lead to explosive disruption of vaporizers (Cohen & Groveman 1966, Thompson 1976). Excessive gas inflow may also occur following failure of a high-pressure reducing valve (Eger & Epstein 1964), although for this to affect the patient the safety relief valve of the regulator must also fail (a combination that has yet to be reported as far as I am aware).

The pipeline system may also deliver too high a pressure (Feeley et al 1975), or alternatively the ventilator may fail in the inspiratory phase allowing pipeline pressure to act on the patient's airway.

Insufficient outflow

If the outflow resistance of the components of the breathing system is too high then, inevitably, the pressure within the breathing system will rise. This may be associated with a normal resistance and a high flow, as in the examples discussed above, or a normal flow and a high expiratory resistance, as discussed below. This obstruction may occur at or within the expiratory limb, at the pressure relief valve or within the anaesthetic gas scavenging system. Finally it may occur within non-rebreathing valves.

Expiratory limb obstruction

Expiratory limb obstruction may be the result of a number of problems, some of which are described below. It has become increasingly popular to use combined bacterial and humidifying filters within the breathing system. By their very nature they collect material that may be present in sufficient quantity to occlude them (Davenport & Keenleyside 1957, Loeser 1978). This may also happen to filters used within the ventilator tube (Anon. 1981b). In circle systems the normal sequence of inspiratory and expiratory valve may be disrupted by exchanging the expiratory valve for an inspiratory valve (Wyant 1979). Misconnection may also occur with the bag and expiratory limb positions on certain ventilators being exchanged (Sellery 1972), with exclusion of the reservoir bag and consequent loss of the pressure buffering facility. Other misconnections have involved anaesthetic machines with dual outlets. Here the breathing system has suffered a disconnection, then been reconnected such that the expiratory limb is not returned to its rightful place, but is instead placed on the occluded 'spare' gas outlet (Wyant 1979). The addition of two sets of valves within a circle system (see above) may also lead to obstructed expiration. Kinking of the expiratory limb has also lead to occlusion. This kinking may be caused by rotation (Taylor & Stoelting 1963) or external compression. Further faults with circle systems and valves have occurred when the expiratory valve has become 'lost' in the system (perhaps displaced [Anon. 1982] following service) and has subsequently been replaced, resulting in occluded expiration at the bag and ventilator connection port.

Barotrauma may also be associated with transtracheal jet ventilation if expiration should become occluded (Van-Besouw 1987, Craft et al 1990), or with PEEP valves, especially if they malfunction (Anagnostou et al 1990).

Pressure relief valve obstruction

The pressure relief valve may cause an obstruction in the breathing system or ventilator. This obstruction may be by sticking (Newton & Adams 1978), omission or malfunction (Dinnick 1973, Thompson 1979). Within the ventilator system, malfunction (Duckett et al 1980) or obstruction (Mason & Tackley 1981) may also occur.

Anaesthetic gas scavenging systems

Obstruction within the scavenging system may, under certain conditions, act as a restriction to gas flow from the breathing system. A particular problem is related to that part between the pressure relief valve and the scavenging interface (Davies & Tarnawsky 1976).

It is common practice within the UK to use 22 mm disposable hose (with an appropriate adaptor) for this purpose. This has the additional hazard that misconnections are made more likely.

Non-rebreathing valve obstruction

Non-rebreathing valves may lock in inspiration, especially if subjected to a high flow of gas, even that caused by a hard squeeze or bump to the inflating bag. Incorrect assembly may also lead to obstruction (Grogono & Poterfield 1970, Munford & Wishaw 1990).

INHALATION OF FOREIGN SUBSTANCES

Foreign substances that enter the airway may have a number of effects. They may lead to obstruction within the airway or breathing system, or cause allergic reactions or direct pulmonary damage. The individual effect will depend on the nature and quantity of substance inhaled.

Use of the Circle system with absorber leads to the generation of absorbent dust. If this is inhaled it may lead to the onset of wheeze, bronchospasm, laryngospasm, cough or decreased lung compliance. Inhalation of this dust is a particular problem when the absorber is placed close to the patient, for example the Waters 'to-and-fro' system, or when high flows are generated through the absorber itself, for example if the bag is on the expiratory side of the absorber.

The use of ethylene oxide for sterilization of apparatus has also been associated with the generation of pulmonary problems when any equipment that has been sterilized by the gas has been insufficiently 'aired'. The presence of water within the system may lead to the generation of ethylene glycol which may be absorbed following inhalation.

Contaminants from within the piped gas system may also be inhaled. These may be in the form of particulate matter or gaseous material (Eichhorn et al 1977, Tingay et al 1978). In hospital compressors used to generate medical grade air, oil mists may form that may subsequently be very difficult to remove (Bushman & Clark 1967). Other contaminants may also enter in this way, particularly if the design of the system has resulted in poor siting of the intake. An elegant study using radioactive tracer (Bjerring & Yberg 1987) has confirmed that this may be a problem with potential contamination of a medical air supply by bacteria aspirated using the hospital suction system.

Nitrous oxide may also be contaminated, either by water or by the higher oxides of nitrogen (nitric oxide and nitrogen dioxide) that have not been removed after the manufacture process (Clutton-Brock 1967). The inhalation of these contaminants will lead to pulmonary oedema and hypoxia.

Other particulate matter may originate from within the anaesthetic machine itself, in the form of flakes from the plating on the inside of components of the anaesthetic machine that have become detached (Austin 1972).

Bacteria may be inhaled by the patient, either as a result of contamination or from another source of infection within the breathing system itself, for instance the tubes of the system or a heated water humidifier.

The anaesthetic agents themselves may break down, either from metabolism by the patient (Sharp et al 1979) or by a heat source within the breathing system, such as a heated humidifier (Karis et al 1980). The accumulation of these products may lead to a high concentration within the circle system, especially if low flows are used.

ANAESTHETIC AGENT OVERDOSE

Anaesthetic overdose may be caused by a wide variety of errors and failures, some of which are discussed below.

Overdose may be caused by the overfilling of a vaporizer. This mainly applies to a type more common in USA practice where the vaporizer is filled from the top and the fill markings are relatively difficult to see. Overfilling in this manner has the effect of allowing liquid agent to overflow into the main gas path, thus saturating the main gas flow.

Tipping of certain types of vaporizer may lead to similar contamination of the main gas pathway. This has become more of a problem following the introduction and widespread use of detachable vaporizers, such as those using the 'Selectatec' mechanism or Penlon 'Off-line' block, particularly those vaporizers with two part 'keyed fillers', where the filler projects below the bottom of the vaporizer.

Calibration errors in flow meters may also create problems, although this is mainly limited to vaporizers with a dedicated flow meter. In fact, there have been case reports where the flow meter has under-read by a factor of six, with a consequent potential for vast overdose (Kelly & Gabel 1970).

The inhalational agent may also be administered inadvertently. This is most commonly related to human error where the anaesthetist using the machine immediately previously has left a vaporizer on, and the next anaesthetist fails to notice this and uses a different agent. Vaporizer interlocking devices prevent this. Alternatively a vaporizer may simply have been turned on without the anaesthetist's knowledge (Austin 1971).

Where two vaporizers are used simultaneously there will, inevitably, be contamination of the 'downstream' vaporizer with vapour from the 'upstream' one. This means that upon subsequent usage the downstream vaporizer will be delivering two agents at the same time (Wickett et al 1974). This is most dangerous when the downstream vaporizer contains a less volatile anaesthetic of a similar potency (i.e. a relatively greater gas flow through the vaporizer). This may lead to an excessive output of the more volatile agent.

Under certain circumstances, vaporizers may 'leak' volatile agent into the main gas flow even though they are turned off.

Inhalational agents may also be absorbed, in moderate quantities, into the black, antistatic rubber from which anaesthetic tubing has traditionally been manufactured. This will then be eluted out when agent-free gas, or gas containing another agent, is passed through the hose, leading to significant exposure of the patient to the first agent (Murray & Fleming 1972). This may be a particular problem with halothane, where repeated exposure at short intervals has been implicated in the genesis of 'halothane hepatitis'.

When using vaporizers of the 'plenum' type, that is those using a splitting of the fresh gas flow, an intermittent alteration in the 'downstream' pressure will, potentially, result in the backward flow of agent into the vaporizer (the 'pumping effect'). This may be caused by minute volume dividers such as the Manley ventilator, or by use of the 'oxygen flush' valve (Zimmerman & Lord 1980).

If an 'agent specific' vaporizer is used with the incorrect vapour, problems will result (Munson 1971). These may include dual delivery of agent and considerable inaccuracy of calibration. This will be a particular problem when an agent of relatively high volatility is placed in a vaporizer designed for use with a low volatility agent. For instance, placing halothane in a Trilene vaporizer will result in vapour output that may be up to four or five times that set (Nichols unpublished observations).

In anaesthetic machines that use a measured flow vaporizer, loss of the main gas flow will lead to less dilution of the vaporizer flow than was intended, thus leading to higher concentrations of vapour than expected (Eldrup-Jorgensen & Sprissler 1977).

In situations where an 'in circuit' vaporizer is used with a spontaneously breathing patient, if rebreathing occurs there is a considerable risk that dangerously high concentrations of inhalational agent will rapidly build up (Morris 1979). A similar effect is seen if such a vaporizer is used with assisted or controlled respiration.

Under certain circumstances, vaporizer inaccuracies may also lead to the delivery of excessive concentrations of inhalational agents. These may result from primary faulty calibrations (Noble 1970), or alteration of output with variations in either the fresh gas flow rate (Paterson et al 1969, Latto 1973) or the composition of the fresh gas flow (Diaz 1976).

A further cause of agent overdose relates to the production of long-lasting and stable foams, with the egress of the foam out of the vaporizer and into the main gas stream. This has occurred when the liquid anaesthetic agent has been contaminated with certain silicone-based substances, such as many lubricants, sealants or leak-detection fluids used in anaesthetic machine maintenance (Rendell-Baker 1977). It is also almost exclusively a problem of 'bubble through' vaporizers rather than the 'flow-over' types, and relates to the stability of the foams produced in this way.

Finally, vaporizers are designed for unidirectional flow. If this flow is reversed for some reason, such as the malconnection of the vaporizer, excessive output may well result (Wyant 1976). This problem is thus mainly confined to those various systems designed for the easy removal and exchange of the vaporizer, such as the Penlon 'off-line' or Ohmeda 'Selectatec' systems.

ANAESTHETIC AGENT UNDERDOSAGE

The effects of anaesthetic agent underdosage may be manifest in two ways: awareness in its several forms or evidence of sympathetic overactivity due to unduly light anaesthesia. The associated hypertension or tachycardia may lead to long-term morbidity from myocardial ischaemia (or infarction), or central nervous system damage in the form of intracranial haemorrhage. Coughing and laryngospasm from too light an anaesthesia may be disastrous. Equipment failures resulting in inadequate anaesthesia may be classified as follows:

- failure of the nitrous oxide supply
- contamination of the nitrous oxide supply
- leaks
- dilution of the fresh gas flow
- flow meter inaccuracies
- empty vaporizers
- incorrect agent delivered
- inaccurate dial settings.

Failure of the nitrous oxide supply

If the nitrous oxide supply fails and this failure goes unnoticed due, perhaps, to oversight, inattention, or distraction, then an important component of the anaesthetic will disappear. This failure may result from leaks and therefore an unexpectedly high rate of use, or from the failure of a pressure gauge to show the correct pressure (Thompson 1978).

Contamination of the nitrous oxide supply

If nitrous oxide becomes contaminated with a non-toxic gas or vapour, the quantity of anaesthetic given will be decreased. Such a failure may occur if a communication develops between the nitrous oxide and oxygen supplies prior to the flow meters. Such a communication may occur following failure of the diaphragm in an oxygen failure safety valve when the oxygen pressure is greater than the nitrous oxide pressure (Puri et al 1987).

Leaks

Leaks may occur within the anaesthetic machine itself. For instance the oxygen flush valve may leak or fail to close following use (Anon. 1981a).

Leaks may arise from within the vaporizer and lead to unnoticed loss of inhalational agent (Mantia 1982).

The breathing system may also leak, the main source of underdosage here relating to the ingress of air to add to the fresh gas flow and thus dilution of the inhaled agents. This may result from an inadequate fresh gas flow and the subsequent entrainment of air through a negative pressure relief valve (as exists on certain ventilators), or a leak in the system, and entrainment of air through this leak as a consequence of negative pressure developed by a ventilator (Bookallil 1967).

Finally the ventilator may itself leak and thus lead to contamination of the breathing system gas by the driving gas of the ventilator, for example the Penlon Nuffield operating with a Bain or Circle system (Hillyer & Johnston 1978).

Dilution of the fresh gas flow

Dilution of the fresh gas flow may occur either from a faulty oxygen flush valve (as discussed above) or from the excessive use, either intentionally or unintentionally, of the same valve in order to maintain a sufficient quantity of gas within the system (Longmuir & Craig 1976).

Flow meter inaccuracies

Certain flow meter inaccuracies also have the potential for underdelivery of inhaled agents. This may involve either under-reading of the nitrous oxide flow meter or an over-reading of the oxygen flow meter (Walts & Inglove, 1964).

Empty vaporizers

Almost all vaporizers have a means to monitor the amount of agent remaining in them, usually in the form of a 'sight glass'. It is possible for these to be inaccurate and to give the impression that agent is still present within the vaporizer when, in fact, it is empty and the wicks have become dry (Barcroft 1989).

Incorrect agent delivered

If an agent-specific vaporizer is incorrectly refilled with the wrong agent then, obviously, the marked calibrations will be inaccurate. If the new agent is of lower volatility than the agent it replaces, underdosage will result (Munson 1971).

Inaccurate dial settings

Certain vaporizers, as a safety feature, automatically disconnect a link between the dial and the control surfaces of the vaporizer. This is usually associated with an alteration in the 'feel' of the control dial. This alteration may, however, go unnoticed by the anaesthetist, and thus lead to no delivery of inhalational agent (Dreissen et al 1990).

It is also necessary to remember that other inaccuracies of output may occur. Traditionally these occurred with some of the earlier vaporizers, such as the Fluotec 2 where the output rose dramatically with decreasing flows. The reverse may also be true, even with modern vaporizers (Slinger et al 1990). The output of vaporizers is also affected by the addition of other substances, such as thymol, where with halothane the output may be half that expected from the dial setting (Gray 1988).

STANDARDIZATION OF ANAESTHETIC EQUIPMENT

Since the first edition of this book there have been some advances, principally with the revision of BS 3849 (1988) and the subsequent Safety Action Bulletin (DOH 1989), such that it now harmonizes with the relevant ISO standard (ISO 5356: 1987).

REPORTING OF HAZARDS

It is essential that knowledge of hazards occurring with our equipment should be widely and reliably disseminated so that any relevant corrective actions may be undertaken. The DOH organizes the distribution of hazard notices and any problems should be reported via the local administration and safety officer. Recommendations for corrective action are provided by the department's 'Health Equipment Information' leaflets and 'Safety Action Bulletins'.

REFERENCES

Allberry R A W 1989 Minireg failure. Anaesth Intensive Care 17: 234–235

Allnutt M F 1987 Human factors in accidents. Br J Anaesth 59: 856–864

Anagnostou J M, Hults S L, Moorthy S S 1990 PEEP valve trauma. Anesth Analg 70: 674–675

Anderson C E, Rendell-Baker L 1982 Exposed oxygen flush hazard. Anesthesiology 56: 328

Anon. 1973 Medical equipment alert: gas leaks in anesthesia machine circuitry. Items Topics April 8

Anon. 1975 Hospital negligent in the supply of oxygen. J Leg Med 3: 12–13

Anon. 1981a Internal leakage from anesthesia unit flush valves. Health Devices 10: 172

Anon. 1981b Ventilator breathing circuits. Health Devices Alerts 5: 2

Anon. 1982 Disc misplacement in anesthesia exhalation check valve. Technol Anesth 34: 1–2

Austin T R 1971 A warning device for the 'Fluotec' Mark II and III. Anaesthesia 26: 368

Austin T R 1972 Metallic flaking: a further hazard of anaesthetic apparatus. Anaesthesia 27: 92–93

Bageant R A, Hoyt J W, Epstein R M 1980 Error in pipeline gas concentration: an unanticipated consequence of a defective check valve. Anesthesiology 54: 166–169

Barasch S T, Booth S, Modell J 1976 Hypercapnia during cyclopropane anesthesia: a case report. Anesth Analg 55: 439–441

Barcroft J P 1989 Is there liquid in the vaporizer? Anaesthesia 44: 939

Bellamy M 1988 Heat and moisture exchangers and closed systems. Anaesthesia 43: 610

Bishop C, Levick C H, Hodbson C 1967 A design fault in the Boyle apparatus. Br J Anaesth 39: 908

Bjerring P, Yberg B 1987 Possible role of vacuum systems and compressed air generators in cross-infection in the ICU. Br J Anaesth 59: 648–650

Bookallil M J 1967 Entrainment of air during mechanical ventilation. Br J Anaesth 39: 184

Boon P E 1990 C-size cylinders. Anaesth Intensive Care 18: 596–597

Bracken A 1976 Deposits in cyclopropane flowmeter tubes. Br J Anaesth 48: 52

Buck N, Devlin H B, Lunn J N 1988 Report of a confidential enquiry into perioperative deaths. King's Fund Publishing Office p 63–84

Bushman J A, Clark P A 1967 Oil mist hazard and piped air supplies. Br Med J 3: 588–590

Caplan R A, Posner K L, Ward R J, Cheney F W 1990 Adverse respiratory events in anesthesia: a closed claims analysis. Anesthesiology 72: 828–833

Chadwick D A 1974 Transposition of rotameter tubes. Anesthesiology 40: 102

Chang J L, Larson C E, Bedger R C, Bleyaert A L 1980 An unusual malfunction of an anesthetic machine. Anesthesiology 52: 446–447

Chopra V, Bovill J G, Spierdijk J 1990 Accidents, near accidents and complications during anaesthesia: a retrospective analysis of a 10-year period in a teaching hospital. Anaesthesia 45: 3–6

Ciobanu M, Meyer J A 1980 Ventilator hazard revealed. Anesthesiology 52: 186–187

Clinical Anesthesia Conference: semi-closed anesthesia 1963 N Y State J Med 63: 2124–2125

Clutton-Brock J 1967 Two cases of poisoning by contamination of nitrous oxide with higher oxides of nitrogen during anaesthesia. Br J Anaesth 39: 388–392

Clutton-Brock J 1976 Static electricity and rotameters. Br J Anaesth 44: 86–90

Cobcroft M D 1978 More misconnected Boyle circuit tubings. Anaesth Intensive Care 6: 170–171

Cohen D D, Groveman J E 1966 'Explosion' in an anesthesia vaporizer. Anesthesiology 27: 331

Cooper J B 1978 Prevention of ventilator hazards. Anesthesiology 48: 299–300

Cooper J B, Newbower R S, Long C D, McPeek B 1978 Preventable anesthesia mishaps: a study of human factors. Anesthesiology 49: 399–406

Cooper J B, Newbower R S, Kitz R J 1984 An analysis of major errors and equipment failures in anaesthesia management: considerations for prevention and detection. Anesthesiology 60(1): 34–42

Cottrell J E, Bernherd W, Turndorf H 1976 Hazards of disposable rebreathing circuits. Anesth Analg 55: 743–744

Coveler L A, Lester R C 1989 Contaminated oxygen cylinder. Anesth Analg 69: 674–676

Craft T M, Chambers P H, Ward M E, Goat V A 1990 Two cases of barotrauma associated with transtracheal jet ventilation. Br J Anaesth 64: 524–527

Craig J, Wilson M E 1981 A survey of anaesthetic misadventures. Anaesthesia 36: 933–936

Cundy J, Baldock G J 1982 Safety check procedures to eliminate faults in anaesthesic machines. Anaesthesia 37: 161–169

Currie M 1989 A prospective survey of anaesthetic critical events in a teaching hospital. Anaesth Intensive Care 17(4): 403–411

Currie M, Pybus D A, Torda T A 1988 A prospective survey of anaesthetic critical events: a report on a pilot study of 88 cases. Anaesth Intensive Care 16(1): 103–107

Davenport H T, Keenleyside H B 1957 Interstitial emphysema and pneumothorax associated with the use of a modified non-rebreathing valve. Can Anaesth Soc J 4: 126 130

Davies G, Tarnawsky M 1976 Letters to the editor. Can Anaesth Soc J 23: 228

DHSS 1982 A confidential enquiry into maternal deaths, 1976–1978. DHSS

DHSS 1987 Carbon dioxide flowmeters on anaesthetic machines: jammed indicator bobbin. Saftey Information Bulletin 32: 4

DHSS 1989 Report on confidential enquiries into maternal deaths in England and Wales 1982–84. p 96–106
Diaz P M 1976 The influence of carrier gas on the output of automatic plenum vaporizers. Br J Anaesth 48: 387–391
Dickson P 1978 The official rules. Arrow, London, p 128–137
Dinnick O P 1973 Hazards of respiratory circuits. Ann R Coll Surg 52: 349–354
DOH 1989 Anaesthetic and respiratory equipment: the use of 22 mm breathing system connections. Safety Action Bulletin 52:
Dolan P F 1976 A simple safety device. Br J Anaesth 48: 499
Dorsch J A, Dorsch S E Hazards of anesthesia machines and breathing systems. In: Understanding anesthesia equipment.
Driessen J J, Eerens J M L G, van Hoonacker G 1990 Problem with vapor vaporizer. Anaesthesia 45: 597
Duckett J E, Hice C, Smith T C 1980 Hazard of a ruptured exhalation mushroom diaphragm. Crit Care Med 8: 750–751
Edwards G, Morton H J V, Park E R, Wylie W D 1956 Deaths associated with anaesthesia. Anaesthesia 11: 194–220
Eger E I, Epstein R M 1964 Hazards of anesthetic equipment. Anesthesiology 25: 490–504
Eger E I, Hykton R R, Irwin R H, Guadagni N 1963 Anesthetic flow meter sequence: a cause for hypoxia. Anesthesiology 24: 396–397
Eichhorn J H, Bancroft M L, Laasberg L H, du Moulin G C, Saubermann A J 1977 Contamination of medical gas and water pipelines in a new hospital building. Anesthesiology 46: 286–289
Elam J O 1958 Channeling and overpacking in carbon dioxide absorbers. Anesthesiology 19: 403–404
Eldrup-Jorgensen S, Sprissler G T 1977 Gas leaks in anesthesia machines. Anesthesiology 46: 439
Esplen J R 1956 A device giving warning of impending failure of the nitrous oxide or oxygen supply. Br J Anaesth 28: 226–227
Feeley T W, Hedley-Whyte J 1976 Bulk oxygen and nitrous oxide delivery systems: design and dangers. Anesthesiology 44: 301–305
Feeley T W, McClelland K J, Malhorta I V 1975 The hazards of bulk oxygen delivery systems. Lancet 1: 1416–1418
Feingold A 1976 Carbon dioxide absorber packaging hazard. Anesthesiology 45: 260
Ferdebar P J, Kettler R E, Jablonski J, Sportiello R 1986 A cause of breathing system leak during closed circuit anesthesia. Anesthesiology 65: 661–663
Finlay J, Penlton D A 1971 Needed: error prevention. Hospitals 45: 64–66
Flannagan J C 1954 The critical incident technique. Psychol Bull 51: 327–358
Forrester A C 1968 Anaesthetists-in-law. Proc R Soc Med 61: 409–416
Frankel D Z N 1983 Adhesive tape obstructing an anesthesia circuit. Anesthesiology 59: 256
Fukunaga A F 1981 Torsion and disconnection of inner tube of coaxial breathing circuit. Br J Anaesth 53: 1106–1107
Gibson O B 1979 Another hazardous pipeline isolator valve. Anaesthesia 34: 213
Goddard J, Abbott T R 1986 Selectatec system: misplaced blood. Anaesthesia 41: 439
Goebel W M 1980 Failure of nitrous oxide and oxygen pin-indexing. Anesthesia Progress 27: 188–191
Goresky G V 1990 Bain circuit delivery tube obstruction. Can J Anaesth 37: 385
Gray W M 1988 Dependence of the output of a halothane vaporizer on thymol concentration. Anaesthesia 43: 1047–1049
Grogono A W, Poterfield J 1970 Ambu valves: danger of wrong assembly. Br J Anaesth 42: 978
Harrison G G 1978 Death attributable to anaesthesia. Br J Anaesth 50: 1041–1046
Hedly-Whyte J 1977 Mechanical failures leading to hypoxia. Audio Digest 19(14):
Hewitt A J, Campbell W 1986 Unusual damage to a Bain system. Anaesthesia 41: 882–883
Higgs B D, Garrett C P 1979 A possible hazard with the Manley ventilator. Anaesthesia 34: 680–681
Hillyer K W, Johnston R R 1978 Unsuspected dilution of anesthetic gases detected by an oxygen analyzer. Anesth Anal 57: 491–492
Holland R 1984 Anesthesia-related mortality in Australia. Int Anesth Clin 22(2): 61–71
Inglis M S 1980 Torsion of the inner tube. Br J Anaesth 52: 705
Jawan B, Lee J H 1990 Cardiac arrest caused by an incorrectly filled oxygen cylinder. Br J Anaesth 64: 749–751
Jayasuriya J P 1986 Another example of Murphy's Law: mix up of pin index valves. Anaesthesia 41: 1164
Johnson D L 1975 Central oxygen supply versus Mother Nature. Respir Care 20: 1043–1044
Jorgensen S 1976 An expired gas collection and disposal system. Br J Anaesth 48: 502–503
Kalra A N, Doughty A G 1963 The wrong gas. Anaesthesia 18: 234–236
Karis J H, O'Neal F, Weitzner S W 1980 Alteration of halothane in heated humidifiers. Anesth Analg 59: 518
Karmann U, Roth F 1982 Prevention of accidents associated with air-oxygen mixers. Anaesthesia 37: 680–682
Keenan R L, Boyan C P 1985 Cardiac arrest due to anesthesia. J Am Med Assoc 253(16): 2373–2377
Kelly J M, Gabel R A 1970 The improperly calibrated flow meter: another hazard. Anesthesiology 33: 467–468
Kemen M, Desai K, Roizen M F, Jennings J 1990 Over fifty percent of disposable circuits leak. Anesth Analg 70: S194
Kerr J H, Evers J L 1958 Carbon dioxide accumulation: valve leaks and inadequate absorption. Can Anaesth Soc J 5: 154–160
Kidner G K, Hunter A R, Donn M C, Constable J 1977 Abridged Report of the Committee of Enquiry Appointed by the Kensington and Chelsea and Westminster Area Health Authority (Teaching).
Klein S L, Lilburn J K 1980 An unusual case of hypercarbia during anesthesia. Anesthesiology 52: 248–250
Lamarche Y 1985 Anaesthetic breathing circuit leak from cracked oxygen sensor connector. Can Anaesth Soc J 32: 682–683
Lane G A 1980 Medical gas outlets: a hazard from interchangeable 'quick connect' couplers. Anesthesiology 52: 85–86
Latto I P 1973 Administration of halothane in the 0–0.5% concentration range with the Fluotec Mark 2 and Mark 3 vaporizers. Br J Anaesth 45: 563–569

Levins F A, Francis R I, Burnley S R 1989 Failure to detect disconnexion by capnography. Anaesthesia 44: 79
Liew P C, Ganedran A 1973 Oxygen failure: a potential danger with air-flowmeters in anesthetic machines with controlled needle valves. Br J Anaesth 45: 1165–1168
Liston A J 1981 Coaxial breathing circuits. Medical devices alert, 40: Health Protection Branch, Health and Welfare, Canada
Loeser E A 1978 Water-induced resistance in disposable respiratory-circuit bacterial filters. Anesth Analg 57: 269–271
Longmuir J, Craig D B 1976 Misadventure with a Boyle's gas machine. Can Anaesth Soc J 23: 671–673
Love J B 1980 Misassembly of a Campbell ventilator causing leakage of the driving gas to a patient. Anaesth Intensive Care 8: 376–377
McQuillan P J, Jackson I J B 1987 Potential leaks from anaesthetic machines. Anaesthesia 42: 1308–1312
Mansell W H 1976 Bain circuit: 'The hazard of the hidden tube.' Can Anaesth Soc J 23: 227
Mantia A M 1982 Gas scavenging systems. Anesth Analg 61: 162–164
Marx G F, Mateo C V, Orkin L R 1973 Computer analysis of post anesthetic deaths. Anesthesiology 39(1): 54–58
Mason J, Tackley R 1981 An acute rise in expiratory resistance due to a blocked ventilator filter. Anaesthesia 36: 335
Mazze R I 1972 Therapeutic misadventures with oxygen delivery systems: the need for continuous in-line oxygen monitors. Anesth Analg 51: 787–792
Meyer J A 1972 Guest discussion. Anesth Analg 51: 790–791
Morris L E 1979 Revell circulator and vapour concentration measurements. In: Aldrete J A, Lowe H G, Virtue R W (eds) Low flow and closed system anesthesia. Grune & Stratton, New York, p 273–276
Morrison A B 1981 Medical gas station outlets and connectors. Health Protection Board, Health and Welfare, Canada, January 14
Mostafa S M, Sutciffe A J 1982 Antipollution expiratory valves: a potential hazard. Anaesthesia 37: 468–469
Munford B J, Wishaw K J 1990 Critical incidents with nonrebreathing valves. Anaesth Intensive Care 18: 560–563
Munson E S 1971 Hazards of agent-specific vaporizers. Anesthesiology 34: 393
Murray W J, Fleming P 1972 Patient exposure to halothane retained in anesthesia machine circuits. Clin Pharmacol Ther 13: 148
Newton N I, Adams A Q 1978 Excessive airway pressure during anaesthesia. Anaesthesia 33: 689–699
Nichols P K T Unpublished observations
Noble W H 1970 Accuracy of halothane vaporizers in clinical use. Can Anaesth Soc J 17: 135–144
Nunn B J, Rosewarne F A 1990 Expiratory valve failure. Anaesth Intensive Care 18: 273–274
Olsson G L, Hallén B 1988 Cardiac arrest during anaesthesia: a computer aided study in 250543 anaesthetics. Acta Anaesthesiol Scand 32: 653–664
Paterson G M, Hulands G H, Nunn J F 1969 Evaluation of a new halothane vaporizer: the Cyprane Fluotec Mark 3. Br J Anaesth 41: 109–119
Peterson W D C 1978 Bain circuit. Can Anaesth Soc J 25: 532
Podraza A, Salem M R, Harris T Z, Moritz H 1991 Effects of bellow leak on anesthesia ventilator function. Anesth Analg 72: S215
Powell J 1981 Leak from an oxygen flow meter. Br J Anaesth 53: 671
Pryn S J, Crosse M M 1989 Ventilator disconnexion alarms failures: the role of ventilator and breathing system accessories. Anaesthesia 44: 978–981
Puri G D, George M A, Singh H, Batra Y K 1987 Awareness under anaesthesia due to a defective gas-loaded regulator. Anaesthesia 42: 539–540
Puttick N 1986 Hazard from the oxygen flush control. Anaesthesia 41: 222–224
Raja S N, Geller H 1986 Another potential source of a major gas leak. Anesthesiology 64: 297–298
Rendell-Baker L 1976 Some gas machine hazards and their elimination. Anesth Analg 55: 26–33
Rendell-Baker L 1977 Equipment standards in anesthesia practice: eliminating the hazards. Clin Trends Anesthesiol 7(2):
Richards C 1989 Failure of a nitrous oxide-oxygen proportioning device. Anesthesiology 71: 997–999
Rolbin S 1977 An unusual cause of ventilator leak. Can Anaesth Soc J 24: 522–524
Rosewarne F, Wells D 1988 Three cases of valve incompetence in a circle system. Anaesth Intensive Care 16: 376–377
Russel G N, Snowdon S L 1986 Medical gas probes. Anaesthesia 41: 968
Saposnick A B 1975 Maintenance and repair of gas, humidity, and aerosol equipment. Respir Care 20: 938–941
Sarnquist F H, Demas K 1982 The silent ventilator. Anesth Analg 61: 713–714
Saunders R J, Calkins J M, Gooden T M 1981 Accuracy in rotameters and linear flowmeters. Anesthesiology 55: A116
Schiller D J 1986 Rusty water in an oxygen flowmeter. Anaesthesia 41: 1061
Sellery J R 1972 Hazards of artificial ventilation in the operating room. Can Med Assoc J 107: 421–423
Sharp J H, Trudell J R, Cohen E N 1979 Volatile metabolites and decomposition products of halothane in man. Anesthesiology 50: 2–8
Shroff P K, Skerman J H 1988 Humidifier malfunction: a cause of anesthesia circuit malfunction. Anesth Analg 67: 710–771
Slinger P D, Scott W A C, Kliffer A P 1990 Intraoperative awareness due to malfunction of a Siemens 900B ventilator. Can J Anaesth 37: 258–261
Smith R H, Volpitto V V 1959 Volume ventilation valve. Anesthesiology 20: 885–886
Sosis M B, Payne M N 1989 Another cause for a leak in a disposable breathing circuit. Anesthesiology 71: 806
Sprague D H, Archer G W 1975 Intraoperative hypoxia from an erroneously filled liquid oxygen reservoir. Anesthesiology 42: 360–363
Spurring P W, Small L F G 1983 Breathing system disconnexions and misconnexions. Anaesthesia 38: 683–688
Taylor C, Stoelting V K 1963 A modified Ayre's T-tube technic-anesthesia for cleft lip and palate. Anesth Analg 42: 55–62
Taylor G, Larson C P, Prestwich R 1976 Unexpected cardiac arrest during anesthesia and surgery. J Am Med Assoc 236(24): 2758–2760
Thompson P W 1976 Safety of anaesthetic apparatus. In: Recent advances in anaesthesia and analgesia. No 12.

Churchill Livingstone, Edinburgh
Thompson P W 1978 Safety of anaesthetic apparatus. Int Anesthesiol Clin 16: 199–223
Thompson P W 1979 Prevention of the hazard of excessive airway pressure. Anaesthesia 34: 593
Thompson P W 1987 Equipment to deliver inhaled gases. In: Taylor T H, Major E (eds) Hazards and complications of anaesthesia. Churchill Livingstone, London
Thorp J M, Railton R 1982 Hypoxia due to air in the oxygen pipeline. Anaesthesia 37: 683–687
Tingay M G, Ilsley A H, Willis R J, Thompson M J, Chalmers A H, Cousins M J 1978 Gas identity hazards and major contamination of medical gas system of a new hospital. Anaesth Intensive Care 6: 202–209
Tiret L, Desmonts J M, Hatton F, Vourc'h G 1986 Complications associated with anaesthesia: a prospective survey in France. Can Anaesth Soc J 33(3): 336–344
Turnbull K W, Fancourt-Smith P F, Banting G C 1980 Death within 48 hours of anaesthesia at the Vancouver General Hospital. Can Anaesth Soc J 27(2): 159–163
Van-Besouw J-P 1987 A hazard of silencers for jet ventilators. Anaesthesia 42: 81
Van-Besouw J-P, Thurlow A C 1987 A hazard of free-standing vaporizers. Anaesthesia 42: 671
Walts L F, Inglove H 1964 Malfunction of a new anesthetic machine. Anesthesiology 25: 867
Waterman P M, Pautler S, Smith R B 1978 Accidental ventilator-induced hyperventilation. Anesthesiology 48: 141
Waters D J 1968 Factors causing awareness during surgery. Br J Anaesth 40: 259–264
Wickett R E, Jenkin L C, Root L S 1974 Downstream contamination of in-series vaporizers. Can Anaesth Soc J 21: 114–116
Wildsmith J A W, Grubb D J 1977 Defective and misused co-axial circuits. Anaesthesia 32: 293
Williamson J A, Webb R K, Pryor G L 1985 Anaesthesia safety and the 'critical incident' technique. Aust Clin Rev 6: 57–61
Wisborg K, Jacebson E 1975 Functional disorders of Ruben and Ambu-E valves after cleaning. Anesthesiology 42: 633–634
Wyant G N 1976 Another hazard of free-standing vaporizers, increased anesthetic concentration with reversed flow of vaporizing gas. Anesthesiology 45: 445–446
Wyant G N 1979 Mechanical misadventures in anaesthesia. University of Toronto Press, Toronto
Zimmerman B L, Lord J 1980 Contamination of an anesthesia system with liquid halothane. Anesthesiology 52: 512–513

43

Electrical equipment

C. J. Hull

INTRODUCTION

The early pioneers of anaesthesia relied on simple clinical observations, such as skin colour, respiratory rate and pulse rate, to monitor the well-being of their patients. Since then a wide range of physiological measurements has become possible and patient monitoring devices have developed accordingly. However, most instruments require skill and understanding if they were to be used effectively, and extraneous influences such as patient movement and electrical interference could at times reduce the output signals to a meaningless jumble. Consequently, most anaesthetists limited their monitoring activity to simple devices.

However, following the recent development of microprocessor technology, the precision, reliability and 'friendliness' of complex patient-monitoring systems have advanced rapidly. Their use has become commonplace and it is widely accepted that the safety of anaesthetized patients has thereby been enhanced. Now it is regarded as foolish or even negligent to anaesthetize a patient without the use of appropriate monitoring. Indeed, our American colleagues are pressed to festoon and invade their patients with monitoring devices for the worst possible reason: that it is medicolegally unsafe to do otherwise.

While it can be argued that any expense on safety is worthwhile, if only for the reason that it also saves money, it must be remembered that every coin has two sides and that the unreasoning proliferation of monitoring devices will bring a new set of problems. As Savarese commented: 'The chief cause of problems is solutions!'

Conversely, some old hazards have diminished. When diethyl ether and cyclopropane were widely used in anaesthesia, the principal electrical hazard was undoubtedly that of explosion, either in the theatre atmosphere or, even worse, in the anaesthetic circuit itself. Today, many anaesthetists would regard the problem to be of historical interest only, although a few diehards cling ferociously to explosive agents. Their patients and colleagues must perforce cling with them.

Today every electrical accident should be regarded as predictable, unnecessary and therefore due to negligence of some kind. It is the responsibility of every practising anaesthetist to be aware of the dangers associated with electrical equipment. He must know how they arise and, by virtue of such knowledge, how they may be prevented, not most of the time but all of the time.

Hazards will be considered according to the following schema:

- the mechanism of electrocution
- the mechanism of the diathermy burn
- the hazard of the 'applied part'
- ignition of flammable gas mixtures
- hazards due to human factors
- hazards caused by misleading or erroneous data.

ELECTROCUTION

Electrocution may be defined as the causing of death by passage of electricity through the body. Electric currents exert their harmful effects by stimulating excitable tissues such as muscle and nerve, and also by the generation of heat. Electrical accidents can be caused by either direct or alternating current, and the mechanisms involved may be asphyxia, disturbance of cardiac rhythm, deep unconsciousness or thermal damage.

Effects of small electric currents on excitable tissues

It has long been recognized (Ferris et al 1936) that the effects of electric currents on excitable tissues such as nerve and muscle are related to the intensity of the *current* flowing through the tissue concerned. Further, it is not so much the total current flowing that matters as the *current density*, which may be expressed in microamperes (μA) per square millimetre of tissue.

If a 50 Hz alternating current is a passed from one hand to the other, all intermediate tissues will be affected, but the nature of the damage (if any) at any point depends on the local current density. At very low currents (less than 1 mA) there will be no adverse effect except for a faint tingling at the points of contact. At approximately 5 mA, local pain will be observed, becoming severe and more widespread as the current increases. Between 10 and 30 mA all subjects experience sustained forearm muscular contraction so that any grasped object cannot be released: the so-called 'let go' threshold (Morse 1959). As the current increases further in the range 25–80 mA, progressively more proximal muscle groups become involved until ultimately (provided the current is not interrupted) sustained contraction of respiratory muscles will lead to death by asphyxia.

However, at the upper end of this range the current density in the heart will be sufficient to cause major disturbances in cardiac performance. These appear first as arrhythmias, progressing to functional pump failure as the conducting system becomes totally disorganized. Finally, at a current of approximately 100 mA, ventricular fibrillation (VF) develops and spontaneous recovery becomes unlikely.

Threshold current for the initiation of ventricular fibrillation

Myocardial excitability varies with the normal cardiac cycle (Wiggers & Wegria 1939), and is maximal during the late repolarization and resting phases. During QRS propagation, each element of the cardiac syncitium becomes refractory as it is depolarized and then passes through a brief phase of relative refractoriness as the resting potential is restored. During this phase a propagating response can be initiated, albeit by a more intense stimulus. Very short (<4 ms) shocks are generally followed by non-repetitive responses (Zoll 1952), and those with a duration of less than 200 ms may fall within the refractory period.

Microshock

Electrodes positioned close to the heart will result in greater cardiac current density than those sited on the extremities, and therefore constitute a hazard at lower current levels. Thus electrodes placed directly in the epicardium can induce ventricular fibrillation at a current of only 1 mA. If the stimulating electrode is placed *inside* the heart the threshold falls even further. A 600 μA alternating current passed through an electrode placed in the right atrium may cause disturbances of cardiac rhythm, although currents exceeding 10 mA may be required to initiate ventricular fibrillation (Raftery et al 1975).

In fact, a small electrode contacting the ventricular endocardium can cause VF in man at currents as low as 60 μA, and dogs have been fibrillated at 30 μA (Watson et al 1973, Roy 1974).

Table 43.1 Approximate thresholds for the provocation of sustained ventricular fibrillation in man by 50 Hz AC current

Current path	Threshold (mA)
Hand-hand	100
Intra-atrial electrode	>10
Small ventricular endocardial electrode	0.05

(from Bruner 1967, Hull 1978, Raftery et al 1975)

If the electrode is free in the ventricular cavity or in the atrium the threshold is significantly higher (Raftery et al 1975). As might be expected, there has been little opportunity to study the problem in man. However, fibrillation thresholds were determined in 22 patients undergoing cardiac surgery (Watson et al 1973, Raftery et al 1975). These studies demonstrated a wide range of fibrillation thresholds, with a log-normal statistical distribution (Hull 1978). It appears that the smallest 50 Hz current likely to present a hazard in man is approximately 50 μA (at which 0.5% of subjects may be expected to be susceptible), but it is re-emphasized that this could occur only by means of a very small electrode having direct contact with the ventricular myocardium (Roy 1974).

Thus the threshold current for the initiation of VF depends on the duration, magnitude and frequency of the myocardial current density, and therefore also on the electrode contact positions and the total current (Bruner 1967).

Heating effects of an electric current

When an electric current passes through a conductor, heat is generated. This can be expressed as:

$$W \text{ (watts)} = V \text{ (volts)} \times I \text{ (amperes)}$$

but in this context it is more usefully expressed as:

$$W = I^2 \times R \text{ or } W = V^2/R$$

where W = power (W, watts), V = voltage (V, volts), I = current (A, amps), R = resistance (Ω, ohms).

It is clear that the rate of heat generation rises with the square of both current and voltage, provided the resistance remains constant. With the passage of current through skin this is likely to apply, at least initially. Normally, the conductive pathway created by a metal–skin contact will have a resistance ranging from 10 to 100 kΩ, depending on the degree of cornification and the presence or absence of sweating.

Electrical burns

The thermal damage caused by an electric current depends on the temperature to which individual tissues are exposed. In turn, the temperature achieved depends on the ratio of heat generation to that dissipated by the medium concerned and the period of exposure.

Skin is a poor thermal conductor, depending heavily on blood flow for equalization with deeper tissues, so that dissipation depends mainly on the adequacy of skin perfusion. It follows that, for a given heating current, dissipation will increase with the surface area of the current source; thus the larger the contact area, the smaller the rise in temperature. A current that would do no harm if applied through a large contact area to well-perfused skin may cause instant charring if applied through a point-contact. An electric current passing through a skin-contact should dissipate no more than 15 mW/mm^2 if thermal damage is to be avoided.

So far as deeper tissues are concerned, the degree of damage depends on the current density in individual zones. The current passes from one contact to another by all possible routes and is 'shared' between alternative routes in proportion to the electrical conductance of the tissues. Each conductance depends on the specific conductivity of the tissue and the cross-sectional area through which the current flows. Thus when a current enters the body at a fingertip, very little will travel proximally through epidermis or bone, both of which have much higher resistance than dermis and subcutaneous tissues (Geddes & Baker 1967). Since these are very limited in cross-sectional area the current density will be high. As the current reaches the forearm the cross-sectional area of conductive tissue increases greatly and the current density decreases accordingly. Thus a current may cause intense charring of the fingertip but no damage to more proximal tissues. Once skin charring has started, the conductivity rises so that the total current may rise also, causing further injury.

The origin of electrocuting currents

Most commonly, electrocuting currents originate from 240 V, 50 Hz mains power sources. Higher voltages may be found in the power circuits for cathode ray tubes (CRT), but these circuit elements are always shielded carefully.

Normally, mains power is supplied to a device by means of two insulated conductors. One of them is grounded at source (neutral), the other (live) carries the full mains voltage. The electrical load is connected across the two and a current flows according to the load impedance. The load is surrounded either by two insulating layers (Class II) or, more commonly, by a metal enclosure (Class I) connected to nearby earth by means of a third conductor.

Leakage current and ground faults

If the insulation between load and enclosure in a Class I device deteriorates, a *leakage current* may flow to ground. This is not a direct hazard since the enclosure voltage will remain very close to ground unless the current is large. In that event a fuse in the live connection will pass sufficient current to melt and the supply will be discontinued. On the other hand the ground connection may be disrupted, usually due to a damaged cable or deterioration of the wall outlet. Here also there is no direct hazard. Only when both faults have developed does the enclosure potential rise to that of the leakage source, that is some voltage between 0 V and 240 V. Now there is a real hazard, since any person contacting both the enclosure and some earthed object will himself become part of the leakage current pathway to ground. The effects will depend on:

- the leakage source voltage
- the route taken through the subject
- the ground-path resistance, which is the sum of the leakage source resistance, the resistance of the pathway through the subject and any further resistance to ground.

The fuse does not offer any useful protection since it is designed to blow when the total current greatly exceeds that normally taken by the load, whereas a lethal leakage current of 400 mA would be most unlikely to raise the total current to the fuse rating.

Application of Ohm's Law (I = V/R) yields the likely current. A subject with dry hands contacting both a 'live' enclosure and grounded metalwork will pass a current of 240/100 000 = 2.4 mA, causing a mild shock. With wet hands and good contact the same subject could have skin resistance of only 1000 Ω, yielding a current of 240 mA. Assuming a contact area of 200 mm^2 the power dissipation would be 288 mW/mm^2 (safe limit 15 mW/mm^2). As a result the subject would experience both contact burns and ventricular fibrillation.

Prevention of electrocution

The safety principle behind the three-wire power delivery system is that two faults must develop before a hazard can arise, so that assiduous maintenance should prevent accidents at all times. Of course, this assumes that maintenance procedures are well-established and rigorously applied. For many years safety standards for electromedical equipment have applied in the UK, originally in a Technical Memorandum (DHSS 1963) but more recently as British Standard 5724 (BSI 1979). BS 5724 specifies many constructional aspects and also states the maximum leakage currents that may flow under normal and fault conditions. Devices that are to make contact with a patient by means of an applied part (type BF) must conform to a more rigorous specification. This includes many monitoring devices. Under the BF specification the patient circuit must not allow more than 0.1 mA current to flow under normal conditions, 0.5 mA with a single fault. These currents are at or below the threshold of sensation and are quite harmless.

These provisions are welcomed. However, the standard specifies that each power lead in a Class I device must be fused. This means that if the neutral fuse blows the load remains live in the presence of some fault condition. There is some doubt as to whether this is good practice. The user must play an important role in the prevention of accidents by applying a sensible code of practice:

1. Ensure that all electrical equipment is subjected to regular testing, as specified in BS5724, and that all results are logged.
2. Do not take any electrical device into the operating theatre if it does not (or even may

not) conform to BS 5724, especially if it has an applied part. If a device cannot be returned to BS compliance by service work, it should formally be destroyed so that return to the clinical arena is impossible.

3. Do not allow a device to be used if the mains cable is damaged or the mains plug shows any sign of deterioration.
4. Do not allow a device to be used if it has been modified in any way by an unauthorized person.
5. Do not allow mains cables to lie in a tangled mass on the floor, and do not allow orderlies to push trolleys (or even worse, radiographers to push mobile X-ray machines) over them.
6. Do not handle electrical equipment with wet hands.
7. Never remove the enclosure cover to investigate a fault. Switch off, disconnect and call for expert assistance.
8. Do not use extension boxes and **never** attach an extension box to an ungrounded anaesthetic machine. To many users who work in operating theatres without overhead pendants the abolition of extension boxes would present a serious problem, since it is equally bad practice to run very long cables to distant mains outlets! Their only recourse is to seek theatre upgrading, however unlikely that may seem in the present financial climate.

THE DIATHERMY BURN

Surgical diathermy is a direct application of the principles set out above, that is that an electric current may generate intense heat at a very small contact area but cause no undesirable effects elsewhere due to the reduction in current density. If diathermy were to operate at line frequency (50 Hz), currents sufficient to produce coagulation or tissue disruption would cause gross stimulation of excitable tissues. However, the threshold for stimulation rises with frequency, so that at 1 MHz large currents can be passed through the body with no excitatory effect on nerve or muscle. Most surgical diathermy sets operate in the radiofrequency range (0.4 to 3 MHz).

Impedance at different frequencies

An alternating current can pass through a capacitor more easily as the frequency rises, but the back-EMF (electromotive force) produced in an inductor is greater at high frequency so that the current passes less easily. Both capacitors and inductors cause 90° phase-shifts between voltage and current, but in opposing directions. In electrical terms the *reactance* of a capacitor falls with frequency, while that of an inductor rises. The units of reactance are ohms, but should not be confused with resistive ohms because of the phase differences. The overall effect of any combination of resistors, capacitors and inductors on an alternating current is the *impedance*, which is also scaled in ohms, and takes into account the phase differences between voltage and current. Since a capacitor consists of two conductors separated by an insulator, numerous 'stray' capacitative pathways exist between the patient and his immediate environment. While not able to pass significant currents at 50 Hz, these pathways may have low impedances at 1 MHz. Also, skin has significant capacitance, its radiofrequency (RF) impedance is lower than at 50 Hz.

Unipolar diathermy

There are two types of diathermy device. *Unipolar diathermy*, which is most commonly used, passes radiofrequency current from an active surgical electrode to a large 'plate' electrode. The principle is that, despite a total power dissipation which may exceed 300 W, the current density under the plate electrode remains sufficiently low to prevent any significant rise in temperature. This return circuit is capacitatively coupled to ground, so that any pathway from the patient to ground (resistive or capacitative) forms a parallel route. Consequently the diathermy return current will 'share' the two (or more) pathways according to their respective impedances at diathermy frequency. Any fault in the 'plate' pathway will greatly increase the current share passing by other routes, and burns may occur at zones of high current density, usually skin contacts with grounded metalwork (Battig 1968, Dobbie 1969, Aronow & Bruner 1975, Spierdijk et al 1976). However, many monitoring devices make physical contact with the patient so that the possibility of an RF pathway to ground, either in normal operation or under fault conditions, must always be considered. This topic is considered in more detail below.

Bipolar diathermy

Bipolar diathermy current flows from one active electrode to another, such as between opposing forcep blades. Consequently, much less current is required, the thermal effects are even more localized and the whole output circuit can be effectively isolated from ground. Thus the hazards of shared return pathways are minimal. Bipolar diathermy is widely used in some surgical disciplines but is slow to find favour in general surgery.

Prevention of diathermy burns

The following is a list of ways in which diathermy burns may be avoided:

1. Encourage surgeons to use bipolar devices.
2. Ensure that the 'plate' electrode is properly applied to the thigh or buttock.
3. Ensure that there is no possible alternative grounding pathway for the diathermy current: keep all skin well away from metal parts and ensure that the applied parts of monitoring devices are not grounded. Any surviving electrocardiogram (ECG) monitor with a grounded 'common' electrode should be destroyed forthwith, since in the operating theatre environment such a device is 'an accident looking for somewhere to happen'.
4. Check that the ECG monitor is protected against diathermy and that it cannot sink RF current to ground. The patient is best protected by either resistors or radiofrequency chokes in each electrode lead (RF chokes are very small inductors that have very low impedance at 50 Hz, but which effectively block radiofrequency currents).

THE HAZARD OF THE APPLIED PART

With very few exceptions, each monitoring device must have some physical interface with the patient. Here the electrical implications of devices that have 'applied parts' are considered.

Surface electrodes

The placement of a skin electrode may cause a variety of problems. There have been reports of dermatitis due to several different constituents of electrode pastes, and of allergy to rubber electrode straps and nickel-plated electrodes (Coskey 1977, Fisher 1977). However, the principal hazard caused by an electrode lies in its very nature: a small surface-area, low-resistance electrical pathway into the body.

50 Hz current

If a 50 Hz current passes from a 250 V source into a grounded patient through an electrode–skin interface, the effects depend largely on the surface area. Large-diameter ECG electrodes have low resistance so that substantial currents may flow and VF is a likely outcome. Miniature electrodes, such as are used for electroencephalography (EEG), may have sufficient resistance to prevent VF, but few would care to put much trust in such protection!

Radiofrequency current

Radiofrequency diathermy currents may find a ground pathway through any electrode system. In practical terms it has been estimated that, if the current through a surface electrode does not exceed 1 mA/mm^2, thermal damage is most unlikely, but is certain to occur at 4 mA/mm^2 (Becker et al 1973, Finlay et al 1974). Since ECG electrodes have low resistance but small surface area, it is not surprising that they have been implicated in a number of incidents involving diathermy burns. As would be anticipated, miniature electrodes are more hazardous than those with large contact areas (Chandra 1982, Finlay et al 1974). EEG electrodes have also been implicated (Neufeld 1983). Clearly, a large electrode offers some measure of protection, since the current density may not be sufficient to cause a burn. Modern ECG monitors have patient circuits that do not provide an RF grounding pathway; the problem is limited to older devices, of which a small number remain in active use.

Internal electrodes

In some cases electrodes are placed inside the body, so that the natural resistance of the skin no longer limits the passage of electric currents to the same degree. As a simple example, hypodermic needles used as ECG electrodes are a potent source of diathermy burns (Marx et al 1968).

Prevention of electrode burns

Wherever possible, use standard-sized ECG electrodes; do not use miniature types; in particular do not use needle electrodes.

Burns due to low voltage, direct current

Under some circumstances (see below), small direct currents from low-voltage sources (<20 V) may flow through surface electrodes. While such a current does not present a thermal or electrocution hazard, it should be appreciated that deep burns can be caused by electrolytic action. If a direct current is applied to skin electrodes, chlorine and hydrochloric acid are released at the anode, sodium hydroxide and hydrogen at the cathode. When the epidermal layers of the skin are destroyed by these substances the electrical resistance of the skin diminishes, the current increases and the rate of electrolysis accelerates further. Anodic and cathodic burns are different in appearance, and their severity is directly related to the magnitude and duration of the current. Even superficial burns of this type are slow to heal, and deep lesions usually require grafting.

A neurosurgical patient (Leeming et al 1970) developed multiple ulcers beneath a surgical diathermy 'plate'. Subsequent investigation showed a 14 V (DC) potential difference between plate and ground. This voltage derived from the plate monitoring circuit and appeared on the plate itself as result of a deteriorated isolating capacitor.

A second instance (A L Brewis personal communication) arose when a very early ECG monitor, attached to a patient, was damaged by the application of DC defibrillation. The next patient to whom the monitor was connected developed deep anodic and cathodic burns at the ECG electrode sites. It was found that the electrode leads from the damaged amplifier applied the power supply voltage (± 12 V DC) to the patient's skin. It is possible that this mechanism was responsible for the 1 cm-wide scalp burn on a fetus caused by a spiral monitoring electrode (Akhter 1976).

Microshock

It was stated above that, if an electrode is passed into the heart itself, the threshold current for the induction of ventricular fibrillation diminishes greatly. There are several substantiated reports of so-called 'microshock' in clinical practice (Nordijk et al 1961, Pengelly & Klassen 1961, Bousvaros et al 1962). It must be noted that the current source can be the intracardiac electrode itself, or simply a contact with any part of the body by the intracardiac electrode (or catheter) simply acting as a current 'sink' to ground.

The incident reported by Bousvaros et al (1962) showed that the intracardiac lead does not have to be a wire connection, since in that case it was a cardiac catheter containing the radio-opaque dye, Hypaque. This dye was estimated to have a resistance of 27 000 Ω, but was sufficiently conductive to pass an estimated 415 μA into the patient.

Hopps (1969) pointed out that a low-resistance intracardiac lead, such as might be provided by a pacing wire, or a cardiac catheter with a metal guide-wire in situ, creates a situation in which the patient may be fibrillated by a potential difference (between the cardiac lead and another contact) of only 100 mV!

Prevention of microshock

BS 5724 defines a category of equipment (type CF) that may be attached to intracardiac electrodes, in which the maximal permissible patient leakage current is 10 μA under normal conditions, 50 μA with a single fault. These values are below the likely minimum threshold for intracardiac electrocution. Unlike the more stringent Australian standard, any other attached equipment need only meet the requirements of type BF. Since microshock currents need two contacts, and the intracardiac lead may simply act as a current sink with the current entering the patient via some other applied device, it is prudent to use only type CF devices when an intracardiac lead is present. Bare wires providing a conductive pathway to the cardiac interior (such as transvenous pacemakers) should be touched only with dry gloved hands. Further, the 'electrically susceptible patient' should be separated from all grounded objects. Those that cannot be removed should be plastic-coated to minimize grounding currents from casual contact. Ideally a cardiac catheter should be of the conductive type. This prevents hazardous current densities near the tip, even when leakage currents are present (Lipton et al 1978).

Other applied parts

It should also be noted that surface-mounted probes, such as for *temperature*, may pass radiofrequency currents to ground and thereby cause diathermy burns (Schneider et al 1977). Similar problems have been reported following the use of oesophageal and rectal temperature probes (Wald et al 1971, Parker 1984). A radiofrequency grounding current through a neuromuscular transmission monitor (using an anal probe) has caused perineal burns (Brock-Utne & Downing 1984), and the originators have advised that it should not be used in the presence of diathermy.

Even insulated devices, such as the encapsulated array of *ultrasonic crystals* used to detect arterial wall movement by the 'Arteriosonde' (Kontron) blood-pressure monitor, can provide an earth pathway. Spierdijk et al (1976) described a diathermy burn of the same size as the transducer capsule which occurred when the unit was operating from mains power. Although it was suggested that lack of insulation was the cause, it appears more probable that the encapsulating plastic, being thin, provided enough capacitance for an RF current to flow. As the authors commented, pressure on the transducer by cuff inflation may have reduced skin perfusion at critical times, thus reducing the current required to cause a burn.

Some devices are capable of causing burns unaided. For instance, the 'Wellcome' *nerve stimulator* is fitted with a pair of small ball-electrodes, beneath which current density may be sufficient to cause superficial burns (Lippmann & Fields 1974). Other nerve stimulators, while not even capable of delivering supramaximal stimuli through surface electrodes, may do so when attached to needle electrodes. Some currently available devices have switched or alternative outputs for surface or needle electrodes, and it would not be surprising if tetanic stimulation of needle electrodes while using the 'surface' setting caused a burn. A report of tissue damage following the use of a simple *photoelectric plethysmograph* (Lebowitz 1970) suggested that heat from the small lightbulb may have been at least partly responsible. While the heat generated was negligible, Lebowitz emphasized the need to consider tissue perfusion before exposing skin to any external heat source.

The *transcutaneous oxygen electrode* has found wide application in monitoring neonates as well as older patients (Eberhard et al 1975), and concern has been raised about the safety margin involved. A thin mylar membrane is applied to the skin and coupled to a Clark oxygen electrode by a layer of electrolyte. The membrane allows the slow diffusion of oxygen into the electrolyte and the electrode measures the oxygen tension, taking into account the tension gradient across the membrane caused by oxygen consumption.

In order that the measured tension might reflect that of arterial blood, the skin adjacent to the membrane is 'arterialized' by direct heating, using an electrical coil mounted in the electrode. The electrode temperature is controlled using a thermistor, also mounted in the electrode, at a level that differs between instruments over the range 42–45°C. If too cool, the electrode does not achieve arterialization and has a slow response time; if too hot, there is a risk of causing thermal burns. In fact, Lofgren & Jacobson (1979) showed that the optimal temperature is 44.5°C, and commented that a transient red mark always developed on the skin beneath the electrode. Other groups (Eberhard et al 1975, Boyle & Oh 1980) have noted that, in preterm infants, more severe lesions may develop, ranging up to the appearance of vesicles, while shocked infants have developed frank blisters (Riegel & Versmold 1979). It may be accepted that such minor lesions are of no great import when the very survival of the patient is at stake. However, the margin of safety must be very narrow, and more serious damage is likely to follow any malfunction of the heating control system.

There are two reported cases of full-thickness burns following overheating of transcutaneous electrodes, one involving a Draeger system (Hardman & Bamford 1980), the other involving Radiometer equipment (Voora et al 1981). In each case the fault was due to failure of the temperature control system. Shaw et al (1980) pointed out that, unless the applied part (i.e the electrode assembly) has a backup thermal cut-out which is non-resetting, the device does not meet the requirements of either British or International Electrotechnical Commission (IEC) standards.

IGNITION OF FLAMMABLE GAS MIXTURES

Ether is most easily ignited at a concentration of 14% in oxygen, but will burn at any concentration in the range 2–82%. Rich mixtures in air will burn with a 'cool' propagating flame which may reach oxygen-enriched zones in which an explosion can occur. In oxygen or oxygen/nitrous oxide mixtures, ether is likely to explode, with the force of detonation increasing as the mixture approaches stoichiometry (3.4%). Similarly, cyclopropane burns in air over the concentration range 2.4–10.3%. Cyclopropane is most easily ignited at 16% in oxygen and detonates in the range 2.5–60% (Hill 1976). Halothane can be ignited in oxygen and nitrous oxide mixtures, but only in high concentration (>6%) and with high ignition energy (Table 43.2). A case of halothane exploding inside a McKesson vaporizer has been reported in which no external energy source was involved (May 1976). Presumably the internal conditions of concentration and pressure allowed a static discharge to ignite the mixture. Under normal working conditions it is not possible to produce a flammable mixture of halothane, oxygen and nitrous oxide in a patient circuit.

It must be assumed that respired mixtures containing diethyl ether or cyclopropane in oxygen are flammable, and that major detonations may occur if the gases are within certain ranges of concentration. Thus the breathing circuit itself must not be exposed to sources of sufficient energy to ignite the gases. The required energy may be very small (1μJ), and static sparks have caused major incidents (Walter 1966). More potent sources of ignition include electrical discharges at the cutting electrode of surgical diathermy or electrical switchgear at mains (or higher) voltages, and surfaces (>300°C) such as may develop in electronic equipment.

An escape of a flammable gas mixture from an anaesthetic breathing system becomes hazardous if an igniting energy source exists close to the point of release. It must be assumed that within 5 cm of the point of escape (usually an expiratory valve) the gas mixture is the same as that in the circuit itself, so that minimal energy may cause ignition. Within a wider range (20 cm) of the escape point the mixture may still be flammable, but need not be assumed to be oxygen-enriched. If the flammable mixture is escaping from a 'push-together' breathing circuit that could become separated, or the valve is on the end of a flexible hose that could reach a wide variety of

Table 43.2 Lower limits of flammability for halogenated anaesthetic vapours

Anaesthetic	% (v/v) in oxygen
Halothane	4.75
Enflurane	5.75
Isoflurane	7.00

positions when disconnected from the patient, the 'flammable zone' should be regarded as including all possible configurations. In my opinion it is naïve to consider only the explosion risk when all components of the breathing circuit are in their 'normal operating positions'. Also it must be remembered that, once an anaesthetic circuit has contained an explosive mixture, it may continue to do so for some time due to the agent leaching out of the rubber (Vickers 1965). Therefore an explosion may occur under the less stringent conditions of maintenance, etc., when least expected.

While the introduction of anaesthetic gas exhaust systems has greatly improved the working environment, and may be of positive benefit to staff, the hazard of explosion is not necessarily eliminated or even reduced. When such equipment is in use, the breathing system now encompasses the entire exhaust pathway which may include electrical pumps with no protection against flammable atmospheres whatever. While an active exhaust system may normally be assumed to dilute the exhaust gases to a considerable extent, this is not the case with a passive system. Here, highly flammable mixtures may be present at the external exhaust point. Few (if any) systems are properly guarded against the casually thrown match in the car park!

Prevention of anaesthetic vapour explosions

The modern operating theatre has become heavily dependent on electrical devices, many of which cannot be used safely in the presence of flammable gas mixtures. It is doubtful whether any gain that might be achieved by the use of ether or cyclopropane would offset the disruption of normal modern working practices, with attendant risk of human error. Indeed, the conditions required for the safe use of agents such as cyclopropane are incompatible with modern concepts of minimal patient monitoring. Since such standards are essential, it follows that explosive agents have no place in modern anaesthetic practice. That said, the antistatic floor has become both unnecessary and redundant. Why such floors should continue to be installed in new operating theatres, regardless of cost, I cannot imagine.

HUMAN FACTORS

The late E A Pask put great emphasis on the need for the clinical anaesthetist to remain continuously in close contact with his patient, and scorned the use of devices that threatened to intervene. He claimed that the best possible monitoring system consisted simply of a dab of glue applied to the anaesthetist's forefingertip, which should then be placed on the patient's temporal pulse. Such a system would be inexpensive and devoid of hazards. It would ensure a constant flow of information and would discourage trips to the anaesthetic room, telephone, coffee room, etc. Those who did not know Pask well regarded this suggestion as evidence of a wry sense of humour.

Complex monitoring systems can be of great value, but are time-consuming in operation and may become a major distraction to the anaesthetist. A single ECG trace on an oscilloscope screen can exert a mesmeric effect on the tired brain; how much worse is the multivariable display with constantly changing data in numerous colours? It is only too easy for the anaesthetist to become entranced by such a device, with the patient relegated to second place in his attention span. Since most anaesthetic disasters are due to fundamental human errors (Cooper et al 1984), Pask's finger would in all likelihood be equally effective, with the added benefit of the anaesthetist's undivided attention.

When the monitoring system is not integrated but consists of a number of separate devices, each with a set of controls and alarm warnings that operate when the measured variable no longer remains within preset limits, hazards multiply. First, there is no consistency of panel design, so that controls of similar function may be found in a variety of forms and colours, and in different positions on the various instruments. This adds to the time taken to make any single reading or adjustment and greatly increases the probability of error. When an alarm is activated, the anaesthetist must locate and identify the source before it can be silenced, then decide whether action is necessary.

When more than one alarm sounds the problem may become acute, since location may now be very difficult. Mixed sounds from more than one source may appear to originate from entirely different directions, and the generation of beat frequencies may change the character of the perceived sound altogether. In my experience it is difficult, if not impossible, to think constructively when surrounded by elusive, insistent and discordant alarms, while further aggravated by friendly surgical inquiries as to whether all this noise is really necessary. Consequently, the response to a life-threatening problem may be delayed appreciably.

Even when the physiological monitoring system is properly integrated, with a global 'silence' switch and a hierarchical alarm status display, the problem will persist, since other monitors, such as those concerned with gas delivery, controlled pulmonary ventilation and ventilator disconnect detection, remain separate (at least at the time of writing). Furthermore, many audible devices in the operating theatre have nothing to do with patient monitoring. These include surgical diathermy, light sources, paging systems, telephones, operating table controls, earth-leakage monitoring and fire alarms. In the absence of a wholly integrated approach to theatre systems, the anaesthetist can only hope that he is able to recognize all possible combinations of audible signals in the theatre.

As monitoring devices increase in number, the range of data formats presented to the anaesthetist increases also. These may take the form of direct analogue signal display, single variable digital readout, trend graphs or histograms. Some systems (such as respiratory mass spectrometers) now present large on-screen tables of both measured variables and derived indices, some of which are vitally important, some not at all. There is a very real danger that the clinician may be presented with so much data that he must spend an appreciable proportion of his time selecting useful information from a morass of irrelevant and gratuitous material. This condition, well-known to those who fly aeroplanes, may be called 'information overload'.

It is to be hoped that the experience gained in designing modern aircraft may be applied to anaesthetic systems, since in that field of human engineering it has long been recognized that the pilot should be presented only with the information he needs at the time. In recent designs, instrument clutter has been reduced to an extraordinary degree, with on-board computers handling much of the low-level information and automatically calculating (and executing) the most fuel-efficient flight plan according to conditions and the known characteristics of the aircraft. The disciplines of ergonomics and anaesthesia have as yet made little contact, but they will.

I was once taught that arrhythmias should be regarded as normal when using trichloroethylene, so that watching the ECG was inclined to make the anaesthetist anxious and likely to take positive action to restore sinus rhythm. Since both were considered undesirable, ECG monitoring was judged both unnecessary and unwise. Although this advice would be regarded as somewhat quaint, it did contain a certain element of very sound common sense, since it encompassed the concept that deviations from normal values do not always demand remedial action. The anaesthetist who responds to every change in heart rate or blood pressure with increments of atropine, propranalol, nitroprusside or dopamine will often be disappointed with the outcome. Here it is not the act, but the uncomprehending use of monitoring that endangers the anaesthetized patient.

MISLEADING AND ERRONEOUS DATA

It is an unfortunate fact that the credibility given to an item of information depends as much on the mode of presentation as its origin. Thus by presenting erroneous data confidently, clearly and unambiguously, a monitoring device may lead the unthinking anaesthetist to embark on a most unwise and hazardous course of action.

Human error

As might be expected, human error is the most frequent cause. Most service engineers have a fund of anecdotes relating emergency calls to instruments that, on examination, operate quite normally, but not necessarily in the manner presumed by the users. Contrary to common belief they do not, when all else fails, read the instructions. A common example is the direct arterial pressure monitor that yields bizarre values because the transducer has not been zeroed in its working position. Similarly, a capnograph that is allowed to conduct its automatic preuse calibration procedure without the sampling tube attached may yield quite surprising results when attached to the patient.

Operation outside design limits

Information may be highly misleading when obtained under conditions outside the design limits of the instrument concerned. For example an automatic oscillometric blood-pressure monitor cannot be expected to yield accurate readings when a standard cuff is applied to the arm of a very obese patient (Maxwell et al 1982). Similarly, the output of a transcutaneous Po_2 monitor will not reflect the arterial Po_2 if the patient is both hypothermic and hypovolaemic with intense peripheral vasoconstriction. Likewise, and end-tidal Pco_2 monitor may be perfectly accurate, but may fail to reflect the arterial Pco_2 due to non-homogeneity of alveolar air or a large alveolar–arterial tension gradient in conditions of low cardiac output. Directly measured radial artery pressures may be correct, but fail to reflect aortic pressure if the artery is compressed proximally. In one instance (Saka et al 1975), spuriously low radial pressures resulted from compression of the subclavian artery by a sternal retractor, and prompted the unnecessary administration of vasopressors during bypass. The authors stressed the importance of corroborative measurements and consideration of distant events as possible causes of measurement error. (See also Chapter 44.)

Design limitations

In some cases the error is due to some limitation in the monitor's capability. For example the displayed values of systolic and diastolic blood pressure by an oscillometric monitor may be incorrect due to the detection of movement artefacts, while surgical diathermy may cause gross errors in an ECG-derived heart rate. Similarly, some oxygen concentration monitors have been found to be affected by the presence of halothane (Maekawa et al 1980). Some peripheral nerve stimulators cannot reliably deliver supramaximal stimuli to the ulnar nerve through surface electrodes over the likely range of electrode impedances, and Mylrea et al (1984) have urged caution in interpreting clinical data obtained by their use. All these examples illustrate the difficulties faced by the instrument designer who works in complete isolation from the field of application.

Design faults may not become apparent until devices are used clinically. For instance, an anaesthetist watched an ECG monitor display progressively 'ischaemic' characteristics with considerable alarm, only to discover that this was due to the built-in batteries losing voltage as they discharged (Bar 1984). Restoration of mains power caused the changes to disappear immediately.

Devices that are intended to warn that a 'disconnect' or ventilator failure has occurred are particularly prone to unpredictable errors (McEwen et al 1980). This follows the almost insuperable problems facing the designer of such a device: he must produce a compact, low-cost instrument that will operate quite independently of the ventilator, but successfully monitor the output of any ventilator that is, or might be, used in clinical practice. If such a device monitors the pressure in the inspiratory limb of a ventilator circuit, the pressures generated *in the absence of any patient connection whatever* may be sufficient to trigger the monitor and thus prevent any warning. This can occur because during 'inspiration' the resistance of the inspiratory hose causes a pressure drop which exceeds the threshold preset by the monitor's manufacturer (Shribman 1982). More obscurely, the ventilator may impose a very brief flow (and therefore pressure) transient at the start of inspiration, which exceeds the monitor's threshold for a few milliseconds only (Mecklenbergh et al 1983). Although this transient is of no significance to the patient, it may completely defeat the disconnect monitor.

Hazards induced by device interactions

Even when a disconnect monitoring function is designed into the ventilator itself, failure may be due to interaction with other devices. For instance, it has been reported that the Servo 900 ventilator used in conjunction with an active gas-scavenging system may fail to report a patient-disconnect (Gray et al 1984). This can occur when the negative pressure induced by the scavenging system causes gas flow in the expiratory limb of the ventilator circuit, thus leading the expiratory flow-sensor to register a positive expired volume. The report emphasized the hazards that may follow the interconnection of devices that, although highly efficient in isolation, interact to function quite differently.

Intrinsic errors

Occasionally, errors are actually designed into the instrument, as in the case of the photoelectric finger pulsemeter (Kneeshaw 1983) which recorded a heart rate of 100 beats/min from a ballpoint pen!

Instrument malfunction

In other cases, instrument or transducer malfunction may result in incorrect data, but this is often due to well-intentioned but disastrous attempts to repair or modify the system. The interactions between electronic and human errors are illustrated by two clinical reports, described below.

Roy et al (1983) described how two DINAMAP oscillometric monitors were found to read consistently low after a period of use. In one case this was due to an electronic fault developing after prolonged use. In the other the fault was primarily due to the users having removed the cuff tubing connectors, subsequently relying on pushing the tubing directly onto the instrument connectors. This resulted in an accumulation of rubber particles in the ports, with eventual failure to empty the cuff during the deflation phase. The residual pressure was then regarded as zero by the microprocessor and subtracted from the subsequent reading, thus giving a spuriously low result.

In another instance it was observed that some thermistor temperature probes read 2–4°C higher in the operating room than on test (Ben-Zvi 1980). It transpired that soaking the probes in Cidex raised the capacitance of the probes. While this procedure did not affect the readings on a DC-excited test bridge, the AC bridge in the monitoring system detected both resistive and capacitative changes and therefore showed a different reading. Ben-Zvi stressed the undesirability of instituting a full-scale regime for malignant hyperpyrexia on account of a faulty temperature monitor.

CONCLUSION

In practice the hazards presented by electrical equipment do not present one at a time, in neatly packaged types as described above; only too often they conspire together so as to confuse and mislead us into believing that all is well. Prevention is the only practical approach towards making the operating theatre a safe place for both patients and staff, and that can be achieved only by technical understanding, constant awareness, and insight into human frailty, especially one's own.

REFERENCES

Akhter M S 1976 An unusual complication of intrapartum fetal monitoring. Am J Obstet Gynecol 126: 657–658

Aronow S, Bruner J M R 1975 Electrosurgery. Anesthesiology 42: 641–644

Bar Z G 1984 The ischaemic ECG monitor. Anaesthesia 39: 611

Battig C G 1968 Electrosurgical burn injuries and their prevention. J Am Med Assoc 204: 91–95

Becker C M, Malhotra I V, Hedley-Whyte J 1973 The distribution of radiofrequency current and burns. Anesthesiology 38: 106–122

Ben-Zvi S 1980 A possible cause of temperature probe failure. Anesthesiology 53: 523

Bousvaros G A, Don C, Hopps J A 1962 An electrical hazard of selective angio-cardiography. Can Med Assoc J 87: 826

Boyle R J, Oh W 1980 Erythema following transcutaneous Po_2 monitoring. Pediatrics 65: 333–334

Brenis A L Personal communication

Brock-Utne J G, Downing J W 1984 Rectal burn after the use of an anal stainless steel electrode/transducer system for monitoring myoneural junction. Anesth Analg 63: 1141–1142

Bruner J M R 1967 Hazards of electrical apparatus. Anesthesiology 28: 396–425

BSI 1979 Specification for safety of medical electrical equipment. I. General requirements. British Standards Institution, London

Chandra P 1982 Severe skin damage from EKG electrodes. Anesthesiology 56: 157–158

Cooper J B, Newbower R S, Kitz R J 1984 An analysis of major errors and equipment failures in anesthesia management: considerations for prevention and detection. Anesthesiology 60: 34–42

Coskey R J 1977 Contact dermatitis caused by ECG electrode jelly. Arch Dermatol 113: 839

DHSS 1963 Technical memorandum No 8. HMSO, London

Dobbie A K 1969 The electrical aspects of surgical diathermy. Biomed Eng 4: 206–216

Eberhard P, Mindt W, Jann F, Hammacher K 1975 Continuous Po_2 monitoring in the neonate by skin electrodes. Medical and Biol Eng 13: 436–442

Ferris L P, King B G, Spence P S, Williams H B 1936 Effect of electric shock on the heart. Electrical Eng 55: 498

Finlay B, Couchie D, Boyce L, Spencer E 1974 Electrosurgery burns resulting from use of miniature ECG electrodes. Anesthesiology 41: 263–269

Fisher A A 1977 Dermatologic hazards of electrocardiography. Cutis 20: 686–695

Geddes L A, Baker L E 1967 The specific resistance of biological material. Med Biol Eng 5: 271

Gray W M, Hall R C, Carter K B, Shaw A, Thomson W J 1984 Medishield A G S system and Servo 900 ventilators: investigation and remedy of hazard caused by defeat of 'low expired minute volume' alarm. Anaesthesia 39: 790–794

Hardman M J, Bamford M 1980 Hazard associated with transcutaneous oxymeter. Lancet 1: 370

Hill D W 1976 Physics applied to anesthesia, 3rd edn. Butterworths, London, ch 9, p 315

Hopps J A 1969 Shock hazards in operating rooms and patient care areas. Anesthesiology 31: 142

Hull C J 1978 Electrocution hazards in the operating theatre. Br J Anaesth 50: 647–657

Kneeshaw J D 1983 A pulsemeter hazard. Anesthesia 38: 1231–1232

Lebowitz M H 1970 Gangrene of a thumb following use of the photoelectric plethysmograph during anaesthesia. Anesthesiology 32: 164–167

Leeming M N, Ray C, Howland W S 1970 Low voltage, direct current burns. J Am Med Assoc 214: 1681–1684

Lippmann M, Fields W A 1974 Burns of the skin caused by a peripheral nerve stimulator. Anesthesiology 40: 82–84

Lipton M J, Ream A K, Hyndman B H 1978. A conductive catheter to improve patient safety during cardiac catheterization. Circulation 58: 1190–1195

Lofgren O, Jacobson L 1979 The influence of different electrode temperatures on the recorded transcutaneous Po_2 level. Pediatrics 64: 892–897

McEwen J A, Small C F, Saunders B A, Jenkins L C 1980 Hazards associated with the use of disconnect monitors. Anesthesiology 53: S391

Maekawa T, Okuda Y, McDowall D G 1980 Effect of low concentrations of halothane on the oxygen electrode. Br J Anaesth 52: 585

Marx G F, Steen S N, Foster E S et al 1968 Burns from needle electrodes of electrocardiogram monitor. N Y State J Med 68: 2083–2084

Maxwell M H, Waks A U, Schroth P C, Karam M, Dornfield L P 1982 Error in blood pressure measurement due to incorrect cuff size in obese patients. Lancet 2: 33

May T W 1976 Explosion during halothane anaesthesia. Br Med J 1: 692

Mecklenbergh J S, Latto I P, Jones P L, Saunders R L 1983 Failure of Penlon IDP alarm. Anaesthesia 38: 703–704

Morse A R 1959 Shock hazards of electric currents. J Engineering Institute of Canada 30: 3

Mylrea K C, Hameroff S R, Calkins J M, Blitt C D, Humphrey L L 1984 Evaluation of peripheral nerve stimulators and relationship to possible errors in assessing neuromuscular blockade. Anesthesiology 60: 464–466

Neufeld G R 1983 Burns and electrocution. In: Orkin R K, Cooperman L H (eds) Complications in anesthesiology. Lippincott, Philadelphia, p 677–688

Nordijk J A, Oey F J I, Tebra W 1961 Myocardial electrodes and the danger of ventricular fibrillation. Lancet 1: 975

Parker E O 1984 Electrosurgical burn at the site of an esophageal temperature probe. Anesthesiology 61: 93–95

Pengelly L D, Klassen G A 1961 Myocardial electrodes and the danger of ventricular fibrillation. Lancet 1: 1234

Raftery E B, Green H L, Yacoub M H 1975 Disturbances in heart rhythm produced by 50 Hz leakage currents in human subjects. Cardiovasc Res 9: 263–265

Riegel K P, Versmold H T 1979 Intra-arterial vs transcutaneous Po_2 monitoring in newborn infants. Biotelem Patient Monit 6: 32–43

Roy O S 1974 Ventricular fibrillation. Med Biol Eng 12: 130

Roy R C, Morgan L, Beamer D E 1983 Factitiously low blood pressure from the DINAMAP. Anesthesiology 59: 258–259

Saka D, Lin Y T, Oka Y 1975 An unusual case of false radial artery blood-pressure readings during cardiopulmonary bypass. Anesthesiology 43: 487–489

Schneider A J L, Apple H P, Braun R T 1977 Electrosurgical burns at skin temperature probes. Anesthesiology 47: 72–74

Shaw A, Mackinson D J, Macauley M 1980 Hazards of overheating in patient connected equipment. Lancet 1: 933

Shribman A J 1982 Failure of a ventilator alarm. Anaesthesia 37: 1044

Spierdijk J, Nandorff A, Van Bijnen A 1976 Burns caused by monitoring equipment during anaesthesia. Resuscitation 5: 127–134

Vickers M D 1965 The duration of the explosion hazard following induction with ether or cyclopropane. Anaesthesia 20: 314

Voora S, Wilks A K, Lilien L D 1981 Transcutaneous Po_2 electrode malfunction resulting in a third-degree burn. Am J Dis Child 135: 271–272

Wald A S, Mazzia V D B, Spencer M D 1971 Accidental burn associated with electrocautery. J Am Med Assoc 217: 916–921

Walter C W 1966 Explosion of an ether vaporizer. Anesthesiology 20: 192
Watson A B, Wright J S, Loughman J 1973 Electrical thresholds for ventricular fibrillation in man. Med J Aust 1: 1179
Wiggers C J, Wegria R 1939 Ventricular fibrillation due to single localized induction and condenser shocks applied during vulnerable phase of ventricular systole. Am J Physiol 128: 500
Zoll P M 1952 Resuscitation of the heart in ventricular standstill by external electrical stimulation. J Am Med Assoc 247: 768

FURTHER READING

Bruner J M R, Leonard P F 1989 Electricity, safety and the patient. Year Book Medical Publishers Inc., Chicago
Mushin W W, Jones P L 1987 Physics for the anaesthetist, 4th edn. Blackwell Scientific, Oxford

44

Avoiding hazards by monitoring

E. Major

Minimum monitoring standards during anaesthesia are becoming increasingly commonplace throughout the Western world. The so-called Harvard standards are probably the best known (Eichhorn et al 1986) of the early recommendations, but these have been followed by others (Association of Anaesthetists 1988).

The presence of a qualified anaesthetist in the operating theatre throughout the operative procedure has been identified as the most important monitor, but it is now recognized that even the very experienced practitioner needs information provided by today's sophisticated monitoring devices if he is to detect problems at an early stage. In fact, speed of detection is probably the most important single advantage that monitors have over the skilled anaesthetist, although, of course, electronic devices have an ability to maintain vigilance well beyond the capabilities of the human. The result is that, if properly set, monitors provide reliable early warning of impending complications. This should allow the anaesthetist to concentrate on monitoring depth of anaesthesia as best he can, for no machine has yet been devised that can outperform the anaesthetist in this respect.

The anaesthetist's other role, of course, is to maintain the patient's physiology in as normal a state as possible in the face of the surgical assault. The ability to predict that the patient is about to bleed profusely from the next surgical manoeuvre is something that comes with experience and which cannot be underestimated in its importance, since early fluid or blood resuscitation will prevent the otherwise inevitable hypotension which, for some patients, might be difficult to reverse. In this instance the human monitor outperforms even invasive blood pressure measurement, but the combination of an alert experienced practitioner and rapid response monitors offers the patient the safest possible surgical environment.

Many of us learned to administer anaesthetics with the aid of fairly rudimentary monitors. Even in the 1970s a finger on the pulse, an electrocardiogram (ECG), an oscillotonometer and maybe an oxygen-supply warning device was all we had, and not every theatre contained an ECG monitor. Other equipment, such as the capnograph, existed but was not generally available. Invasive blood pressure measurement was by no means common and, although the flow-directed pulmonary flotation catheter had been invented (Swan et al 1970), it remained essentially a research device. Since then, of course, inhaled gas analysers have become readily available, carbon dioxide monitors have become reliable and easy to use, the pulse oximeter has arrived, invasive pressure monitoring is commonplace, neuromuscular blockade is easily monitored and temperature probes are universally available, if still underused. It is appropriate, therefore, to review the hazards and complications that might be prevented by the addition of these newer monitoring techniques to the simple methods of old.

Table 44.1 Monitors of gas supply and ventilation

Monitor	False readings due to	Early detection of	Prevention of
Gas analyser	Leaks Kinks Blockage Not calibrated Wrong agent Wrong site	Light anaesthesia Leaks Disconnections Empty vapourizer Wrong agent	Awareness Hypoxaemia
		Agent overdose Wrong setting Inadvertent setting	CVS and respiratory depression
Inspired oxygen (%)	Leaks Kinks Blockage Not calibrated Wrong site	Oxygen failure Disconnection N_2O failure	Hypoxaemia Awareness
Capnograph	Leaks Kinks Blockage Not calibrated Wrong site. N_2O Humidification Slow response time	Oesophageal intubation Disconnection Rebreathing Hypoventilation	Hypoxaemia Hypercarbia Hypertension Excess bleeding Dysrhythmias Raised ICP
		Hyperventilation	Hypocapnia Hypotension Cerebral ischaemia
		MH	Metabolic catastrophe
		Acute acidosis	CVS depression
		Air embolus	Larger embolus
		Pulmonary embolus	
		CVS collapse	
		Dysrhythmias	
		Coughing/hiccup	Patient movement
Airway pressure **Low**	Wrong limits Wrong site High circuit compliance	Disconnection Leak Inadequate volume	Hypoxaemia Awareness
High	Small endotracheal tube	High volume	Barotrauma
	Low circuit compliance	Endobronchial intubation Tube kinked Foreign body	Hypoxaemia Hypoventilation Atelectasis Lung collapse
		Excess secretions Bronchospasm Aspiration Anaphylaxis	
		Pneumothorax	CVS depression Hypoxaemia

ICP = intracranial pressure CVS = cardiovascular system MH = malignant hyperpyrexia

Table 44.2 Physiological signal monitors

Monitor	False readings due to	Early detection of	Prevention of
Pulse oximeter	Carboxyhaemoglobin	Dysrhythmia	
	Methaemoglobin	Hypoxaemia	Detects hypoxaemia only as it occurs
	Dyes	Local ischaemia	Tissue hypoxia
	Hypovolaemia	Hypovolaemia (some	
	Poor perfusion	makes	
	Diathermy		
	Motion artefact		
	Fetal Haemoglobin		
	Optical cross talk		
Temperature probe	Probe in faeces	MH	Metabolic catastrophe
	Too near airway	Thyrotoxic crisis	
	Poor contact	Sepsis	
	Near infusion site	Overheating	Burns
		Hypothermia	Post operative shivering
			Dysrhythmias
		Low cardiac output	Shock/tissue hypoxia
CVP	Ventilation	Hypovolaemia	Shock/tissue hypoxia
	PEEP/CPAP	Fluid overload	Hypoxaemia
	Patient position	Right heart failure	Oedema
	Abdominal distention	Cardiac tamponade	Shock/tissue hypoxia
	Wrong site		
	Incorrect zero		
	Valvular regurgitation		
Pulmonary flotation catheter	Ventilation	Left heart failure	Pulmonary oedema
	PEEP/CPAP	Fluid overload	Myocardial infarct
	Patient position	Myocardial ischaemia	Shock/tissue hypoxia
	Abdominal distention	Hypovolaemia	Shock/tissue hypoxia
	Wrong site	Cardiac tamponade	
	Incorrect zero	CVS depression	
	Valvular regurgitation		
Finger plethysmograph	Movement	Dysrhythmias	
		Poor perfusion	
		Hypovolaemia	
Blood pressure	Cuff size	Low blood pressure	Detects hypovolaemia only as it occurs
Indirect	Cuff position	High blood pressure	Light anaesthesia
	Sensor type		
	Dysrhythmias		
	Movement		
	External pressure		
	Extreme values		
	Kinks and leaks		
Direct	Leaks in system	as above	
	Kink in line	Dysrhythmias	
	Air bubble	Hypovolaemia	
	Thrombus	Poor contractility	
	Choice of artery		
	Overdamping		
ECG	Incorrect electrode positions	Ischaemia	Myocardial infarction
		Dysrhythmias	
	Diathermy		
	Movement		
Train of four	Wrong position	Return of muscle power	Movement
	Nerve damage	Postoperative respiratory failure	Postoperative hypoxaemia
		Nerve damage	

CPAP = continuous positive airways pressure PEEP = positive end expiratory pressure

It is important that the anaesthetist realizes the limitations of his monitoring equipment, since to follow slavishly the advice given by an electronic monitor is to court disaster. Every piece of information is no more than that, a piece of information to be placed in the overall 'data jigsaw'. Many factors may reduce the value of information derived from monitors, and some of the more common pitfalls are listed in Tables 44.1 and 44.2. The first table deals with monitors of respiration and gas supply, whereas the second deals with monitors of physiological signals.

The anaesthetist must also understand exactly what the equipment is monitoring and which monitor is likely to give earliest warning of impending hazards. For example the anaesthetist who relies on an oximeter to warn him of hypoxaemia secondary to disconnection is missing the point. Oximeters do not give early warning of hypoxaemia, they merely report it as it happens. The aim must be to spot a disconnection before hypoxaemia occurs, and in this respect the capnograph or airway pressure alarm is far superior. Similarly, it is not good enough to wait until hypoxaemia signals oesophageal intubation; it should be detected much sooner. In a critical incident survey from Toronto (Mckay & Noble 1988), the pulse oximeter provided first warning of a hazard in only 4% of cases, but of course it is still important to have an oximeter in use since hypoxaemia is such an important complication. In the American Society of Anesthesiologists Closed Claims Analysis (Caplan et al 1990), the reviewers judged that better monitoring would have prevented adverse outcome in 72% of the claims for adverse respiratory events. Pulse oximetry, capnography or both were suggested by the reviewers in 98% of cases. This combination was also the most common reviewers' choice for preventing oesophageal intubation (84%), but pulse oximetry alone was favoured for prevention of adverse outcomes associated with difficult tracheal intubation.

In the tables an attempt is made to highlight which monitors are best for early detection of hazards, but it should be emphasized that the anaesthetist remains the most important monitor.

REFERENCES

Association of Anaesthetists of Great Britain and Ireland 1988 Recommendations for standards of monitoring during anaesthesia and recovery. Association of Anaesthetists, London

Caplan R A, Postner K L, Ward R J, Cheney F W 1990 Adverse respiratory events in anesthesia: a closed claims analysis. Anesthesiology 72: 828–833

Eichhorn J H, Cooper J B, Cullen D J, Maier W R, Philip J H, Seeman R G 1986 Standards for patient monitoring during anaesthesia at Harvard Medical School. J Am Med Assoc 256(8): 1017–1020

Mckay W P, Noble W H 1988 Critical incidents detected by pulse oximetry during anaesthesia. Can J Anaesth 35(3): 265–269

Swan H J C, Ganz W, Forrester J S, Marcus H, Diamond G, Chonette D 1970 Catheterization of the heart in man with the use of a flow-directed balloon-tipped catheter. N Engl J Med 283: 447–451

45

Equipment sterilization and maintenance

T. H. Taylor

INTRODUCTION

When servicing and preparing equipment, instruments and drugs for use in the operating theatre, the safety of the patient is of paramount importance. This is also true when clearing up after an operation. It is expected that these items will present no unforseen hazard to the patient, but equally their production, use and disposal must be safe for the staff that handle them. This is especially important with the disposal of potentially infected materials, including those sharp instruments and broken glass that may cause injury to theatre and other staff.

STERILITY OF ANAESTHETIC EQUIPMENT

All apparatus used during the administration of an anaesthetic must be clean, that is free of all extraneous matter, even if absolute sterility is not required. This includes the removal of any chemicals that may have been applied in an attempt to achieve sterility. Effective scrubbing or thorough washing with a soapy solution is sufficient for many purposes.

The mouth and upper airway are an important source of infection during surgical and anaesthetic procedures. Since it is not possible to sterilize these areas, the patient is at risk from the introduction of organisms into the bronchial tree during intraoral manipulations and intubation. Although the risk cannot be removed, it is important not to increase it by introducing exogenous organisms from dirty apparatus. Patients who are immunosuppressed are particularly at risk, although any patient undergoing surgery, however minor, can suffer adversely from infection introduced from outside sources. Thus it is imperative that the standard of cleanliness of anaesthetic apparatus should be high (Jenkins & Edgar 1964, Lumley 1976, Lumley 1988). This means that parts in direct contact with the patient (endotracheal tubes, airways, laryngoscopes and suckers) should be sterile, and all other apparatus should be free of organic matter and adequately disinfected at the beginning of each case. This can, of course, be achieved by the use of disposable circuits, masks, airways and endotracheal tubes, and this is increasingly common in the UK, although the cost of the first two items still seems to be prohibitive.

More complex anaesthetic circuits and many ventilators need to be effectively decontaminated even if they cannot be sterilized before reuse, and all the smaller items of equipment, such as laryngoscopes, throat sprays, suckers, forceps and tooth guards, also need proper care.

This chapter deals specifically with the hazards to the patient arising from the sterilization or disinfection process, and suggests minimum standards of cleanliness for anaesthetic apparatus. Some suggestions are also made for the routine servicing and preoperative checking of anaesthetic equipment. In addition, some comments are made on potential hazards to theatre and other staff employed on cleaning and maintenance duties.

METHODS AVAILABLE FOR STERILIZATION

Heat sterilization

Heat sterilization is the oldest method and is applicable to many of the smaller items, simply by boiling after a thorough cleansing with soap and water. In the case of airways, endotracheal tubes, tubing and suckers, an efficient method of cleaning the lumen must be devised for the heat to be fully effective, as solid material, such as mucous, may remain as a nidus of infection. Sterilization is enhanced at higher temperatures, thus destroying all bacteria, viruses and spores. This may be achieved by dry heat in a hot air oven, formerly used for glass syringes, or by means of an autoclave.

Modern theatre design and the application of safety standards for staff tends to exclude the provision of boiling water sterilizers, ovens and autoclaves in the operating theatre itself. This is because of the danger of spreading infection by cleaning apparatus within the 'sterile area', and also because of the potential burns injury hazard to both patients and staff. It is thought to be better and safer to entrust the cleaning and recycling process to trained specialist staff in a theatre sterile supplies department (TSSD), and only to keep dry, sterile packs in the theatre itself, together with the commercial 'once only' stores. This arrangement allows the staff of the TSSD to be properly supervised and imposes proper safety standards in a purpose-built workplace. It is probable that this system is cost effective in terms of nurses' and technicians' working time.

Most of the packs are prepared at various temperatures in specialized autoclaves. The cleaned and prepacked equipment is placed in the autoclave chamber and the air is partially exhausted and replaced by steam under pressure (up to 32 lbs pressure, giving a temperature of 134°C). This temperature is held for a period of time to kill not only bacteria, but also their spores. The alterations of pressure inherent in such a device will ensure penetration to all areas of the apparatus in the autoclave if it has been packed correctly. This process is monitored by temperature charts on the outside of the autoclave and also by the use of various heat-sensitive markers within the pack being sterilized, so the user can be sure that the full sterilization cycle has been carried out. The only direct danger to the patient arising from these methods is if a rapid turnover of the instruments does not allow sufficient time for them to cool adequately before use. Repeated heat sterilization does, however, soften rubber, and endotracheal cuffs may be dangerously weakened by the process with consequent dangers for the patient.

Unfortunately, high temperatures also affect plastics, and modern equipment frequently employs this material in its manufacture, making some items unsuitable for heat treatment. Even a lower temperature 'autoclave' with added formaldehyde can still be deleterious, and the formaldehyde vapour needs time to diffuse out of the material, as it is harmful to patients if inhaled.

Certain fibre-optic telescopes may be treated by 'pasteurization', that is heating them in water, after a thorough cleaning, to a temperature of 70°C and maintaining this temperature for a period of 20 min. Any higher temperature would damage the lens system. This method can also be used for rubber apparatus that requires a high degree of cleanliness and not absolute sterility, such as corrugated rubber circuit tubing. There are several commercial washing machines available that effectively do this, and many of their cleaning programmes may be efficient in removing solid material before the 'pasteurizing' sequence if the tubing is suspended in such a way as to allow the flow of water through the lumen.

Chemical sterilization

Chemical sterilization can never be as effective as autoclaving to a high temperature, for resistant organisms and spores may not be killed even if immersion is prolonged. In addition it is difficult to ensure contact with all areas of the apparatus being immersed (George 1975). The chief hazard to the patient from this method is that the chemicals employed can be absorbed onto the anaesthetic apparatus, especially rubber and plastics, and will remain there during use proving harmful to the patient's tissues. Certain chemicals may also give rise to acute reactions in susceptible individuals. Antistatic rubber, which contains carbon, is particularly prone to absorb the chemicals, and chloroxylenol (Dettol) has a bad reputation when used to clean face masks. Formaldehyde vapour is no longer used as a means of chemical sterilization, except to enhance the effectiveness of low-temperature 'autoclaves'.

Glutaraldehyde

Of the substances currently available, glutaraldehyde enjoys some popularity and is effective. It is used in a 2% solution that is activated by alkalinization by the addition of sodium carbonate. Short immersion for 3–5 min kills organisms, and spores are thought to be killed if this time is increased to 3 h. It is advisable that those using the solution to prepare intruments should wear gloves and goggles as both the vapour given off and the solution itself are irritant to the skin and eyes. Excess fluid should be washed off with sterile water before use. If dried in a sterile manner, instruments can be packed for use later, although the efficacy of this has not been confirmed. This form of sterilization is usually carried out in the operating theatre, and is widely used for endoscopes and the television cameras now used in conjunction with them.

Chlorhexidine

Chlorhexidine (0.1% in aqueous solution) is also used, but is not as efficient as glutaraldehyde. A 0.5% solution in 70% alcohol is more bactericidal, and can be used on hard surfaces and articles that do not come into close contact with the patient. It is thought that sodium hypochlorite still has a place in decontamination after apparatus has been used in patients infected with the viruses of hepatitis and AIDS, especially in the presence of blood. Other solutions, such as phenol, iodine and 70% alcohol alone, are now of historical interest only.

Ethylene oxide

Ethylene oxide gas is used for apparatus made of delicate materials or in situations where penetration is important. The gas is very slow in action, difficult to remove from sterilized apparatus, and is explosive and very toxic (Marx et al 1969). It must only be used in special areas equipped for the purpose. The safety requirements during its use are such that the DHSS believes it should only be employed at a few centralized sites in the health service. When the sterilization process is complete it is difficult to remove the residual gas from the sterile pack. This is done either by applying several successive vacuums to the package, insisting on a long-shelf life before use, or both.

Plastic (PVC) and rubber endotracheal tubes that are normally irradiated should not be resterilized by ethylene oxide, as large quantities of the gas may be absorbed and a toxic product may be formed by the process. This will cause damage, not unlike a burn, to the patient's tissues (Marx et al 1969).

Gamma radiation

Many plastic and other delicate articles can be sterilized if prepacked and then subjected to a period of exposure to gamma rays, usually from a cobalt-60 source. The bactericidal dose is of the order of 2.5 Mrads. This process is used frequently in commercial practice for items such as endotracheal tubes, airways, sucker handpieces and tubing, syringes and needles. Many hospitals have the facility to send their own packs for treatment although, as the number of commercially prepared items increases, the need for such a facility diminishes.

Each anaesthetic department will have its own method of cleaning, sterilizing and storing the apparatus required for everyday use in the operating theatre, especially the anaesthetic machines and ventilators. This may be done in a central TSSD, but is often delegated to technicians or unskilled staff. The routines used by these people should be known to and approved of by the consultants in the department. This also applies to the routines for the sterilization of apparatus after use, particularly after it has been used for an infected patient. The Hospital Control of Infections Officer is available for advice and the DHSS lays down many guidelines on particular hazards.

STERILIZATION OF INDIVIDUAL PIECES OF EQUIPMENT

Face masks

Because of their construction of reinforced rubber and the presence, in most patterns, of an air cushion, face masks should not to be autoclaved or heated. Particular care should be exercised in exposing them to chemical solutions, since these substances can be absorbed onto conductive rubber and this can remain in contact with the patient's skin for a long period. Patients that are sensitive to these compounds may then be affected by a contact dermatitis.

After use, masks should be thoroughly cleaned in hot soapy water, then rinsed and allowed to dry. Only after use on an infected case is it necessary to use a solution such as chlorhexidine (0.1% in water) for chemical sterilization. If a mask needs to be autoclaved, the air cushion should be emptied and the spigot left out while this is done. Autoclaving, even at low pressure, does shorten the useful life of rubber goods and may distort their shape, but this may be justified either after use for a particularly infective patient or before use in certain susceptible patients.

Endotracheal tubes and airways

Single-use endotracheal tubes and airways, either made of rubber or plastic, are now commonplace and relatively cheap. They are prepacked and sterilized by gamma radiation, and should be used in most patients, certainly those at greatest risk from infection. Manufacturers now include many reinforced or preformed tubes for various special uses, and endobronchial tubes are available.

It is doubtful whether simple tubes should be reused, but the more complicated and expensive double-lumen endobronchial tubes may have to be. If they are recycled they must be cleaned inside and out with hot, soapy water before being repacked and autoclaved. This process undoubtedly shortens their life and, in the case of cuffed tubes, may render the rubber less elastic, thus causing the cuff to break in use. More dangerous, the softening may be just enough to allow the cuff to herniate without actually breaking. Every tube should be tested immediately before use to obviate these hazards. If it is impossible to autoclave tubes they may be rendered sterile by simple boiling for about 3 min after thoroughly cleaning them, and then allowing them to cool before use. It is vital to ensure the removal of all particulate matter from the lumen before sterilization. Similar methods can be employed for armoured tubes, taking care to see that the lumen of the tube is fully patent before use.

Chemical methods should never be employed to sterilize endotracheal tubes for these are not fully effective and, since the tubes remain in contact with the upper airway for a long time, may give rise to a sensitivity reaction if residual chemical is present in the tube.

Corrugated rubber tubing, expiratory valves, reservoir bags and angle pieces

Disposable circuits of all types are available. These clearly ensure the complete absence of cross-infection, but they are expensive and not in universal use. Single-use tubing and bags should be available for patients greatly at risk, such as the immunocompromised, and also for patients with infections likely to be dangerous to others, as the apparatus can be destroyed after use. In these circumstances, valves and angle pieces can be heat-treated. For other patients it is not strictly necessary to sterilize these articles after every case, although there is evidence that contamination progressively occurs as the tubing is continuously used (Nielsen et al 1978). It is advisable to ensure that the tubes are washed clean between cases, as condensed water and particulate matter left in them may be a source of infection.

At the end of each working day, all machines and ventilators should be stripped and cleaned thoroughly, using a combination of a hard surface disinfectant and either boiling or autoclaving for the other suitable parts. The latter will again shorten the life of the apparatus. There are commercial machines available for washing anaesthetic tubes. These achieve a high degree of sterility by holding the temperature at about 70°C for a period of time. The machine's operating cycle is often long and the tubes thus processed take a long time to cool. Obviously, these washing and pasteurizing machines can be used more frequently, even during the course of a working day, if the amount of tubing available for use is sufficient.

The Bain and the Lack coaxial circuits present particular problems in cleaning, since mechanical washers are unlikely to be completely effective for the central tubing, which in the former carries the fresh gases, in the latter the expired gases. They can be subjected to autoclaving at low temperature, or to ethylene oxide. Before being returned to use they should be checked to ensure that the inner tubing is still connected to the mounts at each end, and that it has not become elongated and therefore possibly kinked. An obstruction to the tube is particularly dangerous in the Bain circuit as it carries the flow of fresh gas from the anaesthetic machine. The inner tube can be easily seen when the outer corrugated tubing is made of semitransparent plastic, and this type of circuit is much safer than those that are opaque.

Laryngoscopes, suckers and forceps

Metallic apparatus can be cleaned and heat-sterilized after each use. Laryngoscopes are an exception because their battery systems and light-bulbs are vulnerable to moisture and heat. These parts must be carefully washed and then treated with antiseptic solutions, although usually the blades can be detached and, after the bulb has been removed, boiled or autoclaved. Again this should be done after each use. Laryngoscope blades from those models with the batteries and bulb in the handle, and a detachable blade with a light projection system to the tip, can be heat treated.

Throat sprays

The Mackintosh and Forrester throat sprays are difficult to clean and sterilize. They have been incriminated in spreading infection (Casewell & Dalton 1977). Preferably either a disposable spray or a fully heat-treatable spray should be used.

Anaesthetic machines and ventilators

As mentioned above, anaesthetic machines and ventilators should be stripped and cleaned at the end of every working day, and additionally after particularly infected cases. The anaesthetic circuit tubing should be sterilized or cleaned as previously described. Ideally the anaesthetic machine should be cleaned by trained staff to minimize the danger of incorrect reassembly. All the working surfaces, which are either of metal or plastic, should be scoured and then washed down with a hard surface disinfectant, such as 0.5% chlorhexidine in spirit.

Circle absorbers are difficult to clean, but the valves can usually be stripped and cleaned with chlorhexidine. The soda-lime canister should be subjected to the same treatment from time to time.

Ventilators are now constructed to allow the major part of the patient's circuit to be autoclaved. This ensures a high standard of decontamination if not sterility and the procedure can be repeated as often as necessary. Older types, however, do not have this facility and need more exacting methods. The work is specialized and should be carried out by trained technicians in a properly equipped workspace, where ethylene oxide, formaldehyde or 'Resiguard' is passed through the apparatus, taking care to eliminate the vapours before returning the machine to use. This may take several hours. Ultrasonic nebulizers can also be used to pass hydrogen peroxide or alcoholic solutions through the non-autoclavable parts of the patient's circuit. Alcohol is explosive when used in this way and again time must be allowed for the elimination of the nebulized agent. With these methods there is often a small part of the ventilator mechanism that is difficult to reach for cleaning. This area may act as a reservoir of infection, thus rapidly recontaminating the whole apparatus. Such machines usually have to be withdrawn from service to protect subsequent patients from infection.

Apparatus for local anaesthetic procedures

This apparatus must be presented in sterile packs, together with the required towels and receptacles. Skin-cleaning solutions are supplied from theatre stock, and the local anaesthetic agents are now available from the manufacturers in sterile packs, thus obviating the need to heat treat these susceptible drugs locally in uncontrolled conditions. Many commercial procedure packs are now available. It is beyond the scope of this chapter to discuss this further, for the choice of these packs must be left to the individual user.

PARTICULAR INFECTIVE HAZARDS

The utmost care and proper regimes are needed at all times in the anaesthetic room and operating theatre, to prevent cross-infection between patients and to stop the transmission of infection from a patient to staff within and without the theatre. Because the disposal of 'clinical waste', including used sharp instruments and broken glass, often employs unskilled workers, special precautions must be taken. The Association of Anaesthetists (1988a) has published guidelines for anaesthetists in respect of AIDS and Hepatitis B. The British Medical Association (BMA) (1990) has issued a document setting out the hazards of the disposal of sharp instruments and suggesting safe procedures.

Virus infections

Hepatitis

There are several pathogens responsible for causing hepatitis. They are rightly feared by theatre staff, especially the virus of Hepatitis B, because it is easily spread through contamination with blood and body secretions, with or without innoculation (Tedder 1983). The risk of infection is related to the magnitude of the contact with infected blood and, of course, also to needle-stick injuries (Hadler et al 1985). The rate of seroconversion in those individuals that suffer needle-stick injuries and consequent inoculation with the virus may be as high as 19–27%.

The virus is very resistant to all forms of disinfection except heat, although hypochlorite solutions are recommended for cleansing hard surfaces that may be contaminated. Protective clothing should be worn and the equipment used for each case should preferably be disposable.

Because of the resistance of the organism and the relative ease of transmission, health workers at risk should be actively immunized against the virus (DOH 1990). If the antibody level is properly monitored and necessary booster doses are given the immunity is excellent, although it may take 6 months to acquire. The BMA (1987) has published a paper detailing the staff at risk who should be immunized. A vaccine (Engerix B: Smith, Kline and French) is available which has been synthetically produced by yeast cells using a recombinant DNA technique (ABPI 1992). The use of this vaccine obviates the small risk of acquiring AIDS infection with vaccines prepared from human sources. If any worker not so immunized is subject to an injury from 'sharps' used on a known infected patient, hepatitis immune globulin should be administered. Many institutions routinely test patients for the virus status on admission, especially for surgery in which major blood loss is expected or power tools are to be employed.

Acquired immunodeficiency syndrome

Of all virus infections the HTLV III virus of acquired immunodeficiency syndrome (AIDS) is most feared by health workers. There are few authenicated cases of infection transmitted in the course of normal work, although needle-stick injuries are relatively common in nurses, anaesthetists and surgeons. Four cases have been reported following accidental inoculation with a previously used needle (Editorial 1984). Roger et al (1989) reported 15 further possible cases.

Because there is a high index of suspicion that HIV-positive individuals are predominantly homosexual or bisexual, or are intravenous drug abusers, the use of appropriate precautions must be compulsory when dealing with these patients. Despite views to the contrary from some legal sources (Sherrard & Gatt 1987), it would seem reasonable that those patients in the high-risk category should be screened before elective surgery is contemplated to ensure the maximum protection for staff. Because the disease has a slow onset (up to 3 months may elapse before tests become positive after infection), testing does not provide full safety for staff. The Association of Anaesthetists (1988a) has issued guidelines for staff liable to infection with both AIDS and hepatitis.

The maximum danger of transmitting infection is through an injury sustained while handling used sharp instruments and broken glass. The BMA has issued through its Board of Science a code of practice on the safe use and disposal of sharps (1990). It suggests risk management techniques and the correct course of action if an injury occurs. The document also suggests that the insertion of a drip or an indwelling cannula at the start of a procedure will enable all subsequent injections to be given without the possibility of contaminating another needle, resulting in only one potentially infected sharp from each case.

It is thought that a considerable volume of blood (perhaps greater than 1 ml) has to be transferred before serum conversion occurs, and this must be intramuscular or deeper. This presupposes that a hollow needle is the offending instrument. If such an injury is sustained from a needle used in a known HIV-positive patient, it is probable that prophylactic treatment with zidovudine should be started immediately, despite the known serious side effects of this drug.

When dealing with a case in which the infection is suspected the health workers should wear proper clothing, including gloves and eyeshields (Waterson 1976). Boiling alone is insufficient to kill the virus. Hypochlorite solution is effective for washing down hard surfaces and, where possible, disposable or autoclavable instruments should be used. Doctors and nurses in contact with the patient or the secretions should wear rubber gloves at all times (Waterson 1976).

Tuberculosis

Tuberculosis bacilli are susceptible to boiling, autoclaving and long exposure to some chemicals, such as chlorhexidine. After apparatus has been used for a patient with active tubercle, a thorough disinfectation should take place and, of course, all possible disposable items should have been used. After a generation unused to the hazard of tuberculosis in the UK there is some evidence that more cases are being admitted, undiagnosed, to hospital.

Pseudomonas infection

Pseudomonas pyocyanea is a very common contaminant of ventilators and breathing circuits if these apparatus are not properly cleansed. Debilitated patients are particularly liable to respiratory infection if exposed to this organism. It is therefore justly feared in the intensive care situation. Great care is needed to prevent it colonizing any anaesthetic apparatus.

MAINTENANCE AND SERVICING OF APPARATUS

Pipelines

Many hospitals are now equipped with pipeline supplies of oxygen, nitrous oxide, compressed air and suction to all areas where these services are required. The provision of anaesthetic gases removes the worry of unobserved emptying of an oxygen cylinder and all the dangers that entails. However, pipelines are not completely free of risk, and need expert supervision and maintenance. These procedures are governed by regulations issued by the DHSS (1977).

The installation of pipeline systems is undertaken by skilled contractors and they are subject to close regulation. It is essential that the system is made from clean and degreased materials, and is tested before use. This testing is undertaken by a responsible officer ('competent person') of the hospital, frequently the pharmacist, and the process may be observed by an anaesthetist. The tests involve quantitative and qualitative estimations, as well as smelling the system to ensure there are no contaminants. All pipework and outlets should be colour coded and particular care should be taken to prevent 'cross-over' connections.

If an established system has to be extended or requires maintenance work, the engineer in charge must obtain a 'permit to work' before starting. This document has six copies which have to be retained in various departments. The original is kept by the 'competent person' for 2 years and includes a signature from a responsible doctor or nurse. The document recognizes three degrees of danger depending on the site of the work. Clearly there is more danger if an existing system is cut, for on completion and bringing the pipeline into service all the tests of quality and quantity have to be reapplied to all outlets. There is obviously increased danger when outlets are to be modified if there is more than one gas present. It is worth noting that hospitals with piped services rarely have on site enough gas cylinders with reducing valves and connections, electrical as opposed to gas-driven ventilators and electrical suckers to cope with a sudden cessation of supply. It would be wise for anaesthetic departments and others involved to have planned methods of obtaining such supplies before the situation arises, especially for the operating theatres and intensive care units.

Apart from the circumstances outlined above, it is assumed that medical and nursing staff need only check that part of the system beyond the terminal outlets in normal usage. This means ensuring that the connections are sound and that gas is flowing at the outlet. Qualitative tests are not thought to be necessary, although whistle discriminators can be used to check the products at the outlet of an anaesthetic machine.

Anaesthetic machines and ventilators

All apparatus should be on a regular maintenance programme, and, if the hospital is not capable of providing this with its own personnel on a proper basis, a contract should be made with the manufacturer. The responsibility for ensuring such a programme lies with the administration of the hospital or nursing home, after consultation with the consultants of the department concerned. It has been suggested by the DOH that one named individual should be responsible in each hospital.

Anaesthetic machines should be serviced quarterly and ventilators half-yearly, unless used excessively. All parts should be stripped and examined for faults before reassembly and any defective parts replaced. The engineer should leave attached to each machine a signed label giving the date of the service so that the first user can be alerted should any problem arise.

Routine preoperative machine checks

The anaesthetist is responsible for ensuring that the apparatus he is about to use for an operating list is in good order. This is frequently quite properly delegated to a trained assistant. The Association of Anaesthetists (1990) has published a 'checklist' for machines before the start of an operating list. The criticism of this list is its length, and it is suggested that compliance may be more complete if it is used in a question and answer form by two people in a similar way to cockpit checks by airline pilots before take off (Crosby 1988).

Oxygen failure warning devices

In addition to the routine checks before a session starts, it should be ascertained at frequent intervals that the machine is capable of delivering gases, especially oxygen, under pressure through the tubing to the patient, and that the vaporizers are full of volatile agent. It is a foolish anaesthetist that delegates these important tasks entirely to a technician, however reliable.

All machines should be fitted with an oxygen failure warning device, which should shut off the other gases if the oxygen supply fails. In the USA it is compulsory to fit an inspired oxygen analyser at the patient outlet to ensure the patient receives adequate oxygen at all times. Many newer models deliver oxygen, not through simple rotameters but, through devices that prevent an anoxic mixture being presented to the patient. This is achieved either by linking the nitrous oxide and oxygen control knobs, or by using a mixing device on which mixtures above 30% oxygen can be set before delivery the required minute volume to the patient.

Before using a machine or ventilator, all vaporizers must be turned off and all circuit switches turned to the correct position. Several serious mishaps have been reported due to the incorrect position of these switches. If there is doubt about the correct functioning of any part of an anaesthetic machine or ventilator it should be removed from service until it can be properly checked.

Vaporizers

Thermally compensated vaporizers require regular maintenance to ensure they deliver the stated concentration and to remove any accumulation of unwanted material from the vaporization chamber. This is usually done by the manufacturer on a contract basis at yearly intervals, and each vaporizer should be labelled with the date of this service. Although modern vaporizers are extremely reliable, if any untoward reaction by a patient is noted the apparatus should be withdrawn for checks, especially on the concentration of volatile agent delivered. The earliest models of some vaporizers did deliver dangerously high doses of halothane in certain circumstances.

Care must be taken when refilling vaporizers. With so many different agents in common use it is important to ensure that the correct liquid is always used. This is done using non-interchangeable filling devices specific for each volatile anaesthetic agent, which are usually colour coded with the vaporizer. There have been sporadic cases where the anaesthetic liquid has been removed and replaced with water by people abusing the drug. The full vaporizer is an ever-present temptation for such people and the anaesthetist must be vigilant to prevent such practices.

Many vaporizers are now interchangeable with others containing the same or different volatile agents on the back bar of the machine. They are located on lugs and then locked into position, thus making a gas-tight joint. If the vaporizer is not properly positioned on the lugs, the joints will leak gas, sometimes even with the locking mechanism apparently correctly set. In these circumstances the vapour is not delivered to the patient and can lead to awareness. The total quantity of gas reaching the patient may also be deficient if the leak is large. The inadvertent exposure of the patient to more than one vapour is now prevented by interlock connections on adjoining vaporizers.

Suction apparatus

No anaesthetic should commence unless the efficiency of the suction apparatus has been determined to the anaesthetist's satisfaction. The sucker should be capable of removing large volumes at high speed and does not necessarily need to develop a high pressure for this. The receptacles for aspirated fluids should be self-sealing and disposable.

During induction of anaesthesia the sucker-end in position should be of a wide-bore pharyngeal type, although all sizes of catheter sucker should be available. Again this apparatus must be subject to regular maintenance and must be replaced between each case.

Separate suction apparatus must be available for the anaesthetist at all times in the anaesthetic room and operating theatre, and must not be shared with the surgeon. Suction apparatus can be arranged to work from an oxygen supply, but this should only be allowed if a pipeline system is in operation.

Electrical apparatus

All electrical apparatus in hospitals should be subjected to routine checks to ensure electrical safety. This is usually carried out by the hospital electrician. A label with the date of the inspection and the signature of the inspector is attached to the equipment. The check includes the safety of the plug and the earthing of the machine. A notice should be fixed to the apparatus warning against the use of the apparatus in close proximity to inflammable anaesthetic vapours, but this hazard is now virtually past as these agents are now very rarely used, indeed, cyclopropane is no longer available in the UK.

Intubation equipment

Each anaesthetic machine should be equipped with two or more laryngoscopes with interchangeable blades of different sizes. Fibre-optic systems are less liable to unexplained fault, but every laryngoscope should be checked just before use. Because it is not always possible to predict the patient that will be difficult to intubate, further instruments should be readily available. These include stylettes, gum-elastic bougies and intubation forceps, as well as a full range of endotracheal tube types and sizes.

Anaesthetists should know where to find and be able to use fibre-optic laryngoscopes. Failure to intubate, or intubation in error of the oesophagus, is still the most common cause of anoxic brain damage and even death during anaesthesia.

In addition to this essential apparatus, working surfaces of anaesthetic machines should hold a range of minor instruments, such as mouth gags, forceps and scissors. Individual departments cater for the tastes of their members, but it is wise to have an agreed schedule of instruments that are regularly checked and put into position for use.

Monitoring equipment

The use of various machine and patient monitors is now recommended for all anaesthetics (Association of Anaesthetists 1988b). Similar recommendations are now almost universally applied throughout the developed world. The equipment required is complex and, while some hospitals have the capacity to maintain their own equipment, many will need to seek the assistance of the manufacturers for this. It is beyond the scope of this chapter to enter into a description of this work.

REFERENCES

ABPI 1992 ABPI data sheet compendium 1991–1992 1456

Association of Anaesthetists 1988a Aids and hepatitis B: guidelines for anaesthetists. Association of Anaesthetists of Great Britain and Ireland, London

Association of Anaesthetists of Great Britain and Ireland 1988b Recommendations for standards of monitoring during anaesthesia and recovery. Association of Anaesthetists, London

Association of Anaesthetists 1990 Checklist for anaesthetic machines. Association of Anaesthetists of Great Britain and Ireland, London

BMA 1987 Immunisation against hepatitis B. Board of Education and Science, British Medical Association, London

BMA 1990 A code of practice on the safe use and disposal of sharps. British Medical Association, London

Casewell M W, Dalton M T 1977 Forrester laryngeal spray as a source of pseudomonas respiratory tract infection. Br Med J 2: 680

Crosby W M 1988 Checking anaesthetic machines, drugs and monitoring devices. Anaesth Intensive Care 16: 32–35

DHSS 1977 Health Technical Memorandum No. 22 (with supplements). DHSS, London

DOH 1990 Immunisation against infectious disease. HMSO, London, p 102

Editorial (1984) Needlestick transmission of HTVL-III from a patient infected in Africa. Lancet 2: 1376–1377

George R H 1975 A critical look at chemical disinfection of anaesthetic apparatus. Br J Anaesth 47: 719–721

Hadler S C, Doto I L, Maynard J E et al 1985 Occupational risks of hepatitis B infection in hospital workers. Infect Control 6: 24

Jenkins J R E, Edgar W M 1964 Sterilisation of anaesthetic equipment. Anaesthesia 19: 177–190

Lumley J 1976 Decontamination of anaesthetic equipment and ventilators. Br J Anaesth 48: 3–7

Lumley J 1988 Some aspects of anaesthetic safety. In: Jewkes D A (ed) Baillière's clinical anaesthesiology. Baillière Tindall, London, Ch 17, p 391–393

Marx G F, Steen S N, Chapira M et al 1969 Hazards associated with ethylene oxide sterilization. N Y State J Med 69: 1319–1323

Nielsen H, Vasegaard M, Stokes D B 1978 Bacterial contamination of anaesthetic gases. Br J Anaesth 50: 811–814

Roger P L, Lantz H C, Henderson D K, Parillo J, Masur H 1989 Admission of AIDS patients to a medical intensive care unit: cause and outcome. Crit Care Med 17: 113–117

Sherrard M, Gatt I 1987 Human immunodeficiency virus (HIV) antibody testing. Br Med J 295: 911–912

Tedder R S 1983 Towards the control of hepatitis B in hospitals. In: Waterson, A P (ed) Recent advances in virology. Churchill Livingstone, Edinburgh, pp 217–287

Waterson A P 1976 Hepatitis B as a hazard in anaesthetic practice. Br J Anaesth 48: 21–23

FURTHER READING

Lowbury E J L, Ayliffe G A J, Geddes A M, Williams J D 1981 Control of hospital infection, 2nd edn. Chapman and Hall, London

SECTION 7

The law

46

The anaesthetist and the law

R. N. Palmer

CRIMINAL AND CIVIL LAW

A detailed consideration of the English legal system is out of place in a book such as this, but a brief description of English Law may assist anaesthetists. The two main divisions within the law are criminal law and civil law.

Criminal law

Criminal law involves offences that the state prohibits, either by statute or by the development of the common law of England and Wales. The common law is that corpus of law created by the judges over the centuries and is binding in the form of legal precedents: murder is a common law crime. Statutory offences are created by Parliament in various Acts and Statutory Instruments, for example theft and conspiracy. The sanction for a criminal matter is a form of punishment (a fine, imprisonment, etc.) that is also intended to act as a deterrent. The object is not to compensate the victim, although the state has instituted a separate scheme in recent years for the compensation of those injured by criminal offences.

Civil law

Civil law deals with private matters between individuals in which the state has no interest, for example trespass, nuisance and negligence. Civil offences may derive from the common law (e.g. negligence) or from statute (e.g. Occupier's Liability Act). The sanction for a civil matter is the award of monetary compensation to the victim by the courts, the object of which is to put the plaintiff into the position he would be in were it not for the civil offence, in so far as this is possible with money. Tort is another word for a civil offence.

Criminal negligence

Confusion about the difference between criminal and civil law leads to much misunderstanding. An allegation of negligence against a medical practitioner is a civil matter, not a criminal offence. The most serious charge that could be brought arising from the practice of anaesthesia is one of murder, but such criminal charges are exceptionally rare. They are likely to involve facts such as an intentional act to hasten death, as in 'euthanasia', and it is important to realize that it is only the doctor's *intentions* that are legally relevant, his motives (however impeccable) are of no interest to the law. Another very serious criminal charge that may arise from the practice of anaesthesia is that of manslaughter, that is causing death by criminal neglect or by reckless disregard of one's professional duties. Prosecutions for manslaughter in the context of medical practice are rare. They are only brought in exceptional cases where the facts demonstrate such gross neglect or misconduct as to take the matter beyond the realms of civil (that is monetary) compensation between individuals into areas requiring retribution by society at large (that is the state).

Only rarely does the practice of anaesthesia result in a prosecution for manslaughter. This occasionally happens in circumstances where the death of a patient has been caused by gross negligence or recklessness on the part of the anaesthetist. In 1990, two anaesthetists were convicted of manslaughter in English courts. In one case an anaesthetist practised in the UK without any postgraduate qualification in anaesthesia and worked for many years in a variety of mainly locum posts. The patient, a healthy man in his thirties, underwent surgery for a detached retina. The anaesthetic was administered by the regular anaesthetist, not the locum, but after approximately 1 h the regular anaesthetist was called away to attend an emergency and he called upon the locum to take over. As well as the change of anaesthetist, the operating department assistant was also changed. Another relevant feature was the dimming of the lighting in the operating theatre to facilitate the visualization of the area of the detachment. The surgeon was unaware of the change of staff. The patient suffered a cardiac arrest. It was discovered that the tubing that delivered the anaesthetic gases to the patient had become disconnected, for the connector had parted from the endotracheal tube. The locum anaesthetist, while in charge of the patient, had apparently not attempted to check the connection between the tubing and the endotracheal tube. It was also alleged that he had left the operating room during the course of the anaesthetic, prior to the arrest.

The patient suffered irreversible brain damage from which he died 6 months later. The subsequent Coroner's Inquest was adjourned while enquiries were made with a view to bringing a criminal prosecution. At the subsequent trial for manslaughter the locum anaesthetist was convicted and sentenced to 6 months imprisonment, suspended for 1 year. The conviction is, at the time of writing, under appeal.

In another case a retired anaesthetist, acting as a locum consultant, was convicted of manslaughter in circumstances in which he connected a patient to a high pressure oxygen source: a cylinder delivering oxygen at 2000 lb per square inch. The patient died from barotrauma. The locum consultant anaesthetist was convicted of manslaughter and sentenced to 6 months imprisonment suspended for 1 year.

If the death of a patient is caused by a standard of care that is so far below that which reasonable clinicians would regard as acceptable, with the facts showing gross negligence or recklessness, it is possible that criminal prosecution will follow. The Crown Prosecution Service would need to be reasonably sure that they would secure a conviction if the matter was tried before a jury. The facts would be likely to be such as to take the issue well beyond compensation between individuals (although that may follow later in subsequent civil proceedings) and into a class of conduct such as to warrant a penalty imposed by the courts on behalf of the state.

NEGLIGENCE

It is important to appreciate that the tort of negligence in no way implies neglect or moral turpitude. The standard of proof required to establish negligence is not the strict criminal standard of proof 'beyond reasonable doubt', but rather the lower civil test of proof on the 'balance of probabilities'. This, of course, is much lower than, say, the standard required for scientific purposes. Anaesthesia is a branch of medicine that is fraught with medico–legal hazards. In a series of 10 000 written reports to the Medical Protection Society from all specialties, 440 were from anaesthetists. The hazards that led to these problems arose before, during and after the anaesthetic, and could be due to a rapid alteration in the condition of the patient.

The legal standards applying to the practice of anaesthesia are not static and immutable. They are, in effect, set by the body of practising anaesthetists, not by lawyers, and they change to reflect the progress and development of the specialty. Before a patient can succeed in a claim for negligence in English civil law, the court must be satisfied of three things. The plaintiff must prove that the anaesthetist owed him a duty of care; he must prove that the anaesthetist failed in that duty; and he must prove that he suffered harm (i.e. damage) as a consequence of that failure. The plaintiff must prove his case by satisfying the test of the civil law mentioned above, that is on the balance of probabilities. The test is whether it was more probable than not that the harm suffered by the patient was occasioned by a failure on the part of the anaesthetist to achieve the standard of care that could reasonably have been expected of colleagues in the specialty with similar training, skill and experience.

Setting the standard of care

A patient who believes he has suffered avoidable harm during an anaesthetic may initiate legal proceedings alleging negligence and/or breach of contract. The culmination of the legal process is a judgment, in the course of which the trial judge will make certain findings, including one about the standard of care in the particular case. The apparent conflict between this statement and the previous statement that the standards of care are set by the profession and not by lawyers can be understood by appreciating how the judge reaches his view.

The trial of an action for medical negligence under English law is usually in two stages. First the facts have to be established; second, expert opinion on those facts is given. The evidence of fact is given by the anaesthetist and others, and in the course of this process great reliance is placed on contempory records, such as notes, charts, radiographs and traces. The importance of making and keeping these records cannot be overemphasized. This evidence is not, however, expert evidence, but merely professional evidence of fact. After the facts have been established, each party to the action, that is the plaintiff and the defendant, will call expert evidence from anaesthetic colleagues and others to support their contentions. The trial judge will listen to this, perhaps ask questions himself, and then possibly have to choose between conflicting opinions. The judge can even ignore opinion evidence where irreconcilable views are expressed and may then make his own findings about the standard of care. However, this situation is very rare and English courts generally adopt the views and opinions of the anaesthetic and other experts who appear before them. When there are two 'schools of thought' on a given aspect of practice the courts will be slow to choose between them, preferring to make a finding compatible with the acceptance of responsibly held differences of anaesthetic opinion.

In practical, pragmatic terms the procedures outlined above mean that a practitioner should adopt a technique that would receive support from a responsible body of professional opinion. The defence of litigation requires support for the course of action adopted by the anaesthetist from distinguished colleagues who are prepared to attend court and give expert evidence on oath which they are prepared to defend under rigorous cross-examination.

The system of setting standards by the profession depends, of course, on each party to litigation calling responsible and respected expert evidence. Only for as long as this continues is it possible to advance the view that, albeit indirectly, the standards of care are set by anaesthetists. The trial judges have the last word and may indeed ignore the expert evidence if to them it seems right to do so: then the lawyers are setting the standard of care.

Duty of care

A practitioner must bring to his work the skill and care that it is reasonable to expect from those of comparable training and experience. The senior house officer is not expected to be able to work at the same standards of skill as a consultant, nor is a consultant expected to achieve the standards of the world's leading authority. An anaesthetist must attain the standards of his average professional peers by working carefully and diligently at all times. This standard, imposed by law, is in fact a high one and requires a thorough, careful and responsible approach. A competent anaesthetist is expected to recognize when he is out of his depth and, knowing his limitations, to call for help from a more experienced colleague when required. He will be expected to ensure that those to whom he delegates responsibility are trained and competent to carry out the tasks. The test in all this is whether he could rely on public support in the courts from distinguished colleagues for his actions.

The reasonable anaesthetist, in the court's view, will practise within the limits of his competence; will not expose his patients to unnecessary risks; and will keep abreast of the important developments in his specialty. He is not expected to have read every journal and he is entitled to follow the practice of one of several schools of thought, even that of a minority school. The practitioner should evaluate fully techniques before changing a safe tried method, but not adhere slavishly to practices that have long been discarded by his peers.

The duty of care and the caring approach

The words 'care' and 'caring' have a different meaning in Medicine and in the Law in some contexts. The standard of care as required by English Law is nothing to do with the caring approach of the health professions. It is not sufficient in law to be 'caring' if in so doing the 'duty of care' is neglected. An example of this may be when a kindly anaesthetist allows himself to be persuaded by a particularly nervous patient to induce anaesthesia with thiopentone in bed in the ward rather than in the safety of the anaesthetic room equipped for the purpose. While this doubtless qualifies the practitioner for the epithet, 'caring', if any harm ensued the courts would regard it as a breach of the 'duty of care'. An action for negligence in such circumstances could be impossible to defend. A perfect anaesthetist will be both caring and fulfil his duty of care, always!

PERSONAL AND VICARIOUS LIABILITY

The principles and standards outlined above apply both to private practice and to practice within the NHS. The anaesthetist remains responsible for his own acts and omissions. However, where the doctor is employed by a Health Authority, the employer is also vicariously liable for the acts and omissions of all its servants and agents, including the medical staff. Where a patient, who alleges he has suffered avoidable harm, initiates litigation, he can select as defendants either the named individual or the employer, the Health Authority, or both. The provider of the indemnity (i.e. the compensation) where negligence has occurred varies according to circumstances. Within the NHS since January 1990 there has been an important change with the introduction of indemnity provided by the hospital and community health sectors (HCHS) of the NHS. This NHS/HCHS indemnity is commonly referred to as 'Crown Indemnity'.

NHS/HCHS ('Crown') Indemnity

Until 1 January 1990, employed medical and dental staff (but not independent contractors, such as general practitioners) in the NHS were required, as a condition of their contracts of employment, to subscribe to one of the recognized medical defence organizations or to take out commercial insurance which the Secretary of State regarded as satisfactory. Defence societies had an agreement with the DOH (in force from 1954 to 1989), the effect of which was that the defence societies paid any compensation due as a result of medical or dental negligence.

By the provisions set out in health department circular HC(89)34 (DOH 1989), the UK health departments introduced new arrangements for dealing with medical and dental negligence claims in the hospital and community health services from 1 January 1990. Health authorities and health boards in the UK now take direct financial responsibility for all claims for compensation attributable to employed staff. General medical practitioners are not directly affected by the new arrangements unless they have a contract of employment with a health authority, for example as a hospital practitioner or part-time medical officer. Health authorities no longer require employed medical and dental staff to subscribe to a recognized defence organization, although they encourage staff to continue to subscribe for the many benefits of membership provided by such organizations other than the indemnity for negligence.

The change in arrangements proved necessary because of the steep increase in medical defence subscriptions in the 1980s, itself the result of an increase in the numbers of claims and in the size of the awards by the courts. Since health authorities, as employers, are vicariously liable for all employed staff in the course of their NHS employment, health authorities and boards now take direct responsibility for costs and damages arising from medical negligence. This includes work performed by university medical staff and other research workers under honorary contracts in the course of NHS duties. However, the indemnity does not extend to preclinical or other university work.

Private practice and NHS/HCHS indemnity

NHS health authories are not responsible for consultants' private practice in any circumstances. However, health authorities may provide some indemnity for junior medical staff who are required to care for private patients in NHS hospitals as part of their contract with the health authority. No category II work is indemnified by the health authority. Nor does the new arrangement provide any assistance in connection with matters such as disciplinary proceedings, General Medical Council hearings, general practice locum work or, indeed, any work outside the scope of the doctor's contract of employment with the health authority. The DOH has made it clear that not even 'good samaritan' acts are included as part of the indemnity provided by the health authorities. However, the defence organizations continue to provide advice and assistance in all these areas for subscribing members.

DELEGATION BY THE ANAESTHETIST

There is both a legal and an ethical duty to ensure that anyone to whom a task is delegated is adequately trained and competent to perform the task. If this duty has been carried out and the person to whom the task has been delegated makes a negligent mistake, then the usual principles of personal and vacarious responsibility apply. If both the delegator and the delegatee are employed, then the employer is vicariously responsible for both.

It is impossible here to deal with all the eventualities of this situation. However, as a broad generalization, if it were shown that the anaesthetist delegated improperly, he would be liable for compensating the patient, although in the NHS the financial burden would be borne by the health authority. If, however, the delegation was correct and the nurse made an error that no such nurse should make, then the nurse, and thus his employer, would be at risk.

The situation is a little different in private practice. An anaesthetist here is vicariously responsible for those whom he employs directly in his own premises. When working in a private clinic the relationship would depend on the exact legal terms of that employment, and that of the clinic's staff. It would also depend on the nature of the contract with the patient. Space does not permit a full discussion here.

In any hospital setting, private or not, the anaesthetist may reasonably expect the hospital authority to engage only adequately trained staff, but he must ensure that they are competent to deal with the particular tasks delegated and to understand what is required of them. This is especially important when delegating for the first time to staff who are unknown, and to those in critical situations such as recovery rooms or intensive care areas.

THE ANAESTHETIST AND EQUIPMENT

Servicing

Medical equipment becomes more sophisticated and the servicing of such equipment more complex. It is clearly essential for the well-being of patients that those who use and service this apparatus should understand it and see that it is properly maintained. Where the equipment is the personal property of the anaesthetist it is his responsibility to see that it is so serviced. In the case of anaesthetic equipment kept at a dental surgery where a doctor attends to administer anaesthetics, a clear and unambiguous agreement should be reached between the doctor and dental surgeon about inspection and maintenance.

When equipment is provided by a hospital or clinic, whether within the NHS or not, there is a clear duty for that organization to provide the service. However, that authority will depend on the users to report faults outside routine maintenance. The anaesthetist should take the item out of service and report the fault.

Familiarity with equipment

It is a legal duty of any person using apparatus to familiarize himself with the equipment before use. In using new machines or when in an unfamiliar environment, extra time must be allowed for this purpose. The defence societies are all too well-acquainted with errors that arise from this cause, ranging from awareness during anaesthesia to brain death from incorrectly connected oxygen supply. A check should be carried out on the anaesthetic machine at the beginning of every list, the contents of cylinders constantly noted and the alarms turned on. Especial care is required in institutions that have pipeline supply in some, but not all, areas.

Small isolated units

Much care and thought is required when anaesthetics are to be given in small hospitals or isolated units that lack the full facilities and staff of a district general hospital. While not wishing to enter into the political debate about the preservation of such places, it is essential that surgeons, anaesthetists and the health authority take all proper steps to ensure the safety and well-being of patients in these hospitals. It is quite improper and legally indefensible to send junior or untrained personnel to situations like this. The patients must be carefully selected in the expectation that their progress will be straightforward. For any doctor in doubt about such a unit, the proper test is the one outlined on page 723. Is there responsible, respected and independent opinion prepared to go to court and to support in the witness box the procedures adopted?

CONSENT FOR THE ADMINISTRATION OF AN ANAESTHETIC

A clinical procedure carried out on a patient without consent is an assault, except in cases of urgent necessity. However, a signature on a consent form is not a valid consent unless it is freely given after a discussion between the patient and the practitioner.

In England, any person of sound mind who has attained the age of 16 years may give legally valid consent to surgical, medical or dental treatment (Family Law Reform Act 1969, Section 8). The House of Lords' decision in the case of Gillick v. West Norfolk and Wisbech Area Health Authority and the DHSS (1985) held that, save where statute otherwise provides, a minor's capacity to make his own decisions depends on his having sufficient understanding and intelligence to make the decision, and is not determined by reference to any judicially fixed age limit. Special statutory rules apply in cases of mental illness and impairment (Mental Health Act 1983) which are too complex to be considered here.

The nature of the explanation to be given to the patient (or parent/guardian) will vary widely for different cases, depending on many factors and calling for fine clinical judgement. Some patients seek a detailed explanation, some prefer to 'leave it to you, Doctor'. English Law does not require that every risk and complication should be mentioned (Sidaway v. Board of Governors of the Bethlem Royal Hospital and the Maudsley Hospital Health Authority and others 1985, House of Lords: The doctor is left to exercise clinical judgement over the warning, just as with treatment). In wide and general terms, the more social and clinically inessential procedures (e.g. cosmetic surgery, sterilizations and dental restorations) require that risks and unwanted effects be stressed, whereas there is less need to dwell on these before acute emergency procedures. The position in English Law is very different from that established in the USA and Canada where there are legal doctrines of Informed Consent with strict duties of full disclosure of material risks.

In the House of Lords it was said that the decision about 'what degree of disclosure of risks is best calculated to assist a particular patient to make a rational choice as to whether or not to undergo a particular treatment must primarily be a matter of clinical judgement'. Another Law Lord said that, at the end of the day, the doctor, bearing in mind the best interests of the patient and the patient's right to information which will enable the patient to make a balanced judgement, must decide what information should be given to the patient and in what terms the information should be couched. However, the House of Lords also stated that, if there is a conflict of medical opinion about how much the patient should be told, the judges would have to resolve such conflict.

A legally valid consent may be given orally or in writing and either expressly or by implication. A written consent is desirable before operative and invasive procedures because it is a permanent documentary record of the patient's agreement following the verbal discussion and is therefore a helpful piece of evidence if litigation ensues. However, the consent form should never be a substitute for a proper discussion between patient and doctor: at best it is an adjunct to such discussions.

When an epidural or other local anaesthetic is intended to be given in the course of a general anaesthetic, it should be mentioned to the patient before induction and preferably at the preanaesthetic assessment. It is unwise to rely entirely on the 'consent to such further or alternative operative measures or treatment as may be necessary', the statement seen on the commonly used standard consent form. Consent to an epidural procedure in an obstetric unit is commonly given orally or by implication by the patient's willing acceptance of the offer of such treatment, following an explanation of its benefits.

Consent for the anaesthetic is usually given with the consent for the procedure for which it is required. However, complaints and litigation may be avoided in large measure by better communication between patient and practitioner. Therefore it is in the best interest of both if a word of explanation about the anaesthetic is given, ideally at the time of the visit for preoperative assessment. The stage has not yet been reached where separate consents are necessary for the anaesthetic and the operative procedure, but it would be the responsibility of the anaesthetist to obtain consent in situations where he was undertaking responsibility for more than just the anaesthetic, such as in pain relief clinics.

Teamwork is essential in the operating theatre and, as the last member of that team to be able to converse with the patient before loss of consciousness, the anaesthetist has a special opportunity and duty to check such matters as consent, identity and the site and side of the procedure.

Problems with consent may arise for certain procedures in some groups of patients. The example usually quoted is the Jehovah's Witnesses who refuse blood transfusion. In the case of an adult, a full and frank disclosure of the consequences of a refusal to agree to standard practices and procedures should be given, preferably in the presence of a witness, perhaps from the nursing staff. If consent is still withheld, the patient should be asked to sign a written statement of his refusal, countersigned by a witness, and an entry should be made in the notes by a senior responsible clinician. Where the patient is a minor or is mentally impaired, and the parents or guardian refuse consent to treatment that is demonstrably in the best interests of the patient, special legal steps can be taken for the protection of the patient.

Research, clinical trials and non-therapeutic procedures pose special legal and ethical problems with respect to consent. The subject is specialized and complex and doctors engaged in such work are urged to take legal advice. The legal case of Re. D (a minor) 1976 is a precedent for the proposition that non-therapeutic procedures on minors may be unlawful if they are irreversible and of no direct benefit to the individual child.

Palmer (1980, 1991) provides a more detailed consideration of the application to medicine of the law of consent.

PREOPERATIVE ASSESSMENT

The proper conduct of an anaesthetic requires a knowledge of the patient gained at a preoperative assessment. There is no law that makes a preoperative visit by the anaesthetist mandatory, but the assessment must be performed by a competent person. Clearly, if the patient suffers avoidable harm, the entire management of the case will be subject to scrutiny and the absence of such a visit may render the matter difficult to defend.

The anaesthetist or doctor making the preoperative assessment will take a complete history and examine the patient. It is not the function of this chapter to detail these matters, but there are a number of points that so frequently give rise to litigation that they are worth mentioning:

1. In the course of the interview the doctor can establish the identity of the patient and the nature, site and side of the operation. If this were routinely done, the elaborate procedures for 'checking' patients seen in many institutions would become superfluous.
2. Questions should be asked specifically about previous anaesthetic experience, good or bad.
3. Previous drug therapy should be noted, especially any untoward incidents. A history of any allergy is important.
4. A full history and examination of the patient's dentition is of prime importance, especially in those who are to be intubated. Damage to teeth, crowns and bridgework is not necessarily negligent in that it may be unavoidable, but to damage them in ignorance of their presence is indefensible.
5. The results of special tests should be scrutinized and, if further tests are ordered, the results should be known to the anaesthetist before induction. Specifically to order a test and then not to check the result before starting an anaesthetic must be difficult to defend unless the case is a grave emergency.
6. Questioning a patient under the influence of a premedicant drug may not lead to valid answers in the matters outlined above, either medically or legally.

Postponement of operations

When seen at a preoperative assessment, the patient's condition may mean that the surgical procedure has to be delayed or abandoned. This must only be done in consultation with the surgeon concerned, and should rarely be done without the patient being seen by the anaesthetist. If there is any doubt, the opinion of a more senior colleague should be sought. This situation frequently arises in emergency surgery and it is often better to postpone than to see 'what one can get away with'. Again the test of proper practice will be the support that can be mustered in court for the procedure adopted.

DRUG AND FLUID ADMINISTRATION

It is the personal responsibility of every practitioner to know the indications, unwanted effects and interactions of any material used in the course of his professional activities. There are no safe drugs, only safe doctors. It is permissible to delegate the preparation of injectable drugs, as frequently happens in anaesthetic practice, but the doctor who injects the substance must assume responsibility for that act. This means proper training in sound procedures for the assistants in the anaesthetic room. The following errors have featured in the cases known to the Medical Protection Society:

1. Mismatched blood, or failure to check properly the identity of the patient to whom it is given.
2. The incorrect substance or the incorrect strength of the right substance has been drawn up. The wrong diluent has been used; for example potassium chloride for saline. Ampoules have been returned to the wrong box.

3. Vaporizers have been charged with the wrong volatile agent, and in draining these the drug has gone into the wrong bottle, for example halothane liquid injected intravenously instead of methohexitone. Water has been substituted for liquids in a vaporizer: halothane is a saleable commodity among the addicted.
4. Mathematical errors have been made in calculating dosage, especially in paediatric practice, or a decimal point may be misplaced on a prescription.
5. Drugs have been given to patients with known and recorded allergies to those drugs, sometimes with fatal results.
6. Many agents, which should be given intravenously, cause intense tissue damage if allowed to extravasate, or if given intraarterially. Especial care is required with certain groups of drugs such as cytotoxic agents.
7. Intramuscular injections may be incorrectly sited and lead to damage to the sciatic or radial nerves, or their branches.
8. Multidose bottles are hazardous because they are potentially infected after the first use. Furthermore they should be discarded after one session and not stored for later use, in case they are incorrectly mixed or contain unwanted substances. Despite the inconvenience and extra cost, the author advocates that only single dose ampoules should be used.

DENTAL DAMAGE

One of the most common causes of litigation in anaesthetic practice is damage to teeth, either natural or false. This has already been mentioned p. 728). It is important to remember that damage to natural teeth is a serious injury that cannot be always be fully restored, and dental crowns and bridges are often very expensive, sometimes costing thousands of pounds. All patients at risk should be warned of the possibility that damage may ensue, and the nature of the warning recorded in the notes before surgery.

If damage does inadvertently occur, despite every possible care, either during the anaesthetic or during recovery, the incident should be recorded in the notes and the patient informed as soon as he can comprehend. This is best done by the anaesthetist concerned. It is of great assistance if the hospital is in a position to offer the help of a dental practitioner in the immediate postoperative period to initiate restoration. If handled in this way a claim for negligence in respect of dental damage is capable of a successful defence.

RELATIONSHIP WITH EMPLOYERS

There is a contractual relationship between a consultant and his employer in the NHS. This contract is usually held by the regional health authority, although in some cases a Trust or the teaching district, university or postgraduate institution holds it. Anaesthetists in training are usually employed by the district health authority. In other forms of practice, including some private clinics, the relationship can be a contract of service (that is employer/employee as in the NHS), or a contract for services in which the anaesthetist is not an employee, but is retained specifically to render the services on terms that are set out in the contract. The laws governing contracts are complicated and will not be discussed further here.

It is more usual in private practice in the UK for the anaesthetist to be engaged by the surgeon on behalf of a named patient to provide specialist services.

The precise contractual relationship is important if there is a problem in the recovery of fees and in other matters, including discipline.

As an employee the practitioner is not in full control of resources, such as the allocation of staff. The employing authority, through its managers, is responsible for these functions. The doctor can do little more than tender professional advice and opinion, unless he holds some administrative post as well as that of a clinician. He is, however, quite entitled to refuse to give an anaesthetic in circumstances in which, in his opinion, the patient would be put at avoidable risk.

CONTROLLED DRUGS

The anaesthetist enjoys no special privileges in the use of controlled drugs, and is governed by the same laws, rules and regulations as other medical practitioners. However he does use controlled drugs, such as opiates, more frequently and in bigger doses that most medical practitioners and must therefore ensure that he complies fully with the legal requirements governing their supply and use. In particular, care is necessary to keep or to assist in keeping a proper drug register and in writing up, in the correct form, all orders and prescriptions for these controlled drugs. This procedure can be found in the Misuse of Drugs Act 1971 and the subsequent Statutory Regulations.

THE SICK ANAESTHETIST: PREVENTION OF HARM TO PATIENTS

Probably because of the relatively easy access to controlled drugs and anaesthetic agents, the anaesthetist is particularly prone to drug, vapour and alcohol abuse. The problem is not confined to anaesthetists, but errors in this field of practice have a rapid and serious consequence for patients in terms of awareness, hypoxic episodes or even cardiorespiratory arrest. The problem may be compounded because of a sense of loyalty and friendship by colleagues, which delays action until indisputable evidence is available. Quite often this evidence is serious harm to a patient. It was just such a situation, in which a patient died in the operating theatre due to neglect by an addicted anaesthetist, that led to the introduction and implementation within the NHS of the guidance circular designed to prevent harm befalling a patient through illness or disability in a member of the medical or dental staff. This document is known, somewhat misleadingly and erroneously, as the 'Three Wise Men' procedure. It was revised in 1982 in NHS Circular HC(82)13 entitled 'Prevention of harm to patients resulting from physical or mental disability of hospital or community medical or dental staff'. Each district health authority is enjoined to set up a special professional panel consisting of senior members of the medical or dental staff from which a subcommittee could at any time be appointed to receive and take action on any report of incapacity due to physical or mental disability, including addiction.

In addition, the Association of Anaesthetists has set up a voluntary scheme for the support and rehabilitation of sick colleagues. Details of this scheme and its mode of operation may be obtained from the Association or from the College of Anaesthetists.

The General Medical Council

Informal voluntary schemes do not always meet with cooperation from a sick doctor, who all too often lacks insight and refuses to seek advice. The General Medical Council now has legal jurisdiction to act in these cases. If the council feels anxiety after receiving information, the doctor is offered a medical examination and counselling. A refusal to accept recommendations or lack of cooperation at any stage may lead to the case being referred to the full Health Committee of the General Medical Council.

DEATHS AND THE CORONER

Deaths on the operating table or in the perioperative period are an inescapable part of anaesthetic practice. While there is strictly no legal duty on a medical practitioner to report any death to one of Her Majesty's Coroners (or in Scotland the Procurators Fiscal), it is in the best interests of all concerned voluntarily to report any death occurring within a few days of an anaesthetic that cannot be clearly ascribed to natural causes. The coroner can then initiate an independent inquiry into the circumstances of the death, in the first instance by arranging with a pathologist for a necropsy. He may then be able to conclude the matter by simply issuing a certificate of the cause of death without holding an inquest.

Where the coroner cannot be satisfied in this way he is likely to hold an inquest. He will usually seek reports from the medical staff and may summon some of them to attend the inquest to give evidence. The decision to hold an inquest does not, of itself, imply criticism of the medical management. However, a doctor who was actively involved in the treatment and who is asked for a statement or called to the inquest is well advised to discuss the matter beforehand with his protection society. The protection society will, if thought necessary, arrange for legal representation at the inquest. Legal representation is usually unnecessary, and even positively contraindicated, especially when the standard of care is beyond reproach. Where, however, a specific attack is anticipated against members of staff by wrathful relatives, it is wise to arrange legal representation. It is also desirable on those occasions where it is known that errors were made, where equipment failed or where criticisms of the patient's management have been made.

It is important to remember that, once a case has been reported to the coroner, nothing may be done with the body without the coroner's consent. Thus organs may not be taken for transplantation nor may matters be discussed with the press or media.

COMPLAINTS BY PATIENTS, RELATIVES AND FRIENDS: INQUIRIES

An increasing awareness of medical matters by the public, gleaned from the press and media, has led to increasing expectations of diagnosis and cure. If complaints are to be avoided it is vital to communicate effectively with the patient and relatives, to explain what the proposed treatment is, to warn of the risks and to make clear what the outcome will be. Anaesthetists should play their part in this process, especially mentioning the trivial discomforts that can be expected, such as a sore throat from intubation. Patients need to be told that they will wake up in different rooms (a recovery or intensive care area) with drips and monitors in place. The presence of an oxygen mask at this point is routine and does not imply that something has gone wrong.

If an untoward incident does occur a careful explanation should be given to the patient and the relatives. Both the surgeon and the anaesthetist should be a party to this and agree beforehand what is to be said. All questions should be factually and simply answered, and speculation should be avoided. The only exception to this is where there are attempts by the relatives to blame someone, and the answers to these queries should be deferred until a report is available following a thorough inquiry.

The NHS makes provision for a variety of official inquiries in many circumstances. Relatives who demand an inquiry can be informed of this and be introduced to the appropriate manager or administrator, who will arrange to start the process. The complainants should be kept informed at intervals of the progress of the inquiry.

Individual departments should endeavour to find the explanation for untoward incidents, even where there is no official inquiry. This is especially important when equipment fails or when other patients may be at risk. These steps should be started promptly, notwithstanding that an official inquiry may yet be set up, although care should be taken that the latter has not been pre-empted or prejudiced. Nor do the foregoing comments apply when a death has been reported to the coroner, for no steps should be taken without the coroner's agreement until his own inquiry is complete.

Complaints about clinical judgment in the NHS are commonly investigated in accordance with the procedure laid down in the guidance circular, HC(88)37 and in the Hospital Complaints Procedure Act 1985.

DISCIPLINARY PROCEDURES

A new NHS hospital disciplinary procedure was introduced by the DOH in March 1990. It replaced the previous disciplinary procedure set out in HM(61)112 which dealt with cases involving personal conduct, professional conduct and professional competence.

The new DOH guidance, set out in circular HC(90)9, consolidates previous guidance following the recommendations of a Joint Working Party on Disciplinary Procedures. The new circular made changes to paragraph 190 of the terms and conditions of service for hospital medical and dental staff in the hospital and community health sectors of the NHS in England and Wales. The new circular introduced two new procedures: professional review machinery whereby a professional panel reviews the conduct of hospital consultants who are alleged to have failed repeatedly to honour their contractual commitments; and a new procedure for dealing with cases of professional misconduct and professional incompetence that warrant disciplinary action short of dismissal. The new circular continues to deal with cases involving personal conduct, professional conduct and professional competence, and describes the procedures to be followed. Any practitioner facing the threat of disciplinary proceedings of any kind is well advised to seek professional advice and assistance from his medical defence organization or professional association.

For cases involving professional conduct and professional competence there is a two-stage procedure. First the facts must be established so as to decide whether or not there is a prima facie case for investigation. Where a prima facie case is established, an investigating panel is set up by the health authority responsible for appointing the practitioner. The detailed workings of the procedure are described in the circular and the procedure has serious implications for the practitioner in that it may result in dismissal from the post held.

THE ROLE OF THE PROTECTION SOCIETIES

Protection societies exist to safeguard the interests of their members in all matters arising from the practice of their profession. They offer a wide range of advice on ethical and medico–legal matters; arrange representation at courts, inquests and inquiries; and, in practice outside the NHS hospital or community service, give indemnity in proven cases of negligence. To assist in this the organizations should be briefed early when potential medico–legal problems come to light. A factual report in chronological order, narrated in the active mood is best, and should be sent to the appropriate office. Further information, or an interview with the secretariat or experts, may later be necessary. No report should be sent out without advice from the defence organization where reputations are at stake, or where large sums of compensation may be sought.

While the protection societies are necessarily pro-doctor they are not anti-patient. They are controlled by medical and dental practitioners whose main raison d'être is the care of patients. If careful consideration of all relevant facts, analysed with the benefit of expert legal and medical opinion, indicates that a patient suffered avoidable harm because of the actions of members, the protection society will seek to achieve an equitable settlement of the plaintiff's claim. However, members of the professions are not the insurers of their patients' misfortunes and will not compensate in circumstances where no negligence occurred. There is no system in the UK to compensate the victims of personal injury by accident without proof of fault, commonly, but misleadingly, called 'no-fault compensation'.

DEATH AND BRAINSTEM DEATH

There is no legal definition of death. On those occasions in the Court of Appeal when the matter of a definition of death has been raised, the Lords' Justices of Appeal have avoided giving a definition. In effect the law at present is that death occurs when the medical profession says it occurs. The criteria for brainstem death, as defined in the Memoranda of the Conference of Medical Royal Colleges and their Faculties in the UK (1979), were known to the Court of Appeal, but were neither accepted nor rejected (Times Law Report, March 17, 1981). Because a definition of death was not essential for the case under consideration, the court reserved the matter for a future occasion.

Death was traditionally diagnosed when irreversible cessation of respiration and heartbeat occurred. This concept is giving way to the definition that death occurs when there is irreversible cessation of brainstem function, sometimes called 'brain death'. It seems reasonable to infer that this definition would find judicial acceptance, provided that in diagnosing brainstem death the criteria laid down by the Conference of Medical Royal Colleges and Faculties were carefully followed.

Anaesthetists will frequently play a part in caring for patients who are maintained on ventilators. The point at which such equipment ceases to be a life-support system and becomes a corpse-ventilation system is seldom clear-cut. Even when brainstem death has occurred it may not be accepted by relatives, although 'death', that is cessation of heartbeat, can usually be expected in these circumstances in about 4 days. This can only be overcome by time-consuming patient explanation. On occassion there is a complete refusal to accept the situation, and one can only hope that time will resolve the matter. If available resources are so limited as to preclude this approach, advice should be sought from more senior colleagues and from the protection societies. The relatives should be informed of the facts, including the fact of irreversible brainstem death, and the need to utilize the limited resources for the benefit of others. The doctor in charge should then tell them of his intention to switch the ventilator off in, say, 24 h time, notwithstanding their objections. The relatives, if dissatisfied, should be encouraged to seek urgent legal advice with a view to an application to the courts to obtain an injunction to restrain the hospital staff from switching off the ventilator. If necessary the matter will then come before the courts for full argument and resolution.

Once a decision is made to discontinue artificial means of support, the physical act of 'switching off' should be undertaken by the most senior member of the team and should not be delegated to the juniors or to the nursing staff.

ORGAN AND TISSUE DONATION

A code of practice for the removal of cadaveric organs for transplantation has been drawn up and published by a working party on behalf of the Health Departments of Great Britain and Northern Ireland (HMSO 1983). This publication also reproduces the Human Tissue Act of 1961 (the statute governing the use of parts of bodies of deceased persons for therapeutic, medical, educational and research purposes) and the colleges' criteria for brainstem death. Under the statutory provisions, only the 'person lawfully in possession of the body' or his designate may authorize the removal of organs or tissue. It is generally believed, but there is no decided case in law, that ordinarily the Health Authority has lawful possession of a body dead on its premises, at least until such time as the body is claimed by a person with a superior right of possession, such as the coroner or the personal representative or next-of-kin of the deceased. The Health Authority will generally delegate its powers to an appropriate named member of staff.

If the deceased patient carried a valid organ donor card, or otherwise gave notice in writing of his wishes, there is no legal requirement to ensure that the relatives do not object to the removal of organs. If the wishes of the deceased were not made known in this way, the delegated representative of the Health Authority may only consent to the removal of organs if: 'having made such reasonable enquiry as may be practicable, he has no reason to believe: (a) that the deceased had expressed an objection to his body being so dealt with after his death, and had not withdrawn it; or (b) that the surviving spouse or any surviving relative of the deceased objects to the body being so dealt with.' (Human Tissue Act, 1961, s. 1(2)).

Once the legal safeguards are fulfilled, parts of the body may be removed, but only by a 'fully registered medical practitioner who must have satisfied himself by personal examination of the body that life is extinct'.

REFERENCES

Conference of Medical Royal Colleges and their Faculties in the UK 1979 Br Med J

DHSS Health circular HC(88)37 Hospital complaints procedures

DHSS 1990 NHS management executive: executive letter EL(90) 1919: Handling claims for medical negligence. 28 September

DOH 1989 Health Circular HC(89)34: Claims of medical negligence against NHS hospital and community doctors and dentists

DOH 1990 Health circular HC(90)9: Disciplinary procedures for hospital and community medical and dental staff

HMSO 1971 Misuse of Drugs Act. Also Statutory Instruments made in pursuance of the Act. HMSO, London

HMSO 1983 Cadaveric organs for transplantation: a code of practice, including the diagnosis of brain death. HMSO, London

NHS DHSS 1982 Health Circular HC(82)13: Prevention of harm to patients resulting from physical or mental disability of hospital or community medical or dental staff

Palmer R N, 1980 Consent. In: Leahy Taylor J (ed) Medical malpractice. Wright, Bristol, ch 3, p 66–75

Palmer R N, 1991 Consent and confidentiality. The Medical Protection Society, London

Regina v. Malcherek and Regina v. Steel 1981 Court of Appeal, Criminal Division. Times Law Report, March 17

Sidaway v. The Board of Governors of the Bethlem Royal Hospital and the Maudsley Hospital Health Authority and others 1985 House of Lords, Times Law Report, February 22, 2 Weekly Law Reports, 480 (HL)

Appendix 1

Antacid regimen

Every anaesthetic department should agree a standardized antacid regimen which can be made known to all medical and nursing staff. It can then be used routinely for all patients in labour, lest the need for an emergency anaesthetic arises, and can also be employed in other emergency and routine situations where there is a possibility of acid regurgitation during induction. These include all obese subjects and patients with such conditions as hiatus hernia and pyloric stenosis. It should theoretically also be used for all mothers that require anaesthesia from early in pregnancy and up to 6 weeks after delivery. However, since ranitidine has not been cleared of causing teratogenic effects in those patients in whom the fetus is to be preserved, it should in these cases be withheld in the first trimester and oral antacids given alone.

The following scheme would be suitable:

1. *Every 6 hours in labour*: Ranitidine 150 mg (in routine cases up to 24 h preoperatively).
2. *Fifteen minutes before induction*: A further dose of ranitidine 50 mg, which can be given intramuscularly or intravenously. The half-life of the drug is about 2 h.
3. *Immediately prior to induction*: A dose of 30 ml of 0.3 sodium citrate. An initial dose can also be given with the premedication.

Ranitidine passes the placental barrier, but has no ill effects on the fetus, and is also excreted in breast milk. The use of a regime of this sort does not eliminate the need for the usual precautions taken for a patient with a full stomach.

Appendix 2

Anaesthetic drugs that react adversely with pre-existing therapy

	Anaesthetic	Interaction
	Induction agents	
1.	Thiopentone	Excessive fall in BP with MAOI and hypotensive agents
	Muscle relaxants	
1.	Suxamethonium (depolarizing)	Antimyasthenic drugs antagonize, for example Ambenonium Azathioprine potentiates Cyclophosphamide potentiates Lithium may delay onset and prolong Thiotepa potentiates Oxytocin antagonizes Ecothiopate eyedrops prolong
2.	Gallamine Pancuronium Atracurium Alcuronium Vecuronium (non-depolarizing)	Antimyasthenic drugs antagonize, for example Ambenonium Aminoglycoside antibiotics potentiate Azathioprine antagonizes Beta blockers potentiate Diazepam increases duration Mustine potentiates Oxytocin potentiates
3.	d-Tubocurarine (non-depolarizing)	As for drugs in (2), except that hypotensive agents may cause a profound fall in blood pressure
	Opiates	
1.	Fentanyl	Not with MAOI
2.	Alfentanil	Not with MAOI Erythromycin can inhibit clearance
3.	Morphine	Possibly hypertension or smaller dose required with MAOI
4.	Pethidine	Extreme caution with MAOI
5.	Phenoperidine	Not with MAOI
	Oxygen	Bleomycin causes fibrosis of lungs Levels of inspired oxygen should be below 25%
	Spinal and epidural	Contraindicated with anticoagulant therapy Prenylamine may cause profound fall in blood pressure

Anaesthetic	Interaction
Volatile agents	
All	Hypotension with calcium channel blockers
1. Enflurane	Prenylamine may cause blood pressure fall
2. Isoflurane	
3. Halothane	Aminophylline may cause arrhythmias Fenfluromine causes arrhythmias Fenoterol and reproterol cause arrhythmias so last dose 8 h before induction Antihypertensives cause blood pressure falls MAOI may cause blood pressure fall Lithium may prolong recovery Phenteramine may cause arrhythmias Prenylamine may cause blood pressure fall

FURTHER INFORMATION

No anaesthetist can reasonably be expected to memorize the approved and proprietary names of all the drugs presently available, and be familiar with all possible interactions. Nevertheless the prevention of potentially serious drug interactions is of paramount importance in the perioperative period. When in doubt about an unfamiliar drug, refer to the ABPI Data Sheet Compendium for the current year. This publication contains the latest information available to the manufacturers on the reported drug interactions. Important information is also contained in the British National Formulary, published jointly by the British Medical Association and the Royal Pharmaceutical Society of Great Britain. The Prescribers' Journal, published periodically by HMSO contains authoritative review articles.

Appendix 3

Specific contraindications to anaesthetic drugs

Caution must be exercised in using the following drugs in the diseases named. Those marked with an asterisk are absolute contraindications.

Anaesthetic	Contraindication
Induction agents	
All	Previous allergy *
	Respiratory obstruction *
	Low fixed cardiac output
	Hepatic failure
	Anticipated difficult intubation
1. Methohexitone	Epilepsy
2. Thiopentone	Porphyria *
	Dystrophia Myotonica
	Chronic disease of the CNS
	Asthma
	Myasthenia gravis
	Huntington's chorea
3. Etomidate	Conditions in which suppresion of cortisol may be hazardous
4. Propofol	Titrate carefully in the elderly
	Disorders of fat metabolism
Muscle relaxants	
All	Previous allergy *
	Respiratory obstruction
	Anticipated difficult intubation
	Dystrophia myotonica
	Myasthenia gravis
	Familial periodic paralysis
	Motor neurone disease
	Muscular dystrophies
1. Suxamethonium	Recent burns
	Malignant hyperpyrexia *
	Abnormal pseudocholinesterase
	Malnutrition
	Dystrophia myotonica *
	Eye injuries
	Familial periodic paralysis
	Huntington's chorea
	Hyperkalaemia
	Spinal cord injuries
	Denervation injuries
	Tetanus

Anaesthetic	Contraindication
2. d-Tubocurarine	Myasthenia gravis *
	Renal failure
	Carcinoid
	Von Recklinghausen's disease
	Asthma
	Malignant hyperpyrexia *
	Hepatic failure
3. Pancuronium	Myasthenia gravis *
	Renal failure
	Tetanus
	Hepatic failure
4. Gallamine	Myasthenia gravis *
	Renal failure *
5. Alcuronium	Myasthenia gravis *
	Renal failure
	Hepatic failure
6. Atracurium	Myasthenia gravis*
7. Vecuronium	Myasthenia gravis *
Opiates	
All	Raised intracranial pressure
	Previous allergy *
	Respiratory depression
	Hepatic failure
1. Morphine	Chronic disease of the CNS
	Asthma
	Hepatic failure
	Pregnancy
	Gross obesity
Papaveretum (Omnopon)	Should not be used in women of child-bearing age
2. Pethidine	Hepatic failure
	Biliary tract disorders
	Gross obesity
3. Fentanyl and Alfentanil	Obstructive airways disease
	Hepatic failure
	Myasthenia gravis
4. Phenoperidine	Obstructive airways disease
Spinal and epidural	
	Central nervous system abnormalities *
	Bleeding diathesis *
	Gut perforations
	Hypovolaemic patients
	Gross obesity
	After trauma
	After large intravenous doses of opioids
Volatile agents	
1. Nitrous oxide	With gas-filled cavities
	Malignant hyperpyrexia *
2. Halothane	Previous idiosyncrasy *
	Malignant hyperpyrexia *
	Obstetric anaesthesia
	Termination of pregnancy
	Repeated administration in 3 months
	Cardiomyopathy
	Raised intracranial pressure
	Recent myocardial infarction

Anaesthetic	Contraindication
3. Enflurane	Epilepsy
	Malignant hyperpyrexia *
	Previous sensitivity *
	Renal failure
	Porphyria
4. Isoflurane	Malignant hyperpyrexia *
	Previous sensitivity *
Other agents	
1. Beta blockers	Asthma
	Diabetes mellitus
	Raynaud's disease
	Hepatic impairment
2. Oxytocin	Renal impairment
	Hepatic impairment
	Hypertension
3. Neostigmine	Asthma
	Intestinal obstruction
	Epilepsy
	Urinary obstruction
4. Atropine	Children with pyrexia
	Known sensitivity
	Severe myocardial ischaemia
5. Glycopyrrolate	Children with pyrexia
	Known sensitivity
	Severe myocardial ischaemia

Index